IMMUNOLOGY

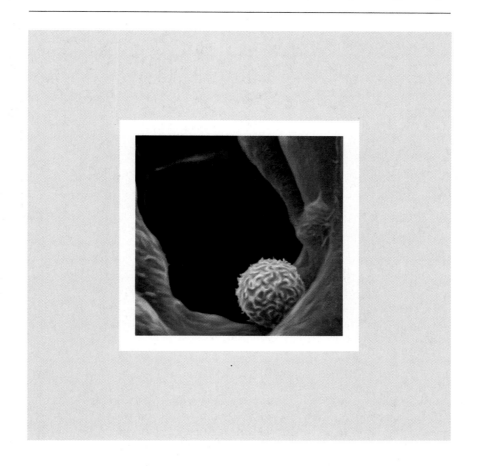

IMMUNOLOGY

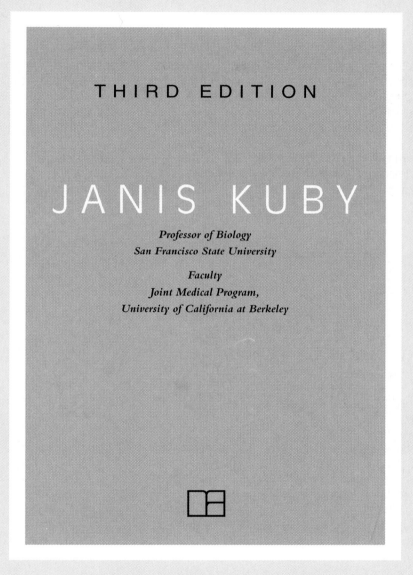

THIRD EDITION

JANIS KUBY

Professor of Biology
San Francisco State University

Faculty
Joint Medical Program,
University of California at Berkeley

W. H. FREEMAN AND COMPANY

New York

SENIOR EDITOR:	Deborah Allen
DEVELOPMENT EDITORS:	Michelle Russel Julet and Diane Cimino Maass
PROJECT EDITOR:	Diane Cimino Maass
LINE EDITOR:	Ruth Steyn
COVER AND TEXT DESIGNER:	Marsha Cohen/ Parallelogram Graphics
ILLUSTRATION COORDINATOR:	Susan Wein
ILLUSTRATION:	Network Graphics
PRODUCTION COORDINATOR:	Sheila E. Anderson
COMPOSITION:	Sheridan Sellers/W. H. Freeman Electronic Publishing Center
MANUFACTURING:	Von Hoffman Press, Inc.

ABOUT THE COVER AND FRONTISPIECE

Interactions of cell adhesion molecules, with different ones involved at different times, are responsible for recruiting leukocytes to inflammatory sites and for their migration through the vascular endothelium. Slowed by vasodilation, leukocytes drift against vessel walls, where selectins are responsible for a loose adherence known as "rolling." This initial step in leukocyte migration is shown in a false-color scanning electron micrograph. (See Chapter 15 for more information.)

Cover and frontispiece images © Morris J. Karnovsky, President and Fellow Harvard College
Cover and frontispiece image colorized by Marie T. Dauenheimer
Cover and frontispiece micrograph © Morris J. Karnovsky, President and Fellow Harvard College

Library of Congress Cataloging-in-Publication Data

Kuby, Janis.
   Immunology / Janis Kuby. — 3rd ed.
     p. cm.
   Includes bibliographical references and index.
   ISBN 0-7167-2868-0
   1. Immunology. I. Title.
   [DNLM: 1. Immune System. 2. Immunity. QW 504 K95i 1997]
   QR181.K83 1997
   616.07´9 — dc21
   DNLM/DLC
   for Library of Congress   96-52442
                                 CIP

Printed in the United States of America

First Printing, 1997

To

My family, David, Rebekah, and Beth,

whose sacrifice and love has made it possible to complete this book.

And to

Violet Kiteley

who was an invaluable source of strength
and inspiration during the most difficult hours.

And to

My mentor, Leon Wofsy,

who instilled in me a love for immunology and teaching
and who taught me, by his example, to always put people first.

And to

all the support from friends, extended family, and the grace of God
that has seen me through an earthquake, a fire, and cancer
during the writing of this book!

CONTENTS

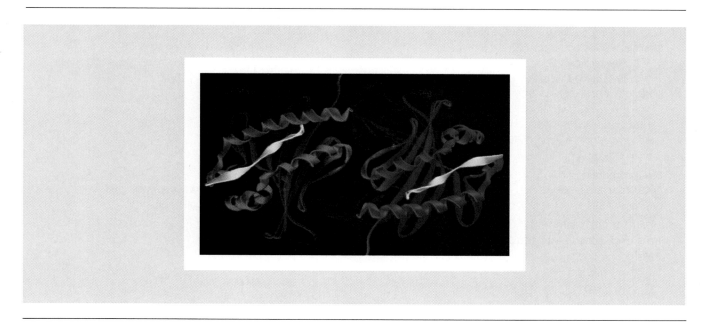

Chapter 3

CELLS AND ORGANS OF THE IMMUNE SYSTEM / 47

PART II

GENERATION OF B-CELL AND T-CELL RESPONSES / 85

Chapter 4

ANTIGENS / 87

C h a p t e r   8

B-CELL MATURATION, ACTIVATION, AND DIFFERENTIATION / 195

C h a p t e r   9

MAJOR HISTOCOMPATIBILITY COMPLEX / 223

PART III

IMMUNE EFFECTOR MECHANISMS / 311

PART IV

THE IMMUNE SYSTEM IN HEALTH AND DISEASE / 441

Chapter 21

IMMUNODEFICIENCY DISEASES / 507

Chapter 22

THE IMMUNE SYSTEM IN AIDS / 523

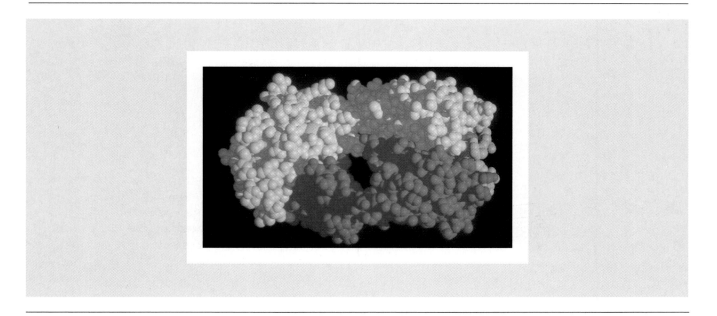

This edition of *Immunology*, as its predecessors, is notable not only for its breadth, clarity and currency in an onrushing and highly complex field, but as a memorable tribute to its author. Readers of the second edition, published in 1994, may have noted Jan's brief allusion to her struggle with cancer. This new edition was prepared with the same energy and care that made the earlier ones so valuable, but also with remarkable personal courage. It was completed literally days before cancer took her life. Jan did her Ph.D. research—studies on the mobility of lymphocyte membrane receptors—in my laboratory at the University of California at Berkeley. She was an outstanding student with a profound interest in the molecular and cell biology of the immune system, and her potential as a creative and inspiring teacher was evident early. Her commitment to science was tested at times by an intensely driven search for a spiritual faith that she could embrace unreservedly. That exploration actually led Jan to suspend her graduate work for a time, but the highest standards of scientific objectivity and integrity in her reserach and studies were unfaltering. Ultimately, Jan Kuby's all too short life was unusually fulfilling—for her, for her husband and daughters and their devoted community, and for her many students and colleagues. She became one of immunology's best teachers and writers. A textbook edition on any phase of modern biology can have a use-life of only a few years. Yet that use-life feeds into an unending stream of students, teachers and scientists. The three editions of *Immunology,* spanning a period of about six years, are testimony to remarkably expanding hopes and possibilities in medical and health sciences. They are also a lasting testimony to an exceptional teacher, Jan Kuby.

Leon Wofsy
Professor Emeritus
Molecular and Cell Biology / Immunology
University of California at Berkeley

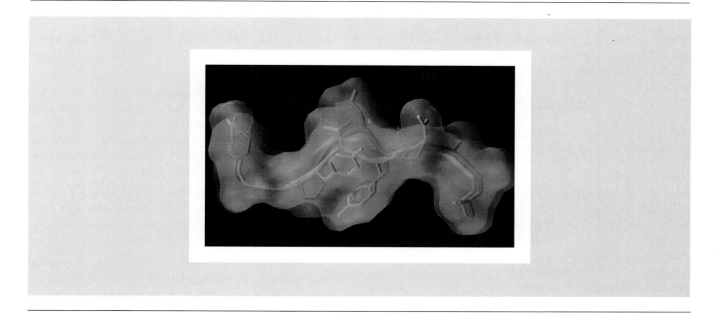

Immunology has been used successfully in scores of introductory courses for both undergraduates and students in clinical medicine. The text's focus on the experimental process conveys much of the excitement of scientific discovery while presenting the relevant facts. Exposure to the landmark experiments that underlay the theoretical framework of immunology enables students to appreciate how current immunologic paradigms evolved. This approach also illustrates how experiments are designed and interpreted to test scientific hypotheses, thus encouraging students to develop the intellectual skills needed to read critically the current immunologic literature.

As a teacher, Jan Kuby recognized the need for a textbook that, first and foremost, emphasizes that immunology is based solidly upon experimental results and, second, that highlights the relationships between basic immunologic principles and their clinical applications. The third edition preserves and builds upon these goals. Discussions of important clinical applications are included throughout the text, and the last seven chapters are devoted to the most important clinically-related subjects. As the AIDS epidemic highlights, these topics are not matters of abstract research interest, but a question of life and death for ever increasing numbers of men, women, and children.

The rapidity and magnitude of exciting developments in immunology pose a rewarding challenge for instructors trying to keep abreast of the tremendous growth spurts that characterize the field. New data and methodology not only contribute to illuminating previously unanswered questions, but may also lead to changes in the interpretation of earlier findings. In this third edition, Dr. Kuby has sought to describe the most recent advances clearly and to relate them to previous concepts. Students thus will have access to the most recent facts, and also see how interpretations may change over time to reflect new data. This approach equips them to synthesize new findings as they are generated.

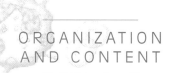

ORGANIZATION AND CONTENT

The first two editions of *Immunology* were enthusiastically received by students and instructors alike. The third edition, therefore, retains much of the original organizational motif. This edition, however, has been divided into four major parts and discussion of several topics has been shifted to maintain these cohesive conceptual units. As a result of this reorganization, the analogies between B-cell and T-cell responses have been clarified, some subjects that were previously discussed in several different chapters have been consolidated into one primary presentation, and the material on monoclonal antibodies, immune regulation, and tolerance has been incorporated into other chapters. This revised approach produces a more integrated, more logical, and more compact presentation without any loss of content.

PART I: INTRODUCTION. As in the previous editions, the first three chapters provide a conceptual framework for the material presented in subsequent chapters. Chapter 1 presents a general, integrated overview of the immune system, introducing many of the key concepts and terminology. Chapter 2 again reviews some of the important experimental systems and techniques used in modern immunology including more extensive discussion about the production of gene-targeted knockout mice. Chapter 3 still includes an introduction to the cells and tissues of the immune system, but information on lymphocyte recirculation has been shifted to a new chapter in Part III.

PART II: GENERATION OF B-CELL AND T-CELL RESPONSES. Part II focuses on how lymphocytes recognize and respond to foreign substances. It begins with a discussion of antigens, particularly the molecular properties that are recognized by B and T cells (Chapter 4). The next four chapters deal with the function of B cells: the structure and function of immunoglobulins (Chapter 5), antigen-antibody interactions (Chapter 6), the organization and expression of immunoglobulin genes (Chapter 7), and a new chapter on the maturation, activation, and differentiation of B cells (Chapter 8). The last four chapters in Part II deal with the function of T cells, beginning with Chapter 9 on the major histocompatibility complex and Chapter 10 on antigen processing and presentation—subjects that are unique to the T-cell response. The extensively updated Chapter 11 on the T-cell receptor and Chapter 12 on the maturation, activation, and differentiation of T cells have been revised to highlight the similarities with analogous B-cell processes.

PART III: IMMUNE EFFECTOR MECHANISMS. Various specific and nonspecific effector mechanisms associated with both humoral and cell-mediated responses are described in Part III. Chapter 13 presents an overview of the numerous cytokines and their effects. Activation of the complement system and the mechanisms by which complement components function in the humoral immune response are covered in Chapter 14. Next comes a new chapter containing a consolidated discussion of leukocyte migration and inflammation (Chapter 15). The major cell-mediated effector mechanisms, the characteristics of primary and secondary humoral effector responses, and regulation of immune effector responses are covered in Chapter 16. Part III concludes with a discussion of the four types of hypersensitive reactions (Chapter 17).

PART IV: THE IMMUNE SYSTEM IN HEALTH AND DISEASE. As in the first and second editions, this edition concludes with a series of clinically-oriented chapters in which the basic concepts discussed in previous chapters are applied to topics of clinical interest. Coverage includes vaccines (Chapter 18), immune response to infectious diseases (Chapter 19), autoimmunity (Chapter 20), immunodeficiency diseases (Chapter 21), AIDS (Chapter 22), transplantation immunology (Chapter 23), and cancer (Chapter 24).

Some of the significant additions and changes to the text of various chapters in the third edition include the following:

• CHAPTER 3, *Cells and Organs of the Immune System,* has been reorganized to include new coverage of cutaneous lymphoid tissue and intestinal lymphoid cells. Sections on hematopoiesis, programmed cell death, dendritic cells, and B- and T-cell activation within the secondary lymphoid organs have been updated and clarified.

• CHAPTER 5, *Immunoglobulins: Structure and Function,* now contains coverage of monoclonal antibodies and their uses. New topics include bioengineering and milk-borne immunity.

• CHAPTER 7, *Organization and Expression of Immunoglobulin Genes,* contains an updated, revised discussion of the molecular mechanisms of gene-segment joining and new material on generation of antibody diversity. The last section describes recent findings about regulation of immunoglobulin-gene transcription in B cells and the inhibition of immunoglobulin-gene expression in T cells.

• CHAPTER 8, *B-Cell Maturation, Activation, and Differentiation,* provides a unified view of the B cell paralleling the similar coverage of the T cell that was added in the second edition. In addition, it includes new information on the bone marrow microenvironment and the negative selection of self-reactive B cells during maturation. This new chapter also includes material on the identity of the B-cell coreceptor complex and much more extensive discussion of intracellular signal-transduction pathways triggered by antigen binding by B cells.

• CHAPTER 9, *Major Histocompatibility Complex,* presents extensive new information on class I and class II MHC molecules and how the structure of these molecules relates to the binding of peptides. The map of the MHC has also been updated.

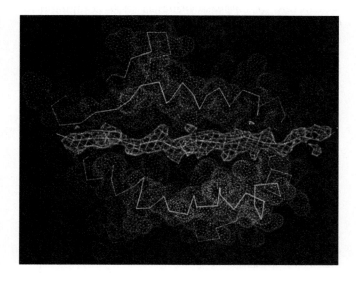

• CHAPTER 10, *Antigen Processing and Presentation,* provides new information on the enzymes and transporters involved in the pathways for handling exogenous and endogenous antigens. Descriptions of the cytosolic proteolytic system, proteasome, and TAP proteins are presented in more detail than in the second edition.

• CHAPTER 11, *T-Cell Receptor,* is extensively updated with new information on the creation of a functional T-cell antigen receptor. It describes the structure of the $\alpha\beta$ and $\gamma\delta$ T-cell receptors and compares their domain structure with the membrane-bound immunoglobulin of B cells. Likewise, the organization of TCR gene segments and their joining into functional genes are compared with analogous processes in B cells, highlighting the similarities in the mechanisms for generating antigen receptors of incredible diversity. Finally, the function of the T-cell coreceptors (CD4 and CD8) is compared with that of the B-cell coreceptor complex, and new information is presented on the role of CD4 and CD8 in T-cell activation.

• CHAPTER 12, *T-Cell Maturation, Activation, and Differentiation,* includes new material on the pre-T cell receptor and the time course of TCR-gene rearrangement during maturation of T cells in the thymus. The section on positive and negative selection during T-cell maturation, including the many unanswered questions about thymic selection, has been extensively revamped. Coverage of T-cell activation and differentiation includes more details about the co-stimulatory signal and signal-transduction pathways; the differences in the ability of dendritic cells, macrophages, and B cells to function as antigen-presenting cells are clearly delineated. Finally, recent findings about ligand recognition by $\gamma\delta$ T cells are presented.

• CHAPTER 13, *Cytokines,* brings a rapidly changing field up to date. The section on the structure and function of cytokine receptors has been substantially expanded, with five receptor families described and illustrated, and new information presented on signal transduction mediated by these receptors. New or updated tables and figures summarize the various effects of cytokines and how they interact with cells and with one another.

• CHAPTER 15, *Leukocyte Migration and Inflammation,* expands the discussion on leukocyte circulation and cell-adhesion molecules and relates it to inflammation. This new chapter presents a more general view of leukocyte circulation, how leukocytes are directed to different tissues, and a detailed picture of neutrophil and lymphocyte extravasation. It also contains a new section on the role of chemokines and other mediators in the inflammatory response.

• CHAPTER 16, *Cell-Mediated and Humoral Effector Responses,* includes new descriptions of the properties of effector T cells as well as soluble and membrane-bound effector molecules. This reorganized chapter also presents new findings concerning the role of apoptosis in target-cell destruction and receptors on natural killer cells that allow them to distinguish normal cells from infected or cancerous cells.

• CHAPTER 17, *Hypersensitive Reactions,* includes updated coverage of intracellular signals involved in mast cell degranulation and expanded discussion of asthma and other manifestations of localized type 1 hypersensitivity.

• CHAPTER 18, *Vaccines,* includes a new section on DNA vaccines, a novel approach that offers several advantages. The discussion of other vaccine types has been updated and clarified.

• CHAPTER 21, *Immunodeficiency Diseases,* describes recent findings about the genetic defects causing several types of X-linked immunodeficiencies and type I bare-lymphocyte syndrome. Updated information also is presented on the progress of gene therapy for severe combined immunodeficiency caused by ADA deficiency.

• CHAPTER 22, *The Immune System in AIDS,* has been reorganized, and discussion of some earlier findings of limited importance has been deleted. The chapter describes the recent discovery of fusin, a G-protein–coupled receptor that is the likely cofactor required for HIV infection of CD4$^+$ T cells. In addition, new information is presented on a possible intriguing link between chemokine levels and susceptibility to infection, as well as the characteristics of long-term survivors.

• CHAPTER 23, *Transplantation Immunology,* includes a new section on xenotransplants, which may become more important in the future as the supply of donor organs continues to fall short of the need.

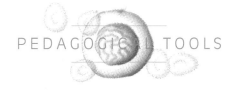

PEDAGOGICAL TOOLS

Words tell only part of the story for today's students. The other part is presented in pictures. Each figure in the previous edition has been carefully reevaluated, and many have been redesigned to improve their graphical appearance and pedagogical effectiveness. In some cases, previous figures were combined to allow a clear comparison of relationships; other figures were simplified so that they portrayed a single important concept.

A significant number of new full-color illustrations have been added to the third edition. These are intended to engage students' attention and help them to better understand complex topics. The use of color not only serves aesthetic purposes but also functions as an additional teaching tool. Color photographs appear throughout this edition, rather than in a single color insert, and thus are located in close proximity to the text points they illustrate.

A number of concepts are crucial for students to develop a firm understanding of immunology. These concepts are illustrated in new key diagrams called "Visualizing Concepts." These figures dramatize important ideas and processes in a way that written text alone cannot convey.

Each of the four parts opens with a brief overview, orienting students to the main topics covered in each chapter. Outlines are placed at the beginning of each chapter in this edition. These provide students with a chapter preview and a guideline to follow as they plan their reading.

Key terms now appear in boldface type within the text. Definitions of many of these terms appear in the revised and updated glossary at the end of the book.

Chapter summaries not only present a concise review of the material but also include references to key illustrations that provide a visual overview of the most important concepts within each chapter.

Updated references are provided at the end of each chapter to enable students to sample the primary literature relating to topics of interest.

Visualizing Concepts

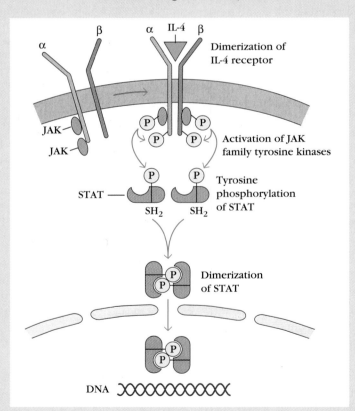

FIGURE 13-9

Model of signal transduction mediated by most class I and class II cytokine receptors. Cytokine binding induces dimerization of the receptor subunits. Association of JAK tyrosine kinases with the dimeric receptor activates the kinases, which then phosphorylate various tyrosine residues, including one or more in STAT transcription factors. After the phosphorylated STATs dimerize, they translocate to the nucleus where they activate transcription of specific genes.

ICONS

Recurring elements—such as various immune system cells and important membrane molecules—are depicted consistently, thereby facilitating the recognition of these elements in different contexts. These recurring elements look more realistic than simple, stylized shapes and provide students with an additional intuitive tool to help them construct a more complete picture of the field of immunology.

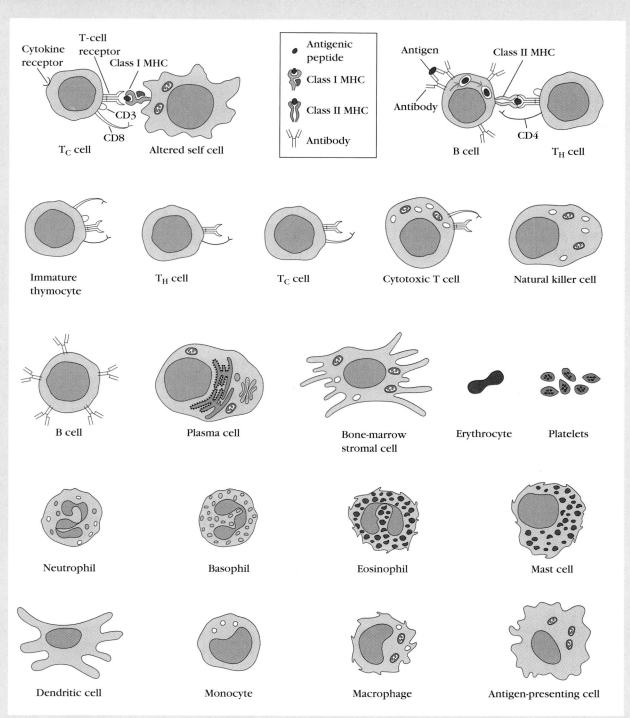

The study questions were a popular feature of earlier editions for both instructors and students. They continue to constitute a useful teaching tool that provides a challenging and thoughtful review for students. Additional questions related to new topics are included in the third edition, and many questions from the previous editions have been rewritten to enhance their clarity. As before, the answers to the study questions are given at the back of the book.

STUDY QUESTIONS

1. Indicate to which branch(es) of the immune system the following statements apply using H for the humoral branch and CM for the cell-mediated branch. Some statements may apply to both branches.
   a. Involves class I MHC molecules
   b. Responds to viral infection
   c. Involves T helper cells
   d. Involves processed antigen
   e. Most likely responds following an organ transplant
   f. Involves T cytotoxic cells
   g. Involves B cells
   h. Involves CD8$^+$ cells
   i. Responds to bacterial infection
2. Name three features of a secondary immune response that make it different from a primary immune response.
3. How does clonal selection contribute to memory in the immune response?
4. Name three features of a secondary immune response that make it different from a primary immune response.

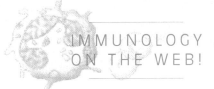

IMMUNOLOGY....
ON THE WEB!

Duane Sears, University of California at Santa Barbara, has created a Web page based upon *Immunology* that brings the subject to life for students and keeps the content refreshed with the latest breaking advances in the field. Many figures from the text, as well as additional images embedded in the Web, are available on the Web site and can be captured for classroom projection or for other use by the instructor.

The Web page also provides links to images, movies, and animations of cells undergoing an immune response, or the dynamic imaging of molecules, such as antibodies and MHC antigens, that mediate immune functions. Students can explore the Web page to discover new areas of immunology that extend beyond the course material, enjoy the visualization of three-dimensional representations of molecules that they can rotate, and access movies and snapshots of immune functions as they appear in our daily news.

To access the Web please use:
http://whfreeman.com/immunology

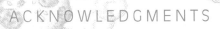

ACKNOWLEDGMENTS

The third edition has benefited greatly from the many reviewers who read all or part of the manuscript. It has become much stronger because of this interaction: Brian Barber, University of Toronto; Nan Carnal, San Francisco State University; Stephen Desiderio, Johns Hopkins University School of Medicine; Jeannine M. Durdik, University of Arkansas; Bryan M. Gebhardt, LSU Eye Center; Paul Gottlieb, University of Texas at Austin; Ted Johnson, St. Olaf College; Richard D. Karp, University of Cinncinati; Doris L. Lefkowitz, Texas Tech University; Hanne Ostergaard, University of Alberta; Charles Pfau, Rensselaer Polytechnic Institute.

Special thanks to Tova Francus, Ph.D., formerly Associate Research Professor of Immunology, Cornell University Medical College and Director, Parasitic Disease Unit, New York City Departament of Health, who was a great help during the final stages of manuscript preparation; Penelope Duerksen-Hughes, who provided a number of the study questions; and finally to Juliet A. Fuhrman, Tufts University, and Andrea M. Mastro, Pennsylvania State University, who reviewed the entire manuscript. Their reviews were truly a labor of love and the book benefited tremendously from their contributions.

We welcome comments and suggestions from users of this text and will make every effort to incorporate them into the next edition. Please direct your letters to Biology Editor, W. H. Freeman and Company, 41 Madison Avenue, New York, New York 10010.

PART I

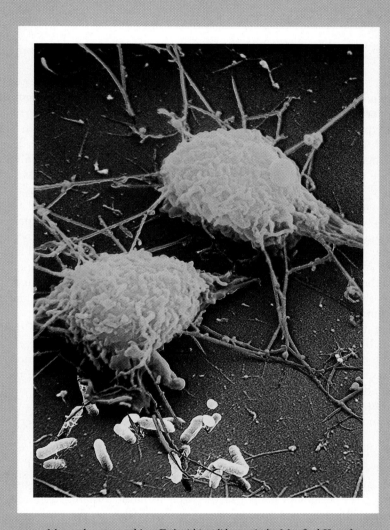

Macrophages attacking *Escherichia coli* bacteria [© Manfred Kage.]

INTRODUCTION

From birth, we are exposed to a continuous stream of microorganisms that can potentially wreak havoc on our bodily processes. Without effective protective mechanisms, each of us would soon succumb to diseases caused by pathogenic microorganisms or to the harmful effects of foreign substances (e.g., toxins) produced by various plants and bacteria. In the battle with microbial invaders, humans and other vertebrates protect themselves by a complex array of defensive measures collectively termed the immune system. Part I provides a framework for understanding the detailed mechanisms that compose the immune system and the experimental techniques used to unravel these mechanisms.

In Chapter 1, we learn about the general properties and development of immunity, the condition of being protected against infection by microorganisms or the effects of foreign molecules. Innate immunity depends on a number of barriers that are effective against a wide variety of pathogens. This nonspecific form of immunity is bolstered and greatly extended by acquired immunity, which is specific for particular microorganisms or foreign molecules. The key cells in acquired immunity are B lymphocytes (B cells) and T lymphocytes (T cells). Two major populations of T cells exist: T helper cells and cytotoxic T cells. T helper cells express the membrane glycoprotein called CD4; when activated, these cells secrete numerous low-molecular-weight proteins called cytokines, which exert various effects on other immune-system cells. T cytotoxic cells express the membrane glycoprotein called CD8; when activated, these cells differentiate into effector cells that can destroy altered self-cells, including virus-infected cells and tumor cells.

An individual contains a large number of immunocompetent clones of B and T lymphocytes. The cells in each clone are capable of recognizing a particular foreign molecule, or antigen, which may be soluble or a cellular component produced by microorganisms. B cells interact with antigen via membrane-bound immunoglobulin (antibody), and T cells interact with antigen via T-cell receptors. Following antigen recognition, lymphocytes proliferate and differentiate, leading to the production of secreted antibodies, which bind to and help eliminate the antigen (humoral response), and to the generation of cells that can destroy the invading pathogen (cell-mediated response). When we are first exposed to a particular pathogen, we normally experience some of the early symptoms of an infection because the immune system needs some time to respond and to destroy the invading pathogen. However, once we have been exposed to a particular pathogen, our immune system "remembers" the encounter and can respond much more quickly to it in subsequent encounters.

Techniques developed in the past few decades, especially recombinant DNA technology, have greatly expanded the range of questions that can be addressed experimentally. Some of the most common experimental systems and techniques used by immunologists are described in Chapter 2. An awareness of the applicability and limitations of these experimental approaches illuminates the experimental data as well as the interpretations of these data presented in later chapters.

The final chapter of Part I, Chapter 3, covers the basic properties of the cells, tissues, and organs that form the immune system. After reviewing the development of blood cells in the bone marrow (hematopoiesis), we examine the general functions of immune-system cells: lymphocytes, macrophages, granulocytes, mast cells, and dendritic cells. (The detailed mechanisms by which these cells participate in immune responses and the ways in which they cooperate with each other are discussed in later chapters.) Finally, the structures of the primary, secondary, and tertiary lymphoid organs—the sites for the maturation of lymphocytes and their activation by antigen—are considered.

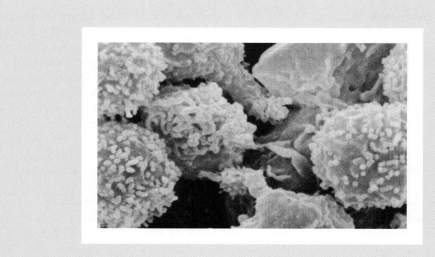

OVERVIEW OF
THE IMMUNE SYSTEM

HISTORICAL PERSPECTIVE

INNATE (NONSPECIFIC) IMMUNITY

ACQUIRED (SPECIFIC) IMMUNITY

The immune system is a remarkably adaptive defense system that has evolved in vertebrates to protect them from invading pathogenic microorganisms and cancer. It is able to generate an enormous variety of cells and molecules capable of specifically recognizing and eliminating an apparently limitless variety of foreign invaders. These cells and molecules act together in an exquisitely adaptable dynamic network whose complexity rivals that of the nervous system.

Functionally, an immune response can be divided into two interrelated activities—**recognition** and **response**. Immune recognition is remarkable for its specificity. The immune system is able to recognize subtle chemical differences that distinguish one foreign pathogen from another. At the same time, the system is able to discriminate between foreign molecules and the body's own cells and proteins. Once a foreign organism is recognized, the immune system enlists the participation of a variety of cells and molecules to mount an appropriate response,

known as an **effector response**, to eliminate or neutralize the organism. In this way the system is able to convert the initial recognition event into different effector responses, each uniquely suited to eliminate a particular type of pathogen. Later exposure to the same foreign organism induces a **memory response**, characterized by a heightened immune reactivity, that serves to eliminate the pathogen and prevent disease.

This chapter presents a broad overview of the cells and molecules that compose the immune system and the mechanisms by which they protect the body against foreign invaders. As is always the case with an overview, the details have been simplified to reveal the essential structure of the immune system. Substantive discussions, experimental approaches, and in-depth definitions are left to the chapters that follow.

HISTORICAL PERSPECTIVE

The discipline of immunology grew out of the observation that individuals who had recovered from certain infectious diseases were thereafter protected from the disease. The Latin term *immunis,* meaning "exempt," is the source of the English word **immunity**, meaning the state of protection from infectious disease.

Perhaps the earliest written reference to the phenomenon of immunity can be traced back to Thucydides, the great historian of the Peloponnesian War. In describing a plague in Athens, he wrote in 430 B.C. that only those who had recovered from the plague could nurse the sick because they would not contract the disease a second time. Although early societies recognized the phenomenon of immunity, almost two thousand years passed before the concept was successfully converted into a medically effective practice.

The first recorded crude attempts to deliberately induce immunity were performed by the Chinese and Turks in the fifteenth century. Various reports suggest that the dried crusts derived from smallpox pustules were either inhaled into the nostrils or inserted into small cuts in the skin (a technique called **variolation**). In 1718 Lady Mary Wortley Montagu, the wife of the British ambassador to Constantinople, observed the positive effects of variolation on the native population and had the technique applied to her own children. The technique was significantly improved by the English physician Edward Jenner in 1798. Intrigued by the fact that milkmaids who contracted cowpox (a mild disease) were subsequently immune to smallpox (a disfiguring and often fatal disease), Jenner reasoned that introducing fluid from a cowpox pustule into people (i.e., inoculating them) might protect them from smallpox. To test this idea, he inoculated an eight-year-old boy with fluid from a cowpox pustule and later intentionally infected the child with smallpox. As predicted, the child did not develop smallpox. Nevertheless, one cannot help but question the ethical implications of such an experiment!

Jenner's technique of inoculating with cowpox to protect against smallpox spread quickly throughout Europe, but it was nearly a hundred years before the technique was applied to other diseases. As so often happens in science, serendipity combined with astute observation led to the next major advance in immunology, the induction of immunity to cholera by Louis Pasteur. Pasteur had succeeded in growing the organism thought to cause fowl cholera in culture and then had shown that chickens injected with the cultured bacterium developed cholera. After returning from a summer vacation, he injected some chickens with an old culture of the bacterium. The chickens became ill, but to Pasteur's surprise they recovered. Pasteur then grew a fresh culture of the bacterium with the intention of injecting it into some fresh chickens. But the story goes, he was low on chickens and therefore used the previously injected chickens. Again to his surprise, the chickens survived and were completely protected from the disease. Pasteur recognized that aging had weakened the virulence of the pathogen and that

such an attenuated strain might be administered to protect against the disease. He called this attenuated strain a **vaccine** (from the Latin *vacca*, meaning "cow") in honor of Jenner's work with cowpox inoculation.

Pasteur extended these findings to other diseases, demonstrating that is was possible to **attenuate**, or weaken, a pathogen and administer the attenuated strain as a vaccine. In a now classical experiment at Pouilly-le-Fort in 1881, Pasteur first vaccinated one group of sheep with heat-attenuated anthrax bacillus; he then challenged the vaccinated sheep and some unvaccinated sheep with a virulent culture of *Bacillus anthracis*. All the vaccinated sheep lived, whereas all unvaccinated animals died. These experiments marked the beginnings of the discipline of immunology. In 1885, Pasteur administered the first vaccine to a human, a young boy who had been bitten repeatedly by a rabid dog (Figure 1-1). The boy, Joseph Meister, lived and later became a custodian at the Pasteur Institute. In 1940, during the Nazi occupation of Paris,

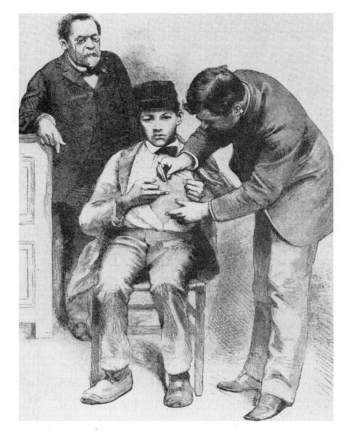

FIGURE 1-1

Wood engraving of Louis Pasteur watching Joseph Meister receive the rabies vaccine. [From *Harper's Weekly* **29**:836, 1885; courtesy of the National Library of Medicine.]

the Nazis asked Meister to give them the keys to Pasteur's crypt. Rather than surrender the keys to the Nazis, Meister took his own life.

Discovery of Humoral and Cellular Immunity

Although Pasteur proved that **vaccination** worked, he did not understand the mechanisms involved. The experimental work of Emil von Behring and Shibasaburo Kitasato in 1890 provided the first insights into the mechanism of immunity, earning von Behring the Nobel prize in medicine in 1901 (Table 1-1). Von Behring and

Kitasato demonstrated that **serum** (the noncellular part of blood) from animals previously immunized to diphtheria could transfer the immune state to unimmunized animals. In search of the protective agent, various researchers during the next decade demonstrated that an active component from immune serum could neutralize toxins, precipitate toxins, rupture (lyse) bacteria, and clump (agglutinate) bacteria. In each case, the active agent was named for the activity it exhibited: antitoxin, precipitin, bacterolysin, and agglutinin, respectively. Initially, a different serum component was thought to be responsible for each activity, but during the 1930s a single substance, called an **antibody**, was shown to be responsible for all of

TABLE 1-1

NOBEL PRIZES FOR IMMUNOLOGIC RESEARCH

YEAR	RECIPIENT	COUNTRY	RESEARCH
1901	Emil von Behring	Germany	Serum antitoxins
1905	Robert Koch	Germany	Cellular immunity to tuberculosis
1908	Elie Metchnikoff Paul Ehrlich	Russia Germany	Role of phagocytosis (Metchnikoff) and antitoxins (Ehrlich) in immunity
1913	Charles Richet	France	Anaphylaxis
1919	Jules Border	Belgium	Complement-mediated bacteriolysis
1930	Karl Landsteiner	U.S.A.	Discovery of human blood groups
1951	Max Theiler	South Africa	Development of yellow fever vaccine
1957	Daniel Bovet	Switzerland	Antihistamines
1960	F. Macfarlane Burnet Peter Medawar	Australia Great Britain	Discovery of acquired immunological tolerance
1972	Rodney R. Porter Gerald M. Edelman	Great Britain U.S.A.	Chemical structure of antibodies
1977	Rosalyn R. Yalow	U.S.A.	Development of radioimmunoassay
1980	George Snell Jean Dausset Baruj Benacerraf	U.S.A. France U.S.A.	Major histocompatibility complex
1984	Cesar Milstein Georges F. Köhler Niels K. Jerne	Great Britain Germany Denmark	Monoclonal antibody Immune regulatory theories
1987	Susumu Tonegawa	Japan	Gene rearrangement in antibody production
1991	E. Donnall Thomas Joseph Murray	U.S.A. U.S.A.	Transplantation immunology
1996	Peter C. Doherty Rolf M. Zinkernagel	Australia Switzerland	The specificity of the cell-mediated immune response

these activities. Because immunity was mediated by antibodies contained in body fluids (known at the time as *humors*), it was called **humoral immunity**.

In 1883, even before the discovery that a serum component could transfer immunity, Elie Metchnikoff demonstrated that cells also contribute to the immune state of an animal. He observed that certain white blood cells, which he termed **phagocytes**, were able to ingest microorganisms and other foreign material. Noting that these phagocytic cells were more active in immunized animals than nonimmunized animals, Metchnikoff hypothesized that cells, rather than serum components, were the major effector of immunity.

In due course, a controversy developed between those who held to the concept of humoral immunity and those who agreed with Metchnikoff's concept of **cell-mediated immunity**. The controversy eventually was resolved when the interrelated roles of humoral and cellular activities were demonstrated and both were shown to be necessary for the immune response. In the 1950s the **lymphocyte** was identified as the cell responsible for both cellular and humoral immunity.

Early Theories of Immunity

One of the greatest enigmas about the antibody molecule facing early immunologists was its specificity for foreign material, or **antigen**. Two major theories were proposed to account for this specificity: the selective theory and the instructional theory.

The earliest conception of the **selective theory** dates to Paul Ehrlich in 1900. In an attempt to explain the origin of serum antibody, Ehrlich proposed that cells expressed a variety of "side-chain" receptors that could react with infectious agents. Binding of an infectious agent to a side-chain receptor was envisioned as a complementary lock-and-key type of interaction. Ehrlich suggested that interaction between an infectious agent and a cell's side-chain receptor would result in release of the side chain and would induce the cell to produce and release more side-chain receptors with the same specificity. According to Ehrlich's theory, the side-chain specificity was determined prior to antigen exposure and antigen selected the appropriate side chain.

In the 1930s and 1940s the selective theory was replaced by various **instructional theories** in which antigen played a central role in determining the specificity of the antibody molecule. According to the instructional theories, a particular antigen would serve as a template around which antibody would fold. The antibody molecule would thereby assume a configuration complementary to that of the antigen template. Such concepts, first postulated by Friedrich Breinl and Felix Haurowitz and later popularized by Linus Pauling, made sense within the limitations of scientific knowledge at that time. But as new information emerged about the structure of DNA, RNA, and protein, the instructional theories were disproved.

In the 1950s, selection theories resurfaced and, through the insights of Niels Jerne, David Talmadge, and F. Macfarlane Burnet, were refined into a theory that came to be known as the **clonal-selection** theory. According to this theory, individual lymphocytes express membrane receptors that are specific for distinct antigens. Each lymphocyte expresses a unique receptor specificity, which is determined prior to antigen exposure. Binding of antigen to a specific receptor activates the cell, resulting in its proliferation into a **clone** of cells, each with the same immunologic specificity as the original parent cell. The clonal-selection theory has been further refined and is now accepted as the underlying paradigm of modern immunology. This theory is examined in more depth later in the chapter.

Components of Immunity

Immunity—the state of protection from infectious disease—has both nonspecific and specific components. **Innate**, or nonspecific, **immunity** refers to the basic resistance to disease that an individual is born with. **Acquired**, or specific, **immunity** requires the activity of a functional immune system, involving cells called lymphocytes and their products. Innate defense mechanisms provide the first line of host defense against invading pathogens until an acquired immune response develops. In general, most of the microorganisms encountered by a healthy individual are readily cleared within a few days by nonspecific defense mechanisms without enlisting a specific immune response. When an invading microorganism eludes the nonspecific host defense mechanisms, a specific immune response then is enlisted. Acquired immunity does not operate independently of innate immunity; rather, the specific immune response supplements and augments the nonspecific defense mechanisms, producing a more effective total response.

INNATE (NONSPECIFIC) IMMUNITY

Innate immunity can be envisioned as comprising four types of defensive barriers: anatomic, physiologic, endocytic and phagocytic, and inflammatory (Table 1-2).

Tissue damage and infection induce leakage of vascular fluid, containing serum proteins with antibacterial activity, and influx of phagocytic cells into the affected area.

Anatomic Barriers

Physical and anatomic barriers that tend to prevent the entry of pathogens are an organism's first line of defense against infection. The **skin** and the surface of **mucous membranes** are included in this category because they provide an effective barrier to the entry of most microorganisms.

The skin consists of two distinct layers: a relatively thin outer layer—the **epidermis**—and a thicker layer—the **dermis**. The epidermis contains several layers of tightly packed epithelial cells. The outer epidermal layer consists of dead cells and is filled with a waterproofing protein called keratin. Old epidermal cells are sloughed from the surface and are replaced by new cells derived from division of cells lying next to the dermis; as a result, the epidermis is completely renewed every 15–30 days. The epidermis does not contain blood vessels, and epidermal cells are instead bathed in nutrients that diffuse from the underlying dermis. The dermis, which is composed of connective tissue, contains blood vessels, hair follicles, sebaceous glands, and sweat glands. The sebaceous glands are associated with the hair follicles and produce an oily secretion called **sebum**. Sebum consists of lactic and fatty acids, maintaining the pH of the skin between 3 and 5, which is inhibitory to the growth of most microorganisms. A few bacteria that metabolize sebum live as commensals on the skin and are responsible for a severe form of acne. One acne drug, isotretinoin (Accutane), is a vitamin A derivative that prevents sebum formation.

Intact skin not only prevents the penetration of most pathogens but also inhibits most bacterial growth due to its low pH. Breaks in the skin, even small ones, resulting from wounds or abrasion are obvious routes of infection. The skin also is penetrated by biting insects (e.g., mosquitoes, mites, ticks, fleas, and sandflies); if these harbor pathogenic organisms, they can introduce the pathogen into the body as they feed. The protozoan that causes malaria, for example, is carried by mosquitoes who deposit it in humans when they take a blood meal. Similarly, bubonic plague is spread by the bite of fleas, and Lyme disease is spread by the bite of ticks.

The conjunctivae and the alimentary, respiratory, and urogenital tracts are lined by mucous membranes, not by the dry, protective skin covering the exterior of the body. These membranes consist of an outer epithelial layer

TABLE 1–2

SUMMARY OF NONSPECIFIC HOST DEFENSES

TYPE	MECHANISM
Atomic barriers	
Skin	Mechanical barrier retards entry of microbes. Acidic environment (pH 3–5) retards growth of microbes.
Mucous membranes	Normal flora compete with microbes for attachment sites and nutrients. Mucus entraps foreign microorganisms. Cilia propel microorganisms out of body.
Physiologic barriers	
Temperature	Body temperature inhibits growth of some pathogens. Fever response inhibits growth of some pathogens.
Low pH	Acidic pH of stomach kills most ingested microorganisms.
Chemical mediators	Lysozyme cleaves bacterial cell wall. Interferon induces antiviral state in uninfected cells. Complement lyses microorganisms or facilitates phagocytosis.
Phagocytic/endocytic barriers	Various cells internalize (endocytose) and break down foreign macromolecules. Specialized cells (blood monocytes, neutrophils, tissue macrophages) internalize (phagocytose), kill, and digest whole microorganisms.
Inflammatory barriers	Tissue damage and infection induce leakage of vascular fluid, containing serum proteins with antibacterial activity, and influx of phagocytic cells into the affected area.

and an underlying connective tissue layer. Although most pathogens enter the body by binding to and penetrating mucous membranes, a number of nonspecific defense mechanisms serve to prevent this entry. For example, saliva, tears, and mucous secretions act to wash away potential invaders and also contain antibacterial or antiviral substances. The viscous fluid called **mucus**, which is secreted by epithelial cells of mucous membranes, entraps foreign microorganisms. In the lower respiratory tract and the gastrointestinal tract, the mucous membrane is covered by **cilia**, hairlike processes projecting from the epithelial cells. The synchronous movement of cilia propel mucousentrapped microorganisms from these tracts. In addition, nonpathogenic organisms tend to colonize the epithelial cells of mucosal surfaces. These **normal flora** generally outcompete pathogens for attachment sites on the epithelial cell surface and for necessary nutrients.

Some organisms have evolved ways to escape this defense mechanism and thus are likely to invade the body through mucous membranes. For example, influenza virus (the agent that causes flu) has a surface molecule that enables it to attach firmly to cells in mucous membranes, preventing the virus from being swept out by the ciliated epithelial cells. Similarly, the organism causing gonorrhea has surface projections that allow it to bind to mucous membrane epithelial cells in the urogenital tract. Adherence of bacteria to mucous membranes involves interactions between hairlike protrusions on a bacterium, called **fimbriae** or **pili**, and certain glycoproteins or glycolipids that are only expressed by some mucous membrane epithelial cells (Figure 1-2). For this reason, some tissues are susceptible to bacterial invasion, whereas others are not.

The importance of anatomic barriers to host defense is vividly illustrated by a group of mice described in a report in *Nature*. These mice appeared to be immune to the parasitic helminth (worm) that causes schistosomiasis, a chronic and debilitating disease affecting more than 300 million people worldwide. After initial infection with this helminth, the mice developed portal hypertension similar to that observed in humans with schistosomiasis. However, when mice were reinfected with the helminth a second time, a very low yield of the helminth was recovered, and the mice appeared to be resistant to the infection. Because the mice had apparently developed immunity to the helminth, they were considered to be a potential animal model for the study of schistosomiasis in humans. After considerable funding was poured into research on this mouse model, the ability to clear the helminth was found to have nothing to do with a specific immune response; instead it resulted from a complex anatomic reorganization in blood vessel architecture that occurred at the time of the second injection. The *Nature* article warned "not to postulate immunological mechanisms

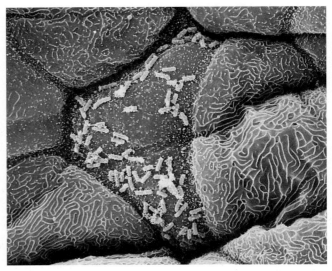

FIGURE 1-2

Electron micrograph of rod-shaped *Escherichia coli* bacteria adhering to surface of epithelial cells of the urinary tract. [From N. Sharon and H. Lis, 1993, *Sci. Am.* **268**(1):85.]

where simple anatomical or physiological explanations might suffice."

Even when a pathogen eludes the anatomic defenses provided by the skin and mucous membranes, it still faces other types of innate defenses including various physiologic, phagocytic, and inflammatory barriers. Only by successfully evading these barriers can a pathogen become established in a host.

Physiologic Barriers

The physiologic barriers that contribute to innate immunity include temperature, pH, oxygen tension, and various soluble factors. Many species are not susceptible to certain diseases simply because their body temperature inhibits pathogen growth. Chickens, for example, display innate immunity to anthrax because their high body temperature inhibits the growth of this pathogen. Gastric acidity also provides an innate physiologic barrier to infection because very few ingested microorganisms can survive the low pH of the stomach. One reason newborns are susceptible to some diseases that do not afflict adults is that their stomach contents are less acid than that of adults.

A variety of soluble factors also contribute to nonspecific immunity. Among these soluble proteins are lysozyme, interferon, and complement. **Lysozyme**, a hydrolytic enzyme found in mucous secretions, is able to cleave the peptidoglycan layer of the bacterial cell wall. **Interferon** comprises a group of proteins produced by virus-infected cells. Among the many functions of the interferons is the ability to bind to nearby cells and induce a generalized antiviral state. **Complement** is a group of serum proteins that circulate in an inactive proenzyme state. These proteins can be activated by a variety of specific and nonspecific immunologic mechanisms that convert the inactive proenzymes into active enzymes. The activated complement components participate in a controlled enzymatic cascade that results in damage to the membranes of pathogenic organisms, either destroying the pathogens or facilitating their clearance.

Endocytic and Phagocytic Barriers

Another important innate defense mechanism is the ingestion of extracellular macromolecules via **endocytosis** and of particulate material via **phagocytosis**. These two internalization processes not only bring different types of extracellular material into the cell, they also differ in several other ways.

In endocytosis, macromolecules within the extracellular tissue fluid are internalized by cells via the invagination (inward folding) and pinching off of small regions of the plasma membrane. The resultant endocytic vesicles are small, approximately 0.1 μm in diameter. Endocytosis occurs through one of two processes: **pinocytosis** or **receptor-mediated endocytosis** (Figure 1-3). In pinocytosis, nonspecific membrane invagination internalizes macromolecules in proportion to their extracellular concentration. In receptor-mediated endocytosis, macromolecules are selectively internalized after binding to specific membrane receptors.

The endocytic vesicles formed by either process fuse with each other and are delivered to **endosomes**, which are intracellular acidic compartments that serve a sorting function. The acidic interior of endosomes facilitates dissociation of macromolecular ligands from their receptors; the latter are then recycled back to the cell surface. Free macromolecules contained within endosomes fuse with

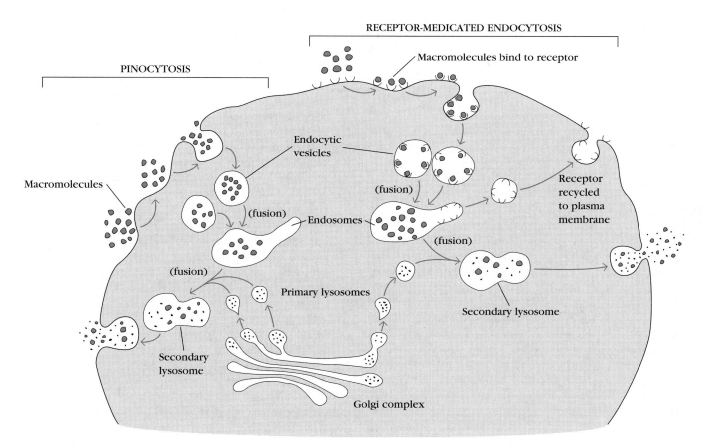

FIGURE 1-3

Endocytosis—the internalization of macromolecules within the extracellular fluid—occurs by pinocytosis or receptor-mediated endocytosis. In both processes, the ingested material is degraded via the endocytic processing pathway.

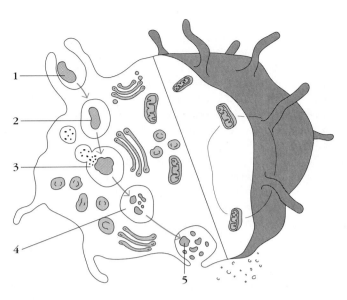

FIGURE 1-4

Phagocytosis of bacteria. Schematic diagram of the steps in phagocytosis: (1) attachment of a bacterium (blue) to long membrane evaginations, called pseudopodia; (2) ingestion of bacterium forming a phagosome, which moves toward a lysosome; (3) fusion of the lysosome and phagosome, releasing lysosomal enzymes into the phagosome; (4) digestion of ingested material; and (5) release of digestion products from the cell.

primary lysosomes to form structures known as **secondary lysosomes**. Primary lysosomes are derived from the Golgi complex and contain large numbers of degradative enzymes, including proteases, nucleases, lipases, and other hydrolytic enzymes. Within secondary lysosomes, the ingested macromolecules are then digested into small breakdown products (e.g., peptides, nucleotides, and sugars), which eventually are eliminated from the cell.

Phagocytosis involves the ingestion of particulate material, including whole pathogenic microorganisms (Figure 1-4). In phagocytosis the plasma membrane expands around the particulate material to form large vesicles called **phagosomes**. These vesicles are roughly 10–20 times larger than endocytic vesicles. The expansion of the membrane in phagocytosis requires participation of microfilaments, which do not take part in endocytosis. Another difference between the two processes is that only specialized cells are capable of phagocytosis, whereas virtually all cells are capable of endocytosis. The specialized phagocytic cells include blood monocytes, neutrophils, and tissue macrophages (see Chapter 3). Once particulate material is ingested into phagosomes, the phagosomes fuse with lysosomes and the ingested material is then digested in the endocytic processing pathway by a process similar to that seen in endocytosis.

Barriers Created by the Inflammatory Response

Tissue damage caused by a wound or by invasion by a pathogenic microorganism induces a complex sequence of events collectively known as the **inflammatory response**. Many of the classic features of the inflammatory response were described as early as 1600 B.C. in Egyptian papyrus writings. In the first century A.D., the Roman physician Celsus described the "four cardinal signs of inflammation" as *rubor* (redness), *tumor* (swelling), *calor* (heat), and *dolor* (pain). In the second century A.D., another physician, Galen, added a fifth sign: *functio laesa* (loss of function).

The cardinal signs of inflammation reflect the three major events that occur during an inflammatory response (Figure 1-5):

1. **Vasodilation**—an increase in the diameter of blood vessels—occurs as the vessels that carry blood away from an affected area constrict, resulting in engorgement of the capillary network. The engorged capillaries are responsible for tissue redness (*erythema*) and an increase in tissue temperature.
2. An **increase in capillary permeability** facilitates an influx of fluid and cells from the engorged capillaries into the tissue. The fluid that accumulates (**exudate**) has a much higher protein content than fluid normally released from the vasculature. Accumulation of exudate contributes to tissue swelling (**edema**).
3. **Influx of phagocytes** from the capillaries into the tissues is facilitated by the increased capillary permeability. The emigration of phagocytes involves a complex series of events including adherence of the cells to the endothelial wall (**margination**) followed by their emigration between the capillary endothelial cells into the tissue (**diapedesis** or **extravasation**) and, finally, their migration through the tissue to the site of the inflammatory response (**chemotaxis**). As phagocytic cells accumulate at the site and begin to phagocytose bacteria, they release lytic enzymes, which can damage nearby healthy cells. The accumulation of dead cells, digested material, and fluid forms a substance called pus.

The events in the inflammatory response are initiated by a complex series of interactions involving a variety of chemical mediators, whose interactions are still only partially understood. Some of these mediators are derived from invading microorganisms, some are released from damaged cells in response to tissue injury, some are generated by several plasma enzyme systems, and some are products of various white blood cells participating in the inflammatory response.

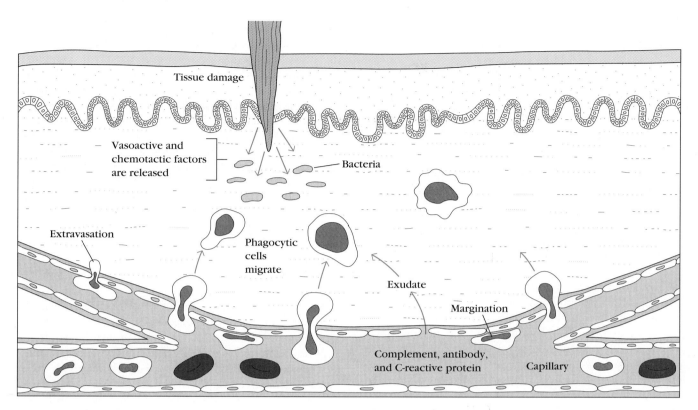

FIGURE 1-5

Major events in the inflammatory response. A bacterial infection causes tissue damage with release of various vasoactive and chemotactic factors. These factors induce increased blood flow to the area, increased capillary permeability, and an influx of white blood cells, including phagocytes and lymphocytes, from the blood into the tissues. The serum proteins contained in the exudate have antibacterial properties, and the phagocytes begin to engulf the bacteria, as illustrated in Figure 1-4.

Among the chemical mediators released in response to tissue damage are various serum proteins called **acute-phase proteins**. The concentrations of these proteins increase dramatically in tissue-damaging infections. C-reactive protein—a major acute-phase protein produced by the liver in response to tissue damage—binds to the C-polysaccharide cell-wall component found on a variety of bacteria and fungi. This binding activates the complement system, resulting in increased clearance of the pathogen either by complement-mediated lysis of the pathogen or by complement-mediated increase in phagocytosis.

One of the principal mediators of the inflammatory response is **histamine**, a chemical released by a variety of cells in response to tissue injury. Histamine binds to receptors on nearby capillaries and venules, causing vasodilation and increased permeability. Another important group of inflammatory mediators, small peptides called **kinins**, are present in an inactive form in blood plasma. Tissue injury induces activation of these peptides, which then cause vasodilation and increased capillary permeabil-

ity. A particular kinin, called bradykinin, also stimulates pain receptors in the skin. This effect probably serves a protective role because pain normally causes an individual to protect the injured area.

Vasodilation and the increase in capillary permeability that occur in an injured tissue also enable enzymes of the blood-clotting system to enter the tissue. These enzymes activate an enzyme cascade that results in the deposition of insoluble strands of **fibrin**, which are the main component of a blood clot. The fibrin clots wall off the injured area from the rest of the body and serve to prevent the spread of infection.

Once the inflammatory response has subsided and most of the debris has been cleared away by phagocytic cells, tissue repair and regeneration of new tissue occur. Tissue repair begins as capillaries grow into the fibrin of a blood clot. New connective tissue cells, called fibroblasts, replace the fibrin as the clot dissolves. As fibroblasts and capillaries accumulate, scar tissue is formed. The inflammatory response is discussed in more detail in Chapter 15.

ACQUIRED (SPECIFIC) IMMUNITY

Acquired, or specific, immunity reflects the presence of a functional immune system that is capable of specifically recognizing and selectively eliminating foreign microorganisms and molecules (i.e., foreign antigens). Unlike innate immune responses, acquired immune responses are adaptive and display four characteristic attributes:

- Antigenic specificity
- Diversity
- Immunologic memory
- Self/nonself recognition

The **antigenic specificity** of the immune system permits it to distinguish subtle differences among antigens. Antibodies can differentiate between two molecules that differ by only a single amino acid. The immune system is capable of generating tremendous **diversity** in its recognition molecules, allowing it to specifically recognize billions of uniquely different structures on foreign antigens. Once the immune system has recognized and responded to an antigen, it exhibits **immunologic memory**; that is, a second encounter with the same antigen induces a heightened state of immune reactivity. Because of this attribute, the immune system can confer life-long immunity to many infectious agents. Finally, the immune system normally responds only to foreign antigens indicating that it is capable of **self/nonself recognition**. The ability of the immune system to distinguish self from nonself and respond only to nonself-molecules is essential, for the outcome of an inappropriate response to self-molecules can be a fatal autoimmune disease.

As noted already, acquired immunity does not occur independently of innate immunity. The phagocytic cells crucial to nonspecific immune responses are intimately involved in activation of the specific immune response. Conversely, various soluble factors, produced during a specific immune response, have been shown to augment the activity of these phagocytic cells. As an inflammatory response develops, for example, soluble mediators are produced that attract cells of the immune system. The immune response will, in turn, serve to regulate the intensity of the inflammatory response. Through the carefully regulated interplay of acquired and innate immunity, the two systems work together to eliminate a foreign invader.

Cells of the Immune System

Generation of an effective immune response involves two major groups of cells: **lymphocytes** and **antigen-presenting cells**. Lymphocytes are one of many types of white blood cells produced in the bone marrow during the process of hematopoiesis (see Chapter 3). Lymphocytes leave the bone marrow, circulate in the blood and lymph system, and reside in various lymphoid organs. Lymphocytes, which possess antigen-binding cell-surface receptors, mediate the defining immunologic attributes of specificity, diversity, memory, and self/nonself recognition. The two major populations of lymphocytes— **B lymphocytes** (**B cells**) and **T lymphocytes** (**T cells**)—are described briefly here and in greater detail in later chapters.

B Lymphocytes

B lymphocytes mature within the bone marrow and leave the marrow expressing a unique antigen-binding receptor on their membrane (Figure 1-6a). The B-cell receptor is a membrane-bound **antibody molecule**. Antibodies are glycoproteins. The basic structure of the antibody molecule consists of two identical heavy polypeptide chains and two identical light polypeptide chains. The chains are held together by disulfide bonds. The amino-terminal ends of each pair of heavy and light chains form a cleft within which antigen binds. When a **naive** B cell, which has not previously encountered antigen, first encounters the antigen for which its membrane-bound antibody is specific, the cell begins to divide rapidly; its progeny differentiate into **memory B cells** and **effector B cells** called **plasma cells**.

Memory B cells have a longer life span and continue to express membrane-bound antibody with the same specificity as the original parent naive B cell. Plasma cells do not express membrane-bound antibody; instead they produce the antibody in a form that can be secreted. Although plasma cells live for only a few days, they secrete enormous amounts of antibody during this time. It has been estimated that a single plasma cell can secrete more than 2000 molecules of antibody per second. Secreted antibodies are the major effector molecule of humoral immunity.

T Lymphocytes

T lymphocytes also arise from hematopoietic stem cells in the bone marrow. Unlike B cells, which mature within the bone marrow, T cells migrate to the thymus gland to mature. During its maturation within the thymus, the T cell comes to express a unique antigen-binding receptor on its membrane, called the **T-cell receptor**. Unlike membrane-bound antibodies on B cells, which can recognize antigen alone, T-cell receptors can only recognize antigen that is associated with cell-membrane proteins known as **major histocompatibility complex (MHC)**

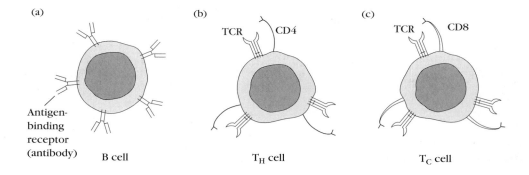

FIGURE 1-6

Distinctive membrane molecules on lymphocytes. (a) B cells have about 10^5 molecules of membrane-bound antibody per cell. All the antibody molecules on a given B cell exhibit the same antigenic specificity and can interact directly with antigen. (b) T cells bearing CD4 only recognize antigen associated with class II MHC molecules. (c) T cells bearing CD8 only recognize antigen associated with class I MHC molecules. In general, CD4⁺ T cells function as helper cells and CD8⁺ cells function as cytotoxic cells. Both types of T cells express about 10^5 identical molecules of the antigen-binding T-cell receptor (TCR) per cell, each with the same antigenic specificity.

molecules. When a naive T cell encounters antigen associated with an MHC molecule on a cell, the T cell proliferates and differentiates into memory T cells and various effector T cells.

There are two well-defined subpopulations of T cells: **T helper (T_H)** and **T cytotoxic (T_C) cells**. Although a third type of T cell, called a T suppressor (T_S) cell, has been postulated, recent evidence suggests that it may not be distinct from the T_H and T_C subpopulations. T helper and T cytotoxic cells can be distinguished from one another by the presence of either membrane glycoproteins **CD4** or **CD8** on their surfaces (Figure 1-6b,c). T cells displaying CD4 generally function as T_H cells, whereas those displaying CD8 generally function as T_C cells (see Chapter 3).

After a T_H cell recognizes and interacts with an antigen–MHC II molecule complex, the cell is activated and becomes an effector cell that secretes various growth factors known collectively as **cytokines**. The secreted cytokines play an important role in activating B cells, T_C cells, macrophages, and various other cells that participate in the immune response. Differences in the pattern of cytokines produced by activated T_H cells results in qualitative differences in the type of immune response that develops.

Under the influence of T_H-derived cytokines, a T_C cell that recognizes an antigen–MHC I molecule complex proliferates and differentiates into an effector cell called a **cytotoxic T lymphocyte** (CTL). In contrast to the T_H cell, the CTL generally does not secrete many cytokines and instead exhibits cytotoxic activity. The CTL has a vital function in monitoring the cells of the body and eliminating any that display antigen, such as virus-infected cells, tumor cells, and cells of a foreign tis-

sue graft. Such cells displaying foreign antigen complexed to an MHC molecule are called **altered self-cells**.

ANTIGEN-PRESENTING CELLS

Activation of both the humoral and cell-mediated branches of the immune system requires cytokines produced by T_H cells. It is essential that activation of T_H cells be carefully regulated because an inappropriate T_H-cell response to self-components can have fatal autoimmune consequences. To ensure carefully regulated activation of T_H cells, they only can recognize antigen that is displayed together with class MHC II molecules on the surface of antigen-presenting cells (APCs). These specialized cells, which include macrophages, B lymphocytes, and dendritic cells, are distinguished by two properties: (1) they express class II MHC molecules on their membrane, and (2) they are able to deliver a co-stimulatory signal that is necessary for T_H-cell activation.

Antigen-presenting cells first internalize antigen, either by phagocytosis or by endocytosis, and then re-express a part of that antigen, together with a class II MHC molecule, on their membrane. The T_H cell recognizes and interacts with the antigen–MHC molecule complex on the membrane of the antigen-presenting cell (Figure 1-7). An additional co-stimulatory signal is then provided by the antigen-presenting cell, leading to activation of the T_H cell.

Functions of Humoral and Cell-Mediated Immune Responses

As mentioned earlier, immune responses can be divided into humoral and cell-mediated responses. The term

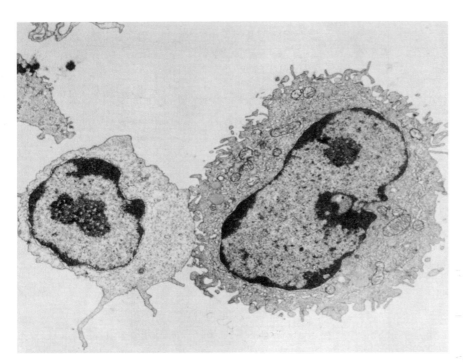

FIGURE 1-7

Electron micrograph of an antigen-presenting macrophage (*right*) associating with a T lymphocyte. [From A. S. Rosenthal et al., 1982, in *Phagocytosis—Past and Future,* Academic Press, p. 239.]

humoral is derived from the Latin *humor,* meaning "body fluid"; thus humoral immunity refers to immunity that can be conferred on a nonimmune individual by administration of serum antibodies from an immune individual. In contrast, cell-mediated immunity can be transferred only by administration of T cells from an immune individual.

The humoral branch of the immune system involves interaction of B cells with antigen and their subsequent proliferation and differentiation into antibody-secreting plasma cells (Figure 1-8). Antibody functions as the effector of the humoral response by binding to antigen and neutralizing it or facilitating its elimination. When an antigen is coated with antibody, it can be eliminated in several ways. For example, antibody can cross-link the antigen, forming clusters that are more readily ingested by phagocytic cells. Binding of antibody to antigen on a microorganism also can activate the complement system, resulting in lysis of the foreign organism. Antibody can also neutralize toxins or viral particles by coating them and preventing their subsequent binding to host cells.

Effector T cells generated in response to antigen are responsible for cell-mediated immunity (see Figure 1-8). Both activated T_H cells and CTLs serve as effector cells in cell-mediated immune reactions. Cytokines secreted by T_H cells can activate various phagocytic cells, enabling them to phagocytose and kill microorganisms more effectively. This type of cell-mediated immune response is especially important in host defense against intracellular bacteria and protozoa. Cytotoxic T lymphocytes (CTLs) participate in cell-mediated immune reactions by killing altered self-cells; they play an important role in the killing of virus-infected cells and tumor cells.

Recognition of Antigen by B and T Lymphocytes

Antigens, which are generally very large and complex, are not recognized in their entirety by lymphocytes. Instead, both B and T lymphocytes recognize discrete sites on the antigen called **antigenic determinants**, or **epitopes**. Epitopes are the immunologically active regions on a complex antigen, the regions that actually bind to B-cell or T-cell receptors.

Although B cells can recognize an epitope alone, T cells can recognize an epitope only when it is associated with an MHC molecule on the surface of a self-cell (either an antigen-presenting cell or altered self-cell). The two branches of the immune system are therefore uniquely suited to recognize antigen in different milieus. The humoral branch (B cells) recognizes an enormous variety of epitopes: those displayed on the surface of bacteria or viral particles, as well as those displayed on soluble proteins, glycoproteins, polysaccharides, or lipopolysaccharides that have been released from invading pathogens. The cell-mediated branch (T cells) recognizes protein epitopes displayed together with MHC molecules on self-cells, including altered self-cells such as virus-infected self-cells and cancerous cells.

Visualizing Concepts

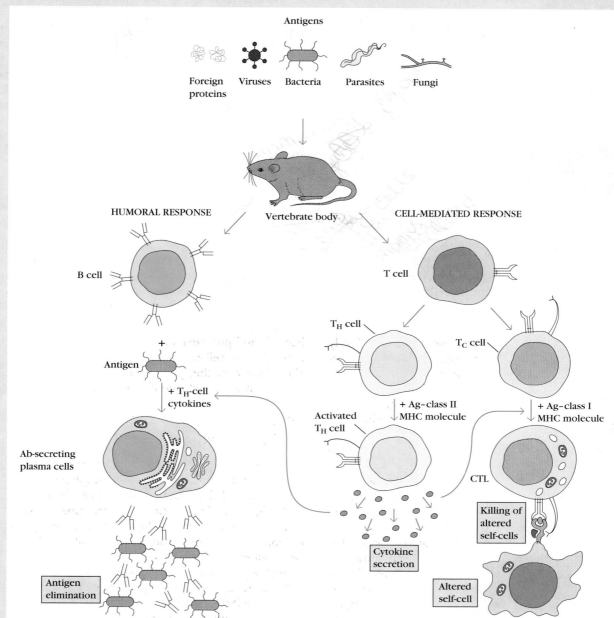

FIGURE 1-8

Overview of the humoral and cell-mediated branches of the immune system. The humoral response involves interaction of B cells with antigen (Ag) and their differentiation into antibody-secreting plasma cells. The secreted antibody (Ab) binds to the antigen and facilitates its clearance from the body. The cell-mediated response involves various subpopulations of T cells that recognize antigen presented on self-cells. T_H cells respond to antigen by producing cytokines. T_C cells respond to antigen by developing into cytotoxic T lymphocytes (CTLs), which mediate killing of altered self-cells (e.g., virus-infected cells).

Thus, four related but distinct cell-membrane molecules are responsible for antigen recognition by the immune system:

- Membrane-bound antibodies on B cells
- T-cell receptors
- Class I MHC molecules present on all nucleated cells
- Class II MHC molecules present on antigen-presenting cells.

Each of these molecules plays a unique role in antigen recognition, ensuring that the immune system can recognize and respond to the different types of antigen that it encounters.

Generation of Lymphocyte Specificity and Diversity

The antigenic specificity of each B cell is determined by the membrane-bound antigen-binding receptor (i.e., antibody) expressed by the cell. The antibody on a B cell can recognize different epitopes on macromolecules with incredible precision. For example, protein antigens that differ by only a single amino acid often can be discriminated from each other. As a B cell matures in the bone marrow, its specificity is generated by random rearrangements of a series of gene segments encoding the antibody molecule (see Chapter 7). As a result of this process, each mature B cell possesses a single functional gene encoding the antibody heavy chain and a single functional gene encoding the antibody light chain; the cell therefore synthesizes and displays antibody with one specificity on its membrane. All 10^5 antibody molecules on a given B lymphocyte have identical specificity, giving each B lymphocyte, and the clone of daughter cells to which it gives rise, a distinct specificity for antigen. The mature B lymphocyte is therefore said to be **antigenically committed**.

The fine specificity of the antibody molecule is coupled to an enormous diversity. The random gene rearrangements that occur during B-cell maturation in the bone marrow generate an enormous number of different antigenic specificities. The resulting B-cell population, which consists of individual B cells each exhibiting antibody with a distinct specificity, is estimated to collectively exhibit more than 10^8 different antigenic specificities. This enormous diversity in the antigenic specificity of the mature B-cell population is later reduced by a selection process in the bone marrow that eliminates any B cells whose membrane-bound antibody recognizes self-components. This process helps to ensure that self-reactive antibodies (auto-antibodies) are not produced.

The attributes of specificity and diversity also characterize the antigen-binding T-cell receptor (TCR) on T

cells. As in B-cell maturation, the process of T-cell maturation involves random rearrangements of a series of gene segments encoding the cell's antigen-binding receptor (see Chapter 11). Each T lymphocyte expresses about 10^5 receptors per cell, and all 10^5 receptors on a cell and its clonal progeny have identical specificity for antigen. The random rearrangement of the TCR genes is capable of generating on the order of 10^{15} unique antigenic specificities. This enormous potential diversity is later diminished through a selection process in the thymus that eliminates any T cell with self-reactive receptors and ensures that only T cells with receptors capable of recognizing antigen associated with MHC molecules will be able to mature (see Chapter 12).

Role of the Major Histocompatibility Complex

The major histocompatibility complex (MHC) is a large genetic complex with multiple loci. The MHC loci encode two major classes of membrane molecules: **class I** and **class II MHC molecules**. As noted previously, T_H cells generally recognize antigen associated with a class II molecule, whereas T_C cells generally recognize antigen associated with class I molecules (Figure 1-9).

Class I MHC molecules are glycoproteins found on the membrane of nearly all nucleated cells, always in association with a small protein called β_2-microglobulin. There are three class I loci in humans (*A*, *B*, and *C*) and two in mice (*K* and *D*). Class II MHC molecules are heterodimeric glycoproteins, consisting of an α and β chain, expressed by the various specialized cells that function as antigen-presenting cells. There are three class II loci in humans (*DR*, *DP*, and *DQ*) and two in mice (*IA* and *IE*). Each class II locus encompasses an α gene and a β gene, which respectively encode the α and β chains of the class II MHC molecule. Both class I and class II MHC genes are highly polymorphic; that is, within a species each gene exists in many different forms, called **alleles**. Because an individual inherits one allele from each parent for each locus, multiple class I MHC molecules are expressed on each nucleated cell in the body; in addition, multiple class II molecules are expressed on antigen-presenting cells.

MHC molecules also function as antigen-recognition molecules, but they do not possess the fine specificity for antigen characteristic of antibodies and T-cell receptors. Rather, individual MHC molecules bind to a spectrum of **antigenic peptides** derived from degradation of antigen molecules. In both class I and class II MHC molecules the distal regions (farthest from the membrane) of different alleles display wide variation in their amino acid sequences. These distal regions form a cleft within which the antigenic peptide sits and is presented to T lympho-

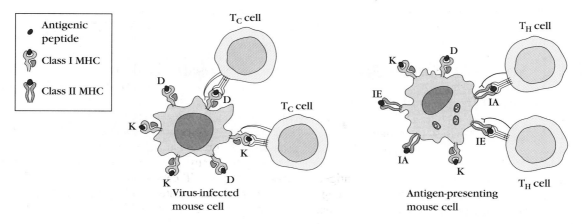

FIGURE 1-9

Role of MHC molecules in antigen recognition by T cells. Class I MHC molecules are encoded by the *K* and *D* loci in mice (*A*, *B*, and *C* loci in humans) and are expressed on nearly all nucleated cells. Class II MHC molecules are encoded by the *IA* and *IE* loci in mice (*DP, DQ,* and *DR* loci in humans) and are expressed only on antigen-presenting cells. CD4$^+$ T cells only recognize antigenic peptides displayed with a class II MHC molecule; they generally function as T helper (T$_H$) cells. CD8$^+$ T cells only recognize antigenic peptides displayed with a class I MHC molecule; they generally function as T cytotoxic (T$_C$) cells.

cytes (see Figure 1-9). Different allelic forms of the genes encoding class I and class II molecules confer different structures on the antigen-binding cleft with different specificity. Thus the ability to present an antigen to T lymphocytes is influenced by the particular set of alleles that an individual inherits.

Processing and Presentation of Antigens

In order for a foreign protein antigen to be recognized by a T cell it must be degraded into small antigenic peptides that form physical complexes with class I or class II MHC molecules. This conversion of proteins into MHC-associated peptide fragments is called antigen processing and presentation. Whether a particular antigen will be processed and presented together with class I MHC or class II MHC molecules appears to be determined by the route that the antigen takes to enter a cell (Figure 1-10).

Exogenous antigen is produced outside of the host cell and enters the cell by endocytosis or phagocytosis. Antigen-presenting cells (macrophages, dendritic cells, and B cells) degrade ingested exogenous antigen into peptide fragments within the endocytic processing pathway. Experiments suggest that class II MHC molecules are expressed within the endocytic processing pathway and that peptides produced by degradation of antigen in this pathway bind to the cleft within the class II MHC molecules. The MHC molecules bearing the peptide then are exported to the cell surface. Since expression of class II MHC molecules is limited to antigen-presenting cells, presentation of exogenous peptide–class II MHC complexes is limited to these cells. T cells displaying CD4 recognize antigen associated with class II MHC molecules and thus are said to be class II MHC restricted. These cells generally function as T helper cells.

Endogenous antigen is produced within the host cell itself. Two common examples are viral proteins synthesized within virus-infected host cells and unique proteins synthesized by cancerous cells. Endogenous antigens are thought to be degraded into peptide fragments that bind to class I MHC molecules within the endoplasmic reticulum. The peptide–class I MHC complex is then transported to the cell membrane. Since all nucleated cells express class I MHC molecules, all cells producing endogenous antigen use this route to process the antigen. T cells displaying CD8 recognize antigen associated with class I MHC molecules and thus are said to be class I MHC restricted. These cells generally function as T cytotoxic cells.

Clonal Selection of Lymphocytes

A mature immunocompetent animal contains a large number of antigen-reactive clones of T and B lymphocytes; the antigenic specificity of each of these clones is determined by the specificity of the antigen-binding receptor on the membrane of the clone's lymphocytes. As noted earlier, the specificity of each T and B lymphocyte

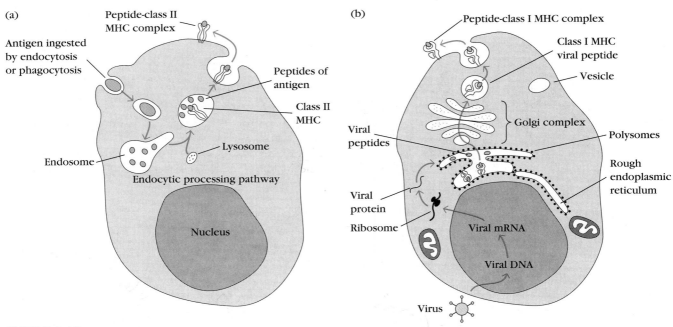

FIGURE 1-10

Processing and presentation of exogenous and endogenous antigens. (a) Exogenous antigen is ingested by endocytosis or phagocytosis and then enters the endocytic processing pathway. Here, within an acidic environment, the antigen is degraded into small peptides, which then are presented with class II MHC molecules on the membrane of the antigen-presenting cell. (b) Endogenous antigen, which is produced within the cell itself (e.g., in a virus-infected cell), is degraded within the cytoplasm into peptides, which move into the endoplasmic reticulum where they bind to class I MHC molecules. The peptide–class I MHC complexes then move via the Golgi complex to the cell surface.

is determined prior to its contact with antigen by random gene rearrangements in the bone marrow or thymus during maturation of lymphocytes.

The role of antigen becomes critical when it interacts with and activates mature, antigenically committed T and B lymphocytes, bringing about expansion of the population of cells with a given antigenic specificity. In this process of **clonal selection**, an antigen binds to and stimulates a particular T or B cell to undergo mitosis and develop into a clone of cells with the same antigenic specificity as the original parent cell (Figure 1-11).

Clonal selection provides a framework for understanding the specificity and self/nonself recognition characteristic of acquired immunity. Specificity is shown because only lymphocytes whose receptors are specific for a given epitope on an antigen will be clonally expanded and thus mobilized for an immune response. Self/nonself discrimination is accomplished by the clonal elimination, during development, of lymphocytes bearing self-reactive receptors or by the functional suppression of these cells in adults.

Immunologic memory also is a consequence of clonal selection. During clonal selection the number of lymphocytes specific for a given antigen is greatly amplified. Moreover, many of these lymphocytes, referred to as memory cells, appear to have a longer life span than the naive lymphocytes from which they arise. The initial encounter of a naive immunocompetent lymphocyte with an antigen induces a **primary response**; a second contact with antigen will induce a more rapid and heightened **secondary response**. The amplified population of memory cells accounts for the more rapid and intense response that characterizes a secondary response and distinguishes it from the initial primary response.

In the humoral branch of the immune system, antigen induces the clonal proliferation of B lymphocytes into antibody-secreting plasma cells and memory B cells. As seen in Figure 1-12a, the initial primary response has a lag of approximately 5–7 days before antibody levels start to rise. This lag is the time required for activation of naive B cells by antigen and T_H cells and for the subsequent proliferation and differentiation of the activated B cells into antibody-secreting plasma cells. Antibody levels peak in the primary response at about day 14 and then begin to drop off as the plasma cells begin to die. In the secondary response the lag is much shorter (only 1–2 days) and antibody levels are much higher and are sustained for a much longer time. The secondary response reflects the response of the clonally expanded population of memory B cells. These memory cells respond to the antigen more rapidly than the naive B cells; in addition, because there are many more memory cells than naive B cells, larger numbers of plasma cells are generated during the secondary response and antibody levels are consequently 100-fold to 1000-fold higher.

In the cell-mediated branch, the recognition of an antigen–MHC complex by a specific mature T lymphocyte induces clonal proliferation into various T cells with effector functions (e.g., T_H cells and CTLs) and into memory T cells. The cell-mediated response to a skin graft is depicted in Figure 1-12b. When skin from a strain

C mouse is grafted onto a strain A mouse, a primary response develops and the graft is rejected in about 10–14 days. If strain C is grafted a second time onto the same mouse, it is rejected much more vigorously and rapidly than the first graft. If a primary graft from a strain B mouse is grafted onto a strain A mouse together with the graft from strain C, the response to strain B is a typical primary response. That is, the graft rejection is a specific immune response. The mouse shows a secondary response to graft C, it gives a primary response to graft B. The increased speed of rejection of graft C reflects the

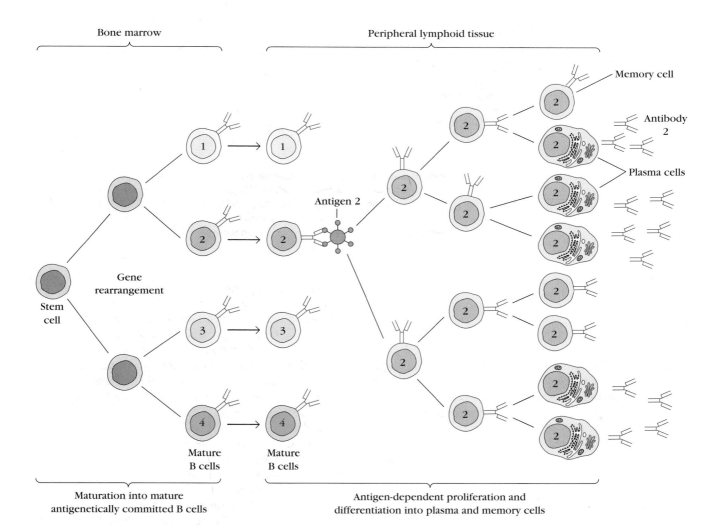

FIGURE 1-11

Maturation and clonal selection of B lymphocytes. Maturation, which occurs in the absence of antigen, produces antigenically committed B cells, each of which expresses antibody with a single antigenic specificity (indicated by 1, 2, 3, and 4). Clonal selection occurs when a given antigen binds to a B cell whose membrane-bound antibody molecules are specific for epitopes on that antigen. Clonal expansion of an antigen-activated B cell (number 2 in this example) leads to a

clone of memory B cells and effector B cells, called plasma cells; all cells in the expanded clone are specific for the original antigen. The plasma cells secrete antibody reactive with the activating antigen. Similar processes occur in the T-lymphocyte population resulting in clones of memory T cells and effector T cells; the latter include activated T_H cells, which secrete cytokines, and cytotoxic T lymphocytes (CTLs).

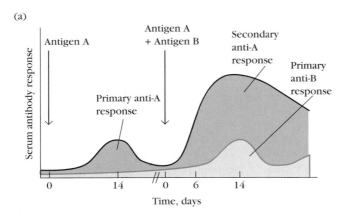

(a)

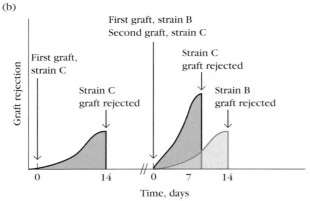

(b)

FIGURE 1-12

Differences in the primary and secondary response to injected anti-gen (humoral response) and to a skin graft (cell-mediated response) reflect the phenomenon of immunologic memory. (a) When an animal is injected with an antigen, it produces a primary serum antibody response of low magnitude and relatively short duration, peaking at about 10–17 days. A second immunization with the same antigen results in a secondary response that is greater in magnitude, peaks in less time (2–7 days), and lasts longer (months to years) than the primary response. (b) When skin from a strain C mouse is grafted onto a strain A mouse, the graft is rejected in about 10–14 days. If a second strain C graft is grafted onto the same mouse, it is rejected much more vigorously and rapidly than the first graft.

presence of a clonally expanded population of memory T_H and T_C cells to the antigens of the foreign graft. This expanded memory population will generate increased numbers of effector cells, resulting in faster graft rejection.

Cellular Interactions Required for Generation of Immune Responses

Both the humoral and the cell-mediated branches of the immune system require interaction among several different types of cells to induce a specific immunologic response. These cells include various antigen-presenting cells, T_H cells, and either B cells for induction of humoral immunity or T_C cells for induction of cell-mediated immunity.

ACTIVATION AND PROLIFERATION OF T HELPER CELLS

The generation of both humoral and cell-mediated immune responses depends on the activation of T_H cells. This process begins when antigen-binding receptors on T_H cells interact with antigenic peptide–class II MHC complexes on antigen-presenting cells (Figure 1-13). This interaction generates a signal that, together with a necessary co-stimulatory signal, leads to activation and proliferation of the T_H cells (Figure 1-14a). The clonally expanded population of antigen-specific T_H cells can now play a role in the activation of the B and T lymphocytes that generate the humoral and cell-mediated responses, respectively.

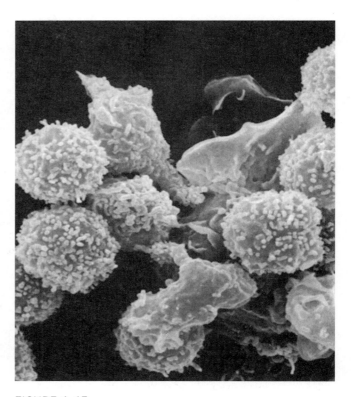

FIGURE 1-13

Scanning electron micrograph reveals numerous T lymphocytes interacting with a single macrophage. The macrophage presents processed antigen associated with class II MHC molecules to the T cells. [From William E. Paul (ed.), 1991, *Immunology: Recognition and Response*, W. H. Freeman and Company, New York; courtesy of Morten H. Nielsen and Ole Werdelin.]

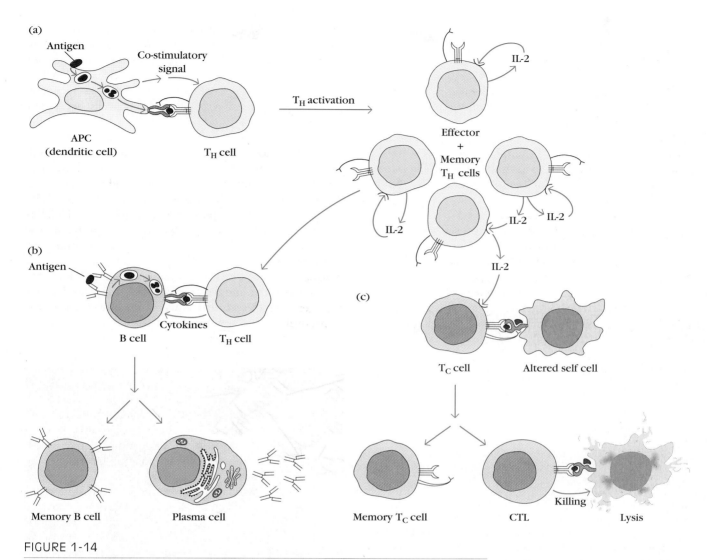

FIGURE 1-14

Cellular interactions involved in induction of immune responses. Activation and proliferation of T$_H$ cells (a) is required for generation of a humoral response (b) and a cell-mediated response to altered self-cells (c). APC = antigen-presenting cell; Ag = antigen. See text for discussion.

GENERATION OF THE HUMORAL RESPONSE

Mature antigen-committed B lymphocytes are seeded out from the bone marrow to circulate in the blood or lymph or to reside in various lymphoid organs. Interaction of the mature B cell with antigen triggers its activation and further proliferation and differentiation. This process begins when antigen cross-links membrane-bound antibody molecules on a B cell. Some of the bound antigen is internalized by receptor-mediated endocytosis. After processing the antigen, the B cell presents the resulting antigenic peptides together with a class II MHC molecule on its membrane. A T$_H$ cell specific

for the presented antigen-MHC complex then binds to the complex; as a result of this interaction, the T$_H$ cell secretes a number of cytokines that stimulate various stages of B-cell division and differentiation. The activated B cell undergoes a series of cell divisions over approximately a 5-day period differentiating into a population of both antibody-secreting plasma cells and memory cells (Figure 1-14b).

GENERATION OF THE CELL-MEDIATED RESPONSE

The cell-mediated response is generated by various subpopulations of T lymphocytes. As in the case of the humoral response, a clonally expanded population of antigen-specific activated T_H cells is required. Cytokines secreted by these T_H cells help to activate various T effector cells responsible for cell-mediated responses. For example, after a T_C cell binds to processed antigen associated with class I MHC molecules on the membrane of an altered self-cell, IL-2 secreted by T_H cells stimulates proliferation and differentiation of the T_C cell. This process generates cytotoxic T lymphocytes (CTLs), which mediate membrane damage to the altered self-cell leading to cell lysis, as well as populations of memory T_H and T_C cells (Figure 1-14c).

The cytokines secreted by activated T_H cells also regulate the proliferation and differentiation of a number of nonspecific effector cells that play various roles in cell-mediated immune responses. These nonspecific effector cells do not possess the immunologic attributes of specificity and memory; instead, their activity is regulated by cytokines secreted by antigen-specific T_H cells. Among the nonspecific effector cells involved in cell-mediated immunity are natural killer (NK) cells and activated macrophages. These are described in Chapter 3, and their role in cell-mediated immunity is covered in Chapter 16.

SUMMARY

1. Immunity is the state of protection against foreign organisms or substances (antigens). Innate (nonspecific) immune responses include anatomic, physiologic, endocytic and phagocytic, and inflammatory barriers that help prevent the entrance and establishment of infectious agents (see Figures 1-3, 1-4, 1-5). When these nonspecific mechanisms fail to effectively combat an invading pathogen, the body mounts an acquired (specific) immune response.

2. Acquired immune responses exhibit four immunologic attributes: specificity, diversity, memory, and self/nonself recognition. Functionally an immune response involves two interrelated events: recognition of antigen and response to that antigen (i.e., generation of effector cells and molecules). Antigen-presenting cells, B lymphocytes, and T lymphocytes are the primary cells involved in generation of immune responses.

3. Both B and T lymphocytes possess antigen-binding receptors in their membrane. The receptors on B cells are antibody molecules, which can recognize and interact directly with antigen. T-cell receptors, in contrast, only recognize antigen that is associated with either class I or class II MHC molecules on the surface of cells. During maturation of B and T lymphocytes, each cell comes to express receptors that recognize a single antigenic determinant (epitope).

4. The two major subpopulations of T lymphocytes are T helper (T_H) cells and T cytotoxic (T_C) cells. In general, T_H cells express CD4, a membrane glycoprotein, and recognize antigen associated with class II MHC cells, whereas T_C cells express CD8 and recognize antigen associated with class I MHC cells (see Figure 1-9).

5. Exogenous (extracellular) antigens are internalized and degraded by antigen-presenting cells (macrophages, B cells, and dendritic cells); the resulting antigenic peptides complexed with class II MHC molecules then are displayed on the cell surface. Endogenous (intracellular) antigens (e.g., viral and tumor proteins produced in altered self-cells) are degraded in the cytoplasm and then displayed with class I MHC molecules on the cell surface. (See Figure 1-10.)

6. Interaction of a mature, immunocompetent lymphocyte with the antigen it recognizes stimulates the cell to proliferate and differentiate into effector cells and memory cells (see Figure 1-11). Such initial exposure to a particular antigen induces a primary response; the expanded population of memory cells permits a more rapid and intense secondary response following subsequent exposure to the same antigen (see Figure 1-12).

7. The immune system produces both humoral and cell-mediated responses. The humoral response is best-suited for elimination of exogenous antigens; the cell-mediated response, for elimination of endogenous antigens. The effector cells of the humoral response are plasma cells, which secrete soluble antibody. The effector cells of the cell-mediated response are activated T_H cells, which secrete various cytokines, and cytotoxic T lymphocytes (CTLs), which arise from T_C cells and can destroy altered self-cells. T_H-cell activation is required for both types of response. (See Figures 1-8 and 1-14.)

REFERENCES

ADA, G. L., AND G. NOSSAL. 1987. The clonal selection theory. *Sci. Am.* **257**(2):62.

ENGELHARD, V. H. 1994. How cells process antigens. *Sci. Am.* **271** (2):54.

GREY, H. M., A. SETTE, AND S. BUUS. 1989. How T cells see antigen. *Sci. Am.* **261**(5):56.

JOHNSON, H. M., F. W. BAZOR, B. E. SZENTE, AND M. A. JARPE. 1994. How interferons fight disease. *Sci. Am.* **270**(5):68.

Life, Death and the Immune System. 1994. Readings from *Scientific American Magazine.* W. H. Freeman and Company.

SHER, A., AND R. AHMED. 1995. Immunity to infection. *Curr. Opin. Immunol.* **7**:471.

STUDY QUESTIONS

1. Indicate to which branch(es) of the immune system the following statements apply, using **H** for the humoral branch and **CM** for the cell-mediated branch. Some statements may apply to both branches.

a. _____ Involves class I MHC molecules

b. _____ Responds to viral infection

c. _____ Involves T helper cells

d. _____ Involves processed antigen

e. _____ Most likely responds following an organ transplant

f. _____ Involves T cytotoxic cells

g. _____ Involves B cells

h. _____ Involves CD8+ T cells

i. _____ Responds to extracellular bacterial infection

j. _____ Involves secreted antibody

k. _____ Kills virus-infected self cells

2. Specific immunity exhibits four characteristic attributes, which are mediated by lymphocytes. List these four attributes and briefly explain how they arise.

3. Name three features of a secondary immune response that distinguish it from a primary immune response.

4. Compare and contrast the four types of antigen-binding molecules utilized by the immune system—antibodies, T-cell receptors, class I MHC molecules, and class II MHC molecules—in terms of the following characteristics:

a. Specificity for antigen

b. Cellular expression

c. Types of antigen recognized

5. Cells can internalize material by endocytosis and phagocytosis. Name four properties that distinguish these two processes.

6. Fill in the blanks in the following statements with the most appropriate terms:

a. _____, _____, and _____ all function as antigen-presenting cells.

b. Antigen-presenting cells deliver a _____ signal to _____ cells.

c. Only antigen-presenting cells express class _____ MHC molecules, whereas nearly all cells express class _____ MHC molecules.

d. _____ antigens are internalized by antigen-presenting cells, degraded in the _____, and displayed with class _____ MHC molecules on the cell surface.

e. _____ antigens are produced in altered self-cells, degraded in the _____, and displayed with class _____ MHC molecules on the cell surface.

7. Briefly describe the three major events in the inflammatory response.

8. The CD8+ T cell is said to be class I restricted. What does this mean?

9. Match each term related to innate immunity (a–p) with the most appropriate description listed below (1–19). Each description may be used once, more than once, or not at all.

Terms:

a. _____ Fimbriae or pili

b. _____ Exudate

c. _____ Sebum

d. _____ Margination

e. _____ Dermis

f. _____ Lysosome

g. _____ Histamine

h. _____ Macrophage

i. _____ Lysozyme

j. _____ Bradykinin

k. _____ Interferon

l. _____ Edema

m. _____ Complement

n. _____ Extravasation

o. _____ C-reactive protein

p. _____ Phagosome

Descriptions:

1) Thin outer layer of skin

2) Layer of skin containing blood vessels and sebaceous glands

3) One of several acute-phase proteins

4) Hydrolytic enzyme found in mucous secretions

5) Migration of a phagocyte through the endothelial wall into the tissues

6) Acidic antibacterial secretion found in the skin

7) Has antiviral activity

8) Induces vasodilation

9) Accumulation of fluid in intercellular space resulting in swelling

10) Large vesicle containing ingested particulate material

11) Accumulation of dead cells, digested material, and fluid

12) Adherence of phagocytic cells to the endothelial wall

13) Structures involved in microbial adherence to mucous membranes

14) Stimulates pain receptors in the skin

15) Phagocytic cell found in the tissues

16) Phagocytic cell found in the blood

17) Group of serum proteins involved in cell lysis and clearance of antigen

18) Cytoplasmic vesicle containing degradative enzymes

19) Protein-rich fluid that leaks from the capillaries into the tissues

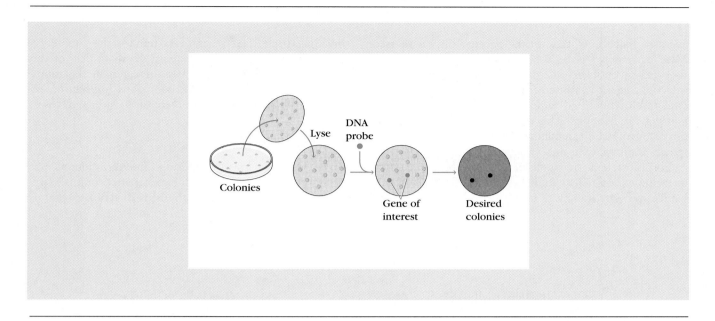

EXPERIMENTAL SYSTEMS

Experimental systems of various types are used to unravel the complex cellular interactions involved in the immune response. The choice of experimental system influences the kinds of data that can be generated and places certain limitations on the interpretation of those data.

In vivo systems, which involve the whole animal, provide the most natural experimental conditions. However, due to their complexity, in vivo systems have a myriad of unknown and uncontrollable cellular interactions that add ambiguity to the interpretation of data. At the other extreme are in vitro systems in which defined populations of lymphocytes are studied under controlled and consequently repeatable conditions; in vitro systems can be simplified to the extent that individual cellular interactions can be studied effectively. Yet in vitro systems have

their own limitations, the most notable of which is their artificiality. One must ask whether a cellular response observed in vitro reflects reality or is a product of the unique conditions generated by the in vitro system itself.

In this chapter some of the experimental systems routinely used by immunologists to study the immune system are described. The chapter also includes a discussion of some recombinant DNA techniques that have revolutionized the study of the immune system in the past decade or so.

EXPERIMENTAL ANIMAL MODELS

The study of the immune system in vertebrates requires suitable animal models. The choice of an animal depends on its suitability for attaining a particular research goal. If large amounts of antiserum are sought, a rabbit, goat, sheep, or horse might be an appropriate experimental animal. If the goal is development of a protective vaccine, the animal chosen must be susceptible to the infectious agent so that the efficacy of the vaccine can be assessed. Mice or rabbits can be used for vaccine development if they are susceptible to the pathogen. But if growth of the infectious agent is limited to humans and primates, vaccine development may require the use of monkeys, chimpanzees, or baboons. The use of primates for research purposes must be carefully regulated to ensure that each species is protected from extinction.

For most basic research in immunology, mice have been the experimental animal of choice. They are easy to handle, are genetically well characterized, and have a rapid breeding cycle. The immune system of the mouse has been characterized more extensively than that of any other species. The value of basic research in the mouse system is highlighted by the enormous impact this research has had on clinical intervention in human disease.

Inbred Strains

To control experimental variation caused by differences in the genetic backgrounds of experimental animals, immunologists often work with **inbred strains**—that is,

TABLE 2-1

SOME INBRED MOUSE STRAINS COMMONLY USED IN IMMUNOLOGY

STRAIN	COMMON SUBSTRAINS	CHARACTERISTICS
A	A/He A/J A/WySn	High incidence of mammary tumors in some substrains
AKR	AKR/J AKR/N AKR/Cum	High incidence of leukemia Thy 1.2 allele in AKR/Cum, and Thy 1.1 allele in other substrains (this gene encodes a T-cell surface protein)
BALB/c	BALB/cj BALB/c AnN BALB/cBy	Sensitivity to radiation Used in hybridoma technology Many myeloma cell lines were generated in these mice
CBA	CBA/J CBA/H CBA/N	Gene (*rd*) causing retinal degeneration in CBA/J Gene (*xid*) causing X-linked immunodeficiency in CBA/N
C3H	C3H/He C3H/HeJ C3H/HeN	Gene (*rd*) causing retinal degeneration High incidence of mammary tumors in many substrains (these carry a mammary-tumor virus that is passed via maternal milk to offspring)
C57BL/6	C57BL/6J C57BL/6By C57BL/6N	High incidence of hepatomas after irradiation High complement activity
C57BL/10	C57BL/10J C57BL/10ScSn C57BL/10N	Very close relationship to C57BL/6 but differences in at least two loci Frequent partner in preparation of congenic mice
C57BR	C57BR/cd*j*	High frequency of pituitary and liver tumors Very resistant to x-irradiation

(continued on the following page)

genetically identical animals produced by inbreeding. The rapid breeding cycle of mice makes them particularly well suited for the production of inbred strains, which are developed by repeated inbreeding between brother and sister littermates. In this way the heterozygosity of alleles that is normally found in randomly outbred mice is replaced by homozygosity at all loci. Repeated inbreeding for 20 generations usually yields an inbred strain whose progeny are homozygous at more than 98% of all loci. More than 150 different inbred strains of mice are available; these are designated by a series of letters and/ or numbers (Table 2-1). Most of these strains are purchased by immunologists from such suppliers as Jackson Laboratory in Bar Harbor, Maine. Inbred strains have also been produced in rats, guinea pigs, hamsters, rabbits, and domestic fowl.

Because inbred animals are genetically identical (**syngeneic**), their immune responses can be studied in the absence of variables introduced by genetic differences among individual animals. Inbred strains are invaluable in the study of immunology. With inbred strains, lymphocyte subpopulations isolated from one animal can be injected

T A B L E   2 - 1   (c o n t i n u e d)

SOME INBRED MOUSE STRAINS COMMONLY USED IN IMMUNOLOGY

STRAIN	COMMON SUBSTRAINS	CHARACTERISTICS
C57L	C57L/J C57L/N	Susceptibility to experimental autoimmune encephalomyelitis (EAE) High frequency of pituitary and reticular cell tumors
C58	C58/J C58/LwN	High incidence of leukemia
DBA/1	DBA/1J DBA/1N	High incidence of mammary tumors
DBA/2	DBA/2J DBA/2N	Low immune response to some antigens Low response to pneumococcal polysaccharide type III
HRS	HRS/J	Hairless (*hr*) gene, usually in heterozygous state
NZB	NZB/BINJ NZB/N	High incidence of autoimmune hemolytic anemia and lupus-like nephritis Autoimmune disease similar to systemic lupus erythematosus (SLE) in F1 progeny from crosses with NZW
NZW	NZW/N	SLE-type autoimmune disease in F1 progeny from crosses with NZB
P	P/J	High incidence of leukemia
SJL	SJL/J	High level of aggression and severe fighting to the point of death, especially in males Tendency to develop certain autoimmune diseases, most susceptible to EAE
SWR	SWR/J	Tendency to develop several autoimmune diseases, especially EAE
129	129/J 129/SvJ	High incidence of spontaneous teratocarcinoma

SOURCE: Adapted from Federation of American Societies for Experimental Biology, 1979, *Biological Handbooks,* Vol. III: Inbred and Genetically Defined Strains of Laboratory Animals.

into another animal of the same strain without eliciting a rejection reaction. This type of experimental system permitted immunologists to first demonstrate that lymphocytes from an antigen-primed animal could transfer immunity to an unprimed syngeneic recipient.

Adoptive-Transfer Systems

In some experiments it is important to eliminate the immune responsiveness of the syngeneic host so that the response of only the transferred lymphocytes can be studied in isolation. This can be accomplished by first exposing the syngeneic host to x-rays and then introducing the donor immune cells, a technique called **adoptive transfer**. Subjecting a mouse that will serve as host to sublethal doses of x-rays (650–750 rads) can kill 99.99% of its lymphocytes, after which the lymphocytes from the spleen of a syngeneic donor can be studied without interference from host lymphocytes. If the host's hematopoietic cells might influence an adoptive-transfer experiment, then higher x-ray levels (900–1000 rads) are used to eliminate the entire hematopoietic system. Mice irradiated with such doses will die unless reconstituted with bone marrow from a syngeneic donor.

The adoptive-transfer system has enabled immunologists to study the development of injected lymphoid stem cells in various organs of the recipient. Adoptive-transfer experiments have also facilitated the study of various populations of lymphocytes and of the cellular interactions required to generate an immune response. Such experiments, for instance, first enabled immunologists to show that a T helper cell is necessary for B-cell activation in the humoral response.

SCID Mice and SCID-Human Mice

An autosomal recessive mutation resulting in **severe combined immunodeficiency disease** (SCID) developed spontaneously in a strain of mice called CB-17. These CB-17 SCID mice fail to develop mature T and B cells and consequently are severely compromised immunologically. The mechanism of the defect in these mice has been determined and is discussed in Chapter 7. SCID mice must be housed in a sterile (germfree) environment if they are to survive, because they cannot fight off microorganisms of even low pathogenicity. The absence of functional T and B cells enables these mice to accept foreign cells and grafts from other strains of mice or even from other species.

Apart from their lack of functional T and B cells, SCID mice appear to be normal in all respects. When normal bone marrow cells are injected into SCID mice, normal T and B cells develop, and the mice are cured of their immunodeficiency. This finding has made SCID mice a valuable model system for the study of immunodeficiency and the process of differentiation of bone-marrow stem cells into mature T or B cells.

Interest in SCID mice mushroomed when it was found that they could be used to study the human immune system. In this system, portions of human fetal liver, thymus, and lymph nodes are implanted in SCID mice (Figure 2-1). Because the mice lack mature T and B cells of their own, they do not reject the transplanted human tissue. The fetal liver contains immature lymphocytes (stem cells), which migrate to the implanted human tissues where they mature into T and B cells, producing a **SCID-human mouse**. Because the human lymphocytes are exposed to mouse antigens while they are still immature, they later recognize mouse cells as self

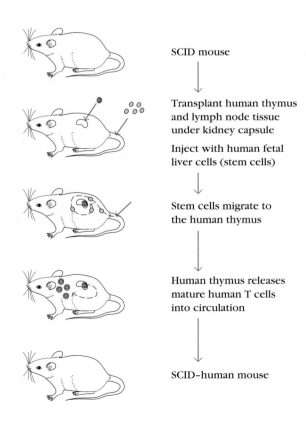

SCID mouse

Transplant human thymus and lymph node tissue under kidney capsule

Inject with human fetal liver cells (stem cells)

Stem cells migrate to the human thymus

Human thymus releases mature human T cells into circulation

SCID-human mouse

FIGURE 2-1

Production of SCID-human mouse. This system permits study of human lymphocytes within an animal model.

and do not mount an immunologic response against the mouse host.

The beauty of the SCID-human mouse is that it enables one to study human lymphocytes within an animal model. As discussed in later chapters, this valuable system has proved useful in research on the development of various lymphoid cells and has also served as an important animal model in AIDS research. There are, however, important ethical considerations that must be addressed concerning the use of human fetal tissue in research.

CELL-CULTURE SYSTEMS

The complexity of the cellular interactions that generate an immune response has led immunologists to rely heavily on various types of in vitro cell-culture systems. A variety of cells can be cultured including primary lymphoid cells, cloned lymphoid cell lines, and hybrid cells.

Primary Lymphoid Cell Cultures

Primary lymphoid cell cultures can be obtained by isolating lymphocytes directly from blood or lymph or from various lymphoid organs by tissue dispersion. The lymphocytes can then be grown in a chemically defined basal medium (containing saline, sugars, amino acids, vitamins, trace elements, and other nutrients) to which various serum supplements are added. For some experiments serum-free culture conditions are employed. Because in vitro culture techniques require from 10- to 100-fold fewer lymphocytes than typical in vivo techniques, they have enabled immunologists to assess the functional properties of minor subpopulations of lymphocytes. It was by means of cell-culture techniques, for example, that immunologists were first able to define the functional differences between CD4$^+$ T helper cells and CD8$^+$ T cytotoxic cells.

Cell-culture techniques have also been used to identify numerous cytokines involved in the activation, growth, and differentiation of various cells involved in the immune response. Early experiments showed that media conditioned by the growth of various lymphocytes or antigen-presenting cells would support the growth of other lymphoid cells. Many of the individual cytokines that characterized various conditioned media have subsequently been identified and purified, and in many cases the genes encoding them have been cloned. These cytokines, which play a central role in the activation and regulation of the immune response, are discussed more fully in Chapter 13 and other chapters.

Cloned Lymphoid Cell Lines

Primary lymphoid cell cultures comprise a heterogeneous group of cells that can be propagated only for a limited time. This heterogeneity complicates interpretation of experiments aimed at understanding the molecular and cellular mechanisms by which lymphocytes generate an immune response. To avoid these problems, immunologists use cloned lymphoid cell lines and hybrid cells.

Normal mammalian cells generally have a finite life span in culture; that is, after a number of population doublings characteristic of the species and cell type, the cells stop dividing. In contrast, normal cells that have undergone **transformation** induced by chemical carcinogens or viruses and tumor cells can be propagated indefinitely in tissue culture; thus they are said to be immortal. Such cells are referred to as **cell lines**.

The first cell line—the **mouse fibroblast L cell**—was derived in the 1940s from cultured mouse subcutaneous connective tissue by exposing the cultured cells to a chemical carcinogen, methylcholanthrene, over a 4-month period. In the 1950s another important cell line, the **HeLa cell**, was derived by culturing human cervical cancer cells. Since these early studies, hundreds of cell lines have been established. Various techniques can be used to ensure that a cell line is derived from a single parent cell. Such a cloned cell line consists of a population of genetically identical (syngeneic) cells that can be grown indefinitely in culture.

A variety of cell lines are used in immunologic research. Table 2-2 lists some of these lines and briefly describes their properties. (Although the meaning of many of the properties described will not become clear until later chapters, the table can serve as a helpful summary.) Some of these cell lines were derived from spontaneously occurring tumors of lymphocytes, macrophages, or other accessory cells involved in the immune response. In other cases the cell line was induced by transformation of normal lymphoid cells with viruses such as Abelson's murine leukemia virus (A-MLV), simian virus 40 (SV40), Epstein-Barr virus (EBV), and human T-cell leukemia virus type 1(HTLV-1).

Lymphoid cell lines differ from primary lymphoid cell cultures in several important ways: They survive indefinitely in tissue culture, they show various abnormal growth properties, and they often have an abnormal number of chromosomes. Cells with more or less than the normal diploid number of chromosomes for a species are said to be **aneuploid**. The big advantage of cloned lymphoid cell lines is that they can be grown for extended periods in tissue culture, enabling immunologists to obtain large numbers of homogeneous cells in culture.

Until the late 1970s immunologists had not succeeded in maintaining normal T cells in tissue culture for extended periods. In 1978 a serendipitous finding led to the observation that conditioned medium containing a T-cell growth factor was required. The essential component of the conditioned medium turned out to be interleukin 2 (IL-2). By culturing normal T lymphocytes with antigen in the presence of IL-2, clones of antigen-specific T lymphocytes could be isolated. These individual clones could be propagated and studied in culture and even frozen for storage. After thawing, the clones continued to grow and express their original antigen-specific functions.

Development of cloned lymphoid cell lines has enabled immunologists to study a number of events that previously could not be examined. For example, research

T A B L E   2 - 2

CELL LINES COMMONLY USED IN IMMUNOLOGIC RESEARCH

CELL LINE	DESCRIPTION
L-929	Mouse fibroblast cell line; often is used in DNA transfection studies and to assay tumor necrosis factor (TNF)
SP2/0	Nonsecreting mouse myeloma; often is used as a fusion partner for hybridoma secretion
P3X63-Ag8.653	Nonsecreting mouse myeloma; often is used as a fusion partner for hybridoma secretion
MPC 11	Mouse IgG2b-secreting myeloma
P3X63 Ag 8	Mouse IgG1-secreting myeloma
MOPC 315	Mouse IgA-secreting myeloma
J558	Mouse IgA-secreting myeloma
ABE-8.1/2	Mouse pre-B cell lymphoma
7OZ/3	Mouse pre-B cell lymphoma; used to study early events in B-cell differentiation
BCL 1	Mouse B-cell leukemia lymphoma that expresses membrane IgM and IgD and can be activated with mitogen to secrete IgM
LBRM-33	Mouse T-cell lymphoma that secretes high levels of IL-2 after mitogen activation; can be used to assay IL-1 activity
CTLL-2	Mouse T-cell line whose growth is dependent on IL-2; often is used to assay IL-2 production
C6VL	Mouse thymoma expressing CD3 and CD4
PU 5-1.8	Mouse monocyte-macrophage line
P338 D1	Mouse monocyte-macrophage line that secretes high levels of IL-1
WEHI 265.1	Mouse monocyte line
P815	Mouse mastocytoma cells; often is used as target to assess killing by cytotoxic T lymphocytes (CTLs)
YAC-1	Mouse lymphoma cells; often is used as target for NK cells
COS-1	African green monkey kidney cells transformed by SV40; often is used in DNA transfection studies

on the molecular events involved in activation of naive lymphocytes by antigen was hampered by the low frequency of naive B and T cells specific for a particular antigen; in a heterogeneous population of lymphocytes, the molecular changes occurring in one responding cell could not be detected against a background of 10^3–10^6 nonresponding cells. T- and B-cell lines with known antigenic specificity have provided immunologists with large, homogeneous cell populations in which to study the membrane and intracellular events involved in antigen recognition. Similarly, the molecular-level genetic changes corresponding to different maturational stages can be studied in cell lines that appear to be "frozen" at different stages of differentiation. Cell lines have also been useful in studying the soluble factors produced by lymphoid cells. Some cell lines secrete large quantities of various cytokines; other lines express membrane receptors for particular cytokines. These cell lines have been used by immunologists to purify and eventually to clone the genes of various cytokines and their receptors.

However, lymphoid cell lines have a number of limitations. Variants arise spontaneously in the course of prolonged culture, necessitating frequent subcloning to limit the cellular heterogeneity that can develop. If variants are selected in subcloning, it is possible that two subclones derived from the same parent clone may represent different subpopulations. Moreover, any cell line derived from tumor cells or transformed cells may have unknown genetic contributions characteristic of the tumor or of the transformed state; because of this possibility, researchers must be cautious when extrapolating results obtained with cell lines to the normal situation in vivo. Nevertheless, transformed cell lines have made a major contribution to the study of the immune response, and a number of molecular events discovered in experiments with transformed cell lines have later been shown to take place in normal lymphocytes.

Hybrid Lymphoid Cell Lines

In somatic-cell hybridization, immunologists fuse normal B or T lymphocytes with tumor cells, obtaining hybrid cells, or **heterokaryons,** containing nuclei from both parent cells. Random loss of some chromosomes and subsequent cell proliferation yield a clone of cells that contain a single nucleus with chromosomes from each of the fused cells; such a clone is called a **hybridoma**.

Historically, cell fusion was promoted with Sendai virus, but now it is generally done with polyethylene glycol. Normal antigen-primed B cells can be fused with cancerous plasma cells, called **myeloma cells** (Figure 2-2). The hybridoma thus formed continues to express the antibody genes of the normal B lymphocyte but is capable of unlimited growth, a characteristic of the

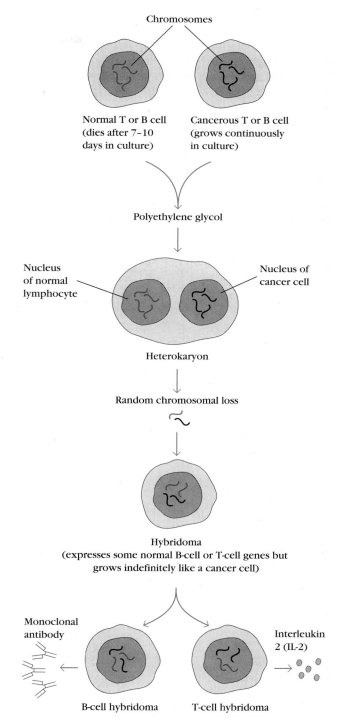

FIGURE 2-2

Production of B-cell and T-cell hybridomas by somatic-cell hybridization. The resulting hybridomas express some of the genes of the original normal B or T cell but also exhibit the immortal-growth properties of the tumor cell. This procedure is used to produce B-cell hybridomas secreting monoclonal antibody and T-cell hybridomas secreting various growth factors.

myeloma cell. B-cell hybridomas that secrete antibody with a single antigenic specificity, called monoclonal antibody, in reference to its derivation from a single clone, have revolutionized not only immunology but biomedical research as well as the clinical laboratory. Chapter 5 discusses the production and uses of monoclonal antibodies in detail.

T-cell hybridomas can also be obtained by fusing T lymphocytes with cancerous T-cell lymphomas. Again, the resulting hybridoma continues to express the genes of the normal T cell but acquires the immortal-growth properties of the cancerous T lymphoma cell. Immunologists have generated a number of stable hybridoma cell lines representing T helper and T cytotoxic lineages.

RECOMBINANT DNA TECHNOLOGY

The various techniques comprising recombinant DNA technology have had an impact on every area of immunologic research. Genes can be cloned, DNA can be sequenced, and recombinant protein products can be produced, providing immunologists with defined components with which to study the structure and function of the immune system at the molecular level. Some of the recombinant DNA techniques commonly employed in immunologic research are briefly described in this section; examples of uses of these techniques are described in subsequent chapters.

Restriction-Endonuclease Cleavage of DNA

A variety of bacteria produce enzymes, called **restriction endonucleases**, that degrade foreign DNA (e.g., bacteriophage DNA) but spare the bacterial cell DNA, which contains methylated residues. The discovery of these bacterial enzymes in the 1970s opened the way to a major technological advance in the field of molecular biology. Before the discovery of restriction endonucleases, double-stranded DNA (dsDNA) could be cut only with DNases. These enzymes do not recognize defined sites and therefore randomly cleave DNA into a variable series of small fragments, which are impossible to order. In contrast, restriction endonucleases recognize and cleave DNA at specific sites, called **restriction sites**, which are short double-stranded sequences containing four to eight nucleotides (Table 2-3).

A restriction endonuclease cuts both DNA strands at a specific point within its restriction site. Some enzymes, like *Hpa*I, cut on the central axis and thus generate blunt-ended fragments. Other enzymes, such as *Eco*RI, cut the DNA off-center from the central axis of the recognition site, producing staggered cleavage products. These staggered fragments have a short single-stranded DNA extension, called a **sticky end**, extending from one of the strands of each double-stranded fragment. When two different DNA molecules are cut with the same restriction enzyme that makes staggered cuts, the sticky ends of the fragments will be complementary; under appropriate conditions, fragments from the two molecules can be joined by base pairing to generate a recombinant DNA molecule. Several hundred different restriction endonucleases have been isolated and many are available commercially, allowing researchers to purchase enzymes that cut DNA at defined restriction sites.

Cloning of DNA Sequences

The development of DNA cloning technology in the 1970s provided a means of amplifying a given DNA fragment to such an extent that unlimited amounts of identical DNA fragments (cloned DNA) could be produced.

CLONING VECTORS

In DNA cloning a given DNA fragment is inserted into an autonomously replicating DNA molecule, called a **cloning vector**, so that the inserted DNA is replicated with the vector. A number of different viruses have been used as vectors including bacterial viruses, insect viruses, and mammalian retroviruses. A common bacterial virus used as a vector is **bacteriophage** λ. If a gene is inserted into bacteriophage λ and the recombinant λ phage is used to infect *E. coli*, the inserted gene will be expressed by the bacteria.

Retroviruses, which can infect virtually any type of mammalian cell, are a common vector used to clone DNA in mammalian cells. Retroviruses are RNA viruses that contain reverse transcriptase, an enzyme that catalyzes conversion of the viral RNA genome into DNA. The viral DNA then integrates into the host chromosomal DNA where it is retained as a provirus, replicating along with the host chromosomal DNA at each cell division. When a retrovirus is used as a vector, most of the retroviral genes are removed so that the vector cannot produce viral particles; the retroviral genes that are left include a strong promoter region, located at the 5′ end of the viral genome, in a sequence called the long terminal repeat (LTR). If a gene is cloned in such a retroviral vector and the vector is then used to infect mammalian cells, the gene will be expressed under the control of the retroviral promoter region.

Plasmids are another common type of cloning vector. A **plasmid** is a small circular, extrachromosomal DNA molecule that can replicate independently in a host cell; the most common host used in DNA cloning is *E. coli*. In general the DNA to be cloned is inserted into a plasmid that contains an antibiotic-resistance gene. After the recombinant plasmid is incubated with bacterial cells, the infected cells containing the recombinant plasmid can be selected by their ability to grow in the presence of the antibiotic.

Another type of vector that is often used for cloning is called a **cosmid vector**. This type of vector is a plasmid that has been genetically engineered to contain the COS sites of λ-phage DNA, a drug-resistance gene, and a replication origin. COS sites are DNA sequences that allow any DNA up to 50 kilobases (kb) in length to be packaged into the λ-phage head.

CLONING OF CDNA AND GENOMIC DNA

Messenger RNA (mRNA) isolated from cells can be transcribed into **complementary DNA** (cDNA) with the enzyme reverse transcriptase. The cDNA can be cloned by inserting it into a plasmid vector carrying a selectable gene that confers resistance to the antibiotic ampicillin. The resulting recombinant plasmid DNA is subsequently transferred into specially treated *E. coli* cells by one of several possible techniques; this transfer process is called **transfection**. If the foreign DNA is incorporated into the host cell and expressed, the cell is said to be **transformed.** When the cells are cultured on agar plates containing ampicillin, only transformed cells containing the ampicillin-resistance gene will survive and grow (Figure 2-3). A collection of DNA sequences within plasmid vectors representing all the mRNA sequences derived from a cell or tissue is called a **cDNA library**.

E. coli plasmid vectors are impractical for cloning of all the **genomic DNA** fragments constituting large genomes because of the relatively low efficiency of *E. coli* transformation and the small number of transformed colonies that can be detected on a typical petri dish. Instead, cloning vectors derived from bacteriophage λ are used to clone genomic DNA fragments obtained by

T A B L E   2 - 3

SOME RESTRICTION ENZYMES AND THEIR RECOGNITION SEQUENCES

MICROORGANISM SOURCE	ABBREVIATION	SEQUENCE* 5′ → 3′ 3′ → 5′
Bacillus amyloliquefaciens H	*Bam* HI	G G A T C C C C T A G G
Escherichia coli RY13	*Eco* RI	G A A T T C C T T A A G
Haemophilus aegyptius	*Hae*III	G G C C G G C C
Haemophilus haemolyticus	*Hha*I	G G C C G G C C
Haemophilus influenzae Rd	*Hin*dIII	A A G C T T T T C G A A
Haemophilus parainfluenzae	*Hpa*I	G T T A A C C A A T T G
Providencia stuartii 164	*Pst*I	G T G C A G G A C G T C
Staphylococcus aureus 3A	*Sau*3A	G A T C C T A G

* Black lines indicate locations of single-strand cuts within the restriction site. Enzymes that make off-center cuts produce fragments with short, single-stranded extensions at their ends.

SOURCE: J. D. Watson et al., 1983, *Recombinant DNA*, W. H. Freeman and Company.

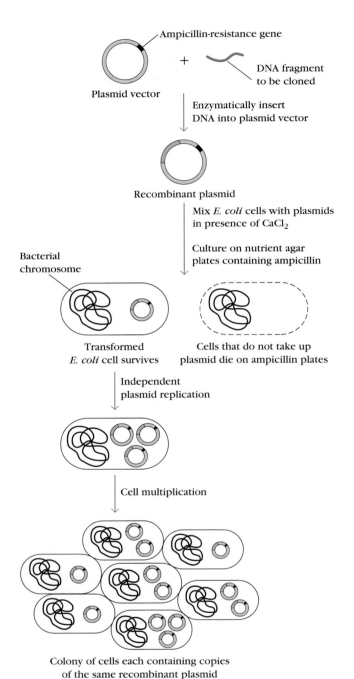

FIGURE 2-3

cDNA cloning using a plasmid vector. A plasmid containing a replication origin and an ampicillin-resistance gene is cut with a restriction endonuclease that produces blunt ends. Following addition of a poly-C tail to the 3′ ends of the cDNA and of a complementary poly-G tail to the 3′ ends of the cut plasmid, the two DNAs are mixed, annealed, and joined by DNA ligase, forming the recombinant plasmid. Uptake of the recombinant plasmid into *E. coli* cells is stimulated by high concentrations of $CaCl_2$. Transformation occurs with a low frequency but the transformed cells can be selected in the presence of ampicillin. [Adapted from Harvey Lodish et al. 1995, *Molecular Cell Biology*, 3rd edition, Scientific American Books.]

cleaving chromosomal DNA with restriction enzymes (Figure 2-4). Bacteriophage λ DNA is 48.5 kb long and contains a central section of about 15 kb that is not necessary for λ replication in *E. coli* and can therefore be replaced with foreign genomic DNA. As long as the recombinant DNA does not exceed the length of the original λ-phage DNA by more than 5%, it can be packaged into the λ-phage head and propagated in *E. coli*. This means that somewhat more than 1.5×10^4 base pairs can be cloned in one λ-phage particle. A collection of λ clones that includes all the DNA sequences of a given species is called a **genomic library**. It has been calculated that about 1 million different recombinant λ-phage particles would be needed to form a complete genomic DNA library representing the entire haploid genome of a mammalian cell, which contains about 3×10^9 base pairs.

Often the 20- to 25-kb stretch of DNA that can be cloned in bacteriophage λ is not long enough to include the regulatory sequences that lie outside the 5′ and 3′ ends of the direct coding sequences of a gene. As noted already, larger genomic DNA fragments—between 30 and 50 kb in length—can be cloned in a cosmid vector. A recombinant cosmid vector, although not a fully functional bacteriophage, can infect *E. coli* and replicate as a plasmid, generating a cosmid library. Recently, a larger *E. coli* virus called **bacteriophage P1** has been packaged with DNA fragments up to 100 kb long. Even larger DNA fragments, approaching a megabase (1000 kb) in length, can be cloned in **yeast artificial chromosomes**, which are linear DNA segments that can replicate in yeast cells (Table 2-4).

Selection of DNA Clones

Once a cDNA or genomic DNA library is prepared, it can be screened to identify a particular DNA fragment by a technique called **in situ hybridization**. The cloned bacterial colonies, yeast colonies, or phage plaques containing the recombinant DNA are transferred onto nitrocellulose or nylon filters by replica plating (Figure 2-5). The filter is then treated with NaOH, which both lyses the bacteria and denatures the DNA, allowing single-stranded DNA (ssDNA) to bind to the filter. The filter with bound DNA then is incubated with a radioactive probe specific for the gene of interest. The probe will hybridize with the colonies or plaques on the filter that contain the sought-after gene, and they can be identified by autoradiography. The position of the positive colonies or plaques on the filter shows where the corresponding clones can be found on the original agar plate.

Various radioactive probes can be used to screen a library. In some cases radiolabeled mRNA or cDNA serves as the probe. When the protein encoded by the gene of interest has been purified and partially sequenced,

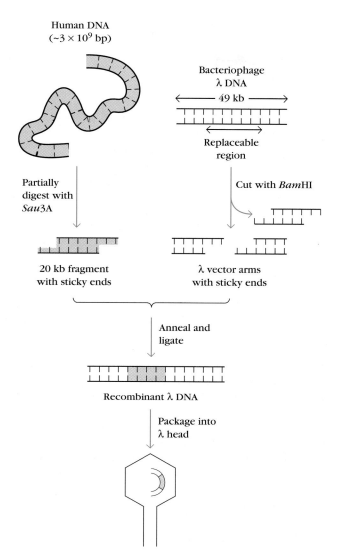

Human DNA
(~3 × 10⁹ bp)

Bacteriophage
λ DNA

← 49 kb →

Replaceable
region

Partially
digest with
*Sau*3A

Cut with *Bam*HI

20 kb fragment
with sticky ends

λ vector arms
with sticky ends

Anneal and
ligate

Recombinant λ DNA

Package into
λ head

FIGURE 2-4

Genomic DNA cloning using bacteriophage λ as the vector. Genomic DNA is partially digested with *Sau*3A, producing fragments with sticky ends. The central 15-kb region of the λ-phage DNA is cut out with *Bam*HI and discarded. These two restriction enzymes produce complementary sticky ends, so the genomic and DNA fragments can be annealed and ligated. After the resulting recombinant DNA is packaged into a λ-phage head, it can be propagated in *E. coli*.

containing a given gene sequence (Figure 2-6). In this technique, called **Southern blotting**, DNA is cut with restriction enzymes and the fragments are separated according to size by electrophoresis on an agarose gel. Then the gel is soaked in NaOH to denature the dsDNA, and the resulting ssDNA fragments are transferred onto a nitrocellulose or nylon filter by capillary action. After transfer, the filter is incubated with an appropriate radiolabeled probe specific for the gene of interest. The probe hybridizes with the ssDNA fragment of interest, and the position of the fragment band is determined by autoradiography. Southern blot analysis played a critical role in unraveling the mechanism by which diversity of antibodies and T-cell receptors is generated.

NORTHERN BLOTTING

Northern blotting (named for its similarity to Southern blotting) is used to detect the presence of specific mRNA molecules. In this procedure the mRNA is first denatured to ensure that it is in an unfolded, linear form. The mRNA molecules are then separated according to size by electrophoresis and transferred to a nitrocellulose filter to which the mRNAs will adhere. The filter is then incubated with a labeled DNA probe and subjected to autoradiography. Northern blot analysis is often used to determine how much of a specific mRNA is expressed in cells under different conditions. Increased levels of

it is possible to work backward from the amino acid sequence to determine the probable nucleotide sequence of the corresponding gene. A known sequence of five or six amino acid residues is all that is needed to synthesize radiolabeled oligonucleotide probes with which to screen a cDNA or genomic library for a particular gene. To cope with the degeneracy of the genetic code, peptides incorporating amino acids encoded by a limited number of codon sequences are usually chosen. Oligonucleotides representing all possible codon sequences for the peptide are synthesized and used as probes to screen the DNA library.

SOUTHERN BLOTTING

DNA fragments generated by restriction-endonuclease cleavage can be separated on the basis of length by agarose gel electrophoresis. The shorter a band is, the faster it moves in the gel. An elegant technique developed by E. M. Southern can be used to identify any fragment band

T A B L E   2 – 4

VECTORS AND MAXIMUM LENGTH OF DNA THAT THEY CAN CARRY

VECTOR TYPE	MAXIMUM LENGTH OF CLONED DNA (KB)
Plasmid	20
Bacteriophage λ	25
Cosmid	45
Bacteriophage P1	100
Yeast artifical chromosome (YAC)	1000

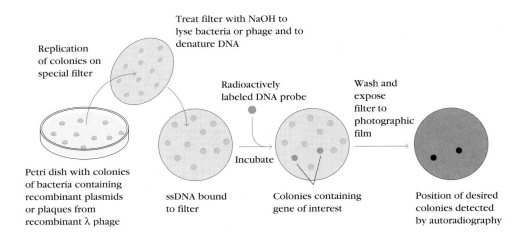

FIGURE 2-5

Selection of specific clones from a cDNA or genomic DNA library by in situ hybridization. A nitrocellulose or nylon filter is placed against the plate to pick up the bacterial colonies or phage plaques containing the cloned genes. After the filter is placed in a NaOH solution and heated, the denatured ssDNA becomes fixed to the filter. A radioactive probe specific for the gene of interest is incubated with the filter. The position of the colonies or plaques containing the desired gene is revealed by autoradiography.

mRNA will bind proportionally more of the labeled DNA probe.

Polymerase Chain Reaction

The **polymerase chain reaction** (PCR) is a powerful technique for amplifying specific DNA sequences even when they are present at extremely low levels in a complex mixture (Figure 2-7). The procedure requires that the DNA sequences flanking the desired DNA sequence be known, so that short oligonucleotide primers can be synthesized. The DNA mixture is denatured into single strands by a brief heat treatment. The DNA is then cooled in the presence of an excess of the oligonucleotide primers, which hybridize with the complementary ssDNA. A temperature-resistant DNA polymerase (called Taq polymerase) is then added, together with the four deoxyribonucleotide triphosphates, and each strand is copied. The newly synthesized DNA duplex is separated by heating and the cycle is repeated. In each cycle there is a doubling of the DNA sequence; in only 25 cycles the desired DNA sequence can be amplified about a million-fold.

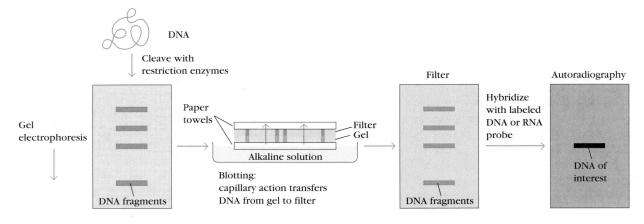

FIGURE 2-6

The Southern blot technique for detecting specific sequences in DNA fragments. The DNA fragments produced by restriction-enzyme cleavage are separated by size by agarose gel electrophoresis. The agarose gel is overlaid with a nitrocellulose or nylon filter and a thick stack of paper towels. The gel is then placed in an alkaline salt solution, which denatures the DNA. As the paper towels soak up the moisture, the solution is drawn through the gel into the filter, transferring each ssDNA band to the filter. This process is called blotting. After heating, the filter is incubated with a radiolabeled probe specific for the sequence of interest; DNA fragments that hybridize with the probe are detected by autoradiography. [Adapted from James Darnell et al., 1990, *Molecular Cell Biology*, 2nd ed., Scientific American Books.]

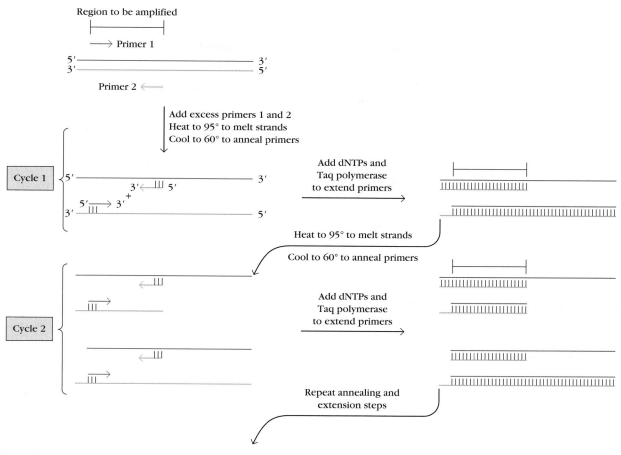

FIGURE 2-7

The polymerase chain reaction (PCR). DNA is denatured into single strands by a brief heat treatment and is then cooled in the presence of an excess of oligonucleotide primers complementary to the DNA sequences flanking the desired DNA segment. Taq polymerase, a heat-resistant DNA polymerase obtained from a thermophilic bacterium, is used to copy the DNA from the 3′ ends of the primers. Because all of the reaction components are heat stable, the heating and cooling cycle can be repeated many times, resulting in alternate DNA melting and synthesis, and rapid amplification of a given sequence. [Adapted from Harvey Lodish et al., 1995, *Molecular Cell Biology*, 3rd ed., Scientific American Books.]

The DNA amplified by the PCR can be further characterized by Southern blotting, restriction-enzyme mapping, and direct DNA sequencing. The PCR has enabled immunologists to amplify genes encoding proteins that are important in the immune response, such as MHC molecules, the T-cell receptor, and immunoglobulins.

ANALYSIS OF DNA REGULATORY SEQUENCES

The transcriptional activity of genes is regulated by **promoter** and **enhancer** sequences. These sequences are cis-acting, meaning that they only regulate genes on the same DNA molecule. The promoter sequence lies upstream from the gene it regulates and includes a TATA box where the general transcription machinery, including RNA polymerase II, binds and begins transcription. The enhancer sequence confers a high rate of transcription on the promoter. Unlike the promoter, which always lies upstream from the gene it controls, the enhancer element can be located anywhere with respect to the gene (5′ of the promoter, 3′ of the gene, or even in an intron of the gene).

The activity of enhancer and promoter sequences is controlled by **transcription factors**, which are DNA-binding proteins. These proteins bind to specific nucleotide sequences within promoters and enhancers and act either to enhance or suppress their activity. Enhancer and promoter sequences and their respective DNA-binding proteins have been identified by a variety of techniques including DNA footprinting, gel-shift analysis, and the CAT assay.

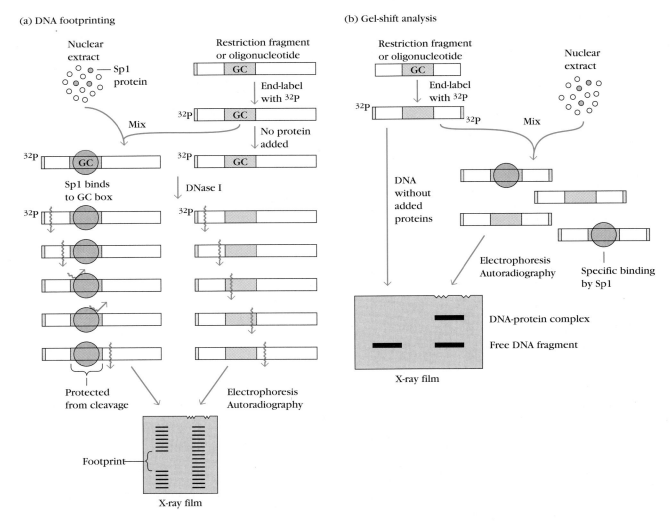

FIGURE 2-8

Identification of DNA sequences that bind protein by DNA-footprinting and gel-shift analysis. (a) In the footprinting technique, labeled DNA fragments containing a putative promoter or enhancer sequence are incubated in the presence and absence of a DNA-binding protein (e.g., Sp1 protein). After the samples are treated with DNase and the strands separated, the resulting fragments are electrophoresed; the gel then is subjected to autoradiography. A blank region (footprint) in the gel pattern indicates that protein has bound to the DNA. (b) In gel-shift analysis, a labeled DNA fragment is incubated with a cellular extract containing transcription factors. The electrophoretic mobility of the DNA-protein complex is slower than that of free DNA fragments. [Adapted from J. D. Watson et al., 1992, *Recombinant DNA*, 2nd ed., W. H. Freeman and Company.]

DNA Footprinting

Identification of the binding sites for DNA-binding proteins on enhancers and promoters can be achieved by a technique called **DNA footprinting** (Figure 2-8a). In this technique a cloned DNA fragment containing a putative enhancer or promoter sequence is first radiolabeled at the 5′ end with ^{32}P. The labeled DNA is then divided into two fractions: One fraction is incubated with a nuclear extract containing a DNA-binding protein; the other DNA fraction is not incubated with the nuclear extract. Both DNA samples are then digested with a nu-

cleare or a chemical that makes random cuts in the phosphodiester bonds of the DNA, and the strands are separated. The resulting DNA fragments are run on a gel to separate fragments of different sizes. In the absence of DNA-binding proteins, a complete ladder of bands is obtained on the electrophoretic gel. When a protein that binds to a site on the DNA fragment is present, it covers some of the nucleotides, protecting that stretch of the DNA from digestion. The electrophoretic pattern of such protected DNA will contain blank regions (or footprints). Each footprint represents the site within an enhancer or promoter that binds a particular DNA-binding protein.

Gel-Shift Analysis

When a protein binds to DNA, forming a DNA-protein complex, the electrophoretic mobility of the DNA is reduced, producing a shift in its gel band. This phenomenon is the basis of **gel-shift analysis**. In this technique radioactively labeled cloned DNA containing an enhancer or a promoter sequence is incubated with a nuclear extract containing a DNA-binding protein (Figure 2-8b). The DNA-protein complex is then electrophoresed and its electrophoretic mobility is compared to that of DNA alone. A shift in the mobility indicates that a protein is bound to the DNA, retarding its migration on the electrophoretic gel.

CAT Assay

One way to assess promoter activity is to engineer and clone a DNA sequence containing a **reporter gene** and a promoter of interest. When this sequence, or construct, is introduced into eukaryotic cells, transcription will be initiated from the promoter. If the promoter is active, the reporter gene will be transcribed and its protein product can be measured.

Most reporter genes encode proteins that can be easily measured, such as the enzyme **chloramphenicol acetyltransferase** (CAT), which transfers the acetyl group from acetyl–CoA to the antibiotic chloramphenicol (Figure 2-9). The more active the promoter is, the more CAT will be produced within the transfected cell. By introducing mutations into promoter sequences and then assaying for promoter activity with the corresponding reporter gene, conserved sequence motifs have been identified within promoters that are necessary for promoter activity.

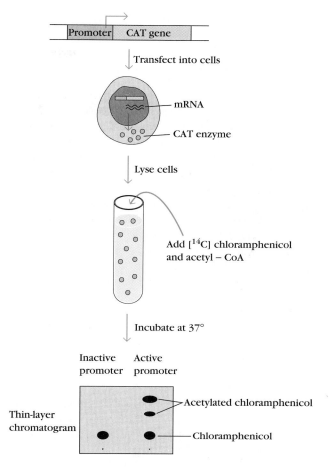

FIGURE 2-9

CAT assay for assessing functional activity of a promoter sequence. In this assay a DNA construct consisting of the promoter of interest and the reporter gene encoding chloramphenicol acetyltransferase (CAT) is introduced (transfected) into eukaryotic cells. If the promoter is active, the CAT gene will be transcribed and the CAT enzyme will be produced within the transfected cell. The presence of the enzyme can easily be detected by lysing the cell and incubating the cell lysate with [^{14}C]chloramphenicol and acetyl-CoA. If present, the CAT enzyme will transfer the acetyl group from acetyl–CoA to the chloramphenicol forming acetylated chloramphenicol, which can be easily detected by thin-layer chromatography. [Adapted from J. D. Watson et al., 1992, *Recombinant DNA*, 2nd ed., W. H. Freeman and Company.]

GENE TRANSFER INTO MAMMALIAN CELLS

A variety of genes involved in the immune response have been isolated and cloned by use of recombinant DNA techniques. The expression and regulation of these genes has been studied by introducing them into cultured cells and, more recently, into the **germ line** of animals.

Transfer of Cloned Genes into Cultured Cells

Diverse techniques have been developed for introducing, or **transfecting**, genes into cells. A common technique involves the use of a retrovirus in which a viral structural gene has been replaced with the cloned gene to be transfected. The altered retrovirus is then used as a vector for introducing the cloned gene into cultured cells. Because of the properties of retroviruses, the recombinant DNA integrates into the cellular genome with a high frequency. In an alternative method, the cloned gene of interest is complexed with calcium phosphate. The calcium phosphate–DNA complex is slowly precipitated onto the cells and the DNA is taken up by a small percentage of them. In another transfection method, called electroporation, an electric current creates pores in cell membranes through which the cloned DNA is taken up. In both of these latter methods, the transfected DNA integrates, apparently at random sites, into the DNA of a small percentage of treated cells.

Generally the cloned DNA being transfected is engineered to contain a selectable marker gene, such as one conferring resistance to neomycin. Following transfection the cells are cultured in the presence of neomycin. Because only the transfected cells are able to grow, the relatively small number of transfected cells in the total cell population can be identified and selected.

Transfection of cloned genes into cells has proved to be a highly effective technique in immunologic research. By transfecting genes involved with the immune response into cells lacking those genes, the product of a specific gene can be studied apart from interacting proteins encoded by other genes. For example, transfection of MHC genes into a mouse fibroblast cell line (L929 or simply L cells) has enabled immunologists to study the role of MHC molecules in antigen presentation to T cells (Figure 2-10). Transfection of the gene encoding the T-cell receptor has provided information about the antigen-MHC specificity of the T-cell receptor.

Transfer of Cloned Genes into Mouse Embryos

Development of techniques to introduce cloned foreign genes (called **transgenes**) into mouse embryos has permitted immunologists to study the effects of immune-system genes in vivo. If the introduced gene integrates stably into the germ-line cells, it will be transmitted to the offspring. Two techniques for producing transgenic mice are discussed in this section; one of these has been used to produce **knockout mice**, which cannot express a particular gene product (Table 2-5).

TRANSGENIC MICE

The first step in producing transgenic mice is injection of foreign cloned DNA into a fertilized egg. In this technically demanding process, fertilized mouse eggs are held under suction at the end of a pipet and the transgene is microinjected into one of the pronuclei with a fine needle. The transgene integrates into the chromosomal DNA of the pronucleus and is passed on to the daughter cells of eggs that survive the process. The eggs then are implanted in the oviduct of "pseudo-pregnant" females, and transgenic pups are born after 19 or 20 days of gestation (Figure 2-11). In general the efficiency of this procedure is low, with only one or two transgenic mice produced for every 100 fertilized eggs collected.

With transgenic mice immunologists have been able to study the expression of a given gene in a living animal. Although all the cells in a transgenic animal contain the transgene, differences in the expression of the transgene in

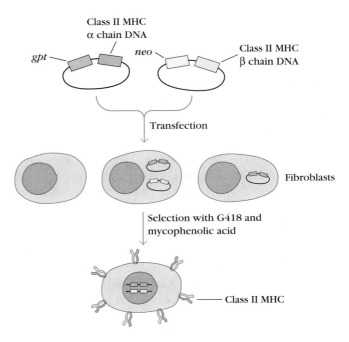

FIGURE 2-10

Transfection of the genes encoding the class II MHC α chain and β chain into mouse fibroblast L cells, which do not produce these proteins. Two constructs containing one of the MHC genes and a selectable gene were engineered: the α-chain gene with the guanine phosphoribosyl transferase gene (*gpt*), which confers resistance to the drug G418, and the β-chain gene with a neomycin gene (*neo*), which confers resistance to mycophenolic acid. Following transfection, the cells are placed in medium containing both G418 and mycophenolic acid. Only those fibroblasts containing both the *neo* and *gpt* genes (and consequently the genes encoding the class II MHC α and β chains) will survive this selection. These fibroblasts will express both class II MHC chains on their membrane.

different tissues has shed light on mechanisms of tissue-specific gene expression. By constructing a transgene with a particular promoter, researchers can control the expression of a given transgene. For example, the metallothionein promoter is activated by zinc. Transgenic mice carrying a transgene linked to a metallothionein promoter express the transgene only if zinc is added to their water supply. Other promoters are functional only in certain tissues; the insulin promoter, for instance, promotes transcription only in pancreatic cells. Transgenic mice carrying a transgene linked to the insulin promoter, therefore, will express the transgene in the pancreas but not in other tissues.

Because a transgene is integrated into the chromosomal DNA within the one-celled mouse embryo, it will be integrated into both somatic cells and germ-line cells. The resulting transgenic mice thus can transmit the transgene to their offspring as a mendelian trait. In this way it

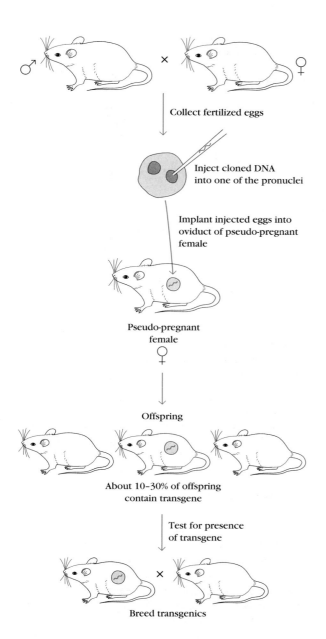

Collect fertilized eggs

Inject cloned DNA into one of the pronuclei

Implant injected eggs into oviduct of pseudo-pregnant female

Pseudo-pregnant female ♀

Offspring

About 10–30% of offspring contain transgene

Test for presence of transgene

Breed transgenics

FIGURE 2-11

General procedure for producing transgenic mice. Fertilized eggs are collected from a pregnant female mouse. Cloned DNA (referred to as the transgene) is microinjected into one of the pronuclei of a fertilized egg. The eggs are then implanted into the oviduct of pseudo–pregnant foster mothers (obtained by mating a normal female with a sterile male). The transgene will be incorporated into the chromosomal DNA of about 10%–30% of the offspring and will be expressed in all of their somatic cells. If a tissue-specific promoter is linked to a transgene, then tissue-specific expression of the transgene will result.

has been possible to produce lines of transgenic mice in which every member of a particular line contains the same transgene. A variety of such transgenic lines are currently available and are widely used in immunologic research today. Included among these are lines carrying transgenes that encode immunoglobulin, T-cell receptor, class I and class II MHC molecules, various foreign antigens, and a number of cytokines. Several lines carrying oncogenes as transgenes also have been produced.

GENE-TARGETED KNOCKOUT MICE

One of the limitations with transgenic mice is that the transgene is integrated randomly within the genome. To circumvent this limitation, researchers have developed a technique in which a desired gene is targeted to specific sites within the germ line of a mouse. The primary use of this technique has been to replace a normal gene with a mutant allele or a disrupted form of the gene, thus knocking out the gene's function. Transgenic mice carrying such a disrupted gene, called knockout mice, have been extremely helpful to immunologists trying to understand how the removal of a particular gene product affects the immune system. A variety of knockout mice are being used in immunologic research, including mice lacking particular cytokines or MHC molecules.

TABLE 2-5

COMPARISON OF TRANSGENIC AND KNOCKOUT MICE

CHARACTERISTIC	TRANSGENIC MICE	KNOCKOUT MICE
Cells receiving DNA	Zygote	Embryonic stem (ES) cells
DNA constructs used	Natural gene or cDNA	Mutated gene
Means of delivery	Microinjection into zygote and implantation into foster mother	Transfer of ES cells to blastocyst and implantation into foster mother
Outcome	Gain of a gene	Loss of a gene

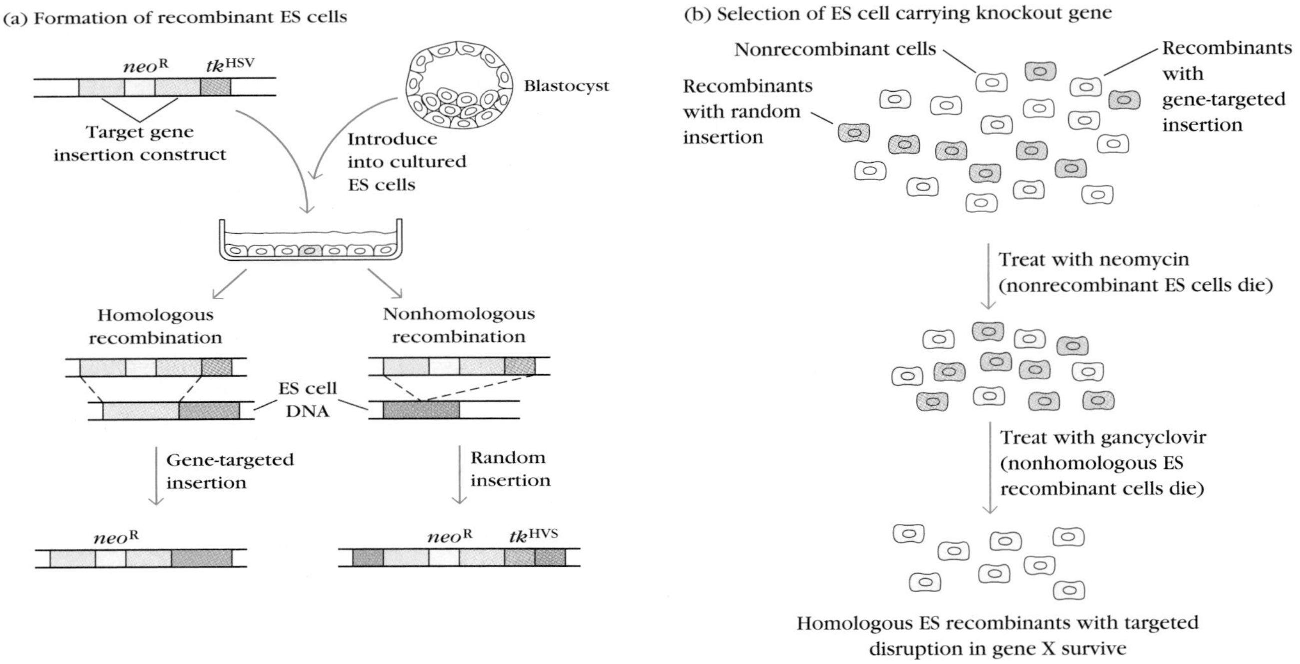

(a) Formation of recombinant ES cells

(b) Selection of ES cell carrying knockout gene

FIGURE 2-12

Formation and selection of mouse recombinant ES cells in which a particular target gene is disrupted. (a) In the engineered insertion construct, the target gene is disrupted with the neo^R gene and the thymidine kinase tk^{HSV} gene is located outside the target gene. The construct is transfected into cultured ES cells. If homologous recombination occurs, only the target gene and the neo^R gene will be inserted into the chromosomal DNA of the ES cells. If nonhomologous recombination occurs, all three genes will be inserted. Recombination occurs in only about 1% of the cells, with nonhomologous recombination much more frequent than homologous recombination. (b) Selection with the neomycin-like drug G418 will kill any nonrecombinant ES cells. Selection with gancyclovir will kill the nonhomologous recombinants carrying the tk^{HSV} gene, which confers sensitivity to gancyclovir. Only the homologous ES recombinants will survive this selection scheme. [Adapted from Harvey Lodish et al., 1995, *Molecular Cell Biology,* 3rd ed., Scientific American Books.]

Production of gene-targeted knockout mice involves the following steps:

- Isolation and culturing of **embryonic stem (ES) cells** from the inner cell mass of a mouse blastocyst.
- Introduction of a mutant or disrupted gene into the cultured ES cells and selection of **homologous recombinant cells** in which the gene of interest has been knocked out (i.e., replaced by a nonfunctional form of the gene).
- Injection of gene-targeted recombinant ES cells into a recipient mouse blastocyst and surgical implantation of the blastocyst into a pseudopregnant mouse.
- Mating of chimeric offspring heterozygous for the disrupted gene to produce homozygous knockout mice.

The ES cells used in this procedure are obtained by culturing the inner cell mass of a mouse blastocyst on a feeder layer of fibroblasts or in the presence of leukemia inhibitory factor. Under these conditions, the stem cells grow but remain pluripotent and capable of later differentiating in a variety of directions, generating distinct cellular lineages (e.g., germ cells, myocardium, blood vessels, myoblasts, nerve cells). One of the advantages of ES cells is the ease with which they can be genetically manipulated. Cloned DNA containing a desired gene can be introduced into ES cells in culture by various transfection techniques. The introduced DNA will be inserted by recombination into the chromosomal DNA of a small number of ES cells.

The insertion constructs introduced into ES cells contain three genes: the **target gene** of interest and two **selection genes** such as neo^R, which confers neomycin resistance, and the thymidine kinase gene from herpes simplex virus (tk^{HSV}), which confers sensitivity to gancyclovir, a cytotoxic nucleotide analog (Figure 2-12a). The construct often is engineered with the target-gene sequence disrupted by the neo^R gene and the tk^{HSV} gene at one end, beyond the sequence of the target gene. Most constructs will insert at random by nonhomologous recombination rather than by gene-targeted insertion

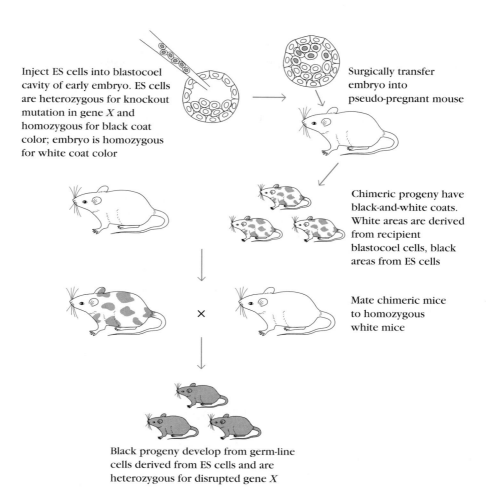

Inject ES cells into blastocoel cavity of early embryo. ES cells are heterozygous for knockout mutation in gene *X* and homozygous for black coat color; embryo is homozygous for white coat color

Surgically transfer embryo into pseudo-pregnant mouse

Chimeric progeny have black-and-white coats. White areas are derived from recipient blastocoel cells, black areas from ES cells

Mate chimeric mice to homozygous white mice

×

Black progeny develop from germ-line cells derived from ES cells and are heterozygous for disrupted gene *X*

FIGURE 2-13

General procedure for producing homozygous knockout mice. ES cells homozygous for a marker gene (e.g., black coat color) and heterozygous for a disrupted target gene (see Figure 2-12) are injected into an early embryo homozygous for an alternate marker (e.g., white coat color). The chimeric transgenic offspring, which have black-and-white coats, then are mated with homozygous white mice. The all-black progeny from this mating have ES-derived cells in their germ line. Mating of these mice with each other produces animals homozygous for the disrupted target gene, that is, knockout mice. [Adapted from M. R. Capecchi, 1989, *Trends Genet.* **5**:70.]

via homologous recombination. As illustrated in Figure 2-12b, a two-step selection scheme is used to obtain those ES cells that have undergone homologous recombination whereby the disrupted gene replaces the target gene.

The ES cells obtained by this procedure are heterozygous for the knockout mutation in the target gene. These cells are clonally expanded in cell culture and then injected into a mouse blastocyst, which subsequently is implanted into a pseudo-pregnant female. The transgenic offspring that develop are chimeric, composed of cells derived from the genetically altered ES cells and cells derived from normal cells of the host blastocyst. When the germ-line cells are derived from the genetically altered ES cells, the genetic alteration can be passed on to the offspring. If the recombinant ES cells are homozygous for black coat color (or other visible marker) and

they are injected into a blastocyst homozygous for white coat color, then the chimeric progeny that carry the heterozygous knockout mutation in their germ line can be easily identified (Figure 2-13). When these are mated with each other, the offspring will be homozygous for the knockout mutation.

SUMMARY

1. Inbred mouse strains allow immunologists to work routinely with syngeneic, or genetically identical, animals. With these strains, aspects of the immune response can be studied uncomplicated by unknown variables that could be introduced by genetic differences between animals.

2. In adoptive-transfer experiments, lymphocytes are transferred from one mouse to a syngeneic recipient mouse that has been exposed to a sublethal (or potentially lethal) dose of x-rays. The irradiation inactivates the immune cells of the recipient, so that one can study the response of only the transferred cells.

3. With in vitro cell-culture systems, populations of lymphocytes can be studied under more-defined conditions than are possible with in vivo animal systems. Such systems include primary cultures of lymphoid cells, cloned lymphoid cell lines, and hybrid lymphoid cell lines. Unlike primary cultures, cell lines are immortal and homogeneous. With cell lines, the intracellular events and cell products associated with individual subpopulations of lymphocytes can be investigated (see Table 2-2). Such studies are difficult, if not impossible, with the heterogeneous populations typical of primary cultures.

4. The ability to identify, clone, and sequence immune-system genes, using recombinant DNA techniques, has revolutionized the study of all aspects of the immune response. Both cDNA, which is prepared by transcribing mRNA with reverse transcriptase, and genomic DNA can be cloned. Generally, cDNA is cloned using a plasmid vector; the recombinant DNA containing the gene to be cloned is propagated in *E. coli* cells (see Figure 2-3). Genomic DNA can be cloned within a bacteriophage λ vector or cosmid vector, both of which are propagated in *E. coli* (see Figure 2-4). Even larger genomic DNA fragments can be cloned within bacteriophage P1 vectors, which can replicate in *E. coli*, or yeast artificial chromosomes, which can replicate in yeast cells (see Table 2-4).

5. Transcription of genes is regulated by promoter and enhancer sequences; the activity of these sequences is controlled by DNA-binding proteins. Footprinting and gel-shift analysis can be used to identify DNA-binding proteins and their binding sites within the promoter or enhancer sequence (see Figure 2-8). Promoter activity can be assessed by the CAT assay (see Figure 2-9).

6. Cloned genes can be transfected (transferred) into cultured cells by several methods. Commonly, immune-system genes are transfected into cells that do not express the gene of interest. Cloned genes also can be incorporated into the germ-line cells of mouse embryos, yielding transgenic mice, which can transmit the incorporated transgene to their offspring (see Figure 2-11). With transgenic mice, expression of a given gene can be studied in a living animal. Knockout mice are transgenics in which a particular target gene has been replaced by a nonfunctional form of the gene, so the gene product is not expressed (see Table 2-5).

REFERENCES

BELL, J. 1989. The polymerase chain reaction. *Immunol. Today* **10**:351.

CAMPER, S. A. 1987. Research applications of transgenic mice. *Biotechniques* **5**:638.

CAPECCHI, M. R. 1989. Altering the genome by homologous recombination. *Science* **244**: 1288.

DENIS, K. A., AND O. N. WITTE. 1989. Long-term lymphoid cultures in the study of B cell differentiation. In *Immunoglobulin Genes.* Academic Press, p. 45.

DEPAMPHILIS, M. L., ET AL. 1988. Microinjecting DNA into mouse ova to study DNA replication and gene expression and to produce transgenic animals. *Biotechniques* **6**(7):622.

KOLLER, B. H., AND O. SMITHIES. 1992. Altering genes in animals by gene targeting. *Annu. Rev. Immunol.* **10**:705.

McCUNE, J. M., ET AL. 1988. The SCID-Hu mouse; murine model for analysis of human hematolymphoid differentiation and function. *Science* **241**:1632.

MEINL, E., ET AL. 1995. Immortalization of human T cells by *herpesvirus saimiri. Immunol. Today* **16**: 55.

MELTON, D. W. 1994. Gene targeting in the mouse. *BioEssays* **16**:633.

SCHLESSINGER, D. 1990. Yeast artificial chromosomes: tools for mapping and analysis of complex genomes. *Trends Genet.* **6**(8):254.

SHARPE, A. H. 1995. Analysis of lymphocyte costimulation in vivo using transgenic and knockout mice. *Curr. Opin. Immunol.* **7**:389.

WATSON, J., ET AL. 1992. *Recombinant DNA,* 2nd ed. W. H. Freeman and Company.

STUDY QUESTIONS

1. Explain why the following statements are **false**.

a. The amino acid sequence of a protein can be determined from the nucleotide sequence of a genomic clone encoding the protein.

b. Transgenic mice can be prepared by microinjection of DNA into a somatic-cell nucleus.

c. Primary lymphoid cultures can be propagated indefinitely and are useful in studies on specific subpopulations of lymphocytes.

2. Fill in the blanks in the following statements with the most appropriate terms:

a. In inbred mouse strains, all or nearly all genetic loci are _____; such strains are said to be _____ .

b. SCID mice have a genetic defect that prevents development of functional _____ and _____ cells.

c. B-cell hybridomas are formed by fusion of _____ with _____. They are capable of _____ growth and are used to produce _____.

d. A normal lymphoid cell that undergoes _____ can give rise to a cell line, which has an _____ life span.

3. The gene diagrammed below contains one leader (L), three exons (E), and three introns (I). Illustrate the primary transcript, mRNA, and the protein product that could be generated from such a gene.

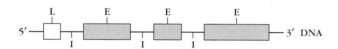

4. The term *transfection* refers to which of the following:

a. Synthesis of mRNA from a DNA template
b. Synthesis of protein based on an mRNA sequence
c. Introduction of foreign DNA into a cell
d. The process by which a normal cell becomes malignant
e. Transfer of a signal from outside a cell to inside a cell

5. Which of the following are required to carry out the PCR?

a. Short oligonucleotide primers
b. Thermostabile DNA polymerase
c. Antibodies directed against the encoded protein
d. A method for heating and cooling the reaction mixture periodically
e. All of the above

6. Why is it necessary to include a selectable marker gene in transfection experiments?

7. What would be the result if a transgene were injected into one cell of a four-cell mouse zygote rather than into a fertilized mouse egg before it divides?

8. A circular plasmid was cleaved with *Eco*RI, producing a 5.4-kb band on a gel. A 5.4-kb band was also observed when the plasmid was cleaved with *Hind*III. Cleaving the plasmid with both enzymes simultaneously resulted in a single band 2.7 kb in size. Draw a diagram of this plasmid showing the relative location of its restriction sites. Explain your reasoning.

9. DNA footprinting is a suitable technique for identifying which of the following?

a. Particular mRNAs in a mixture
b. Particular tRNAs in a mixture
c. Introns within a gene
d. Protein-binding sites within DNA
e. Specific DNA sites at which restriction endonucleases cleave the nucleotide chain

10. Explain briefly how you might go about cloning a gene for interleukin 2 (IL-2). Assume that you have available a monoclonal antibody specific for IL-2.

11. You have a sample of a mouse DNA-binding protein and of the mRNA that encodes it. Assuming you have a mouse genomic library available, briefly describe how you could first select a clone carrying a DNA fragment that contains the binding site and then identify the short binding sequence.

12. What are the major differences between transgenic mice and knockout mice and in the procedures for producing them.

13. For each term related to recombinant DNA technology (a–i), select the most appropriate description (1–10) listed below. Each description may be used once, more than once, or not at all.

Terms:

a. _____ Yeast artificial chromosome
b. _____ Restriction endonuclease
c. _____ cDNA
d. _____ COS sites
e. _____ Retrovirus
f. _____ Plasmid
g. _____ cDNA library
h. _____ Sticky ends
i. _____ Genomic library

Descriptions:

1) Cleaves mRNA at specific sites.

2) Cleaves double-stranded DNA at specific sites.

3) Circular genetic element that can replicate in *E. coli* cells.

4) Used to clone DNA in mammalian cells.

5) Formed from action of reverse transcriptase.

6) Collection of DNA sequences within plasmid vectors representing all of the mRNA sequences derived from a cell.

7) Produced by action of certain DNA-cleaving enzymes.

8) Used to clone very large DNA sequences.

9) Used to introduce larger-than-normal DNA fragments in λ-phage vectors.

10) Collection of λ clones that includes all the DNA sequences of a given species.

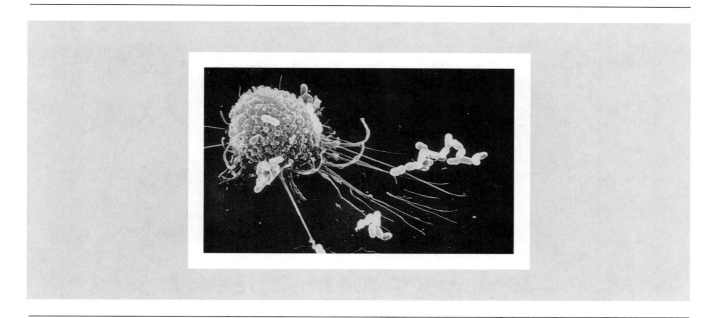

CELLS AND ORGANS
OF THE IMMUNE SYSTEM

HEMATOPOIESIS

IMMUNE-SYSTEM CELLS

ORGANS OF THE IMMUNE SYSTEM

The immune system consists of many structurally and functionally diverse organs and tissues that are widely dispersed throughout the body. These organs can be classified on the basis of functional differences into two main groups. The **primary lymphoid organs** provide appropriate microenvironments for lymphocyte maturation. The **secondary lymphoid organs** trap antigen from defined tissues or vascular spaces and provide sites where mature lymphocytes can interact effectively with that antigen. The blood vasculature and lymphatic systems interconnect these organs, uniting them into a functional whole.

Carried within the blood and lymph and populating the various lymphoid organs are a variety of white blood cells, or **leukocytes**, that participate in development of the immune response (Figure 3-1). Of these cells, only the lymphocytes possess the attributes of diversity, speci-

ficity, memory, and self/nonself recognition, the hallmarks of an immune response. All the other cells play accessory roles, serving to activate lymphocytes, to increase the effectiveness of antigen clearance by phagocytosis, or to secrete various immune effector molecules. In this chapter, the formation of blood cells is described first; then the properties of the various immune-system cells are presented. Finally, the functions of the lymphoid organs are examined.

HEMATOPOIESIS

In humans, **hematopoiesis**, the formation and development of red and white blood cells from **stem cells**, begins in the yolk sac in the first weeks of embryonic development. Here yolk-sac stem cells differentiate into primitive erythroid cells containing embryonic hemoglobin. In the third month of gestation, the stem cells migrate from the yolk sac to the fetal liver and then to the spleen; these two organs have major roles in hematopoiesis from the third to the seventh months of

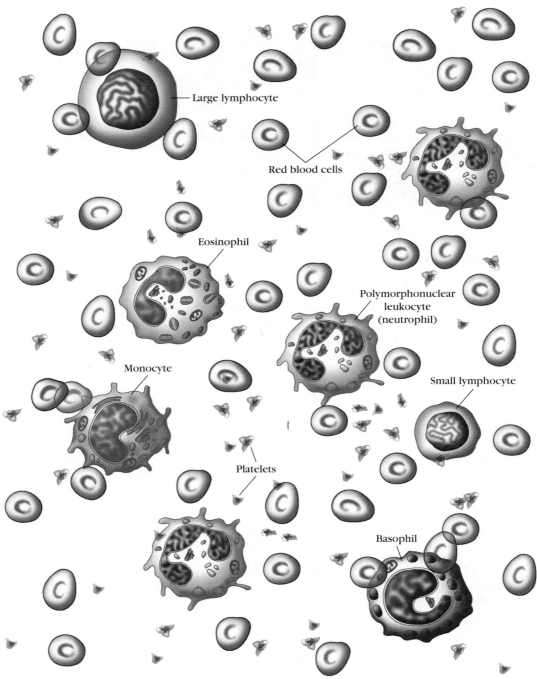

FIGURE 3-1

Morphology and staining characteristics of various types of blood cells. Red blood cells and platelets, which both lack nuclei, are the most numerous. Among the leukocytes responsible for immune responses, the neutrophil is the predominant cell type.

gestation. As gestation continues, the bone marrow becomes the major hematopoietic organ; by birth hematopoiesis has ceased within the liver and spleen.

It is remarkable that every functionally specialized, mature blood cell is derived from a common stem cell.

In contrast to a unipotent cell, which differentiates into a single cell type, a hematopoietic stem cell is **pluripotent**, able to differentiate along a number of pathways and thereby generate erythrocytes, granulocytes, monocytes, mast cells, lymphocytes, and megakaryocytes. These stem cells are few in number, occurring with a frequency of one stem cell per 10^4 bone marrow cells.

The study of stem cells has been hampered by their low frequency and the inability of researchers to maintain them in tissue culture. As a result, little is known about the regulation of their proliferation and differentiation. By virtue of their capacity for self-renewal, stem cells are maintained at homeostatic levels throughout adult life; however, when there is an increased demand for hematopoiesis, stem cells display an enormous proliferative capacity. This can be demonstrated in mice whose hematopoietic systems have been completely destroyed by a lethal dose (950 rads) of x-rays. Such irradiated mice will die within 10 days unless they are infused with normal bone marrow cells from a syngeneic (genetically identical) mouse. Although a normal mouse has 3×10^8 bone marrow cells, infusion of only 10^4–10^5 donor bone marrow cells (i.e., 0.01%–0.1% of the normal level) is sufficient to completely restore the hematopoietic system, demonstrating the enormous proliferative and differentiative capacity of the few stem cells in the donor bone marrow.

Early in hematopoiesis, a pluripotent stem cell differentiates along one of two pathways, giving rise to either a **lymphoid stem cell** or a **myeloid stem cell** (Figure 3-2). The types and amounts of growth factors present in the microenvironment in which a particular stem cell resides control its differentiation. Lymphoid and myeloid stem cells differentiate into **progenitor cells,** which have lost the capacity for self-renewal and are committed to a given cell lineage. The lymphoid stem cell generates T and B progenitor lymphocytes. The myeloid stem cell generates progenitor cells for red blood cells (erythrocytes), the various white blood cells (neutrophils, eosinophils, basophils, monocytes, mast cells), and platelets. Progenitor commitment depends on the acquisition of responsiveness to particular growth factors. When the appropriate growth factors are present, progenitor cells proliferate and differentiate, giving rise to the corresponding type of mature red or white blood cells.

In adult bone marrow, the hematopoietic cells grow and mature on a meshwork of **stromal cells**, which are nonhematopoietic cells that support the growth and differentiation of the hematopoietic cells. Stromal cells include fat cells, endothelial cells, fibroblasts, and macrophages. Stromal cells influence hematopoietic stem-cell differentiation by providing a **hematopoietic-inducing microenvironment** consisting of a cellular matrix and either membrane-bound or diffusible growth factors. As hematopoietic stem cells differentiate in this microenvironment, their membranes acquire deformability, allowing the mature cells to pass through the sinusoidal wall into the sinuses of the bone marrow, whence they enter the circulation.

Hematopoietic Growth Factors

Development of cell-culture systems that can support the growth and differentiation of lymphoid and myeloid stem cells led to identification of numerous hematopoietic growth factors. In these in vitro systems, bone-marrow stromal cells are cultured to form a layer of adherent cells; freshly isolated bone-marrow hematopoietic cells placed on this layer will grow and produce large visible colonies (Figure 3-3). If the cells are cultured on semisolid agar, the clonal progeny will be immobilized and can be analyzed for cell types. Colonies containing stem cells can be replated, producing mixed colonies containing a number of differentiated cell types; progenitor cells, which cannot be replated, produce lineage-restricted colonies.

Various growth factors are required for the survival, proliferation, differentiation, and maturation of hematopoietic cells in culture. These growth factors, or **cytokines**, were originally detected in serum or in conditioned medium from in vitro cell cultures. Subsequently they were defined on the basis of their ability to stimulate the formation of hematopoietic cell colonies in bone marrow cultures. Among the cytokines detected by this method was a family of acidic glycoproteins, the **colony-stimulating factors** (CSFs), named for their ability to induce the formation of distinct hematopoietic cell lineages.

Four distinct colony-stimulating factors have been identified: **multilineage CSF** (multi-CSF), also known as interleukin 3 (IL-3); **granulocyte-macrophage CSF** (GM-CSF); **macrophage CSF** (M-CSF); **granulocyte CSF** (G-CSF). Another important hematopoietic cytokine detected by this method is a glycoprotein called **erythropoietin** (EPO); produced by the kidney, this cytokine induces terminal erythrocyte development and regulates red blood cell production. Hematopoiesis also depends on several **interleukins**, as indicated in Table 3-1. Many of the hematopoietic cytokines are secreted by bone-marrow stromal cells, activated T helper (T_H) cells, and activated macrophages.

The various growth factors involved in hematopoiesis exert their biological activity at concentrations as low as 10^{-12} M. Biochemical purification of these cytokines was initially hampered by their low physiologic concentrations. A major breakthrough came when the genes encoding hematopoietic growth factors were cloned. By transfecting these cloned genes into cultured cells, researchers have obtained sufficient quantities of the various hematopoietic growth to determine their target cells and biological effects (see Table 3-1).

The colony-stimulating factors act in a stepwise manner, inducing proper maturation of the hematopoietic

Visualizing Concepts

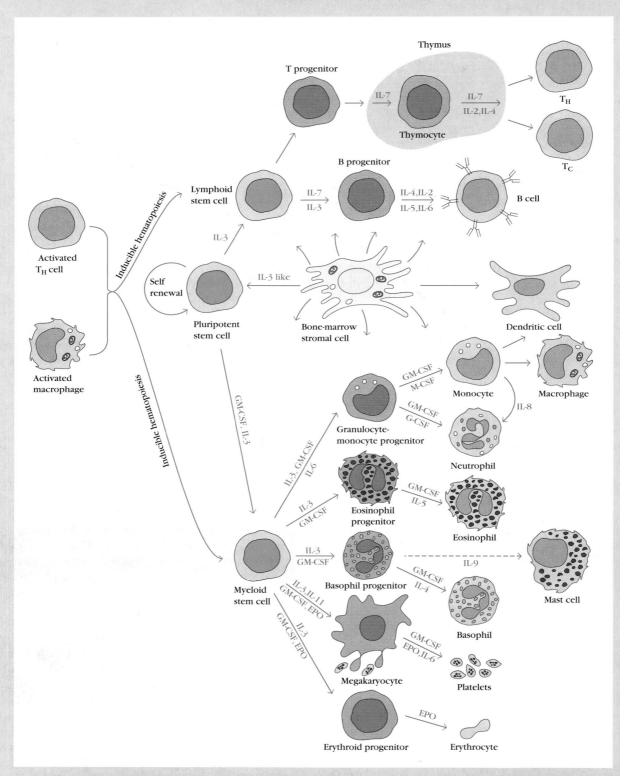

◄ FIGURE 3-2

Regulation of hematopoiesis by cytokines that stimulate the proliferation and/or differentiation of various hematopoietic cells. In the absence of infection, bone-marrow stromal cells are the major source of hematopoietic cytokines. In the presence of infection, cytokines produced by activated macrophages and T_H cells induce additional hematopoietic activity, resulting in rapid expansion of the population of white blood cells that participate in fighting infection. IL = interleukin; CSF = colony-stimulating factor; EPO = erythropoietin. Stem cells are shown in blue; progenitor and immature cells in purple; stromal cell in yellow; and mature differentiated cells in tan.

cells. Multi-CSF (IL-3) acts early in differentiation, possibly even at the level of the pluripotent stem cell, to induce formation of all the nonlymphoid blood cells, including erythrocytes, monocytes, granulocytes (neutrophils, eosinophils, and basophils), and megakaryocytes. GM-CSF acts at a slightly later stage, but it also induces formation of all the nonlymphoid blood cells. M-CSF and G-CSF act still later to promote the formation of monocytes and neutrophils, respectively.

The commitment of a progenitor cell to a given differentiation pathway is associated with the expression on the cell of membrane receptors that are specific for particular cytokines. The macrophage progenitor cell, for example, bears specific receptors for M-CSF; the binding of M-CSF to these receptors stimulates cellular proliferation and differentiation in a concentration-dependent manner.

Regulation of Hematopoiesis

Hematopoiesis is a continuous process that generally maintains a steady state in which the production of ma-

ture blood cells equals their loss (principally as the cells age). The average erythrocyte has a life span of 120 days before it is phagocytosed and digested by macrophages in the spleen. The various white blood cells have life spans ranging from days for neutrophils to as long as 20–30 years for some T lymphocytes. To maintain steady-state levels, the average human must produce an estimated 3.7×10^{11} cells per day.

Hematopoiesis is regulated by complex mechanisms that affect all of the individual cell types. These regulatory mechanisms provide steady-state levels of the various blood cells and yet have enough built-in flexibility so that production of blood cells can rapidly increase tenfold to twentyfold in response to hemorrhage or infection. Steady-state regulation of hematopoiesis is accomplished by the controlled production of cytokines by bone-marrow stromal cells. These cells have been shown to produce GM-CSF, M-CSF, G-CSF, IL-4, IL-6, and IL-7. Although multi-CSF (IL-3) is the earliest-acting cytokine, it has not been detected in stromal cells, but only in activated T_H cells. It is thought that some other, as yet unidentified, cytokine must be produced by

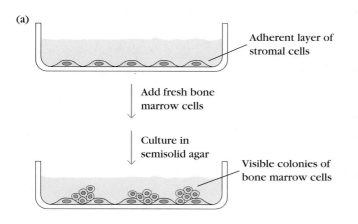

(a)

Adherent layer of stromal cells

Add fresh bone marrow cells

Culture in semisolid agar

Visible colonies of bone marrow cells

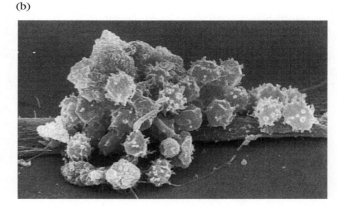

(b)

FIGURE 3-3

(a) Experimental scheme for culturing hematopoietic cells. Adherent bone-marrow stromal cells form a matrix on which the hematopoietic cells proliferate. Cells can be transferred to semisolid agar for colony growth, and the colonies analyzed for differentiated cell types.

(b) Scanning electron micrograph of cells in long-term culture of human bone marrow. [Photograph from M. J. Cline and D. W. Golde, 1979, *Nature* **277**:180.]

bone-marrow stromal cells to maintain steady-state levels of the pluripotent stem cells.

In response to infection, localized influxes of white blood cells generate an inflammatory reaction that can limit the infection. The hematopoietic system is capable of rapid expansion and maturation of specific cell lineages to provide the necessary cells for such a localized inflammatory response. This inducible hematopoietic activity is regulated by activated T_H cells and activated macrophages, which secrete a number of cytokines that stimulate proliferation and differentiation of different white blood cells involved in the immune response. The concerted actions of these factors induce localized hematopoietic activity to meet the needs of the immune system to fight infection.

Production of different hematopoietic lineages can be regulated by changes in the local concentrations of cytokines or by differential expression of the receptors for the various cytokines in different lineages. Very little is known about how cytokine concentrations are regulated because the stromal-cell matrix in bone marrow, which creates unique microenvironments for the developing hematopoietic cells, has not been duplicated and studied in vitro. Likewise, although expression of cytokine receptors is known to vary among different hematopoietic lineages, the events determining this differential expression are not understood.

The effect of differential expression of cytokine receptors can be illustrated by the M-CSF receptor. Cells of the erythroid, lymphoid, eosinophilic, and megakaryocytic lineages lack M-CSF receptors, cells of the neutrophilic lineage express low levels of M-CSF receptors, and cells of the monocyte-macrophage lineage express high levels of M-CSF receptors. Since the level of receptor expression governs the responsiveness of a lineage to M-CSF concentrations, only cells of the monocyte-macrophage lineage respond to low concentrations of M-CSF; cells of the neutrophil lineage require much higher concentrations of M-CSF to induce a response, and the other hematopoietic lineages do not respond to M-CSF at all.

The binding of a CSF to its receptor causes some of the receptors to be internalized by the cell; internalization serves to down-modulate receptor expression by the cell.

T A B L E   3 - 1

EFFECT OF CYTOKINES ON HEMATOPOIETIC CELLS

TARGET CELLS ACTED ON IN BONE MARROW	CYTOKINES											
	MULTI-CSF (IL-3)	GM-CSF	G-CSF	M-CSF (CSF-1)	IL-4	IL-5	IL-6	IL-7	IL-8	IL-9	IL-10	EPO
Pluripotent stem cell	+	+	–	–	–	–	–	–	–	–	–	–
Myeloid stem cell	+	+	–	–	–	–	+	–	–	–	–	–
Granulocyte-monocyte progenitor	+	+	+	+	–	–	–	–	–	–	–	–
Monocyte progenitor	+	+	–	+	–	–	–	–	–	–	–	–
Neutrophil progenitor	+	+	+	–	–	–	–	–	+	–	–	–
Eosinophil progenitor	+	+	–	–	–	+	–	–	–	–	–	–
Basophil progenitor	–	+	–	–	+	–	–	–	–	–	–	–
Mast cell	+	+	–	–	+	–	–	–	–	+	+	–
Megakaryocyte	+	+	–	–	–	–	–	–	–	–	–	+/–
Erythroid progenitor	+/–	+/–	–	–	–	–	–	–	–	–	–	+
Lymphoid stem cell B progenitor	–	–	–	–	+	–	–	+	–	–	–	–
T progenitor (thymus)	–	–	–	–	–	–	–	+	–	–	–	–

KEY: (+) indicates cytokine acts on the indicated target cell to stimulate its proliferation and differentiation; (–) indicates no effect of the cytokine on the indicated cell. See Figure 3-2 for the position of the various target cells in the overall pathway of hematopoiesis.

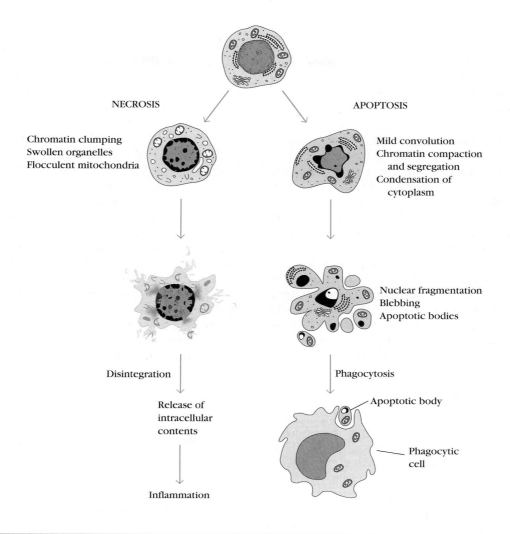

NECROSIS   APOPTOSIS

Chromatin clumping   Mild convolution
Swollen organelles   Chromatin compaction
Flocculent mitochondria   and segregation
                                            Condensation of
                                               cytoplasm

                                            Nuclear fragmentation
                                            Blebbing
                                            Apoptotic bodies

Disintegration   Phagocytosis

                                            Apoptotic body

Release of
intracellular
contents   Phagocytic
                                            cell

Inflammation

FIGURE 3-4

Comparison of morphologic changes that occur in apoptosis and necrosis. Apoptosis, which is associated with the programmed cell death of hematopoietic cells, does not induce a localized inflammatory response. In contrast, necrosis, the process leading to death of injured cells, results in release of the intracellular contents, which induce a localized inflammatory response.

With fewer receptors on its membrane, the cell becomes progressively less responsive to the CSF, and proliferation of the lineage slows down. This down-modulation of CSF-receptor expression can even be induced by the binding of unrelated CSFs to their receptors. For example, when GM-CSF binds to its receptor, it induces the cell to down-modulate the expression of G-CSF and M-CSF receptors as well. This down-modulation of G-CSF and M-CSF receptors causes the lineages bearing these receptors to become less responsive to these CSFs.

Hematopoiesis can also be regulated by degradation of a CSF following its binding to a receptor. Experiments suggest that binding of M-CSF to its receptor results in degradation of the cytokine. As monocyte numbers increase, there is a corresponding increase in M-CSF receptors, leading to increased M-CSF degradation. Thus the

M-CSF concentration falls as cell numbers increase, thereby slowing further proliferation and differentiation of this lineage as long as the number of monocytes remains high.

PROGRAMMED CELL DEATH

In order for steady-state levels of the various hematopoietic cells to be maintained, cell division and differentiation in each of the lineages is balanced by a process called **programmed cell death**. Cells undergoing programmed cell death often exhibit distinctive morphologic changes, collectively referred to as **apoptosis** (Figure 3-4). These changes include a pronounced decrease in cell volume, modification of the cytoskeleton resulting in pronounced membrane blebbing, a condensation of the chromatin, and degradation of the DNA into oligonucleosomal fragments. Following these morphologic changes, an apoptotic cell sheds tiny membrane-bound apoptotic bodies containing intact organelles. Macrophages quickly phagocytose apoptotic bodies, ensuring that their intracellular contents, including proteolytic and other lytic enzymes, cationic proteins, and oxidizing molecules are not released into the surrounding tissue. In this way apoptosis occurs without inducing a localized inflammatory response. Apoptosis differs markedly from **necrosis**, the changes associated with cell death arising from injury. In necrosis the injured cell swells and bursts, releasing its intracellular contents, which are cytotoxic to other cells in the tissue; as a result, an inflammatory response develops.

Each of the cells produced by hematopoiesis has a characteristic life span and then dies by programmed cell death. In the adult human, for example, there are about 5×10^{10} neutrophils in the circulation. These cells have a life span of only 1 day and then die by programmed cell death. This death, coupled with constant neutrophil production, maintains steady-state levels of these cells. If programmed cell death fails to occur, a leukemic state may develop. Programmed cell death also plays a role in maintaining proper levels of hematopoietic progenitor cells. For example, when colony-stimulating factors are removed, progenitor cells undergo programmed cell death.

The expression of several genes has been associated with the regulation of apoptosis in hematopoietic cell lineages (Table 3-2). Some of these gene products induce apoptosis, whereas other gene products inhibit apoptosis. The *bcl-2* (B-cell lymphoma 2) gene, for example, encodes a protein product that inhibits apoptosis. This gene was originally identified at the breakpoint of a chromosomal translocation in a human B-cell lymphoma. This translocation moved the *bcl-2* gene into the immunoglobulin heavy-chain locus, resulting in transcriptional activation of the *bcl-2* gene and overproduction of the encoded Bcl-2 protein by the lymphoma cells. The resulting high levels of Bcl-2 are thought to contribute to transformation of lymphoid cells into cancerous lymphoma cells by inhibiting the normal signals that would induce apoptotic cell death.

Bcl-2 levels have been found to play an important role in regulating the normal life span of various hematopoietic cell lineages, including lymphocytes. A normal adult has about 5 L of blood with about 2000 lymphocytes/mm³, for a total of about 10 billion lymphocytes. During acute infection the lymphocyte count increases by 4- to 15-fold, giving a total lymphocyte count of 40-150 billion. Because the immune system cannot sustain such a massive increase in cell numbers for an extended period, the system needs a means to eliminate unneeded activated lymphocytes once the antigenic threat has passed. Activated lymphocytes have been found to express lower levels of Bcl-2 and therefore are more susceptible to apoptotic death than naive lymphocytes or memory cells. If the lymphocytes continue to be activated by antigen, then the signals received during activation bypass the apoptotic signal. As antigen levels subside, so does activation of the lymphocytes and they begin to die by apoptosis (Figure 3-5).

REGULATORY ABNORMALITIES AND LEUKEMIA

Abnormalities in the expression of hematopoietic cytokines or their receptors may result in some leukemias. Colony-stimulating factors are secreted by a limited number of cells, including activated T lymphocytes, macrophages, endothelial cells, and bone-marrow stromal cells. As mentioned above, each factor induces the proliferation and differentiation of only those hematopoietic stem cells and progenitor cells that bear its receptor. Expression of receptors for a particular growth factor appears to be linked to cellular differentiation following proliferation induced by earlier-acting growth factors. A defect in regulation of expression of either the growth factor or its receptor could lead to unregulated cellular proliferation.

For example, failure to down-modulate receptor expression following GM-CSF activation may lead to a leukemic state. The binding of GM-CSF induces downmodulation of both G-CSF and M-CSF receptors on normal hematopoietic cells but not on leukemic cells (Figure 3-6a, b). This failure of GM-CSF to downmodulate the G-CSF or M-CSF receptors on leukemic cells may allow leukemic cells to respond to low levels of

TABLE 3 - 2

GENES THAT REGULATE APOPTOSIS

GENE	FUNCTION	ROLE IN PROGRAMMED CELL DEATH
bcl-2	Prevents apoptosis	Prevents
bax	Opposes *bcl-2*	Promotes
bcl-X^L (long)	Prevents apotosis	Prevents
bcl-X^S (short)	Opposes *bcl-X^L*	Promotes
ICE *	Protease	Promotes
fas/apo-1	Promotes apoptosis	Promotes

* Gene encoding the interleukin 1β–converting enzyme.

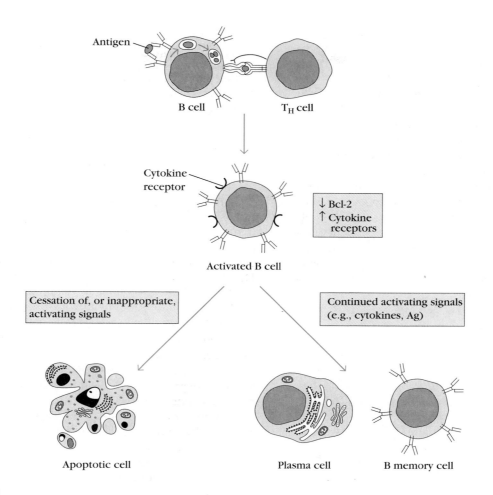

Antigen

B cell   T$_H$ cell

Cytokine receptor

↓ Bcl-2
↑ Cytokine receptors

Activated B cell

Cessation of, or inappropriate, activating signals

Continued activating signals (e.g., cytokines, Ag)

Apoptotic cell   Plasma cell   B memory cell

FIGURE 3-5

Regulation of activated B-cell numbers by apoptosis. Activation of B cells induces increased expression of cytokine receptors and decreased expression of Bcl-2. Since Bcl-2 prevents apoptosis, its reduced level in activated B cells makes them more susceptible to programmed cell death than naive or memory B cells. A reduction in activating signals quickly leads to destruction of excess activated B cells by apoptosis. Similar processes occur with T cells.

CSFs that would not induce proliferation of normal down-modulated hematopoietic cells.

Likewise, inappropriate expression of a hematopoietic cytokine by a cell bearing a receptor for that cytokine could lead to unregulated cancerous proliferation. Some findings suggest that this phenomenon occurs in certain leukemias. For example, leukemic cells from some patients with acute myeloid leukemia have been shown to secrete GM-CSF, whereas normal myeloid cells do not secrete this growth factor (Figure 3-6c). Similarly, when normal myeloid cell lines bearing receptors for GM-CSF are transfected with cloned GM-CSF cDNA, they auto-stimulate their own growth in the absence of added GM-CSF (Figure 3-6d); if these transfected cells are injected into mice, the animals develop leukemias.

Perhaps the strongest evidence that such abnormal autostimulation can lead to cancerous proliferation comes from the human adult T-cell leukemia associated with the HTLV-1 retrovirus, which infects human T cells and transforms them into leukemic cells. T cells infected with HTLV-1 begin to express the IL-2 receptor in the absence of previous antigen activation. Secretion of IL-2 by these same cells allows unregulated cellular proliferation resulting in leukemia. The molecular basis for this transformation is discussed in the chapter on cytokines (see Figure 13-13).

Enrichment of Hematopoietic Stem Cells

I. L. Weissman and colleagues developed a novel way of enriching mouse pluripotent stem cells, which constitute only 0.05% of all bone marrow cells in mice. Their approach involved reacting bone marrow samples with

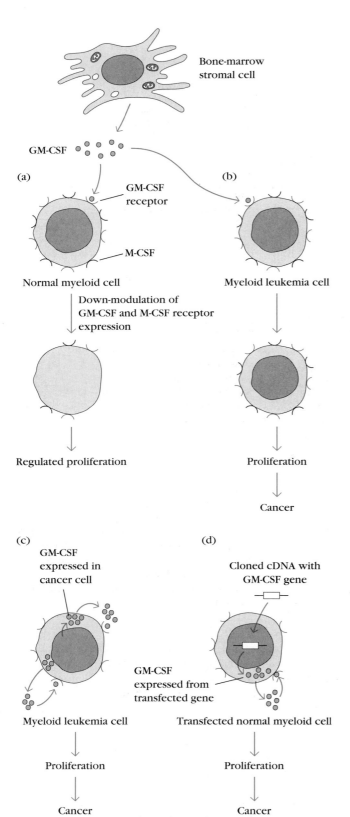

FIGURE 3-6

Possible role of regulatory abnormalities in hematopoiesis in generation of leukemia. (a) Down-modulation of expression of receptors for M-CSF and GM-CSF following GM-CSF activation of a normal myeloid stem cell results in regulated proliferation of monocyte and granulocyte lineages. (b) The absence of this down-modulation in myeloid leukemia cells might lead to leukemia. (c) Secretion of GM-CSF has been demonstrated in some myeloid leukemia cells. Such secretion, which does not occur in normal myeloid cells, might lead to autostimulation and unregulated proliferation. (d) Transfection of cDNA encoding GM-CSF has been shown to cause unregulated proliferation of the transfected cells. Injection of these transfected cells into mice results in leukemia.

fluorescent monoclonal antibodies specific for the **differentiation antigens** expressed on the surface of mature red and white blood cells (Figure 3-7). The labeled cells were then removed by flow cytometry with a fluorescence-activated cell sorter. After each sorting, the remaining cells were assayed for their ability to restore hematopoiesis in a lethally x-irradiated mouse; this assay indicates the relative number of stem cells in a bone marrow sample. As long as the pluripotent stem cell was being progressively enriched, fewer and fewer cells were needed to restore hematopoiesis in this system. By removing those hematopoietic cells that express known differentiation antigens, these researchers were able to obtain a 50- to 200-fold enrichment of pluripotent stem cells. To further enrich the pluripotent stem cell, the remaining cells were incubated with various monoclonal antibodies raised against cells likely to represent early differentiation stages in hematopoiesis. One of these monoclonal antibodies recognized a differentiation antigen called stem-cell antigen 1 (Sca-1). Treatment with this monoclonal antibody yielded a preparation so enriched in pluripotent stem cells that an aliquot containing only 30–100 cells could restore hematopoiesis in a lethally x-irradiated mouse, whereas $1–3 \times 10^4$ nonenriched bone marrow cells were needed for restoration.

Efforts are presently under way to identify and enrich the pluripotent stem cell in humans. One membrane molecule, called CD34, has been shown to be present on a small population (1%–3%) of hematopoietic cells that can reconstitute the entire hematopoietic system, suggesting that the pluripotent stem cell is among the CD34$^+$ cell population. The next step is to further enrich the pluripotent stem cell from the CD34$^+$ population.

One of the obstacles in identifying and characterizing the human pluripotent stem cell is the lack of an in vivo assay system comparable to that in mice. One experimental system that is being used to study the human pluripotent stem cell is SCID mice implanted with frag-

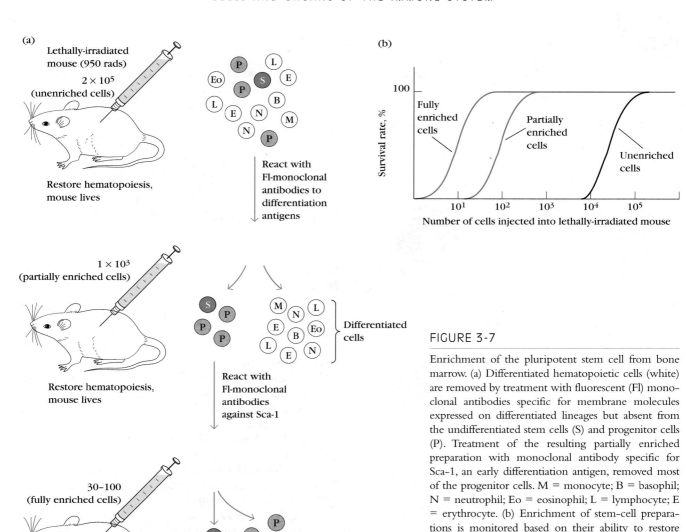

FIGURE 3-7

Enrichment of the pluripotent stem cell from bone marrow. (a) Differentiated hematopoietic cells (white) are removed by treatment with fluorescent (Fl) monoclonal antibodies specific for membrane molecules expressed on differentiated lineages but absent from the undifferentiated stem cells (S) and progenitor cells (P). Treatment of the resulting partially enriched preparation with monoclonal antibody specific for Sca-1, an early differentiation antigen, removed most of the progenitor cells. M = monocyte; B = basophil; N = neutrophil; Eo = eosinophil; L = lymphocyte; E = erythrocyte. (b) Enrichment of stem-cell preparations is monitored based on their ability to restore hematopoiesis in lethally irradiated mice. Only animals in which hematopoiesis occurs survive. Progressive enrichment of stem cells is indicated by the decrease in the number of injected cells needed to restore hematopoiesis. A total enrichment of about 1000-fold is possible by this procedure.

ments of human thymus and bone marrow (see Figure 2-1). Different subpopulations of CD34+ human bone marrow cells are injected into these SCID-human mice, and the development of various lineages of human cells in the bone marrow fragment is subsequently assessed. In the absence of human growth factors, only low numbers of granulocyte-macrophage progenitors develop. However, when human IL-3, GM-CSF, erythropoietin, and mast cell growth factor are administered along with CD34+ cells, progenitor and mature cells of the myeloid, lymphoid, and erythroid lineages develop. This system has enabled researchers to study subpopulations of CD34+ cells and to determine the effect of human growth factors on the differentiation of different hematopoietic lineages.

Clinical Uses of Pluripotent Stem Cells

Identification and enrichment of the pluripotent stem cell in humans promises to have a profound impact on the treatment of blood and immune-system diseases.

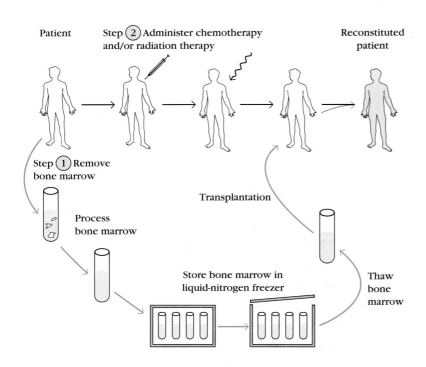

Patient　　Step ② Administer chemotherapy
　　　　　　and/or radiation therapy

Reconstituted
patient

Step ① Remove
bone marrow

Process
bone marrow

Transplantation

Store bone marrow in
liquid-nitrogen freezer

Thaw
bone
marrow

FIGURE 3-8

Autologous transplantation of bone marrow can be used to reconstitute the hematopoietic system of cancer patients whose blood cells have been injured by radiation and/or chemotherapy. Bone marrow is removed from the patient before treatment, stored, and reinfused at a later time. The amount of bone marrow that must be removed would be greatly reduced if a procedure for enriching and expanding pluripotent stem-cell populations was available.

TRANSPLANTATION OF BONE MARROW

Individuals with hematopoietic and immune-system dysfunctions caused by congenital disorders, cancer, chemotherapy, or radiation therapy often require bone marrow transplantation for survival. In this procedure an unrelated donor and the recipient must be carefully matched for identity within the MHC, but the probability of such a match is less than one in a million. Even with an MHC match, marrow from an unrelated donor fails to engraft about 10%–20% of the time. In addition, the grafted bone marrow can cause **graft-versus-host disease** (GVHD) in which lymphocytes in the donor bone marrow begin to attack the recipient's cells. Transplantation of stem cells, rather than whole bone marrow, might increase acceptance of the foreign cells and decrease the incidence of GVHD. A recent advance in bone marrow transplantation is the availability of recombinant CSFs. Administration of recombinant GM-CSF or G-CSF along with the donor bone marrow dramatically increases stem-cell engraftment.

With new technologies for freezing human bone marrow in liquid nitrogen, individuals can donate their own bone marrow and receive it back at a later time. This procedure, known as **autologous transplantation**, has been used with cancer patients, permitting doctors to administer much higher doses of chemotherapy or radiation—doses that destroy the hematopoietic system. The frozen bone marrow is later reinfused into

the patient where it reconstitutes the hematopoietic system (Figure 3-8).

At the present time large volumes of bone marrow must be extracted and frozen to ensure that sufficient numbers of stem cells are present to reconstitute the hematopoietic system. If techniques for enriching and expanding populations of the pluripotent stem cell are developed, autologous transplantation would be feasible with much smaller samples of bone marrow. In May 1992, CellPro Inc. reported significant enrichment of CD34$^+$ stem cells with a monoclonal antibody specific for CD34 (Figure 3-9). The stem-cell preparations obtained by the CellPro procedure have been used successfully in autologous bone marrow transplantation. Clinical trials in patients with metastatic breast cancer and lymphoma are currently under way.

GENE THERAPY WITH ENGINEERED STEM CELLS

Advances in genetic engineering may soon make gene therapy a realistic treatment for individuals with genetic disorders involving blood cells (e.g., sickle cell anemia, thalassemia, and various forms of severe combined immunodeficiency disease). In this approach, hematopoietic stem cells removed from an affected individual would be transfected with functional genes; the engineered stem cells then would be reinjected into the individual. Obviously, the ability to enrich stem cells would be helpful in this type of therapy.

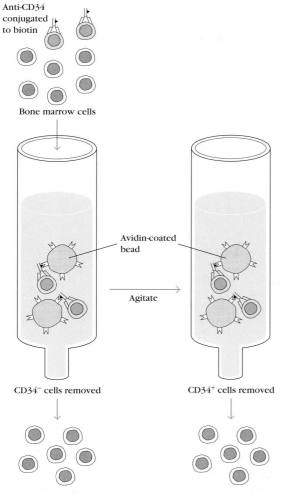

FIGURE 3-9

Enrichment of hematopoietic stem cells by affinity chromatography. CD34 is expressed on stem cells (blue) but not on other bone marrow cells. Bone marrow cells are incubated with an anti-CD34 monoclonal antibody that is conjugated to biotin (black triangle) and then are passed through a column packed with avidin-coated beads. Because avidin binds strongly to biotin, the antibody-coated stem cells are retained on the column, while the CD34$^-$ cells pass through. After washing, the CD34$^+$ stem cells are removed by mechanical agitation.

In an NIH study, CD34$^+$ cells were purified from pooled white blood cells from an individual with a severe combined immunodeficiency disease (SCID) resulting from a defect in the gene encoding adenosine deaminase (ADA). The isolated cells were engineered with a good *ADA* gene. If some of the engineered CD34$^+$ cells are pluripotent stem cells, then all the white blood cells originating from these stem cells will be healthy. The advantage of using stem cells, rather than

mature blood cells, in gene therapy is that they are self-renewing. In theory, patients will have to receive only a single injection of engineered stem cells, whereas gene therapy with engineered mature lymphocytes or other blood cells will require periodic injections because these cells are not capable of self-renewal.

IMMUNE-SYSTEM CELLS

As we've seen, lymphocytes are the central cells of the immune system, responsible for acquired immunity and the immunologic attributes of diversity, specificity, memory, and self/nonself recognition. The other types of white blood cells play ancillary roles, engulfing and destroying microorganisms, presenting antigens, and secreting cytokines.

Lymphoid Cells

Lymphocytes constitute 20%–40% of the body's white blood cells and 99% of the cells in the lymph (Table 3-3). There are approximately 10^{10}–10^{12} lymphocytes in the human body, the equivalent in cellular mass to that of the brain or liver! These lymphocytes continuously circulate in the blood and lymph and are capable of migrating into the tissue spaces and lymphoid organs, thereby providing a high degree of cellular integration to the immune system as a whole.

The lymphocytes can be broadly subdivided on the basis of function and cell-membrane components into three populations: B cells, T cells, and null cells. All three cell types are small, motile, nonphagocytic cells, which cannot be distinguished morphologically. B and T lymphocytes that have not interacted with antigen—referred

TABLE 3-3

NORMAL ADULT BLOOD-CELL COUNTS

CELL TYPE	CELLS/MM^3	%
Red blood cells	5.0×10^6	
Platelets	2.5×10^5	
Leukocytes	7.3×10^3	
Neutrophil		50–70
Lymphocyte		20–40
Monocyte		1–6
Eosinophil		1–3
Basophil		<1

(a)

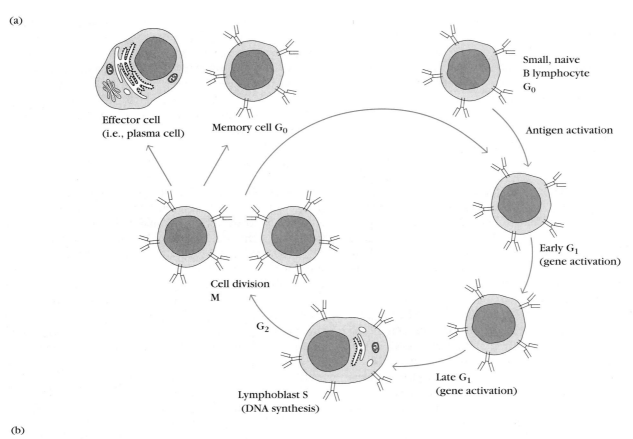

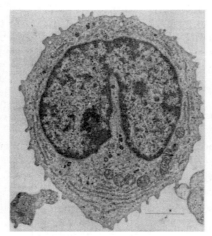

(b)

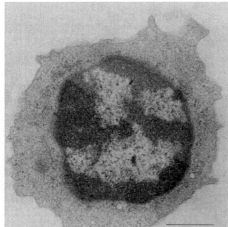

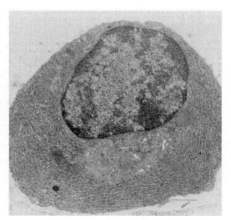

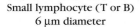

Small lymphocyte (T or B)
6 µm diameter

Blast cell (T or B)
15 µm diameter

Plasma cell (B)
15 µm diameter

FIGURE 3-10

Fate of antigen–activated small lymphocytes. (a) A small resting (unprimed or naive) lymphocyte resides in the G_0 phase of the cell cycle. At this stage, B and T lymphocytes cannot be distinguished morphologically. Following antigen activation, a B or T cell enters the cell cycle and enlarges into a lymphoblast, which undergoes several rounds of cell division and eventually generates effector cells and memory cells. Shown here are B-cell lineage cells. (b) Electron micrographs of a small lymphocyte (*left*) showing condensed chromatin indicative of a resting cell, an enlarged lymphoblast (*center*) showing decondensed chromatin, and a plasma cell (*right*) showing abundant endoplasmic reticulum arranged in concentric circles. The three cells are shown at different magnifications. [Part (b) courtesy of Dr. Joseph R. Goodman, Dept. of Pediatrics, University of California at San Francisco.]

to as **naive**, or unprimed—are resting cells in the G_0 phase of the cell cycle. Known as **small lymphocytes**, these cells are only about 6 μm in diameter; their cytoplasm forms a barely discernible rim around the nucleus. Small lymphocytes have densely packed chromatin, few mitochondria, and a poorly developed endoplasmic reticulum and Golgi apparatus. The naive lymphocyte is generally thought to have a short life span, although recently some researchers have suggested that some naive cells may have much longer life spans. Interaction of small lymphocytes with antigen, in the presence of certain cytokines discussed later, induces these cells to enter the cell cycle by progressing from G_0 into G_1 and subsequently into S, G_2, and M (Figure 3-10a). As they progress through the cell cycle, lymphocytes enlarge into 15-mm-diameter blast cells, called **lymphoblasts**; these cells have a higher cytoplasm:nucleus ratio and more organellar complexity than small lymphocytes.

Lymphoblasts proliferate and eventually differentiate into **effector cells** or into **memory cells**. Effector cells function in various ways to eliminate the antigen. These cells have short life spans, generally ranging from a few days to a few weeks. Plasma cells—the effector cell of the B-cell lineage—have a characteristic cytoplasm developed for active secretion with abundant endoplasmic reticulum arranged in concentric layers and many Golgi vesicles (Figure 3-10b). The effector cells of the T-cell lineage include the cytokine-secreting T_H cell and the cytotoxic T lymphocyte (CTL). Some of the progeny of B and T lymphoblasts differentiate into memory cells. The persistence of this population of cells is responsible for the life-long immunity observed for many pathogens. Memory cells appear morphologically as small lymphocytes but can be distinguished from naive cells by the presence or absence of certain cell-membrane molecules. Although it has been a widely held belief that memory cells are extremely long lived, recent evidence suggests that this may not be true of all memory cells. Rather, some memory cells may be short-lived cells that undergo continuous activation by persisting antigen or by cross-reacting environmental antigens.

Different lineages or maturational stages of lymphocytes can be distinguished by their expression of membrane molecules recognized by particular monoclonal antibodies. All of the monoclonal antibodies that react with a particular membrane molecule are grouped together as a **cluster of differentiation** (CD). Each new monoclonal antibody that recognizes a leukocyte membrane molecule is analyzed to determine if it falls within a recognized CD designation; if it does not, it is given a new CD designation reflecting a new membrane molecule. Although the CD nomenclature was originally developed for human leukocyte membrane molecules, the homologous membrane molecules found in other spe-cies, such as mice, are commonly referred to by the same CD designations. Table 3-4 lists some common CD molecules found on human lymphocytes.

The general characteristics and functions of B and T lymphocytes were discussed in Chapter 1 and are reviewed briefly in the following sections. These central cells of the immune system are examined in more detail in later chapters.

B LYMPHOCYTES

The B lymphocyte derived its name from its site of maturation in the bursa of Fabricius in birds; the name turned out to be apt, for its major site of maturation in mammals is the bone marrow. Mature B cells can be distinguished from other lymphocytes by the presence of membrane-bound immunoglobulin (antibody) molecules, which serve as receptors for antigen. Each of the approximately 1.5×10^5 molecules of antibody on the membrane of a single B cell have an identical binding site for antigen. Among the other molecules expressed on the membrane of mature B cells are the following:

- **B220** (or CD45), the earliest marker of the B-cell lineage, which first appears during maturation on the precursor B cell, remains throughout the life span of the B cell, and functions in signal transduction
- **Class II MHC molecules**, which permit the B cell to function as an antigen-presenting cell (APC)
- **CR1** (CD35) and **CR2** (CD21), which are receptors for certain complement products
- **FcγRII** (CD32), a receptor for the carboxyl-terminal (Fc) region of IgG
- **B7**, a co-stimulatory molecule that interacts with CD28 on T_H cells

Other important B-cell membrane molecules are discussed in later chapters.

Appropriate interaction between antigen and the membrane-bound antibody on a naive B cell, together with T-cell and macrophage interactions, induces clonal selection of the B cell. In this process, the B cell divides repeatedly and differentiates, over a 4- to 5-day period generating a population of plasma cells and memory cells (see Figure 1-11). Plasma cells, which lack membrane-bound antibody, actively secrete one of the five classes of antibody. All clonal progeny from a given B cell secrete antibody molecules with the same antigen-binding specificity. Most plasma cells are a terminally differentiated cell type, and die within 1–2 weeks. Production of the memory B cell is somewhat controversial. Some theories suggest that unequal division of an activated B cell generates both plasma and memory cells. Other theories suggest that the memory B cell may be a separate lineage that clonally expands following primary antigen exposure (see Chapter 8).

T LYMPHOCYTES

T lymphocytes derive their name from their site of maturation in the thymus. Like B lymphocytes, these cells have membrane receptors for antigen. Although the antigen-binding T-cell receptor is structurally distinct from immunoglobulin, it does share some common structural features with the immunoglobulin molecule, most notably in the structure of its antigen-binding site. Unlike the membrane-bound antibody on B cells, the T-cell receptor recognizes antigen only when the antigen is associated with a self-molecule encoded by genes within the major histocompatibility complex (MHC). Thus, as discussed in Chapter 1, a fundamental difference between the humoral and cell-mediated branches of the immune system is that the B cell is capable of binding soluble antigen, whereas the T cell is restricted to binding antigen displayed on self-cells. This antigen must be

T A B L E 3 - 4

COMMON CD ANTIGENS USED TO DISTINGUISH FUNCTIONAL LYMPHOCYTE SUBPOPULATIONS

CD DESIGNATION*	FUNCTION	B CELL	T CELL T_H	T CELL T_C	NK CELL
CD2	Adhesion molecule; signal transduction	−	+	+	+
CD3	Signal transduction element of T-cell receptor	−	+	+	−
CD4	Adhesion molecule that binds to class II MHC molecules; signal transduction	−	+ (usually)	− (usually)	−
CD5	Unknown	+ (subset)	+	+	−
CD8	Adhesion molecule that binds to class I MHC molecules; signal transduction	−	− (usually)	+ (usually)	+ (variable)
CD11a/CD18 (LFA-1)	Adhesion molecule that binds to ICAM-1 and ICAM-2	+	+	+	+
CD16 (FcγRIII)	Low-affinity receptor for Fc region of IgG	−	−	−	+
CD21 (CR2)	Receptor for complement (C3d) and Epstein–Barr virus	+	−	−	−
CD28	Receptor for co-stimulatory B7 molecule on antigen-presenting cells	−	+	+	−
CD32 (FcγRII)	Receptor for Fc region of IgG	+	−	−	−
CD35 (CR1)	Receptor for complement (C3b)	+	−	−	−
CD40	Signal transduction	+	−	−	−
CD45	Signal transduction	+	+	+	+
CD54 (ICAM-1)	Adhesion molecule that binds to CD11a/CD18 (LFA-1)	+	+	+	+
CD56	Adhesion molecule	−	−	−	+

* Synonyms are shown in parentheses.

displayed together with MHC molecules on the surface of antigen-presenting cells or on virus-infected cells, cancer cells, and grafts (see Figure 1-9). The T-cell system has developed to eliminate these altered self-cells, which pose a threat to the normal functioning of the body.

Like B cells, T cells express distinctive membrane molecules. All T-cell subpopulations express the T-cell receptor, but they can be distinguished by the presence of one or the other of two membrane molecules, CD4 and CD8. In addition, all mature T cells express the following membrane molecules:

- **Thy-1**, the earliest marker of the T-cell lineage, which is first expressed during maturation in the thymus and remains throughout the life span of the cell
- **CD3**, a membrane complex associated with the T-cell receptor
- **CD28**, a receptor for the co-stimulatory B7 molecule present on antigen-presenting cells
- **CD45**, a signal-transduction molecule

T cells that express CD4 recognize antigen associated with class II MHC molecules, whereas T cells expressing CD8 recognize antigen associated with class I MHC molecules. Thus the expression of CD4 versus CD8 corresponds to the MHC restriction of the T cell. In general, expression of CD4 and of CD8 also defines two major functional subpopulations of T lymphocytes. $CD4^+$ T cells generally function as T helper (T_H) cells and are class II restricted; $CD8^+$ T cells generally function as T cytotoxic (T_C) cells and are class I restricted. Thus the ratio of T_H to T_C cells in a sample can be determined by assaying for the number of $CD4^+$ and $CD8^+$ T cells. This ratio is approximately 2:1 in normal human peripheral blood, but it may be significantly altered in immunodeficiency diseases, autoimmune diseases, and other disorders.

T_H cells are activated following recognition of an antigen–class II MHC complex on an antigen-presenting cell. Following activation the T_H cell begins to divide and gives rise to a clone of effector cells, each specific for the same antigen–class II MHC complex (see Figure 1-14). These T_H cells secrete various cytokines, which play a central role in the activation of B cells, T_C cells, and a variety of other cells that participate in the immune response. Changes in the pattern of cytokines produced by T_H cells can result in qualitative changes in the type of immune response that develops. A response, designated as the **T_H1 response**, results in a cytokine profile that activates mainly T cytotoxic cells and macrophages, whereas the **T_H2 response** activates mainly B cells.

T_C cells are activated by interaction with an antigen–class I MHC complex on the surface of an altered self-cell (e.g., virus-infected cell) in the presence of appropriate cytokines (see Figure 1-14). This activation results in differentiation of the T_C cell into an effector cell, called a **cytotoxic T lymphocyte** (CTL). In contrast to T_H cells, CTLs generally secrete few cytokines. Instead, CTLs acquire cytotoxic activity and function to recognize and eliminate altered self-cells.

Another subpopulation of T lymphocytes—called **T suppressor** (T_S) cells—has been postulated. It is clear that some T cells mediate suppression of the humoral and the cell-mediated branches of the immune system, but no actual T_S cell has been isolated and cloned. For this reason, immunologists are still unsure whether T_S cells constitute a separate subpopulation or whether the observed suppression is simply the result of suppressive activities of the T_H and T_C subpopulations.

The classification of $CD4^+$, class II–restricted cells as T_H cells and $CD8^+$, class I–restricted cells as T_C cells is not absolute. Some functional T_H cells have been shown to express CD8 and recognize antigen associated with class I MHC, and some functional T_C cells are class II restricted and express CD4. Even the functional classification is not absolute. For example, many T_C cells have been shown to secrete a variety of cytokines and exert effects on other cells comparable to that exerted by T_H cells. The distinction between T_H and T_C cells, then, is not always clear; there can be ambiguous functional activities. However, because these ambiguities are the exception and not the rule, the general description of T helper cells as being $CD4^+$ and class II restricted and of T cytotoxic cells as being $CD8^+$ and class I restricted is adhered to, unless otherwise specified, throughout this text.

NULL CELLS

A small group of peripheral-blood lymphocytes, called **null cells**, fail to express the membrane molecules that distinguish T- and B-cell lineages. These cells also fail to display antigen-binding receptors of either the T- or B-cell lineage and therefore lack the attributes of immunologic specificity and memory. One functional population of null cells called **natural killer** (NK) cells are large, granulated lymphocytes; these cells constitute 5%–10% of the peripheral-blood lymphocytes in humans.

The natural killer cell was first described in 1976, when it was shown that certain null cells display cytotoxic activity against a wide range of tumor cells in the absence of any previous immunization with the tumor. NK cells were subsequently shown to play an important role in host defense against tumor cells. NK cells can interact with tumor cells in two different ways. In some cases, an NK cell makes direct membrane contact with a tumor cell in a nonspecific, antibody-independent process. Some NK cells, however, express CD16, a membrane

(a) Monocyte

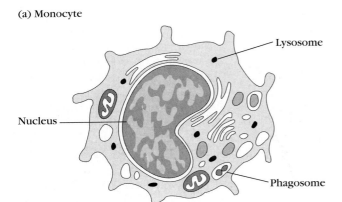

(b) Macrophage

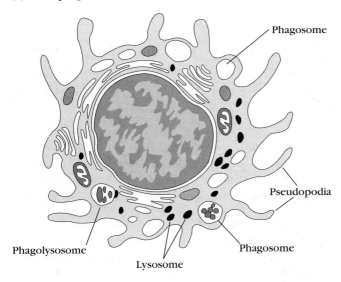

FIGURE 3-11

Drawings showing typical morphology of a monocyte and macrophage. Macrophages are five- to tenfold larger than monocytes and contain more organelles, especially lysosomes.

receptor for the carboxyl-terminal end of the IgG molecule, called the Fc region. These NK cells can bind to antitumor antibodies bound to the surface of tumor cells and subsequently destroy the tumor; this specific process is called **antibody-dependent cell-mediated cytotoxicity** (ADCC). The exact mechanism of tumor-cell killing by NK cells, the focus of much current experimental study, is discussed further in Chapter 16.

Several lines of evidence suggest that NK cells play an important role in host defense against tumors. For example, in humans **Chediak-Higashi syndrome**—an autosomal recessive disorder—is associated with an ab-

sence of NK cells and an increased incidence of lymphomas. Likewise, mice with an autosomal mutation called *beige* lack NK cells; these mutants are more susceptible than normal mice to tumor growth following injection with live tumor cells.

Mononuclear Cells

The mononuclear phagocytic system consists of circulating **monocytes** in the blood and **macrophages** in the tissues. During hematopoiesis in the bone marrow, granulocyte-monocyte progenitor cells differentiate into promonocytes, which leave the bone marrow and enter the blood, where they further differentiate into mature monocytes. Monocytes circulate in the bloodstream for about 8 h, during which time they enlarge; they then migrate into the tissues and differentiate into specific tissue macrophages (Figure 3-11).

Differentiation of a monocyte into a tissue macrophage involves a number of changes: The cell enlarges five- to tenfold; its intracellular organelles increase in both number and complexity; and it acquires increased phagocytic ability, produces higher levels of lytic enzymes, and begins to secrete a variety of soluble factors. Macrophages are dispersed throughout the body. Some take up residence in particular tissues becoming fixed macrophages, whereas others remain motile and are called free, or wandering, macrophages. Free macrophages move by amoeboid movement throughout the tissues. Fixed macrophages serve different functions in different tissues and are named to reflect their tissue location:

- **Alveolar macrophages** in the lung
- **Histiocytes** in connective tissues
- **Kupffer cells** in the liver
- **Mesangial cells** in the kidney
- **Microglial cells** in the brain

Although normally in a resting state, macrophages are activated by a variety of stimuli in the course of an immune response. Phagocytosis of particulate antigens serves as an initial activating stimulus. However, macrophage activity can be further enhanced by cytokines secreted by activated T_H cells, by mediators of the inflammatory response, and by bacterial cell-wall products. One of the most potent activators of macrophages is interferon gamma (IFN-γ) secreted by activated T_H cells.

Compared with resting macrophages, activated macrophages are more effective in eliminating potential pathogens because they exhibit greater phagocytic activity, increased secretion of inflammatory mediators, and an increased ability to activate T cells. In addition, activated macrophages, but not resting ones, secrete various cytotoxic proteins that help them eliminate a broad range of

(a)

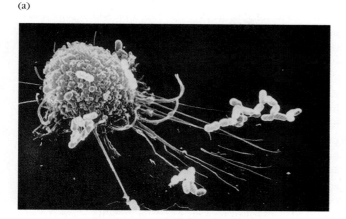

(b)

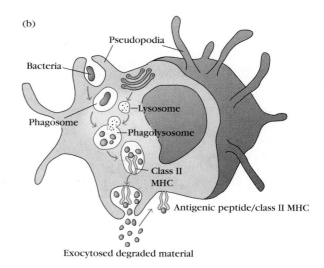

FIGURE 3-12

Macrophages can ingest and degrade particulate antigens, including bacteria. (a) Scanning electron micrograph of a macrophage. Note the long pseudopodia extending toward and making contact with bacterial cells, an early step in phagocytosis. (b) Phagocytosis and processing of exogenous antigen by macrophages. Most of the products resulting from digestion of ingested material are exocytosed, but some peptide products interact with class II MHC molecules, forming complexes that move to the cell surface where they are presented to T_H cells. See text for details. [Photograph by Lennart Nilsson; courtesy of Boehringer Ingelheim International GmbH.]

pathogens, including virus-infected cells, tumor cells, and intracellular bacteria. Activated macrophages also express higher levels of class II MHC molecules, allowing them to function more effectively as antigen-presenting cells. Thus macrophages and T_H cells exhibit an interacting relationship during the immune response with each facilitating activation of the other.

PHAGOCYTOSIS

Macrophages are actively phagocytic cells capable of ingesting and digesting exogenous antigens such as whole microorganisms, insoluble particles, injured and dead host cells, cellular debris, and activated clotting factors. In the first step in phagocytosis, macrophages are attracted by and move toward a variety of substances generated in an immune response; this process is called **chemotaxis**. The next step in phagocytosis involves adherence of the antigen to the macrophage cell membrane. (Complex antigens, such as whole bacterial cells or viral particles, tend to adhere well and are readily phagocytosed; isolated proteins and encapsulated bacteria tend to adhere poorly and are less readily phagocytosed.) Adherence induces membrane protrusions, called **pseudopodia**, to extend around the attached material (Figure 3-12a). Fusion of the pseudopodia encloses the material within a membrane-bound structure called a **phagosome**, which then enters the endocytic processing pathway. In this pathway, a phagosome moves toward the cell interior, where it fuses with a **lysosome** to form a **phagolysosome**. Lysosomes contain hydrogen peroxide, oxygen-free radicals, peroxidase, lysozyme, and various hydrolytic enzymes, which digest the ingested material. The digested contents of the phagolysosome are then eliminated in a process called **exocytosis** (Figure 3-12b).

The macrophage membrane possesses receptors for certain classes of antibody and certain complement components, both of which also can bind to antigen. When an antigen (e.g., a bacterium) is coated with the appropriate antibody or complement component, the antigen binds more readily to the macrophage membrane; as a result, phagocytosis is enhanced. In one study, for example, the rate of phagocytosis of an antigen was 4000-fold higher in the presence of specific antibody to the antigen than in its absence. Thus antibody and complement function as **opsonins**, molecules that bind to both antigen and macrophages and enhance phagocytosis. The process by which particulate antigens are rendered more susceptible to phagocytosis is called **opsonization**.

ANTIMICROBIAL AND CYTOTOXIC ACTIVITIES

A number of antimicrobial and cytotoxic substances produced by activated macrophages are responsible for the intracellular destruction of phagocytosed microorganisms (Table 3-5). In addition, these toxic substances

TABLE 3-5

MEDIATORS OF ANTIMICROBIAL AND CYTOTOXIC ACTIVITY OF MACROPHAGES AND NEUTROPHILS

OXYGEN-DEPENDENT KILLING	OXYGEN-INDEPENDENT KILLING
Reactive oxygen intermediates	Defensins
O_2^- (superoxide anion)	Tumor necrosis factor α
$OH^\cdot$ (hydroxyl radicals)	(macrophage only)
$^1O_2$ (singlet oxygen)	Lysozyme
H_2O_2 (hydrogen peroxide)	Hydrolytic enzymes
$HOCl$ (hypochlorous acid)	
NH_2Cl (monochloramine)	
Reactive nitrogen intermediates	
NO (nitric oxide)	
NO_2 (nitrogen dioxide)	
HNO_2 (nitrous acid)	

can be released from macrophages to mediate potent anti-tumor activity. The toxic effects of these substances involve both oxygen-dependent and oxygen-independent mechanisms.

Oxygen-Dependent Killing Mechanisms Activated phagocytes produce a number of **reactive oxygen intermediates** (ROIs) and **reactive nitrogen intermediates** (RNIs) that have potent antimicrobial activity. During phagocytosis a metabolic process known as the **respiratory burst** occurs in activated macrophages. This process results in the activation of a membrane-bound oxidase that catalyzes the reduction of oxygen to superoxide anion, a reactive oxygen intermediate that is extremely toxic to ingested microorganisms. The superoxide anion also generates other powerful oxidizing agents, including hydroxyl radicals, singlet oxygen, and hydrogen peroxide. As the lysosome fuses with the phagosome, myeloperoxidase together with a halide ion act on the hydrogen peroxide to produce longer-lived oxidants, including hypochlorite, which are toxic.

When macrophages are activated with bacterial cell-wall lipopolysaccharide (LPS) or muramyl dipeptide (MDP) together with a T-cell–derived cytokine (IFN-γ), they begin to express high levels of nitric oxide synthetase, which oxidizes L-arginine to yield citrulline and **nitric oxide**, a reactive radical. Nitric oxide itself has potent antimicrobial activity; it also can combine with the superoxide anion to yield even more potent antimi-

crobial substances. Recent evidence suggests that much of the antimicrobial activity of macrophages against bacterial, fungal, helminthic, and protozoal pathogens is due to nitric oxide and substances derived from it.

Oxygen-Independent Killing Mechanisms Activated macrophages also synthesize **lysozyme** and various hydrolytic enzymes whose degradative activities do not involve oxygen. In addition, activated macrophages produce a group of antimicrobial and cytotoxic peptides, commonly known as **defensins**. These molecules are cysteine-rich cationic peptides containing 29–35 amino acid residues. Each peptide, which contains six invariant cysteines, forms a circular molecule that is stabilized by intramolecular disulfide bonds. These circularized defensin peptides have been shown to form ion-permeable channels in bacterial and mammalian cell membranes. Defensins can kill a variety of bacteria, including *Staphylococcus aureus, Streptococcus pneumoniae, Escherichia coli, Pseudomonas aeruginosa*, and *Haemophilus influenzae*. Activated macrophages also secrete **tumor necrosis factor α** (TNF-α), which is cytotoxic for tumor cells but not to normal cells.

Resistant Pathogens Most phagocytosed microorganisms are killed by the lysosomal contents that are released into phagosomes. Some microorganisms, however, can survive and multiply within macrophages. These **intracellular pathogens** include *Listeria monocytogenes, Salmonella typhimurium, Neisseria gonorrhoeae, Mycobacterium avium, Mycobacterium tuberculosis, Mycobacterium leprae, Brucella abortus*, and *Candida albicans*.

Some intracellular pathogens prevent lysosome-phagosome fusion and proliferate within phagosomes; others have cell-wall components that render them resistant to the contents of lysosomes; and still others survive by escaping from phagosomes and proliferating within the cytoplasm of infected macrophages. These intracellular pathogens, which have developed a clever defense against the nonspecific phagocytic defense system, are shielded from a specific immunologic response. A unique cell-mediated immunologic defense mechanism, called **delayed-type hypersensitivity** (DTH), combats such pathogens; this mechanism is discussed in Chapter 16.

ANTIGEN PROCESSING AND PRESENTATION

Not all of the antigen ingested by macrophages is degraded and eliminated by exocytosis. Experiments with radiolabeled antigens have demonstrated the presence of labeled antigen components on the macrophage membrane after most of the antigen has been digested and eliminated. As depicted in Figure 3-12b, phagocytosed antigen is degraded within the endocytic processing pathway into peptides that associate with class II MHC molecules; these peptide–class II MHC complexes then move to the macrophage membrane. Activation of macrophages induces increased expression of both class II MHC molecules and the co-stimulatory B7 membrane molecule, thereby rendering the macrophages more effective in activating T_H cells. This processing and presentation of antigen, examined in detail in Chapter 10, are critical to T_H-cell activation, a central event in the development of both humoral and cell-mediated immune responses.

SECRETION OF FACTORS

A number of important proteins central to development of immune responses are secreted by activated macrophages (Table 3-6). These include **interleukin 1** (IL-1), which acts on T_H cells and provides a co-stimulatory signal for activation following antigen recognition. Interleukin 1 also acts on vascular endothelial cells, thus influencing the inflammatory response, and affects the thermoregulatory center in the hypothalamus, leading to the fever response.

Activated macrophages secrete a variety of other factors involved in the development of an inflammatory response. These include a group of **complement proteins**, which assist in eliminating foreign pathogens and the ensuing inflammatory reaction. The hydrolytic enzymes contained within their lysosomes also can be secreted by activated macrophages. The buildup of these enzymes within the tissues contributes to the inflammatory response and can, in some cases, lead to extensive tissue damage. Activated macrophages also secrete soluble factors, such as tumor necrosis factor α, that can kill a variety of cells. The secretion of these cytotoxic factors has been shown to contribute to tumor destruction by macrophages. Finally, as discussed earlier, activated macrophages secrete a number of cytokines that stimulate inducible hematopoiesis.

Granulocytic Cells

The **granulocytes** are classified as neutrophils, eosinophils, or basophils on the basis of cellular morphology and cytoplasmic staining characteristics (Figure 3-13; see also Figure 3-1). The **neutrophil** has a multilobed nucleus and a granulated cytoplasm that stains with both acid and basic dyes; it is often called a polymorphonuclear leukocyte (PMN) for its multilobed nucleus. The **eosinophil** has a bilobed nucleus and a granulated cytoplasm that stains with the acid dye eosin Y (hence its name). The **basophil** has a lobed nucleus and heavily granulated cytoplasm that stains with the basic dye methylene blue. Both neutrophils and eosinophils are phagocytic, whereas basophils are not. Neutrophils, which constitute 50%–70% of the circulating white blood cells, are much more numerous than eosinophils (1%–3%) or basophils (<1%).

NEUTROPHILS

Neutrophils are produced in the bone marrow during hematopoiesis. They are released into the peripheral blood and circulate for 7–10 h before migrating into the tissues where they have a 3-day life span. In response to many types of infections the bone marrow releases more than the usual number of neutrophils. The resulting transient increase in the number of circulating neutrophils, called **leukocytosis**, is used medically to indicate the presence of an infection.

Neutrophils generally are the first cell to arrive at a site of inflammation. Movement of circulating neutrophils into tissues, called **extravasation**, involves several steps: the cell first adheres to the vascular endothelium, then penetrates the gap between adjacent endothelial

---

T A B L E   3 - 6

SOME FACTORS SECRETED BY ACTIVATED MACROPHAGES

FACTOR	FUNCTION
Interleukin 1 (IL-1)	Induces activation of T_H cells following interaction with antigen-MHC complexes; promotes inflammatory response and fever
Complement proteins	Promote elimination of pathogens and of inflammatory response
Hydrolytic enzymes	Promote inflammatory response
Interferon alpha (IFN-α)	Activates cellular genes resulting in the production of proteins that confer an antiviral state on the cell
Tumor necrosis factor (TNF-α)	Kills tumor cells
Interleukin 6 (IL-6) GM-CSF G-CSF M-CSF	Promote inducible hematopoiesis

(a) Neutrophil

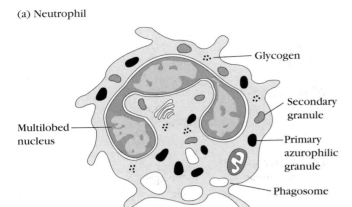

Multilobed nucleus

Glycogen

Secondary granule

Primary azurophilic granule

Phagosome

(b) Eosinophil

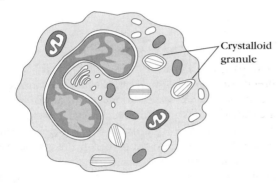

Crystalloid granule

(c) Basophil

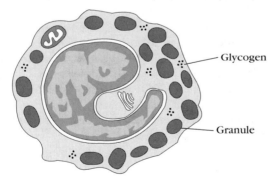

Glycogen

Granule

FIGURE 3-13

Drawings showing typical morphology of granulocytes. Note differences in the shape of the nucleus and in the number and shape of cytoplasmic granules.

cells lining the vessel wall, and finally penetrates the vascular basement membrane, moving out into the tissue spaces. (This process is discussed in detail in Chapter 15.) A number of substances generated in an inflammatory reaction serve as **chemotactic factors** that promote accumulation of neutrophils at an inflammatory site. Among these chemotactic factors are some of the complement components, components of the blood-clotting system, and several cytokines secreted by activated T_H cells and macrophages (e.g., IL–1, IL–8, and transforming growth factor β).

Like macrophages, neutrophils are active phagocytic cells. The process of phagocytosis by neutrophils is similar to that described for macrophages, except that neutrophils contain lytic enzymes and bactericidal substances within primary and secondary granules (see Figure 3-13a). The larger, denser primary (or azurophilic) granules are a type of lysosome containing peroxidase, lysozyme, and various hydrolytic enzymes. The smaller, secondary granules contain collagenase, lactoferrin, and lysozyme. Both primary and secondary granules fuse with the phagosome, whose contents are then digested and eliminated much as they are in macrophages.

Neutrophils also employ both oxygen-dependent and oxygen-independent pathways to generate antimicrobial substances. Neutrophils are in fact much more likely than macrophages to kill ingested microorganisms. Neutrophils exhibit a larger respiratory burst than macrophages and consequently are able to generate more reactive oxygen intermediates and reactive nitrogen intermediates (see Table 3-5). In addition, neutrophils express higher levels of defensins than macrophages.

EOSINOPHILS

Eosinophils, like neutrophils, are motile, phagocytic cells that can migrate from the blood into the tissue spaces. Their phagocytic role is significantly less important than that of neutrophils, and it is thought that their major role is in defense against parasitic organisms (see Chapter 19). The secretion of the contents of eosinophilic granules results in damage to the parasite membrane.

BASOPHILS

Basophils are nonphagocytic granulocytes that function by releasing pharmacologically active substances contained within their cytoplasmic granules. Release of the contents of their granules plays a major role in certain allergic response. Basophils are discussed in detail in Chapter 17 in the section on type I hypersensitive reactions.

Mast Cells

Mast cell precursors, which are formed in the bone marrow during hematopoiesis, are released into the blood as undifferentiated precursor cells and do not differentiate until they leave the blood and enter the tissues. Mast cells can be found in a wide variety of tissues, including the skin, connective tissues of various organs, and mucosal epithelial tissue of the respiratory, genitourinary, and digestive tracts. Like circulating basophils, these cells have large numbers of cytoplasmic granules containing histamine and other pharmacologically active substances. Mast cells, together with blood basophils, play an important role in the development of allergies and are discussed in more detail in Chapter 17.

Dendritic Cells

The **dendritic cell** acquired its name because it is covered with a maze of long membrane processes resembling dendrites of nerve cells. Dendritic cells have been very difficult to study because conventional procedures for isolating lymphocytes and accessory immune-system cells tend to damage their long dendritic processes, so that the cells fail to survive. Use of gentler dispersion techniques with enzymes has facilitated isolation of these cells for in vitro study.

Most dendritic cells process and present antigen to T_H cells (Table 3-7). These cells can be classified based on their location:

- **Langerhans cells** found in the epidermis and mucous membranes
- **Interstitial dendritic cells,** which populate most organs (e.g., heart, lungs, liver, kidney, gastrointestinal tract)
- **Interdigitating dendritic cells** present in T-cell areas of secondary lymphoid tissue and the thymic medulla
- **Circulating dendritic cells** including those in the blood, which constitute 0.1% of the blood leukocytes, and those in the lymph (known as **veiled cells**)

The dendritic cells in each of these locations have morphologic and functional differences. Despite their differences, all of these dendritic cells constitutively express high levels of both class II MHC molecules and the co-stimulatory B7 molecule. For this reason, they are more potent antigen-presenting cells than macrophages and B cells, both of which need to be activated before they can function as APCs. After capturing antigen in the tissues by phagocytosis or by endocytosis, dendritic cells migrate into the blood or lymph and circulate to various lymphoid organs where they present the antigen to T lymphocytes.

Whether these dendritic cells belong to the monocyte/macrophage lineage or develop from an entirely separate lineage is still an unresolved question. Two possible development pathways are depicted in Figure 3-14. In

TABLE 3-7

DENDRITIC CELLS

LOCATION	CELL TYPE
Nonlymphoid organs	
Skin, mucous membranes	Langerhans cells
	Interstitial dendritic cells
Organs	
Lymphoid organs	
T-cell areas	Interdigitating dendritic cells
B-cell areas	Follicular dendritic cells
Circulation	
Blood	Blood dendritic cells
Lymph	"Veiled" cells

one pathway, dendritic cells develop from a myeloid precursor in the bone marrow, appearing in the blood as an immature cell that completes its differentiation into a dendritic cell in the tissues. In the alternative pathway, a late monocytic stage (indeterminate cell) differentiates in the tissues to generate either a macrophage or dendritic cell. Some evidence suggests that mature macrophages and dendritic cells may interconvert, although this has yet to be confirmed. The striking morphologic and functional differences among Langerhans cells and interstitial, interdigitating, and circulating dendritic cells is thought to reflect different maturational states of the cells and the different microenvironments in which they reside.

Another type of dendritic cell, the **follicular dendritic cell**, appears to have a different origin and function from the antigen-presenting dendritic cells described above. Follicular dendritic cells do not express class II MHC molecules and therefore do not function as antigen-presenting cells for T_H-cell activation. These dendritic cells were named for their exclusive location in organized structures of the lymph node, called lymph follicles, which are rich in B cells. Although they do not express class II molecules, follicular dendritic cells express high levels of membrane receptors for antibody and complement. Binding of circulating antibody-antigen complexes by these receptors is thought to facilitate B-cell activation in lymph nodes. These complexes have been shown to be retained on the dendritic-cell membrane for very long periods of time, ranging from weeks to months or even years (Figure 3-15). The presence of antigen-antibody complexes on the membrane of follicular dendritic cells is thought to play a role in the development of memory B cells within the follicle.

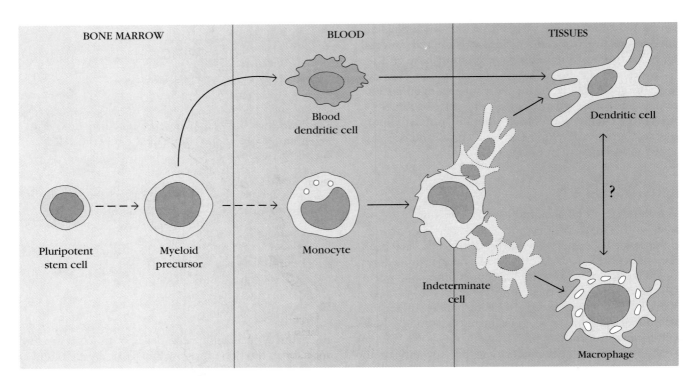

FIGURE 3-14

Two proposed pathways for development of dendritic cells (exclusive of follicular dendritic cells). The dendritic-cell lineage may branch from the monocyte/macrophage lineage at the myeloid precursor stage in the bone marrow. Alternatively, dendritic cells and macro-phages may arise from a common late intermediate stage (indeterminate cell). The interconversion of mature dendritic cells and macro-phages is suggested by some evidence but is not confirmed as yet. [Adapted from J. H. Peters et al., 1996, *Immunol. Today* **17**:273.]

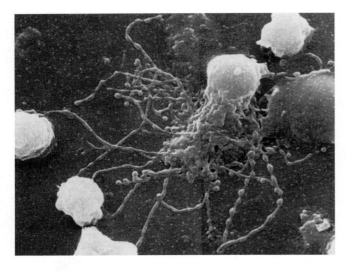

FIGURE 3-15

Scanning electron micrograph of follicular dendritic cells showing long "beaded" dendrites. The beads are coated with antigen-antibody complexes. The dendrites emanate from the cell body. [From A. K. Szakal et al., 1985, *J. Immunol.* **134**:1353. American Association of Immunologists. Reprinted with permission.]

ORGANS OF THE IMMUNE SYSTEM

A number of morphologically and functionally diverse organs and tissues have various functions in the development of immune responses. These can be divided on the basis of function into the **primary** and **secondary lymphoid organs** (Figure 3-16). The thymus and bone marrow constitute the primary (or central) lymphoid organs, where maturation of lymphocytes occurs. The lymph nodes, spleen, and various mucosal-associated tissues (MALT) compose the secondary (or peripheral) lymphoid organs, which trap antigen and provide sites for mature lymphocytes to interact with that antigen. In addition, **tertiary lymphoid tissues**, which normally contain few lymphoid cells, can import lymphoid cells during an inflammatory response. Most prominent of these are cutaneous-associated lymphoid tissue. Once mature lymphocytes are generated in the primary lymphoid organs, they circulate in the blood and **lymphatic system**.

FIGURE 3-16

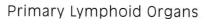

The human lymphoid system. The primary organs (bone marrow and thymus) are shown in red; secondary organs and tissues, in blue. These structurally and functionally diverse lymphoid organs and tissues are interconnected by the blood vessels (not shown) and lymphatic vessels (purple) through which lymphocytes circulate. Only one bone is shown, but all major bones contain marrow and thus are part of the lymphoid system. [Adapted from Harvey Lodish et al., 1995, *Molecular Cell Biology,* 3rd ed., Scientific American Books.]

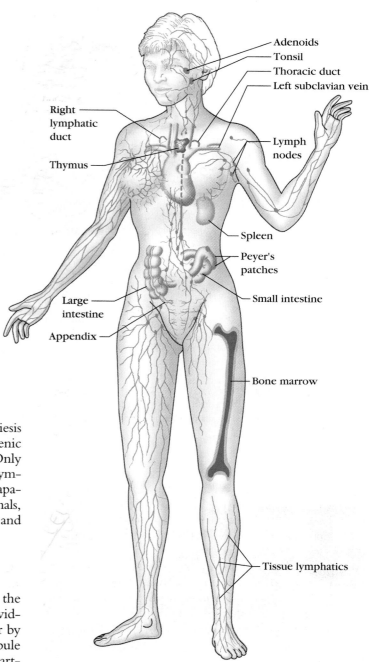

Primary Lymphoid Organs

Immature lymphocytes generated during hematopoiesis mature and become committed to a particular antigenic specificity within the primary lymphoid organs. Only after a lymphocyte has matured within a primary lymphoid organ is the cell **immunocompetent** (i.e., capable of mounting an immune response). In mammals, B-cell maturation occurs in the **bone marrow** and T-cell maturation occurs in the **thymus**.

THYMUS

The thymus is a flat, bilobed organ situated above the heart. Each lobe is surrounded by a capsule and is divided into lobules, which are separated from each other by strands of connective tissue called trabeculae. Each lobule is organized into two compartments: the outer compartment, or **cortex**, is densely packed with immature T cells, called thymocytes, whereas the inner compartment, or **medulla**, is sparsely populated with thymocytes.

The actual sequence of T-cell maturation within the thymus is not completely understood. After progenitor T cells formed during hematopoiesis enter the thymus, they are thought to multiply rapidly within the cortex; this rapid proliferation of thymocytes is coupled to an enormous rate of cell death. A small subset of more mature thymocytes are then thought to migrate from the cortex to the medulla where they continue to mature

and finally leave the thymus via postcapillary venules. There appear to be exceptions to this sequence, with some studies showing that a small subpopulation of cortical thymocytes can mature and leave the thymus without ever entering the medulla.

Both the cortex and medulla of the thymus are crisscrossed by a three-dimensional stromal-cell network composed of epithelial cells, interdigitating dendritic cells, and macrophages, which make up the framework

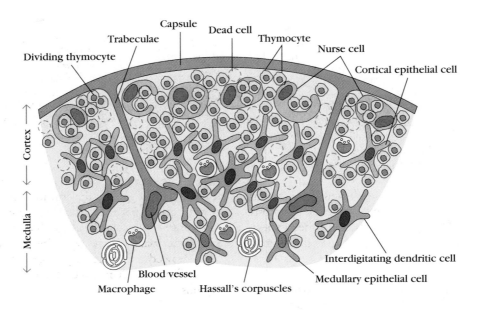

FIGURE 3-17

Diagrammatic cross-section of a portion of the thymus, showing several lobules separated by connective tissue strands (trabeculae). The densely populated outer cortex is thought to contain many immature thymocytes (blue), which undergo rapid proliferation coupled with an enormous rate of cell death. Also present in the outer cortex are thymic nurse cells (gray), which are specialized epithelial cells with long membrane processes that surround up to 50 thymocytes. The medulla is sparsely populated and is thought to contain more mature thymocytes. During their stay within the thymus, thymocytes interact with various stromal cells including cortical epithelial cells (light red), medullary epithelial cells (tan), interdigitating dendritic cells (purple), and macrophages (yellow). These cells produce thymic hormones and express high levels of class I and class II MHC molecules. Hassall's corpuscles found in the medulla contain concentric layers of degenerating epithelial cells. [Adapted from W. van Ewijk, 1991, *Annu. Rev. Immunol.* **9**:591.]

of the organ and contribute to thymocyte maturation. Many of these stromal cells physically interact with the developing thymocytes (Figure 3-17). Some thymic epithelial cells in the outer cortex, called **nurse cells**, have long membrane processes that surround as many as 50 thymocytes, forming large multicellular complexes. Other cortical epithelial cells have long interconnecting cytoplasmic processes that form a network and have been shown to interact with numerous thymocytes as they traverse the cortex. Interdigitating dendritic cells, which are located at the junction of the cortex and medulla, also have long processes that interact with developing thymocytes.

Maturation and Selection of T Cells Thymic epithelial cells secrete several hormonal factors necessary for the differentiation and maturation of thymocytes into the various types of mature T cells. Four such hormonal factors that have been characterized are α_1-thymosin, β_4-thymosin, thymopoietin, and thymulin. When bone marrow cells are cultured with these factors, membrane molecules characteristic of the T-cell lineage have been shown to appear, although the role of each of these factors in T-cell maturation remains unknown. Thymic stromal cells also secrete interleukin 7 (IL-7), which stimulates growth of thymocytes.

In the course of thymocyte maturation within the thymus, the antigenic diversity of the T-cell receptor is generated by a series of random gene rearrangements (see Chapter 11). After developing thymocytes begin to express antigen-binding receptors, they are subjected to a two-step selection process, so that only T cells recognizing antigenic peptides in the context of self-MHC molecules are released from the thymus. Thymic stromal cells, which express high levels of class I and class II MHC molecules, play a role in this selection process. During this selection process any developing thymocytes that are unable to recognize self-MHC molecules or that have a high affinity for self-antigen plus self-MHC (or self-MHC alone) are eliminated by programmed cell death. Thus only those cells whose receptor recognizes a self-MHC molecule plus foreign antigen are allowed to mature. A detailed discussion of thymic selection is presented in Chapter 12.

An estimated 95%–99% of all thymocyte progeny undergo programmed cell death within the thymus without ever maturing. This high death rate probably results primarily from the elimination of thymocytes that cannot recognize foreign antigenic peptides displayed by self-MHC molecules and of thymocytes that recognize self-peptides displayed by self-MHC molecules. It is not known whether some sort of external signal (e.g., the presence or absence of a factor) initiates programmed cell death in those thymocytes. Some have suggested that the death of most nonselected thymocytes may be induced by endogenous glucocorticoids. It has been known for some time that cortical thymocytes, especially in rodents, are extremely sensitive to glucocorticoids, whereas mature T cells are not. For instance, when mouse thymocytes are incubated with high physiologic levels of glucocorticoids, the cells begin to die within 1–2 h by apoptosis. Injection of glucocorticoids into rats and other experimental animals leads to marked atrophy of the thymus (Figure 3-18).

Relation Between Thymic and Immune Function The first evidence implicating the thymus in immune function came from experiments involving neonatal thymectomy in which the thymus was surgically removed from newborn mice. These thymectomized mice showed a dramatic decrease in circulating lymphocytes of the T-cell lineage and an absence of cell-mediated immunity. A congenital birth defect in humans (**DiGeorge's syndrome**) and in certain mice (**nude mice**) that involves failure of the thymus to develop provides further evidence. In both cases there is an absence of circulating T cells and of cell-mediated immunity and an increase in infectious disease.

The decline in immune functions that accompanies aging, leading to an increase in infections, autoimmunity, and cancer, probably results primarily from changes in the T-cell component of the immune system. The thymus reaches its maximal size at puberty and then atrophies, with a significant decrease in both cortical and medullary cells and an increase in the total fat content of the organ. Whereas the average weight of the thymus is 70 g in infants, its average weight is only 3 g in the elderly. This thymic involution, with the associated decrease in cortical size, medullary size, and hormonal production, precedes the decrease in immune function that is seen with aging.

A number of experiments have been designed to look at the effect of age on the immune function of the thymus. In one experiment the thymus from a 1-day-old or 33-month-old mouse was grafted into thymectomized adult littermates. Mice receiving the newborn thymus graft showed a significantly larger improvement in immune function than mice receiving the 33-month-old thymus.

BONE MARROW

In birds a lymphoid organ called the bursa of Fabricius is the primary site of B-cell maturation. There is no bursa in mammals and no single counterpart to it as a primary lymphoid organ. Instead, regions of the bone marrow and possibly of other lymphoid tissues serve as the "bursal equivalent" where B-cell maturation occurs.

Immature B cells proliferate and differentiate within the microenvironment of the bone marrow. Stromal cells within the bone marrow interact directly with the B cells and secrete various cytokines that are required for the B-cell developmental process. Similar to thymic selection during T-cell maturation, a selection process

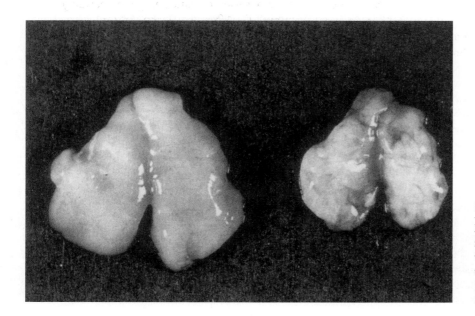

FIGURE 3-18

Effects of glucocorticosteroids on the rat thymus gland. A normal thymus *(left)* compared with the thymus of a rat 48 h following injection of a corticosteroid (5 mg/kg body weight). [From M. M. Compton and J. A. Cidlowski, 1992, *Trends Endocrinol. Metabol.* **3**:17.]

within the bone marrow eliminates B cells with self-reactive antibody receptors. This process is covered in more detail in Chapter 8.

Lymphatic System

As blood circulates under pressure, the fluid component of the blood (**plasma**) seeps through the thin wall of the capillaries into the surrounding tissue. Much of this fluid, called **interstitial fluid**, returns to the blood through the capillary membranes. The remainder of the interstitial fluid, now called **lymph**, flows from the connective tissue spaces into a network of tiny open lymphatic capillaries and then into a series of progressively larger collecting vessels called **lymphatic vessels** (Figure 3-19).

The largest lymphatic vessel, the **thoracic duct**, empties into the left subclavian vein near the heart (see Figure 3-16). In this way the lymphatic system functions to capture fluid lost from the blood and return it to the blood, thus ensuring steady-state levels of fluid within the circulatory system. The heart does not pump the lymph through the lymphatic system; instead the flow of lymph is achieved as the lymph vessels are squeezed by movements of the body's muscles. A series of one-way valves along the lymphatic vessels ensure that lymph flows only in one direction.

When a foreign antigen gains entrance into the tissues, it is picked up by the lymphatic system (which drains all the tissues of the body) and is carried to various organized lymphoid tissues, which trap the foreign antigen. As lymph passes from the tissues to lymphatic vessels, it becomes progressively enriched in lymphocytes. Thus, the lymphatic system also serves as a means of transporting lymphocytes and antigen from the connective tissues to organized lymphoid tissues where the lymphocytes may interact with the trapped antigen.

Secondary Lymphoid Organs

Various types of organized lymphoid tissues are located along the vessels of the lymphatic system. Some lymphoid tissue in the lung and lamina propria of the intestinal wall consists of diffuse collections of lymphocytes and macrophages. Other lymphoid tissue is organized into structures called lymphoid follicles, which consist of aggregates of various cells surrounded by a network of draining lymphatic capillaries. In the absence of antigen activation, a lymphoid follicle—called a **primary follicle**—comprises a network of follicular dendritic cells and small resting B cells. Following an antigenic challenge, a primary follicle becomes a larger **secondary follicle**—a ring of concentrically packed B lymphocytes surrounding a center (the **germinal center**) in which proliferat-

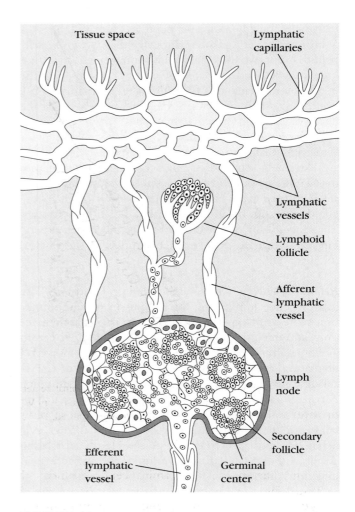

FIGURE 3-19

Lymphatic vessels. Small lymphatic capillaries opening into the tissue spaces pick up interstitial tissue fluid and carry it into progressively larger lymphatic vessels, which carry the fluid, now called lymph, into regional lymph nodes. As lymph leaves the nodes, it is carried through larger efferent lymphatic vessels, which eventually drain into the circulatory system at the thoracic duct or right lymph duct (see Figure 3-16).

ing B lymphocytes, memory B cells, and plasma cells are interspersed with macrophages and follicular dendritic cells (Figure 3-20).

The germinal center is a site of intense B-cell activation and contains large numbers of blast cells, called **centroblasts**. B cells that interact with antigen displayed on the membrane of follicular dendritic cells are induced to proliferate and differentiate into plasma and memory cells. In the absence of antigen activation, the B cells appear to undergo programmed cell death within the germinal center. The process of B-cell activation, prolifer-

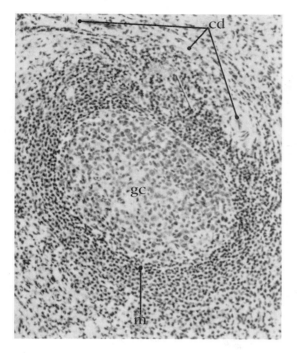

FIGURE 3-20

A secondary lymphoid follicle consisting of a large germinal center (gc) surrounded by a dense mantle of small lymphocytes. [From W. Bloom and D. W. Fawcett, 1975, *Textbook of Histology*, 10th ed., W. B. Saunders Co.]

ation, and differentiation in germinal centers is discussed more fully in Chapter 8.

Lymph nodes and the **spleen** are the most highly organized of the secondary lymphoid organs; in addition to lymphoid follicles, they possess distinct regions of T-cell and B-cell activity and are surrounded by a fibrous capsule. Less organized lymphoid tissue, collectively called mucosal-associated lymphoid tissue (MALT), occurs in various body sites. MALT includes Peyer's patches in the small intestine, the tonsils, and the appendix, as well as numerous lymphoid follicles within the lamina propria of the intestines and in the mucous membranes lining the upper airways, bronchi, and genital tract.

LYMPH NODES

Lymph nodes are encapsulated bean-shaped structures containing a reticular network packed with lymphocytes, macrophages, and dendritic cells. Clustered at junctions of the lymphatic vessels, lymph nodes are the first organized lymphoid structure to encounter antigens that enter the tissue spaces. As lymph percolates through a node, any particulate antigen that is brought in with the lymph will be trapped by the cellular network of phago-

cytic cells and dendritic cells (follicular and interdigitating). The overall architecture of a lymph node provides an ideal microenvironment for lymphocytes to effectively encounter and respond to trapped antigens.

Morphologically, a lymph node can be divided into three roughly concentric regions: the cortex, paracortex, and medulla each of which provides a distinct microenvironment (Figure 3-21). The outermost layer, the **cortex**, contains lymphocytes (mostly B cells), macrophages, and follicular dendritic cells arranged in primary follicles. Following antigenic challenge, the primary follicles enlarge into secondary follicles, each containing a germinal center. Intense B-cell activation and differentiation into plasma and memory B cells occurs in the germinal centers of lymph nodes. (In children with B-cell deficiencies, the cortex lacks primary follicles and germinal centers.) Beneath the cortex is the **paracortex**, which is populated largely with T lymphocytes and also contains interdigitating dendritic cells thought to have migrated from tissues to the node. These interdigitating dendritic cells express high levels of class II MHC molecules, which are necessary for antigen presentation to T_H cells. Lymph nodes taken from neonatally thymectomized mice show a severe depletion of cells in the paracortical region; the paracortex is therefore sometimes referred to as a **thymus-dependent area** in contrast to the cortex, which is a **thymus-independent area**. The innermost layer of a lymph node, the **medulla**, is more sparsely populated with lymphocytes, but many of these are plasma cells actively secreting antibody molecules.

As antigen is carried into a regional node by the lymph, it is trapped, processed, and presented together with class II MHC molecules by interdigitating dendritic cells in the paracortex, resulting in T_H-cell activation. The initial activation of B cells is also thought to take place within the T-cell–rich paracortex. Once activated, T_H and B cells form small foci consisting largely of proliferating B cells at the edges of the paracortex. Some B cells within the foci differentiate into plasma cells secreting IgM and IgG. These foci reach maximum size within 3–4 days of antigen challenge.

Within 4–7 days of antigen challenge a few B cells, together with a few T_H cells, migrate to the primary follicles of the cortex. It is not known what causes these cells to migrate to the primary follicles. Within a primary follicle, cellular interactions between follicular dendritic cells, B cells, and T_H cells take place, leading to development of a secondary follicle with a central germinal center. Follicular dendritic cells, which make up the cellular meshwork of the germinal center, trap antigen complexed with antibody and retain the antigen-antibody complexes on the membrane for long periods of time (see Figure 3-15). Antigen trapped on the membrane of these cells is thought to be particularly effective in activating

(a)

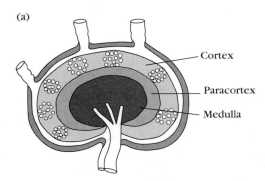

FIGURE 3-21

Structure of a lymph node. (a) The three layers of a lymph node provide distinct microenvironments. (b) The left side depicts the arrangement of reticulum and lymphocytes within the various regions of a lymph node. Macrophages and dendritic cells, which trap antigen, are present in the cortex and paracortex. T_H cells are concentrated in the paracortex; B cells are located primarily in the cortex within follicles and germinal centers. The medulla is populated largely by antibody-producing plasma cells. Lymphocytes circulating in the lymph are carried into the node via afferent lymphatics; they either enter the reticular matrix of the node or pass through it and leave via the efferent lymphatic vessel. The right side of (b) depicts the lymphatic artery and vein and the postcapillary venules. Lymphocytes in the circulation can pass into the node from the postcapillary venules by a process called extravasation (*inset*).

(b)

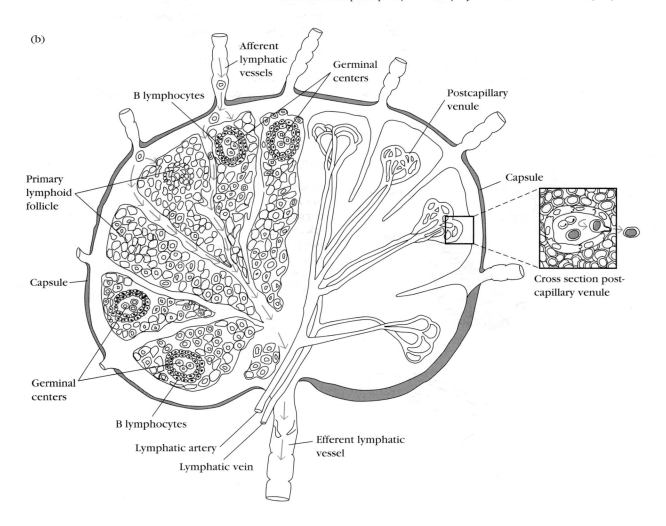

B cells. Follicular dendritic cells also produce growth factors that are essential for B-cell activation. The activated B cells in the germinal center divide rapidly and either differentiate into plasma and memory B cells or die by programmed cell death. Some of the cell death occurring within the germinal center is due to a process of selection to remove self-reactive B cells. This process, as well as other events taking place within the germinal center, are discussed more fully in Chapter 8. Plasma cells leave the germinal centers and migrate to the medulla where they secrete large quantities of antibody.

Afferent lymphatic vessels pierce the capsule of a lymph node at numerous sites and empty lymph into the subcapsular sinus (see Figure 3-21b). Lymph coming from the tissues percolates slowly inward through the cortex, paracortex, and medulla, allowing phagocytic cells and dendritic cells to trap any bacteria or particulate material (e.g., antigen-antibody complexes) carried by the lymph.

Following infection or introduction of other antigens into the body, the lymph leaving a node through its single efferent lymphatic vessel is enriched with antibodies newly secreted by medullary plasma cells and also has a 50-fold higher concentration of lymphocytes than the afferent lymph.

The increase in lymphocytes in lymph leaving a node is due in part to lymphocyte proliferation within the node in response to antigen. Most of the increase, however, represents blood-borne lymphocytes that migrate into the node by passing between specialized endothelial cells lining the **postcapillary venules** of the node. Estimates are that 25% of the lymphocytes leaving a lymph node have migrated across this endothelial layer and entered the node from the circulation. Because antigenic stimulation within a node can increase this migration tenfold, the concentration of lymphocytes in nodes involved in an active immune response can increase greatly, resulting in visible swelling of the nodes. Factors released in lymph nodes during antigen stimulation are thought to facilitate this increased lymphocyte migration.

SPLEEN

The spleen is a large, ovoid secondary lymphoid organ situated high in the left abdominal cavity. Unlike lymph nodes, which are specialized to trap localized antigen from regional tissue spaces, the spleen is adapted to filtering blood and trapping blood-borne antigens, and thus can respond to systemic infections. The spleen is surrounded by a capsule that sends a number of projections (trabeculae) into the interior to form a compartmentalized structure. The compartments are of two types, the red pulp and white pulp, which are separated by a diffuse marginal zone (Figure 3-22). The splenic **red pulp** consists of a network of sinusoids populated with

(a)

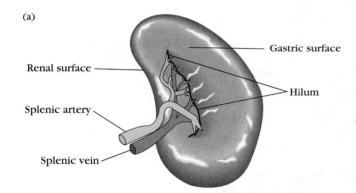

(b)

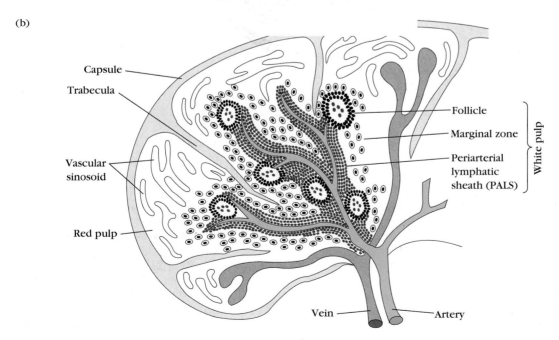

FIGURE 3-22

Structure of the spleen. (a) The spleen, which is about 5 inches long in adults, is the largest secondary lymphoid organ. It is specialized for trapping blood-borne antigens. (b) Diagrammatic cross section of the spleen. The arteriole blood supply pierces the capsule and divides into progressively smaller arterioles, ending in vascular sinusoids that drain back into the splenic vein. The erythrocyte-filled red pulp surrounds the sinusoids. The white pulp forms a sleeve, the periarteriolar lymphoid sheath (PALS) around the arterioles; this sheath contains numerous T cells. Closely associated with the PALS is the marginal zone, a B-cell–rich area containing lymphoid follicles that can develop into germinal centers.

macrophages and numerous red blood cells (erythrocytes); it is the site where old and defective red blood cells are destroyed and removed. Many of the macrophages within the red pulp contain engulfed red blood cells or iron pigments from degraded hemoglobin. The splenic **white pulp** surrounds the arteries, forming a **periarteriolar lymphoid sheath** (PALS) populated mainly by T lymphocytes. The **marginal zone**, located peripheral to the PALS, is rich in B cells organized into primary lymphoid follicles.

The initial activation of B and T cells takes place in the T-cell–rich PALS. Here interdigitating dendritic cells capture antigen and present it with class II MHC molecules to T_H cells. Once activated these T_H cells can then activate B cells. The activated B cells, together with some T_H cells, then migrate to primary follicles in the marginal zone. Upon antigenic challenge, these primary follicles develop into characteristic secondary follicles containing germinal centers (like those in the lymph nodes) where rapidly dividing B cells (centroblasts) and plasma cells are surrounded by dense clusters of concentrically arranged lymphocytes.

The effects of splenectomy on the immune response depends on the age at which the spleen is removed. In children, splenectomy often leads to an increased incidence of bacterial sepsis caused primarily by *Streptococcus pneumoniae, Neisseria meningitidis,* and *Haemophilus influenzae.* Splenectomy in adults has less adverse effects, although it leads to some increase in blood-borne bacterial infections (**bacteremia**).

Unlike the lymph nodes, the spleen is not supplied by afferent lymphatics draining the tissue spaces. Instead, blood-borne antigens are carried into the spleen through the splenic artery, which empties into the marginal zone. As antigen enters the marginal zone, it is trapped by interdigitating dendritic cells, which carry the antigen to the periarteriolar lymphoid sheath. Lymphocytes in the blood also enter sinuses in the marginal zone and migrate to the periarteriolar lymphoid sheath. Experiments with radioactively labeled lymphocytes show that more recirculating lymphocytes pass daily through the spleen than through all the lymph nodes combined.

MUCOSAL-ASSOCIATED LYMPHOID TISSUE

The mucous membranes lining the digestive, respiratory, and urogenital systems have a combined surface area of about 400 m^2, and are the major sites of entry for most pathogens. The defense of these vulnerable membrane surfaces is provided by a group of organized lymphoid tissues known collectively as **mucosal-associated lymphoid tissue** (MALT). Structurally these tissues range from loose clusters of lymphoid cells with little organization in the lamina propria of intestinal villi to organized structures such as the tonsils, **appendix**, and Peyer's

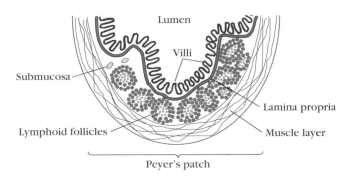

FIGURE 3-23

Cross-sectional diagram of the mucous membrane lining the intestine showing nodule of lymphoid follicles constituting a Peyer's patch in the submucosa. The intestinal lamina propria contains loose clusters of lymphoid cells and diffuse follicles.

patches (see Figure 3-16). The functional importance of MALT in the body's defense is attested to by its large population of antibody-producing plasma cells, whose number far exceeds that of plasma cells in the spleen, lymph nodes, and bone marrow combined.

The **tonsils** are found in three locations: lingual at the base of the tongue; palatine at the side of the back of the mouth; and nasopharyngeal (adenoids) in the roof of the nasopharynx. All three tonsil groups are nodular structures consisting of a meshwork of reticular cells and fibers interspersed with lymphocytes, macrophages, granulocytes, and mast cells. The B cells are organized into follicles and germinal centers; the latter are surrounded by regions showing T-cell activity. The tonsils play a role in defense against antigens entering through the nasal and oral epithelial routes.

The best studied of the mucous membranes is that lining the gastrointestinal tract. Lymphoid cells are found in three regions within this tissue. The outer mucosal epithelial layer contains so-called **intraepithelial lymphocytes** (IELs). The majority of these lymphocytes are CD8$^+$ T cells that express unusual T-cell receptors ($\gamma\delta$ TCRs), which exhibit limited diversity for antigen. It is thought that this population of T cells may be uniquely suited to encounter antigens that enter through the intestinal mucous epithelium. The lamina propria, which lies under the epithelial layer, contains large numbers of B cells, plasma cells, activated T_H cells, and macrophages in loose clusters. Histologic sections have revealed more than 15,000 lymphoid follicles within the intestinal lamina propria of a healthy child. Finally, within the submucosal layer of the intestinal lining are nodules consisting of 30–40 organized lymphoid follicles, called **Peyer's patches** (Figure 3-23). Like lymphoid follicles present in other sites, those composing Peyer's patches can develop into secondary follicles with germinal centers.

(a)

(b)

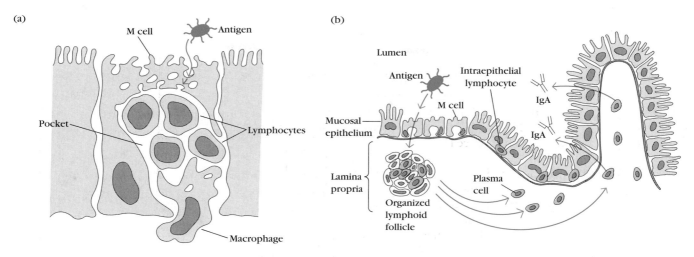

FIGURE 3-24

Structure of M cells and production of IgA at inductive sites. (a) M cells, located in mucous membranes, endocytose antigen present in the lumen of the digestive, respiratory, and urogenital tracts. The antigen is transported across the cell and released into the large basolateral pocket. (b) Antigen transported across the epithelial layer by M cells at an inductive site activates B cells in the underlying lymphoid follicles. The activated B cells differentiate into IgA-producing plasma cells, which migrate along the submucosa. The outer mucosal epithelial layer contains intraepithelial lymphocytes, which often are CD8+ T cells expressing $\gamma\delta$ TCRs with limited receptor diversity for antigen.

The epithelial cells of mucous membranes play an important role in promoting the immune response by delivering small samples of foreign antigen from the lumina of the respiratory, digestive, and urogenital tracts to the underlying mucosal-associated lymphoid tissue. This antigen transport is carried out by specialized cells, called **M cells**. The structure of the M cell is striking: these cells are flattened epithelial cells, lacking the microvilli that characterize the rest of the mucous epithelium. In addition, M cells contain a deep invagination, or pocket, in the basolateral plasma membrane; this pocket is filled with a cluster of B cells, T cells, and macrophages (Figure 3-24a). Luminal antigens are endocytosed into vesicles that are transported from the luminal membrane to the underlying pocket membrane. The vesicles then fuse with the pocket membrane, delivering the antigens to the clusters of lymphocytes contained within the pocket. M cells express class II MHC molecules, but it is not known whether antigen is processed within the endocytic vesicles and then is presented with class II MHC to the T_H cells contained within the pocket.

M cells are located in so-called **inductive sites**—small regions of a mucous membrane that lie over organized lymphoid follicles (Figure 3-24b). Antigens transported across the mucous membrane by M cells activate B cells within these lymphoid follicles. The activated B cells differentiate into plasma cells, which leave the follicles and secrete the IgA class of antibodies. These antibodies then are transported across the epithelial cells and released as **secretory IgA** into the lumen where they can interact with antigens present in the lumen.

As discussed in Chapter 1, mucous membranes provide an effective barrier to the entrance of most pathogens, thereby contributing to nonspecific immunity. One reason for this is that the mucosal epithelial cells are cemented to one another by tight junctions that make it difficult for pathogens to penetrate. Interestingly, some enteric pathogens, including both bacteria and viruses, have exploited the M cell as an entry route through the mucous-membrane barrier. In some cases the pathogen is internalized by the M cell and transported into the pocket. In other cases the pathogen specifically binds to the M cell and disrupts the cell, allowing entry of the pathogen. Among the pathogens that utilize M cells as a site of invasion are several invasive *Salmonella* species, *Vibrio cholerae*, and the polio virus.

Cutaneous-Associated Lymphoid Tissue

The skin provides an important anatomic barrier to the external environment and its large surface area makes this tissue important in nonspecific (innate) defenses. The outer epidermal layer of the skin is composed largely of specialized epithelial cells called keratinocytes. These cells secrete a number of cytokines that may function to induce a local inflammatory reaction. In addition, keratinocytes can be induced to express class II MHC

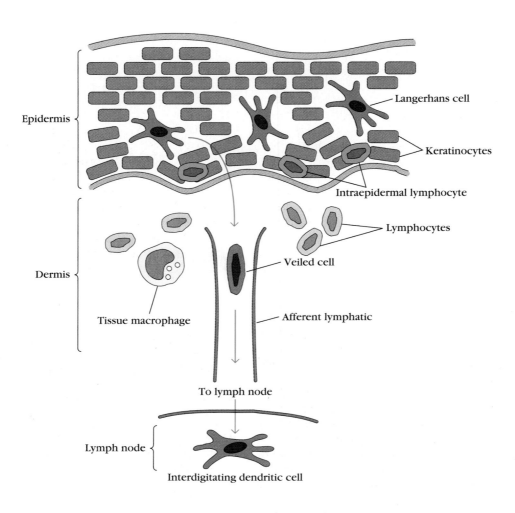

FIGURE 3-25

Cutaneous-associated lymphoid tissue. Keratinocytes, the major cells of the epidermis, secrete cytokines that may induce an inflammatory response. Langerhans cells in the skin internalize antigen and move in the lymph (as veiled cells) to lymph nodes where they differentiate into interdigitating dendritic cells; these function as potent antigen-presenting cells. Intraepidermal lymphocytes are predominantly CD8$^+$ T cells expressing the $\gamma\delta$ T-cell receptor.

molecules and may function as antigen-presenting cells. Scattered among the epithelial-cell matrix of the epidermis are **Langerhans cells,** a type of dendritic cell, which internalize antigen by phagocytosis or endocytosis. The Langerhans cells then migrate from the epidermis to regional lymph nodes where they differentiate into interdigitating dendritic cells (Figure 3-25). These cells express high levels of class II MHC molecules and function as potent activators of naive T$_H$ cells.

The epidermis also contains so-called **intraepidermal lymphocytes**. These are similar to the intraepithelial lymphocytes of MALT in that they are largely CD8$^+$ T cells, with a high proportion expressing $\gamma\delta$ T-cell receptors and limited diversity for antigen. It is thought that these intraepidermal T cells may be uniquely suited to combat antigens that enter through the skin. The underlying dermal layer of the skin contains scattered CD4$^+$ and CD8$^+$ T cells and macrophages. Most of these dermal T cells were either previously activated cells or are memory cells.

SUMMARY

1. The cells that participate in the immune response are white blood cells, or leukocytes (see Figure 3-1). The lymphocyte—the central cell of the immune system—is the only cell to possess the immunologic attributes of specificity, diversity, memory, and self/nonself recognition.

2. All of the white blood cells develop from a common pluripotent stem cell during hematopoiesis. Various hematopoietic growth factors (cytokines) induce proliferation and differentiation of the different blood cells (see Figure 3-2). This process is closely regulated to assure steady-state levels of each of the different types of blood cells. Cell division and differentiation of each of the lineages is balanced by programmed cell death by apoptosis (see Figure 3-4).

3. Lymphoid cells can be subdivided into B lymphocytes, T lymphocytes, and null cells (e.g., NK cells); the latter are much less abundant than B and T cells and also lack an antigen-binding receptor. Although morphologically indistinguishable, the three types of lymphoid cells can be distinguished on the basis of function and the presence of various membrane molecules (see Table 3-4).

4. Naive B and T lymphocytes, which have not encountered antigen, are small resting cells in the G_0 phase of the cell cycle. After interacting with antigen, these cells enlarge into lymphoblasts, which proliferate and eventually differentiate into effector cells and memory cells (see Figure 3-10).

5. Macrophages and neutrophils are the accessory cells of the immune system that phagocytose and degrade antigens (see Figure 3-12b). Phagocytosis is facilitated by opsonins such as antibody and complement, which increase the attachment of antigen to the membrane of the phagocyte. Activated macrophages also secrete various factors which are involved in development of the immune and the inflammatory responses (see Table 3-6). Basophils and mast cells are nonphagocytic cells that release a variety of pharmacologically active substances; these cells are critical in hypersensitivity responses.

6. Dendritic cells, which capture antigen, are classified based on their location in the body (see Table 3-7). With the exception of follicular dendritic cells, these cells express high levels of class II MHC molecules. Along with macrophages and B cells, these dendritic cells play an important role in T_H-cell activation by processing and presenting antigen in association with class II MHC molecules and by providing the required co-stimulatory signal. Follicular dendritic cells, unlike the others, facilitate B-cell activation but play no role in T-cell activation.

7. The primary lymphoid organs provide sites where lymphocytes mature and become antigenically committed. T lymphocytes mature within the thymus (see Figure 3-17), and B lymphocytes mature within the bursa of Fabricius in birds and largely in the bone marrow in mammals. In both cases, a selection process eliminates immature lymphocytes that react with self-antigens; in addition, thymocytes that do not recognize self-MHC molecules are eliminated.

8. The secondary lymphoid organs function to capture antigen and to provide sites where lymphocytes interact with that antigen and undergo clonal proliferation and differentiation into effector cells. The lymphatic system drains the tissue spaces and interconnects many organized lymphoid tissues (see Figure 3-19). Lymph nodes are specialized to trap antigen from regional tissue spaces (see 3-21), whereas the spleen is adapted to trapping blood-borne antigens (see Figure 3-22). Less organized lymphoid tissue is associated with mucous membranes including Peyer's patches (see Figure 3-23), loose clusters of lymphoid follicles in the intestinal lamina propria. Cutaneous-associated lymphoid tissue constitutes the most important tertiary lymphoid tissue (see Figure 3-25).

REFERENCES

CAUX, C. Y., J. LIU, AND J. BANCHEREAU. 1995. Recent advances in the study of dendritic cells and follicular dendritic cells. *Immunol. Today* **16**:2.

CORY, S. 1995. Regulation of lymphocyte survival by the BCL-2 gene family. *Annu. Rev. Immunol.* **12**:513.

DEXTER, T. M., AND E. SPOONCER. 1987. Growth and differentiation in the hemopoietic system. *Annu. Rev. Cell Biol.* **3**:423.

DORSHKIND, K. 1990. Regulation of hematopoiesis by bone marrow stromal cells and their products. *Annu. Rev. Immunol.* **8**:111.

ECKMANN, L., M. F. KAGNOFF, AND J. FLERER. 1995. Intestinal epithelial cells as watchdogs for the natural immune system. *Trends Microbiol.* **3**:118.

GOLDE, D. W. 1991. The stem cell. *Sci. Am.* **255** (Dec.):86.

GORDON, S., ET AL. 1995. Molecular immunobiology of macrophages: recent progress. *Curr. Opin. Immunol.* **7**:24.

JONES, B., L. PASCOPELLA, AND S. FALKOW. 1995. Entry of microbes into the host: using M cells to break the mucosal barrier. *Curr. Opin. Immunol.* **7**:474.

LAPIDOT, T., ET AL. 1992. Cytokine stimulation of multilineage hematopoiesis from immature human cells engrafted in SCID mice. *Science* **255**:1137.

LEHRER, R. I., A. K. LICHTENSTEIN, AND T. GANZ. 1993. Defensins: antimicrobial and cytotoxic peptides of mammalian cells. *Annu. Rev. Immunol.* **11**:105.

MacLennan, I. C. M. 1994. Germinal centers. *Annu. Rev. Immunol.* **12**:117.

Moore, M. A. S. 1991. The clinical use of colony stimulating factors. *Annu. Rev. Immunol.* **9**:159.

Nathan, C. F., and J. B. Hibbs. 1991. Role of nitric oxide synthesis in macrophage antimicrobial activity. *Curr. Opin. Immunol.* **3**:65.

Neutra, M. R., and J. P. Kraehenbühl. 1992. Transepithelial transport and mucosal defense I: the role of M cells. *Trends Cell Biol.* **2**:134.

Nuñez, G., and M. F. Clarke. 1994. The Bcl-2 family of proteins: regulators of cell death and survival. *Trends Cell Biol.* **4**:399.

Nuñez, G., et al. 1994. Bcl-2 and Bcl-x: regulatory switches for lymphoid death and survival. *Immunol. Today* **15**:582.

Russell, D. G. 1995. Of microbes and macrophages: entry, survival and persistence. *Curr. Opin. Immunol.* **7**:479.

Schmidt, H. H., and U. Walter. 1994. NO at work. *Cell* **78**:919.

Spangrude, G. J. 1994. Biological and clinical aspects of hematopoietic stem cells. *Annu. Rev. Med.* **45**:93.

Steinman, R. M. 1991. The dendritic cell system and its role in immunogenicity. *Annu. Rev. Immunol.* **9**:271.

Van den Dobbelsteen, G. P., and E. P. van Rees. 1995. Mucosal immune response to pneumococcal polysaccharides: implications for vaccination. *Trends Microbiol.* **3**:155.

Van Ewijk, W. 1991. T-cell differentiation is influenced by thymic microenvironments. *Annu. Rev. Immunol.* **9**:591.

STUDY QUESTIONS

1. Explain why each of the following statements is false.

a. All T_H cells express CD4 and only recognize antigen associated with class II MHC molecules.

b. The pluripotent stem cell is one of the most abundant cell types in the bone marrow.

c. Activation of macrophages increases their expression of class I MHC molecules, making the cells more effective in antigen presentation.

d. Lymphoid follicles are present only in the spleen and lymph nodes.

e. Infection has no influence on the rate of hematopoiesis.

f. Follicular dendritic cells can process and present antigen to T lymphocytes.

g. All lymphoid cells possess antigen-binding receptors on their membrane.

2. For each of the following situations, indicate which type(s) of lymphocytes would be expected to proliferate rapidly in lymph nodes and where in the nodes they would do so.

a. Normal mouse immunized with a soluble protein antigen

b. Normal mouse with a viral infection

c. Neonatally thymectomized mouse immunized with a protein antigen

d. Neonatally thymectomized mouse immunized with the thymus-independent antigen bacterial lipopolysaccharide (LPS), which does not require the aid of T_H cells to activate B cells

3. Do monocyte progenitor cells secrete M-CSF; do they express receptors for M-CSF? What would be the consequences to the cell if both M-CSF and the receptor for M-CSF were expressed?

4. List the primary lymphoid organs and summarize their functions in the immune response?

5. List the secondary lymphoid organs and summarize their functions in the immune response.

6. What are the two primary characteristics that distinguish hematopoietic stem cells and progenitor cells.

7. What do nude mice and humans with DiGeorge's syndrome have in common?

8. What cell types compose the stroma of the thymus? List two important functions of the thymic stromal cells.

9. Describe the processes of antigenic commitment and clonal selection. Indicate where these processes occur and how they contribute to the specificity and memory of the immune response.

10. At what age does the thymus reach its maximal size in an individual?

a. During the first year of life

b. Teenage years (puberty)

c. Between 40 and 50 years of age

d. After 70 years of age

11. Preparations enriched in pluripotent stem cells would be useful for research and in clinical practice.

a. In Weissman's method for enriching pluripotent stem cells, why is it necessary to use lethally irradiated mice?

b. Describe briefly the CellPro method for enriching pluripotent stem cells by affinity chromatography.

12. What effect does thymectomy have on a neonatal mouse? On an adult mouse? Explain why these effects differ.

13. What effect would removal of the bursa of Fabricius (bursectomy) have on chickens?

14. Some microorganisms (e.g., *Neisseria gonorrhoeae, Mycobacterium tuberculosis,* and *Candida albicans*) are classi-fied as intracellular pathogens. Define this term and ex-plain why the immune response to these pathogens differs from that to common pathogens such as *Staphylo-coccus aureus* and *Streptococcus pneumoniae.*

15. Indicate whether each of the following statements about the spleen is true or false. If you think a statement is false, explain why.

a. It filters antigens out of the blood.

b. The marginal zone is rich in T cells, and the periar-teriolar lymphoid sheath (PALS) is rich in B cells.

c. It contains germinal centers.

d. It functions to remove old and defective red blood cells.

e. Lymphatic vessels draining the tissue spaces enter the spleen.

16. For each type of cell indicated (a–l), select the most appropriate description (1–15) listed below. Each de-scription may be used once, more than once, or not at all.

Cell Types:

a. _____ Myeloid stem cells

b. _____ Monocytes

c. _____ Eosinophils

d. _____ Veiled cells

e. _____ Natural killer (NK) cells

f. _____ Kupffer cells

g. _____ Langerhans cells

h. _____ Mast cells

i. _____ Neutrophils

j. _____ M cells

k. _____ Bone-marrow stromal cells

l. _____ Intraepithelial lymphocytes

Descriptions:

1) Circulating dendritic cells

2) Specialized epithelial cells found in MALT

3) Phagocytic cells important in body's defense against parasitic organisms

4) Macrophages found in the liver

5) Give rise to red blood cells

6) Dendritic cells found exclusively in lymph nodes

7) Generally first cells to arrive at site of inflammation

8) Secrete colony-stimulating factors (CSFs)

9) Give rise to thymocytes

10) Circulating blood cells that differentiate into macro-phages in the tissues

11) A type of null cell involved in antibody-dependent cell-mediated toxicity

12) Dendritic cells found in the epidermis and mucous membranes

13) CD8$^+$ cells that may be important in combating intestinal pathogens

14) Nonphagocytic granulocytic cells that release vari-ous pharmacologically active substances

15) White blood cells that migrate into the tissues and play an important role in development of allergies

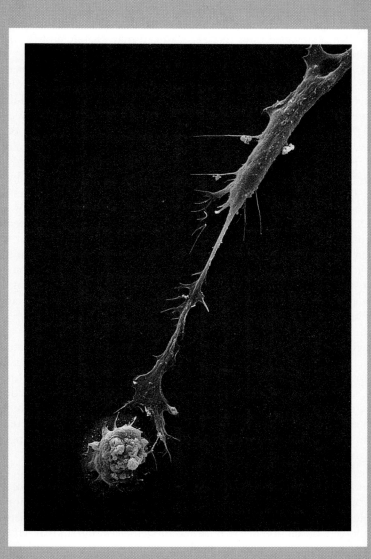

Dendritic cells and T cells interact to initiate
an immune response. [© David Scharf]

GENERATION OF B-CELL
AND T-CELL RESPONSES

In Part II we take a closer look at how lymphocyte progenitor cells develop into mature B and T cells, how these mature cells recognize foreign substances, and the consequences of such recognition. Although there are many similarities between B and T cells, they exhibit fundamental differences in how they recognize antigen.

We begin in Chapter 4 by focusing on the properties that contribute to immunogenicity, that is, the ability to induce an immune response. Lymphocytes do not recognize, or interact with, an entire antigen molecule, but only with discrete, relatively small sites (epitopes) on the macromolecule. B and T cells recognize quite distinct epitopes because of their different mechanisms of antigen recognition. In addition to the nature of the antigen itself, certain other factors influence whether a particular antigen will induce an immune response in an individual.

Chapter 5 describes the structure of immunoglobulins, or antibodies, the recognition and effector molecules of humoral immunity. Naive B cells express membrane-bound antibody and an associated signal-transducing membrane-protein complex, which together form the antigen-binding B-cell receptor. Secreted antibody is produced by plasma cells, which are generated from naive B cells that have interacted with antigen. The sequence of the antigen-binding region of the antibody molecule is highly variable, allowing for recognition of a great diversity of antigen molecules. The remainder of the antibody molecule, the constant region, has one of a small number of different sequences, which mediate different effector functions. Finally, the production and uses of monoclonal antibody, which is specific for a single antigenic determinant (epitope), are discussed.

The characteristics of antigen-antibody interactions are covered in Chapter 6. The association between an antibody and an antigen involves a large number of noncovalent interactions and is highly specific. Although these interactions produce no chemical changes in either the antigen or antibody, they can lead to precipitation of soluble antigens and agglutination (visible clumping) of particulate antigens. The exquisite specificity of antigen-antibody interactions has allowed development of both qualitative and highly sensitive quantitative assays for detecting either antigen or antibody.

We learn in Chapter 7 how the organization of germ-line immunoglobulin DNA permits the generation of an incredibly large number of genes encoding antibodies specific for different epitopes. As discussed in Chapter 8, during maturation of a progenitor B cell in the bone marrow, rearrangement of the germ-line DNA generates a single functional immunoglobulin gene. The resulting mature B cell expresses antibody specific for one or more closely related epitopes. Mature B cells leave the bone marrow and circulate within the bloodstream and lymphatic system. Binding of antigen by the membrane immunoglobulin on a circulating mature B cell and its interaction with an activated T_H cell may occur within the specialized environment of secondary lymphoid organs. These events generate intracellular signals that cause changes in gene expression, leading to activation, proliferation, and differentiation of a naive B cell into memory B cells and antibody-secreting plasma cells. During the initial response to an antigen, the class of antibodies produced may change and the affinity of the antibodies for antigen increases.

In the remaining four chapters in Part II, we explore the analogous processes involving T cells. Unlike B cells, T cells do not recognize soluble antigen; instead they recognize small peptides, derived from protein antigens, that are displayed on the surface of other body cells in association with membrane molecules encoded by the major histocompatibility complex (MHC) described in Chapter 9. Thus antigen recognition by T cells is self-MHC restricted. Chapter 10 discusses the two pathways by which endogenous and exogenous antigens are processed and presented with MHC molecules so that they can be recognized by T cells.

In Chapter 11, we examine the heterodimeric T-cell receptor, which recognizes antigen. Unlike antibodies, T-cell receptors exist only as membrane-bound molecules. But like the antibody molecule, the TCR molecule contains a variable region, which interacts with antigen, and a constant region. Also like membrane-bound antibody, the T-cell receptor is associated with a signal-transducing membrane-protein complex, as well as other accessory molecules that strengthen the association with antigen and assist in signal transduction. A further similarity between B and T cells is exhibited in the organization of the germ-line DNA encoding their antigen-binding molecules and in the rearrangement of this DNA to generate functional genes.

As we see in Chapter 12, T-cell maturation, activation, and differentiation are similar in many ways to analogous processes in B cells. Activation of T cells requires formation of a ternary complex between the T-cell receptor, an antigenic peptide, and an MHC molecule on an antigen-presenting cell or altered self-cell. This interaction generates a TCR-mediated signal and co-stimulatory signal that induce changes in gene expression, leading to activation, proliferation, and differentiation of T cells into effector and memory T cells. The vast majority of mature T cells express the $\alpha\beta$ T-cell receptor; these cells recirculate extensively and are primarily responsible for cell-mediated immune responses. About 5%–10% of the peripheral T cells express the alternative $\gamma\delta$ T-cell receptor; these cells are located primarily in the skin and intestinal epithelium, do not recirculate, and may form a primitive surveillance system for guarding the body's surfaces against invasion by microorganisms.

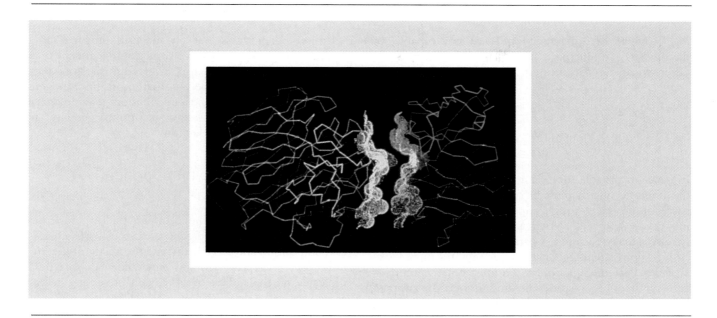

ANTIGENS

Substances capable of inducing a specific immune response commonly are referred to as antigens. The molecular properties of antigens and the way in which these properties ultimately contribute to immune activation are central to our understanding of the immune system. Some of the molecular features of antigens recognized by B or T cells are described in this chapter. The contribution made by the biological system to immunogenicity is also explored; ultimately the biological system determines whether a molecule that can bind to a B or T cell's antigen-binding receptor subsequently can induce an immune response. Fundamental differences in the way T and B lymphocytes recognize antigen determine which molecular features of an antigen are recognized by each branch of the immune system. These differences also are examined in this chapter.

IMMUNOGENICITY VERSUS ANTIGENICITY

Immunogenicity and antigenicity are related, but distinct, immunologic properties that sometimes are confused. **Immunogenicity** is the ability to induce a humoral and/or cell-mediated immune response:

B cells + antigen → effector B cells + memory B cells
(plasma cells)

T cells + antigen → effector T cells + memory T cells
(e.g., CTLs)

Although a substance that induces a specific immune response is usually called an **antigen**, it is more appropriately called an **immunogen**.

Antigenicity is the ability to combine specifically with the final products of the above responses (i.e., antibodies and/or cell-surface receptors). Although all molecules possessing the property of immunogenicity also possess the property of antigenicity, the reverse is not true. Some small molecules, referred to as **haptens**, possess the property of antigenicity but are not capable, by themselves, of inducing a specific immune response. In other words, they lack immunogenicity.

FACTORS THAT INFLUENCE IMMUNOGENICITY

In order to provide protection against infectious disease, the immune system must be able to recognize bacteria, bacterial products, fungi, parasites, and viruses as immunogens. Closer analysis has shown that the immune system actually recognizes particular macromolecules of an infectious agent, generally either proteins or polysaccharides. Proteins function as the most potent immunogens, with polysaccharides ranking second. In contrast, lipids and nucleic acids of an infectious agent generally do not serve as immunogens unless they are complexed to proteins or polysaccharides. Immunologists tend to use soluble proteins or polysaccharides as immunogens in most experimental studies of humoral immunity (Table 4-1). For cell-mediated immunity, only proteins serve as immunogens. These proteins are not recognized directly; instead they must first be processed into small peptides and then presented in association with MHC molecules on the membrane of a cell before they can be recognized as immunogens (see Figure 1-9).

TABLE 4-1

MOLECULAR WEIGHT OF SOME COMMON EXPERIMENTAL ANTIGENS USED IN IMMUNOLOGY

ANTIGEN	APPROX. MOLECULAR MASS (Da)
Bovine gamma globulin (BGG)	150,000
Bovine serum albumin (BSA)	69,000
Flagellin (monomer)	40,000
Hen egg-white lysozyme (HEL)	15,000
Keyhole limpet hemocyanin (KLH)	> 2,000,000
Ovalbumin (OVA)	44,000
Sperm whale myoglobin (SWM)	17,000
Tetanus toxoid (TT)	150,000

Immunogenicity is not an intrinsic property of a macromolecule but rather is a condition dependent on a number of interrelated factors involved in the total biological system. The properties that most immunogens share in common and the contribution the biological system makes to the expression of immunogenicity are discussed in the next two sections.

Contribution of the Immunogen to Immunogenicity

Immunogenicity is determined, in part, by four properties of the immunogen: its foreignness, molecular size, chemical composition and complexity, and the ability of the immunogen to be processed and presented with an MHC molecule on the surface of an antigen-presenting cell or altered self-cell.

FOREIGNNESS

In order to elicit an immune response, a molecule must be recognized as nonself by the biological system. The ability to recognize self-molecules is thought to arise during development by exposure of immature lymphocytes to self-components. Any molecule that is not exposed to immature lymphocytes during this critical period is later recognized as nonself, or foreign, by the immune system. When an antigen is introduced into an organism, the degree of its immunogenicity depends on the degree of its foreignness. Generally, the greater the phylogenetic distance between two species, the greater the genetic (and therefore the antigenic) disparity between them.

For example, the common experimental antigen bovine serum albumin (BSA) is not immunogenic when injected into a cow, but is an excellent immunogen when injected into a rabbit. Moreover, BSA would be expected to exhibit greater immunogenicity in a chicken than in a goat, which is more closely related to bovines. There are some exceptions to this rule: Some macromolecules (e.g., collagen and cytochrome *c*) were highly conserved throughout evolution and therefore display very little immunogenicity across diverse species lines. Conversely, some self-components (e.g., corneal tissue and sperm) are effectively sequestered from the immune system, so that if these tissues are injected even into the animal from which they originated, they will function as immunogens.

MOLECULAR SIZE

There is a correlation between the size of a macromolecule and its immunogenicity. The best immunogens tend to have a molecular mass approaching 100,000 daltons

– Lys – Ala – His – Gly – Lys – Lys – Val – Leu

(amino acid sequence
of polypeptide chain)

PRIMARY STRUCTURE

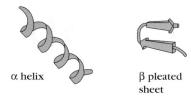

α helix   β pleated
sheet

SECONDARY STRUCTURE

FIGURE 4-1

The four levels of protein organizational structure. The linear arrangement of amino acids constitutes the primary structure. Folding of parts of a polypeptide chain into regular structures (e.g., α helices and β pleated sheets) generates the secondary structure. Tertiary structure refers to the folding of regions between secondary features to give the overall conformation of the molecule or portions of it (domains) with specific functional properties. Quaternary structure results from association of two or more polypeptide chains into a single polymeric protein molecule.

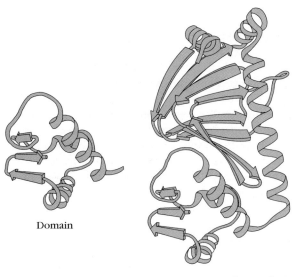

Domain

Monomeric polypeptide
molecule

TERTIARY STRUCTURE

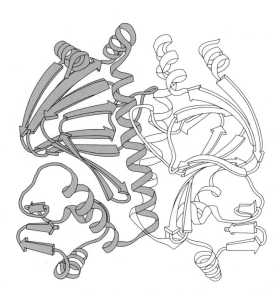

Dimeric protein molecule

QUATERNARY STRUCTURE

(Da). Generally, substances with a molecular mass less than 5000–10,000 Da are poor immunogens; however, in a few instances substances with a molecular mass less than 1000 Da have proven to be immunogenic.

CHEMICAL COMPOSITION AND HETEROGENEITY

Size and foreignness are not, by themselves, sufficient to make a molecule immunogenic; other properties are needed as well. For example, synthetic homopolymers (polymers composed of a single amino acid or sugar) tend to lack immunogenicity regardless of their size. Studies with copolymers composed of different amino acids has shed light on the contribution of chemical complexity to immunogenicity. Copolymers of sufficient size, containing two or more different amino acids, are immunogenic. The addition of aromatic amino acids, such as tyrosine or phenylalanine, has a profound effect on the immunogenicity of these synthetic polymers. For example, a synthetic copolymer of glutamic acid and lysine requires a minimum molecular weight of 30,000–40,000 for immunogenicity. The addition of tyrosine to the copolymer reduces the minimum molecular weight required for immunogenicity to between 10,000 and 20,000, and the addition of both tyrosine and phenylalanine reduces the minimum molecular weight for immunogenicity to 4000. All four levels of protein organization—primary, secondary, tertiary, and quaternary—contribute to the structural complexity of a protein and hence affect its immunogenicity (Figure 4-1).

SUSCEPTIBILITY TO ANTIGEN PROCESSING AND PRESENTATION

The development of both humoral and cell-mediated immune responses requires interaction of T cells with antigen that has been processed and presented in association with MHC molecules. For T_H cells the antigen must be presented with class II MHC molecules on an antigen-presenting cell; for T_C cells, the antigen must be presented with class I MHC molecules on an altered self-cell. Macromolecules that cannot be degraded and presented with MHC molecules are poor immunogens. This can be illustrated by polymers of D-amino acids, which are stereoisomers of the naturally occurring L-amino acids. Because the degradative enzymes within antigen-presenting cells can only degrade proteins containing L-amino acids, polymers of D-amino acids cannot be processed and thus are poor immunogens.

Large, insoluble macromolecules generally are more immunogenic than small, soluble ones because they are more readily phagocytosed and processed. Intermolecular chemical cross-linking, heat aggregation, and attachment to insoluble matrices have been routinely used to increase the insolubility of macromolecules, thereby facilitating their phagocytosis and increasing their immunogenicity.

Contribution of the Biological System to Immunogenicity

Even when a macromolecule has the properties that contribute to immunogenicity, its ability to induce an immune response will depend on certain properties of the biological system that the antigen encounters.

GENOTYPE OF THE RECIPIENT ANIMAL

The genetic constitution (**genotype**) of an immunized animal influences the type of immune response the animal manifests, as well as the degree of the response. For example, Hugh McDevitt showed that two different inbred strains of mice exhibited very different responses to a synthetic polypeptide immunogen. Following exposure to the immunogen, one strain produced high levels of serum antibody, whereas the other strain produced low levels. When the two strains were crossed, the F_1 generation showed an intermediate response to the immunogen. By backcross analysis, the gene controlling **immune responsiveness** was mapped to a subregion of the major histocompatibility complex (MHC). Numerous experiments with simple defined immunogens have demonstrated genetic control of immune responsiveness, largely confined to genes within the MHC (Table 4-2). These

TABLE 4-2

EFFECT OF MHC HAPLOTYPE ON THE ANTIBODY RESPONSE TO THE SYNTHETIC COPOLYMERS (H,G)-A-L AND (T,G)-A-L IN MICE

MHC HAPLOTYPE*	REPRESENTATIVE MOUSE STRAINS	ANTIBODY RESPONSE TO (H,G)-A-L[†]	ANTIBODY RESPONSE TO (T,G)-A-L[‡]
H-2^b	C57BL/6	Low	High
H-2^b	C3H.SW	Low	High
H-2^d	BALB/c	Intermediate	Intermediate
H-2^d	DBA/2	Intermediate	Intermediate
H-2^k	CBA	High	Low
H-2^k	C3H/HeJ	High	Low
H-2^s	B10.S	Low	Low
H-2^s	SJL	Low	Low

* The MHC haplotype is the entire set of closely linked MHC alleles inherited from the mother or the father. The haplotype is indicated by arbitrary superscripts. Since inbred strains are homozygous at each MHC locus (called H-2 in the mouse), a single superscript defines their haplotype.

[†] Copolymer consists of polylysine backbone with polyalanine side chains to which histidine and glutamic acid residues are attached at the end.

[‡] Copolymer consists of polylysine backbone with polyalanine side chains to which tyrosine and glutamic acid residues are attached at the end (see Figure 4-5).

data indicate that MHC gene products, which function to present processed antigen to T cells, play a central role in determining the degree of immune responsiveness to an antigen.

The response of an animal to an antigen is also influenced by the genes encoding B-cell and T-cell receptors and by genes encoding various proteins involved in immune regulatory mechanisms. Genetic variability in all of these genes affects the immunogenicity of a given macromolecule in different animals. These genetic contributions to immunogenicity are discussed more fully in later chapters.

IMMUNOGEN DOSAGE AND ROUTE OF ADMINISTRATION

Each experimental immunogen exhibits a particular dose-response curve, which is determined by measuring the immune response with various doses and administration routes. Some combination of optimal dosage and route of administration will induce a peak immune response in a given animal.

An insufficient dose will not stimulate an immune response either because it fails to activate enough lymphocytes or because it induces a nonresponsive state. Conversely, an excessively high dose also can fail to induce a response because it causes lymphocytes to enter a nonresponsive state. In mice the immune response to the purified pneumococcal capsular polysaccharide illustrates the importance of dose. A 0.5-mg dose of antigen fails to induce an immune response in mice, whereas a thousand-fold lower dose of the same antigen (5×10^{-4} mg) induces a humoral antibody response. This phenomenon of "immunologic unresponsiveness," or **tolerance**, is discussed in Chapter 16. A single dose of most experimental immunogens will not induce a strong response; rather, repeated administration over a period of weeks is required to stimulate a strong immune response. Such repeated administrations, or **boosters**, increase the clonal proliferation of antigen-specific T cells or B cells.

Experimental immunogens are generally administered **parenterally** (*para*, around; *enteric*, gut)—that is, by routes other than the digestive tract. The following administration routes are common:

- Intravenous: into a vein
- Intradermal: into the skin
- Subcutaneous: beneath the skin
- Intramuscular: into a muscle
- Intraperitoneal: into the peritoneal cavity

The administration route determines which immune organs and cell populations will be involved in the response. Antigen administered intravenously is carried first to the spleen, whereas antigen administered subcutaneously moves first to local lymph nodes. Differences in the lymphoid cells populating these organs generate differences in the quality of the subsequent immune response.

ADJUVANTS

Adjuvants (from Latin *adjuvare*, to help) are substances that, when mixed with an antigen and injected with it, serve to enhance the immunogenicity of that antigen. Adjuvants are often used to boost the immune response when an antigen has low immunogenicity or when only small amounts of an antigen are available, limiting the immunizing dosage. For example, the antibody response in mice following immunization with BSA can be increased fivefold or more if the BSA is administered with an adjuvant. Precisely how adjuvants augment the immune response is not entirely known, but they appear to exert one or more of the following effects (Table 4-3):

- Prolong antigen persistence
- Enhance co-stimulatory signal
- Induce granuloma formation
- Stimulate lymphocyte proliferation nonspecifically

Aluminum potassium sulfate (alum) acts to increase antigen persistence. When an antigen is mixed with alum, the salt precipitates the antigen. Injection of this alum precipitate results in a slower release of antigen from the injection site, so that the effective time of exposure to the antigen increases from a few days without adjuvant to several weeks with the adjuvant. The alum precipitate also increases the size of the antigen, thus increasing the likelihood of phagocytosis.

Freund's water-in-oil adjuvants also function to prolong antigen persistence. **Freund's incomplete adjuvant** contains antigen in aqueous solution, mineral oil, and an emulsifying agent such as mannide monooleate, which disperses the oil into small droplets surrounding the antigen; the antigen is then released very slowly from the site of injection. **Freund's complete adjuvant**, which contains heat-killed *Mycobacteria* in the water-in-oil emulsion, also has this effect. In addition, a muramyl dipeptide component of the mycobacterial cell wall activates macrophages, making Freund's complete adjuvant more potent than the incomplete form. Compared with unactivated macrophages, activated macrophages are more phagocytic, express higher levels of class II MHC molecules and the B7 membrane molecule, and secrete increased levels of interleukin 1 (IL-1). Both B7 and IL-1 bind to T_H cells, triggering a **co-stimulatory signal** necessary for T_H-cell activation. Thus, antigen presentation and the requisite co-stimulatory signal may be generated more easily in the presence of adjuvant than in its absence.

Alum and both Freund's adjuvants also stimulate a local, chronic inflammatory response with an increase in phagocytic cells as well as in lymphocytes. This cellular infiltration at the site of the adjuvant injection often results in formation of a dense, macrophage-rich mass of cells called a **granuloma**. Because the macrophages in a granuloma are activated, this mechanism also enhances T_H-cell activation.

Other adjuvants (e.g., synthetic polyribonucleotides and bacterial lipopolysaccharides) stimulate nonspecific lymphocyte proliferation and thus increase the likelihood of antigen-induced clonal selection of lymphocytes.

EPITOPES

As mentioned in Chapter 1, immune cells do not interact with, or recognize, an entire immunogen molecule; instead, lymphocytes recognize discrete sites on the macromolecule called **epitopes**, or **antigenic determinants**. Epitopes are the immunologically active regions of an immunogen that bind to antigen-specific membrane receptors on lymphocytes or to secreted antibodies. Studies using small antigens have revealed that B and T cells recognize different epitopes on the same antigenic molecule. For example, when mice are immunized with glucagon, a small human hormone of 29 amino acids, antibody is elicited to epitopes in the amino-terminal portion,

whereas the T cells respond only to epitopes in the carboxyl-terminal portion.

Interaction between lymphocytes and a complex antigen may involve several levels of antigen structure. In the case of protein antigens, an epitope may involve elements of the primary, secondary, tertiary, and even quaternary structure of the protein (see Figure 4-1). In the case of polysaccharide antigens, extensive side-chain branching via glycosidic bonds affects the overall three-dimensional conformation of individual epitopes.

T cells and B cells exhibit fundamental differences in antigen recognition (Table 4-4). B cells recognize soluble antigen when it binds to their membrane-bound antibody. Because B cells bind antigen that is free in solution, the epitopes they recognize tend to be highly accessible sites on the exposed surface of the immunogen. As noted previously, T cells only recognize processed peptides associated with MHC molecules on the surface of antigen-presenting cells and altered self-cells. Because T cells exhibit MHC-restricted antigen recognition, T-cell epitopes cannot be considered apart from their associated MHC molecules.

Properties of B-Cell Epitopes

Several generalizations have emerged about properties of B-cell epitopes from studies with immunogens in which the conformation of the epitope recognized by B cells has been determined.

The size of a B-cell epitope is determined by the size of the antigen-binding site on the antibody molecules displayed by B

TABLE 4 – 3

POSTULATED MODE OF ACTION OF SOME COMMONLY USED ADJUVANTS

ADJUVANT	POSTULATED MODE OF ACTION			
	PROLONGS ANTIGEN PERSISTENCE	ENHANCES CO-STIMULATORY SIGNAL	INDUCES GRANULOMA FORMATION	STIMULATES LYMPHOCYTES NONSPECIFICALLY
Freund's incomplete adjuvant	+	+	+	−
Freund's complete adjuvant	+	+ +	+ +	−
Insoluble aluminum salts (alum)	+	?	+	−
Mycobacterium tuberculosis	−	?	+	−
Bordetella pertussis	−	?	−	+
Bacterial lipopolysaccharide (LPS)	−	+	−	+
Synthetic polynucleotides (poly IC/poly AU)	−	?	−	+

cells. The binding of an antibody to an epitope involves weak noncovalent interactions, which operate only over short distances. In order for a strong interaction to occur, the antibody's binding site and the epitope must have a complementary conformation. The size of the epitope recognized by a B cell thus is determined by the size, shape, and amino acid residues of the antibody's binding site. A detailed picture of B-cell epitope structure has emerged from x-ray crystallographic analyses of complexes between monoclonal antibody and various types of antigens.

Smaller ligands such as carbohydrates, nucleic acids, peptides, and haptens often bind to an antibody within a deep concave pocket. For example, angiotensin II, a small octapeptide hormone, binds within a deep and narrow groove (725 Å^2) of monoclonal antibody specific for the hormone (Figure 4-2). Within this groove, the bound peptide hormone is folded into a compact structure with two turns, which brings its amino and carboxyl termini close together. All eight amino acid residues of the octapeptide are involved in van der Waals contacts with 14 residues of the antibody's groove.

A quite different picture of epitope structure emerges from x-ray crystallographic analyses of monoclonal antibodies bound to globular protein antigens such as hen egg–white lysozyme (HEL) or neuraminidase (an envelope glycoprotein of influenza). In this case the antibody makes contact with the protein antigen across a large planar face (Figure 4-3). The interacting face between antibody and epitope has been observed as a somewhat flat to undulating surface in which protrusions on the epitope or antibody are matched by corresponding depressions on the respective antibody or epitope. These studies have revealed that 15–22 amino acids on the surface of the protein antigen make contact with a similar number of

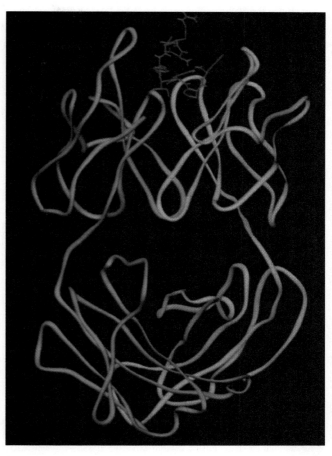

FIGURE 4-2

Three-dimensional structure of an octapeptide hormone (angiotensin II) complexed to a monoclonal antibody Fab fragment. The angiotensin II peptide is shown in red, the heavy chain in blue, and the light chain in purple. [From K. C. Garcia et al., 1992, *Science* **257**:502.]

T A B L E 4 – 4

COMPARISON OF ANTIGEN RECOGNITION BY T CELLS AND B CELLS

CHARACTERISTIC	B CELLS	T CELLS
Interaction with antigen	Involves binary complex of membrane Ig and Ag	Involves ternary complex of T-cell receptor, Ag, and MHC molecule
Binding of soluble antigen	Yes	No
Involvement of MHC molecules	None required	Required to display processed antigen
Chemical nature of antigens	Protein, polysaccharide, lipid	Only protein
Epitope properties	Accessible, hydrophilic, mobile peptides containing sequential or nonsequential amino acids	Internal linear peptides produced by processing of antigen and capable of binding to MHC molecules

(a)

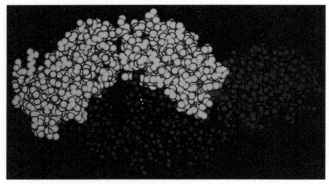

(b)

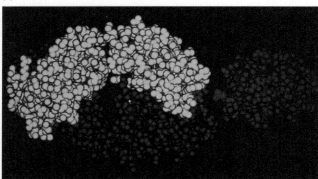

(c)

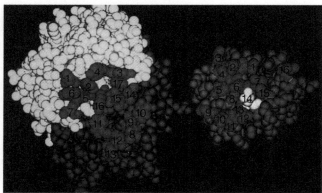

FIGURE 4-3

(a) Model of interaction between hen egg–white lysozyme (HEL) and Fab fragment of anti-HEL antibody based on x-ray diffraction analysis. HEL is shown in green, the Fab heavy chain in blue, and the Fab light chain in yellow. A glutamine residue of lysozyme (red) fits into a pocket in the Fab fragment. (b) Representation of HEL and the Fab fragment when pulled apart showing complementary surface features. (c) View of the interacting surfaces of the Fab fragment and HEL obtained by rotating each of the molecules. The contacting residues are numbered and shown in red with the protruding glutamine (#14) in HEL now shown in white. [From A. G. Amit, et al., 1986, *Science* **233**:747.]

narrow cleft. In Chapter 5 the nature of the interaction of the epitope with the antigen-binding site of the antibody is examined in more detail.

B-cell epitopes in native proteins generally are hydrophilic amino acids on the protein surface that are topographically accessible to membrane-bound or free antibody. A B-cell epitope must be accessible in order to be able to bind to an antibody. Amino acid sequences that are hidden within the interior of a protein cannot function as B-cell epitopes unless the protein is first denatured.

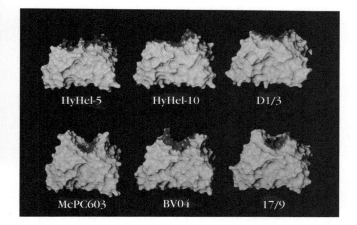

residues in the antibody's binding site; the surface area of this large complementary interface is between 650 and 900 Å². For these globular protein antigens, then, the epitope is entirely dependent on the tertiary conformation of the native protein.

Thus globular protein antigens and small peptide antigens interact with antibody in distinct ways (Figure 4-4). Epitopes on globular protein antigens appear to be considerably larger and occupy a more extensive surface area on the antibody than do small antigens. In contrast a small antigen, such as angiotensin II, folds into a compact structure that interacts with the antibody within a deep and

FIGURE 4-4

Models of the variable domains of six Fab fragments with their antigen-binding regions shown in purple. The top three antibodies are specific for lysozyme, a large globular protein. The lower three antibodies are specific for smaller molecules: McPC603 for phosphocholine; BV04 for single-stranded DNA; and 17/9 for a peptide from hemagglutinin, an envelope protein from influenza. In general, the binding sites for small molecules appear as deep pockets, whereas binding sites for large proteins appear as flatter, more undulating surfaces. [From I. A. Wilson and R. L. Stanfield, 1993, *Curr. Opin. Struc. Biol.* **3**:113.]

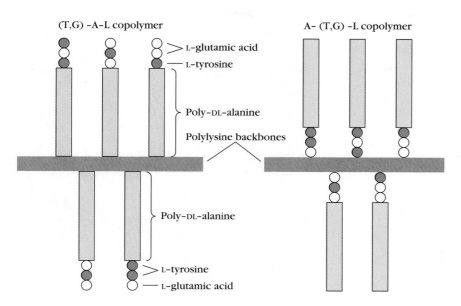

(T,G) -A-L copolymer

L-glutamic acid
L-tyrosine

Poly-DL-alanine

Polylysine backbones

Poly-DL-alanine

L-tyrosine
L-glutamic acid

A- (T,G) -L copolymer

FIGURE 4-5

Antibodies elicited by immunization with the (T,G)-A-L copolymer (*left*) react largely with the exposed tyrosine and glutamic acid residues. Anti-(T,G)-A-L antibodies do not react with the A-(T,G)-L copolymer (*right*) in which the tyrosine and glutamic acid residues are buried. [Adapted from M. Sela, 1969, *Science* **166**:1365.]

Michael Sela demonstrated the importance of this topographical accessibility in experiments with synthetic branched copolymers in which the accessible amino acids attached to the backbone polypeptide chain were varied. One copolymer, designated (T,G)-A-L, consisted of a poly-L-lysine backbone with poly D,L-alanine side chains whose N-termini were capped with variable amounts of glutamic acid and/or tyrosine (Figure 4-5). Antibody to (T,G)-A-L reacted largely with the accessible tyrosine and glutamic acid residues at the end of each side chain. Furthermore, the related synthetic copolymer A-(T,G)-L, in which poly D,L-alanine residues were in the accessible terminal positions and the glutamic acid and tyrosine residues were in a less accessible position, did not react with the antibody to (T,G)-A-L.

The entire surface of globular protein antigens is thought to be potentially antigenic. In general, regions that tend to protrude on the surface of the protein are often recognized as epitopes. Because the residues are accessible, they are often hydrophilic. In the crystallized antigen-antibody complexes analyzed to date, the interface between antibody and antigen possesses numerous complementary protrusions and depressions (Figure 4-6). Between 15 and 22 amino acids on the antigen contact

(a)

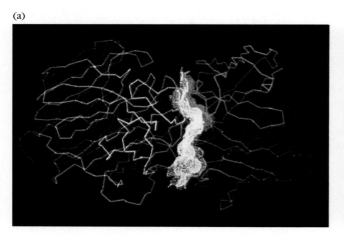

(b)

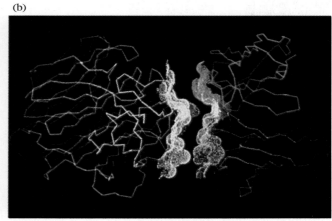

FIGURE 4-6

Computer simulation of an antibody-antigen interaction between antibody and influenza virus antigen, a globular protein. (a) The antigen (yellow) is shown interacting with the antibody molecule (*right*); the variable heavy chain is red, and the variable light chain is blue.

(b) The complementarity of the two molecules is revealed by separating the antigen from the antibody by a distance of 8 Å. Simulation is based on x-ray crystallography data collected by P. M. Colman and W. R. Tulip. [From G. J. V. H. Nossal, 1993, *Sci. Am.* **269**(3):22.]

(a)

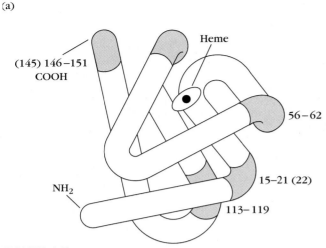

Heme

(145) 146–151
COOH

56–62

NH₂

15–21 (22)

113–119

(b)

FIGURE 4-7

Protein antigens usually contain both sequential and nonsequential B-cell epitopes. (a) Diagram of sperm whale myoglobin showing locations of five sequential B-cell epitopes (light blue). (b) Ribbon diagram of hen egg-white lysozyme showing residues that compose one nonsequential (conformational) epitope. Residues contacting antibody light chains, heavy chains, or both are shown in red, blue, and white, respectively. These residues are widely spaced in the amino acid sequence but are brought into proximity by folding of the protein. [Part (a) adapted from M. Z. Atassi and A. L. Kazim, 1978, *Adv. Exp. Med. Biol.* **98**:9; part (b) from W. G. Laver et al., 1990, *Cell* **61**:554.]

the antibody via 75–120 hydrogen bonds as well as ionic and hydrophobic interactions.

B-cell epitopes can contain sequential or nonsequential amino acids. Epitopes may be composed of sequential contiguous residues along the polypeptide chain or nonsequential residues from segments of the chain brought together by the folded conformation of an antigen. Most antibodies elicited by globular protein antigens bind to the protein only when it is in its native conformation. Because denaturation of such antigens usually results in loss of the topographical structure of their epitopes, antibodies to the native protein do not bind to the denatured protein.

Sperm whale myoglobin, which has an abundance of α-helical regions, contains five distinct **sequential epitopes,** each containing six to eight contiguous amino acids. Each of these epitopes is on the surface of the molecule at bends between the α-helical regions (Figure 4-7a). Sperm whale myoglobin also contains several **nonsequential epitopes,** or **conformational determinants.** The residues constituting these epitopes are far apart in terms of the primary amino acid sequence but close together in the tertiary structure of the molecule. Such epitopes are dependent on the native protein conformation for their topographical structure. One well-characterized nonsequential epitope present in hen egg-white lysozyme is shown in Figure 4-7b. Although the amino acid residues that compose this epitope of HEL are far apart in the primary amino acid sequence, they are brought together by the tertiary folding of the protein.

Sequential and nonsequential epitopes generally behave differently when a protein is fragmented or reduced. For example, appropriate fragmentation of sperm whale myoglobin can yield five fragments, each retaining one sequential epitope, as demonstrated by the observation that antibody can bind to each fragment. On the other hand, fragmentation of a protein or reduction of its disulfide bonds often destroys any nonsequential epitopes that it contains. For example, HEL has four intrachain disulfide bonds, which determine the final protein conformation. Antibodies to HEL recognize eight different epitopes, most of which are conformational determinants dependent on the overall structure of the protein. If the intrachain disulfide bonds of HEL are reduced with mercaptoethanol, the nonsequential epitopes are lost; for this reason, antibody to native HEL does not bind to reduced HEL. The inhibition experiment described in Figure 4-8 also demonstrates the importance of these disulfide bonds in determining the structure of HEL epitopes.

B-cell epitopes tend to be located in flexible regions of an immunogen and display site mobility. John A. Tainer and his colleagues analyzed the epitopes on a number of protein antigens (myohemerytherin, insulin, cytochrome *c*, myoglobin, and hemoglobin) by comparing the positions of the known B-cell epitopes with the atomic mobility of the same residues. Their analysis revealed that the major antigenic determinants in these proteins generally were located in the most mobile regions. These investigators proposed that site mobility of epitopes maximizes complementarity with the antibody's binding site, permitting

(a) Hen egg-white lysozyme

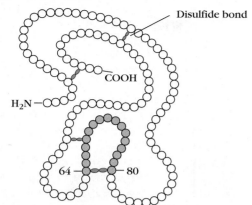

(b) Synthetic loop peptides

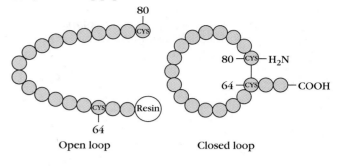

Open loop   Closed loop

(c) Inhibition of reaction between HEL loop and anti-loop antiserum

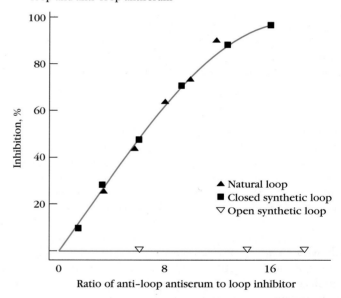

FIGURE 4-8

Experimental demonstration that binding of antibody to conformational determinants in hen egg-white lysozyme (HEL) depends on maintenance of the tertiary structure of the epitopes by intrachain disulfide bonds. (a) Diagram of HEL primary structure in which balls represent amino acid residues. The loop (blue balls) formed by the disulfide bond between the cysteine residues at positions 64 and 80 constitutes one of the conformational determinants in HEL. (b) Synthetic open-loop and closed-loop peptides corresponding to the HEL loop epitope. (c) Inhibition of reaction between HEL loop epitope and anti-loop antiserum. Anti-loop antiserum was first incubated with the natural loop sequence, the synthetic closed-loop peptide, or the synthetic open-loop peptide; the ability of the antiserum to bind the natural loop sequence then was determined. The absence of any inhibition by the open-loop peptide indicates that it does not bind to the anti-loop antiserum. [Adapted from D. Benjamin et al., 1984, *Annu. Rev. Immunol.* **2**:67.]

an antibody to react with an epitope that it might not otherwise react with if it were rigid. However, due to the loss of entropy involved in binding to a flexible site, the binding of antibody to a flexible epitope is generally of lower affinity than that of an antibody binding to a rigid epitope.

Complex proteins contain multiple overlapping B-cell epitopes, some of which are immunodominant. For many years it was dogma in immunology that a given globular protein had a small number of epitopes, each confined to a highly accessible region and determined by the overall conformation of the protein. However, it has been shown more recently that most of the surface of a globular protein is potentially antigenic. This has been demonstrated by comparing the antigen-binding profiles of different monoclonal antibodies to various globular pro-

teins. For example, when 64 different monoclonal antibodies to BSA were compared for their ability to bind to a panel of 10 different mammalian albumins, 25 different overlapping antigen-binding profiles emerged, suggesting that these 64 different antibodies recognized a minimum of 25 different epitopes on BSA. Similar findings have emerged for other globular proteins, such as myoglobin and HEL.

The surface of a protein, then, must present a large number of potential antigenic sites. The subset of antigenic sites on a given protein that is recognized by the immune system of an individual animal is much smaller than the potential antigenic repertoire, and it varies from species to species and even among individual members of a given species. Within a given animal, certain epitopes of a particular antigen are recognized as immunogenic, whereas others are not. Furthermore, some epitopes, referred to as **immunodominant**, induce a more pronounced immune response than other epitopes in a particular animal. It is thought that intrinsic topographical properties of the epitope as well as the animal's regulatory mechanisms influence the immunodominance of particular epitopes.

Properties of T-Cell Epitopes

Early studies by P. G. H. Gell and Baruj Benacerraf in 1959 suggested that there was a qualitative difference between the T-cell and the B-cell response to protein antigens. Gell and Benacerraf compared the humoral and cell-mediated responses to a series of native and denatured protein antigens (Table 4-5). They found that when primary immunization was with a native protein, only native protein, not denatured protein, could elicit a secondary antibody (humoral) response. In contrast, both native and denatured protein could elicit a secondary cell-mediated response. The finding that a secondary T-cell–mediated response was induced by denatured protein, even when the primary immunization had been with native protein, initially puzzled immunologists. In the 1980s, however, it became clear that T cells do not recognize soluble native antigen but rather recognize antigen that has been processed into **antigenic peptides**, which are presented in association with MHC molecules. For this reason, destruction of the conformation of a protein by denaturation does not affect its T-cell epitopes.

Because the T-cell receptor does not bind an epitope directly, experimental systems for studying T-cell epitopes must include antigen-presenting cells or target cells that can display the epitope together with an MHC molecule. In some systems, synthetic peptides are first allowed to interact with MHC molecules on antigen-presenting cells, and then T-cell proliferation is measured.

Antigenic peptides recognized by T cells form trimolecular complexes with a T-cell receptor and an MHC molecule. Before a T cell can be activated, a trimolecular complex must form between its antigen-binding receptor, an MHC molecule, and an antigenic peptide. Antigens recognized by T cells must, therefore, possess two distinct interaction sites: one, the **epitope**, interacts with the T-cell receptor, and the other, called the **agretope**, interacts with an MHC molecule. The three-dimensional structure of a TCR-peptide-MHC trimolecular complex has not yet been determined. However, cocrystallization of class I or class II MHC molecules with defined T-cell antigenic peptides has revealed that the peptide binds to a cleft in the MHC molecule (see Figure 9-8). This interaction primarily involves certain anchor residues of the peptide, which protrude into complementary pockets in the cleft of the MHC molecule (Figures 9-11 and 9-13). Unlike B-cell epitopes, which can be viewed strictly in terms of their ability to interact with antibody, T-cell epitopes must be viewed in terms of a trimolecular complex involving a T-cell receptor, an antigenic peptide, and an MHC molecule (Figure 4-9).

The antigen-binding cleft on an MHC molecule interacts with multiple oligomeric peptides, which function as T-cell epitopes. The antigen-binding cleft on an MHC molecule determines the nature and size of the peptide(s) that it can bind and consequently the maximal size of the T-cell epitope. Studies of the binding of peptides to class I MHC molecules have revealed that peptides of nine amino acid residues (nonamers) bind most strongly; peptides of 8–11 residues also bind but generally with lower affinity than nonamers. In the case of class II MHC molecules, peptides of 12–25 amino acid residues are preferentially bound.

The binding of an MHC molecule to an antigenic peptide does not appear to have the kind of fine specificity exhibited in the interaction between an antibody and its epitope. Instead, a given MHC molecule can selectively bind a variety of different peptides. For example, the class

TABLE 4-5

ANTIGEN RECOGNITION BY T AND B LYMPHOCYTES REVEALS QUALITATIVE DIFFERENCES

| | | SECONDARY IMMUNE RESPONSE | |
PRIMARY IMMUNIZATION	SECONDARY IMMUNIZATION	ANTIBODY PRODUCTION	CELL-MEDIATED T_{DTH} RESPONSE*
Native protein	Native protein	+	+
Native protein	Denatured protein	−	+

* T_{DTH} refers to a subset of $CD4^+$ T_H cells that mediate a type of cell-mediated response known as delayed-type hypersensitivity (see Chapter 16).

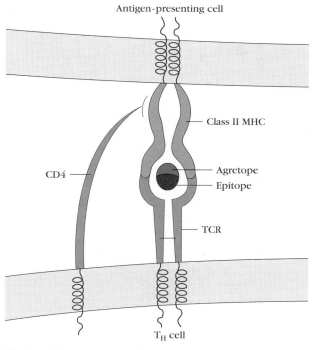

FIGURE 4-9

Schematic diagram of the ternary complex formed between a T-cell receptor (TCR) on a T_H cell, an antigen, and class II MHC molecule. Antigens that are recognized by T cells have two distinct interaction sites: an agretope, which interacts with an MHC molecule, and an epitope, which interacts with the T-cell receptor. As discussed in later chapters, CD4 on T_H cells also interacts with MHC molecules. T_C cells form similar ternary complexes with class I MHC molecules on target cells.

II MHC molecule designated IA^d can bind peptides from ovalbumin (residues 323–339), hemagglutinin (residues 130–142), and lambda repressor (residues 12–26). This broad, but selective, interaction suggests that the agretopes on these various peptides may share certain structural features, enabling them to bind to the same MHC molecule. Studies revealing common structural features, or motifs, among different peptides that bind to a single MHC molecule are discussed in Chapter 9.

Antigen processing is required to generate peptides that interact specifically with MHC molecules. As mentioned in Chapter 1, endogenous antigens and exogenous antigens appear to be processed by different intracellular pathways (see Figure 1-10). Endogenous antigens are processed into peptides within the cytoplasm, while exogenous antigens are processed within the endocytic pathway. Processing yields antigenic peptides that associate with class I or class II MHC molecules; the resulting peptide-MHC complexes are then presented on the cell surface where they can be recognized by T cells. The details of antigen processing and presentation are described in Chapter 10.

Epitopes recognized by T cells are often internal. T cells tend to recognize internal peptides that are exposed during processing within antigen-presenting cells or altered self-cells. J. Rothbard analyzed the tertiary conformation of hen egg-white lysozyme and sperm whale myoglobin to determine which amino acids protruded. He then mapped the major T-cell epitopes for both proteins and found that in each case the T-cell epitopes exhibited minimum protrusion; that is, they tend to be on the "inside" of the protein molecule (Figure 4-10).

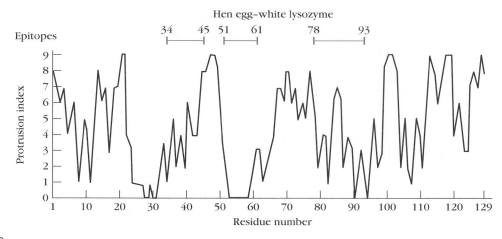

FIGURE 4-10

Experimental evidence that T_H cells tend to recognize internal peptides of antigens. This plot shows the relative protrusion of amino acid residues in the tertiary conformation of hen egg-white lysozyme. The known T-cell epitopes in HEL are indicated by the blue bars at the top. Notice that the amino acid residues corresponding to the T-cell epitopes exhibit little protrusion. [From J. Rothbard et al., 1987, *Mod. Trends Hum. Leuk.*, vol. 7.]

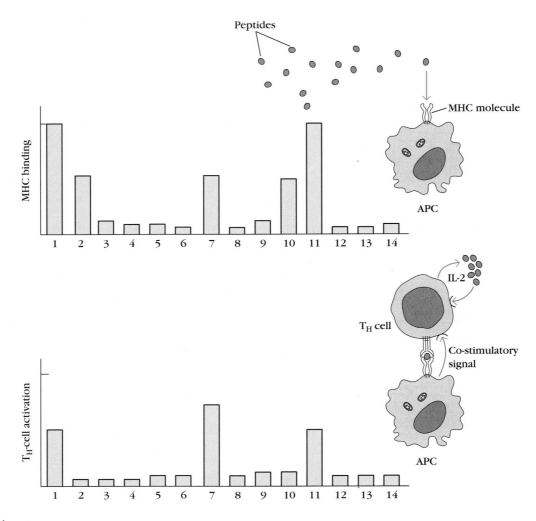

FIGURE 4-11

Correlation of MHC-binding ability and T-cell–activating ability of 14 synthetic peptides representing overlapping sequences of an immunogenic protein. Of the five peptides that bound to MHC molecules on mouse antigen-presenting cells (*top*), three also stimulated T-cell activation (*bottom*). These data suggest that binding to an MHC molecule is necessary, but not sufficient, for a peptide to induce an immune response. [Adapted from H. M. Grey et al., 1989, *Sci. Am.* **261**(5):59.]

Immunodominant T-cell epitopes are determined in part by the set of MHC molecules expressed by an individual. Various types of experiments have suggested that the MHC plays a significant role in determining which T-cell epitopes in a given antigen will be immunodominant in a given individual. For example, S. Buus and coworkers found a correlation between the ability of a peptide to bind to a particular MHC molecule and the T-cell response to that peptide. These researchers analyzed 14 synthetic peptides, representing overlapping sequences of the entire length of an immunogenic protein. Of these 14 peptides, the three that activated T_H cells also bound to a class II MHC molecule expressed by the same strain of mice (Figure 4-11).

HAPTENS AND THE STUDY OF ANTIGENICITY

The pioneering work of Karl Landsteiner in the 1920s and 1930s provided a simple, chemically defined system for studying the binding of an individual antibody to a unique epitope on a complex protein antigen. Landsteiner employed various **haptens**, small organic molecules that are antigenic but not immunogenic. Chemical coupling of a hapten to a large protein, called a **carrier**, yields an immunogenic **hapten–carrier conjugate**. Animals immunized with such a conjugate produce antibodies specific for (1) the hapten determinant, (2) unaltered epitopes on the carrier protein, and (3) new epitopes formed by combined parts of both the hapten and carrier (Figure 4-12). By itself a hapten cannot function as an immunogenic epitope. But when multiple molecules of a single hapten are coupled to a carrier protein (or nonimmunogenic homopolymer), the hapten becomes accessible to the immune system and functions as the **immunodominant determinant**.

The beauty of the hapten-carrier system is that it provides immunologists with a chemically defined determinant that can be subtly modified by chemical means to determine the effect of various chemical structures on immune specificity. In his studies, Landsteiner immunized rabbits with a hapten-carrier conjugate and then tested the reactivity of the rabbit's immune sera with that hapten and with closely related haptens coupled to a different carrier protein. Thus he could measure, specifically, the reaction of the antihapten antibodies in the immune serum and not that of antibodies to the original carrier epitopes. Landsteiner tested whether an antihapten antibody could bind to other haptens having a slightly different chemical structure. If a reaction occurred, it was referred to as a **cross-reaction**. By observing which hapten modifications prevented or permitted cross-reactions, Landsteiner was able to gain insight into the specificity of antigen-antibody interactions.

Using various derivatives of aminobenzene as haptens, Landsteiner found that the overall configuration of a hapten plays a major role in determining whether it can react with a given antibody. For example, antiserum specific for aminobenzene or one of its carboxyl derivatives (o-aminobenzoic acid, m-aminobenzoic acid, and p-aminobenzoic acid) reacted only with the original immunizing hapten and did not cross-react with any of the haptens (Table 4-6, *top*). In contrast, if the overall configuration of the hapten was kept the same and the hapten was modified in the para position with various nonionic derivatives, then the antisera showed varying degrees of cross-reactivity (Table 4-6, *bottom*). In addition to demonstrating the specificity of the immune system, Landsteiner's work also demonstrated the enormous diversity of epitopes that the immune system is capable of recognizing.

Many biologically important substances, including drugs, peptide hormones, and steroid hormones, can function as haptens. Conjugates composed of these haptens and large protein carriers can be used to produce hapten-specific antibodies. These antibodies are useful for measuring the presence of various substances in the body. For instance, the original home pregnancy test kit employed antihapten antibodies in a **hapten-inhibition assay**. This assay determined whether a woman's urine

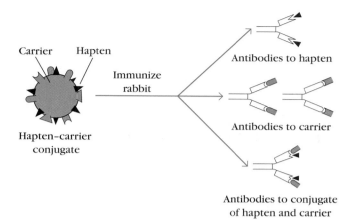

Injection with:	Antibodies formed:
Hapten (DNP)	None
Protein carrier (BSA)	Anti-BSA
Hapten-carrier conjugate (DNP-BSA)	Anti-DNP (major) Anti-BSA (minor) Anti-DNP/BSA (minor)

FIGURE 4-12

A hapten-carrier conjugate contains multiple copies of the hapten—a small nonimmunogenic organic compound such as dinitrophenol (DNP)—chemically linked to a large protein carrier such as bovine serum albumin (BSA). Immunization with DNP alone elicits no anti-DNP antibodies, but immunization with DNP-BSA elicits three types of antibodies. Of these, anti-DNP antibody is predominant, indicating that the hapten is the immunodominant epitope in a hapten-carrier conjugate.

contained human chorionic gonadotropin (HCG), which is a sign of pregnancy (Figure 4-13).

MITOGENS

Mitogens are agents capable of inducing cell division in a high percentage of T or B cells. Unlike an immunogen, which only activates lymphocytes bearing receptors specific for that immunogen, a mitogen can activate many clones of T or B cells irrespective of their antigen specificity. Because of this ability, mitogens are known as **polyclonal activators**.

A variety of agents function as mitogens. Several common mitogens are sugar-binding proteins called **lectins**, which bind specifically to different glycoproteins on the surface of various cells, including lymphocytes. Binding of lectin molecules to membrane glycoproteins often leads to agglutination, or clustering, of the cells, which

T A B L E   4 – 6

REACTIVITY OF ANTISERA WITH VARIOUS HAPTENS

REACTIVITY WITH

ANTISERUM AGAINST	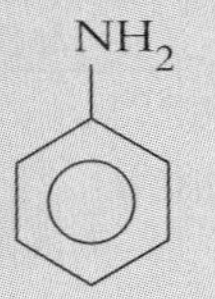 AMINOBENZENE (ANILINE)	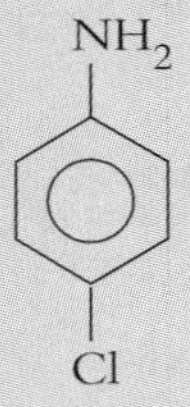 o-AMINOBENZOIC ACID	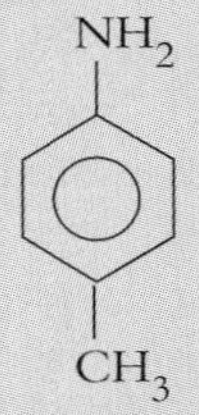 m-AMINOBENZOIC ACID	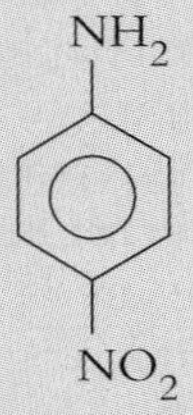 p-AMINOBENZOIC ACID
Aminobenzene	+++	0	0	0
o-aminobenzoic acid	0	+++	0	0
m-aminobenzoic acid	0	0	++++	0
p-aminobenzoic acid	0	0	0	+++±

REACTIVITY WITH

ANTISERUM AGAINST	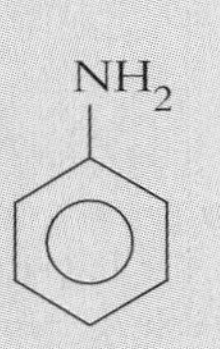 AMINOBENZENE (ANILINE)	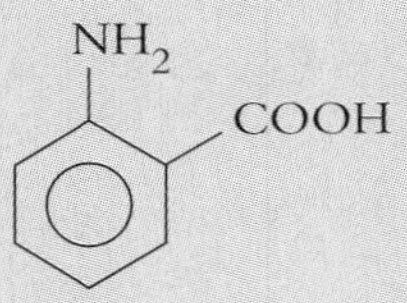 P-CHLOROAMINO-BENZENE	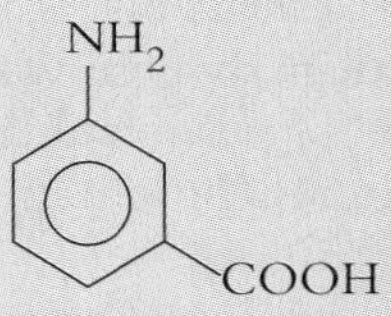 P-TOLUIDINE	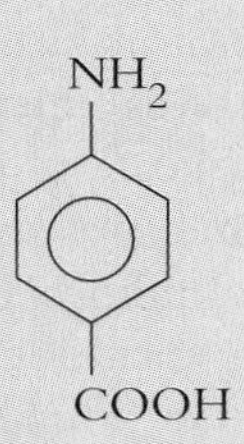 P-NITROAMINO-BENZENE
Aminobenzene	+ ∴ ++	+	+±	+
p-chloroaminobenzene	+++	++	++	+±
p-toluidine	+±	++	++	+
p-nitroaminobenzene	+	++	+±	+

KEY: 0 indicates no reactivity; +++ and ++++ indicate strong reactivity; +±, and ++ indicate lesser degrees of reactivity

SOURCE: Based on K. Landsteiner, 1962, *The Specificity of Serologic Reaction,* Dover Press.
Modified by J. Klein, 1982, *Immunology: The Science of Self-Nonself Discrimination,* John Wiley Publishers.

may trigger cellular activation and proliferation. Some mitogens preferentially activate B cells, some preferentially activate T cells, and some activate both populations. Three common lectins with mitogenic activity are **concanavalin A** (Con A), **phytohemagglutinin** (PHA), and **pokeweed mitogen** (PWM). Each of these mitogens binds to different carbohydrate residues in glycoproteins; Con A and PHA activate T cells, and pokeweed mitogen activates both T and B cells (Table 4-7).

Not all mitogens are lectins. The **lipopolysaccharide** (LPS) component of the gram-negative bacterial cell wall functions as a B-cell mitogen. The mitogenic activity of LPS is due to its lipid moiety, which is thought to interact with the plasma membrane, resulting in a cellular activation signal through as-yet-unknown mechanisms.

An unusual group of substances, known as **superantigens**, are among the most potent T-cell mitogens known. Superantigens bind to residues in the V (variable)

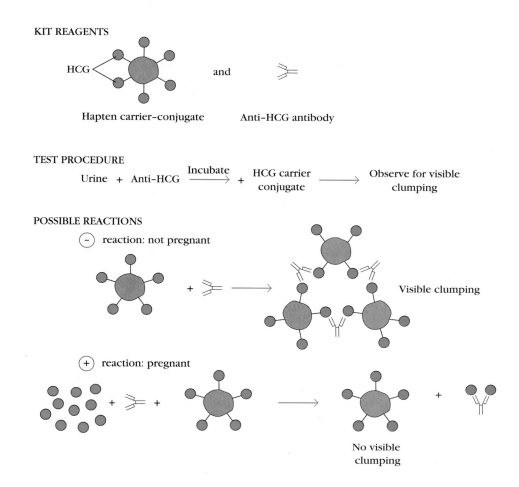

KIT REAGENTS

HCG

Hapten carrier-conjugate

and

Anti-HCG antibody

TEST PROCEDURE

Urine + Anti-HCG $\xrightarrow{\text{Incubate}}$ + HCG carrier conjugate $\longrightarrow$ Observe for visible clumping

POSSIBLE REACTIONS

(–) reaction: not pregnant

+ $\longrightarrow$ Visible clumping

(+) reaction: pregnant

+ + $\longrightarrow$ No visible clumping +

FIGURE 4-13

The early home pregnancy test kit employed hapten inhibition to determine the presence or absence of human chorionic gonadotropin (HCG). The original test kits used the presence or absence of visible clumping to determine if HCG was present. If a woman was not pregnant, her urine would not contain HCG; in this case, the anti-HCG antibodies and HCG-carrier conjugate in the kit would react, producing visible clumping. If a woman was pregnant, the HCG in her urine would bind to the anti-HCG antibodies, thus inhibiting the subsequent binding of the antibody to the HCG-carrier conjugate. Because of this inhibition, no visible clumping occurred if a woman was pregnant. The kits currently on the market use ELISA-based assays (see Figure 6-14).

T A B L E   4 – 7

CHARACTERISTICS OF THREE LECTIN MITOGENS

CHARACTERISTIC	CONCANAVALIN A (CON A)	PHYTOHEMAGGLUTININ (PHA)	POKEWEED MITOGEN (PWM)
Source	Jack beans	Kidney beans	Pokeweed
Molecular structure	Tetramer	Tetramer	Polymeric
Ligand	α-D-mannose and α-D-glucose	N-acetylgalatosamine	di-N-acetylchitobiose
Target cell(s)	T cells	T cells	T cells and B cells

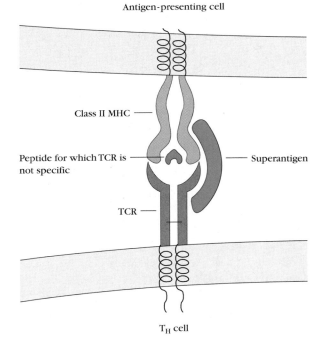

Antigen-presenting cell

Class II MHC

Peptide for which TCR is
not specific

Superantigen

TCR

T$_H$ cell

FIGURE 4-14

Schematic diagram of ternary complex formed between a T-cell receptor (TCR), superantigen, and MHC molecule. Superantigens bind to common sequences in class II MHC molecules and T-cell receptors that lie outside the normal antigen-binding sites (see Figure 4-9). T-cell activation by superantigens is not limited by the antigenic specificity of the T cell.

domain of the T-cell receptor and to residues in class II MHC molecules outside of the antigen-binding cleft (Figure 4-14). In this way a superantigen can cross-link a T cell to a class II MHC molecule even when the TCR does not recognize the bound antigenic peptide, leading to activation of the T cell. Thus a superantigen can activate all T cells expressing the V domain to which that superantigen binds.

Common superantigens include the staphylococcal enterotoxins (SEs) and toxic shock syndrome toxin 1 (TSST1), which is produced by the gram-positive bacterium *Staphylococcal aureus*. These toxins appear to activate large numbers of T$_H$ cells by cross-linking the T-cell receptors with any class II MHC molecule expressed on an antigen-presenting cell. Estimates are that one out of every five T cells can be activated by a superantigen, resulting in the release of abnormally high levels of cytokines. The high levels of cytokines released can lead to shock and death, seen most dramatically in tampon-related toxic shock syndrome caused by TSST1. These superantigens are discussed more fully in later chapters.

SUMMARY

1. Immunogenicity is the ability of an antigen to induce an immune response within either the humoral or the cell-mediated branch of the immune system. Antigenicity is the ability of an antigen simply to interact specifically with free antibody and/or with antigen-binding receptors on lymphocytes. B cells and T cells recognize small sites called antigenic determinants, or epitopes, on a complex immunogen.

2. The foreignness, molecular size, chemical composition and complexity, and susceptibility to antigen processing and presentation influence the immunogenicity of a substance. In addition, several properties of the biological system that an antigen encounters affect its immunogenicity; these include the genotype of the recipient animal, particularly its set of MHC genes; the immunogen dosage; the route of administration; and the presence or absence of adjuvants.

3. The size of B-cell epitopes—those epitopes recognized by membrane-bound antibody and free antibody—is determined by the size of an antibody's antigen-binding site. B-cell epitopes tend to be amino acid sequences within an antigen that are accessible, usually hydrophilic, and mobile. In general, a small peptide antigen interacts with a deep, narrow groove in the antibody molecule; a protein antigen interacts with a larger, flatter complementary surface on the antibody molecule (see Figures 4-2 to 4-4). Sequential B-cell epitopes consist of contiguous amino acid residues along the polypeptide chain. In contrast, nonsequential B-cell epitopes, also called conformational determinants, are formed from noncontiguous segments of the polypeptide chain that are brought into proximity by the three-dimensional folding of a protein.

4. T-cell epitopes—those epitopes recognized by T-cell receptors—generally consist of internal amino acid sequences. T-cell epitopes are rendered accessible to the immune system by antigen processing, which fragments the protein into small peptides that interact with class I MHC or class II MHC molecules. The resulting peptide-MHC complexes are then displayed on the surface of altered self-cells or antigen-presenting cells. Activation of T cells requires formation of a ternary complex between the T-cell receptor, MHC molecule, and antigenic peptide (see Figure 4-9).

5. MHC molecules have an antigen-binding cleft that selectively binds multiple antigenic peptides. The T-cell epitopes within an antigen that are immunodominant are determined in part by the particular MHC molecules expressed by an individual.

6. Haptens are small molecules that can bind to antibodies but cannot by themselves induce an immune

response. The conjugate formed by coupling a hapten to a large carrier protein is immunogenic and elicits production of antihapten antibodies when injected into an animal (see Figure 4-12). The study of haptens has allowed immunologists to learn about the structural basis of antibody specificity. Antihapten antibodies can be used in assays for nonimmunogenic biological substances including drugs, peptide hormones, and steroid hormones (see Figure 4-13).

7. Mitogens nonspecifically induce proliferation of cells, especially lymphocytes. Various mitogens preferentially activate B cells, T cells, or both. Several bacterial toxins, called superantigens, are potent T-cell mitogens. They bind to both T_H cells and class II MHC molecules (see Figure 4-14).

REFERENCES

ABRAHMSEN, L. 1995. Superantigen engineering. *Curr. Opin. Struc. Biol.* **5**:464.

AREVALO, J. H., M. J. TAUSSIG, AND I. A. WILSON. 1993. Molecular basis of crossreactivity and the limits of antibody-antigen complementarity. *Nature* **365**:859.

BERZOFSKY, J. A., ET AL. 1987. Protein antigenic structures recognized by T cells: potential applications to vaccine design. *Immunol. Rev.* **98**:9.

BERZOFSKY, J., S. BRETT, H. STREICHER, AND H. TAKAHASHI. 1988. Antigen processing for presentation to T lymphocytes: function, mechanisms and implications for the T cell repertoire. *Immunol. Rev.* **106**:5.

BUUS, S., A. SETTE., AND H. M. GREY. 1987. The interaction between protein–derived immunogenic peptides and IA. *Immunol. Rev.* **98**:115.

DEMOTZ, S., H. M. GREY, E. APPELLA, AND A. SETTE. 1989. Characterization of a naturally processed MHC class II-restricted T cell determinant of hen egg lysozyme. *Nature* **342**:682.

GREENSPAN, M. S. 1992. Epitopes, paratopes, and other topes: Do immunologists know what they are talking about? *Bull. Inst. Pasteur* **90**:267.

GREY, H. M., A. SETTE, AND S. BUUS. 1989. How T cells see antigen. *Sci. Am.* **261**(5):56.

HERMAN, A., J. W. KAPPLER, P. MARRACK, AND A. M. PULLEN. 1991. Superantigens: mechanism of T-cell stimulation and role in immune responses. *Annu. Rev. Immunol.* **9**:745.

HUNT, D. F., et al. 1992. Characterization of peptides bound to the class I MHC molecule HLA-A2.1 by mass spectrometry. *Science* **255**:1261.

LAVER, W. G., G. M. AIR, R. G. WEBSTER, AND S. J. SMITH-GILL. 1990. Epitopes on protein antigens: misconceptions and realities. *Cell* **61**:553.

MADDEN, D. R., J. G. GORGA, J. L. STROMINGER, AND D. C. WILEY. 1992. The three-dimensional structure of HLA-B27 at 2.1 Å resolution suggests a general mechanism for tight peptide binding to MHC. *Cell* **70**:1035.

ROTHBARD, J. B., AND M. L. GEFTER. 1991. Interactions between immunogenic peptides and MHC proteins. *Annu. Rev. Immunol.* **9**:527.

SILVER, M. L., H. C. GUO, J. L. STROMINGER, AND D. C. WILEY. 1992. Atomic structure of a human MHC molecule presenting an influenza virus peptide. *Nature* **360**:367.

STANFIELD, R. L., AND I. A. WILSON. 1995. Protein-peptide interactions. *Curr. Opin. Struc. Biol.* **5**:103.

TAINER, J. A., ET AL. 1985. The atomic mobility component of protein antigenicity. *Annu. Rev. Immunol.* **3**:501.

STUDY QUESTIONS

1. Indicate whether each of the following statements is true or false. If you think a statement is false, explain why.

a. Most antigens induce a polyclonal response.

b. A large protein antigen generally can combine with many different antibody molecules.

c. A hapten can stimulate antibody formation but cannot combine with antibody molecules.

d. MHC genes play a major role in determining the degree of immune responsiveness to an antigen.

e. T-cell epitopes tend to be accessible amino acid residues that can interact with the T-cell receptor.

f. B-cell epitopes are often nonsequential amino acids brought together by the tertiary conformation of a protein antigen.

g. Both T_H and T_C cells recognize antigen that has been processed and presented with an MHC molecule.

h. Each MHC molecule binds a unique peptide.

i. All antigens also are immunogens.

2. An antigenic peptide derived from hemagglutinin induces potent proliferation of T_H cells in mice expressing the class II MHC molecule designated IA^k. Would this peptide also induce potent T_H-cell proliferation in mice expressing IA^d? Explain your answer.

3. Two vaccines are described below. Would you expect either or both of them to activate T_C cells? Explain your answer.

a. A UV-inactivated ("killed") viral preparation that has retained its antigenic properties but cannot replicate.

b. An attenuated viral preparation that has low virulence but can still replicate within host cells.

4. For each pair of antigens listed below indicate which is likely to be most immunogenic. Explain your answer.

a. Native bovine serum albumin (BSA)

   Heat-denatured BSA

b. Hen egg-white lysozyme (HEL)

   Hen collagen

c. A protein with a molecular weight of 30,000

   A protein with a molecular weight of 150,000

d. A synthetic copolymer of two nonaromatic amino acids

   A similar copolymer that also includes tyrosine residues

5. Indicate which of the following statements regarding haptens and carriers are **true**.

a. Haptens are large protein molecules such as BSA.

b. When a hapten-carrier complex containing multiple hapten molecules is injected into an animal, most of the induced antibodies are specific for the hapten.

c. Carriers are needed only if one wants to elicit a cell-mediated response.

d. It is necessary to immunize with a hapten-carrier complex in order to obtain antibodies directed against the hapten.

e. Carriers include small molecules such as dinitrophenol and penicillinic acid.

6. Various disorders are related to overproduction or underproduction of thyroxine (T_4), the primary hormone produced by the thyroid gland:

Thyroxine (T_4)

Even though T_4 is nonimmunogenic, how might serum T_4 levels be measured immunologically?

7. For each of the following statements, indicate whether it is true only of B-cell epitopes (B), only of T-cell epitopes (T), or both types of epitopes (BT) within a large antigen.

a. They *always* consist of a linear sequence of amino acid residues.

b. They generally are located in the interior of a protein antigen.

c. They generally are located on the surface of a protein antigen.

d. They lose their immunogenicity when a protein antigen is subjected to heat denaturation.

e. Immunodominant epitopes are determined in part by the MHC molecules expressed by an individual.

f. They are present only in protein antigens.

g. Multiple different epitopes may occur in the same antigen.

h. Their immunogenicity may depend on the three-dimensional structure of the antigen.

i. The immune response to them may be enhanced by co-administration of Freund's complete adjuvant.

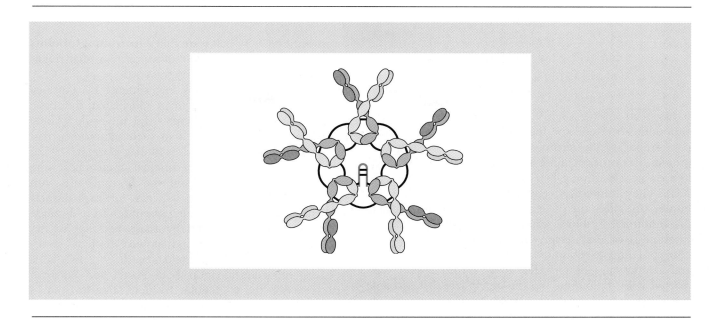

IMMUNOGLOBULINS:
STRUCTURE AND FUNCTION

Immunoglobulins function as antibodies, the antigen-binding proteins present on the B-cell membrane and secreted by plasma cells. Membrane-bound antibody confers antigenic specificity on B cells; antigen-specific proliferation of B-cell clones depends on interaction of membrane antibody and antigen. Secreted antibodies circulate in the blood and serve as the effectors of humoral immunity by searching out and neutralizing or eliminating antigens. All immunoglobulins share certain structural features, bind to antigen, and participate in a limited number of effector functions. Most of this chapter focuses on how the primary, secondary, and tertiary structure of immunoglobulins contribute to both their specificity and their effector functions.

The serum antibodies produced in response to a particular antigen are heterogeneous because of the presence of multiple B-cell epitopes on protein antigens. Although the polyclonal antibody produced in vivo is beneficial to the organism, it has numerous disadvantages for immunologic research. The last section of this chapter describes the production and uses of monoclonal antibody, which is specific for a single epitope. In addition to their use in research, monoclonal antibodies have many diagnostic and therapeutic applications.

BASIC STRUCTURE OF IMMUNOGLOBULINS

It has been known since the turn of the century that antibodies—the effector molecules of humoral immunity—reside in the serum. Identification of the serum-protein fraction containing antibodies was accomplished in a classic experiment by A. Tiselius and E. A. Kabat in 1939. They immunized rabbits with the protein ovalbumin (the albumin of egg whites), and then divided the immunized rabbits' serum into two aliquots. Electrophoresis of one serum aliquot revealed four peaks corresponding to albumin and the alpha (α), beta (β), and gamma (γ) globulins. The other serum aliquot was reacted with ovalbumin and the precipitate that formed was removed; the remaining serum proteins, which did not react with the antigen, were then electrophoresed. A comparison of the electrophoretic profiles of these two serum aliquots revealed that there was a significant drop in the γ-globulin peak in the aliquot that had been subjected to precipitation with antigen (Figure 5-1). Thus the **γ-globulin** fraction was identified as containing

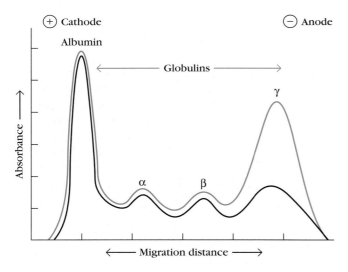

FIGURE 5-1

Experimental demonstration that antibodies are present in the γ-globulin fraction of serum proteins. After rabbits were immunized with ovalbumin (OVA), their antisera were pooled and electrophoresed, which separates the serum proteins based on electric charge. The blue line shows the electrophoretic pattern of untreated antiserum. The black line shows the pattern of antiserum that was incubated with OVA to remove anti-OVA antibody and then electrophoresed. [Adapted from A. Tiselius and E. A. Kabat, 1939, *J. Exp. Med.* **69**:119.]

serum antibodies, which were called **immunoglobulins** to distinguish them from any other proteins that might be contained in the γ-globulin fraction.

In the 1950s and 1960s experiments by Rodney Porter and by Gerald Edelman elucidated the basic structure of the immunoglobulin (Ig) molecule. (These experiments were considered of such significance that the two investigators shared a Nobel prize in 1972.) Edelman's and Porter's experimental approaches were quite different. Porter cleaved the Ig molecule with enzymes to obtain fragments, whereas Edelman dissociated the molecule by reducing the interchain disulfide bonds. The results attained by these two approaches complemented each other and allowed the basic structure of the Ig molecule to be elucidated.

Using ultracentrifugation, both Porter and Edelman first separated the γ-globulin fraction of serum into a high–molecular-weight fraction with a sedimentation constant of 19S and a low–molecular-weight fraction with a sedimentation constant of 7S. They used the 7S fraction, containing a 150,000-MW γ-globulin designated as immunoglobulin G, or IgG, for their studies. Porter subjected IgG to brief digestion with the enzyme **papain** and separated the fragments. Although papain has general, nonspecific proteolytic activity and will eventually digest the entire IgG molecule, brief treatment cleaves only the most susceptible bonds. Papain digestion of IgG produced two identical fragments (each with a MW of 45,000) called **Fab fragments**, because they retained their "antigen-binding" activity, and one fragment (MW of 50,000) called the **Fc fragment**, because it was found to crystallize during cold storage (Figure 5-2). A similar experimental approach, but with the enzyme **pepsin**, was taken by Alfred Nisonoff. Brief pepsin digestion generated a single 100,000-MW fragment composed of two Fab-like fragments and designated **F(ab′)$_2$**. Like the Fab fragments, the F(ab′)$_2$ fragment was also able to visibly precipitate antigens. However, after pepsin digestion, the Fc fragment was not recovered because it had been digested into multiple fragments.

The chain structure of IgG was first suggested by experiments of Edelman and his colleagues and later confirmed by Porter. Porter subjected IgG to mercaptoethanol reduction and alkylation, a chemical treatment that irreversibly cleaves disulfide bonds. The sample was then chromatographed on a column that separates molecules on the basis of size. This experiment revealed that the 150,000-MW IgG molecule was composed of two 50,000-MW polypeptide chains, designated as **heavy (H) chains**, and two 25,000-MW chains, designated as **light (L) chains** (see Figure 5-2).

The remaining puzzle was to determine how the enzyme digestion products—Fab, F(ab′)$_2$, and Fc—were related to the heavy-chain and light-chain reduction

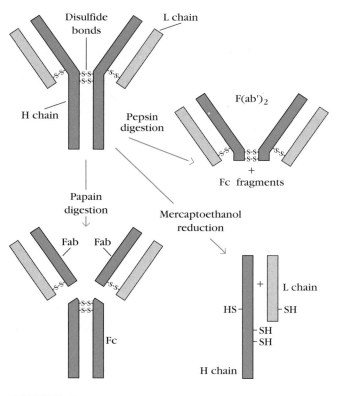

FIGURE 5-2

Prototype structure of IgG, proposed by Rodney Porter in 1962, showing chain structure and interchain disulfide bonds. The fragments produced by various treatments are also indicated. Light (L) chains are in gray and heavy (H) chains in blue.

Initial attempts to determine the amino acid sequence of the Ig heavy and light chains were unsuccessful because sufficient amounts of homogeneous protein were unavailable. Although the basic structure and chemical properties of different antibodies are similar, their antigen-binding specificities, and therefore their exact amino acid sequences, are very different. The γ-globulin fraction consists of a heterogeneous spectrum of antibodies that reflect all the different antigens that have induced an immune response in an animal. Even if immunization is done with a hapten-carrier conjugate, the antibodies formed just to the hapten alone are heterogeneous: they recognize different epitopes of the hapten and have different binding affinities. This heterogeneity of serum immunoglobulin rendered it unsuitable for sequencing studies.

Role of Multiple Myeloma

Sequencing analysis finally became feasible with the discovery of **multiple myeloma**, a cancer of antibody-producing plasma cells. The plasma cells in a normal individual are end-stage cells that secrete specific antibody for a few days and then die. In contrast, the plasma cells in an individual with multiple myeloma are not end-stage cells; rather, they divide over and over in an unregulated way without requiring any activation by antigen to induce clonal proliferation. Although such a cancerous plasma cell, called a **myeloma cell**, has been transformed, its protein-synthesizing machinery and secretory functions are not altered; thus the cell continues to secrete specific antibody. This antibody is indistinguishable from normal antibody molecules but is referred to as **myeloma protein** to denote its source.

In a patient afflicted with multiple myeloma, myeloma protein can account for 95% of the serum immunoglobulins. Most patients with multiple myeloma also secrete large amounts of excess light chains from their myeloma cells. These excess light chains were first discovered in the urine of myeloma patients and were named **Bence-Jones proteins** for their discoverer.

Multiple myeloma also occurs in other animals. In mice it can arise spontaneously, as it does in humans, or can be induced by injecting mineral oil into the peritoneal cavity. The clones of malignant plasma cells that develop are called **plasmacytomas** and are designated MOPCs, denoting the mineral-oil induction of plasmacytoma cells. A large number of mouse MOPC lines secreting different immunoglobulin classes are presently

products. Porter answered this question by using antisera from goats that had been immunized with the Fab fragments and Fc fragments of rabbit IgG. He found that antibody to the Fab fragment could react with both the H and the L chains, whereas antibody to the Fc fragment reacted only with the H chain. These observations led to the conclusion that Fab consists of portions of a heavy and a light chain and that Fc contains only heavy-chain components. Based on these results, Porter and Edelman proposed the prototype structure for IgG shown at the top of Figure 5-2. According to this model, the IgG molecule consists of two identical H chains and two identical L chains, which are linked by disulfide bridges. The enzyme papain cleaves just above the interchain disulfide bonds linking the heavy chains, whereas the enzyme pepsin cleaves just below these disulfide bonds, so that the two proteolytic enzymes generate different digestion products. Mercaptoethanol reduction and alkylation allow separation of the individual heavy and light chains.

(a)

(b)

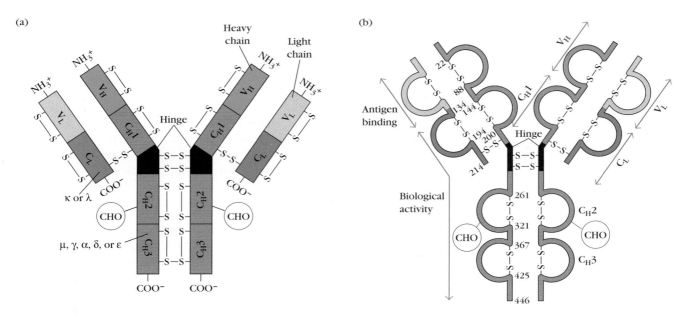

FIGURE 5-3

Schematic diagram of structure of immunoglobulins derived from amino acid sequencing studies. (a) Each heavy and light chain in an immunoglobulin molecule contains an amino-terminal variable (V) region (aqua and tan, respectively) that consists of 100–110 amino acids and differs from one antibody to the next. The remainder of the molecule—the constant (C) region (red and purple)—exhibits limited variation that defines the two light-chain subtypes and the five heavy-chain subclasses. Some heavy chains (γ, δ, and α) also contain a pro-line-rich hinge region (black). (b) Heavy and light chains are folded into domains, each containing about 110 amino acid residues and an intrachain disulfide bond that forms a 60-amino acid loop. The amino-terminal domains, corresponding to the V regions, function in antigen binding; effector functions are mediated by the other domains. The μ and ε heavy chains, which lack a hinge region (black), contain an additional domain in the central portion of the molecule.

carried by the American-type culture collection, a repository of cell lines commonly used in research. Some MOPC lines are listed in Table 2-2.

Light-Chain Sequencing

When the amino acid sequences of several Bence-Jones proteins (light chains) were compared, a striking pattern emerged. The amino-terminal half of the chain, consisting of 100–110 amino acids, was found to vary among different Bence-Jones proteins. This region was called the **variable (V) region**. The carboxyl-terminal half of the molecule, called the **constant (C) region**, had two basic amino acid sequences, which were designated **kappa (κ)** and **lambda (λ)** (Figure 5-3a). In humans 60% of the light chains are kappa, and 40% are lambda, whereas in mice 95% of the light chains are kappa, and only 5% are lambda. A single antibody molecule contains either κ light chains or λ light chains but never both.

A comparison of the amino acid sequences of λ light chains revealed minor differences on the basis of which λ light chains are classified into subtypes. In mice there are three subtypes ($\lambda 1$, $\lambda 2$, and $\lambda 3$); in humans there are four subtypes. Single amino acid interchanges at two or three positions are responsible for the subtype differences.

Heavy-Chain Sequencing

For heavy-chain sequencing studies, myeloma proteins were reduced with mercaptoethanol and alkylated, and the heavy chains were separated by gel filtration in a denaturing solvent. When the amino acid sequences of several myeloma protein heavy chains were compared, a pattern similar to that observed with the light chains emerged. The amino-terminal, consisting of 100–110 amino acids, showed great sequence variation from one myeloma heavy chain to the next and was therefore called the variable (V) region. The remaining part of the protein revealed five basic amino acid sequence patterns (μ, δ, γ, ε, and α) corresponding to five different heavy-chain constant (C) regions (see Figure 5-3a). Each of the different heavy-chain constant-region sequences is called an **isotype**. The length of the constant regions is approximately 330 amino acids for δ, γ, and α and 440 amino acids for μ and ε. The heavy chains of a given antibody molecule determine the class of that antibody:

T A B L E   5 – 1

CHAIN COMPOSITION OF THE FIVE IMMUNOGLOBULIN CLASSES IN HUMANS

CLASS	HEAVY CHAIN	LIGHT CHAIN	SUBCLASSES	MOLECULAR FORMULA
IgG	γ	κ or λ	$\gamma 1$, $\gamma 2$, $\gamma 3$, $\gamma 4$	$\gamma 2 \kappa 2$ $\gamma 2 \lambda 2$
IgA	α	κ or λ	$\alpha 1$, $\alpha 2$,	$(\alpha 2 \kappa 2)_n$ $(\alpha 2 \lambda 2)_n$ $n = 1, 2,$ 3, or 4
IgM	μ	κ or λ	None	$(\mu 2 \kappa 2)_n$ $(\mu 2 \lambda 2)_n$ $n = 1$ or 5
IgD	δ	κ or λ	None	$\delta 2 \kappa 2$ $\delta 2 \lambda 2$
IgE	ε	κ or λ	None	$\varepsilon 2 \kappa 2$ $\varepsilon 2 \lambda 2$

IgM, IgG, IgA, IgD, or IgE. Each class can have either κ or λ light chains. A single antibody molecule has two identical heavy chains and two identical light chains (Table 5-1).

Minor differences in the amino acid sequences of the α and the γ heavy chains led to further classification of the heavy chains into subclasses. In humans there are two subclasses of α heavy chains ($\alpha 1$ and $\alpha 2$) and four subclasses of γ heavy chains ($\gamma 1$, $\gamma 2$, $\gamma 3$, and $\gamma 4$); in mice there are four subclasses of γ heavy chains ($\gamma 1$, $\gamma 2a$, $\gamma 2b$, and $\gamma 3$).

IMMUNOGLOBULIN FINE STRUCTURE

The structure of the immunoglobulin molecule is determined by its primary, secondary, tertiary, and quaternary protein structure. The primary amino acid sequence accounts for the variable and constant regions of the heavy and light chains. The secondary structure is formed as the extended polypeptide chain folds back and forth upon itself forming an antiparallel β pleated sheet (Figure 5-4). The chains are then folded into a tertiary structure of compact globular domains, which are connected to neighboring domains by narrow, more exposed areas. Finally, the globular domains of adjacent heavy and light polypeptide chains interact in the quaternary structure, forming functional domains that enable the molecule to specifically bind antigen and, at the same time, perform a limited number of biological effector functions (Figures 5-3b and 5-5).

Immunoglobulin Domains

Careful analysis of the amino acid sequences of immunoglobulin heavy and light chains showed that both chains contain several homologous units of about 110 amino acid residues. Within each unit, termed a **domain**, an intrachain disulfide bond forms a loop of about 60 amino acids. Light chains contain one variable

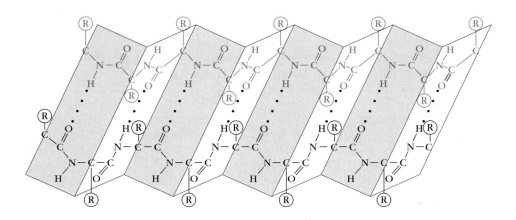

FIGURE 5-4

Structural formula of a β pleated sheet containing two antiparallel β strands. The structure is held together by hydrogen bonds between peptide bonds in neighboring chains. The amino acid side groups (R) are arranged perpendicular to the plane of the sheet. [Adapted from J. Darnell et al., 1990, *Molecular Cell Biology*, page 50, Scientific American Books, New York.]

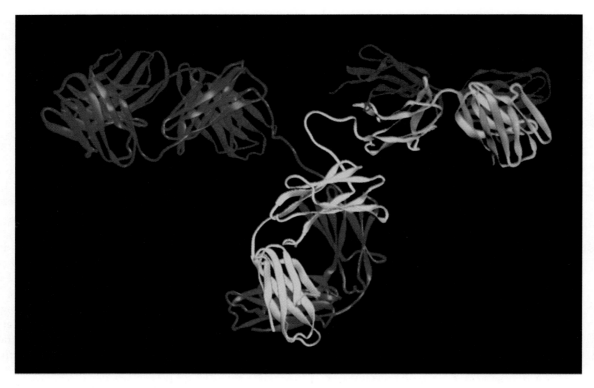

FIGURE 5-5

Ribbon representation of an intact monoclonal antibody depicting the heavy chains (yellow and blue) and light chains (red). The domains of the molecule composed of β pleated sheets are readily visible as is the extended conformation of the hinge region. [The laboratory of A. McPhearson provided this image based on x-ray crystallography data determined by L. J. Harris, 1992, *Nature* **360**:369.]

domain (V_L), and one constant domain (C_L); heavy chains contain one variable domain (V_H), and either three or four constant domains (C_H1, C_H2, C_H3, and C_H4), depending on the antibody class (see Figure 5-3).

X-ray crystallographic analysis revealed that immunoglobulin domains are folded into a characteristic compact structure known as the **immunoglobulin fold**. This structure consists of a "sandwich" of two β pleated sheets, each containing antiparallel β strands of amino acids, which are connected by loops of varying lengths (Figure 5-6). The β strands within a sheet are stabilized by hydrogen bonds that connect the −NH groups in one strand with a carboxyl group in an adjacent strand (see Figure 5-4). The β strands are characterized by alternating hydrophobic and hydrophilic amino acids whose side chains are arranged perpendicular to the plane of the sheet; the hydrophobic amino acids are oriented toward the interior and the hydrophilic amino acids face outward.

The two β sheets within an immunoglobulin fold are stabilized by the hydrophobic interactions between them and by the conserved disulfide bond. An analogy has been made to two pieces of bread, the butter between them, and a toothpick holding the slices together. The bread slices represent the two β pleated sheets; the butter represents the hydrophobic interactions between them; and the toothpick represents the intrachain disulfide bond. Although variable and constant domains have a similar structure, there are subtle differences between them. The V domain is slightly longer than the C domain and contains an extra pair of β strands within the β-sheet structure, as well as an extra loop sequence connecting this pair of β strands (see Figure 5-6).

The basic structure of the immunoglobulin fold contributes to the quaternary structure of immunoglobulins by facilitating noncovalent interactions between domains across the faces of the β sheets (Figure 5-7). Interactions occur between identical domains (e.g., C_H2/C_H2, C_H3/C_H3, and C_H4/C_H4), and between nonidentical domains (e.g., V_H/V_L and C_H1/C_L). The structure of the immunoglobulin fold also allows for variable lengths and sequences of amino acids that form the loops connecting the β strands. As discussed in the next section, some of the loop sequences of the V_H and V_L domains contain variable amino acids and constitute the antigen–binding site of the molecule.

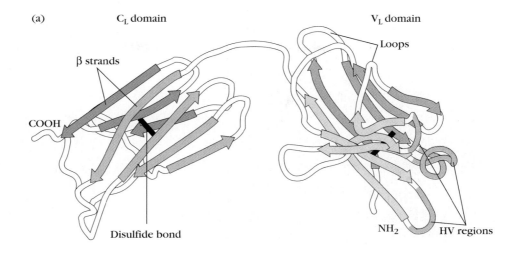

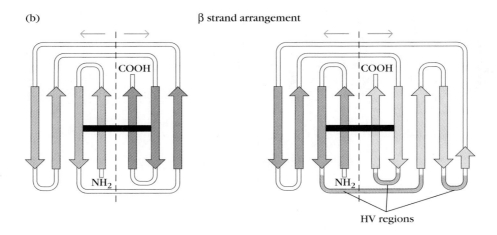

FIGURE 5-6

(a) Diagram of immunoglobulin light chain depicting the immuno-globulin-fold structure of its variable and constant domains. The two β pleated sheets in each domain are held together by hydrophobic interactions and the conserved disulfide bond. The β strands compos-ing each sheet are shown in different colors. The amino acid sequence in three loops of each variable domain show considerable variation; these hypervariable (HV) regions (blue) make up the antigen-binding site. Heavy-chain domains have the same characteristic structure. (b) The β pleated sheets are opened out to reveal the relationship of the individual β strands and joining loops. Note that the variable domain contains two more β strands than the constant domain. [Part (a) adapted from M. Schiffer et al., 1973, *Biochemistry* **12**:4620; part (b) adapted from Williams and Barclay, 1988, *Annu. Rev. Immunol.* **6**:381.]

Variable-Region Domains

Detailed comparisons of the amino acid sequences of V_L and V_H domains revealed that the sequence vari-ability is concentrated in several **hypervariable (HV) regions** (Figure 5-8). Three such hypervariable regions are present in each mouse and human heavy and light chain, constituting 15%–20% of the variable domain. The remainder of the V_L and V_H domains exhibit far less variation; these stretches are referred to as the **frame-work regions** (FRs). The hypervariable regions form the antigen-binding site of the antibody molecule. Be-cause the antigen-binding site is complementary to the structure of the epitope, the hypervariable regions are also called **complementarity-determining regions** (CDRs).

High-resolution x-ray crystallography has been used to determine the three-dimensional structure of the framework regions and hypervariable regions (or CDRs). The more conserved sequence of the framework regions generates the basic β pleated sheet structure of the V_H and V_L domains. The three heavy-chain and

(a)

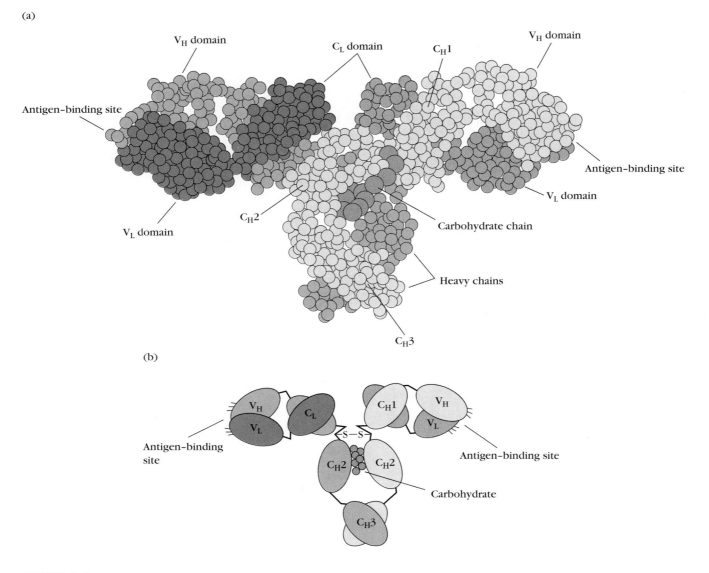

(b)

FIGURE 5-7

Interactions between domains in the separate chains of an immuno-globulin molecule are critical to its quaternary structure. (a) Model of IgG molecule, based on x-ray crystallographic analysis, showing associations between domains. Each solid ball represents an amino acid residue. The two light chains are shown in shades of red; the two heavy chains, in shades of blue. (b) A schematic diagram showing the interacting heavy- and light-chain domains. Note that the C_H2/C_H2 domain protrudes due to the presence of carbohydrate (tan) in the interior. The protrusion makes this domain more accessible, enabling it to interact with molecules such as certain complement components. [Part (a) from E. W. Silverton et al., 1977, *Proc. Nat. Acad. Sci. USA* **74**:5140.]

three light-chain HV regions are located on the loops that connect the β strands of the V_H and V_L domains (see Figure 5-6, *right*). The wide range of specificities exhibited by antibodies is a function of variations in the length and amino acid composition of the six hypervariable loops in each Fab fragment. The framework region thus acts as a scaffold supporting these six loops. The framework re-gions of virtually all of the antibodies analyzed to date can be superimposed on one another; in contrast, the hy-pervariable loops (i.e., the CDRs) show different orien-tations in different antibodies. The three-dimensional structure of the immunoglobulin variable region thus provides a rigid framework, which is necessary for overall antibody function; at the same time an enormous spec-

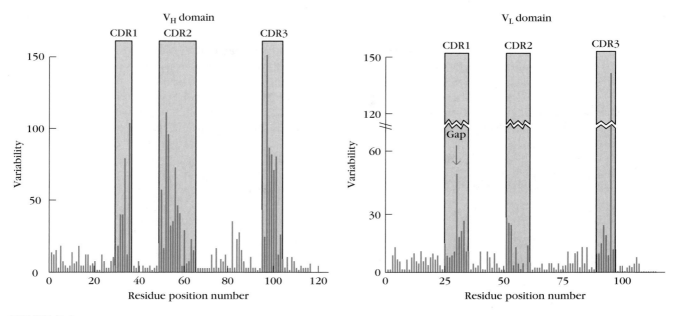

FIGURE 5-8

Relative variability of amino acid residues in the V_L and V_H domains of human antibodies with different specificities. Three hypervariable (HV) regions, also called complementarity-determining regions (CDRs), are present in both heavy- and light-chain V domains (blue). As shown in Figure 5-6 (*right*), the three HV regions in the light-chain V domain are brought into proximity in the folded structure. The same is true of the heavy-chain V domain. [Based on E. A. Kabat et al., 1977, *Sequence of Immunoglobulin Chains*, U.S. Dept. of Health, Education, and Welfare.]

trum of antigen-binding specificities is achieved by the diversity within the six CDRs.

CDRs and Antigen Binding

The earliest evidence demonstrating the role of the hypervariable regions in binding antigen was obtained by L. Wofsy, H. Metzger, and S. J. Singer using an experimental technique called **affinity labeling**. This technique used a chemically reactive hapten as a labeling reagent that could bind specifically to an antibody, forming a covalent bond with neighboring residues within the antibody's binding site. Identification of the amino acids covalently bound to the affinity label revealed that hypervariable amino acids within light- and heavy-chain CDRs constitute the antigen-binding site.

The three-dimensional structure of the antigen-binding site and the role of the CDRs in the binding of antigen have also been investigated by high-resolution x-ray crystallography. To date, crystallographic analysis has been completed for over 50 Fab fragments of monoclonal antibodies complexed either to large globular protein antigens or to a number of smaller antigens including carbohydrates, nucleic acids, peptides, and small haptens. In addition, complete x-ray pictures have recently been obtained for several intact monoclonal antibodies.

The results of these crystallographic studies have provided valuable insights into the structure of the V_H and V_L domains and the interactions between antigen and antibody. As discussed in the previous chapter, a large globular protein antigen contacts the antibody molecule across a rather flat, undulating face (see Figure 4-6). In the area of contact, protrusions or depressions on the antigen are matched by complementary depressions or protrusions on the respective antibody. The surface area of this large complementary face ranges from about 650 $Å^2$ to more than 900 $Å^2$ in the antibody; within this area some 15–22 amino acids in the antibody contact a similar number of residues in the protein antigen (see Figure 4-3). In antibodies that bind smaller antigens (e.g., the hapten phosphocholine or the octapeptide hormone angiotensin II), the antigen-binding site is generally smaller and appears more like a deep pocket in which the ligand is largely buried (see Figures 4-2 and 4-4).

Computer analysis of x-ray crystallographic data for various antigen-Fab complexes yields the values for contact-area parameters shown in Table 5-2. These values clearly illustrate the differences in the binding of small and large antigens to antibodies. In particular, 60% or more of the contact area in small antigens is "buried" within the antibody's binding site; in contrast, less than 15% of the contact area in globular protein antigens is buried.

Further analysis of antigen–Fab complexes has shown that a minimum of four of the six CDRs in a Fab fragment make contact with the antigen's epitope (Table 5-3). In the case of some antibodies, including that to angiotensin II, all six CDR loops in the Fab fragment contact the antigen (Figure 5-9). In general, more residues in the heavy-chain CDRs appear to contact antigen than in the light-chain CDRs. Thus, the V_H domain generally contributes more to antigen binding than the V_L domain (see Table 5-3, right-hand columns). The dominant role of the heavy chain in antigen binding was demonstrated in a study in which a single heavy chain specific for a glycoprotein antigen of the human immunodeficiency virus (HIV) was combined with various light chains of different antigenic specificity. All of the resulting hybrid antibodies exhibited affinity for the HIV glycoprotein antigen, indicating that the heavy chain alone was sufficient to confer specificity.

Recent experiments have shown that the framework region makes a small contribution to antigen binding and that three of the six CDRs account on average for 73% of the interactions between an antibody and anti-

TABLE 5-2

CONTACT AREA BETWEEN FAB FRAGMENTS AND ANTIGEN*

FAB	FAB CONTACT AREA ($Å^2$)	ANTIGEN	AG MOLECULAR WEIGHT (KDA)	AG CONTACT AREA ($Å^2$)	AG BURIED CONTACT AREA ($Å^2$)	% ANTIGEN BURIED
SMALL ANTIGENS						
McPC603	161	Phosphocholine	169	169	137	81
DB3	286	Progesterone	314	277	246	89
Se155-4	297	Dodecasaccharide	1416	378	248	66
4-4-20	308	Fluoroscein	334	282	266	94
AN02	350	Dinitrophenyl spin-label	392	344	232	67
17/9	468	HA peptide	1055	742	436	59
BV04	515	d(pT)₃	932	687	454	66
B13/2	560	C-helix peptide	818	701	462	66
131	725	Angiotensin II	1046	ND	620	ND
GLOBULAR PROTEIN ANTIGENS						
D1.3	690	Lysozyme	14000	5564	680	12
HyHEL-10	721	Lysozyme	14000	5414	774	14
HyHEL-5	746	Lysozyme	14000	5436	750	14
NC41	916	Neuraminidase	50000	14638	899	6

* Contact area determined by computer analysis of x-ray crystallographic data of Fab fragments bound to their respective antigens.

KEY: Ag = antigen; HA = hemagglutinin; ND = not determined.

SOURCE: Adapted from I. A. Wilson and R. L. Stanfield, 1993, *Curr. Opin. Struc. Biol.* **3**:113.

gen. The average contributions to the overall binding interactions are as follows:

- Heavy-chain CDR3: 29%
- Heavy-chain CDR2: 23%
- Light-chain CDR3: 21%
- Heavy-chain CDR1: 10%
- Light-chain CDR1: 9%
- Light-chain CDR2: 4%
- Framework residues: 4%

As illustrated in Figure 5-9a, heavy- and light-chain CDR1s and CDR2s are positioned at the ends of the

antigen-binding site with the heavy and light CDR3s in between in the center of the site. Because of their central position, the CDR3s make the majority of contacts with the epitope. As discussed in Chapter 7, the CDR3s are also the most variable of the CDRs and therefore contribute the most to the specificity of an antibody for its antigen.

CONFORMATIONAL CHANGES INDUCED BY ANTIGEN BINDING

As more x-ray crystallographic analyses of Fab fragments were completed, it became clear that in some cases binding of antigen induces conformational changes in the

TABLE 5 - 3

HYPERVARIABLE LOOPS USED IN ANTIGEN BINDING*

FAB FRAGMENT	LIGHT CHAIN			HEAVY CHAIN			CONTRIBUTION TO AG BINDING (%)	
	CDR1	CDR2	CDR3	CDR1	CDR2	CDR3	V_L	V_H
B1312	+	−	+	+	+	+	22	78
17/9	+	−	+	−	+	+	26	74
DB3	+	−	+	+	+	+	35	65
4-4-20	+	−	+	+	+	+	40	60
Se155-4	+	−	+	+	+	+	40	60
HyHEL-5	+	+	+	+	+	+	41	59
131	+	−	+	+	+	+	41	57
BV04	+	+	+	+	+	+	43	57
HyHEL-10	+	+	+	+	+	+	43	57
D1.3	+	+	+	+	+	+	43	57
NC41	−	+	+	+	+	+	46	54
McPC603	−	−	+	+	+	+	47	53
AN02	+	+	+	−	−	+	61	39
Total	11	6	13	11	12	13		

*A + = that at least one residue in the CDR loop is involved in binding antigen; a − = that no residue in the CDR loop is involved in binding. The percentage contribution of the variable light-chain (V_L) and heavy-chain (V_H) domains to antigen binding was calculated from crystallographic data. See Table 5-2 for antigens bound by the listed Fab fragments.

SOURCE: Adapted from I. A. Wilson and R. L. Stanfield, 1993, *Curr. Opin. Struc. Biol.* **3**:113.

(a)

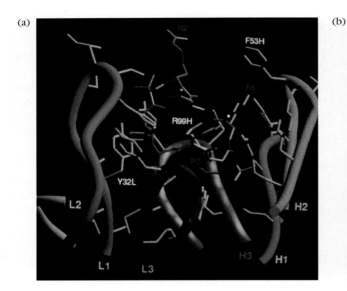

(b)

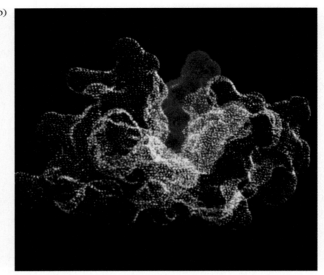

FIGURE 5-9

(a) Side view of the three-dimensional structure of the combining site of an angiotensin II–Fab complex. The peptide is in red. The three heavy-chain CDRs (H1, H2, H3) and three light-chain CDRs (L1, L2, L3) are each shown in a different color. All six CDRs contain side chains, shown in yellow, that are within van der Waals contact of the angiotensin peptide. (b) Side view of the van der Waals dot surface contact between angiotensin II and Fab fragment. [From K. C. Garcia et al., 1992, *Science* **257**:502.]

antibody, antigen, or both. Formation of the antigen-antibody complex between neuraminidase and anti-neuraminidase is accompanied by a conformational change in the orientation of side chains in both the epitope and the antigen-binding site of the antibody. This conformational change results in a closer fit between the epitope and the antibody's binding site.

In some cases more significant conformational changes have been observed in the CDRs upon antigen binding. For example, comparison of an anti-hemagglutinin Fab fragment before and after binding to a hemagglutinin peptide antigen has revealed a visible conformational change in the heavy-chain CDR3 loop following binding (Figure 5-10) and in the accessible surface of the binding site (Figure 5-11). Thus, variability in the length and amino acid composition of the hypervariable loops, coupled with significant changes in the conformation of these loops upon antigen binding, enables a given antibody to assume more effectively a structure complementary to that of the epitope.

Constant-Region Domains

The immunoglobulin constant-region domains are associated with various biological functions that are determined by the amino acid sequence of each domain.

C_H1 AND C_L DOMAINS

The C_H1 and C_L domains serve to extend the Fab arms of the antibody molecule, thereby facilitating interaction with antigen and increasing the maximum rotation of the Fab arms. These constant-region domains also help to hold the V_H and V_L domains together by virtue of the interchain disulfide bond between them (see Figure 5-3).

The C_H1 and C_L domains also may contribute to antibody diversity by allowing more random associations between V_H and V_L domains than would occur if this association were driven by the V_H/V_L interaction alone. Reassociation experiments have provided some support for this concept. For instance, when V_H and V_L domains from two antibodies having different known specificities (*a* and *b*) were prepared separately and then mixed, each domain reassociated almost exclusively with its original partner to form homogeneous V_La/V_Ha or V_Lb/V_Hb complexes. In another experiment Fab fragments from antibody *a* and antibody *b* were mildly reduced and denatured to obtain V_HC_H1 and V_LC_L fragments from each antibody. Mixing of these longer fragments yielded not only homogeneous complexes containing heavy and light chains from antibody *a* (V_LaC_La/V_HaC_H1a) or heavy and light chains from antibody *b* but also hybrid complexes with one chain from antibody *a* and one from antibody *b* (e.g., V_LaC_La/V_HbC_H1b).

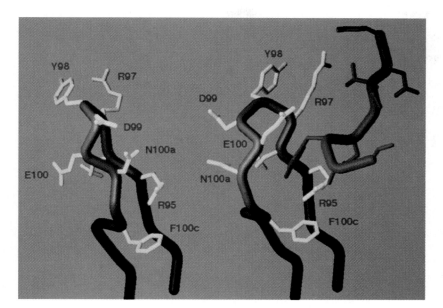

FIGURE 5-10

Model of the heavy-chain CDR3 loops in an unbound (*left*) and bound (*right*) anti-hemagglutinin Fab fragment. Note the major rearrangement in the heavy-chain CDR3 loop (green) that accompanies binding of hemagglutinin peptide (red). The side chains in the CDR3 loop are shown in yellow. [From J. M. Rini et al., 1992, *Science* **255**:959.]

As is discussed in Chapter 7, random rearrangements of the immunoglobulin genes generate unique V_H and V_L sequences for the heavy and light chains expressed by each B lymphocyte; association of the V_H and V_L sequences then generates a unique antigen-binding site. The presence of C_H1 and C_L domains appears to increase the number of stable V_H and V_L interactions that are possible, thus contributing to the overall diversity of antibody molecules that can be expressed by an animal.

HINGE REGION

The γ, δ, and α heavy chains contain an extended peptide sequence between the C_H1 and C_H2 domains that has no homology with the other domains (see Figure 5-3). This region, called the **hinge region**, is rich in proline residues and is flexible, giving IgG, IgD, and IgA segmental flexibility. As a result, the two Fab arms can assume various angles relative to each other when antigen is bound. This flexibility of the hinge region can be

(a)

(b)

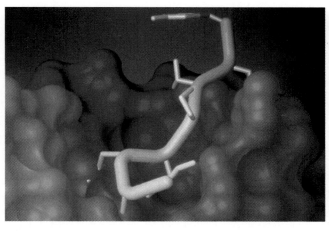

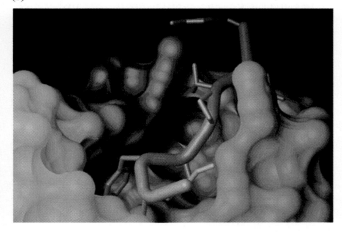

FIGURE 5-11

Model of the solvent-accessible surface of an unbound and bound anti-hemagglutinin Fab fragment showing that peptide binding is accommodated by an alteration in the shape of the antibody's binding pocket. (a) The free hemagglutinin peptide (light blue) is positioned over an open, basin-shaped pocket in the unbound Fab fragment. (b) The bound Fab fragment has a prominent channel that interacts with the extended peptide and a pocket that interacts with the tyrosine residue. [From J. M. Rini et al., 1992, *Science* **255**:959.]

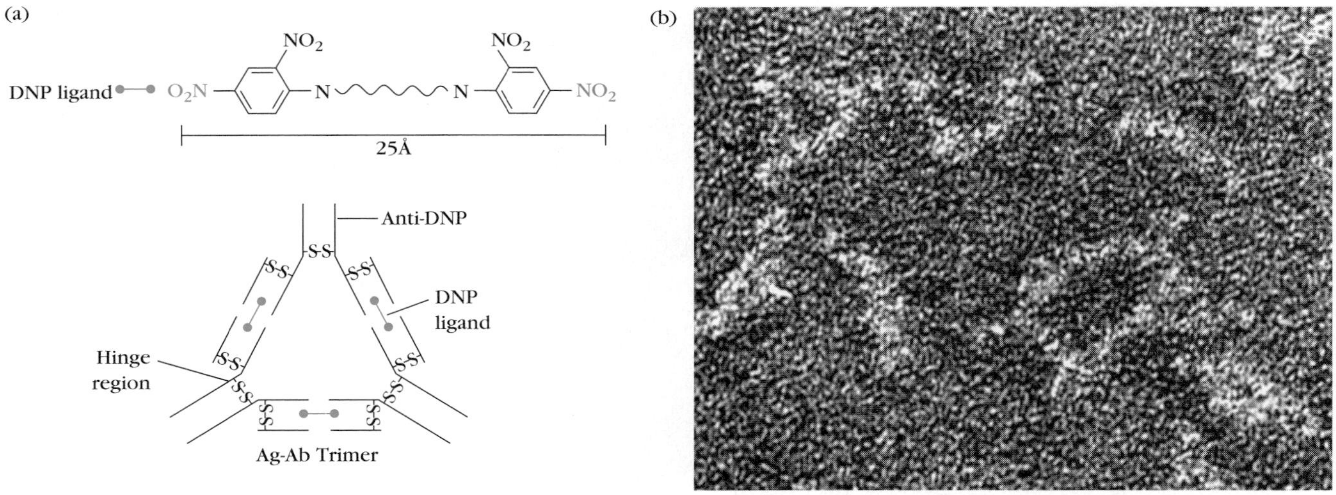

(a)

(b)

FIGURE 5-12

Experimental demonstration of the flexibility of the hinge region in antibody molecules. (a) A divalent dinitrophenol (DNP) hapten reacts with anti-DNP antibodies to form trimers, tetramers, and other larger antigen-antibody complexes. A trimer is shown schematically. (b) In an electron micrograph of a negatively stained preparation of these com-plexes, several trimers, as well as a tetramer and pentamer, are visible. The antibody protein stands out as a light structure against the electron-dense background. Because of the flexibility of the hinge region, the angle between the arms of the antibody molecules varies. [Photograph from R. C. Valentine and N. M. Green, 1967, *J. Mol. Biol.* **27**:615.]

visualized in electron micrographs of antigen-antibody complexes. For example, when a molecule containing two dinitrophenol (DNP) groups reacts with anti-DNP antibody and the complex is captured on a grid, nega-tively stained, and observed with electron microscopy, large complexes (e.g., dimers, trimers, tetramers) are seen. The angle between the arms of the Y-shaped antibody molecules varies in the different complexes, reflecting the flexibility of the hinge region (Figure 5-12).

X-ray crystallographic analysis of an entire mono-clonal antibody specific for canine lymphoma-cell mem-brane antigen has revealed that the hinge region serves as a sort of tether that allows the Fab components and the Fc to move relative to each other (see Figure 5-5). In this way the Fab arms can move and twist to align the CDRs with epitopes displayed on cell surfaces, and the Fc can move to maximize various effector functions such as complement activation or binding to cell-surface recep-tors specific for the Fc region.

Two prominent amino acids in the hinge region are proline and cysteine. The large number of proline resi-dues in the hinge region confers an extended poly-peptide conformation on it, making the hinge region particularly vulnerable to cleavage by proteolytic en-zymes; it is this region that is cleaved with papain or pepsin (see Figure 5-2). The cysteine residues form inter-chain disulfide bonds that hold the two heavy chains together. The number of interchain disulfide bonds in the hinge region varies considerably among different classes of antibodies and between species. Although μ and ε chains lack a hinge region, they have an additional 110-amino acids domain (C_H2/C_H2) that has hingelike features.

OTHER CONSTANT-REGION DOMAINS

As noted already, the heavy chains in IgE and IgM (ε and μ, respectively) contain four constant-region domains but lack a hinge region, whereas the heavy chains IgA, IgD, and IgG (α, δ, and γ, respectively) contain three constant-region domains and a hinge region. The cor-responding domains in the sequences of the two groups are as follows:

IgA, IgD, IgG	IgE, IgM
C_H1/C_H1	C_H1/C_H1
Hinge region	C_H2/C_H2
C_H2/C_H2	C_H3/C_H3
C_H3/C_H3	C_H4/C_H4

Although the C_H2/C_H2 domains in IgE and IgM occur in the same position in the polypeptide chains as the hinge region in the other classes of immunoglobu-lin, the function of this extra domain has not yet been determined.

X-ray crystallographic analyses have revealed that the two C_H2 domains of IgA, IgD, and IgG (and the C_H3 domains of IgE and IgM) are separated by oligosaccharide side chains; as a result these two globular domains are much more accessible than the other domains to the aqueous environment (see Figure 5-7). This accessibility accounts for the important biological activity of these domains in the activation of complement components by the IgG and IgM classes of antibody molecules.

The carboxyl-terminal domain is designated C_H3/C_H3 in IgA, IgD, and IgG and C_H4/C_H4 in IgE and IgM. **Secreted immunoglobulin** (sIg) has a hydrophilic amino acid sequence of varying lengths at the carboxyl-terminal end. The functions of this domain in the various classes of antibody secreted by plasma cells are discussed later.

The carboxyl-terminal domain in **membrane-bound immunoglobulin** (mIg) differs in both structure and function from the corresponding domain in secreted immunoglobulin. In mIg the carboxyl-terminal domain contains three regions:

- An extracellular hydrophilic "spacer" sequence composed of 26 amino acid residues
- A hydrophobic transmembrane sequence
- A short cytoplasmic tail

Although the length of the transmembrane sequence is constant among all immunoglobulin isotypes, the lengths of the extracellular spacer sequence and cytoplasmic tail vary.

Each of the five immunoglobulin classes and their subclasses can be expressed as membrane-bound antibody. B cells express different classes of mIg at different developmental stages. The immature B cell, called a pre-B cell, expresses only mIgM; mIgD appears later in maturation and is the predominant class on mature resting B cells. A memory B cell can express a variety of classes, including combinations of mIgM, mIgG, mIgA, and mIgE. Even when different classes are expressed on a single cell, however, the antigenic specificity of all the membrane antibody molecules is identical, so that each antibody molecule binds to the same epitope. The genetic mechanism that allows a single B cell to express multiple immunoglobulin isotypes all with the same antigenic specificity is discussed in Chapter 7.

B-CELL RECEPTOR

Immunologists have long been puzzled about how mIg mediates an activating signal after contact with an antigen. The dilemma is that all isotypes of mIg have very short cytoplasmic tails: the mIgM and mIgD cytoplasmic tails contain only 3 amino acids; the mIgA tail, 14 amino acids; and the mIgG and mIgE tails, 28 amino acids. In each case, the cytoplasmic tail is too short to be able to associate with intracellular signaling molecules (e.g., tyrosine kinases and G proteins).

The apparent answer to this puzzle is that mIg does not constitute the entire antigen-binding receptor on B cells. The **B-cell receptor** (BCR) is a transmembrane protein complex composed of mIg and a disulfide-linked heterodimer called **Ig-α/Ig-β**. It is thought that two molecules of this heterodimer associate with one mIg molecule to form a single BCR (Figure 5-13). The Ig-α chain has a long cytoplasmic tail containing 61 amino acids; the tail of the Ig-β chain contains 48 amino acids. The tails in both Ig-α and Ig-β are long enough to interact with intracellular signaling molecules. Discovery of the Ig-α/Ig-β heterodimer has substantially furthered understanding of B-cell activation, which is discussed in detail in Chapter 8.

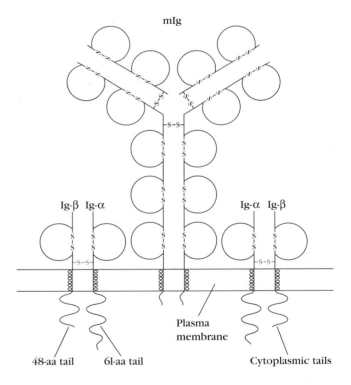

FIGURE 5-13

General structure of the B-cell receptor (BCR). This antigen-binding receptor is composed of membrane-bound immunoglobulin (mIg) and a disulfide-linked heterodimer called Ig-α/Ig-β. The heterodimer contains the immunoglobulin-fold structure and cytoplasmic tails much longer than those in mIg. As depicted, each mIg molecule is thought to be associated with two heterodimer molecules. [Adapted from A. D. Keegan and W. E. Paul, 1992, *Immunol. Today* **13**:63, and M. Reth, 1992, *Annu. Rev. Immunol.* **10**:97.]

ANTIGENIC DETERMINANTS ON IMMUNOGLOBULINS

Since antibodies are glycoproteins, they can themselves function as potent immunogens to induce an antibody response. Such anti-Ig antibodies are powerful tools for the study of B-cell development and humoral immune responses. The antigenic determinants, or epitopes, on immunoglobulin molecules fall into three major categories: **isotypic**, **allotypic**, and **idiotypic** determinants, which are located in characteristic portions of the molecule (Figure 5-14).

Isotypic Determinants

Isotypic determinants are constant-region determinants that collectively define each heavy-chain class and subclass and each light-chain type and subtype within a species (see Figure 5-14a). Each isotype is encoded by a separate constant-region gene, and all members of a species carry the same constant-region genes. Within a species, each normal individual will express all isotypes in their serum. Different species inherit different constant-region genes and therefore express different isotypes. Therefore, when an antibody from one species is injected into another species, the isotypic determinants will be recognized as foreign, inducing an antibody response to the isotypic determinants on the foreign antibody. Anti-isotype antibody is routinely used for research purposes to determine the class or subclass of serum antibody produced during an immune response or to characterize the class of membrane-bound antibody present on B cells.

Allotypic Determinants

Although all members of a species inherit the same set of isotype genes, multiple alleles exist for some of the genes (see Figure 5-14b). These alleles encode subtle amino acid differences, called allotypic determinants, that occur in some, but not all, members of a species. In humans, **allotypes** have been characterized for all four IgG subclasses, for one IgA subclass, and for the κ light chain. The γ-chain allotypes are referred to as **Gm markers**. To date, 25 different Gm allotypes have been identified; they are designated by the class and subclass followed by the allele number, for example, G1m(1), G2m(23), G3m(11), G4m(4a). Of the two IgA subclasses, only the IgA2 subclass has allotypes, designated as A2m(1) and A2m(2). The κ light chain has three allotypes, designated κm(1), κm(2), and κm(3). Each of these allotypic determinants represents differences in one to four amino acids that are encoded by different alleles.

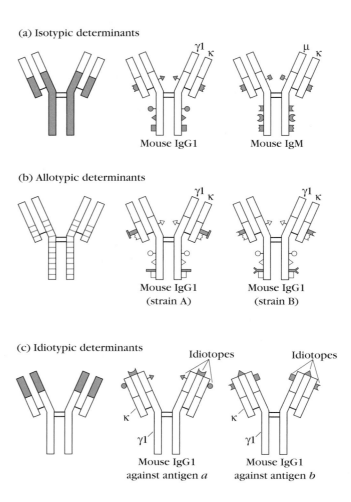

(a) Isotypic determinants

Mouse IgG1   Mouse IgM

(b) Allotypic determinants

Mouse IgG1
(strain A)   Mouse IgG1
(strain B)

(c) Idiotypic determinants

Idiotopes   Idiotopes

Mouse IgG1
against antigen *a*   Mouse IgG1
against antigen *b*

FIGURE 5-14

Antigenic determinants of immunoglobulins. For each type of determinant, the general location of determinants within the antibody molecule is shown (*left*) and two examples are illustrated (*center* and *right*). (a) Isotypic determinants are constant-region determinants that distinguish each Ig class and subclass within a species. (b) Allotypic determinants are subtle amino acid differences encoded by different alleles of isotype genes. Allotypic differences can be detected by comparing the same antibody class among different inbred strains. (c) Idiotypic determinants are generated by the conformation of the amino acid sequences of the heavy- and light-chain variable region specific for each antigen. Each individual determinant is called an idiotope, and the sum of the individual idiotopes is the idiotype.

Antibody to allotypic determinants can be produced by injecting antibodies from one member of a species into another member of the same species who carries different allotypic determinants. Antibody to allotypic determinants sometimes is produced by a mother during pregnancy in response to paternal allotypic determinants on the fetal immunoglobulins. Antibodies to allotypic determinants can also arise following a blood transfusion.

Idiotypic Determinants

The unique amino acid sequence of the V_H and V_L domains of a given antibody can function not only as an antigen-binding site but also as an antigenic determinant. The idiotypic determinants are generated by the conformation of the heavy- and light-chain variable regions. Each individual antigenic determinant of the variable region is referred to as an **idiotope** (see Figure 5-14c). In some cases an idiotope may be the actual antigen-binding site, and in some cases an idiotope may comprise variable-region sequences outside of the antigen-binding site. Each antibody will present multiple idiotopes; the sum of the individual idiotopes is called the **idiotype** of the antibody.

Because the antibodies produced by individual B cells derived from the same clone have identical variable-region sequences, they all have the same idiotype. Anti-idiotype antibody is produced by minimizing isotypic or allotypic differences, so that the idiotypic difference can be recognized. Often a homogeneous antibody such as myeloma protein or monoclonal antibody is used. Injection of such an antibody into a syngeneic recipient will result in the formation of anti-idiotype antibody to the idiotypic determinants. According to one theory, anti-idiotype antibody produced naturally during the course of an immune response plays an important role in regulating the immune response; this phenomenon is discussed in Chapter 16.

IMMUNOGLOBULIN CLASSES

The various immunoglobulin classes, or isotypes, have been mentioned briefly already. In this section, the structure and effector functions of each class are discussed in more detail. Each class is distinguished by unique amino acid sequences in the heavy-chain constant region that confer class-specific structural and functional properties. The structures of the five major classes are diagrammed in Figure 5-15. The molecular properties and biological activities of the immunoglobulin classes are listed in Table 5-4. The effector functions of each class results from interactions between its heavy-chain constant regions and other serum proteins or cell-membrane receptors.

Immunoglobulin G (IgG)

IgG, the most abundant class in serum, constitutes about 80% of the total serum immunoglobulin. The IgG molecule is a monomer consisting of two γ heavy chains and two κ or two λ light chains. There are four IgG subclasses in humans, numbered in accordance with their decreas-ing average serum concentrations: IgG1 (9 mg/ml), IgG2 (3 mg/ml), IgG3 (1 mg/ml), and IgG4 (0.5 mg/ml).

The four IgG subclasses are encoded by different germ-line C_H genes whose DNA sequences are 90%–95% homologous. The structural characteristics that distinguish these subclasses from one another are the size of the hinge region and the number and position of the interchain disulfide bonds between the heavy chains (Figure 5-16). The subtle amino acid differences between subclasses of IgG affect the biological activity of the molecule:

- IgG1, IgG3, and IgG4 readily cross the placenta and play an important role in protecting the developing fetus.
- IgG3 is the most effective complement activator, followed by IgG1; IgG2 is relatively inefficient at complement activation, and IgG4 is not able to activate complement at all.
- IgG1 and IgG3 bind with a high affinity to **Fc receptors** on phagocytic cells; IgG4 has an intermediate affinity, and IgG2 has an extremely low affinity. Fc binding permits IgG to function as an opsonin.

Immunoglobulin M (IgM)

IgM accounts for 5%–10% of the total serum immunoglobulin with an average serum concentration of 1.5 mg/ml. Monomeric IgM, with a molecular weight of 180,000, is expressed as membrane-bound antibody on B cells. IgM is secreted by plasma cells as a pentamer in which five monomer units are held together by disulfide bonds linking their carboxyl-terminal ($C_\mu4/C_\mu4$) domains and $C_\mu3/C_\mu3$ domains (see Figure 5-15e). The five monomer subunits are arranged with their Fc regions in the center of the pentamer and the 10 antigen-binding sites on the periphery of the molecule. Each pentamer contains an additional Fc-linked polypeptide called the **J (joining) chain**, which is disulfide-bonded to the carboxyl-terminal cysteine residue of 2 of the 10 μ chains. The J chain appears to be required for polymerization of the monomers to form pentameric IgM; it is added just before secretion of the pentamer.

IgM is the first immunoglobulin class produced in a primary response to an antigen, and it is also the first immunoglobulin to be synthesized by the neonate. Because of its pentameric structure with 10 antigen-binding sites, serum IgM has a higher **valency** than the other isotypes. An IgM molecule can bind 10 small hapten molecules; however, because of steric hindrance, only 5 molecules of larger antigens can be bound simultaneously. Because of its high valency, pentameric IgM is more efficient than other isotypes in binding such

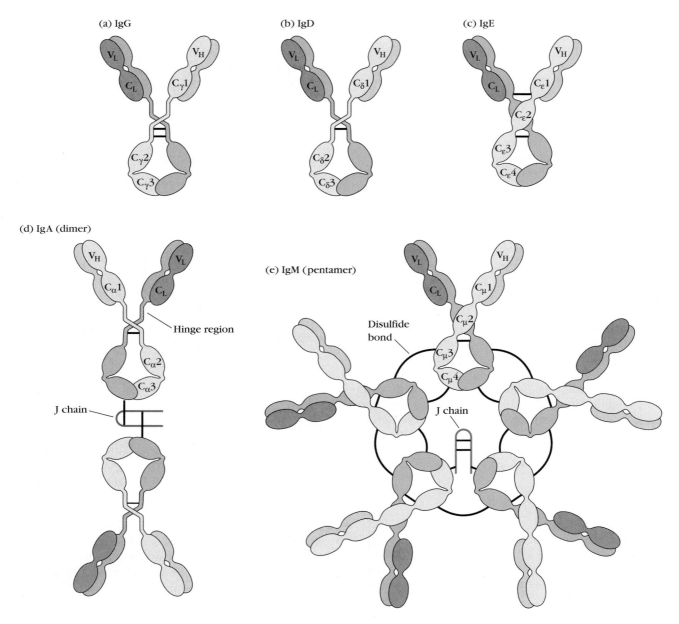

(a) IgG

V$_L$ C$_L$ V$_H$ C$_\gamma$1 C$_\gamma$2 C$_\gamma$3

(b) IgD

V$_L$ C$_L$ V$_H$ C$_\delta$1 C$_\delta$2 C$_\delta$3

(c) IgE

V$_L$ C$_L$ V$_H$ C$_\varepsilon$1 C$_\varepsilon$2 C$_\varepsilon$3 C$_\varepsilon$4

(d) IgA (dimer)

V$_H$ C$_\alpha$1 V$_L$ C$_L$ Hinge region C$_\alpha$2 C$_\alpha$3 J chain

(e) IgM (pentamer)

V$_L$ C$_L$ V$_H$ C$_\mu$1 C$_\mu$2 C$_\mu$3 C$_\mu$4 Disulfide bond J chain

FIGURE 5-15

General structures of the five major classes of secreted antibody. Light chains are shown in shades of gray and heavy chains in shades of blue; disulfide bonds are indicated by thick black lines. Note that the IgG, IgA, and IgD heavy chains contain four domains and a hinge region, whereas the IgM and IgE heavy chains contain five domains but no hinge region. The polymeric forms of IgM and IgA contain a polypeptide, known as the J chain, that is linked by two disulfide bonds to the Fc region in two different monomers. Serum IgM is always a pentamer; most serum IgA exists as a monomer, although some dimers, trimers, and even tetramers sometimes are present. Not shown in these figures are intrachain disulfide bonds and disulfide bonds linking light and heavy chains (see Figure 5-3).

multidimensional antigens as viral particles and red blood cells (RBCs). For example, when RBCs are incubated with specific antibody, they clump together into large aggregates in a process called **agglutination**. It takes 100 to 1000 times more molecules of IgG than of IgM to achieve the same level of agglutination. A similar phenomenon occurs with viral particles: less IgM than IgG is required to neutralize viral infectivity. IgM is also more efficient than IgG at complement activation. Complement activation requires two Fc regions in close proximity, and the pentameric structure of a single molecule of IgM fulfills this requirement.

Because of its large size, IgM does not diffuse well and therefore is found in very low concentrations in the intercellular tissue fluids. The presence of the J chain allows IgM to bind to receptors on secretory cells, which transport it across epithelial linings to the external secretions that bathe mucosal surfaces. Although IgA is the major isotype found in these secretions, IgM plays an important accessory role as a secretory immunoglobulin.

Immunoglobulin A (IgA)

Although IgA constitutes only 10%–15% of the total immunoglobulin in serum, it is the predominant immunoglobulin class in external secretions such as breast milk, saliva, tears, and mucus of the bronchial, genitourinary, and digestive tracts. In serum, IgA exists primarily as a monomer, although polymeric forms such as dimers, trimers, and even tetramers are sometimes seen. The IgA of external secretions, called **secretory IgA**, consists of a dimer or tetramer, a J-chain polypeptide,

T A B L E   5 – 4

PROPERTIES AND BIOLOGICAL ACTIVITIES*
OF CLASSES AND SUBCLASSES OF HUMAN SERUM IMMUNOGLOBULINS

PROPERTY/ACTIVITY	IgG1	IgG2	IgG3	IgG4	IgA1	IgA2	IgM‡	IgE	IgD
Molecular weight†	150,000	150,000	150,000	150,000	150,000–600,000	150,000–600,000	900,000	190,000	150,000
Heavy-chain component	$\gamma1$	$\gamma2$	$\gamma3$	$\gamma4$	$\alpha1$	$\alpha2$	μ	ε	δ
Normal serum level (mg/ml)	9	3	1	0.5	3.0	0.5	1.5	0.0003	0.03
In vivo serum half life (days)	23	23	8	23	6	6	5	2.5	3
Activates classical complement pathway	+	+/–	++	–	–	–	+++	–	–
Crosses placenta	+	+/–	+	+	–	–	–	–	–
Present on membrane of mature B cells	–	–	–	–	–	–	+	–	+
Binds to macrophage Fc receptors	++	+/–	++	+	–	–	+	–	–
Present in secretions	–	–	–	–	++	++	+	–	–
Induces mast-cell degranulation	–	–	–	–	–	–	–	+	–

* Activity levels indicated as follows: ++ = high, + = moderate; +/– = minimal; and – = none.

† IgG, IgE, and IgD always exist as monomers; IgA can exist as a monomer, dimer, trimer, or tetramer. Membrane-bound IgM is a monomer, but secreted IgM in serum is a pentamer.

‡ IgM is the first isotype produced by the neonate and during a primary immune response.

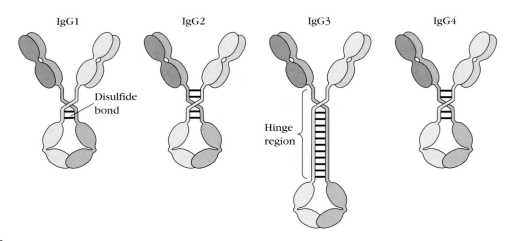

FIGURE 5-16

General structure of the four subclasses of human IgG, which differ in the number and arrangement of the interchain disulfide bonds (thick black lines) linking the heavy chains. The hinge region in IgG3 is four times as long as the hinge region in the other IgG subclasses and contains 11 interchain disulfide bonds.

and a polypeptide chain called **secretory component** (Figure 5-17a). The J-chain polypeptide is identical to that found in pentameric IgM and serves a similar function in facilitating the polymerization of both serum IgA and secretory IgA. The secretory component is a 70,000-MW polypeptide produced by epithelial cells of mucous membranes. It consists of five immunoglobulin-like domains that bind to the Fc region domains of the IgA dimer. This interaction is stabilized by a disulfide bond between the fifth domain of the secretory component and one of the chains of the dimeric IgA.

Surprisingly, daily production of secretory IgA is greater than that of any other immunoglobulin class. IgA-secreting plasma cells are concentrated along mucous membrane surfaces. Along the jejunum of the small intestines, for example, there are more than 2.5×10^{10} IgA-secreting plasma cells—a number that surpasses the total plasma cells of the bone marrow, lymph, and spleen combined! Each day humans secrete 5–15 g of secretory IgA into mucous secretions.

The plasma cells that produce IgA preferentially migrate (home) to subepithelial tissue, where the secreted IgA binds tightly to a receptor for polymeric immunoglobulin molecules (Figure 5-17b). This **poly-Ig receptor** is expressed on the basolateral surface of most mucosal epithelia (e.g., the lining of the digestive, respiratory, and genital tracts) and on glandular epithelia in the mammary, salivary, and lacrimal glands. After polymeric IgA binds to the poly-Ig receptor, the receptor-IgA complex is transported across the epithelial barrier to the lumen. Transport of the poly-Ig receptor/IgA complex involves receptor-mediated endocytosis into coated pits and directed transport of the vesicle across the

epithelial cell to the luminal membrane, where the vesicle fuses with the plasma membrane. The poly-Ig receptor is then cleaved enzymatically from the membrane and becomes the secretory component, which is bound to and released together with polymeric IgA into the mucous secretions. The secretory component masks sites susceptible to protease cleavage in the hinge region of secretory IgA, allowing the polymeric molecule to exist for a longer period of time in the protease-rich mucosal environment than would be possible otherwise. Pentameric IgM is also transported into mucous secretions by this mechanism, although it accounts for a much lower percentage of antibody in the mucous secretions than does IgA. It is thought that the poly-Ig receptor recognizes the J chain associated with both polymeric IgA and IgM antibodies.

Secretory IgA serves an important effector function at mucous membrane surfaces, which are the main entry sites for most pathogenic organisms. Because it is polymeric, secretory IgA can cross-link large antigens with multiple epitopes. Binding of secretory IgA to bacterial and viral surface antigens prevents attachment of the pathogens to the mucosal cells. Once attachment is blocked, viral infection and bacterial colonization are inhibited. Complexes of secretory IgA and antigen are easily entrapped in mucous and then eliminated by the ciliated epithelial cells of the respiratory tract or by peristalsis of the gut. Secretory IgA has been shown to provide an important line of defense against bacteria such as *Salmonella, Vibrio cholerae, Neisseria gonorrhoeae,* and viruses such as polio, influenza, and reovirus.

Breast milk contains several types of leukocytes, secretory IgA, and many other molecules that help protect

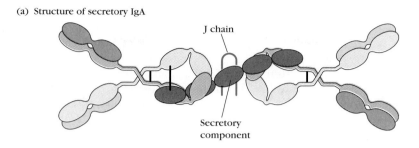

(a) Structure of secretory IgA

J chain

Secretory
component

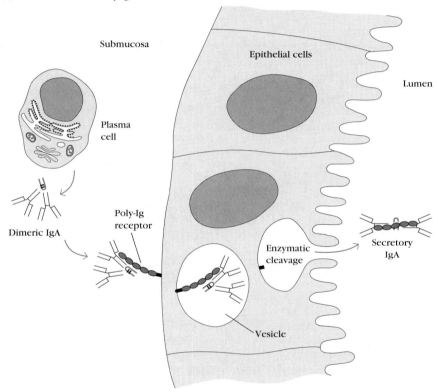

(b) Formation of secretory IgA

Submucosa

Epithelial cells

Lumen

Plasma
cell

Poly-Ig
receptor

Dimeric IgA

Enzymatic
cleavage

Secretory
IgA

Vesicle

FIGURE 5-17

Structure and formation of secretory IgA. (a) Secretory IgA consists of at least two IgA molecules, which are covalently linked via a J chain and covalently associated with the secretory component. The secretory component contains five Ig-like domains and is linked to dimeric IgA by a disulfide bond between its fifth domain and one of the IgA heavy chains. (b) Secretory IgA is formed during transport through mucous membrane epithelial cells. Dimeric IgA binds to a poly-Ig receptor on the basolateral membrane of an epithelial cell and is internalized by receptor-mediated endocytosis. After transport of the receptor-IgA complex to the luminal surface, the poly-Ig receptor is enzymatically cleaved, releasing the secretory component bound to the dimeric IgA.

the newborn against infection during the first month of life (Table 5-5). Because the immune system of infants is not fully functional, breast-feeding plays an important role in maintaining the health of newborns.

Immunoglobulin E (IgE)

The potent biological activity of IgE allowed it to be identified in serum despite its extremely low average serum concentration (0.3 μg/ml). IgE antibodies mediate the immediate hypersensitivity reactions that are responsible for the symptoms of hay fever, asthma, hives, and anaphylactic shock. The presence of a serum component responsible for allergic reactions was first demonstrated in 1921 by K. Prausnitz and H. Kustner, who injected serum from an allergic person intradermally into a non-allergic individual. When the appropriate antigen was later injected at the site of injection, a wheal and flare reaction (analogous to hives) developed there. This reaction, called the **P-K reaction**, was the basis for the earliest biological assay for IgE activity.

Actual identification of IgE was accomplished by K. and T. Ishizaka in 1966. They obtained serum from an allergic individual and immunized rabbits with it to prepare anti-isotype antiserum. The rabbit antiserum was then allowed to react with each class of human antibody known at that time (i.e., IgG, IgA, IgM, and IgD). In this way, each of the known anti-isotype antibodies was precipitated and removed from the rabbit anti-serum. What remained was an anti-isotype antibody specific for an unidentified class of antibody. This anti-isotype antibody turned out to completely block the P-K reaction.

T A B L E   5 – 5

IMMUNE BENEFITS OF BREAST MILK

COMPONENT	ACTION
WHITE BLOOD CELLS	
B cells	Give rise to antibodies targeted against specific microbes.
Macrophages	Kill microbes outright in the baby's gut, produce lysozyme and activate other components of the immune system.
Neutrophils	May act as phagocytes, ingesting bacteria in baby's digestive system.
T cells	Kill infected cells directly or send out chemical messages to mobilize other defenses. They proliferate in the presence of organisms that cause serious illness in infants. They also manufacture compounds that can strengthen a child's own immune response.
MOLECULES	
Antibodies of secretory IgA class	Bind to microbes in baby's digestive tract and thereby prevent them from passing through walls of the gut into body's tissues.
B_{12} binding protein	Reduces amount of vitamin B_{12}, which bacteria need in order to grow.
Bifidus factor	Promotes growth of *Lactobacillus bifidus,* a harmless bacterium, in baby's gut. Growth of such nonpathogenic bacteria helps to crowd out dangerous varieties.
Fatty acids	Disrupt membranes surrounding certain viruses and destroy them.
Fibronectin	Increases antimicrobial activity of macrophages; helps to repair tissues that have been damaged by immune reactions in baby's gut.
Hormones and growth factors	Stimulate baby's digestive tract to mature more quickly. Once the initially "leaky" membranes lining the gut mature, infants become less vulnerable to microorganisms.
Interferon (IFN-γ)	Enhances antimicrobial activity of immune cells.
Lactoferrin	Binds to iron, a mineral many bacteria need to survive. By reducing the available amount of iron, lactoferrin thwarts growth of pathogenic bacteria.
Lysozyme	Kills bacteria by disrupting their cell walls.
Mucins	Adhere to bacteria and viruses, thus keeping such microorganisms from attaching to mucosal surfaces.
Oligosaccharides	Bind to microorganisms and bar them from attaching to mucosal surfaces.

SOURCE: J. Newman, 1995, How breast milk protects newborns. *Sci. Am.* 273(**6**): 76.

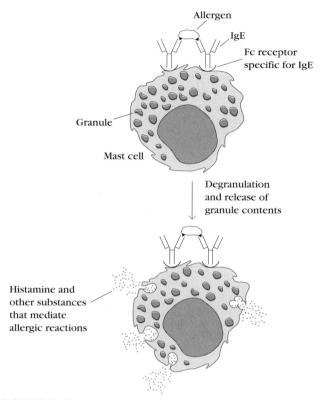

FIGURE 5-18

Allergen cross-linkage of receptor-bound IgE on mast cells induces degranulation, causing release of substances (blue dots) that mediate allergic manifestations.

The new antibody was called IgE (in reference to the E antigen of ragweed pollen, which is a potent inducer of this class of antibody).

IgE binds to Fc receptors on the membranes of blood basophils and tissue mast cells. Cross-linkage of receptor-bound IgE molecules by antigen (**allergen**) induces degranulation of basophils and mast cells; as a result, a variety of pharmacologically active mediators present in the granules are released, giving rise to allergic manifestations (Figure 5-18). Localized mast-cell degranulation induced by IgE also may release mediators that facilitate a buildup of various cells necessary for antiparasitic defense (see Chapter 19).

Immunoglobulin D (IgD)

IgD was first discovered when a patient developed a multiple myeloma whose myeloma protein failed to react with anti-isotype antisera against the then-known isotypes: IgA, IgM, and IgG. When rabbits were immunized with this myeloma protein, the resulting antisera identified this same class of antibody at low levels in normal human serum. This new class, called IgD, has a serum concentration of 30 μg/ml and constitutes about 0.2%

of the total immunoglobulin in serum. IgD, together with IgM, is the major membrane-bound immunoglobulin expressed by mature B cells, and it is thought to function in the activation of B cells by antigen. No biological effector function has been identified for IgD.

THE IMMUNOGLOBULIN SUPERFAMILY

The structures of the various immunoglobulin heavy and light chains described earlier share several features, suggesting that they have a common evolutionary ancestry. In particular, all heavy- and light-chain classes have the immunoglobulin-fold domain structure (see Figures 5-3b and 5-6). The presence of this characteristic structure in all immunoglobulin heavy and light chains suggests that the genes encoding them arose from a common primordial gene encoding a polypeptide of about 110 amino acids. Gene duplication and later divergence could then have generated the various heavy- and light-chain genes.

Large numbers of membrane proteins have been shown to possess one or more regions homologous to an immunoglobulin domain. Each of these membrane proteins is classified as a member of the **immunoglobulin superfamily**. The term *superfamily* is used to denote proteins whose corresponding genes derived from a common primordial gene encoding the basic domain structure. These genes have evolved independently and do not share genetic linkage or function. The following proteins, in addition to the immunoglobulins themselves, are members of the immunoglobulin superfamily (Figure 5-19):

- Ig-α/Ig-β heterodimer, part of the B-cell receptor
- Poly-Ig receptor, which contributes the secretory component to secretory IgA and IgM
- T-cell receptor
- T-cell accessory proteins including CD2, CD4, CD8, CD28, and the γ, δ, and ε chains of CD3
- Class I and class II MHC molecules
- β_2-microglobulin, an invariant protein associated with class I MHC molecules
- Various cell-adhesion molecules including VCAM-1, ICAM-1, ICAM-2, and LFA-3
- Platelet-derived growth factor

Numerous other proteins, some of them discussed in other chapters, belong to the immunoglobulin superfamily.

X-ray crystallographic analysis has not been accomplished for most members of the immunoglobulin superfamily. Nonetheless, the primary amino acid sequence of these proteins suggests that they all contain typical

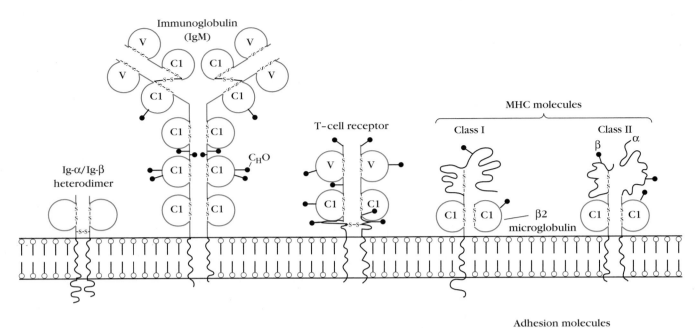

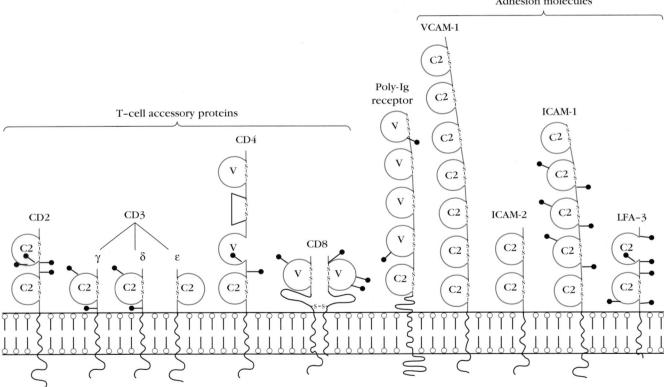

FIGURE 5-19

Some members of the immunoglobulin superfamily, a group of struc-turally related, usually membrane-bound glycoproteins. The loops shown in blue represent those portions of the molecule with the characteristic Ig-fold structure. In all cases the carboxyl-terminal end of the molecule is anchored in the membrane. Domains labeled C2 are shorter than the classical immunoglobulin constant-region domain (labeled C1) and exhibit equal homology with both variable- and constant-region domains.

immunoglobulin-fold domains consisting of about 110 amino acids, arranged in pleated sheets of antiparallel β strands, usually with an invariant intrachain disulfide bond spanning 50–70 residues.

Most members of the immunoglobulin superfamily cannot bind antigen. Thus, the characteristic Ig-fold structure found in so many membrane proteins must have some function other than antigen binding. One possibility is that the immunoglobulin fold may facilitate interactions between membrane proteins. As discussed earlier, interactions can occur between the faces of β pleated sheets in homologous immunoglobulin domains (e.g., C_H2/C_H2 interaction) and those in nonhomologous domains (e.g., V_H/V_L and C_H1/C_L interactions). The observed associations between some members of the Ig superfamily may depend on similar interactions between nonhomologous Ig-fold domains such as the following:

- CD4 and a class II MHC molecule
- CD8 and a class I MHC molecule
- T-cell receptor and either a class I or class II MHC molecule
- Poly-Ig receptor and polymeric IgA or IgM
- Ig-α/Ig-β heterodimer and membrane-bound immunoglobulin on B cells

MONOCLONAL ANTIBODIES

As noted in Chapter 4, most antigens possess multiple epitopes and therefore induce proliferation and differentiation of a variety of B-cell clones. The resulting serum antibodies are heterogeneous, comprising a mixture of antibodies each specific for one epitope (Figure 5-20). Such a **polyclonal** antibody response facilitates the localization, phagocytosis, and complement-mediated lysis of antigen; it thus has clear advantages for the organism in vivo. Unfortunately, the antibody heterogeneity that increases immune protection in vivo often reduces the efficacy of an antiserum for various in vitro uses. For most research, diagnostic, and therapeutic purposes, **monoclonal antibodies**, derived from a single clone and thus specific for a single epitope, are preferable.

Direct biochemical purification of a monoclonal antibody from a polyclonal antibody preparation is not feasible. In 1975, Georges Köhler and Cesar Milstein devised a method for preparing monoclonal antibody, which was described briefly in Chapter 2. By fusing a normal activated, antibody-producing B cell with a myeloma cell (a cancerous plasma cell), they were able to generate a hybrid cell, called a **hybridoma**, that possessed the immortal-growth properties of the myeloma cell and

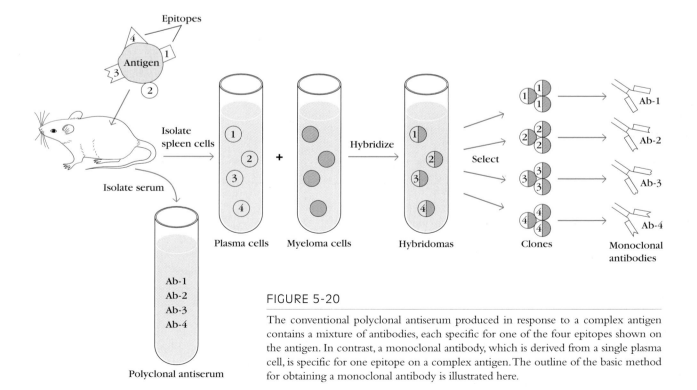

FIGURE 5-20

The conventional polyclonal antiserum produced in response to a complex antigen contains a mixture of antibodies, each specific for one of the four epitopes shown on the antigen. In contrast, a monoclonal antibody, which is derived from a single plasma cell, is specific for one epitope on a complex antigen. The outline of the basic method for obtaining a monoclonal antibody is illustrated here.

secreted the antibody produced by the B cell (see Figure 5-20). The resulting clones of hybridoma cells, which secrete large quantities of monoclonal antibody, can be cultured indefinitely. The development of techniques for producing monoclonal antibody gave immunologists (and molecular biologists in general) a powerful and versatile research tool. The significance of the work by Köhler and Milstein was acknowledged when each was awarded a Nobel Prize in 1984.

Formation and Selection of Hybrid Cells

Since the early 1970s it has been possible to fuse one somatic cell with another to form a hybrid cell called a **heterokaryon**. Fusion can be achieved by incubating a suspension of two cell types with an inactivated enveloped virus called Sendai virus or with polyethylene glycol, both of which promote the fusion of plasma membranes. In this way the plasma membranes, cytoplasm, and nuclei of two separate cells are brought together into a single hybrid cell. Initially A heterokaryon is multinucleated, having two to five separate nuclei. In the course of cell division the nuclear membranes disintegrate, and a single large nucleus is formed containing the chromosomes of both parent cells. At this stage the hybrid cell is unstable, and as it continues to divide, it loses a variable number of chromosomes from one or both parent cells until the fused cell stabilizes. Sometimes this random chromosome loss results in loss of a chromosome that is necessary for cell survival, and these hybrids die off (see Figure 2-2).

Only a small percentage of the cells actually fuse, and some of the fused cells are homogeneous parent cells, A–A or B–B, rather than the desired A–B hybrid. Thus, the A–B hybrid cells must be separated from unfused parent cells as well as from the homogeneous fused cells. One common method of selecting for the A-B hybrid cells requires the use of parent cells that are deficient (by mutation) for one of the nucleotide synthesis pathways. The fused cells are then grown in **HAT medium** (named for its three components—**h**ypoxanthine, **a**minopterin, and **t**hymidine) in which neither of the parent cells can survive, but the A-B fusion cells can.

HAT selection depends on the fact that mammalian cells can synthesize nucleotides by two different pathways: the **de novo** and the **salvage pathways** (Figure 5-21). The de novo pathway, in which a methyl or formyl group is transferred from an activated form of tetrahydrofolate, is blocked by **aminopterin**, a folic acid analog. When the de novo pathway is blocked, cells utilize the salvage pathway, which bypasses the aminopterin block by converting purines and pyrimidines directly into DNA. The enzymes catalyzing the salvage pathway include hypoxanthine-guanine phosphoribosyl transferase (HGPRT) and thymidine kinase (TK). A mutation in either of these two enzymes blocks the salvage pathway. HAT medium contains aminopterin to block the de novo pathway and hypoxanthine and thymidine to allow growth via the salvage pathway. When two types of cells, one with a mutation in TK and the other with a mutation in HGPRT, are fused, only the hybrid cells will contain the full complement of necessary enzymes for growth on HAT medium via the salvage pathway. Thus only hybrid cells will grow in HAT medium; unfused cells and homogeneous heterokaryons will not survive.

Production of Monoclonal Antibodies

The production of a given monoclonal antibody involves three basic steps:

1. Generating B-cell hybridomas by fusing antigen-primed B cells and myeloma cells and selecting for fused clones
2. Screening the resulting clones for those that secrete antibody with the desired antigenic specificity
3. Propagating the desired hydridomas

In their innovative method for producing monoclonal antibodies, Köhler and Milstein applied the techniques of cell fusion and HAT selection of hybrid cells to gen-

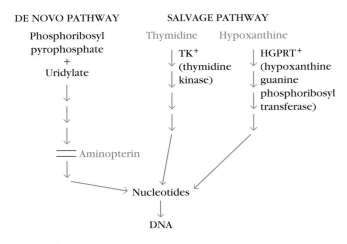

FIGURE 5-21

Aminopterin blocks DNA synthesis by the de novo pathway. It acts as an analog of dihydrofolic acid and binds with a high affinity to dihydrofolate reductase inhibiting purine synthesis. In the presence of aminopterin, cells must use the salvage pathway to produce DNA.

erate B-cell hybridomas. The general procedure is outlined in Figure 5-22.

Myeloma cells that are both HGPRT⁻ and Ig⁻ are used as one fusion partner. These cells, which contribute immortal-growth properties to the fused cells, cannot grow in HAT medium or secrete antibody. The other fusion partner is made up of spleen cells, which contain primed B cells that are HGPRT⁺ and Ig⁺. Because unfused spleen cells are terminally differentiated cells and thus only capable of limited growth in vitro, they do not need to carry a selection gene.

After the cell fusion step, aliquots are cultured in wells containing HAT medium. After 7–10 days, most of the wells contain dead cells, but a few wells contain small clusters of viable cells, which can be visualized by using an inverted phase contrast microscope. Each cluster represents clonal expansion of a hybridoma. Single cells from these clusters are transferred and cultured in separate wells in an effort to ensure the monoclonality of any secreted antibody. Subclones derived from single cells are then screened for the presence of antibody in the supernatant; antibody-positive clones are subcultured at low cell densities, again to ensure clonal purity in each microwell.

Once pure clones of antibody-secreting hybridomas are obtained, they must be screened for the desired antigenic specificity. Although some hybridomas will produce antibody specific for the antigen used for immunization, others will be specific for unwanted antigens. The supernatant of each hybridoma culture contains its secreted antibody and can be assayed for a particular antigenic specificity in various ways. Two of the most common screening techniques are ELISA and RIA, which are described in Chapter 6.

Following identification of a hybridoma secreting a monoclonal antibody of the desired specificity, the hybridoma is recloned by limiting dilution to ensure that the culture is truly monoclonal. The cloned hybridoma can then be propagated in one of several ways to produce the desired monoclonal antibody. When a hybridoma is grown in tissue-culture flasks, the antibody is secreted into the medium at fairly low concentrations (10–100 µg/ml). A hybridoma can also be propagated in the peritoneal cavity of histocompatible mice, where it secretes the monoclonal antibody into the ascites fluid at much higher concentrations (1–25 mg/ml); the antibody can be purified from the mouse ascites fluid by chromatography. To meet the increased demand for monoclonal antibodies, several techniques for obtaining increased yields from hybridomas have been developed.

The production of human monoclonal antibodies has been hampered by a number of technical difficulties. First and foremost is the difficulty of obtaining antigen-primed B cells in humans (equivalent to the mouse spleen cells shown in Figure 5-22). Human hybridomas must be prepared from human peripheral blood, which contains few activated B cells engaged in an immune response. It is possible to obtain B cells primed to the antigens in accepted vaccines, but human volunteers cannot be immunized with the range of antigens that can be given to mice or other animals. To overcome this difficulty, cultured human cells are sometimes primed with antigen in vitro. However, the in vitro system cannot mimic the normal microenvironment of lymphoid tissue; as a result the B cells usually produce only low-affinity IgM antibody.

One way to avoid the need for in vitro priming of human B cells is to incorporate genes encoding human antibody within mice. **SCID-human mice**, for example, contain human B and T cells (see Figure 2-1). Following immunization of these mice, activated human B cells can be isolated from the spleen and used to produce human monoclonal antibodies. Using another approach, GenPharm International has knocked out the heavy- and light-chain genes within mice and then introduced yeast artificial chromosomes engineered with large DNA sequences containing human heavy- and light-chain genes. The resulting transgenic mice produce human antibodies exclusively.

Another major difficulty in producing human monoclonal antibodies by the procedure outlined in Figure 5-22 has been the lack of human myeloma cells that exhibit immortal growth, are susceptible to HAT selection, and do not secrete antibody. As an alternative to conferring immortality on human B cells through fusion to myeloma cells, normal human B lymphocytes can be transformed with Epstein-Barr virus (EBV). When lymphocytes are cultured with antigen in the presence of EBV, some of the B cells acquire the immortal-growth properties of a transformed cell while continuing to secrete antibody. Cloning of such primed, transformed cells has permitted production of human monoclonal antibody.

Clinical Uses for Monoclonal Antibodies

Monoclonal antibodies are proving to be very useful as diagnostic, imaging, and therapeutic reagents in clinical medicine. Initially, monoclonal antibodies were used primarily as in vitro diagnostic reagents. Among the many monoclonal antibody diagnostic reagents now available are products for detecting pregnancy, diagnosing numerous pathogenic microorganisms, measuring the blood levels of various drugs, matching histocompatibility antigens, and detecting antigens shed by certain tumors.

Radiolabeled monoclonal antibodies can also be used in vivo for detecting tumor antigens, permitting earlier diagnosis of some primary or metastatic tumors in

Visualizing Concepts

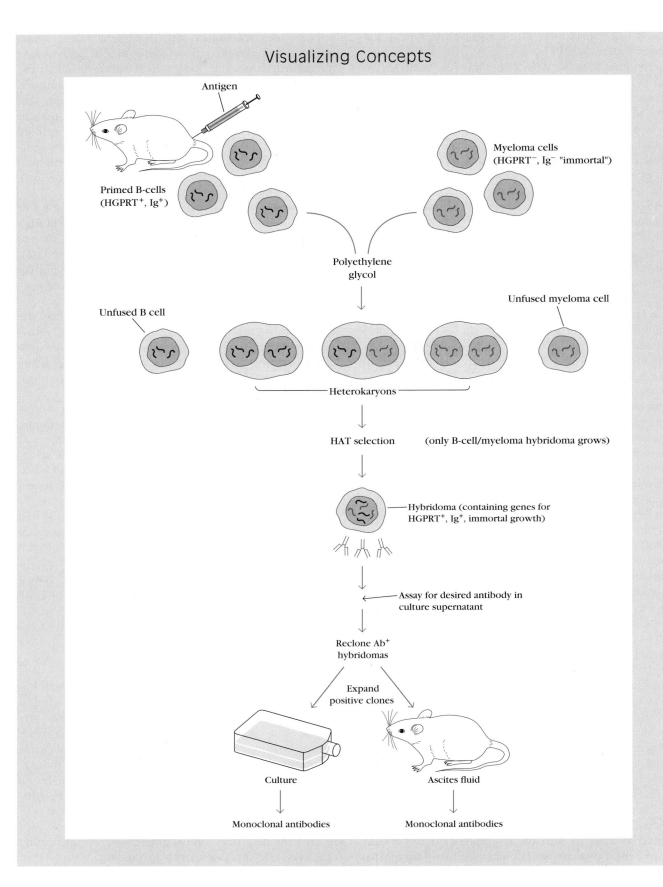

Antigen

Myeloma cells
(HGPRT⁻, Ig⁻ "immortal")

Primed B-cells
(HGPRT⁺, Ig⁺)

Polyethylene
glycol

Unfused B cell

Unfused myeloma cell

Heterokaryons

HAT selection   (only B-cell/myeloma hybridoma grows)

Hybridoma (containing genes for
HGPRT⁺, Ig⁺, immortal growth)

Assay for desired antibody in
culture supernatant

Reclone Ab⁺
hybridomas

Expand
positive clones

Culture

Ascites fluid

Monoclonal antibodies

Monoclonal antibodies

patients. For example, monoclonal antibody to breast-cancer cells labeled with iodine-131 has been introduced into the blood to detect tumor spread to regional lymph nodes. This monoclonal imaging technique can detect breast-cancer metastases that would be undetected by other scanning techniques.

Immunotoxins composed of tumor-specific monoclonal antibodies coupled to lethal toxins are potentially valuable therapeutic reagents. The toxins used in preparing immunotoxins include ricin, *Shigella* toxin, and diphtheria toxin, all of which inhibit protein synthesis. These toxins are so potent that a single molecule has been shown to kill a cell. Each of these toxins consists of two types of functionally distinct polypeptide components, an inhibitory (toxin) chain and one or more binding chains, which interact with receptors on cell surfaces; without the binding polypeptide(s) the toxin cannot get into cells and therefore is harmless. An immunotoxin is prepared by replacing the binding polypeptide(s) with a monoclonal antibody having specificity for a particular tumor cell (Figure 5-23a). In theory, the attached monoclonal antibody will target the toxin chain specifically to tumor cells, where it will cause death by inhibiting protein synthesis (Figure 5-23b). A number of phase I or phase II clinical trials using immunotoxins have been completed or are currently ongoing. In general, the clinical responses in leukemia and lymphoma patients have been quite promising, whereas the responses in patients with large tumors have been disappointing to date.

Engineered Monoclonal Antibodies

When mouse monoclonal antibodies are introduced into humans they are recognized as foreign and evoke an antibody response. The induced human anti–mouse antibodies quickly reduce the effectiveness of the mouse monoclonal antibody by clearing it from the bloodstream. In addition, circulating complexes of mouse and human antibodies can cause allergic reactions. In some cases the buildup of these complexes in organs such as the kidney can cause serious and even life-threatening reactions.

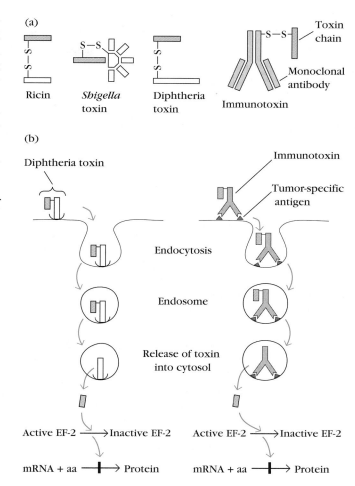

FIGURE 5-23

(a) Toxins used to prepare immunotoxins include ricin, *Shigella* toxin, and diphtheria toxin. Each toxin contains an inhibitory toxin chain (blue) and a binding component (white). To make an immunotoxin, the binding component of the toxin is replaced with a monoclonal antibody (gray). (b) Diphtheria toxin binds to a cell-membrane receptor (*left*) and a diphtheria-immunotoxin binds to a tumor-associated antigen (*right*). In either case the toxin is internalized in an endosome. The toxin chain is then released into the cytoplasm, where it inhibits protein synthesis by catalyzing the inactivation of elongation factor 2 (EF-2).

◀ FIGURE 5-22

The procedure for producing monoclonal antibodies specific for a given antigen developed by G. Kohler and C. Milstein. Spleen cells (HGPRT$^+$ and Ig$^+$) from an antigen-primed mouse are fused with mouse myeloma cells (HGPRT$^-$ and Ig$^-$). The spleen cell provides the necessary enzymes for growth on HAT medium, while the myeloma cell provides immortal-growth properties. Unfused myeloma cells or myeloma/myeloma fusions fail to grow due to lack of HGPRT. Unfused spleen cells have limited growth capabilities in vitro and will die within a few days.

These undesirable reactions place limitations on the use of mouse monoclonal antibodies for clinical purposes in humans. Clearly, one way to overcome at least some of these complications is to use human monoclonal antibodies. However, as discussed previously, preparation of human monoclonal antibodies has been hampered by numerous technical problems. Because of the difficulty of producing human monoclonal antibodies and the complications resulting from use of mouse monoclonal antibodies in humans, researchers have begun engineering monoclonal antibody using recombinant DNA technology.

CHIMERIC AND HYBRID MONOCLONAL ANTIBODIES

One approach to engineering an antibody is to clone recombinant DNA containing the promoter, leader, and variable-region sequences from a mouse antibody gene and the constant-region exons from a human antibody gene (Figure 5-24). The antibody encoded by such a recombinant gene is a mouse-human **chimera**, commonly known as a **humanized antibody**. Its antigenic specificity, which is determined by the variable region, is derived from the mouse DNA; its isotype, which is determined by the constant region, is derived from the human DNA (Figure 5-25a). Because their constant regions are encoded by human genes, these chimeric antibodies have fewer mouse antigenic determinants and are far less immunogenic than mouse monoclonal antibodies when administered to humans. Another advantage of a chimeric antibody is that it retains the biological effector functions of the human antibody and is more likely to trigger complement activation or Fc receptor binding.

Because the mouse variable region in these humanized antibodies can also induce an antibody response in humans, chimeric antibodies containing only mouse CDRs have been developed. In this novel approach, the CDRs of a mouse antibody are grafted to human framework regions to construct a variable region retaining the human β-strand framework (Figure 5-25b). These antibodies are less immunogenic in humans than humanized antibodies containing the entire mouse variable region. Since the CDRs compose the antigen-binding site, some CDR-grafted antibodies retain their ability to bind antigen. Often, however, CDR-grafted antibodies exhibit reduced binding affinity. In some cases, this can be corrected by introducing small mutations in the framework region that induce small changes in the three-dimensional configuration of the CDRs resulting in improved antibody affinity. CDR-grafted antibodies have many potential therapeutic uses. Table 5-6 lists some of the CDR-grafted monoclonal antibodies that are presently being assessed in clinical trials. In one study, for example, clinical remission was obtained in two patients

with non-Hodgkin's lymphoma who received daily injections of CDR-grafted monoclonal antibody specific for a cell-membrane antigen on the lymphoma cells.

Chimeric monoclonal antibodies that function as immunotoxins can also be prepared. In this case, the terminal constant-region domain in a tumor-specific monoclonal antibody is replaced with toxin chains (Figure 5-25c). Because these immunotoxins lack the terminal Fc domain, they are not able to bind to cells bearing Fc receptors. These immunotoxins could bind only to tumor cells, making them more efficient as a therapeutic reagent.

Heteroconjugates are hybrids of two different antibody molecules (Figure 5-25d). Various heteroconjugates have been designed in which one half of the

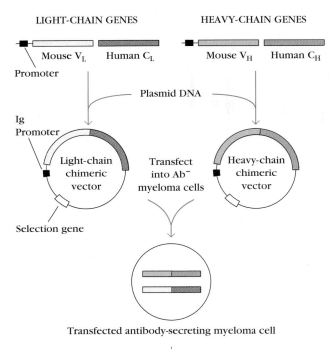

LIGHT-CHAIN GENES   HEAVY-CHAIN GENES

Mouse V_L Human C_L Mouse V_H Human C_H

Promoter

Plasmid DNA

Ig Promoter

Light-chain chimeric vector   Transfect into Ab⁻ myeloma cells   Heavy-chain chimeric vector

Selection gene

Transfected antibody-secreting myeloma cell

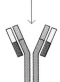

Chimeric mouse-human antibody

FIGURE 5-24

Production of chimeric mouse-human monoclonal antibodies. Chimeric mouse-human heavy- and light-chain expression vectors are produced. These vectors are transfected into Ab⁻ myeloma cells. Culture in ampicillin medium selects for transfected myeloma cells, which secrete the chimeric antibody. [Adapted from M. Verhoeyen and L. Reichmann, 1988, *BioEssays* **8**:74.]

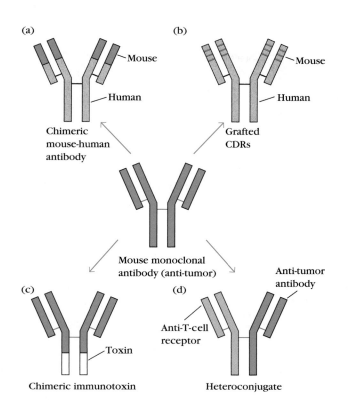

FIGURE 5-25

Chimeric and hybrid monoclonal antibodies engineered by recombinant DNA technology. (a) Chimeric mouse-human monoclonal antibody containing the V_H and V_L domains of a mouse monoclonal antibody (blue) and the C_L and C_H domains of a human monoclonal antibody (gray). (b) A chimeric monoclonal antibody containing only the CDRs of a mouse monoclonal antibody (blue bands) grafted within the framework regions of a human monoclonal antibody. (c) A chimeric monoclonal antibody in which the terminal Fc domain is replaced by a toxin chain (white). (d) A heteroconjugate in which one-half of the mouse antibody molecule is specific for a tumor antigen and the other half is specific for the CD3/T-cell receptor complex.

antibody has specificity for a tumor and the other half has specificity for a surface molecule on an immune effector cell, such as an NK cell, an activated macrophage, or a cytotoxic T lymphocyte (CTL). The heteroconjugate thus serves to cross-link the immune effector cell to the tumor. Some heteroconjugates have been designed to activate the immune effector cell when it is cross-linked to the tumor cell so that it begins to mediate destruction of the tumor cell.

T A B L E   5 - 6

THERAPEUTIC USES FOR CDR-GRAFTED ANTIBODIES

TARGET ANTIGEN	CLINICAL POTENTIAL
Cdw52 (surface molecule on leukocytes)	Lymphomas, systemic vasculitis, rheumatoid arthritis
CD3 (T-cell marker)	Organ transplantation
CD4 (T-cell marker)	Organ transplantation, rheumatoid arthritis, Crohn's disease
Receptor for interleukin 2	Leukemias and lymphomas, organ transplantation, graft-versus-host disease
Tumor necrosis factor α	Septic shock
Human immunodeficiency virus (HIV)	AIDS
Rous sarcoma virus (RSV)	Respiratory syncytial virus infection
Herpes simplex virus (HSV)	Neonatal, ocular, and genital herpes infection
Receptor for human epidermal growth factor (EGF)	Cancer
Placental alkaline phosphatase	Cancer
Carcinoembryonic antigen	Cancer

SOURCE: Adapted from G. Winter and W. J. Harris, 1993, *Immunol. Today* **14**:243.

MONOCLONAL ANTIBODIES CONSTRUCTED FROM IG-GENE LIBRARIES

A quite different approach for generating monoclonal antibodies employs the polymerase chain reaction (PCR) to amplify the DNA encoding antibody heavy-chain and light-chain Fab fragments from hybridoma cells or plasma cells (see Figure 2-7). A promoter region and *Eco*RI site are added to the amplified sequences, and the resulting constructs are inserted into bacteriophage λ, yielding separate heavy- and light-chain libraries. Cleavage with *Eco*RI and random joining of the heavy- and light-chain genes yield numerous novel heavy-light constructs (Figure 5-26).

This procedure generates an enormous diversity of antibody specificities; clones containing these random combinations of H + L chains can be rapidly screened for those secreting antibody to a particular antigen. For example, in one study a million clones were screened in just 2 days, with over 100 clones being identified that produced antibody specific for the desired antigen. The technique has the potential of producing an enormous repertoire of antibody specificities without the limitations of antigen priming and hybridoma technology that currently complicate the production of monoclonal antibodies.

CATALYTIC MONOCLONAL ANTIBODIES (ABZYMES)

The binding of an antibody to its antigen is similar in many ways to the binding of an enzyme to its substrate. In both cases the binding involves weak, noncovalent interactions and exhibits high specificity and often high affinity. What distinguishes an antibody-antigen interaction from an enzyme-substrate interaction is that the antibody does not alter the antigen, whereas the enzyme catalyzes a chemical change in its substrate. The enzyme uses its binding energy to stabilize the transition state of the substrate, thus reducing the activation energy for chemical modification of the bound substrate.

Because of the similarities between antigen-antibody interactions and enzyme-substrate interactions, R. A. Lerner and his colleagues wondered whether some antibodies might behave like enzymes and catalyze chemical reactions. To investigate this possibility, they produced a hapten-carrier complex in which the hapten structurally resembled the transition state of an ester undergoing hydrolysis. Using this conjugate, they generated antihapten monoclonal antibodies. When these monoclonal antibodies were incubated with an ester substrate, some of them accelerated hydrolysis by about 1000-fold; that is, they acted like the enzyme that normally catalyzes the substrate's hydrolysis. The catalytic activity of these anti-

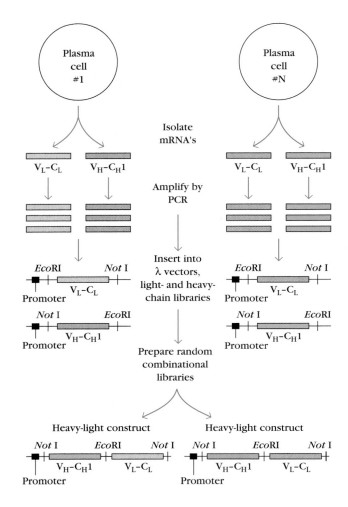

FIGURE 5-26

General procedure for producing gene libraries encoding Fab fragments. In this procedure isolated mRNA heavy and light chains are amplified by the polymerase chain reaction (PCR) and cloned in λ vectors. Random combinations of heavy and light chain genes generate an enormous number of heavy-light constructs encoding Fab fragments with different antigenic specificity. [Adapted from W. D. Huse et al., 1989, *Science* **246**:1275.]

bodies was highly specific; that is, they hydrolyzed only esters whose transition-state structure closely resembled that of the hapten in the immunizing conjugate. These catalytic antibodies have been called **abzymes** in reference to their dual role as antibody and enzyme.

In order to screen large numbers of different antibodies for catalytic activity, Lerner pioneered use of immunoglobulin-gene libraries to produce an enormous antibody repertoire without the requirement of antigen priming. As more and more abzymes are identified, it may be possible to assemble a battery of abzymes that cut peptide bonds at specific amino acid residues, much as restriction enzymes cut DNA at specific sites. Such abzymes would be invaluable tools in facilitating structural and functional analysis of proteins. Additionally, it may be possible to generate abzymes with the ability to dissolve blood clots or to cleave viral glycoproteins at specific sites, thus blocking viral infectivity. Abzymes are likely to represent a major technological advance that will impact on various branches of science in the coming years.

SUMMARY

1. The basic structure of an antibody molecule consists of two identical light chains and two identical heavy chains, which are linked by disulfide bonds (see Figure 5-3). The amino-terminal 110 amino acids in each heavy and light chain constitute a variable (V_H and V_L) sequence. The remainder of each light chain consists of a single constant sequence (C_L); the remainder of each heavy chain contains three or four constant sequences (C_H).

2. In any given antibody molecule, the constant region contains one of five basic heavy-chain sequences (μ, γ, δ, α, or ε) and one of two basic light-chain sequences (κ or λ). These sequences are called isotypes. The heavy-chain isotypes determine the five classes of antibody (IgM, IgG, IgD, IgA, and IgE) and the effector functions of the molecule.

3. Each of the domains in the immunoglobulin molecule has a characteristic tertiary structure called the immunoglobulin fold (see Figure 5-6). The Ig-fold structure is also present in a large group of membrane proteins (see Figure 5-19). Except for antibodies and T-cell receptors, the members of the immunoglobulin superfamily do not bind antigen. The basic Ig-fold structure may facilitate homologous and nonhomologous interactions between members of this family.

4. Within the amino-terminal variable domain of each heavy and light chain are three hypervariable regions, also called complementarity-determining regions (CDRs). These are present in some of the loops connecting the β strands composing these domains (see Figures 5-6b). In the three-dimensional conformation of an antibody molecule, these regions are brought into proximity, forming its antigen-binding site and determining its specificity (see Figure 5-9).

5. Immunoglobulins are expressed in two forms: secreted antibody produced by plasma cells and membrane-bound antibody present on the surface of B cells. Membrane-bound immunoglobulin associates with a heterodimer called Ig-α/Ig-β to form the B-cell receptor (see Figure 5-13). The antigenic specificity of a B cell is determined by the membrane-bound antibody that it expresses. The Ig-α/Ig-β heterodimer of the B-cell receptor mediates the intracellular signals that lead to B-cell activation following interaction with antigen.

6. The five antibody classes differ in their ability to carry out various effector functions, in their average serum concentrations and their half-life (see Table 5-4). IgG, the most abundant class in serum, is particularly important in antigen clearance by various mechanisms; it also is the only class that can cross the placenta. Serum IgM exists as a pentamer; because of its high valency, IgM is more effective than other classes in viral neutralization, bacterial agglutination, and complement activation (Figure 5-15). IgA is the predominant class in external secretions including breast milk and mucus. In these secretions, secretory IgA exists as a dimer or tetramer linked by disulfide bonds to the J chain and secretory component (Figure 5-17). IgD and IgE are the two least abundant classes in serum. IgD (along with IgM) is the major membrane-bound antibody on mature B cells, and IgE mediates mast-cell degranulation (see Figure 5-18).

7. Unlike polyclonal antibodies, a monoclonal antibody is a homogeneous preparation specific for a single epitope on a complex antigen (see Figure 5-20). In a common procedure for producing monoclonal antibodies, primed splenic B cells (HGPRT$^+$, Ig$^+$) are fused with mouse myeloma cells (HGPRT$^-$, Ig$^-$). These hybrid cells, called B-cell hybridomas, continue to secrete the specific antibody of the primed B cell but possess the immortal-growth properties of the myeloma cell (see Figure 5-22).

8. Recombinant DNA technology has been used to engineer chimeric monoclonal antibodies consisting of mouse variable regions or CDRs and human constant regions (see Figures 5-24 and 5-25). These chimeras do not elicit an anti-isotype response when injected into humans. Chimeric immunotoxins and heteroconjugate antibodies can be engineered by similar techniques (see Figure 5-25).

9. Monoclonal Fab fragments have been produced by random combination of heavy- and light-chain gene libraries constructed in bacteriophage λ (see Figure 5-26). This procedure allows the production of monoclonal Fab antibodies without antigen priming or hybridoma technology. Several catalytic monoclonal antibodies, or abzymes, have been identified. Future screening of large numbers of monoclonal antibodies generated from immunoglobulin-gene libraries may identify other abzymes with useful catalytic functions.

REFERENCES

ABRAHMSEN, L. 1995. Superantigen engineering. *Curr. Opin. Struc. Biol.* **5**:464.

AREVALO, J. H., E. A. STURA, M. J. TUSSIG, AND I. A. WILSON. 1993. Three-dimensional structure of an anti-steroid Fab and progesterone-Fab complex. *J. Mol. Biol.* **231**:103.

AREVALO, J. H., M. J. TAUSSIG, AND I. A. WILSON. 1993. Molecular basis of crossreactivity and the limits of antibody-antigen complementarity. *Nature* **365**:859.

BARBAS, C. F. 1995. Synthetic human antibodies. *Nature Medicine* **1**:837.

BRANDEN, C., AND J. TOOZE. 1991. *Introduction to Protein Structure.* Gezland Pub.

DAVIS, D. R, E. A. PADLAN, AND S. SHERIFF. 1991. Antibody-antigen complexes. *Annu. Rev. Biochem.* **59**:439.

GARCIA, K. C., ET AL. 1992. Three-dimensional structure of an angiotensin II-Fab complex at 3 Å: hormone recognition by an anti-idiotypic antibody. *Science* **257**:502.

GREENSPAN, N. S., AND C. A. BONA. 1993. Idiotypes: structure and immunogenicity. *FASEB* **7**:437.

HARRIS, L. J., ET AL. 1992. The three-dimensional structure of an intact monoclonal antibody for canine lymphoma. *Nature* **360**:369.

HUSE, W. D., ET AL. 1989. Generation of a large combinatorial library of the immunoglobulin repertoire in phage lambda. *Science* **246**:1275.

KOHLER, G., AND C. MILSTEIN. 1975. Continuous cultures of fused cells secreting antibody of predefined specificity. *Nature* **256**:495.

KRAEHENBUHL, J. P., AND M. R. NEUTRA. 1992. Transepithelial transport and mucosal defence II: secretion of IgA. *Trends Cell Biol.* **2**:134.

NEWMAN, J. 1995. How breast milk protects newborns. *Sci. Am.* **273**(6):76.

RETH, M. 1992. Antigen receptors on B lymphocytes. *Annu. Rev. Immunol.* **10**:97.

RETH, M. 1995. The B-cell antigen receptor complex and co-receptor. *Immunol. Today* **16**:310.

STANFIELD, R. L., AND I. A. WILSON. 1994. Antigen-induced conformational changes in antibodies: a problem for structural prediction and design. *Trends Biotech.* **12**:275.

STANFIELD, R. L., AND I. A. WILSON. 1995. Protein-peptide interactions. *Curr. Opin. Struc. Biol.* **5**:103.

TORMO, J., ET AL. 1994. Crystal structure of a human rhinovirus neutralizing antibody complexed with a peptide derived from viral capsid protein VP2. *EMBO J.* **13**:2247.

TULIP, W. R., et al. 1992. Refined crystal structure of the influenza virus N9 neuraminidase-NC41 Fab complex. *J. Mol. Biol.* **227**:122.

UNDERDOWN, B. J., AND J. M. SCHIFF. 1986. Immunoglobulin A: strategic defence initiative at the mucosal surface. *Annu. Rev. Immunol.* **4**:389.

WILSON, I. A., AND R. L. STANFIELD. 1995. Antibody-antibody interactions: new structures and new conformational changes. *Curr. Opin. Struc. Biol.* **4**:857.

WINTER, G., AND W. J. HARRIS. 1993. Humanized antibodies. *Immunol. Today* **14**:243.

ZHOU, G. W., ET AL. 1994. Crystal structure of a catalytic antibody with a serine protease active site. *Science* **265**:1059.

STUDY QUESTIONS

1. Indicate whether each of the following statements is true or false. If you think a statement is false, explain why.

a. A rabbit immunized with human IgG3 will produce antibody that reacts with all subclasses of IgG in humans.

b. An HGPRT$^-$ myeloma cell requires hypoxanthine for growth.

c. All immunoglobulin molecules on the surface of a given B cell have the same idiotype.

d. All immunoglobulin molecules on the surface of a given B cell have the same isotype.

e. All myeloma protein molecules derived from a single myeloma clone have the same idiotype and allotype.

f. When a heterokaryon initially is formed, it is multinucleated.

g. The hypervariable regions make significant contact with the epitope.

h. IgG functions more effectively than IgM in bacterial agglutination.

i. Chromosome loss from heterokaryons occurs randomly.

j. Hypoxanthine is added to HAT medium to prevent cell growth by the salvage pathway.

k. All isotypes are normally found in each individual of a species.

l. The heavy-chain variable region (VH) is twice as long as the light-chain variable region (VL).

m. An HGPRT⁺ revertant myeloma cell would be a good fusion partner for production of B-cell hybridomas because it would not be able to grow in HAT medium.

2. An energetic immunology student has isolated protein X, which he believes is a new isotype of human immunoglobulin.

a. What structural features would protein X have to have in order to be classified as an immunoglobulin?

b. You prepare rabbit antisera to whole human IgG, human κ chain, and human γ chain. Assuming protein X is, in fact, a new immunoglobulin isotype, to which of these antisera would it bind? Why?

c. Devise an experimental procedure for preparing an antiserum that is specific for protein X.

3. According to the clonal selection theory, all the immunoglobulin molecules on a single B cell have the same antigenic specificity. Explain why the presence of both IgM and IgD on the same B cell does not violate the unispecificity implied by clonal selection.

4. IgG, which contains γ heavy chains, developed much more recently during evolution than IgM, which contains μ heavy chains. Describe two advantages and two disadvantages that IgG has in comparison with IgM.

5. Although the five immunoglobulin isotypes share many common structural features, the differences in their structures affect their biological activities.

a. Draw a schematic diagram of a typical IgG molecule and label each of the following parts: H chains, L chains, interchain disulfide bonds, intrachain disulfide bonds, hinge, Fab, Fc, and all the domains. Indicate which domains are involved in antigen binding.

b. How would you have to modify the diagram of IgG to depict an IgA molecule isolated from saliva?

c. How would you have to modify the diagram of IgG to depict serum IgM?

6. Fill out the accompanying table relating to the properties of IgG molecules and their various parts. Insert a (+) if the molecule or part exhibits the property; a (−) if it does not; and a (+/−)if it does so only weakly.

Property	Whole IgG	H chain	L chain	Fab	F(ab′)$_2$	Fc
Binds antigen						
Bivalent antigen binding						
Binds to Fc receptors						
Fixes complement in presence of antigen						
Has V domains						
Has C domains						

7. Because immunoglobulin molecules possess antigenic determinants, they can function as immunogens, inducing formation of antibody. For each of the following immunization scenarios, indicate whether anti-immunoglobulin antibodies would be formed to isotypic (IS), allotypic (AL), or idiotypic (ID) determinants:

a. Anti-DNP antibodies produced in a BALB/c mouse are injected into a C57BL/6 mouse.

b. Anti-BGG monoclonal antibodies from a BALB/c mouse are injected into another BALB/c mouse.

c. Anti-BGG antibodies produced in a BALB/c mouse are injected into a rabbit.

d. Anti-DNP antibodies produced in a BALB/c mouse are injected into an outbred mouse.

e. Anti-BGG antibodies produced in a BALB/c mouse are injected into the same mouse.

8. Write YES or NO in the accompanying table to indicate whether the rabbit antisera listed at the top reacts with the mouse antibody components listed at the left.

	Rabbit antisera to mouse antibody component				
	γ chain	κ chain	IgG Fab fragment	IgG Fc fragment	J chain
Mouse γ chain					
Mouse κ chain					
Mouse IgM whole					
Mouse IgM Fc fragment					

9. The myeloma cells used in production of B-cell hybridomas have three properties that make them suitable fusion partners. List these properties and explain why they are necessary for the production of hybridomas that secrete B-cell antibodies.

10. The characteristic structure of immunoglobulin domains, termed the immunoglobulin fold, also occurs in the numerous membrane proteins belonging to the immunoglobulin superfamily.

a. Describe the typical features that define the immunoglobulin-fold domain structure.

b. List three membrane proteins that belong to the immunoglobulin superfamily. How might the presence of the immunoglobulin-fold domain structure in these proteins facilitate their function?

11. Where are the hypervariable regions located on an antibody molecule and what are their functions?

12. What would be the consequences if you omitted aminopterin from the HAT medium used to select hybridomas in the standard procedure for producing monoclonal antibodies?

13. You prepare an immunotoxin by conjugating diphtheria toxin with a monoclonal antibody specific for a tumor antigen.

a. If this immunotoxin is injected into an animal, will any normal cells be killed? Explain.

b. If the antibody part of the immunotoxin is degraded so that the toxin is released, will normal cells be killed? Explain.

14. A technician wanted to make a rabbit antiserum specific for mouse IgG. She injected a rabbit with purified mouse IgG and obtained an antiserum that reacted strongly with mouse IgG. To her dismay, however, the antiserum also reacted with each of the other mouse isotypes. Explain why she got this result. How could she make the rabbit antiserum specific for mouse IgG?

15. You fuse spleen cells having a normal genotype for immunoglobulin heavy chains (H) and light chains (L) with three myeloma-cell preparations differing in their immunoglobulin genotype as follows: (a) H^+, L^+; (b) H^-, L^+; and (c) H^-, L^-. For each hybridoma, predict how

many unique antigen-binding sites, composed of one H and one L chain, theoretically could be produced and show the chain structure of the possible antibody molecules. For each possible antibody molecule indicate whether the chains would originate from the spleen (S) or from the myeloma (M) fusion partner (e.g., $H_S L_S / H_M L_M$).

16. For each immunoglobulin isotype (a–e) select the description(s) listed below (1–13) that are true about that isotype. Each description may be used once, more than once, or not at all; more than one description may apply to some isotypes.

Isotypes:

a. _____ IgA

b. _____ IgD

c. _____ IgE

d. _____ IgG

e. _____ IgM

Descriptions:

1) Secreted form is a pentamer of the basic $H_2 L_2$ unit

2) Binds to Fc receptors on mast cells

3) Multimeric forms have J chain

4) Present on the surface of mature, unprimed B cells

5) The most abundant isotype in serum

6) Major antibody in secretions such as saliva, tears, and breast milk

7) Present on the surface of immature B cells

8) The first serum antibody made in a primary immune response

9) Plays an important role in immediate hypersensitivity

10) Plays primary role in protecting against pathogens that invade through the gut or respiratory mucosa

11) Multimeric forms may contain a secretory component

12) Can fix complement by the classical pathway

13) Least abundant isotype in serum

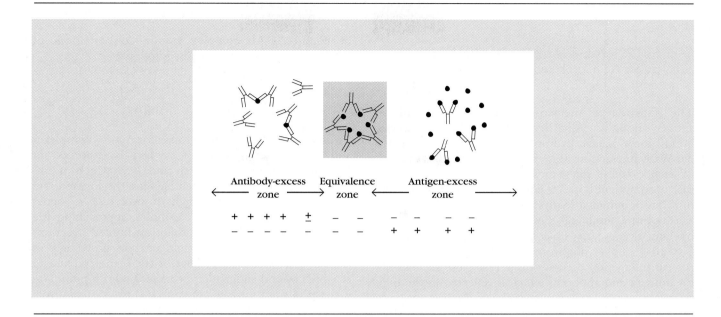

ANTIGEN-ANTIBODY
INTERACTIONS

The antigen–antibody interaction is a bimolecular association similar to an enzyme-substrate interaction but with the important distinction that it does not lead to an irreversible chemical alteration in either the antibody or antigen and therefore is reversible. The interaction between an antibody and an antigen involves various non-covalent interactions between the antigenic determinant, or epitope, of the antigen and the variable-region (V_H/V_L) domain of the antibody molecule, particularly the hypervariable regions, or complementarity-determining regions (CDRs). The exquisite specificity of antigen–antibody interactions has led to the development of a variety of immunologic assays. These assays can be used to detect the presence of either antibody or antigen and have played vital roles in diagnosing diseases, monitoring the level of the humoral immune response, and identifying molecules of biological or medical interest. These assays differ in their speed and their sensitivity; some are strictly qualitative, and others are quantitative. In this chapter, the nature of the antigen–antibody interaction is examined, and various immunologic assays that measure this interaction are described.

STRENGTH OF ANTIGEN-ANTIBODY INTERACTIONS

The noncovalent interactions that form the basis of antigen-antibody (Ag-Ab) binding include hydrogen bonds, ionic bonds, hydrophobic interactions, and van der Waals interactions (Figure 6-1). Because the strength of each of these interactions is weak (compared with that of a covalent bond), a large number of such interactions are required to form a strong Ag-Ab interaction. Furthermore, each of these noncovalent interactions operates over a very small distance, generally less than 1×10^{-7} mm (1 angstrom, Å); consequently, a strong Ag-Ab interaction depends on a very close fit between the antigen and antibody, which is reflected in the high degree of specificity characteristic of antigen-antibody interactions.

Antibody Affinity

The strength of the total noncovalent interactions between a *single* antigen-binding site on an antibody and a *single* epitope is the **affinity** of the antibody for that epitope. Low-affinity antibodies bind antigen weakly and tend to dissociate readily, whereas high-affinity antibodies bind antigen more tightly and remain bound longer. The association between a binding site on an antibody (Ab) with a monovalent antigen (Ag) can be described by the equation

$$Ag + Ab \underset{k_{-1}}{\overset{k_1}{\rightleftharpoons}} Ab - Ag$$

where k_1 is the forward (association) rate constant and k_{-1} is the reverse (dissociation) rate constant. The ratio of k_1/k_{-1} is the association constant K, a measure of affinity. It can be calculated from the ratio of the concentration

of bound Ag-Ab complex to the concentrations of unbound antigen and antibody, as follows:

$$K = \frac{k_1}{k_{-1}} = \frac{[Ag - Ag]}{[Ab][Ag]}$$

The value of K varies for different Ag-Ab complexes and depends upon both k_1, which is expressed in liters/mole/second (L/mol/s), and k_{-1}, which is expressed in 1/second. For small haptens, the forward rate constant can be extremely high; in some cases k_1 values can be as high as 4×10^8 L/mol/s, approaching the theoretical upper limit of diffusion-limited reactions (10^9 L/mol/s). For larger protein antigens, however, k_1 is smaller, with values in the range of 10^5 L/mol/s. The rate at which bound antigen leaves an antibody's binding site (i.e., the dissociation rate constant, k_{-1}) plays a major role in determining the antibody's affinity for an antigen.

Table 6-1 illustrates the role of k_{-1} in determining the association constant K for several Ag-Ab interactions. For example, the k_1 for the DNP-L-lysine system is about one-fifth that for the fluorescein system, but its k_{-1} is 200 times greater; consequently, the K for the fluorescein system is about a thousandfold higher than K for the DNP-L-lysine system. Low-affinity Ag-Ab complexes have K values between 10^4 and 10^5 L/mol; high-affinity complexes can have K values as high as 10^{11} L/mol.

The association constant K can be determined by **equilibrium dialysis**. In this procedure a dialysis chamber containing two equal compartments separated by a semipermeable membrane is used. Antibody is placed in one compartment, and a radioactively labeled ligand that is small enough to pass through the semipermeable membrane is placed in the other compartment (Figure 6-2). Suitable ligands include haptens as well as oligosaccharides and oligopeptides composing the epitope of complex polysaccharide or protein antigens. In the ab-

TABLE 6-1

FORWARD (k_1) AND REVERSE (k_{-1}) RATE CONSTANTS AND ASSOCIATION CONSTANT (K) OF THREE LIGAND-ANTIBODY INTERACTIONS

ANTIBODY	LIGAND	k_1 (L/MOL/S)	k_{-1} (S^{-1})	K (L/MOL)
Anti-DNP	ε-DNP-L-lysine	8×10^7	1	10^8
Anti-flourescein	Flourescein	4×10^8	5×10^{-3}	10^{11}
Anti-bovine serum albumin (BSA)	Dansyl-BSA	3×10^5	2×10^{-3}	1.7×10^8

SOURCE: Adapted from H. N. Eisen, 1990, *Immunology*, 3rd ed., Harper and Row Publishers.

Visualizing Concepts

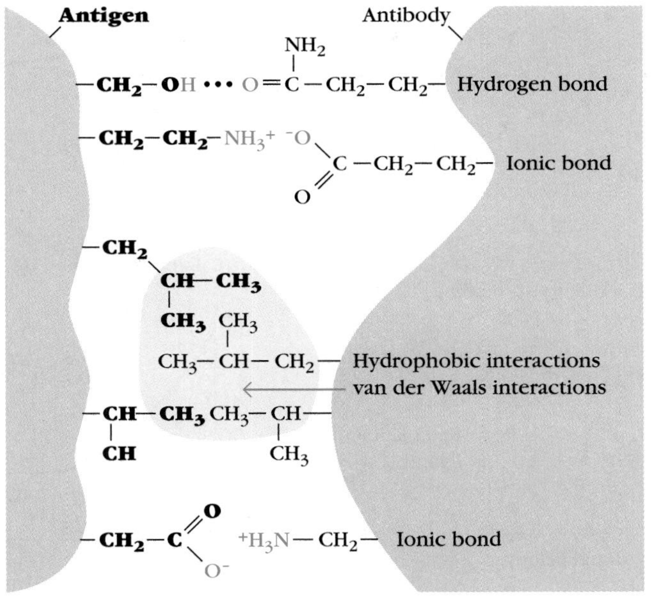

FIGURE 6-1

The interaction between an antibody and an antigen (shown here in bold type) depends on four types of noncovalent forces: (1) hydrogen bonds in which a hydrogen atom is shared between two electronegative atoms, (2) ionic bonds between oppositely charged residues, (3) hydrophobic interactions in which water forces hydrophobic groups together to maximize hydrogen bonding of water molecules, and (4) van der Waals interactions between the outer electron clouds of two atoms. In an aqueous environment noncovalent interactions are extremely weak and depend upon close structural complementarity between antibody and antigen.

sence of antibody, ligand added to compartment B will equilibrate on both sides of the membrane (Figure 6-2a). In the presence of antibody, however, part of the labeled ligand will be bound to the antibody at equilibrium, and the unbound ligand will be equally distributed in both compartments. Thus the total concentration of ligand will be greater in the compartment containing antibody (Figure 6-2b). The difference in the ligand concentration in the two compartments represents the concentration of ligand bound to the antibody (i.e., the concentration of Ag-Ab complex). The higher the affinity of the antibody, the more ligand that is bound.

Since the total concentration of antibody in the equilibrium dialysis chamber is known, the equilibrium equation can be rewritten as:

$$K = \frac{[Ab - Ag]}{[Ab][Ag]} = \frac{r}{(n - r)\,(c)}$$

where r = the ratio of the concentration of bound ligand to total antibody concentration, c = concentration of free ligand, and n = number of binding sites per antibody molecule. This expression can be rearranged to give the **Scatchard equation**:

$$\frac{r}{c} = Kn - Kr$$

Values for r and c can be obtained by repeating the equilibrium dialysis with the same concentration of antibody but with different concentrations of ligand. If K is

(a)

Control: No antibody present
(ligand equilibrates on both sides equally)

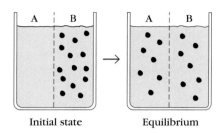

Experimental: Antibody in A
(at equilibrium more ligand in A due to Ab binding)

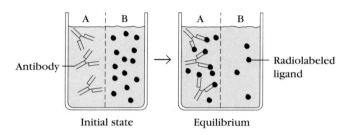

(b)

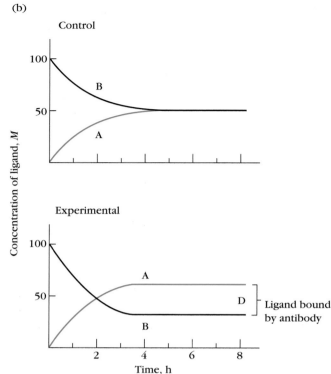

FIGURE 6-2

Determination of antibody affinity by equilibrium dialysis. (a) The dialysis chamber contains two compartments (A and B) separated by a semipermeable membrane. Antibody is added to one compartment and a radiolabeled ligand to another. At equilibrium the concentration of radioactivity in both compartments is measured. (b) Plot of concentration of ligand in each compartment with time. At equilibrium the difference in the concentration of radioactive ligand in the two compartments represents the amount of ligand bound to antibody.

a constant, that is, if all the antibodies within the dialysis chamber have the same affinity for the ligand, then a Scatchard plot of r/c versus r will yield a straight line with a slope of $-K$ (Figure 6-3a). As the concentration of unbound ligand c increases, r/c approaches 0, and r approaches n, the **valency**.

For most antibody preparations, K is not a constant because antibodies (unless they are monoclonal) are heterogeneous and have a range of affinities. A Scatchard plot of heterogeneous antibody yields a curved line whose slope is constantly changing, reflecting the antibody heterogeneity (Figure 6-3b). With this type of Scatchard plot, it is possible to determine the average affinity constant K_0 by determining the value of K when half of the antigen-binding sites are filled:

$$K_0 = \frac{1}{(2-1)c} = \frac{1}{c}$$

Antibody Avidity

The affinity at one binding site does not always reflect the true strength of the antibody-antigen interaction. When complex antigens containing multiple, repeating antigenic determinants are mixed with antibodies containing multiple binding sites, the interaction of antibody with antigen at one site will increase the probability of reaction at a second site. The strength of such multiple interactions between a multivalent antibody and antigen is called the **avidity**. The avidity of an antibody is a better measure of its binding capacity within biological systems (e.g., the reaction of an antibody with antigenic determinants on a virus or bacterial cell) than is the affinity of its individual binding sites. High avidity can compensate for low affinity. For example, secreted pentameric IgM often has a lower affinity than IgG, but the high avidity of IgM, resulting from its multivalence, enables it to bind antigen effectively.

(a) Homogeneous antibody

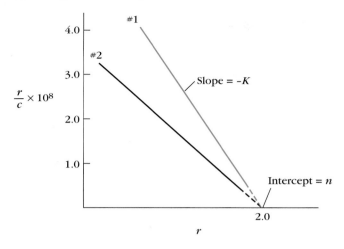

(b) Heterogeneous antibody

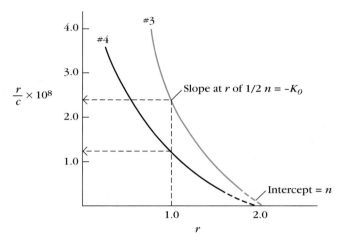

FIGURE 6-3

Scatchard plots are based on repeated equilibrium dialyses with a constant concentration of antibody and varying concentration of ligand. In these plots, r = moles bound ligand/mole antibody and c = free ligand. From a Scatchard plot, both the equilibrium constant (K) and the number of binding sites per antibody molecule (n), or its valency, can be obtained. (a) If all antibodies have the same affinity, then a Scatchard plot yields a straight line with a slope of $-K$. The Y intercept is the valence of the antibody, which is 2 for IgG. In this graph antibody #1 has a higher affinity than antibody #2. (b) If the antibodies have a range of affinities, a Scatchard plot yields a curved line, whose slope is constantly changing. The average affinity constant K_0 can be calculated by determining the value of K when one half of the binding sites are occupied (i.e., when $r = 1$). In this graph antisera #3 has a higher affinity ($K_0 = 2.4 \times 10^8$) than antisera #4 ($K_0 = 1.25 \times 10^8$).

CROSS-REACTIVITY

Although Ag-Ab reactions are highly specific, in some cases antibody elicited by one antigen can cross-react with an unrelated antigen. Such **cross-reactivity** occurs if two different antigens share an identical epitope or if antibodies specific for one epitope also bind to an unrelated epitope possessing similar chemical properties. In the latter case the antibody's affinity for the cross-reacting epitope is usually less than that for the original epitope.

Cross-reactivity is often observed among polysaccharide antigens that contain similar oligosaccharide residues. The **ABO blood-group antigens**, for example, are glycoproteins expressed on red blood cells. Subtle differences in the terminal sugar residues distinguish the A and B blood-group antigens (see Figure 17-12). An individual lacking one or both of these antigens will have serum antibodies to the missing antigen(s). A type O individual thus has anti-A and anti-B antibodies; a type A individual has anti-B; and a type B individual has anti-A (Table 6-2). Cross-reactivity is the basis for the presence of these blood-group antibodies, which are induced in an indi-

vidual not by exposure to red blood cell antigens but by exposure to cross-reacting microbial antigens present on common intestinal bacteria. These cross-reacting microbial antigens induce the formation of antibodies in individuals lacking these antigens. The blood-group antibodies, although elicited by microbial antigens, will cross-react with similar oligosaccharides on red blood cells.

A number of viruses and bacteria possess antigenic determinants identical or similar to normal host-cell components. In some cases these microbial antigens have been shown to elicit antibody that cross-reacts with the

TABLE 6 – 2

ABO BLOOD TYPES

BLOOD TYPE	ANTIGENS ON RBCs	SERUM ANTIBODIES
A	A	Anti-B
B	B	Anti-A
AB	A and B	Neither
O	Neither	Anti-A and anti-B

host-cell components, resulting in a tissue-damaging autoimmune reaction. The bacterium *Streptococcus pyogenes*, for example, expresses cell-wall proteins called M antigens. Antibodies produced to streptococcal M antigens have been shown to cross-react with several myocardial and skeletal muscle proteins and have been implicated in heart and kidney damage following streptococcal infections. The role of other cross-reacting antigens in the development of autoimmune diseases is discussed in Chapter 20.

Some vaccines also exhibit cross-reactivity. For instance, vaccinia virus, which causes cowpox, expresses cross-reacting epitopes with variola virus, the causative agent of smallpox. This cross-reactivity was the basis of Jenner's method of using vaccinia virus to induce immunity to smallpox, as mentioned in Chapter 1.

PRECIPITATION REACTIONS

The interaction between an antibody and a soluble antigen in aqueous solution forms a lattice that eventually develops into a visible precipitate. Antibodies that thus aggregate soluble antigens are called **precipitins.** Although formation of the soluble Ag-Ab complex occurs within minutes, formation of the visible precipitate occurs more slowly and often takes a day or two to reach completion. The precipitate develops as neighboring antibody molecules within the lattice form ionic bonds with each other, causing the lattice to lose its charge and thus become insoluble.

Formation of an Ag-Ab lattice depends on the valency of both the antibody and antigen:

- The antibody must be bivalent; a precipitate will not form with monovalent Fab fragments.
- The antigen must either be bivalent or polyvalent; that is, it must have at least two copies of the same epitope, or have different epitopes that react with different antibodies present in polyclonal antisera.

Myoglobin illustrates the requirement that protein antigens be bivalent or polyvalent for a precipitin reaction to occur. Myoglobin precipitates well with specific polyclonal antisera but fails to precipitate with a specific monoclonal antibody because it contains multiple, distinct epitopes but only a single copy of each epitope (see Figure 4-7a). Myoglobin thus can form a cross-linked lattice structure with polyclonal antisera but not with monoclonal antisera. Several common immunologic assays are based on precipitation reactions; the sensitivity of these assays varies considerably, as shown in Table 6-3.

Precipitation Reactions in Fluids

A quantitative precipitation reaction can be performed by placing a constant amount of antibody in a series of tubes and adding increasing amounts of antigen to the tubes. After the precipitate forms, each tube is centrifuged to pellet the precipitate, the supernatant is poured off, and the amount of precipitate is measured. Plotting the amount of precipitate against increasing antigen concentrations yields a precipitin curve. As Figure 6-4 shows, excess of either antibody or antigen interferes with maximal precipitation, which occurs in the so-called **equivalence zone**, when the ratio of antibody to antigen is optimal. As a large multimolecular lattice is formed at equivalence, the complex increases in size and precipitates out of solution. In the region of **antibody**

T A B L E   6 - 3

SENSITIVITY OF VARIOUS IMMUNOASSAYS

ASSAY	SENSITIVITY * (μG ANTIBODY N/ML)
Precipitation reaction in fluids	3–30
Precipitation reactions in gels	
Mancini radial immunofusion	0.2–1.0
Ouchterlony double immunofusion	3–20
Immunoelectrophoresis	3–20
Rocket electrophoresis	0.2
Agglutination reactions	
Direct	0.05
Passive agglutination	0.001–0.01
Agglutination inhibition	0.001–0.01
Radioimmunoassay	0.0001–0.001
Enzyme-linked immunosorbent assay (ELISA)	0.0001–0.001
Immunofluorescence	1.0

* The sensitivity depends upon the affinity of the antibody as well as the epitope density and distribution.

SOURCE: Adapted from N. R. Rose et al. (eds.), 1986, *Manual of Clinical Laboratory Immunology,* American Society for Microbiology, Washington, D.C.

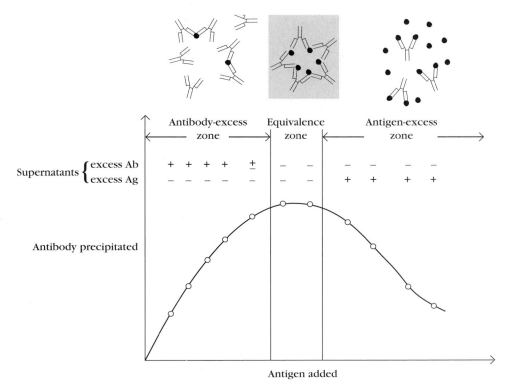

FIGURE 6-4

A precipitation curve for a system of one antigen and its antibodies. This plot of the amount of antibody precipitated versus increasing antigen concentrations (at constant total antibody) reveals three zones: a zone of antibody excess in which precipitation is inhibited and excess antibody can be detected in the supernatant; an equiva-

lence zone of maximal precipitation in which antibody and antigen form large insoluble complexes (shaded in blue) and neither antibody nor antigen can be detected in the supernatant; and a zone of antigen excess in which precipitation is inhibited and excess antigen can be detected in the supernatant.

excess, unreacted antibody is found in the supernatant along with small soluble complexes consisting of multiple molecules of antibody bound to a single molecule of antigen. In the region of **antigen excess**, unreacted antigen can be detected and small complexes are again observed, this time consisting of one or two molecules of antigen bound to a single molecule of antibody. Although the quantitative precipitation reaction is seldom used experimentally today, the principles of antigen excess, antibody excess, and equivalence apply to many Ag–Ab reactions.

The precipitation reaction can also be used as a rapid test for the presence of antibody or antigen. The **interfacial (ring) precipitin test** is performed by adding antiserum to a small tube and layering antigen on top. If the antiserum contains antibodies specific for the test antigen, then the antibody and antigen diffuse toward each other and form a visible band of precipitation at the interface within a few minutes (Figure 6-5).

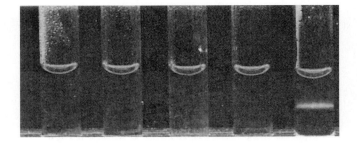

FIGURE 6-5

The interfacial (ring) precipitin test is a rapid, qualitative method for determining the presence of antibody or antigen. The antiserum is placed in the bottom of a tube, and then the antigen solution is carefully layered on top. Formation of a visible line of precipitation in the tube at the extreme right indicates a positive reaction. The other four tubes are various controls (e.g., normal serum with antigen and antiserum with buffer). [From J. S. Garvey et al., 1977, *Methods in Immunology*, 3d ed., W. A. Benjamin Inc., Advanced Book Program.]

Precipitation Reactions in Gels

Immune precipitates can form not only in solution but also in an agar matrix. When antigen and antibody diffuse toward one another in agar or when antibody is incorporated into the agar and antigen diffuses into the antibody-containing matrix, a visible line of precipitation will form. As in a precipitation reaction in fluid, visible precipitation occurs in the region of equivalence, whereas no visible precipitate forms in regions of antibody or antigen excess. These **immunodiffusion reactions** can be used to determine relative concentrations of antibodies or antigens, to compare antigens, or to determine the relative purity of an antigen preparation. Two frequently used immunodiffusion techniques are **radial immunodiffusion** (Mancini method) and **double immuno-**

diffusion (Ouchterlony method); both are carried out in a semisolid medium like agar (Figure 6-6).

RADIAL IMMUNODIFFUSION (MANCINI METHOD)

The relative concentrations of an antigen can be determined by a simple quantitative assay in which an antigen sample is placed in a well and allowed to diffuse into agar containing a suitable dilution of an antiserum. As the antigen diffuses into the agar, the region of equivalence is established and a ring of precipitation forms around the well (see Figure 6-6). The area of the precipitin ring is proportional to the concentration of antigen. By comparing the area of the precipitin ring with a standard curve (obtained by measuring the precipitin areas of known concentrations of the antigen), the concentration of the antigen sample can be determined.

The Mancini method is routinely used to quantitate serum levels of IgM, IgG, and IgA by incorporating class-specific anti-isotype antibody into the agar (Figure 6-7). The technique is also applied to determine the concentrations of complement components in serum. The Mancini method cannot detect antigens present in concentrations below 5–10 μg/ml; this moderate sensitivity is the major limitation of the radial immunodiffusion method.

DOUBLE IMMUNODIFFUSION (OUCHTERLONY METHOD)

In the Ouchterlony method both antigen and antibody diffuse radially from wells toward each other, thereby establishing a concentration gradient. As equivalence is reached, a visible line of precipitation forms (see Figure 6-6). This simple technique is an effective *qualitative* tool for determining the relationship between antigens and the number of different Ag-Ab systems present.

The pattern of the precipitin lines that form when two different antigen preparations are placed in adjacent wells indicates whether or not they share epitopes (Figure 6-8):

- **Identity** occurs when two antigens share identical epitopes. The antiserum forms a single precipitin line with each antigen that grow toward each other and fuse to give a single curved line of identity.
- **Nonidentity** occurs when two antigens are unrelated (i.e., share no common epitopes). The antiserum forms independent precipitin lines that cross.
- **Partial identity** occurs when two antigens share some epitopes but one or the other has a unique epitope(s). The antiserum forms a line of identity with the common epitope(s) and a curved spur with the unique epitope(s).

RADIAL IMMUNODIFFUSION

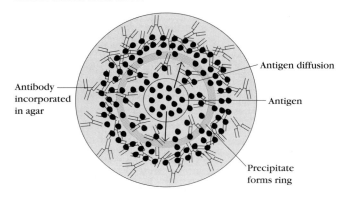

Antibody incorporated in agar

Antigen diffusion

Antigen

Precipitate forms ring

DOUBLE IMMUNODIFFUSION

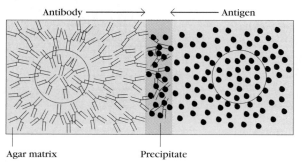

Antibody →   ← Antigen

Agar matrix   Precipitate

FIGURE 6-6

Diagrammatic representation of radial (Mancini) and double immunodiffusion (Ouchterlony) in a gel. In both cases, large insoluble complexes form in the agar in the zone of equivalence, which are visible as a line of precipitation (blue region). Only the antigen diffuses in radial immunodiffusion, whereas both the antibody and antigen diffuse in double immunodiffusion.

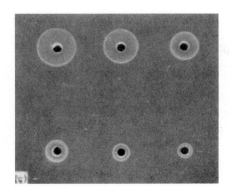

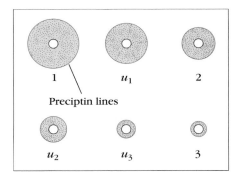

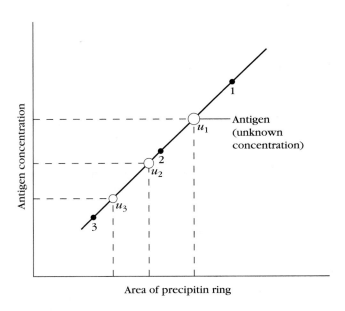

FIGURE 6-7

Determination of antigen concentration by radial immunodiffusion. The area of the ring of precipitation is proportional to the concentration of antigen. A standard curve can be obtained from the results with known concentrations of antigen (wells 1–3). From the standard curve, the antigen concentration can be determined in samples of unknown concentration (wells u_1, u_2, and u_3). [Photograph from D. M. Weir (ed.), 1986, *Handbook of Experimental Immunology,* Blackwell Scientific Publications.]

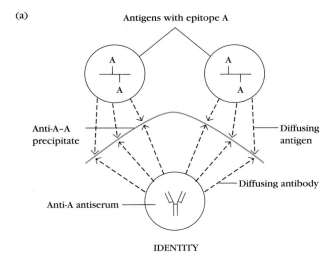

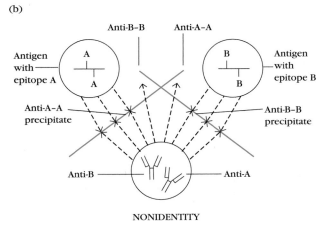

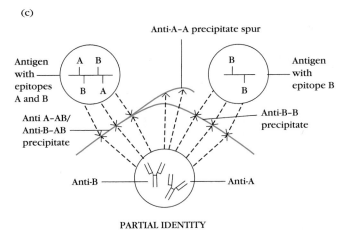

FIGURE 6-8

Diagrams of possible precipitin patterns obtained in double immunodiffusion (Ouchterlony method) of antiserum with two different antigen preparations. The pattern of lines (blue) indicates whether the two antigens have identical epitopes (identity), partially identical epitopes (partial identity), or no epitopes in common (nonidentity).

(a)

(b)

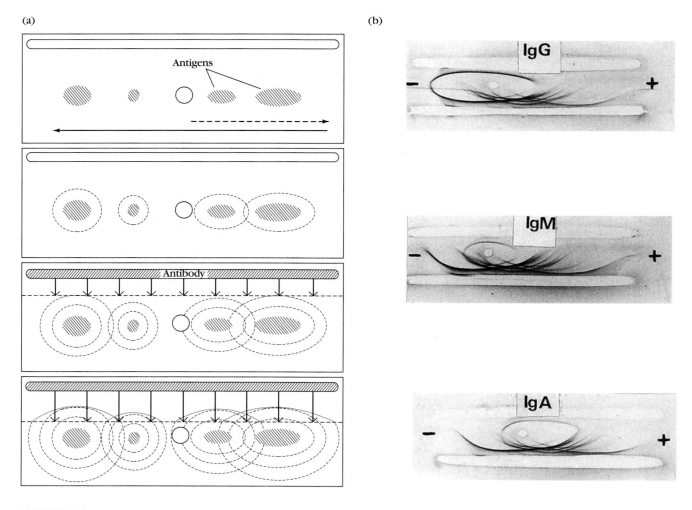

FIGURE 6-9

Immunoelectrophoresis of an antigen mixture. (a) An antigen preparation is first electrophoresed, which separates the component antigens on the basis of charge. Antiserum is then added to troughs on one or both sides of the separated antigens and allowed to diffuse; in time, lines of precipitation (blue curves) form where specific antibody and antigen interact. (b) Immunoelectrophoretic patterns of human serum. Goat antibody to whole human serum was placed in the bottom trough of each slide; goat antibody to human IgG, IgM, or IgA was placed in the top trough of each slide. After electrophoresis, the IgG, IgM, and IgA antibodies form a single line of precipitation with their respective antisera. The position of the human IgG, IgM, and IgA in the electrophoresed whole human serum sample can be determined by comparing the position of the single band at the top of each slide with the complex band pattern of the whole serum sample. [Part (b) J. S. Garvey et al., 1977, *Methods in Immunology*, 3d ed., W. A. Benjamin Inc., Advanced Book Program.]

In the nonidentity pattern, the precipitin lines cross because the unrelated antigen and antibody do not precipitate and therefore are free to diffuse past the precipitin lines; as a result, the precipitin line of each related antigen-antibody system extends beyond that of the other (see Figure 6-8b). In the partial identity pattern, antibodies to the unique epitope(s) diffuse past the common precipitin line to form a precipitin line (spur) with the unique epitope(s) of the more complex antigen (see Figure 6-8c).

IMMUNOELECTROPHORESIS

The technique of **immunoelectrophoresis** combines separation by electrophoresis with identification by double immunodiffusion (Figure 6-9a). An antigen mixture is first electrophoresed and separated by charge. Troughs are then cut into the agar gel parallel to the direction of the electric field, and antiserum is added to the troughs. The agar gel is then incubated in a humid chamber during which time antigen and antibody diffuse toward each other. The formation of precipitin bands with poly-

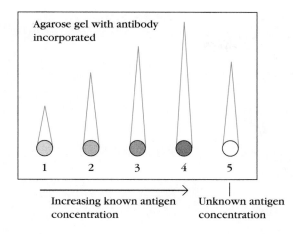

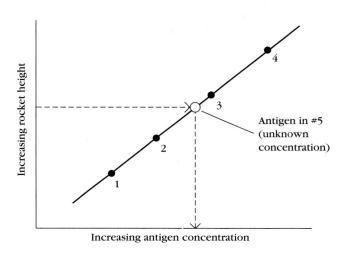

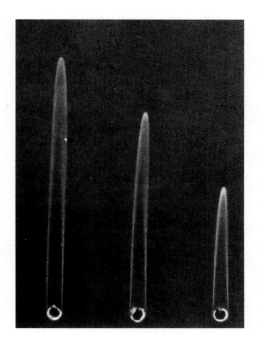

FIGURE 6-10

In rocket electrophoresis, antigen is electrophoresed in an agarose gel in which antibody has been incorporated. The height of the rocket-shaped line of precipitation that forms following electrophoresis for 2–3 h is proportional to the concentration of antigen. A sample of unknown antigen concentration (well 5) can be quantitated by reference to a standard curve. [Photograph from D. M. Weir (ed.), 1986, *Handbook of Experimental Immunology,* Blackwell Scientific Publications.]

valent or specific antiserum identifies individual antigen components.

Immunoelectrophoresis is widely used in clinical laboratories to detect the presence or absence of proteins in the serum. The serum proteins are electrophoresed, and the individual serum components are identified with antisera specific for a given protein or immunoglobulin class (Figure 6-9b). This technique is useful in determining whether a patient produces abnormally low amounts of one or more isotypes, characteristic of certain immunodeficiency diseases. It can also show if a patient overproduces some serum protein, such as albumin, immunoglobulin, or transferrin. The immunoelectrophoretic pattern of serum from patients with multiple myeloma, for example, shows a heavy distorted arc caused by the large amount of myeloma protein, which is monoclonal and therefore uniformly charged.

Immunoelectrophoresis is a strictly *qualitative* technique that can detect antibody concentrations of 3–20 μg/ml. It is useful for detecting quantitative anomalies

only when the departure from normal is striking, as in immunodeficiency and immunoproliferative disorders. The related technique of rocket electrophoresis permits quantitation of antigen levels as low as 0.2 μg/ml.

In **rocket electrophoresis** a negatively charged antigen is electrophoresed in a gel containing antibody. The precipitate formed between antigen and antibody has the shape of a rocket, the height of which is proportional to the concentration of antigen in the well (Figure 6-10). One limitation of rocket electrophoresis is the need for the antigen to be negatively charged for electrophoretic movement within the agar matrix. Some proteins, such as immunoglobulins, are not sufficiently charged to be quantitated by rocket electrophoresis; nor is it possible to quantitate several antigens in a mixture at the same time.

Several antigens in a complex mixture can be quantitated simultaneously with a modification of rocket electrophoresis called **two-dimensional immunoelectrophoresis**. In this technique antigen is first separated into components by electrophoresis. The gel is then laid over

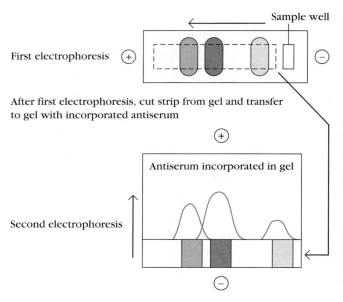

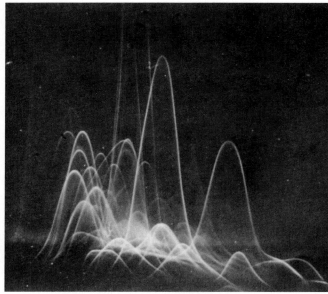

FIGURE 6-11

Several antigens in a complex antigen mixture can be quantitated by two-dimensional immunoelectrophoresis. The antigen sample is first electrophoresed; after the gel is laid over another gel containing antiserum, it is electrophoresed at right angles. The heights of the pre-cipitin peaks (blue curves) in the second electrophoresis are proportional to the antigen concentrations, which can be determined by reference to standard curves. [Photograph from D. M. Weir (ed.), 1986, *Handbook of Experimental Immunology,* Blackwell Scientific Publications.]

another agar gel containing antiserum, and electrophoresis is repeated at right angles to the first direction, forming precipitin peaks similar to those obtained with rocket electrophoresis. Measurement of the size of the peaks allows quantitation of a number of proteins in a complex antigen mixture (Figure 6-11).

AGGLUTINATION REACTIONS

The interaction between antibody and a particulate antigen results in visible clumping called **agglutination**. Antibodies that produce such reactions are called **agglutinins.** Agglutination reactions are similar in principle to precipitation reactions. Just as antibody excess inhibits precipitation reactions, an excess of antibody inhibits agglutination reactions; this inhibition is called the **prozone effect**.

Several mechanisms can cause the prozone effect. First, high levels of antibody increase the likelihood that a single antibody molecule will bind to two or more epitopes on a single particulate antigen rather than cross-linking epitopes on two or more particulate antigens. The prozone effect can also occur at high concentrations of antibodies that bind to the antigen but do not induce agglutination; these antibodies, called **incomplete anti-**

bodies, are often of the IgG class. At high concentrations of IgG, incomplete antibodies may occupy all of the antigenic sites, thus blocking access by IgM, which is a good agglutinin. The lack of agglutinating activity of an incomplete antibody may be due to restricted flexibility in the hinge region, making it difficult for the antibody to assume the required angle for optimal cross-linking of epitopes on two or more particulate antigens. Alternatively, the density of epitope distribution or the location of some epitopes in deep pockets of a particulate antigen may make it difficult for antibodies, specific for these epitopes, to agglutinate certain particulate antigens.

Hemagglutination

Agglutination reactions are routinely performed to type red blood cells (RBCs). In typing for the ABO antigens, RBCs are mixed on a slide with antisera to the A and B blood-group antigens. If the antigen is present on the cells, they agglutinate, forming a visible clump on the slide (see Table 6-2). Determination of which antigens are present on donor and recipient RBCs is the basis for matching blood types for transfusions.

At neutral pH, red blood cells are surrounded by a negative ion cloud that makes the cells repel one another; this repulsive force is called the **zeta potential**. Because of its size and pentameric nature, IgM can overcome the zeta potential and cross-link red blood cells, leading to agglutination. The smaller size and bivalency of IgG makes it less able to overcome the zeta potential. For this reason, IgM is more effective than IgG in agglutinating red blood cells. Antibodies to some RBC antigens (e.g., the Rh antigen) are of the IgG class exclusively. In order to agglutinate Rh^+ red blood cells with anti-Rh antibody, the zeta potential must be reduced. This is commonly done by placing the red blood cells in serum albumin, which has a high net negative charge that reduces the effect of the negative ion cloud surrounding the red blood cells, thus allowing anti-Rh antibody to agglutinate Rh^+ cells.

Bacterial Agglutination

A bacterial infection often elicits the production of serum antibodies specific for surface antigens on the bacterial cells. The presence of such antibodies can be detected by bacterial agglutination reactions. Serum from a patient thought to be infected with a given bacterium is serially diluted in a series of tubes to which the bacteria is added. The last tube showing visible agglutination will reflect the serum antibody **titer** of the patient. The agglutinin titer is defined as the reciprocal of the last serum dilution that elicits a positive agglutination reaction. For example, if serial twofold dilutions of serum are prepared and if the dilution of 1/640 shows agglutination but the dilution of 1/1280 does not, then the agglutination titer of the patient's serum is 640. In some cases serum can be diluted up to 1/50,000 and still show agglutination of bacteria.

The agglutinin titer of an antiserum can be used to diagnose a bacterial infection. Patients with typhoid fever, for example, show a significant rise in the agglutination titer to *Salmonella typhi*. Agglutination reactions also provide a way to type bacteria. For instance, different species of the bacterium *Salmonella* can be distinguished by agglutination reactions with a panel of typing antisera.

Passive Agglutination

The sensitivity and simplicity of agglutination reactions can be extended to soluble antigens by the technique of **passive hemagglutination**. In this technique, a soluble antigen is mixed with red blood cells that have been treated with tannic acid or chromium chloride, both of which promote adsorption of the antigen to the surface of the cells. Serum containing antibody is serially diluted into microtiter plate wells, and the antigen-coated red blood cells are added to each well; agglutination is assessed by the size of the characteristic spread pattern of agglutinated red blood cells on the bottom of the well (Figure 6-12).

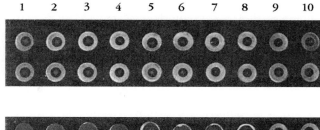
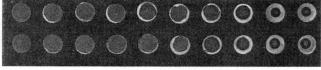

FIGURE 6-12

Passive hemagglutination test to detect antibodies against BSA-conjugated sheep red blood cells (SRBCs). (*Top*) The control wells contain only SRBCs, which settle into a solid "button." (*Bottom*) The experimental wells (in duplicate) contain a constant number of BSA-conjugated SRBCs plus serial dilutions of anti-BSA serum. The spread pattern in the experimental series indicates positive hemagglutination through tube 7, with a slightly positive reaction persisting at the next dilution in tube 8. [From J. S. Garvey et al., 1977, *Methods in Immunology*, 3d ed., W. A. Benjamin Inc., Advanced Book Program.]

Passive hemagglutination is far more sensitive than precipitation reactions and can detect antibody concentrations as low as 0.001 μg/ml. The sensitivities of precipitation and hemagglutination can be compared by testing an antiserum to hen ovalbumin in a tube-precipitation reaction and in passive hemagglutination with ovalbumin-coated red blood cells. Dilution of the antiserum by 1 : 5 results in loss of precipitation ability, whereas the antiserum still functions in passive agglutination out to a dilution of 1 : 10,000. Passive agglutination also can be performed with antigen-coated particles of latex or the mineral colloid bentonite.

Agglutination Inhibition

A modification of the agglutination reaction, called **agglutination inhibition**, provides a highly sensitive assay to detect small quantities of an antigen. For example, one of the early types of home pregnancy test kits included latex particles coated with human chorionic gonadotropin (HCG) and antibody to HCG (see Figure 4-13). The addition of urine from a pregnant woman, which contained HCG, inhibited agglutination of the latex particles when the anti-HCG antibody was added; thus the absence of agglutination indicated pregnancy.

Agglutination inhibition assays also can be used to determine if an individual is using certain types of illegal drugs such as cocaine or heroin. A urine or blood sample containing the suspected drug is first incubated with antibody specific for the drug. Then red blood cells or other particles coated with the drug are added. If the red blood cells are not agglutinated by the antibody, then it suggests that the individual may have been using the illicit drug. One problem with these tests is that some legal drugs have chemical structures similar to those of illicit drugs, and these legal drugs may cross-react with the antibody giving a false-positive reaction. For this reason a positive reaction must be confirmed by a nonimmunologic method.

Agglutination inhibition assays are widely used in clinical laboratories to determine if an individual has been exposed to certain types of viruses that cause agglutination of red blood cells. If an individual's serum contains specific antiviral antibodies, then the antibodies will bind to the virus and interfere with hemagglutination by the virus. This technique is commonly used in premarital testing to determine the immune status of women to rubella virus. The reciprocal of the last serum dilution to show inhibition of rubella hemagglutination is the titer of the serum. A titer greater than 10 (1 : 10 dilution) indicates that a woman is immune to rubella, whereas a titer of less than 10 is indicative of a lack of immunity and the need for immunization with the rubella vaccine.

RADIOIMMUNOASSAY

One of the most sensitive techniques for detecting antigen or antibody is **radioimmunoassay** (RIA). The technique was first developed by two endocrinologists, S. A. Berson and Rosalyn Yalow, in 1960 to determine levels of insulin–anti-insulin complexes in diabetics. Although their original attempts to publish a report of this research met with some resistance from immunologists, the technique soon proved its own value for quantitating hormones, serum proteins, drugs, and vitamins at concentrations of 0.001 μg or less. In 1977, some years after Berson's death, the significance of the technique was acknowledged by the award of a Nobel Prize to Yalow.

The principle of RIA involves competitive binding of radiolabeled antigen and unlabeled antigen to a high-affinity antibody. The antigen is generally labeled with a gamma-emitting isotope such as ^{125}I. The labeled antigen is mixed with antibody at a concentration that just saturates the antigen-binding sites of the antibody molecule, and then increasing amounts of unlabeled antigen of unknown concentration are added. The antibody does not distinguish labeled from unlabeled antigen, and so the two kinds of antigen compete for available binding sites on the antibody. With increasing concentrations of unlabeled antigen, more labeled antigen will be displaced from the binding sites. By measuring the amount of

labeled antigen free in solution, it is possible to determine the concentration of unlabeled antigen.

Several methods have been developed for separating the bound antigen from the free antigen in RIA. One method involves precipitating the Ag-Ab complex with a secondary anti-isotype antiserum. For example, if the Ag-Ab complex contains rabbit IgG antibody, then goat anti-rabbit IgG can precipitate the complex. Another method makes use of the fact that protein A of *Staphylococcus aureus* has high affinity for IgG. If the complex contains an IgG antibody, the complex can be precipitated by mixing with formalin-killed *S. aureus*. After removal of the complex by either of these methods, the amount of free labeled antigen remaining in the supernatant can be quantitated in a gamma counter. A standard curve is then plotted of the percentage of bound labeled antigen versus known concentrations of unlabeled antigen. Once a standard curve had been plotted, unknown concentrations of the unlabeled antigen can be determined from the standard curve.

Various solid-phase RIAs have been developed that make it easier to separate the Ag-Ab complex from the unbound antigen. In some cases the antibody is covalently cross-linked to Sepharose beads. The amount of radiolabeled antigen bound to the beads can be quantitated after the beads have been centrifuged and washed. Alternatively, the antibody can be immobilized on polystyrene or polyvinylchloride and the amount of free labeled antigen in the supernatant can be determined in a gamma counter. In another approach, the antibody is immobilized on the walls of microtiter wells. This procedure is well suited for determining the concentration of a particular antigen in large numbers of samples. For example, a microtiter RIA has been widely used to screen for the presence of the hepatitis B virus (Figure 6-13). RIA screening of donor blood has sharply reduced the incidence of hepatitis B infections in recipients of blood transfusions.

ENZYME-LINKED IMMUNOSORBENT ASSAY

Enzyme-linked immunosorbent assay, commonly known as **ELISA** (or EIA), is similar in principle to RIA but depends on an enzyme rather than a radioactive label. An enzyme conjugated to an antibody reacts with a colorless substrate to generate a colored reaction product. A number of enzymes have been employed for ELISA, including alkaline phosphatase, horseradish peroxidase, and *p*-nitrophenyl phosphatase. When mixed with suitable substrate, each of these enzymes generates a colored reaction product. These assays approach the

(a)

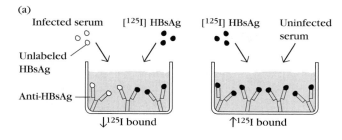

FIGURE 6-13

A solid-phase radioimmunoassay (RIA) to detect hepatitis B virus in blood samples. (a) Microtiter wells are coated with a constant amount of antibody specific for HBsAg, the surface antigen on hepatitis B virions. A serum sample and [^{125}I]HBsAg are then added. After incubation, the supernatant is removed and the amount of radioactivity bound to the antibody is determined. If the sample is infected, the amount of label bound will be less than in controls with uninfected serum. (b) A standard curve is obtained by adding increasing concentrations of unlabeled HBsAg to a fixed quantity of [^{125}I]HBsAg and specific antibody. From the plot of the percentage of labeled antigen bound versus the concentration of unlabeled antigen, the concentration of HBsAg in unknown serum samples can be determined from the linear portion of the curve.

(b)

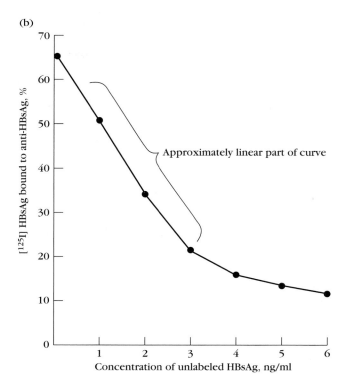

sensitivity of RIAs and have the advantage of being safer and less costly.

A number of variations of ELISA have been developed, allowing detection and quantitation of either antigen or antibody. Each type of ELISA can be used qualitatively to detect the presence of antibody or antigen. Alternatively, a standard curve based on known concentrations of antibody or antigen is prepared from which the unknown concentration of a sample can be determined.

Indirect ELISA

Antibody can be detected or quantitated with an indirect ELISA (Figure 6-14a). Serum or some other sample containing primary antibody (Ab$_1$) is added to an antigen-coated microtiter well and allowed to react with the bound antigen. After any free Ab$_1$ is washed away, the presence of antibody bound to the antigen is detected by adding an enzyme-conjugated secondary anti-isotype antibody (Ab$_2$), which binds to the primary antibody. Any free Ab$_2$ then is washed away, and a substrate for the enzyme is added. The colored reaction product that forms is measured by specialized spectrophotometric plate readers, which can measure the absorbance of a 96-well plate in less than a minute.

Indirect ELISA has been the method of choice to detect the presence of serum antibodies against human immunodeficiency virus (HIV), the causative agent of AIDS. In this assay recombinant envelope and core proteins of HIV are adsorbed as solid-phase antigens to microtiter wells. Individuals infected with HIV will produce serum antibodies to epitopes on these viral proteins. Generally, serum antibodies to HIV can be detected by indirect ELISA within 6 weeks of infection.

Sandwich ELISA

Antigen can be detected or quantitated by a sandwich ELISA (Figure 6-14b). In this technique the antibody (rather than the antigen) is immobilized on a microtiter well. A sample containing antigen is added and allowed to react with the bound antibody. After the well is washed, a second enzyme-linked antibody specific for a different epitope on the antigen is added and allowed to react with the bound antigen. After any free second antibody is removed by washing, substrate is added and the colored reaction product is measured.

Competitive ELISA

Another variation for quantitating antigen is competitive ELISA (Figure 6-14c). In this technique antibody is first incubated in solution with a sample containing antigen. The antigen–antibody mixture is then added to an

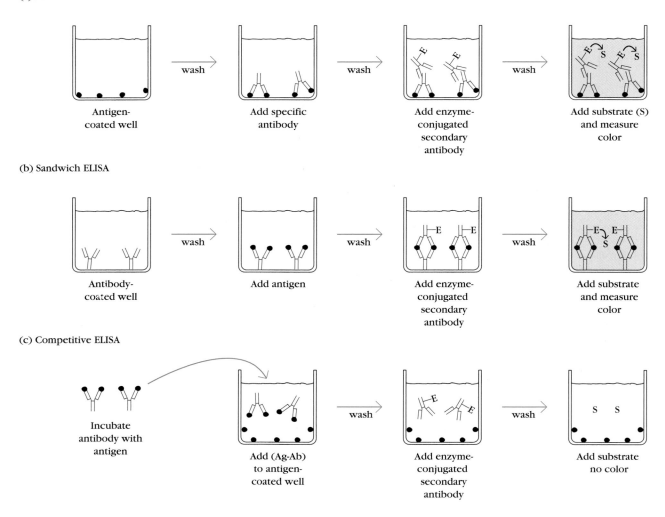

(a) Indirect ELISA

Antigen-
coated well → wash → Add specific
antibody → wash → Add enzyme-
conjugated
secondary
antibody → wash → Add substrate (S)
and measure
color

(b) Sandwich ELISA

Antibody-
coated well → wash → Add antigen → wash → Add enzyme-
conjugated
secondary
antibody → wash → Add substrate
and measure
color

(c) Competitive ELISA

Incubate
antibody with
antigen → Add (Ag-Ab)
to antigen-
coated well → wash → Add enzyme-
conjugated
secondary
antibody → wash → Add substrate
no color

FIGURE 6-14

Variations in the enzyme-linked immunosorbent assay (ELISA) technique allow determination of antibody or antigen. Each assay can be used qualitatively or quantitatively by comparison with standard curves prepared with known concentrations of antibody or antigen. Antibody can be determined with an indirect ELISA (a), whereas antigen can be determined with a sandwich ELISA (b) or competitive ELISA (c). In the competitive ELISA, which is an inhibition-type assay, the concentration of antigen is inversely proportional to the color produced.

antigen–coated microtiter well. The more antigen present in the sample, the less free antibody will be available to bind to the antigen-coated well. Addition of an enzyme-conjugated secondary antibody (Ab_2) specific for the isotype of the primary antibody can be used to quantitate the amount of primary antibody bound to the well as in an indirect ELISA. In the competitive assay, however, the higher the concentration of antigen in the original sample, the lower the absorbance.

WESTERN BLOTTING

Identification of a specific protein in a complex mixture of proteins can be accomplished by a technique known as **Western blotting**, named for its similarity to Southern blotting, which detects DNA fragments, and Northern blotting, which detects mRNAs. In Western blotting a protein mixture is electrophoretically separated

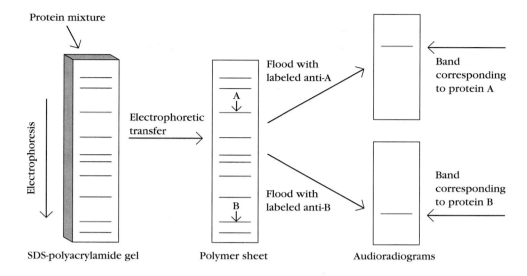

Protein mixture

Electrophoresis

Electrophoretic transfer

A

B

Flood with labeled anti-A

Flood with labeled anti-B

Band corresponding to protein A

Band corresponding to protein B

SDS-polyacrylamide gel

Polymer sheet

Audioradiograms

FIGURE 6-15

In Western blotting a protein mixture is separated by electrophoresis, and the protein bands are transferred by electrophoresis onto a nitrocellulose or other polymer sheet. After the sheet is flooded with radiolabeled specific antibodies, the various protein bands can be visualized by autoradiography.

on a polyacrylamide slab gel in the presence of sodium dodecyl sulfate (SDS), a dissociating agent. The protein bands are transferred to a nitrocellulose membrane by electrophoresis and the individual protein bands are identified by flooding the nitrocellulose membrane with radiolabeled polyclonal or monoclonal antibody specific for the protein of interest. The Ag-Ab complexes that form are visualized by autoradiography (Figure 6-15). If labeled specific antibody is not available, Ag-Ab complexes can be detected by adding a secondary anti-isotype antibody that is either radiolabeled or enzyme-labeled; in this case the band is visualized by autoradiography or substrate addition.

Western blotting can also identify a specific antibody in a mixture. In this case, the separated antibody bands are visualized with a labeled antigen. For example, this technique has been used to identify the envelope and core proteins of HIV and the antibodies to these components in the serum of HIV-infected individuals.

IMMUNOFLUORESCENCE

Antibodies that are bound to cells or tissue sections can be visualized by tagging the antibody molecules with a fluorescent dye, or **fluorochrome**. In this technique, known as **immunofluorescence**, the most commonly used fluorescent dyes are fluorescein and rhodamine. Both dyes can be conjugated to the Fc region of an antibody molecule without affecting the specificity of the antibody. Each of these dyes absorbs light at one wavelength and emits light at a longer wavelength:

- **Fluorescein** absorbs blue light (490 nm) and emits an intense yellow-green fluorescence (517 nm).
- **Rhodamine** absorbs in the yellow-green range (515 nm) and emits a deep red fluorescence (546 nm).

The emitted light is generally viewed with a fluorescence microscope, which is equipped with a UV light source and excitation filters. By conjugating fluorescein to one antibody and rhodamine to another antibody, one can visualize two cell-membrane antigens simultaneously on the same cell.

Fluorescent-antibody staining of cell-membrane molecules or tissue sections can be direct or indirect (Figure 6-16). In **direct** staining the specific antibody (called the primary antibody) is directly conjugated with fluorescein; in **indirect** staining the primary antibody is unlabeled and is detected with an additional fluorochrome-labeled reagent. A number of reagents have been developed for indirect staining. The most common is **fluorochrome-labeled anti-isotype antibody,** such as fluorescein-labeled goat anti-mouse immunoglobulin. Another reagent is **fluorochrome-labeled protein A** from *Staphylococcus aureus*; this pro-

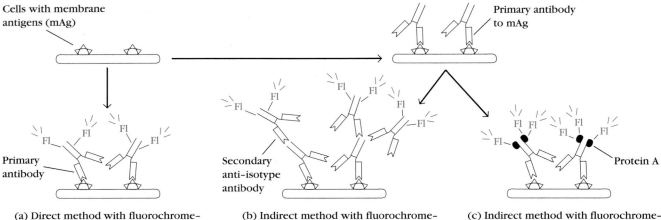

Cells with membrane
antigens (mAg)

Primary antibody
to mAg

Primary
antibody

Secondary
anti-isotype
antibody

Protein A

(a) Direct method with fluorochrome-
labeled antibody to mAg

(b) Indirect method with fluorochrome-
labeled anti-isotype antibody

(c) Indirect method with fluorochrome-
labeled protein A

FIGURE 6-16

Direct and indirect immunofluorescence staining of membrane antigen (mAg). Cells are affixed to a microscope slide. In the direct method (a), cells are stained with anti-mAg antibody that is labeled with a fluorochrome (Fl). In the indirect methods (b and c), cells are first incubated with unlabeled anti-mAg antibody and then stained with a fluorochrome-labeled secondary reagent that binds to the primary antibody. Observation under a fluorescence microscope indicates whether the cells have been stained.

tein binds with high affinity to the Fc region of IgG antibody molecules. A third indirect approach involves use of a secondary biotin-conjugated anti-isotype antibody followed by addition of fluorochrome-conjugated avidin, a protein that binds to biotin with extremely high affinity.

Indirect immunofluorescence staining has two advantages over direct staining. First, the primary antibody does not need to be conjugated with label. Because the supply of primary antibody is often a limiting factor, indirect methods avoid the loss of antibody that usually occurs during radiolabeling. Second, indirect methods increase the sensitivity of staining because multiple fluorochrome reagents will bind to each primary antibody molecule.

Immunofluorescence has been applied to identify a number of subpopulations of lymphocytes, notably the CD4$^+$ and CD8$^+$ T-cell subpopulations. The technique is also suitable for identifying bacterial species, detecting Ag-Ab complexes in autoimmune disease, detecting complement components in tissues, and localizing hormones and other cellular products stained in situ.

Subpopulations of lymphocytes labeled with fluorochrome-conjugated antibody can be analyzed and sorted on the basis of the intensity of staining in a specialized flow cytometer called a **fluorescence-activated cell sorter** (FACS), as illustrated in Figure 6-17. The FACS permits separation of fluorescein-stained and rhodamine-stained subpopulations as well as high-, medium-, and low-staining cells. Flow cytometry also makes it possible to analyze three fluorochromes on a single stained sample.

IMMUNOELECTRON MICROSCOPY

The fine specificity of antibodies has made them powerful tools for visualizing specific intracellular tissue components by **immunoelectron microscopy**. In this technique an electron-dense label is either conjugated directly to the Fc portion of an antibody molecule or an indirect staining technique is employed in which the electron-dense label is conjugated to an anti-immunoglobulin reagent. A number of electron-dense labels have been employed including ferritin and colloidal gold. As the electron-dense label absorbs electrons, it can be visualized with the electron microscope as small black dots. In the case of immunogold labeling, different antibodies can be conjugated with different sizes of gold

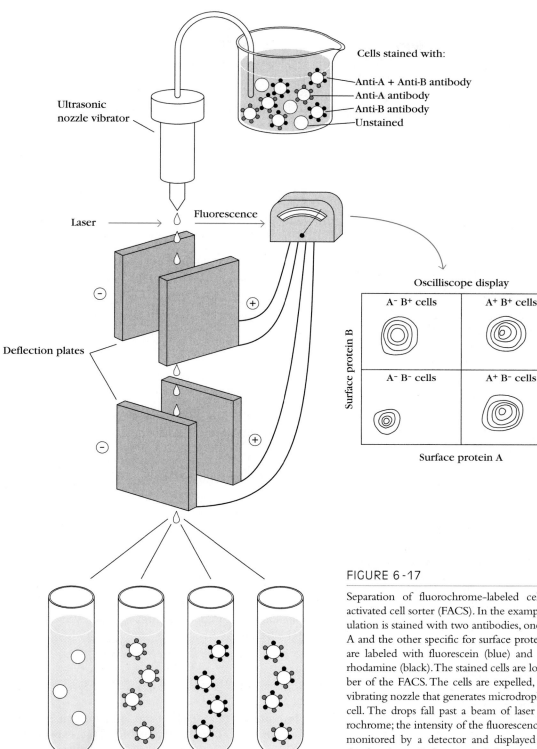

Cells stained with:

Anti-A + Anti-B antibody
Anti-A antibody
Anti-B antibody
Unstained

Ultrasonic nozzle vibrator

Laser

Fluorescence

Deflection plates

Oscilliscope display

A⁻ B⁺ cells   A⁺ B⁺ cells

A⁻ B⁻ cells   A⁺ B⁻ cells

Surface protein B

Surface protein A

A⁻ B⁻
cells

A⁺ B⁻
cells

A⁻ B⁺
cells

A⁺ B⁺
cells

FIGURE 6-17

Separation of fluorochrome-labeled cells with the fluorescence-activated cell sorter (FACS). In the example shown, a mixed cell population is stained with two antibodies, one specific for surface protein A and the other specific for surface protein B. The anti-A antibodies are labeled with fluorescein (blue) and the anti-B antibodies with rhodamine (black). The stained cells are loaded into the sample chamber of the FACS. The cells are expelled, one at a time, from a small vibrating nozzle that generates microdroplets, each containing a single cell. The drops fall past a beam of laser light that excites the fluorochrome; the intensity of the fluorescence emitted by each droplet is monitored by a detector and displayed on an oscilloscope. Those droplets that emit fluorescent light are electrically charged in proportion to their fluorescence; the charged droplets then are separated as they flow past the deflection plates. Based on surface proteins A and B, this mixture of cells contains four subpopulations: A^+B^-, A^-B^+, A^+B^+, and A^-B^-.

particles, allowing identification of several intracellular antigens within a cell by the size of the electron-dense gold particle attached to the antibody. These techniques have played an important role in demonstrating that class I and class II MHC molecules may be sequestered along different intracellular processing routes.

SUMMARY

1. The Ag-Ab interaction depends on noncovalent interactions including hydrogen bonds, ionic bonds, hydrophobic interactions, and van der Waals interactions (see Figure 6-1). The strength of this interaction depends on the number of these weak noncovalent interactions between antigen and antibody. The affinity of an antibody for an antigen refers to the strength of the noncovalent interactions between the antibody and antigen at a single binding site; the avidity reflects the overall strength of the interactions between a multivalent antibody and multivalent antigen at multiple sites.

2. The interaction of a soluble antigen and precipitating antibody (precipitin) forms an Ag-Ab complex that has a lattice structure and precipitates out of solution. Precipitation reactions can be performed in liquids or gels. Most are useful primarily for qualitative comparison of antibodies or antigens (see Figure 6-8), although some versions can quantitate antibodies or antigens (see Figure 6-7). Electrophoresis can be combined with precipitation in gels in a technique called immunoelectrophoresis. A variety of immunoelectrophoretic techniques have been developed, including rocket electrophoresis and two-dimensional electrophoresis (see Figures 6-9, 6-10, and 6-11).

3. The interaction between a particulate antigen and agglutinating antibody (agglutinin) produces visible clumping, or agglutination. In some cases the antigen is a membrane protein on a bacterial cell or red blood cell. In other cases the antigen may be attached to a latex particle or adsorbed on the surface of a red blood cell. Agglutination reactions are more sensitive than precipitin reactions and can often detect 100- or 1000-fold lower levels of antigen or antibody than can be detected with a precipitin reaction.

4. Radioimmunoassay (RIA) utilizes radioactively labeled antigen or antibody and is therefore a highly sensitive technique. Liquid-phase RIA is based on the principle of competition between labeled and unlabeled antigen for a limited amount of antibody. In solid-phase RIA, antigen (or antibody) is immobilized on a solid matrix (see Figure 6-13). The main advantage of this technique over liquid-phase RIA is its simplicity of performance and the ease with which bound Ag-Ab complex can be separated from unreacted antigen. Both types of RIA can be used to quantitate antibody or antigen.

5. The enzyme-linked immunosorbent assay (ELISA) involves principles similar to those of RIA but depends on an enzyme-substrate reaction that generates a colored reaction product rather than a radiolabel. An indirect ELISA detects antibody, whereas sandwich ELISA and competitive ELISA detect antigen (see Figure 6-14).

6. In Western blotting, a protein mixture is separated by electrophoresis; then the protein bands are electrophoretically transferred onto nitrocellulose and identified with labeled antibody or labeled antigen (see Figure 6-15).

7. Fluorescent-antibody staining can visualize antigen on cells. Various direct and indirect immunofluorescence staining techniques have been developed (see Figure 6-16). The fluorescence-activated cell sorter analyzes and sorts cells labeled with fluorescent antibody (see Figure 6-17).

REFERENCES

AXELSEN, N. H. 1983. *Handbook of Immunoprecipitation-in-Gel Techniques.* Blackwell Scientific Publications.

EDWARDS, R. 1985. *Immunoassay: An Introduction.* Heinemann Medical Books.

JOHNSTONE, A. (ED.). 1989. Immunological techniques. *Curr. Opin. Immunol.* **1**:927.

JOHNSTONE, A., AND R. THORPE. 1987. *Immunochemistry in Practice,* 2d ed. Blackwell Scientific Publications.

POLAK, J. M., AND S. VANNOORDEN. 1987. *An Introduction to Immunocytochemistry: Current Techniques and Problems.* Oxford Science Publishers.

WEIR, D. M. (ED.). 1986. *Handbook of Experimental Immunology,* 4th ed. Vols. I and II. Blackwell Scientific Publications.

STUDY QUESTIONS

1. Indicate whether each of the following statements is true or false. If you think a statement is false, explain why.

a. Indirect immunofluorescence is a more sensitive technique than direct immunofluorescence.

b. Most antigens induce a polyclonal response.

c. A papain digest of anti-SRBC antibodies can agglutinate sheep red blood cells (SRBCs).

d. A pepsin digest of anti-SRBC antibodies can agglutinate SRBCs.

e. Indirect immunofluorescence can be performed using a Fab fragment as the initial nonlabeled antibody.

f. For precipitation to occur, both antigen and antibody must be multivalent.

g. The Ouchterlony technique is a quantitative precipitin technique.

h. Precipitation tests are generally more sensitive than agglutination tests.

2. Briefly outline the ELISA test for HIV infection indicating which antigen and antibody are used.

3. You have obtained a preparation of purified albumin from normal bovine serum. To determine whether any other serum proteins remain in this preparation of BSA, you decide to use immunoelectrophoresis.

a. What antigen would you use to prepare the antiserum needed to detect impurities in the BSA preparation?

b. Assuming that the BSA preparation is pure, draw the immunoelectrophoretic pattern you would expect if the assay was performed with bovine serum in one well, the BSA sample in a second well, and the antiserum you prepared in (a) in the trough between the wells.

4. The labels from four bottles (A, B, C, and D) of hapten-carrier conjugates were accidentally removed. However, it was known that each bottle contained either hapten 1-carrier 1 (H1-C1), hapten 1-carrier 2 (H1-C2), hapten 2-carrier 1 (H2-C1), or hapten 2-carrier 2 (H2-C2). Double-immunodiffusion (Ouchterlony) assays with either anti–H1-C2 or anti–H2-C2 were performed. From the precipitin patterns shown below, determine which conjugate is in each bottle.

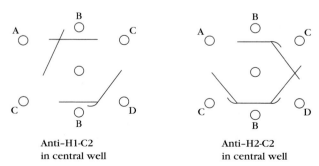

Anti-H1-C2
in central well

Anti-H2-C2
in central well

5. The concentration of a hapten can be determined by which of the following assays: (a) ELISA, (b) Ouchterlony method, (c) rocket electrophoresis, and (d) RIA.

6. You perform an Ouchterlony assay in which the central well contains goat antiserum against the F(ab')$_2$ fragment of pooled mouse IgG and the surrounding wells (A–F) contain six different test antigens. The resulting precipitin pattern is shown below.

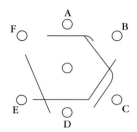

Based on this pattern, indicate which well contains each of the following test antigens:

a. _____ Fab fragment from an IgG myeloma protein ($\gamma_2\kappa_2$)

b. _____ Kappa (κ) light chains

c. _____ Gamma (γ) heavy chains

d. _____ Lambda (λ) light chains

e. _____ Fc fragment from IgG myeloma protein ($\gamma_2\lambda_2$)

f. _____ A mixture of γ heavy chains and κ light chains

7. You have a myeloma protein X whose isotype is unknown and several other myeloma proteins of known isotype (e.g., IgG, IgM, and IgA).

a. How could you produce anti-isotype antibodies that could be used to determine the isotype of myeloma protein X?

b. How could you use this anti-isotype antibody to measure the level of myeloma protein X in normal serum?

8. For each antigen or antibody listed below, indicate an appropriate assay method and the necessary test reagents. Keep in mind the sensitivity of the assay and the expected concentration of each protein.

a. IgG in serum

b. Insulin in serum

c. IgE in serum

d. Complement component C3 on glomerular basement membrane

e. Anti-A antibodies to blood-group antigen A in serum

f. Horsemeat contamination of hamburger

g. Syphilis spirochete in a smear from a chancre

9. Which of the following does *not* participate in the formation of antigen-antibody complexes?

a. Hydrophobic bonds

b. Covalent bonds

c. Electrostatic interactions

d. Hydrogen bonds

e. van der Waals forces

10. Explain the difference between antibody affinity and antibody avidity. Which of these properties of an antibody better reflects its ability to contribute to the humoral immune response to invading bacteria.

11. You want to develop a sensitive immunoassay for a hormone that occurs in the blood at concentrations around 10^{-7} M. You are offered a choice of three different antisera whose affinities for the hormone have been determined by equilibrium dialysis. The results are shown in the following Scatchard plots.

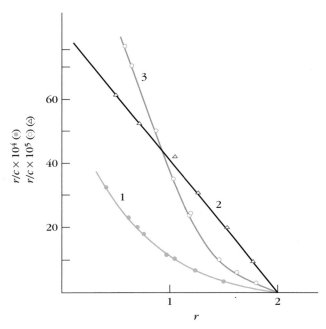

a. What is the value of K_0 for each antiserum?

b. What is the valence of each of the antibodies?

c. Which of the antisera might be a monoclonal antibody?

d. Which of the antisera would you use for your assay? Why?

12. In preparing a demonstration for her immunology class, an instructor purified IgG antibodies to sheep red blood cells (SRBCs) and digested some of the antibodies into Fab, Fc, and F(ab')$_2$ fragments. She placed each preparation in a separate tube, labeled the tubes with a water-soluble marker, and left them in an ice bucket. When the instructor returned for her class period, she discovered that the labels had smeared and were unreadable. Determined to salvage the demonstration, she relabeled the tubes 1, 2, 3, and 4 and proceeded. Based on the test results described below, indicate which preparation was contained in each tube and explain why you so identified the contents.

a. The preparation in tube 1 agglutinated SRBCs but did not lyse them in the presence of complement.

b. The preparation in tube 2 did not agglutinate SRBCs or lyse them in the presence of complement. However, when this preparation was added to SRBCs before the addition of whole anti-SRBC, it prevented agglutination of the cells by the whole anti-SRBC antiserum.

c. The preparation in tube 3 agglutinated SRBCs and also lysed the cells in the presence of complement.

d. The preparation in tube 4 did not agglutinate or lyse SRBCs and did not inhibit agglutination of SRBCs by whole anti-SRBC antiserum.

13. You are given two solutions, one containing protein X and the other antibody to this protein. When you add 1 ml of anti-X to 1 ml of protein X, a precipitate forms. But when you dilute the antibody solution 100-fold and then mix 1 ml of the diluted anti-X with 1 ml of protein X, no precipitate forms.

a. Explain why no precipitate formed with the diluted antibody.

b. Which species (protein X or anti-X) would likely be present in the supernatant of the antibody-antigen mixture in each case?

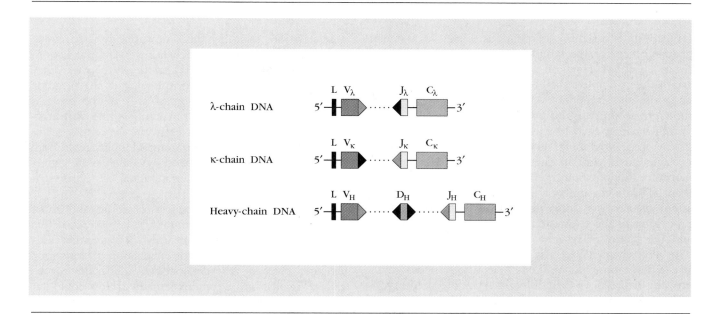

ORGANIZATION AND EXPRESSION
OF IMMUNOGLOBULIN GENES

One of the most remarkable features of the vertebrate immune system is its ability to respond to an apparently limitless array of foreign antigens. As immunoglobulin (Ig) sequence data accumulated, virtually every antibody molecule studied was found to contain a unique amino acid sequence in its variable region but only one of a limited number of invariant sequences in its constant region. The genetic basis of such tremendous variation coupled with constancy in a single protein molecule lies in the organization of the immunoglobulin genes.

In germ-line DNA, multiple gene segments encode a single immunoglobulin heavy or light chain. These gene segments are carried in the germ cells but cannot be transcribed and translated into heavy and light chains until they are arranged into functional genes. During B-cell maturation in the bone marrow, these gene segments are randomly shuffled by a dynamic genetic system capable of generating more than 10^8 specificities. This process is carefully regulated: the progression of a progenitor B cell into a mature cell involves an ordered sequence of Ig-gene rearrangements. By the end of this process a mature, immunocompetent B cell will contain a single, functional variable-region DNA sequence encoding an Ig heavy chain and a single, functional variable-region DNA sequence encoding an Ig light chain, so that the individual B cell is antigenically committed to a specific epitope. After antigenic stimulation of a mature B cell in peripheral lymphoid organs, further rearrangement of constant-region gene segments can generate changes in the isotype expressed, producing changes in the associated biological effector functions without changing the specificity of the immunoglobulin molecule. Thus mature B cells contain chromosomal DNA that is no longer identical to germ-line

DNA. While we think of genomic DNA as a stable genetic blueprint, the lymphocyte cell lineage does not retain an intact copy of this blueprint. Genomic rearrangement is an essential feature of lymphocyte differentiation, and no other vertebrate cell type has been shown to accomplish this process.

This chapter first describes the detailed organization of the immunoglobulin genes, the process of Ig-gene rearrangement, and the mechanisms by which the dynamic immunoglobulin genetic system generates more than 10^8 different antigenic specificities. Then the mechanism of class switching, the role of differential RNA processing in the expression of immunoglobulin genes, and regulation of Ig-gene transcription are discussed. The next chapter covers in detail the entire process of B-cell development from the first gene rearrangement in progenitor B cells to final differentiation into memory B cells and antibody-secreting plasma cells. Figure 7-1 outlines the sequential stages in B-cell development.

GENETIC MODEL COMPATIBLE WITH IG STRUCTURE

The results of the immunoglobulin-sequencing studies discussed in Chapter 5 revealed a number of features of immunoglobulin structure that were difficult to reconcile with classic genetic models. Any viable model of the immunoglobulin genes had to account for the following properties of antibodies:

- The vast diversity of antibody specificities
- The presence of a variable region at the amino-terminal end and of a constant region at the carboxyl-terminal end of Ig heavy and light chains
- The existence of isotypes with the same antigenic specificity, which result from the association of a given variable region with different heavy-chain constant regions

Germ-Line and Somatic-Variation Models

It has been estimated that the mammalian immune system can generate more than 10^8 different antibody specificities, allowing an animal to respond to a vast number of potential antigens. Since antibodies are proteins and proteins are encoded by genes, it follows that this tremendous diversity in antibody structure must arise from a genetic system capable of generating enormous diversity. For several decades immunologists sought to imagine a genetic mechanism that might generate such diversity. Two very different sets of theories emerged. The **germ-line** theories maintained that the genome contains a large repertoire of immunoglobulin genes sufficient to generate more than 10^8 different antibody specificities; thus no special genetic mechanisms were invoked to account for antibody diversity in these theories. They argued that the immense survival value of the immune system justified the dedication of 15% of the genome to the coding of antibodies. In contrast, the **somatic-variation** theories maintained that the genome contains a relatively small number of immunoglobulin genes from which a large number of antibody specificities are generated in the somatic cells by mutational or recombinational mechanisms.

As the amino acid sequences of more and more immunoglobulins were determined, it became clear that there must be mechanisms not only for generating antibody diversity but also for maintaining constancy. Whether diversity was generated by germ-line or by somatic mechanisms, a paradox remained: How could stability be maintained in the constant (C) region while some kind of diversifying mechanism generated the variable (V) region?

Neither the germ-line nor the somatic variation proponents could offer a reasonable explanation of this central feature of immunoglobulin structure. Germ-line proponents found it difficult to account for an evolutionary mechanism that could generate diversity in the variable part of each gene while preserving the constant region unchanged. Somatic-variation proponents found it difficult to conceive of a mechanism that could diversify the variable region of a single gene in the somatic cells without allowing a single alteration in the amino acid sequence encoded by the constant region.

A third structural feature of immunoglobulins requiring an explanation emerged when amino acid sequencing of the human myeloma protein called Ti1 revealed that identical variable-region sequences were associated with both γ and μ heavy-chain constant regions. A similar phenomenon was observed in rabbits by C. Todd, who found that a particular allotypic marker in the heavy-chain variable region could be associated with α, γ, and μ heavy-chain constant regions. Considerable additional evidence has confirmed that a single variable-region sequence, defining a particular antigenic specificity, can be associated with multiple heavy-chain constant region sequences; in other words, different classes, or **isotypes**, of antibody (e.g., IgG, IgM) can be expressed having identical variable-region sequences.

Dryer and Bennett Two-Gene Model

In an attempt to develop a genetic model consistent with these findings about the structure of immunoglobulins, W. Dryer and J. Bennett suggested, in their classic theoretical paper of 1965, that two separate genes encode a single immunoglobulin heavy or light chain, one gene encoding the V region and one gene encoding the C

Visualizing Concepts

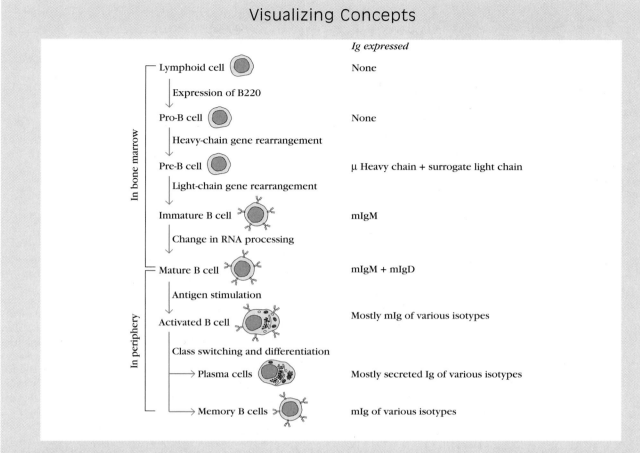

FIGURE 7-1

Overview of B-cell development. The events that occur during maturation in the bone marrow do not require antigen, whereas activation and differentiation of mature B cells in peripheral lymphoid organs require antigen. mIgM, mIgD, and mIgG refer to membrane-associated Igs.

region. They suggested that these two genes must somehow come together at the DNA level to form a continuous message that can be transcribed and translated to yield a single Ig heavy or light chain. Moreover, they proposed that hundreds or thousands of V-region genes were carried in the germ line, whereas only single copies of C-region class and subclass genes need exist.

The strength of this type of recombinational model (which combined elements of the germ-line and somatic-variation theories) was that it could account for those immunoglobulins in which a single V region was combined with various C regions. By postulating a single constant-region gene for each immunoglobulin class and subclass, the model also could account for the conservation of necessary biological effector functions while

allowing for evolutionary diversification of variable-region genes.

At first, support for the Dryer and Bennett hypothesis was indirect. Early studies of DNA hybridization kinetics using a radioactive constant-region DNA probe indicated that the probe hybridized with only one or two genes, confirming the model's prediction that only one or two copies of each constant-region class and subclass gene existed. Not only was the evidence in support of the Dryer and Bennett model initially indirect, there was stubborn resistance to their hypothesis in the scientific community. The suggestion that two genes coded a single polypeptide contradicted the existing one gene–one polypeptide principle and was without precedent in any known biological system.

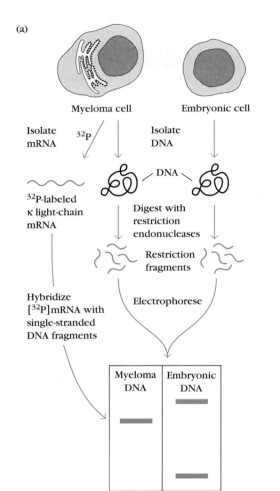

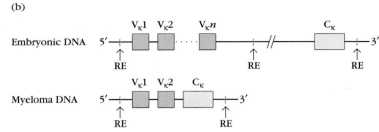

FIGURE 7-2

Experimental demonstration that genes encoding κ light chains are rearranged during B-cell development. (a) DNA from embryonic cells and myeloma cells (equivalent to differentiated plasma cells) was digested with several restriction endonucleases, and the digests were subjected to agarose gel electrophoresis. After the gels were cut into slices and eluted, the eluted samples were treated to denature the double-stranded DNA fragments into single-stranded DNA, and then incubated with ^{32}P-labeled mRNA encoding κ light chains. The mRNA probe hybridized with two bands from the germ-line embryonic DNA but with only a single band from the differentiated myeloma DNA. (b) Structure of embryonic and myeloma κ light-chain DNA compatible with the experimental results supports the Dryer and Bennett two-gene model. During development of B cells, κ exons (V_{κ} and C_{κ}) are brought closer together and the restriction-endonuclease (RE) site between them is eliminated. [Adapted from N. Hozumi and S. Tonegawa, 1976, *Proc. Natl. Acad. Sci. USA* **73**:3628.]

As so often is the case in science, theoretical and intellectual understanding of Ig-gene organization progressed ahead of the available methodology. Although the Dryer and Bennett model provided a theoretical framework for reconciling the dilemma between Ig-sequence data and gene organization, actual validation of their hypothesis had to wait for several major technological advances in the field of molecular biology. In time, the Dryer and Bennett hypothesis was proven to be essentially correct. Indeed, far more complex genetic mechanisms have been shown to be involved than could have been imagined at the time that Dryer and Bennett published their paper.

Verification of the Dryer and Bennett Hypothesis

In 1976 S. Tonegawa and N. Hozumi provided the first direct evidence that separate genes encode the V and C regions of immunoglobulins and that the genes are rearranged in the course of B-cell differentiation. This work changed not only the field of immunology, but all of the biological sciences. In 1987 Tonegawa was awarded the Nobel Prize for this work.

Using various restriction endonucleases, Tonegawa and Hozumi cleaved DNA from embryonic cells and from adult myeloma cells into fragments. These fragments were separated by size on agarose gel electrophoresis and were analyzed for their ability to hybridize with a radiolabeled κ-chain mRNA probe. Two separate restriction fragments from the embryonic DNA hybridized with the mRNA, whereas only a single restriction fragment of the myeloma DNA hybridized with the same probe (Figure 7-2a). Tonegawa and Hozumi suggested that during differentiation of lymphocytes from the embryonic state to the fully differentiated plasma-cell stage (represented in their system by myeloma cells), the V and C genes undergo rearrangement. In the embryo the V and C genes are separated by a large DNA segment containing a restriction-endonuclease site; during differentiation the V and C genes are brought closer together and the intervening DNA sequence containing the restriction site is eliminated (Figure 7-2b).

Subsequently, researchers took an approach similar to that of Tonegawa and Hozumi but used the newly developed technique of Southern blotting, thus eliminating the need to elute the separated restriction DNA fragments from the gel slices (see Figure 2-6). Southern-blot analyses permitted comparisons of the light-chain and heavy-chain gene arrangement in non-B cells (e.g., embryonic cells and liver cells) and in myeloma cells, which represent fully differentiated B cells. These results, analogous to those in Figure 7-2, demonstrated that the Dryer and Bennett two-gene model—one gene encoding the variable region and one gene encoding the constant region—applied to both heavy- and light-chain genes.

MULTIGENE ORGANIZATION OF IG GENES

As cloning and sequencing of the light- and heavy-chain DNA was accomplished, even greater complexity was revealed than had been predicted by Dryer and Bennett. The κ and λ light chains and the heavy chains are encoded by separate multigene families situated on different chromosomes (Table 7-1). In germ-line DNA, each of these multigene families contains several coding sequences, called **gene segments**, separated by noncoding regions. During B-cell maturation, these gene segments are rearranged and brought together to form functional immunoglobulin genes.

The κ and λ light-chain families contain **V**, **J**, and **C** gene segments; the rearranged VJ segments encode the variable region of the light chains. The heavy-chain family contains **V**, **D**, **J**, and **C** gene segments; the rearranged VDJ gene segments encode the variable region of the

heavy chain. The C gene segments encode the constant regions. Each V gene segment is preceded at its 5′ end by a small exon that encodes a short **signal** or **leader** (L) peptide that guides the heavy or light chain through the endoplasmic reticulum. The signal peptide is cleaved from the nascent light and heavy chains before assembly of the finished immunoglobulin molecule. Thus amino acids encoded by this leader sequence do not appear in the immunoglobulin molecule.

λ-Chain Multigene Family

The first evidence that the light-chain variable region was actually encoded by two gene segments was provided when Tonegawa cloned the germ-line DNA encoding the variable region of mouse λ light chain and determined its complete nucleotide sequence. When the nucleotide sequence was compared with the known amino acid sequence of the λ-chain variable region, an unusual discrepancy was observed. Although the first 97 amino acids of the λ-chain variable region corresponded to the nucleotide codon sequence, the remaining 13 carboxyl-terminal amino acids of the protein's variable region did not correspond to the sequential nucleotide sequence. It turned out that many base pairs away a separate, 39-bp gene segment, called **J** for **joining**, encoded the remaining 13 amino acids of the λ-chain variable region. Thus a functional λ variable-region gene contains two coding segments—a 5′ V segment and a 3′ J segment—which are separated by a noncoding DNA sequence in unrearranged germ-line DNA.

The λ multigene family in the mouse contains two V_λ gene segments, four J_λ gene segments, and four C_λ gene segments (Figure 7-3a). The $J_\lambda 4$ and $C_\lambda 4$ gene segments are defective genes, called **pseudogenes**, which are indicated with the psi symbol (ψ). The V_λ and J_λ gene segments encode the variable region of the light chain, and the three functional C_λ gene segments encode the constant regions of the three λ-chain subtypes ($\lambda 1$, $\lambda 2$, and $\lambda 3$). In humans there are an estimated 100 V_λ gene segments, 6 J_λ segments, and 6 C_λ segments.

κ-Chain Multigene Family

The κ-chain multigene family in the mouse contains approximately 300 V_κ gene segments, each with an adjacent leader sequence a short distance upstream (i.e., on the 5′ side). There are five J_κ gene segments (one of which is a nonfunctional pseudogene) and a single C_κ gene segment (Figure 7-3b). As in the λ multigene family, the V_κ and J_κ gene segments encode the variable region of the κ light chain, and the C_κ gene segment encodes the constant region. Since there is only one C_κ gene segment, there are no subclasses of κ light chains.

TABLE 7-1

CHROMOSOMAL LOCATIONS OF IMMUNOGLOBULIN GENES IN HUMAN AND MOUSE

	CHROMOSOME	
GENE	HUMAN	MOUSE
λ Light chain	22	16
κ Light chain	2	6
Heavy chain	14	12

Visualizing Concepts

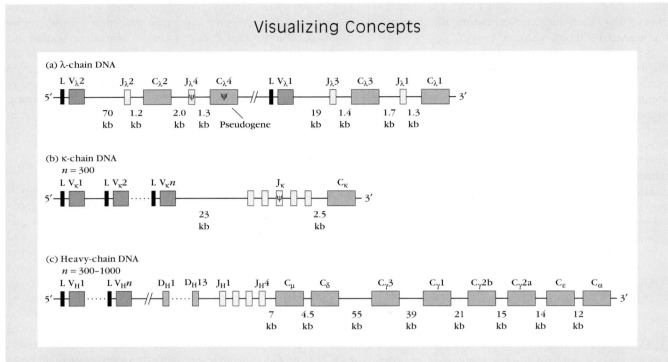

FIGURE 7-3

Organization of immunoglobulin germ-line gene segments in the mouse: (a) λ light chain, (b) κ light chain, and (c) heavy chain. The λ and κ light chains are encoded by V, J, and C gene segments. The heavy chain is encoded by V, D, J, and C gene segments. The distances in kilobases (kb) separating the various gene segments in mouse germ-line DNA are shown below each chain diagram.

Comparison of Figure 7-3a and b shows that the arrangement of the gene segments is quite different in the κ and λ gene families. The κ-chain multigene family in humans, which is similar to that in the mouse, contains approximately 100 V_κ gene segments, 5 J_κ segments, and a single C_κ segment.

Heavy-Chain Multigene Family

The organization of the mouse immunoglobulin heavy-chain genes is similar to, but more complex than, that of the κ and λ light-chain genes (Figure 7-3c). An additional gene segment encodes part of the heavy-chain variable region. The existence of this gene segment was first proposed by Leroy Hood and his colleagues, who compared the heavy-chain variable region amino acid sequence with the V_H and J_H nucleotide sequences. The V_H gene segment was found to encode amino acids 1 to 94 and the J_H gene segment was found to encode

amino acids 98 to 113; however, neither of these gene segments carried the information to encode amino acids 95 to 97. When the nucleotide sequence was determined for a rearranged myeloma DNA and compared with the germ-line DNA sequence, an additional nucleotide sequence was observed between the V_H and J_H gene segments. This nucleotide sequence corresponded to amino acids 95 to 97 of the heavy chain.

Based on these results, Hood proposed that a third germ-line gene segment must join with the V_H and J_H gene segments to encode the entire variable region of the heavy chain. This gene segment, which encoded amino acids within the third complementarity-determining region (CDR3), was designated **D** for **diversity**, because of its contribution to the generation of antibody diversity. Tonegawa and his colleagues located the D gene segments within mouse germ-line DNA with a cDNA D-region probe, which hybridized with a stretch of DNA lying between the V_H and J_H gene segments.

The heavy-chain multigene family on chromosome 12 in the mouse has an estimated 300–1000 V_H gene segments, located upstream from a cluster of about 13 D_H gene segments. As with the light-chain genes, each V_H gene segment has a leader sequence a short distance upstream from it. Downstream from the D_H gene segments are four J_H gene segments, followed by a series of C_H gene segments. Each C_H gene segment encodes the constant region of an immunoglobulin heavy-chain isotype. The C_H gene segments are organized into a series of coding **exons** and noncoding **introns**. Each exon encodes a separate domain of the heavy-chain constant region (see Figure 5-3). A similar heavy-chain gene organization is found in humans with an estimated 100 V_H gene segments, 30 D_H segments, and 6 functional J_H segments followed by a series of C_H segments.

The conservation of important biological effector functions of the antibody molecule is maintained by the limited number of heavy-chain constant-region genes. In the mouse the C_H gene segments are arranged sequentially in the following order: C_μ-C_δ-$C_\gamma3$-$C_\gamma1$-$C_\gamma2b$-$C_\gamma2a$-C_ε-C_α (see Figure 7-3c). This sequential arrangement is no accident; it is generally related to the developmental appearance of the immunoglobulin classes in the course of an immune response. During B-cell differentiation there are sequential changes in the classes of immunoglobulin expressed, while the antibody specificity remains the same. The changes are accomplished by DNA rearrangements mediating class switching, which are discussed in a later section.

VARIABLE-REGION GENE REARRANGEMENTS

The previous sections have shown that the assembly of functional genes encoding immunoglobulin light and heavy chains involves recombinational events at the DNA level. These recombination events are the only known form of site-specific DNA rearrangement in vertebrates. Variable-region gene rearrangements occur in an ordered sequence during B-cell maturation in the bone marrow. The heavy-chain variable-region genes rearrange first, then the light-chain variable-region genes. At the end of this process, each B cell contains a single, functional variable-region DNA sequence for its heavy chain and a single, functional variable-region DNA sequence for its light chain.

This process of variable-region gene rearrangement thus leads to generation of mature, **immunocompetent** B cells; each such cell is **antigenically committed** to a *single* epitope and expresses membrane-bound anti-

body on its surface. As discussed later, subsequent rearrangement of heavy-chain constant-region genes generates changes in the immunoglobulin class (isotype) expressed by a B cell without changing its antigenic specificity. Although variable-region gene rearrangements occur in an ordered sequence, they are random events that result in the random determination of B-cell specificity. The order, mechanism, and consequences of these rearrangements are described in this section.

V-J Rearrangements in Light-Chain DNA

Expression of both κ and λ light chains requires rearrangement of the variable-region V and J gene segments. In the case of the mouse λ light-chain DNA, rearrangement can join the $V_\lambda1$ gene segment with either the $J_\lambda1$ or $J_\lambda3$ gene segments, or the $V_\lambda2$ gene segment can be joined with the $J_\lambda2$ gene segment. In the case of the mouse κ light-chain DNA, any one of the estimated 300 V_κ gene segments can be joined with any one of the four functional J_κ gene segments.

Rearranged κ and λ genes contain the following regions in order from the 5′ to 3′ end: a short leader (L) exon, a noncoding sequence (intron), a joined VJ gene segment, a second intron, and a C gene segment. Upstream from each leader gene segment is a promoter sequence. The rearranged light-chain sequence is transcribed by RNA polymerase from the L exon through the C segment to the stop signal, generating a light-chain primary RNA transcript (Figure 7-4). The introns in the primary transcript are removed by RNA-processing enzymes, and the resulting light-chain messenger RNA then exits from the nucleus. The light-chain mRNA binds to ribosomes and is translated into the light-chain protein. The leader sequence at the amino terminus pulls the growing polypeptide chain into the lumen of the rough endoplasmic reticulum and is then cleaved, so it is not present in the finished light-chain protein product.

V-D-J Rearrangements in Heavy-Chain DNA

Generation of a functional immunoglobulin heavy-chain gene requires two separate rearrangement events within the variable region. As illustrated in Figure 7-5, a D_H gene segment first joins to a J_H segment; the resulting $D_H J_H$ segment then moves next to and joins a V_H segment to generate a $V_H D_H J_H$ unit that encodes the entire variable region. In heavy-chain DNA, variable-region rearrangement produces a rearranged gene consisting of the following sequences starting from the 5′ end: a short L exon, an intron, a joined VDJ segment, another intron,

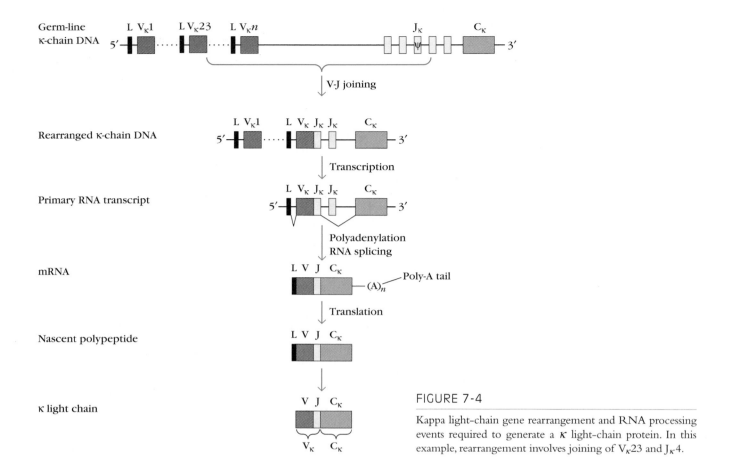

FIGURE 7-4

Kappa light-chain gene rearrangement and RNA processing events required to generate a κ light-chain protein. In this example, rearrangement involves joining of $V_\kappa 23$ and $J_\kappa 4$.

and a series of C gene segments. As with the light-chain genes, a promoter sequence is located a short distance upstream from each heavy-chain leader sequence.

Once heavy-chain gene rearrangement is accomplished, RNA polymerase can bind to the promoter sequence and transcribe the entire heavy-chain gene, including the introns. Initially, both C_μ and C_δ gene segments are transcribed. Differential polyadenylation and RNA splicing remove the introns and process the primary transcript to generate mRNA, encoding either C_μ or C_δ. These two mRNAs then are translated, and the leader peptide of the resulting nascent polypeptide is cleaved, generating finished μ and δ chains. Since two different heavy-chain mRNAs are produced following heavy-chain variable-region gene rearrangement, a mature, immunocompetent B cell expresses *both* IgM and IgD with identical antigenic specificity on its surface.

Mechanism of Variable-Region DNA Rearrangements

Now that we've seen the results of variable-region gene rearrangements, let's examine in detail how this process occurs during maturation of B cells.

RECOMBINATION SIGNAL SEQUENCES

Discovery of two closely related conserved sequences in variable-region germ-line DNA paved the way toward fuller understanding of the mechanism of gene rearrangements. DNA sequencing studies revealed the presence of unique **recombination signal sequences** (RSSs) flanking each germ-line V, D, and J gene segment. One RSS is located 3' to each V gene segment, 5' to each J gene segment, and on both sides of each D gene segment. These sequences function as signals for the recombination process. Each RSS contains a conserved palindromic heptamer and a conserved AT-rich nonamer sequence separated by an intervening sequence of 12 or 23 base pairs (Figure 7-6a). Leroy Hood observed that the intervening 12- and 23-bp sequences correspond, respectively, to one and two turns of the DNA helix; for this reason the sequences are referred to as **one-turn signal sequences** and **two-turn signal sequences**.

The V_κ signal sequence has a one-turn spacer, and the J_κ signal sequence has a two-turn spacer. In λ light-chain DNA this order is reversed; that is, the V_λ signal sequence has a two-turn spacer, and the J_λ signal sequence has a

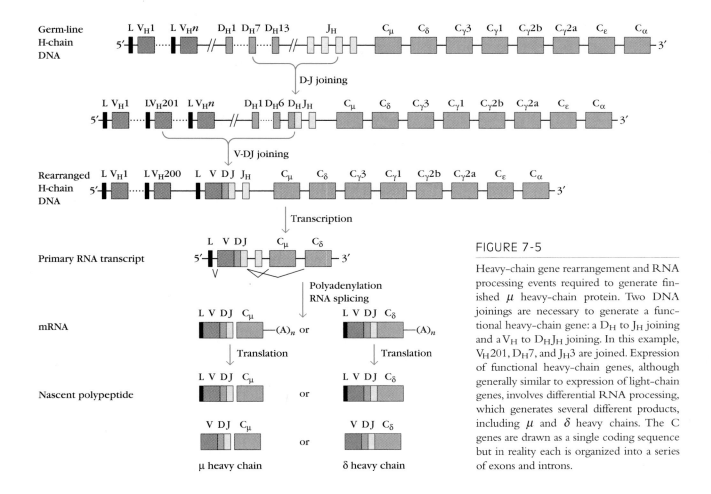

FIGURE 7-5

Heavy-chain gene rearrangement and RNA processing events required to generate finished μ heavy-chain protein. Two DNA joinings are necessary to generate a functional heavy-chain gene: a D_H to J_H joining and a V_H to $D_H J_H$ joining. In this example, $V_H 201$, $D_H 7$, and $J_H 3$ are joined. Expression of functional heavy-chain genes, although generally similar to expression of light-chain genes, involves differential RNA processing, which generates several different products, including μ and δ heavy chains. The C genes are drawn as a single coding sequence but in reality each is organized into a series of exons and introns.

one-turn spacer. In heavy-chain DNA, a two-turn spacer occurs in the signal sequences of the V_H and J_H gene segments, and a one-turn spacer occurs in the signals on either side of the D_H gene segment (Figure 7-6b). Signal sequences having a one-turn spacer can only join with sequences having a two-turn spacer (the so-called **one-turn/two-turn joining rule**). This joining rule ensures that a V_L segment only joins to a J_L segment and not to another V_L segment; the rule likewise ensures that V_H, D_H, and J_H segments join in proper order and that segments of the same type do not join each other.

ENZYMATIC JOINING OF GENE SEGMENTS

V-(D)-J recombination, which takes place at the junctions between RSSs and coding sequences, is catalyzed by enzymes collectively referred to as **V(D)J recombinase**. Recombination results in the formation of a **coding joint**, formed by joining of the coding sequences, and a **signal joint**, formed by joining of the RSSs. The relative transcriptional orientation of the gene segments to be joined determines the fate of the signal joint and intervening DNA. When the two gene segments are in the

same transcriptional orientation, joining results in **deletion** of the signal joint and intervening DNA as a circular excision product (Figure 7-7). Less frequently, the two gene segments have opposite orientations. In this case joining occurs by **inversion** of the DNA resulting in the retention of both the coding joint and the signal joint (and intervening DNA) on the chromosome. In the human κ locus about half of the V_κ gene segments are inverted with respect to J_κ and joining is therefore by inversion.

Identification of the enzymes involved in recombination of V, D, and J gene segments began in the late 1980s and is still ongoing. In 1990 David Schatz, Marjorie Oettinger, and David Baltimore first reported identification of two **recombination-activating genes,** designated *RAG-1* and *RAG-2,* whose encoded proteins act synergistically to mediate V-(D)-J joining. The **RAG-1** and **RAG-2 proteins** and the enzyme **terminal deoxynucleotidyl transferase** (Tdt) are the only lymphoid-specific gene products that are required for V-(D)-J rearrangement.

Current evidence suggests that recombination of variable-region gene segments is a multistep process

(a) Nucleotide sequence of RSSs

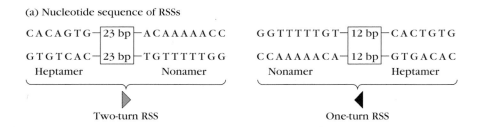

Two-turn RSS

One-turn RSS

(b) Location of RSSs in germ-line immunoglobulin DNA

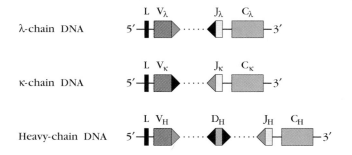

FIGURE 7-6

Two conserved sequences in light-chain and heavy-chain DNA function as recombination signal sequences (RSSs). (a) Both signal sequences consist of a conserved palindromic heptamer and conserved AT-rich nonamer; these are separated by nonconserved spacers of 12 or 23 base pairs. (b) The two types of RSS—designated one-turn RSS and two-turn RSS—have characteristic locations within λ-chain, κ-chain, and heavy-chain germ-line DNA. During DNA rearrangement, gene segments adjacent to the one-turn RSS can join only with segments adjacent to the two-turn RSS.

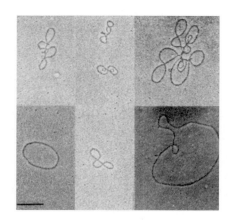

FIGURE 7-7

Circular DNA isolated from thymocytes in which the DNA encoding the chains of the T-cell receptor (TCR) undergoes rearrangement in a process analogous to that involving the immunoglobulin genes. Isolation of this circular excision product is direct evidence for the mechanism of deletional joining shown in Figure 7-8. [From K. Okazki et al., 1987, *Cell* **49**:477.]

involving a number of recombinase enzymes and the following sequence of events (Figure 7-8):

- Recognition of recombination signal sequences (RSSs) by recombinase enzymes, followed by synapsis in which two signal sequences and the adjacent coding sequences (gene segments) are brought into proximity of each other
- Cleavage of one strand of DNA by RAG–1 and RAG–2 at the juncture of the signal sequence and coding sequence
- Transesterification reaction catalyzed by RAG–1/2 in which the free 3′-OH group on the cut DNA strand attacks the phosphodiester bond linking the opposite strand to the signal sequence, simultaneously producing a hairpin structure at the cut end of the coding sequence and a flush, 5′-phosphorylated double-strand break at the signal sequence
- Cutting of the hairpin to generate **P-nucleotides** followed by the trimming of a few nucleotides from the coding sequence by a single-strand endonuclease

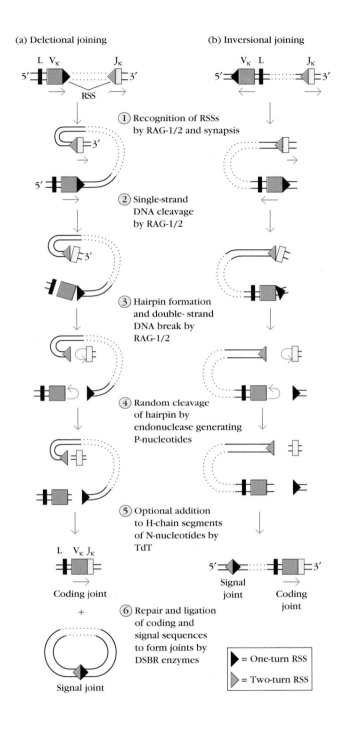

(a) Deletional joining

(b) Inversional joining

① Recognition of RSSs by RAG-1/2 and synapsis

② Single-strand DNA cleavage by RAG-1/2

③ Hairpin formation and double-strand DNA break by RAG-1/2

④ Random cleavage of hairpin by endonuclease generating P-nucleotides

⑤ Optional addition to H-chain segments of N-nucleotides by TdT

⑥ Repair and ligation of coding and signal sequences to form joints by DSBR enzymes

Coding joint

Signal joint

Signal joint

Coding joint

▶ = One-turn RSS

▷ = Two-turn RSS

FIGURE 7-8

Model depicting the general process of recombination of immunoglobulin gene segments is illustrated with V_κ and J_κ. (a) Deletional joining occurs when the gene segments to be joined have the same transcriptional orientation (indicated by horizontal blue arrows). This process yields two products: a rearranged VJ unit that includes the coding joint and a circular excision product consisting of the recombination signal sequences (RSSs), signal joint, and intervening DNA. (b) Inversional joining occurs when the gene segments have opposite transcriptional orientations. In this case, the RSSs, signal joint, and intervening DNA are retained, and the orientation of one of the joined segments is inverted. In both types of recombination, a few nucleotides may be deleted from or added to the cut ends of the coding sequences before they are rejoined. See text for further discussion.

One of the striking features of gene-segment recombination is the diversity of the coding joints that are formed between any two gene segments. This junctional diversity at the V-J and V-D-J coding joints is generated by a number of mechanisms: variation in cutting of the hairpin to generate P-nucleotides, variation in trimming of the coding sequences, variation in N-nucleotide addition, and flexibility in joining the coding sequences. As discussed later, this variation contributes greatly to the diversity of the CDR3 region of the antigen-binding site.

EXPERIMENTAL IDENTIFICATION OF *RAG-1* AND *RAG-2* GENES

When Schatz, Oettinger, and Baltimore set out to identify the *RAG-1* and *RAG-2* genes, they first had to develop an assay system for demonstrating recombination between immunoglobulin gene segments. Their novel approach employed a retroviral construct containing a promoter sequence, V and J gene segments with flanking signal sequences, and a gene that confers resistance to mycophenolic acid (Figure 7-9). The genes were arranged in an unusual way so that the promoter was oriented in the opposite transcriptional orientation from that of the gene for mycophenolic acid resistance. If the V and J gene segments were rearranged by inversional joining, then the orientation of the gene for mycophenolic acid resistance would also be inverted, placing the gene in the correct 5′ to 3′ orientation to be transcribed from the promoter. Cells transfected with this construct thus would acquire resistance to mycophenolic acid if they could rearrange the V and J gene segments, whereas transfected cells that could not rearrange the V and J gene segments would not be resistant to mycophenolic acid.

When a variety of cell types were tested in this system, only pre-B cells and pre-T cells were able to

- Optional addition of up to 15 nucleotides, called **N-nucleotides**, at the cut ends of the V, D, and, J coding sequences of the heavy chain by an enzyme called terminal deoxynucleotidyl transferase (TdT)
- Repair and ligation to join the coding sequences and the signal sequences catalyzed by normal **double-strand break repair (DSBR) enzymes**

Retroviral construct:

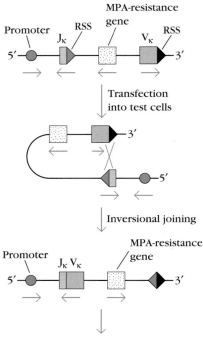

FIGURE 7-9

Assay system for demonstrating recombination of immunoglobulin gene segments. If the test cells possess all the enzymes required for inversional joining, then the transfected cells will be resistant to mycophenolic acid (MPA), as shown. If the test cells lack one or more of these enzymes, the MPA-resistance gene will not be expressed because its transcriptional orientation (horizontal blue arrows) is opposite to that of the promoter.

rearrange the V and J gene segments. (As is discussed in Chapter 11, the pre-T cell employs the same recombinase enzymes and signal sequences in rearranging the genes for the T-cell receptor, which is why it also proved to be positive in this assay.) Mature B and T cells were unable to rearrange the retroviral construct, indicating that the recombinase activity is limited to an early stage in the maturation of both B and T cells.

Once these researchers established that the retroviral construct could be rearranged in pre-B cells, they then set out to isolate the recombinase genes. First fibroblasts were transfected with the retroviral construct. Since fibroblasts do not express the recombinase genes, the transfected cells could not rearrange the construct. Assuming that the recombinase genes were located on a single locus, the researchers then transfected genomic DNA from pre-B cells into fibroblasts containing the retroviral construct. The presence of activated recombinase genes in the genomic DNA could be detected

by the rearrangement of the retroviral construct, which conferred resistance to mycophenolic acid upon the transfected fibroblasts. With this experimental system the researchers identified *RAG-1* and *RAG-2*, two closely linked genes, both of which were needed to mediate recombination of the retroviral construct at a high frequency. RAG-1 and RAG-2 mRNA was shown to be present in pre-B cells and pre-T cells but absent in mature B and T cell stages.

DEFECTS IN IG-GENE REARRANGEMENTS

Several strains of mice with defects in various recombination genes have been developed and are proving valuable in unraveling the various steps in the recombination process. For example, knockout mice lacking either *RAG-1* or *RAG-2* are unable to initiate the recombination process because they cannot introduce double-strand DNA breaks between the recombination signal sequences (RSSs) and coding sequences in germ-line immunoglobulin DNA (Figure 7-10). As a result of this defect, the V, D, and J gene segments remain unrearranged. Since both B and T cells utilize the same recombination machinery, the RAG-1⁻ and RAG-2⁻ knockout mice lack mature T and B cells and consequently exhibit a **severe combined immunodeficiency** (SCID). In humans, mutations in the *RAG* genes, located on chromosome 11, have been linked to several different cases of autosomal SCIDs (see Chapter 21).

Another recombination defect is found in CB-17 SCID mice. These mice have an autosomal recessive mutation that impairs the V-(D)-J recombination process. SCID mice have a general absence of mature functional T and B cells and, like RAG⁻ mice, manifest a severe combined immunodeficiency. Unlike the RAG mutants, SCID mice begin the recombination process normally: synapsis occurs between the D and J gene segments; double-strand DNA breaks are properly introduced at the juncture of the recombination signal sequences and coding sequences; and the signal sequences are then rejoined. Joining of the coding sequences, however, occurs some distance from the D and J gene segments, resulting in deletion of one or both of the coding sequences (see Figure 7-10). These SCID mice have functional RAG-1 and RAG-2 enzymes; their defect is instead in one or more double-strand break repair (DSBR) enzymes that rejoin the cut DNA.

PRODUCTIVE AND NONPRODUCTIVE REARRANGEMENTS

Although the double-strand DNA breaks that initiate V-(D)-J rearrangements are introduced precisely at the

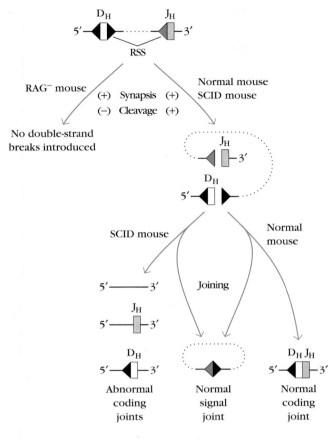

FIGURE 7-10

Recombination defects have been identified in RAG-deficient mice and SCID mice. Mice that lack a functional RAG-1 or RAG-2 cannot even start the recombination process. In contrast, SCID mice can carry out synapsis between D_H and J_H gene segments, introduce double-strand breaks to produce normal recombination intermediates, and form a normal signal joint. However, SCID mice cannot properly join the coding sequences. Both types of defective mice lack mature B and T cells and thus exhibit a severe combined immunodeficiency. [Adapted from F. W. Alt et al., 1992, *Immunol. Today* **13**:306.]

tained. In such a **productive rearrangement**, the resulting VJ or VDJ unit can be translated in its entirety, yielding a complete variable-region polypeptide.

If one allele rearranges nonproductively, a B cell can then rearrange the other allele and may generate a productive rearrangement. If an in-phase rearranged heavy-chain and light-chain gene is not produced, the B cell dies by apoptosis. It is estimated that only one in three attempts at V_L-J_L, D_H-J_H, and V_H-$D_H J_H$ joining are productive. As a result, only about 8% of the pre-B cells in the bone marrow progress to maturity and leave the bone marrow as mature, immunocompetent B cells.

ALLELIC EXCLUSION

B cells, like all somatic cells, are diploid and contain both maternal and paternal chromosomes. Even though a B cell is diploid, it expresses the rearranged heavy-chain genes from only one chromosome and the rearranged light-chain genes from only one chromosome. This

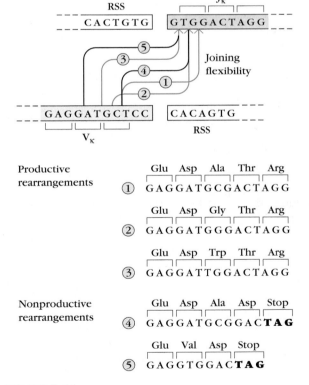

FIGURE 7-11

Junctional flexibility in the joining of immunoglobulin gene segments is illustrated with V_κ and J_κ. In-phase joining (arrows 1, 2, and 3) generates a productive rearrangement, which can be translated into protein. Out-of-phase joining (arrows 4 and 5) leads to a nonproductive rearrangement, which contains stop codons and is not translated into protein.

junctions of signal sequences and coding sequences, the subsequent joining of the coding sequences exhibits some flexibility. This flexibility in the joining process helps generate antibody diversity by contributing to the hypervariability of the antigen-binding site. (This phenomenon is covered in more detail in the section on generation of antibody diversity.)

Another consequence of joining flexibility is that gene segments may be joined out of phase, so that the triplet reading frame for translation is not preserved. In such a **nonproductive rearrangement**, the resulting VJ or VDJ unit will contain numerous stop codons, which interrupt translation (Figure 7-11). When gene segments are joined in phase, the reading frame is main-

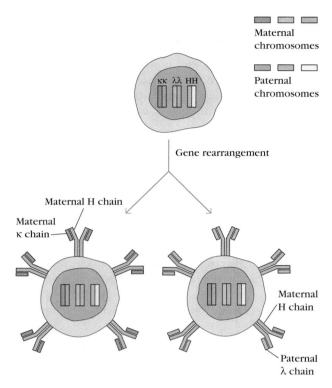

Maternal
chromosomes

Paternal
chromosomes

Gene rearrangement

Maternal H chain

Maternal
κ chain

Maternal
H chain

Paternal
λ chain

FIGURE 7-12

Because of allelic exclusion, the immunoglobulin heavy- and light-chain genes of only one parental chromosome are expressed per cell. This process ensures that a single B cell will be specific for a given epitope. The selection of which allele of each pair is rearranged to produce a functional gene is random. Thus the expressed immunoglobulin may contain one maternal and one paternal chain or both chains may derive from only one parent. Only B cells and T cells exhibit allelic exclusion.

process, called **allelic exclusion**, ensures that functional B cells never contain more than one $V_H D_H J_H$ and one $V_L J_L$ unit (Figure 7-12). This is, of course, essential for the antigenic specificity of the B cell, because the expression of both alleles would render the B cell multispecific. The phenomenon of allelic exclusion suggests that once a productive V_H-D_H-J_H rearrangement and a productive V_L-J_L rearrangement have occurred, the recombination machinery is turned off, so that the heavy- and light-chain genes on the homologous chromosomes are not expressed.

G. D. Yancopoulos and F. W. Alt have proposed a model to account for allelic exclusion (Figure 7-13). They suggest that once a productive rearrangement is attained, its encoded protein is expressed and the presence of this protein acts as a signal to prevent further gene rearrangement. According to their model, the presence of μ heavy chains signals the maturing B cell to turn off rearrangement of the other heavy-chain allele and to turn on rearrangement of the κ light-chain genes.

If a productive κ rearrangement occurs, κ light chains are produced and then pair with μ heavy chains to form a complete antibody molecule. The presence of this antibody then turns off further light-chain rearrangement. If κ rearrangement is nonproductive for both alleles, rearrangement of the λ-chain genes begins. If neither λ allele rearranges productively, the B cell presumably ceases to mature and soon dies by apoptosis.

Two studies with transgenic mice have supported the hypothesis that the protein products encoded by rearranged heavy- and light-chain genes regulate rearrangement of the remaining alleles. In one study, transgenic mice carrying a rearranged μ heavy-chain transgene were prepared (see Figure 2-11). The μ transgene product was expressed by a large percentage of the B cells, and rearrangement of the endogenous immunoglobulin heavy-chain genes was blocked. Similarly, cells from a transgenic mouse carrying a κ light-chain transgene did not rearrange the endogenous κ-chain genes when the κ transgene was expressed and was associated with a heavy chain to form complete immunoglobulin. These studies suggest that expression of the heavy- and light-chain proteins may indeed prevent gene rearrangement of the remaining alleles and thus account for allelic exclusion. Further discussion of allelic exclusion is presented later in the chapter.

GENERATION OF ANTIBODY DIVERSITY

As the organization of the immunoglobulin genes was deciphered, the sources of the vast diversity in the variable region began to become clear. The germ-line theory, mentioned earlier, argued that the entire variable-region repertoire is encoded in the germ line of the organism and is transmitted from parent to offspring via the germ cells (egg and sperm). The somatic-variation theory held that the germ line contains a limited number of variable genes, which are diversified in the somatic cells by mutational or recombinational events during development of the immune system. With the cloning and sequencing of the immunoglobulin genes, both models were partially vindicated.

To date, seven mechanisms have been shown to generate antibody diversity in the mouse:

- Multiple germ-line gene segments
- Combinatorial V-(D)-J joining
- Junctional flexibility
- P-region nucleotide addition
- N-region nucleotide addition
- Somatic hypermutation
- Combinatorial association of light and heavy chains

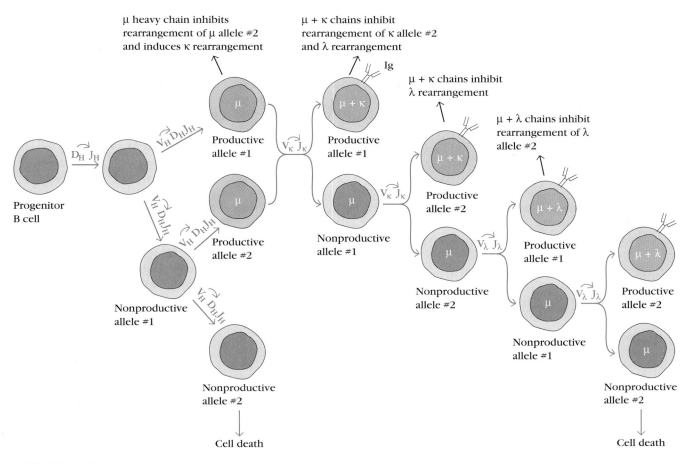

FIGURE 7-13

Model to account for allelic exclusion. Heavy-chain genes rearrange first, and once a productive heavy-chain gene rearrangement occurs, the μ protein product prevents rearrangement of the other heavy-chain allele and initiates light-chain gene rearrangement. In the mouse, rearrangement of κ light-chain genes precedes rearrangement of the λ genes, as shown here. In humans, however, either κ or λ rearrangement can proceed once a productive heavy-chain rearrangement has occurred. Formation of a complete immunoglobulin inhibits further light-chain gene rearrangement. If a nonproductive rearrangement occurs for one allele, then the cell attempts rearrangement of the other allele. [Adapted from G. D. Yancopoulos and F. W. Alt, 1986, *Annu. Rev. Immunol.* **4**:339.]

The same sources of diversity are thought to operate in humans. Although the exact contribution of each source of diversity to the total antibody diversity is not known, the number of different antibody specificities that can be generated by the mammalian immune system is estimated to range from a low of 10^8 to a high of 10^{11} (Table 7-2).

Multiple Germ-Line V, D, and J Gene Segments

DNA hybridization studies have demonstrated that mouse germ-line DNA contains about 300 V_κ gene segments and 300–1000 V_H gene segments but only two V_λ gene segments. The existence of multiple J_L, D_H, and J_H segments expands the germ-line contribution to diver-

sity. In the mouse, there appear to be 4 functional J_H, 4 functional J_κ, 3 functional J_λ, and an estimated 13 D_H gene segments. Although the numbers of germ-line genes are far fewer than predicted by early proponents of the germ-line model, multiple germ-line V, D, and J genes clearly do contribute to diversity of the antigen-binding sites in antibodies.

Combinatorial V-J and V-D-J Joining

The contribution of multiple germ-line gene segments to antibody diversity is magnified by the random re-arrangement of these segments in somatic cells. The ability of any of the 300–1000 V_H gene segments to combine with any of the 13 D_H segments and any of the

$4 J_H$ segments allows an enormous amount of diversity to be generated ($300 \times 13 \times 4 = 1.6 \times 10^4$ minimum possible combinations). Similarly, $300 \text{ } V_\kappa$ gene segments randomly combining with $4 J_\kappa$ segments has the potential of generating 1.2×10^3 possible combinations. With only $2 \text{ } V_\lambda$ and $3 \text{ } J_\lambda$ gene segments, the combinatorial diversity of the mouse λ light-chain DNA is much less.

Junctional Flexibility

The enormous diversity generated by means of V, D, and J combinations is further augmented by a phenomenon known as junctional flexibility. As discussed earlier, the process of recombination involves both the joining of recombination signal sequences to form a signal joint and the joining of coding sequences to form a coding joint (see Figure 7-8). Although the signal sequences are always joined precisely, joining of the coding sequences often is imprecise. In one study, for example, joining of

the $V_\kappa21$ and $J_\kappa1$ coding sequences was analyzed in several pre-B cell lines. Sequence analysis of the signal and coding joints revealed precise joining of the signal sequences but flexible joining of the coding sequences (Figure 7-14).

As illustrated previously, this junctional flexibility leads to many nonproductive rearrangements, but it also generates several productive combinations encoding alternative amino acids at each coding joint (see Figure 7-11), thereby increasing antibody diversity. The amino acid sequence variation generated by junctional flexibility in the coding joints has been shown to fall within the third hypervariable region (CDR3) in immunoglobulin heavy-chain and light-chain DNA (Table 7-3). Since the CDR3 hypervariable region makes a major contribution to antigen binding by the antibody molecule (see Table 5-3), an amino acid change generated by junctional flexibility can have major impact in generating antibody diversity.

TABLE 7-2

CUMULATIVE GENERATION OF MINIMUM ANTIBODY DIVERSITY IN THE MOUSE

MECHANISM OF DIVERSITY	HEAVY CHAIN	LIGHT CHAINS	
		κ	λ
ESTIMATED NUMBER OF SEGMENTS *			
Multiple germ-line gene segments:			
V	300–1000	300	2
D	13	0	0
J	4	4	3
POSSIBLE NUMBER OF COMBINATIONS †			
Combinatorial V-J and V-D-J joining	$300 \times 13 \times 4 = 1.6 \times 10^4$	$300 \times 4 = 1.2 \times 10^3$	$2 \times 3 = 6$
Junctional flexibility	+	+	+
P-region nucleotide addition	+	+	+
N-region nucleotide addition	+	–	–
Somatic mutation	+	+	+
Combinatorial association of heavy and light chains	$>1.6 \times 10^4 \times (>1.2 \times 10^3 + >6) = \gg 1.9 \times 10^7$		

* The estimated number of variable-region segments in human DNA is as follows: 100 V_H, 30 D_H, and 6 functional J_H; 100 V_κ and 5 J_κ; 100 V_λ, and 6 J_λ . The sources of antibody diversity in humans are identical to those in the mouse.

† (+) indicates mechanism makes a significant contribution to diversity but to an unknown extent. (–) indicates mechanism does not operate.

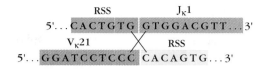

FIGURE 7-14

Experimental evidence for junctional flexibility in immunoglobulin-gene rearrangement. The nucleotide sequences flanking the coding joints between V$_\kappa$21 and J$_\kappa$1 and of the corresponding signal joints were determined in four pre-B cell lines. The sequence constancy in the signal joints contrasts with the sequence variability in the coding joints. Pink and blue screens indicate nucleotides derived from V$_\kappa$21 and J$_\kappa$1, respectively, and green and yellow screens indicate nucleotides from the two CSSs.

P-Nucleotide Addition

As described earlier, following the initial single-strand DNA cleavage at the junction of a variable-region gene segment and attached signal sequence, the nucleotides at the end of the coding sequences are thought to turn back to form a hairpin structure (see Figure 7-8a). This hairpin is later cleaved by an endonuclease. Cleavage sometimes occurs at a position that leaves a short single-stranded region at the end of the coding sequences. These regions are referred to as **P-nucleotides**, because subsequent addition of complementary nucleotides by repair enzymes generates palindromic sequences in the coding joint (Figure 7-15a). Variation in the position at which the hairpin is cut thus leads to variation in the sequence of the coding joint.

N-Region Nucleotide Addition

Variable-region coding joints in rearranged heavy-chain genes have been shown to contain short amino acid sequences that are not encoded by the V, D, or J gene

T A B L E   7 - 3

SOURCES OF SEQUENCE VARIATION IN COMPLEMENTARITY-DETERMINING REGIONS OF IMMUNOGLOBULIN HEAVY- AND LIGHT-CHAIN GENES

SOURCE OF VARIATION	CDR1	CDR2	CDR3
Sequence encoded by:	V segment	V segment	V$_L$-J$_L$ junction
			V$_H$-D$_H$-J$_H$ junctions
Junctional flexibility	−	−	+
P-nucleotide addition	−	−	+
N-nucleotide addition*	−	−	+
Somatic hypermutation	+	+	+

* N-nucleotide addition occurs only in heavy-chain DNA.

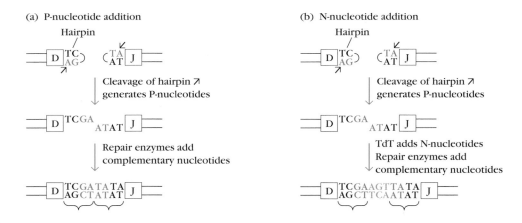

FIGURE 7-15

P-nucleotide and N-nucleotide addition during deletional joining. (a) If cleavage of the hairpin intermediate yields a double-stranded end on the coding sequence, then P-nucleotide addition does not occur. In many cases, however, cleavage yields a single-stranded end, generating a P-nucleotide (dark blue). During subsequent repair complementary nucleotides are added, producing palindromic sequences (indicated by brackets). In this example, an extra four base pairs (light blue) are present in the coding joint as the result of P-nucleotide addition. (b) Besides P-nucleotide addition, addition of random N-nucleotides (light blue) by TdT can occur during joining of heavy-chain coding sequences.

segments. These amino acids are encoded by **N-nucleotides** that are added during the joining process in a reaction catalyzed by terminal deoxynucleotidyl transferase (TdT) (Figure 7-15b). Evidence that TdT is responsible for N-nucleotide addition has come from transfection studies in fibroblasts. When fibroblasts were transfected with the *RAG-1* and *RAG-2* genes, V-D-J rearrangement occurred but no N-nucleotides were present in the coding joints. However, when the fibroblasts were also transfected with the gene encoding TdT, then V-D-J rearrangement was accompanied by addition of N-nucleotides at the coding joints.

Up to 15 N-nucleotides can be added to both the D_H-J_H and V_H-$D_H J_H$ joints. Thus a complete heavy-chain variable region is encoded by a $V_H N D_H N J_H$ unit. The additional heavy-chain diversity generated by N-region nucleotide addition is quite large because N regions appear to consist of wholly random sequences. Since this diversity occurs at V-D-J coding joints, it is localized in the CDR3 of the heavy-chain genes.

Somatic Hypermutation

All the antibody diversity discussed so far stems from mechanisms that operate during formation of specific variable regions by gene rearrangement. The implicit assumption throughout this chapter has been that once a functional variable-region gene unit is formed, it is not altered. This assumption turns out to be false, and additional antibody diversity is generated in rearranged variable-region gene units by a process called **somatic hypermutation**. As a result of somatic hypermutation, individual nucleotides in VJ or VDJ units are replaced with alternative bases, thus potentially altering the specificity of the encoded immunoglobulins.

Somatic hypermutation is targeted to the V-region segments located within a DNA sequence, containing about 1000 nucleotides, that includes the whole of the VJ or VDJ segments. Somatic hypermutation occurs at a frequency approaching 10^{-3} per base pair per generation. This rate is a million-fold higher than the spontaneous mutation rate in other genes (hence the name hypermutation). Since the combined length of the H-chain and L-chain variable-region genes is about 600 bp, then an average of one mutation will be introduced by somatic hypermutation in every one to two cell divisions.

The mechanism of somatic hypermutation has not yet been determined. It has been suggested that mutations are introduced by an error-prone DNA polymerase that is specifically targeted to the VJ or VDJ locus. Most of the mutations are nucleotide substitutions rather than deletions or insertions. Somatic hypermutation introduces these nucleotide substitutions in a largely, but not completely, random fashion. Recent evidence suggests that certain nucleotide motifs and palindromic sequences within V_H and V_L may be especially susceptible to somatic hypermutation.

Because the process of somatic hypermutation is largely random, it will generate antibodies with varying affinity for antigen. Following exposure to antigen, those B cells with higher affinity receptors will be preferentially selected because of their greater ability to bind to the antigen. This process, called **affinity maturation**, takes place within the germinal center and is discussed more fully in Chapter 8. Somatic hypermutations are clustered within the CDRs of the V_H and V_L sequences. This clustering reflects the role of antigen in selecting B cells with higher affinity receptors during affinity maturation. Because the CDRs are directly involved in antigen recognition, mutation within the CDRs is more likely to influence the overall affinity for antigen.

Claudia Berek and Cesar Milstein obtained experimental evidence demonstrating somatic hypermutation during the course of an immune response to a hapten-carrier conjugate. These researchers were able to sequence the mRNA encoding antihapten antibodies produced in response to primary, secondary, or tertiary immunization with a hapten-carrier conjugate. The hapten that they chose was 2-phenyl-5-oxazolone (phOx) coupled to a protein carrier. They chose this hapten because it had previously been shown to induce production of a majority of antibodies encoded by a single germ-line V_H and V_κ gene segment (i.e., antibodies against a single epitope). Berek and Milstein immunized mice with the phOx-carrier conjugate and then used the mice spleen cells to prepare hybridomas secreting

monoclonal antibodies specific for the phOx hapten. The mRNA sequence for the H chain and κ light chain of each hybridoma was then determined to identify deviations from the germ-line sequences.

The results of this experiment are depicted in Figure 7-16. Of the 12 hybridomas obtained from mice seven days after a primary immunization, all used the V_H Ox-1 gene and all but one used the V_κ Ox-1 gene. Moreover, only a few mutations from the germ-line sequence were present in these hybridomas. By day 14 after primary immunization, analysis of eight hybridomas revealed that six continued to use the germ-line V_H Ox-1 gene and all continued to use the V_κ Ox-1 gene. Now, however, all of these hybridomas included one or more mutations from the germ-line sequence. Hybridomas analyzed from the secondary and tertiary responses showed a larger percentage utilizing germ-line V_H genes other than the V_H Ox-1 gene. In those hybridoma clones that utilized the V_H Ox-1 and V_κ Ox-1 gene segments, most of the mutations were clustered in the CDR1 and CDR2 hypervariable regions. The number of mutations in the anti-phOx hybridomas progressively increased following primary, secondary, and tertiary immunizations, as did the overall affinity of the antibodies for phOx (see Figure 7-16).

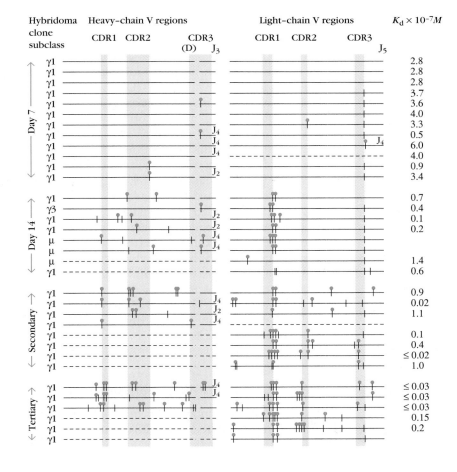

FIGURE 7-16

Experimental evidence for somatic mutation in variable regions of immunoglobulin genes. The diagram compares the mRNA sequences of the heavy and light chains from hybridomas specific for the phOx hapten. The horizontal solid lines represent the germ-line V_H and V_κ Ox-1 sequences; dashed lines represent sequences derived from other germ-line genes. Vertical lines show the position of mutations; the blue circles with vertical lines indicate mutations that encode a different amino acid than the germ-line sequence. These data show that the frequency of mutation (1) increases in the course of the primary response (day 7 vs. day 14) and (2) is higher after secondary and tertiary immunizations than after primary immunization. Moreover, the dissociation constant (K_D) of the anti-phOx antibodies decreases in going from the primary to tertiary response, indicating an increase in the overall affinity of the antibody. Note also that most of the mutations are clustered within CDR1 and CDR2 of both the heavy and light chains. [Adapted from C. Berek and C. Milstein, 1987, *Immunol. Rev.* **96**:23.]

Association of Heavy and Light Chains

The final source of antibody diversity is the combinatorial association of heavy and light chains. Because the specificity of an antibody's antigen-binding site is determined by the variable regions in both its heavy and light chains, combinational association of H and L chains also can generate diversity. As shown in Table 7-2, a minimum of 1.6×10^4 heavy-chain genes and 1.2×10^3 light-chain genes can be generated in the mouse as a result of the variable-region gene rearrangements. Assuming that any one of the possible heavy-chain and light-chain genes can occur randomly in the same cell, the minimum number of possible heavy- and light-chain combinations is 1.9×10^7.

However, the actual number of possible antigenic specificities is considerably greater because of the unknown but significant number of nucleotide sequences introduced by junctional flexibility, P-nucleotide addition, N-region nucleotide addition, and somatic hypermutation. Although estimates of the quantitative contribution of these mechanisms to antibody diversity are very imprecise, nonetheless they significantly increase the number of possible specificities that can be generated. Some have estimated that total antibody diversity may be as high as 10^{11}.

CLASS SWITCHING AMONG CONSTANT-REGION GENES

Following antigenic stimulation of a B cell, the heavy-chain DNA can undergo a further rearrangement in which the $V_H D_H J_H$ unit can combine with any C_H gene segment. The exact mechanism of this process, called **class (isotope) switching** is unclear, but evidence suggests that DNA flanking sequences (termed **switch sites**) located 2–3 kb upstream from each C_H segment (except C_δ) are involved. These switch sites, though rather large, are composed of multiple copies of short repeated sequences. One hypothesis is that a series of class-specific recombinase proteins bind to these switch sites and facilitate DNA recombination. The particular immunoglobulin class that is expressed thus may depend on the specificity of the recombinase protein expressed.

Various cytokines secreted by activated T_H cells have been shown to induce B cells to class-switch to a particular isotype. Interleukin 4 (IL-4), for example, induces class switching from C_μ to $C_\gamma 1$ or C_ε. K. Yoshida, H. Sakano, and colleagues have demonstrated that IL-4 induces class switching in a successive manner: first from C_μ to $C_\gamma 1$ and then from $C_\gamma 1$ to C_ε (Figure 7-17). They were able to demonstrate this by identifying the circular excision products produced during class switching. The class switch from C_μ to $C_\gamma 1$ was shown to generate a circular excision product containing C_μ together with the 5′ end of the $\gamma 1$ switch site ($S_\gamma 1$) and the 3′ end of the μ switch site (S_μ). The switch from $C_\gamma 1$ to C_ε was shown to generate two circular excision products containing $C_\gamma 1$ together with portions of the μ, γ, and ε switch sites. The role of cytokines in immunoglobulin class switching is discussed more fully in Chapters 8 and 13.

EXPRESSION OF IG GENES

As in the expression of other genes, post-transcriptional processing of immunoglobulin primary transcripts is required to produce functional mRNAs (see Figures 7-4 and 7-5). The first step in this RNA processing, which occurs while transcription is proceeding, is addition of a 7-methylguanosine residue to the 5′ end of the primary transcript. This forms the 5′ cap structure, which plays a role in translation of mRNA on the polyribosomes. Once transcription is completed, the primary RNA transcript is cleaved some 15–30 nucleotides downstream of a highly conserved AAUAAA sequence (called the polyadenylation signal). An enzyme called poly-A polymerase recognizes this signal sequence and adds sequential adenylate residues derived from ATP to the 3′ end of the primary transcript, forming a poly-A tail of about 250 residues.

The primary transcripts produced from rearranged heavy-chain and light-chain genes contain intervening DNA sequences, which include noncoding introns and J gene segments not lost during V-(D)-J rearrangement. In addition, as noted earlier, the heavy-chain C gene segments are organized as a series of coding exons and noncoding introns. Each exon of a C_H gene segment corresponds to a domain or hinge region of the heavy polypeptide chain. Following capping and polyadenylation of the primary transcript, the intervening DNA sequences are excised and their flanking exons are connected by a process called RNA splicing. Short, moderately conserved splice sequences, or splice sites, which are located at the intron-exon boundaries within a primary transcript, signal the positions at which splicing occurs. Processing of the primary transcript in the nucleus removes each of these intervening sequences to yield the final mRNA product. The mRNA is then exported from the nucleus and goes to polyribosomes for translation into complete H or L chains.

Differential RNA Processing of Heavy-Chain Primary Transcripts

Processing of an immunoglobulin heavy-chain primary transcript can yield different mRNAs. Such differential

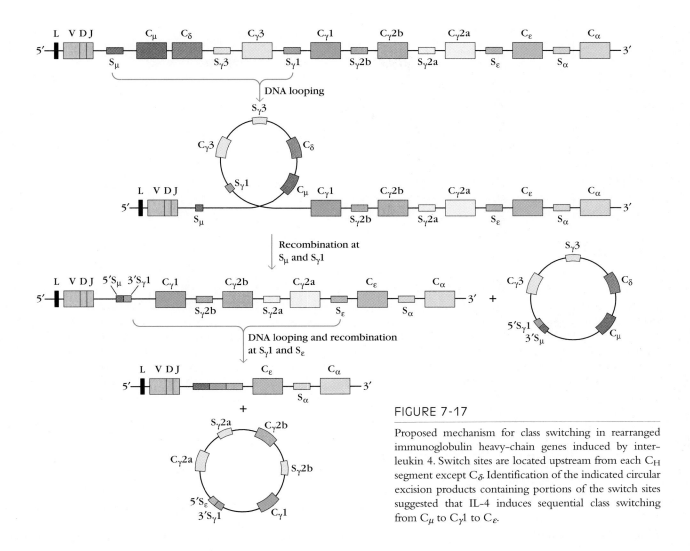

FIGURE 7-17

Proposed mechanism for class switching in rearranged immunoglobulin heavy-chain genes induced by inter-leukin 4. Switch sites are located upstream from each C_H segment except C_δ. Identification of the indicated circular excision products containing portions of the switch sites suggested that IL-4 induces sequential class switching from C_μ to $C_\gamma 1$ to C_ε.

RNA processing of heavy-chain transcripts explains the production of secreted or membrane-bound forms of a particular immunoglobulin and the simultaneous expression of IgM and IgD by a single B cell.

EXPRESSION OF MEMBRANE OR SECRETED IMMUNOGLOBULIN

As discussed in Chapter 5, a particular immunoglobulin can exist in a membrane-bound form or in a secreted form. The two forms differ in the amino acid sequence of the heavy-chain carboxyl-terminal domains (C_H3/C_H3 in IgA, IgD, and IgG and C_H4/C_H4 in IgE and IgM). The secreted form has a hydrophilic sequence of about 20 amino acids in the carboxyl-terminal domain; this is replaced in the membrane-bound form with a sequence of about 40 amino acids containing a hydrophilic segment, a hydrophobic transmembrane segment,

and a short hydrophilic cytoplasmic segment at the carboxyl terminus (Figure 7-18a). For some time the existence of these two forms seemed inconsistent with the structure of germ-line heavy-chain DNA, which had been shown to contain a single C_H gene segment corresponding to each class and subclass.

The explanation of this apparent paradox came from DNA sequencing of the C_μ gene segment, which consists of four exons ($C_\mu 1$, $C_\mu 2$, $C_\mu 3$, and $C_\mu 4$) corresponding to the four domains of the IgM molecule. The $C_\mu 4$ exon contains a nucleotide sequence (S) at its 3′ end that encodes the hydrophilic sequence in the C_H4 domain of secreted IgM. Two additional exons called M1 and M2 are located just 1.8 kb downstream from the 3′ end of the $C_\mu 4$ exon. The M1 exon encodes the transmembrane segment, and M2 encodes the cytoplasmic segment of the C_H4 domain in membrane-bound IgM. Later DNA sequencing revealed that all the C_H gene segments have

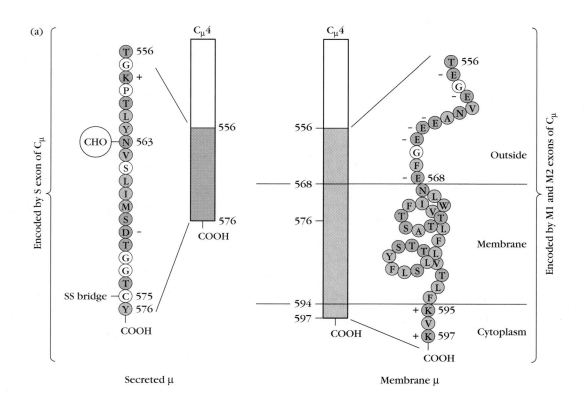

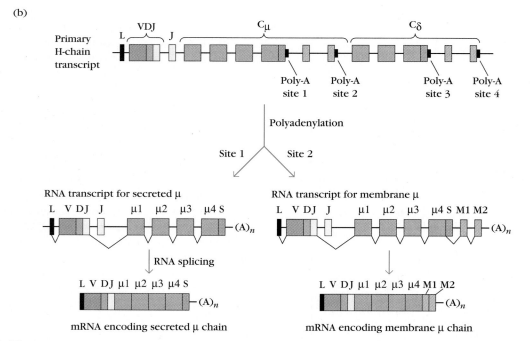

FIGURE 7-18

Expression of secreted and membrane forms of the heavy chain by alternative RNA processing. (a) Amino acid sequence of the carboxyl-terminal end of secreted and membrane μ heavy chains. Residues are indicated by the single-letter amino acid code. Hydrophilic residues and regions are shaded purple; hydrophobic residues and regions are shaded orange. Charged amino acids are indicated with a + or −. The rest of the sequence is identical in both forms. (b) Structure of the primary transcript of a rearranged heavy-chain gene showing the C_μ exons and poly-A sites. Polyadenylation of the primary transcript at either site 1 or site 2 and subsequent splicing (indicated by V-shaped lines) generates mRNAs encoding secreted or membrane μ chains.

two additional downstream M1 and M2 exons encoding the transmembrane and cytoplasmic segments.

The primary transcript produced by transcription of a rearranged μ heavy-chain gene contains two polyadenylation signal sequences, or **poly-A sites**. Site 1 is located at the 3′ end of the $C_\mu 4$ exon and site 2 at the 3′ end of the M2 exon (Figure 7-18b). If cleavage of the primary transcript and addition of the poly-A tail occurs at site 1, the M1 and M2 exons are lost. Excision of the introns and splicing of the remaining exons then produces mRNA encoding the secreted form of the heavy chain. If cleavage and polyadenylation of the primary transcript occurs instead at site 2, then a different pattern of splicing occurs. In this case, splicing removes the S sequence at the 3′ end of the $C_\mu 4$ exon, which encodes the hydrophilic carboxyl-terminal end of the secreted form, and joins the remainder of the $C_\mu 4$ exon with the M1 and M2 exons, producing mRNA for the membrane form of the heavy chain.

Production of the secreted or membrane form of an immunoglobulin thus depends on differential processing of a common primary transcript. As noted previously,

mature naive B cells produce only membrane-bound antibody, whereas differentiated plasma cells produce secreted antibodies. Presumably some mechanism exists in naive B cells and in plasma cells that directs RNA processing preferentially toward the production of mRNA encoding either the membrane form or secreted form of an immunoglobulin.

SIMULTANEOUS EXPRESSION OF IgM AND IgD

The phenomenon of differential RNA processing also explains the simultaneous expression of membrane-bound IgM and IgD by mature B cells. As mentioned already, transcription of rearranged heavy-chain genes in mature B cells produces primary transcripts containing both the C_μ and C_δ gene segments. One explanation for this is that the close proximity of C_μ and C_δ, which are only about 5 kb apart, and the lack of a switch site between them permits the entire $VDJC_\mu C_\delta$ region to be transcribed into a long primary RNA transcript, about 15 kb long, which contains four poly-A sites (Figure 7-19a). Sites 1 and 2 are associated with C_μ, as described in

(a) H-chain primary transcript

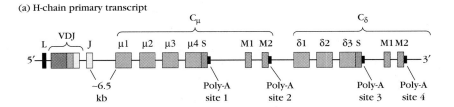

(b) Polyadenylation of primary transcript at site 2 → μ_m

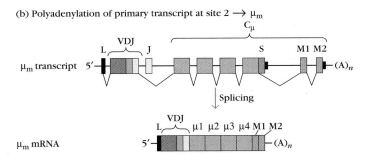

FIGURE 7-19

Expression of membrane forms of μ and δ heavy chains by alternative RNA processing. (a) Structure of rearranged heavy-chain gene showing C_μ and C_δ exons and poly-A sites. (b) Structure of μ_m transcript and μ_m mRNA resulting from polyadenylation at site 2 and splicing. (c) Structure of δ_m transcript and δ_m mRNA resulting from polyadenylation at site 4 and splicing. Both processing pathways can proceed in any given B cell.

(c) Polyadenylation of primary transcript at site 4 → δ_m

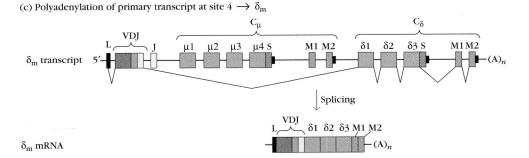

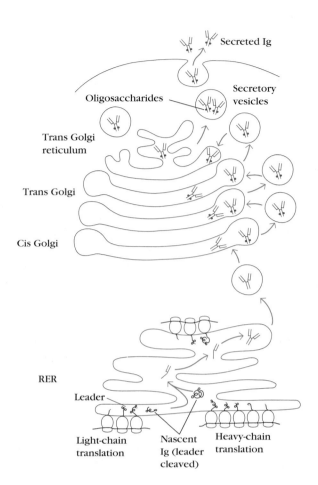

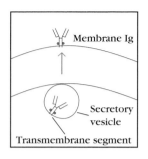

FIGURE 7-20

Synthesis, assembly, and secretion of the immunoglobulin molecule. The heavy and light chains are synthesized on separate polyribosomes (polysomes). The assembly of the chains to form the disulfide-linked and glycosylated immunoglobulin molecule occurs as the chains pass through the cisternae of the rough endoplasmic reticulum (RER) into the Golgi apparatus and then into secretory vesicles. The main figure depicts assembly of a secreted antibody. The inset depicts a membrane-bound antibody, which contains the carboxyl-terminal transmembrane segment. This form becomes anchored in the membrane of secretory vesicles and then is inserted into the cell membrane when the vesicle fuses with the membrane.

the previous section; sites 3 and 4 are located at similar places in the C_δ gene segment.

If the heavy-chain transcript is cleaved and polyadenylated at site 2 after the C_μ exons, then the mRNA will encode the membrane form of the μ heavy chain (Figure 7-19b); if polyadenylation is instead further downstream at site 4 after the C_δ exons, then RNA splicing will remove the intervening C_μ exons and produce mRNA encoding the membrane form of the δ heavy chain (Figure 7-19c). Since the mature B cell expresses both IgM and IgD on its membrane, processing by both pathways must occur simultaneously. Likewise, cleavage and polyadenylation of the primary heavy-chain transcript at poly-A site 1 or 3 in plasma cells and subsequent splicing will yield the secreted form of the μ or δ heavy chains, respectively (see Figure 7-18b).

Synthesis, Assembly, and Secretion of Immunoglobulins

Immunoglobulin heavy- and light-chain mRNAs are translated on separate polyribosomes of the rough endo-

plasmic reticulum (RER). Newly synthesized chains contain an amino-terminal leader sequence, which serves to guide the chains into the lumen of the RER where it is then cleaved off. The assembly of light (L) and heavy (H) chains into the disulfide-linked and glycosylated immunoglobulin molecule occurs as the chains pass through the cisternae of the RER. The complete molecules are transported to the Golgi apparatus and then into secretory vesicles, which fuse with the plasma membrane (Figure 7-20).

The order of chain assembly varies among the immunoglobulin classes. In the case of IgM, the H and L chains assemble within the RER to form half-molecules, and then two half-molecules assemble to form the complete molecule. In the case of IgG, two H chains assemble, then an H_2L intermediate is assembled, and finally the complete H_2L_2 molecule is formed. Interchain disulfide bonds are formed, and the polypeptides are glycosylated as they move through the Golgi apparatus.

If the molecule contains the transmembrane sequence of the membrane form, it becomes anchored in the membrane of a secretory vesicle and is inserted into the plasma membrane as the vesicle fuses with the plasma membrane (see Figure 7-20, insert). If the molecule contains the hydrophilic sequence of secreted immunoglobulins, it is transported as a free molecule in a secretory vesicle and is released from the cell when the vesicle fuses with the plasma membrane.

REGULATION OF IG-GENE TRANSCRIPTION

The immunoglobulin genes are expressed only in B-lineage cells, and even within this lineage, the genes are expressed at different rates during different developmental stages. As with other eukaryotic genes, three major classes of cis regulatory sequences in DNA regulate transcription of immunoglobulin genes:

- **Promoters:** relatively short nucleotide sequences, extending about 200 bp upstream from the transcription initiation site, that promote initiation of RNA transcription in a specific direction
- **Enhancers:** nucleotide sequences situated some distance upstream or downstream from a gene that activate transcription from the promoter sequence in an orientation-independent manner
- **Silencers:** nucleotide sequences that down-regulate transcription, operating in both directions over a distance

The locations of the three types of regulatory elements in germ-line immunoglobulin DNA are shown in Figure 7-21.

Each V_H and V_L gene segment has a promoter located just upstream from the leader sequence. Like other promoters, the immunoglobulin promoters contain a highly conserved AT-rich sequence, called the TATA box, to which RNA polymerase II binds. After binding to the TATA box, the RNA polymerase starts transcribing the DNA from the initiation site, located about 25–35 bp downstream of the TATA box.

The mechanism by which enhancers and silencers modulate transcription is still not fully understood. It is thought that DNA-binding factors bound to an enhancer may alter chromatin structure in the vicinity, thereby facilitating the formation of a stable transcription-initiation complex at the promoter site. Similarly, silencer-binding proteins may interact directly with histones, causing the chromatin structure to become inaccessible for transcription.

One heavy-chain enhancer is located within the intron between the last (3′) J gene segment and the first (5′) C gene segment (C_μ), which encodes the μ heavy chain. Because this heavy-chain enhancer (E_μ) is located 5′ of the S_μ switch site near to C_μ, it can continue to function after class switching has occurred. Another heavy-chain enhancer ($3'\alpha E$) has been detected 3′ of the C_α gene segment. One κ light-chain enhancer (E_κ) is located between the J_κ segment and the C_κ segment, and another enhancer ($3'\kappa E$) is located 3′ of the C_κ segment. The λ light-chain enhancers are located 3′ of $C_\lambda 4$ and

(a) H-chain DNA

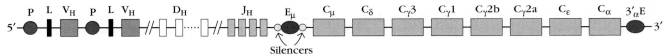

(b) κ-chain DNA

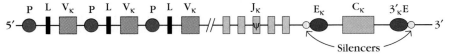

(c) λ-chain DNA

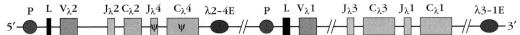

FIGURE 7-21

Location of promoters (dark red), enhancers (green), and silencers (yellow) in mouse heavy-chain, κ light-chain, and λ light-chain germ-line DNA. Variable-region DNA rearrangement moves an enhancer close enough to a promoter so that the enhancer can activate transcription from the promoter.

$3'$ of $C_\lambda 1$. Silencers have been identified in heavy-chain and κ-chain DNA, adjacent to enhancers, but not in λ-chain DNA.

Effect of DNA Rearrangement on Transcription

The promoters associated with the immunoglobulin V gene segments bind RNA polymerase II very weakly. For this reason, the rate of transcription of V_H and V_L coding regions is almost negligible in unrearranged germ-line DNA. In germ-line DNA, the variable-region enhancers are about 250–300 kb away from the promoters. Variable-region gene rearrangement brings a promoter and enhancer within 2 kb of each other, close enough for the enhancer to influence transcription from the nearby promoter. As a result, the rate of transcription of a rearranged $V_L J_L$ or $V_H D_H J_H$ unit is as much as 10^4 times the rate of transcription of unrearranged V_L or V_H segments. For example, in one study, B cells transfected with rearranged heavy-chain genes from which the enhancer had been deleted did not transcribe the genes, whereas B cells transfected with similar genes that contained the enhancer transcribed the transfected genes at a high rate. These findings highlight the importance of enhancers in the normal transcription of immunoglobulin genes.

Genes that regulate cellular proliferation or cell death, called cellular **oncogenes**, sometimes translocate to the immunoglobulin heavy- or light-chain loci. Here, under the influence of an immunoglobulin enhancer, the normally silent oncogene is activated, leading to increased expression of the oncogene product. Translocations of the c-*myc* and *bcl-2* oncogenes have each been associated with malignant B-cell lymphomas. The translocation of c-*myc* leads to constitutive expression of c-Myc and an aggressive B-cell lymphoma called Burkitt's lymphoma. The translocation of *bcl-2* leads to suspension of programmed cell death in B cells, resulting in follicular B-cell lymphoma. This topic is covered in greater detail in Chapter 24.

Inhibition of Ig-Gene Expression in T Cells

As noted earlier, germ-line DNA encoding the T-cell receptor (TCR) undergoes V-(D)-J rearrangement to generate functional TCR genes. Rearrangement of both immunoglobulin and TCR germ-line DNA occurs by a similar recombination process mediated by RAG-1 and RAG-2 and involving recombination signal sequences with one-turn or two-turn spacers (see Figure 7-8). Despite this common process, complete Ig-gene rearrangement of H and L chains occurs only in B cells and complete TCR-gene rearrangement is limited to T cells.

Recently, Hitoshi Sakano and coworkers have obtained results suggesting that a sequence within the κ-chain $3'$ enhancer ($3'\kappa$E) serves to regulate V_κ to J_κ joining in B and T cells. When a sequence known as the PU.1 binding site within the $3'$ κ-chain enhancer was mutated, these researchers found that V_κ-J_κ joining occurred in T cells as well as B cells. They propose that binding of a protein expressed by T cells, but not B cells, to this κ-chain enhancer prevents V_κ-J_κ joining in T cells. The nature of this DNA-binding protein in T cells remains to be determined. Similar processes may prevent rearrangement of heavy-chain and λ-chain DNA in T cells.

SUMMARY

1. Immunoglobulin κ and λ light chains and heavy chains are encoded by three separate multigene families located on different chromosomes. In germ-line DNA, each multigene family contains numerous gene segments (see Figure 7-3). The variable-region gene segments are designated V and J in light-chain DNA and V, D, and J in heavy-chain DNA. Multiple constant-region (C) gene segments are also present.

2. Functional light-chain and heavy-chain genes are generated by random rearrangement of the variable-region gene segments in germ-line DNA. Conserved DNA sequences, termed recombination signal sequences, flank each V, D, and J gene segment and direct the joining of segments. Each recombination signal contains a conserved heptamer sequence, a conserved nonamer sequence, and either a 12-bp (one-turn) or 23-bp (two-turn) spacer; the length, but not the nucleotide sequence, of these spacers is conserved (see Figure 7-6). During rearrangement, gene segments flanked by a one-turn spacer join only to segments flanked by a two-turn spacer. This one-turn/two-turn joining rule assures proper V_L-J_L and V_H-D_H-J_H joining. The multistep recombination process is mediated by several enzymes including RAG-1, RAG-2, terminal deoxynucleotidyl transferase (in heavy-chain rearrangement), and double-strand break repair (DSBR) enzymes (see Figure 7-8).

3. Immunoglobulin-gene rearrangements occur in sequential order, with heavy-chain rearrangements occurring first followed by light-chain rearrangements (see Figure 7-13). These rearrangements are carefully regulated so that the immunoglobulin DNA of only one parental chromosome is rearranged to form a functional light-chain or heavy-chain gene. This allelic

exclusion is necessary to assure that a mature B cell expresses immunoglobulin with a single antigenic specificity.

4. The various mechanisms contributing to antibody diversity are estimated to generate 10^8–10^{11} possible combinations in mammals. Major sources of antibody diversity are the random joining of multiple V, J, and D germ-line gene segments and the random association of a given heavy-chain and light-chain in a particular cell (see Table 7-2). Other mechanisms that augment antibody diversity by a significant but unknown extent are junctional flexibility, P-nucleotide addition, and N-region nucleotide addition, which produce variability in the nucleotide sequences at the coding joints between gene segments, as well as somatic mutation following antigenic stimulation.

5. After antigenic stimulation of mature B cells, additional rearrangement of their heavy-chain C gene segments can occur (see Figure 7-17). Such class switching results in expression of different classes of antibody (IgG, IgA, and IgE) with the same antigenic specificity.

6. Differential RNA processing of the immunoglobulin heavy-chain primary transcript generates membrane-bound antibody in mature B cells and secreted antibody in plasma cells (see Figure 7-18). Differential processing is also responsible for the simultaneous expression of IgM and IgD by mature B cells (see Figure 7-19).

7. Transcription of immunoglobulin genes is regulated by three types of DNA regulatory sequences: promoters, enhancers, and silencers. A promoter is located just upstream of the leader sequence associated with each V_H and V_L gene segment, whereas enhancers and silencers are located considerable distances from the transcription start site (see Figure 7-21). In germ-line DNA, transcription of V_H and V_L gene segments is negligible; gene rearrangement brings enhancers close to the promoter they influence, greatly increasing the transcription rate of rearranged $V_L J_L$ and $V_H D_H J_H$ units.

REFERENCES

ALT, F. W., ET AL. 1992. VDJ recombination. *Immunol. Today* **13**:306.

CHEN, J., AND F. W. ALT. 1993. Gene rearrangement and B-cell development. *Curr. Opin. Immunol.* **5**:194.

COOK, G. P., AND I. M. TOMLINSON. 1995. The human immunoglobulin V_H repertoire. *Immunol. Today* **16**: 237.

DRYER, W. J. AND J. C. BENNETT. 1965. The molecular basis of antibody formation. *Proc. Natl. Acad. Sci. USA.* **54**:864.

HARRIMAN, W., ET AL. 1993. Immunoglobulin class switch recombination. *Annu. Rev. Immunol.* **11**:361.

HIRAMATSU, R., ET AL. 1995. The 3′ enhancer region determines the B/T specificity and pro-B/pre-B specificity of immunoglobulin V_κ-J_κ joining. *Cell* **83**:1.

HOZUMI, N., AND S. TONEGAWA. 1976. Evidence for somatic rearrangement of immunoglobulin genes coding for variable and constant regions. *Proc. Natl. Acad. Sci. USA* **73**:3628.

LEWIS, S. M. 1994. The mechanisms of V(D)J rejoining: lessons from molecular, immunological, and comparative analysis. *Adv. Immunol.* **56**:27.

LIN, W. C., AND S. DESIDERIO. 1995. V(D)J recombination and the cell cycle. *Immunol. Today* **16**:279.

OETTINGER, M. A. 1992. Activation of V(D)J recombination by *RAG1* and *RAG2*. *Trends Genet.* **8**:413.

OETTINGER, M. A., ET AL. 1990. *RAG-1* and *RAG-2*, adjacent genes that synergistically activate V(D)J recombination. *Science* **248**:1517.

RETH, M. 1992. Antigen receptors on B lymphocytes. *Annu. Rev. Immunol.* **10**:97.

ROTH, D. B., ET AL. 1992. V(D)J recombination: broken DNA molecules with covalently sealed (hairpin) coding ends in SCID mouse thymocytes. *Cell* **70**: 983.

SCHATZ, D. G., M. A. OETTINGER, AND M. S. SCHLISSEL. 1992. V(D)J recombination: molecular biology and regulation. *Annu. Rev. Immunol.* **10**:359.

TACCIOLI, G. E., AND F. W. ALT. 1995. Potential targets for autosomal SCID mutations. *Curr. Opin. Immunol.* **7**:436.

TONEGAWA, S. 1983. Somatic generation of antibody diversity. *Nature* **302**:575.

VAN GENT, D. C., ET AL. 1995. Initiation of V(D)J recombination in a cell-free system. *Cell* **81**:925.

YANCOPOULOS, G. D., AND F. W. ALT. 1986. Regulation of the assembly and expression of variable-region genes. *Annu. Rev. Immunol.* **4**:339.

STUDY QUESTIONS

1. Indicate whether each of the following statements is true or false. If you think a statement is false, explain why.

a. V_κ gene segments sometimes join to C_λ gene segments.

b. Immunoglobulin class switching usually is mediated by DNA rearrangements.

c. Separate exons encode the transmembrane portion of each membrane immunoglobulin.

d. Although each B cell carries two alleles encoding the immunoglobulin heavy and light chains, only one allele is expressed.

e. Primary transcripts are processed into functional mRNA by removal of introns, capping, and addition of a poly-A tail.

f. The primary transcript is an RNA copy of the DNA and includes both introns and exons.

2. Explain why a V_H segment cannot join directly with a J_H segment in heavy-chain gene rearrangement.

3. Considering only combinatorial joining of gene segments and association of light and heavy chains, how many different antibody molecules potentially could be generated from germ-line DNA containing 500 V_L and 4 J_L gene segments and 300 V_H, 15 D_H, and 4 J_H gene segments?

4. For each incomplete statement below (a–g), select the phrase(s) that correctly completes the statement. More than one choice may be correct.

a. Recombination of immunoglobulin gene segments serves to

1) promote Ig diversification

2) assemble a complete Ig coding sequence

3) allow changes in coding information during B-cell maturation

4) increase the affinity of immunoglobulin for antibody

5) all of the above

b. Somatic mutation of immunoglobulin genes accounts for

1) allelic exclusion

2) class switching from IgM to IgG

3) affinity maturation

4) all of the above

5) none of the above

c. The frequency of somatic mutation in Ig genes is greatest during

1) differentiation of pre-B cells into mature B cells

2) differentiation of pre-T cells into mature T cells

3) generation of memory B cells

4) antibody secretion by plasma cells

5) none of the above

d. Kappa and lambda light-chain genes

1) are located on the same chromosome

2) associate with only one type of heavy chain

3) can be expressed by the same B cell

4) all of the above

5) none of the above

e. Generation of combinatorial diversity among immunoglobulins involves

1) mRNA splicing

2) DNA rearrangement

3) recombination signal sequences

4) one-turn/two-turn joining rule

5) switch sites

f. A B cell becomes immunocompetent

1) following productive rearrangement of variable-region heavy-chain gene segments in germ-line DNA

2) following productive rearrangement of variable-region heavy-chain and light-chain gene segments in germ-line DNA

3) following class switching

4) during affinity maturation

5) following binding of T_H cytokines to their receptors on the B cell

g. The mechanism that permits immunoglobulins to be synthesized in either a membrane-bound or secreted form is

1) allelic exclusion

2) codominant expression

3) class switching

4) one-turn/two-turn joining rule

5) differential RNA processing

5. What mechanisms generate the three hypervariable regions (complementarity-determining regions) of immunoglobulin heavy and light chains? Why is the third hypervariable region (CDR3) more variable than the other two (CDR1 and CDR2)?

6. You have been given a cloned myeloma cell line that secretes IgG with the molecular formula $\gamma_2\lambda_2$. Both the heavy and light chains in this cell line are encoded by genes derived from allele 1. Indicate the form(s) in which each of the genes listed below would occur in this cell line using the following symbols: G = germ-line form; R = productively rearranged form; NP = nonproductively rearranged form. State the reason for your choice in each case.

a. Heavy-chain allele 1

b. Heavy-chain allele 2

c. κ-chain allele 1

d. κ-chain allele 2

e. λ-chain allele 1

f. λ-chain allele 2

7. You have a B-cell lymphoma that has made nonproductive rearrangements for both heavy-chain alleles. What is the arrangement of its κ light-chain DNA? Why?

8. Indicate whether each of the class switches indicated below can occur (Yes) or cannot occur (No).

a. IgM to IgD

b. IgM to IgA

c. IgE to IgG

d. IgA to IgG

e. IgM to IgG

9. Describe one advantage and one disadvantage of N-nucleotide addition during the rearrangement of immunoglobulin heavy-chain gene segments.

10. X-ray crystallographic analyses of over two dozen antibody molecules bound to their respective antigens have revealed that in every case the CDR3 of both the heavy and light chains make contact with the epitope. Moreover, sequence analyses reveal that the variability of CDR3 is greater than that of either CDR1 or CDR2. What mechanisms account for the greater diversity in CDR3 than in the rest of the variable region?

11. You wish to study the effect of the *RAG-1* gene on B-cell development in the bone marrow. You have available FITC-labeled anti-IgM monoclonal antibodies and rhodamine-labeled anti-IgD monoclonal antibodies. After treating bone marrow cells from normal mice and *RAG-1*⁻ mice with both antibodies, you subject each sample to FACS analysis. In the following diagrams, below, draw the FACS staining pattern you would expect with bone marrow cells from the (a) normal mice and (b) mice lacking the *RAG-1* gene. In both cases, label the cell population in each quadrant.

(a) Normal mice

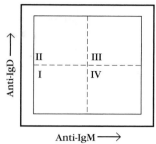

(b) *RAG-1*⁻ mice

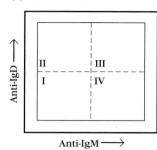

12. How many chances does a developing B cell have to generate a functional immunoglobulin light-chain gene?

13. Select the description(s) listed below (1–11) that are true about each of the following terms (a–h). Each description may be used once, more than once, or not at all; more than one description may apply to some terms.

Terms

a. _____ RAG-1 and RAG-2

b. _____ Double-strand break repair (DSBR) enzymes

c. _____ Coding joints

d. _____ RSSs

e. _____ P-nucleotides

f. _____ N-nucleotides

g. _____ Promoters

h. _____ Enhancers

Descriptions

1) Junctions between immunoglobulin gene segments formed during rearrangement

2) Source of diversity in antibody heavy chains

3) DNA regulatory sequences

4) Conserved DNA sequences, located adjacent to V, D, and J segments, that help direct gene rearrangement

5) Enzymes expressed in developing B cells

6) Enzymes expressed in mature B cells

7) Nucleotide sequences located close to each leader segment in immunoglobulin genes to which RNA polymerase binds

8) Product of endonuclease cleavage of hairpin intermediates in Ig-gene rearrangement

9) Enzymes that are defective in SCID mouse

10) Nucleotide sequences that greatly increase the rate of transcription of rearranged immunoglobulin genes compared with germ-line DNA

11) Nucleotides added by TdT enzyme

14. For each immunoglobulin heavy-chain or light-chain DNA, mRNA, or polypeptide (a–g) described below, select the corresponding schematic diagram (1–9) in the figure below.

a. _____ Heavy-chain DNA in a liver cell

b. _____ λ-Chain DNA in a liver cell

c. _____ Heavy-chain DNA in a mature B cell

d. _____ Primary RNA transcript encoding heavy chain in a mature B cell

e. _____ mRNA encoding light chain in a mature B cell

f. _____ Heavy-chain proteins observed on the membrane of a mature B cell before any class switching

g. _____ Heavy-chain DNA in a plasma cell secreting IgE

For use with Question 14.

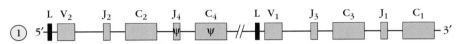
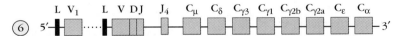
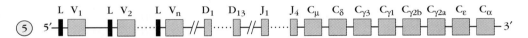
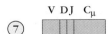
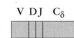

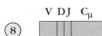
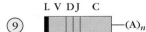

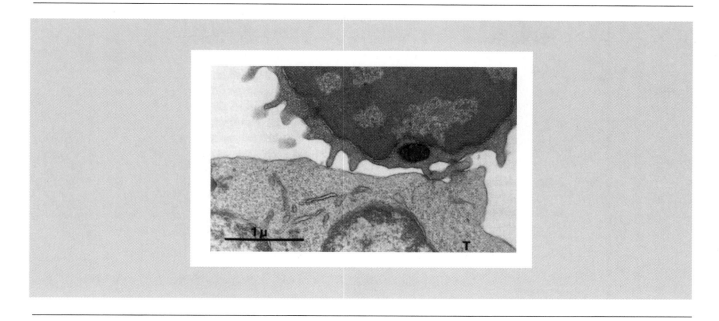

B-CELL MATURATION, ACTIVATION, AND DIFFERENTIATION

The developmental process that results in generation of plasma cells and memory B cells can be divided into three broad stages: generation of mature, immunocompetent B cells (maturation), activation of mature B cells by interaction with antigen, and differentiation of activated B cells into plasma cells and memory B cells. B-cell maturation, which occurs in the bone marrow, involves an orderly sequence of Ig-gene rearrangements and progresses in the absence of antigen. This is the **antigen-independent phase** of B-cell development.

A mature B cell leaves the bone marrow expressing membrane-bound immunoglobulin (mIgM and mIgD) with a single antigenic specificity. These **naive** B cells, which have not encountered antigen, circulate in the blood and lymph and are carried to the secondary lymphoid organs, most notably the spleen and lymph nodes (see Chapter 3). If a B cell is activated by interacting with the antigen for which its membrane-bound antibody is specific, the cell undergoes proliferation (clonal expansion) and differentiation, generating a population of antibody-secreting plasma cells and memory B cells. Affinity maturation and class switching occur during these stages. Since B-cell activation and differentiation in the periphery require antigen, these stages comprise the **antigen-dependent phase** of development.

Large numbers of B cells are produced in the bone marrow throughout life, but very few of these cells become mature recirculating B cells. In mice the size of the recirculating pool of B cells is about 2×10^8 cells. The majority of these cells circulate as naive B cells, which have a life span of approximately 4–8 weeks. Given that the immune system is able to generate a total antibody diversity approaching 10^{11}, clearly only a small fraction of the antigen-binding specificities are displayed by membrane immunoglobulin on recirculating B cells. Indeed, throughout the life span of an individual animal, only a small fraction of the possible antibody diversity is ever expressed.

Visualizing Concepts

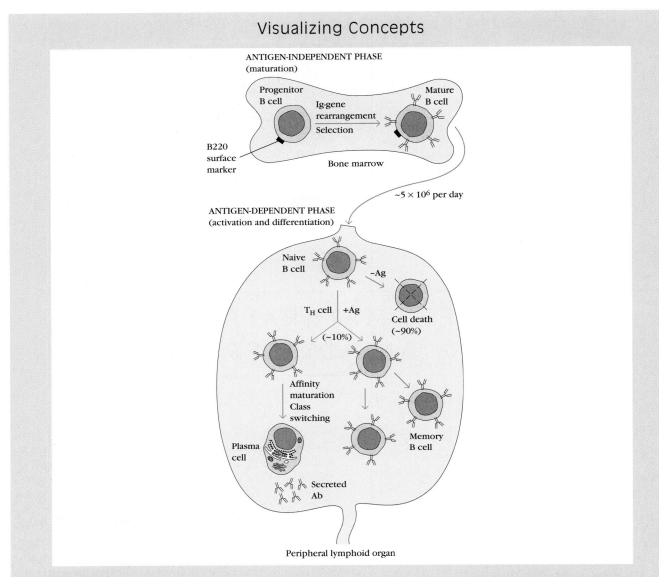

FIGURE 8-1

Overview of B-cell development. During the antigen-independent maturation phase, immunocompetent B cells expressing membrane IgM and IgD are generated in the bone marrow. Only about 10% of the potential B cells reach maturity and exit the bone marrow. In the absence of antigen-induced activation, naive B cells in the periphery die within a few days. In the presence of soluble protein antigen and activated T$_H$ cells, B cells are activated and proliferate within secondary lymphoid organs. Those bearing high-affinity mIg differentiate into plasma cells and memory B cells, which may express different isotypes.

We've referred to some aspects of B-cell developmental processes in previous chapters. The overall pathway, beginning with the earliest distinctive B-lineage cell, is discussed in sequence in this chapter. Figure 8-1 presents an overview of the major events. After these developmental events are described, recent evidence concerning the regulation of B-cell development at various stages is presented.

B-CELL MATURATION

The generation of mature B cells first occurs in the embryo and continues throughout life. Before birth, the yolk sac, fetal liver, and fetal bone marrow are the major sites of B-cell maturation; after birth, generation of mature B cells occurs in the bone marrow.

FIGURE 8-2

Bone-marrow stromal cells are required for maturation of progenitor B cells into precursor B cells. Pro-B cells bind to stromal cells by means of an interaction between VCAM-1 on the stromal cell and VLA-4 on the pro-B cell. This interaction promotes the binding of c-Kit, on the pro-B cell, to stem cell factor (SCF) on the stromal cell. This interaction triggers a signal, mediated via the tyrosine kinase activity of c-Kit, that stimulates the pro-B cell to express receptors for IL-7. IL-7 released from the stromal cell then binds to the IL-7 receptors, inducing the pro-B cell to mature into a pre-B cell. Pre-B cells then detach from the stromal cells and begin proliferating under the stimulus of IL-7, eventually differentiating into immature B cells.

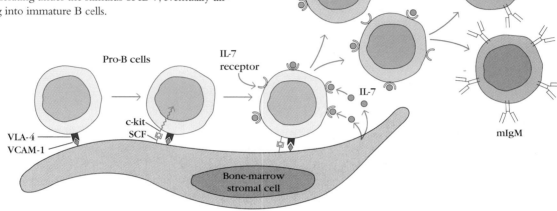

Bone Marrow Environment

B-cell development begins as lymphoid stem cells differentiate into the earliest distinctive B-lineage cell—the **progenitor B cell** (pro-B cell)—which expresses a transmembrane tyrosine phosphatase called CD45R in humans (or B220 in mice). Pro-B cells proliferate within the bone marrow, filling the extravascular spaces between large sinusoids in the shaft of a bone. Proliferation and differentiation of pro-B cells into **precursor B cells** (pre-B cells) requires the microenvironment provided by the bone-marrow stromal cells. If pro-B cells are removed from the bone marrow and cultured in vitro, they will not develop into more mature B-cell stages unless stromal cells are present. The stromal cells play two important roles: They interact directly with pro-B and pre-B cells, and they secrete various cytokines, notably IL-7, that support the developmental process.

At the earliest developmental stage, pro-B cells require direct contact with stromal cells in the bone marrow. This interaction is mediated by several cell-adhesion molecules, including VLA-4 on the pro-B cell and its ligand, VCAM-1, on the stromal cell (Figure 8-2). After initial contact is made, a receptor on the pro-B cell, called c-Kit, interacts with a stromal-cell surface molecule known as stem-cell factor (SCF). This interaction activates c-Kit, which has tyrosine kinase activity, and the

pro-B cell begins to divide and differentiate into a pre-B cell expressing a receptor for IL-7. The IL-7 secreted by the stromal cells drives the maturation process, eventually inducing down-regulation of the adhesion molecules on the pre-B cells, so that the proliferating cells can detach from the stromal cells. At this stage pre-B cells no longer require direct stromal-cell contact but continue to require IL-7 for growth and maturation.

Ig-Gene Rearrangements

B-cell maturation depends on gene rearrangement of the immunoglobulin DNA present in the hematopoietic stem cells. The mechanisms involved in Ig-gene rearrangement were described in Chapter 7. First to occur in the pro-B cell stage is a heavy-chain D_H to J_H gene rearrangement; this is followed by a V_H to $D_H J_H$ rearrangement (Figure 8-3). If the first heavy-chain rearrangement is not productive, then V_H-D_H-J_H rearrangement continues on the other chromosome. Upon completion of heavy-chain rearrangement the cell is now classified as a pre-B cell. Continued development of a pre-B cell into an **immature B cell** requires a productive light-chain gene rearrangement. Because of allelic exclusion, only one light-chain isotype is expressed on the membrane of a B cell (see Figure 7-12). Completion of a productive light-chain rearrangement

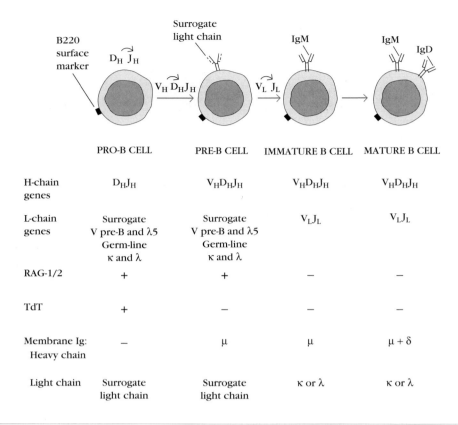

	PRO-B CELL	PRE-B CELL	IMMATURE B CELL	MATURE B CELL
H-chain genes	$D_H J_H$	$V_H D_H J_H$	$V_H D_H J_H$	$V_H D_H J_H$
L-chain genes	Surrogate V pre-B and λ5 Germ-line κ and λ	Surrogate V pre-B and λ5 Germ-line κ and λ	$V_L J_L$	$V_L J_L$
RAG-1/2	+	+	−	−
TdT	+	−	−	−
Membrane Ig: Heavy chain	−	μ	μ	μ + δ
Light chain	Surrogate light chain	Surrogate light chain	κ or λ	κ or λ

FIGURE 8-3

Sequence of events and characteristics of cell stages in B-cell maturation in the bone marrow. The pre-B cell expresses a membrane immunoglobulin consisting of a μ heavy (H) chain and surrogate light chain; the latter is encoded by two genes, Vpre-B and λ5. Changes in the RNA processing of heavy-chain transcripts following the pre-B cell stage lead to synthesis of both membrane-bound IgM and IgD by mature B cells. See text for details. RAG-1/2 = two enzymes encoded by recombination-activating genes; TdT = terminal deoxyribonucleotidyl transferase.

commits the now immature B cell to a particular antigenic specificity determined by the cell's heavy-chain VDJ sequence and light-chain VJ sequence. Immature B cells express IgM on the cell surface.

As would be expected, the recombinase enzymes RAG-1 and RAG-2, which are required for both heavy-chain and light-chain gene rearrangements, are expressed during the pro-B and pre-B cell stages (see Figure 8-3). The enzyme terminal deoxyribonucleotidyl transferase (TdT), which catalyzes insertion of N-nucleotides at the D_H-J_H and V_H-$D_H J_H$ coding joints, is active only during the pro-B cell stage. Because TdT expression is turned off at the pre-B cell stage, when light-chain rearrangement occurs, N-nucleotides are not found in the V_L-J_L coding joints.

Further development of immature B cells leads to the coexpression of IgD and IgM on the membrane, which characterizes **mature B cells**. This progression involves a change in RNA processing of the heavy-chain primary transcript to permit production of two mRNAs, one encoding the membrane form of the μ chain and the other encoding the membrane form of the δ chain (see Figure 7-18). The earliest mature cells in the bone marrow express low levels of IgD. These cells are exported from the bone marrow to peripheral lymphoid organs where the expression of membrane IgD increases.

Pre-B Cell Receptor

Recent evidence has shown that in the pre-B cell the membrane μ chain is associated with an unusual light-chain molecule called a **surrogate light chain**. The surrogate light chain consists of two proteins: a V-like sequence (called **Vpre-B**) and a C-like sequence (called **λ5**), which associate noncovalently to form a light chain–like structure. The genes encoding Vpre-B and λ5 are located at an unknown distance from the λ light-chain genes in mouse and human DNA.

The surrogate light chain is first expressed on the membrane of the pro-B cell complexed with two other glycoproteins (gp130/gp55) and without the μ heavy chain. The function of this membrane glycoprotein remains unknown. Later the surrogate light chain appears on the pro-B cell with a truncated heavy-chain protein encoded by $D_H J_H C_\mu$, and finally it appears with a complete $V_H D_H J_H C_\mu$ chain in the pre-B cell stage. The complex consisting of the membrane-bound μ heavy chain and surrogate light chain is associated with the Ig-α/Ig-β heterodimer to form a **pre-B cell receptor** (Figure 8-4). Only pre-B cells that are able to express membrane-bound μ heavy chains in association with surrogate light chains are able to proceed along the maturation pathway.

The function of the pre-B cell receptor has not yet been determined, but there is speculation that this receptor may recognize a ligand on the stromal-cell membrane, thereby transmitting a signal that prevents V_H to $D_H J_H$ rearrangement of the other heavy-chain allele leading to allelic exclusion. There is also evidence to suggest that the signal generated through the pre-B cell receptor causes proliferation of the pre-B cells. The progeny of these pre-B cells may then rearrange different light-chain gene segments, thereby increasing the overall diversity of the antibody repertoire.

The critical role of the pre-B cell receptor was demonstrated with knockout mice in which the $\lambda5$ gene of the pre-B receptor was disrupted. B-cell development in these mice was shown to be blocked at the pre-B cell stage. This finding suggests that a signal generated through the pre-B cell receptor is necessary for maturation to proceed from the pre-B cell stage to the immature B-cell stage.

Selection of Immature Self-Reactive B Cells

It is estimated that the bone marrow produces about 5×10^7 B cells/day but only 5×10^6 (or about 10%) actually are recruited into the recirculating B-cell pool. This means that 90% of the B cells produced each day die without ever leaving the bone marrow. Some of this loss is attributable to **negative selection** and subsequent elimination (**clonal deletion**) of immature B cells expressing autoantibodies against self-antigens present in the bone marrow.

NEGATIVE SELECTION

It has long been established that the cross-linkage of mIgM on immature B cells can cause the cells to die within the bone marrow. This has been demonstrated experimentally by treating immature B cells with antibody against the μ constant region. This treatment causes cross-linking of mIgM molecules and results in the death of the immature B cells by apoptosis. A similar process is thought to occur in vivo when immature B cells expressing self-reactive mIgM bind to self-antigens in the bone marrow.

Experiments with transgenic mice have helped to shed light on the process of negative selection. These experiments have revealed that when immature B cells encounter self-antigens within the bone marrow, the immature B cells die, presumably by apoptosis. For

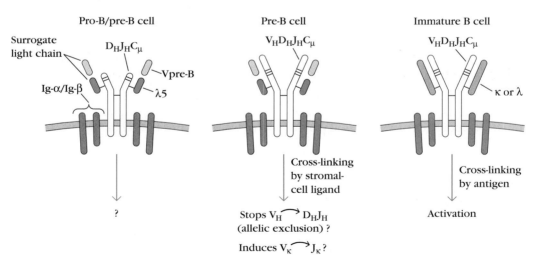

FIGURE 8-4

Schematic diagram of sequential expression of membrane immunoglobulin and surrogate light chain at different stages of B-cell differentiation in the bone marrow. The pre-B cell receptor contains a surrogate light chain consisting of a Vpre-B polypeptide and a $\lambda5$ polypeptide, which are noncovalently associated. The surrogate light chain is expressed at the pro-B/pre-B cell stage with a truncated heavy-chain protein ($D_H J_H C_\mu$). Later the surrogate light chain appears with a complete μ heavy chain. The immature B cell no longer expresses the surrogate light chain and instead expresses the κ or λ light chain together with the μ heavy chain.

example, D. A. Nemanzee and K. Burki introduced a transgene encoding an IgM antibody specific for K^k, an $H-2^k$ class I MHC molecule, into $H-2^d$ and into $H-2^{d/k}$ mice (Figure 8-5a,b). Since class I MHC molecules are expressed on the membrane of all nucleated cells, the endogenous $H-2^k$ and $H-2^d$ class I MHC molecules would be present on bone-marrow stromal cells in the transgenic mice. In the $H-2^d$ mice, which do not express K^k, 25%–50% of the mature, peripheral B cells express the transgene-encoded anti-K^k both as a membrane antibody and as secreted antibody. In contrast, in the $H-2^{d/k}$ mice, which express K^k, no mature, peripheral B cells expressed the transgene-encoded antibody to $H-2^k$ (Table 8-1). These results suggest that the presence of a self-antigen (e.g., the K^k molecule in $H-2^{d/k}$ transgenics) on stromal cells leads to the cross-linking of the corresponding membrane autoantibodies on immature B cells and to their subsequent death.

RESCUE BY EDITING OF LIGHT-CHAIN GENES

Later work by other researchers, using the transgenic system described by Nemazee and Burki, showed that negative selection of immature B cells does not always result in their immediate deletion (Figure 8-5c). Instead, maturation of the self-reactive cell is arrested while the B cell "edits" its receptor. In this case, the $H-2^{d/k}$ transgenics produced a few mature B cells expressing mIgM containing transgene-encoded μ chains but different, endogenous light chains. This experimental finding suggests that a change in the expression of the light chain can convert self-reactive immature B cells into nonself-reactive cells, thereby rescuing the cells from programmed cell death.

One explanation for these results is that when some immature B cells bind a self-antigen, maturation is arrested; the cells up-regulate RAG-1 and RAG-2 expression and begin further rearrangement of their endogenous light-chain DNA. Some of these cells succeed in replacing the κ light chain of the self-antigen with a λ chain encoded by endogenous λ-chain gene segments.

As a result, these cells will begin to express an "edited" mIgM with a different specificity that is not self-reactive. Because these cells are no longer self-reactive, they will escape negative selection and leave the bone marrow as mature B cells bearing the edited, nonself-reactive mIgM. The importance of this process for rescuing potentially self-reactive cells is not yet clear.

B-CELL ACTIVATION AND PROLIFERATION

Following export of mature B cells from the bone marrow, the subsequent steps in B-cell development—activation, proliferation, and differentiation—occur in the periphery and require antigen. In the absence of antigen-induced activation, naive B cells in the periphery have a short life span, dying within a few weeks by apoptosis (see Figure 8-1). Antigen-driven activation and clonal selection of naive B cells leads to generation of plasma cells and memory B cells.

Thymus-Dependent and Thymus-Independent Antigens

Depending on the nature of the antigen, B-cell activation proceeds by two different routes: one that is dependent upon T_H cells and one that is independent of T_H cells. The B-cell response to **thymus-dependent (TD) antigens** requires direct contact with T_H cells, not simply exposure to T_H-derived cytokines. Antigens that activate B cells in the absence of T_H cells are known as **thymus-independent (TI) antigens**. TI antigens can be divided into two types, which activate B cells by different mechanisms. Some bacterial cell-wall components, including lipopolysaccharide (LPS), function as type 1 thymus-independent (TI-1) antigens. Type 2 thymus-independent (TI-2) antigens are highly repetitious

TABLE 8-1

EXPRESSION OF TRANSGENE ENCODING IgM ANTIBODY TO H-2^k CLASS I MHC MOLECULES

| EXPERIMENTAL ANIMAL | NO. ANIMALS TESTED | EXPRESSION OF TRANSGENE | |
		AS MEMBRANE AB	AS SECRETED AB (μG/ML)
Nontransgenic	13	(−)	<0.3
$H-2^d$ Transgenics	7	(+)	93.0
$H-2^{d/k}$ Transgenics	6	(−)	<0.3

SOURCE: Adapted from D. A. Nemazee and K. Burki, 1989, *Nature* **337**:562.

(a) H-2$^{d/k}$ transgenics

Immature B cells

Anti-K^k

Anti-K^k

No mature B cells express anti-K^k

K^d

K^k

Bone-marrow
stromal cell

(b) H-2^d transgenics

25–50% of mature B cells express anti -K^k

K^d

(c) H-2$^{d/k}$ transgenics

Light-chain editing

A few mature B cells with new
light chains no longer bind K^k

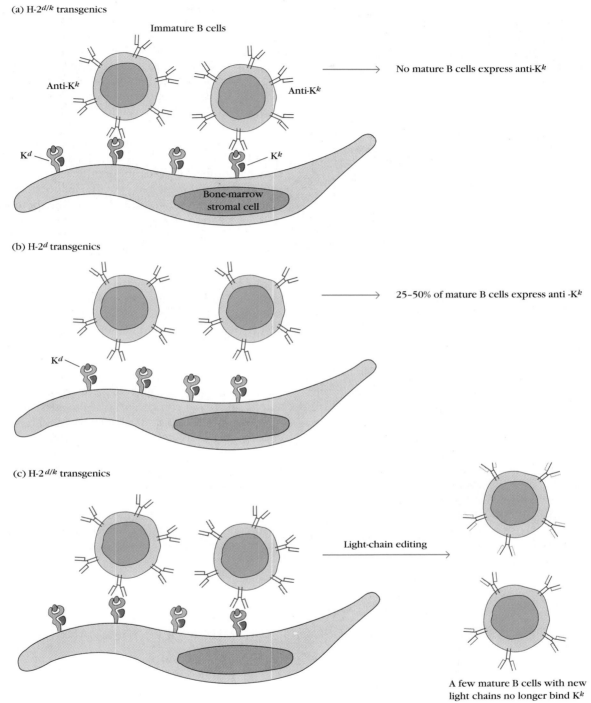

FIGURE 8-5

Experimental evidence for negative selection (clonal deletion) of self-reactive B cells during maturation in the bone marrow. The presence of mature peripheral B cells expressing a transgene-encoded IgM against the H–2 class I molecule K^k was determined in H-2$^{d/k}$ mice (a) and H-2^d mice (b). In the H-2$^{d/k}$ transgenics, the immature B cells recognized the self-antigen (K^k) and were deleted by negative selection. In the H-2^d transgenics, the immature B cells did not bind to a self-antigen and consequently went on to mature, so that 25%–50% of the splenic B cells expressed the transgene-encoded anti-K^k as membrane Ig. More detailed analysis of the H-2$^{d/k}$ transgenics revealed a few peripheral B cells that expressed the transgene-encoded μ chain but a different light chain (c). Apparently, a few immature B cells underwent light-chain editing, so they no longer bound the K^k molecule and consequently escaped negative selection. [Adapted from D. A. Nemazee and K. Burki, 1989, *Nature* **337**: 562; S. L. Tiegs et al. 1993, *JEM* **177**:1009.]

molecules such as bacterial cell-wall polysaccharides with repeating polysaccharide units and polymeric proteins (e.g., bacterial flagellin).

Most TI-1 antigens are polyclonal B-cell activators (**mitogens**); that is, they are able to activate B cells regardless of their antigenic specificity. At high concentrations, some TI-1 antigens will stimulate proliferation and antibody secretion by as many as one third of all B cells. The mechanism by which TI-1 antigens activate B cells is not understood well. When B cells are exposed to lower concentrations of TI-1 antigens, only those B cells specific for epitopes of the antigen will be activated. These antigens can stimulate antibody production in nude mice (which lack a thymus) and thus are truly T cell–independent antigens. The prototypic TI-1 antigen is **lipopolysaccharide** (LPS), a major component of the cell walls of gram-negative bacteria. At low concentrations LPS stimulates specific antibody production. At high concentrations, it is a polyclonal B-cell activator, stimulating proliferation and differentiation of large numbers of B cells, regardless of their antigenic specificity.

TI-2 antigens activate B cells by extensively cross-linking the mIg receptor. Although the B-cell response to TI-2 antigens does not require direct T_H-cell involvement, cytokines derived from T_H cells are required for efficient B-cell proliferation and for class switching to isotypes other than IgM.

The humoral response to thymus-independent antigens is different from the response to thymus-dependent antigens (Table 8-2). The response to TI antigens is generally weaker, no memory cells are formed, and IgM is the predominant antibody secreted, reflecting a lack of class switching. These differences highlight the important role played by T_H cells in generating memory B cells, affinity maturation, and class switching to other isotypes.

Origin of Activating Signals

Naive, or resting, B cells are nondividing cells in the G_0 stage of the cell cycle. Activation drives the resting cell into the cell cycle, progressing through G_1 into the S phase, in which DNA is replicated (see Figure 3-10). The G_1-to-S transition represents a critical restriction point in the cell cycle. Once a cell has reached S, it completes the cell cycle, moving through G_2 and into mitosis (M).

After analyzing the events involved in the progression of lymphocytes from G_0 to the S phase, Ken Ichi Arai noted a number of similarities with events that had been identified in fibroblast cells. He divided these events into competence and progression signals. **Competence signals** are envisioned to drive the B cell from G_0 into early G_1, rendering the cell competent to receive the next level of signals. **Progression signals** then drive the cell from G_1 into S and ultimately to cell division and differentiation. The competence signal is not a single signaling event but rather consists of at least two distinct events that are designated **signal 1** and **signal 2**. These signaling events are generated by different pathways with thymus-independent antigens and thymus-dependent antigens.

Because of their multivalent nature, TI antigens induce a strong stimulation by cross-linking B-cell mIg molecules (signal 1). In addition, TI-1 antigens are thought to contain an additional component that provides an additional signaling event (signal 2) (Figure 8-6a). The extensive cross-linking of mIg provided by TI-2 antigens is thought to generate an effective competence signal. In the B-cell response to TI-1 antigens, cytokine binding provides a progression signal, which is required for extensive proliferation. A progression signal apparently is not required for proliferation of B cells stimulated by TI-2 antigens.

In contrast, TD antigens, which are either divalent or oligovalent, induce a relatively weak signal 1 when they

T A B L E 8 - 2

PROPERTIES OF THYMUS-DEPENDENT AND THYMUS-INDEPENDENT ANTIGENS

PROPERTY	TD ANTIGENS	TI ANTIGENS	
		TYPE 1	TYPE 2
Chemical nature	Soluble protein	Bacterial cell-wall components (e.g., LPS)	Polymeric protein antigens; capsular polysaccharides
Humoral response to:			
Isotype switching	Yes	No	Limited
Affinity maturation	Yes	No	No
Immunologic memory	Yes	No	No
Polyclonal activation	No	Yes (high doses)	No

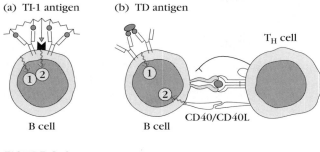

FIGURE 8-6

An effective competence signal for B-cell activation involves two distinct signals induced by membrane events. Binding of a type 1 thymus-independent (TI-1) antigen to a B cell provides both signals. A thymus-dependent (TD) antigen provides signal 1 by cross-linking mIg, but a separate interaction between CD40 on the B cell and CD40L on an activated T_H cell is required to generate signal 2.

interact with B-cell mIg. An additional signal (signal 2) is then provided through interaction of CD40 on the B-cell membrane with a stimulating molecule, called CD40L, expressed on the membrane of the T_H cell (Figure 8-6b). Once the B cell has acquired an effective competence signal in early activation, it begins to express membrane receptors for a variety of cytokines. The interaction of these cytokines with the B-cell membrane receptors provides the progression signal, inducing proliferation and differentiation of the B cell in response to TD antigens.

Transduction of Activating Signals

Immunologists have long puzzled about how mIg mediates an activating signal after contact with an antigen.

The problem is that all isotypes of mIg have very short cytoplasmic tails. Both mIgM and mIgD on B cells extend into the cytoplasm by only three amino acids; the mIgA tail consists of 14 amino acids; and the mIgG and mIgE tails contains 28 amino acids. In each case, the cytoplasmic tail is too short to be able to associate with intracellular signaling molecules (e.g., tyrosine kinases and G proteins).

The puzzle was solved when it was discovered that membrane Ig is associated with a disulfide-linked heterodimer (Ig-α/Ig-β) forming the **B-cell receptor** (BCR). Two molecules of the Ig-α/Ig-β heterodimer associate with one mIg to form a single BCR (see Figure 5-13). Thus the BCR is functionally divided into the ligand-binding immunoglobulin molecule and the signal-transducing Ig-α/Ig-β heterodimer. The Ig-α chain has a long cytoplasmic tail containing 61 amino acids; the tail of the Ig-β chain contains 48 amino acids. The cytoplasmic tails of Ig-α/Ig-β function to transduce the stimulus produced by cross-linking of mIg molecules into an effective intracellular signal.

The cytoplasmic tail of both Ig-α and Ig-β contain an 18-residue motif, termed the **immunoreceptor tyrosine-based activation motif** (ITAM). These sites have been shown to associate with several members of the Src family of tyrosine kinases and with Syk tyrosine kinase. ITAM sites are also present in several other leukocyte receptor molecules, including CD3, which is associated with the T-cell receptor, and the IgE receptor on mast cells. In resting B cells only a small percentage of the BCR complexes are associated with tyrosine kinases. Antigenic stimulation of B cells causes these tyrosine kinases to associate with the BCR and induces their activation. The activated kinases phosphorylate tyrosine residues in the Ig-α/Ig-β heterodimer (Figure 8-7).

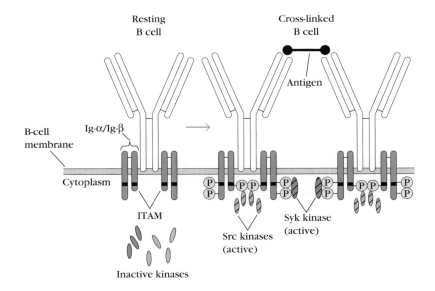

FIGURE 8-7

The B-cell receptor (BCR) comprises an antigen-binding mIg and two signal-transducing Ig-α/Ig-β heterodimers. Following antigen cross-linkage of the BCR, the immunoreceptor tyrosine-based activation motifs (ITAMs) interact with several members of the Src family of tyrosine kinases (Lyn, Blk, Lck, and Fyn) and with Syk kinase, activating the kinases. The activated enzymes phosphorylate tyrosine residues on the cytoplasmic tails of the Ig-α/Ig-β heterodimer.

Visualizing Concepts

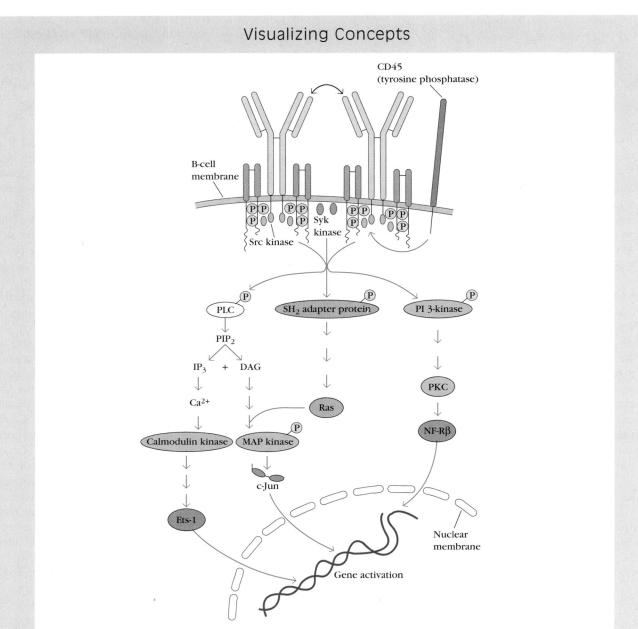

FIGURE 8-8

Overview of signal-transduction pathways triggered by cross-linkage of the B-cell receptor by thymus–independent antigens. CD45 tyrosine phosphatase is thought to remove specific inhibitory phosphates from the Src-family tyrosine kinases, thereby aiding in their activation. Once these kinases and the Syk kinase are activated, they transduce the membrane signal along at least three pathways that involve protein/protein interactions, serine/threonine phosphorylation, and generation of second messengers (e.g., IP_3, DAG, and Ca^{2+}). The final outcome of the three pathways is the activation of various transcription factors that stimulate transcription of specific genes. Note that PIP_2 is a membrane phospholipid; one of its hydrolysis products, DAG, remains in the membrane, while the other, IP_3, diffuses into the cytosol. PLC = phospholipase C; PI = phosphatidylinositol; PIP_2 = phosphatidylinositol bisphosphate; IP_3 = inositol trisphosphate; DAG = diacylglycerol; PKC = protein kinase C.

As noted previously, interaction of both TI-1 and TI-2 antigens with mIg produces an effective competence signal. In the case of TD antigens, however, generation of an effective competence signal requires both mIg cross-linkage and interaction with a T_H cell, as described in detail later. Once an effective competence signal is generated, it triggers a complex cascade of biochemical and cellular responses, ultimately leading to changes in gene expression that characterize the activated B cell (Figure 8-8).

Within minutes of mIg cross-linkage by TI antigens, tyrosine kinase and tyrosine phosphatase activities are released; tyrosine phosphorylation can be detected by 30 s and peaks within 3–5 min of cross-linkage. As tyrosines are phosphorylated and dephosphorylated, a number of more-or-less parallel signal-transduction pathways are activated. One pathway involves activation of phospholipase C, which subsequently hydrolyzes phosphatidylinositol bisphosphate (PIP$_2$) to inositol 1,4,5-trisphosphate (IP$_3$) and diacylglycerol (DAG). IP$_3$ and DAG act as second messengers that either individually or synergistically induce a number of biochemical events, including mobilization of Ca^{2+} from intracellular stores, activation of protein kinase C (PKC), and activation of the $Ca^{2+}/$calmodulin-dependent kinase. These pathways ultimately generate active transcription factors, which translocate to the nucleus where they stimulate or inhibit transcription of specific genes.

B-Cell Coreceptor Complex

Although many naive B cells express mIg with relatively low affinity for antigen, they are able to respond to low concentrations of antigen in a primary response. (As discussed later, response to an antigen can lead to affinity maturation, resulting in higher average affinity of the B-cell population.) Recent research has identified an additional component of the B-cell membrane, called the **B-cell coreceptor**, which can intensify the activating signal resulting from cross-linkage of the BCR. The B-cell coreceptor is a complex of three proteins: CD19, CR2, and TAPA-1. CD19, a member of the immunoglobulin superfamily, has a long cytoplasmic tail and three Ig-fold structures in its extracellular domain. The CR2 component is a receptor for the complement component C3b; it also functions as a receptor for a membrane molecule, CD23, found on the membrane of follicular dendritic cells in germinal centers. TAPA-1 is a transmembrane protein that spans the membrane four times.

As shown in Figure 8-9, the CR2 component of the coreceptor complex binds to complement-coated antigen that has been captured by the mIg on the B cell. This cross-links the coreceptor to the BCR and allows the CD19 component of the coreceptor to interact with the

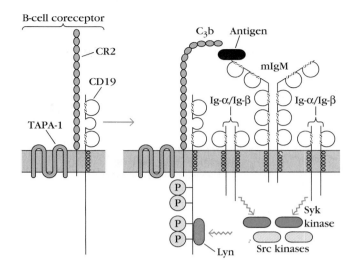

FIGURE 8-9

The B-cell coreceptor is a complex of three cell membrane molecules: TAPA-1, CR2, and CD19. Binding of the CR2 component to C3b-coated antigen captured by mIg results in the phosphorylation of CD19. The Src-family tyrosine kinase Lyn binds to phosphorylated CD19. The resulting activated Lyn can trigger the signal-transduction pathways that begin with phospholipase C and phosphatidylinositol 3-kinase (PI 3-kinase), which are shown in Figure 8-8.

Ig-α/Ig-β component of the BCR. CD19 contains six tyrosine residues in its long cytoplasmic tail and is a major substrate of the protein tyrosine kinase activity that is mediated by engagement of the BCR. Phosphorylation of CD19 permits it to bind and activate the Src-family tyrosine kinase Lyn, which in turn activates two intracellular enzymes involved in B-cell activation pathways: phospholipase C and phosphatidylinositol 3′-kinase (see Figure 8-8). In this way the coreceptor complex serves to amplify the activating signal transmitted through the BCR. In one experimental in vitro system, for example, 10^4 molecules of mIgM had to be engaged by antigen for B-cell activation to occur when the coreceptor was not involved. But when CD19 was cross-linked to the BCR, only 10^2 molecules of mIgM had to be engaged for B-cell activation.

Role of T_H Cells in Humoral Response

As noted already, activation of B cells by soluble protein antigens requires involvement of T_H cells. In this case, binding of antigen to the mIg does not induce an effective competence signal, and additional interaction with membrane molecules on the T_H cell is needed to induce B-cell activation. In addition, a cytokine-mediated progression is required for B-cell proliferation. Figure 8-10 outlines the probable sequence of events in B-cell

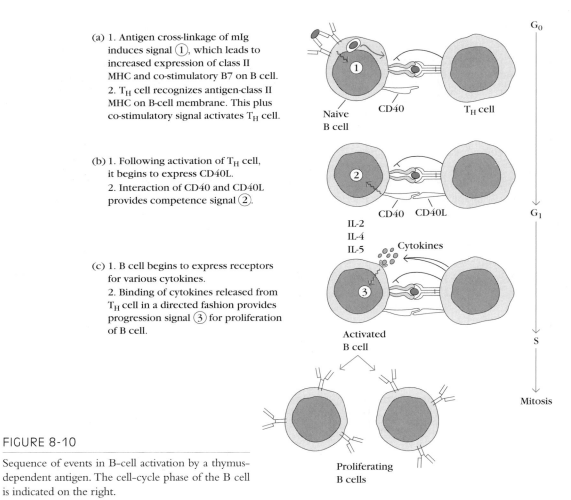

(a) 1. Antigen cross-linkage of mIg induces signal ①, which leads to increased expression of class II MHC and co-stimulatory B7 on B cell.
2. T$_H$ cell recognizes antigen-class II MHC on B-cell membrane. This plus co-stimulatory signal activates T$_H$ cell.

(b) 1. Following activation of T$_H$ cell, it begins to express CD40L.
2. Interaction of CD40 and CD40L provides competence signal ②.

(c) 1. B cell begins to express receptors for various cytokines.
2. Binding of cytokines released from T$_H$ cell in a directed fashion provides progression signal ③ for proliferation of B cell.

FIGURE 8-10

Sequence of events in B-cell activation by a thymus-dependent antigen. The cell-cycle phase of the B cell is indicated on the right.

activation by a TD antigen. This process is considerably more complex than activation induced by TI antigens.

FORMATION OF T-B CONJUGATE

Following binding of antigen by mIg on B cells, the antigen is internalized by receptor-mediated endocytosis and processed within the endocytic pathway into peptides (see Figure 1-10a). Antigen binding also provides competence signal 1 and appears to induce the B cell to up-regulate a number of cell-membrane molecules, including class II MHC molecules and the co-stimulatory ligand B7 (see Figure 8-10a). Increased expression of both of these membrane proteins enhances the ability of the B cell to function as an antigen-presenting cell in T$_H$-cell activation, which is discussed in detail in Chapter 12. The antigenic peptides produced within the endocytic processing pathway associate with class II MHC molecules and are presented on the B-cell membrane to the T$_H$ cell, inducing its activation. It generally takes 30–60 min fol-

lowing internalization of antigen for processed antigenic peptides to be displayed on the B-cell membrane associated with class II MHC molecules. Presumably this is the time required for antigen processing and association with MHC molecules within B cells.

Because a B cell recognizes antigen specifically, by way of its membrane-bound Ig, a B cell is able to present antigen to T$_H$ cells at antigen concentrations that are 100- to 10,000-times lower than what is required for presentation by macrophages or dendritic cells. When antigen concentrations are high, macrophages and dendritic cells serve as effective antigen-presenting cells, but as antigen levels drop, B cells take over as the major presenter of antigen to T$_H$ cells.

Once a T$_H$ cell recognizes a processed antigenic peptide displayed by a class II MHC molecule on the membrane of a B cell, the two cells interact, forming a **T-B conjugate** (Figure 8-11). Micrographs of T-B conjugates reveal that the T$_H$ cells in antigen-specific conjugates exhibit a reorganization of the Golgi apparatus and

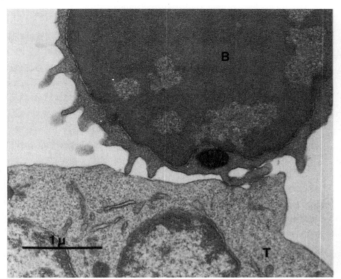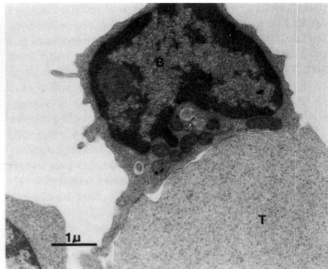

FIGURE 8-11

Transmission electron micrographs of initial contact between a T cell and B cell (*left*) and of a T-B conjugate (*right*). Note the broad area of membrane contact between the cells following conjugate formation. The bar = 1 μm. [From V. M. Sanders et al., 1986, *J. Immunol.* **137**: 2395.]

the microtubular-organizing center toward the junction with the B cell. This reorganization of the Golgi apparatus may provide a mechanism for the directed release of cytokines toward the antigen-specific B cell. Formation of a T-B conjugate not only leads to the directional release of T_H-cell cytokines, but also to the activation-dependent expression of a new T_H-cell membrane protein, CD40L, that is necessary for B-cell activation.

CONTACT-DEPENDENT HELP MEDIATED BY CD40/CD40L INTERACTION

Naive B cells express the membrane glycoprotein CD40, which belongs to a family of cell-surface proteins that regulate cell proliferation and programmed cell death by apoptosis. On activation, T_H cells express a ligand for CD40, known as CD40L. Interaction of CD40L with CD40 on the B cell delivers competence signal 2 to the B cell; this signal plus signal 1 generated by mIg cross-linkage constitutes an effective competence signal that drives the B cell into G_1 (see Figure 8-10b). The competence signal is transduced via intracellular signaling pathways leading to changes in gene expression. The nature of the signal-transduction pathways have not been fully demonstrated in the case of T_H-dependent B-cell activation, but they probably are similar to those involved in T_H-independent activation (see Figure 8-8). For example, following the CD40/CD40L interaction phosphorylation of proteins, including the Src tyrosine kinase Lyn, has been shown to occur in B cells.

The role of an inducible T_H-cell membrane protein in B-cell activation initially was revealed by experiments in which naive B cells were incubated with antigen and plasma membranes prepared either from activated T_H-cell clones or from resting T_H-cell clones. Only the membranes from the activated T_H cells induced B-cell proliferation, suggesting that one or more molecules expressed on the membrane of an activated T_H cell engage receptors on the B cell to provide contact-dependent help.

Several lines of evidence have identified the CD40/CD40L interaction as the one involved in contact-dependent help. For example, when antigen-stimulated B cells are treated with anti-CD40 monoclonal antibodies in the absence of T_H cells, they become activated and proliferate. Thus engagement of CD40, whether by antibodies to CD40 or by CD40L, is critical in providing signal 2 to the B cell. If cytokines also are provided in this experimental system, then the proliferating B cells will differentiate into plasma cells. Conversely, antibodies to CD40L have been shown to block B-cell activation by blocking the CD40/CD40L interaction.

PROGRESSION SIGNALS INDUCED BY T_H-CELL CYTOKINES

Although B cells stimulated with membranes from activated T_H cells are able to proliferate, they fail to differentiate unless cytokines also are present; this finding suggests that both a membrane-contact signal and cytokine

(a)

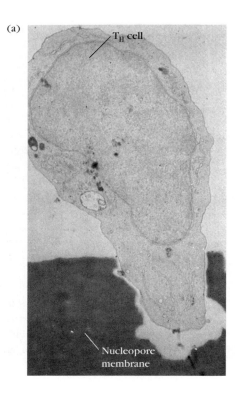

(b)

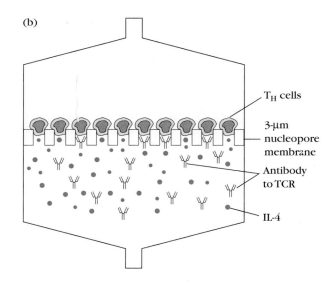

FIGURE 8-12

Experimental demonstration of directional release of cytokines from activated T_H cells. (a) Electron micrograph of a T_H cell centrifuged onto nucleopore membrane. Note how the cell completely blocks the pore. (b) Diagram of culture system. Addition of monoclonal antibody specific for the idiotype of the T-cell receptors resulted in T_H-cell activation and release of IL-4 on one side of the membrane only. [From W. J. Poo et al., 1988, *Nature* **332**:378.]

signal are necessary to induce B-cell proliferation and differentiation. As noted already, electron micrographs of T-B conjugates reveal that the antigen-specific interaction between a T_H and a B cell induces a redistribution of T_H-cell membrane proteins and cytoskeletal elements that may result in the polarized release of cytokines toward the interacting B cell.

In a simple, yet ingenious experiment, W. J. Poo and C. A. Janeway sought to determine whether cytokines are released from T_H cells in a directional manner. They worked with a T_H-cell clone that secreted IL-4 in response to binding of a clonotypic monoclonal antibody specific for the idiotype of the T-cell receptor. This T_H clone was centrifuged onto a nucleopore membrane having 3-μm pores. Since the cells were larger than 3 μm, they completely plugged the pores. The cell-packed membrane was then suspended between two chambers, and the anti-TCR monoclonal antibody was added to one chamber (Figure 8-12). Measurement of IL-4 in both chambers showed that IL-4 was released toward the chamber containing the activating monoclonal antibody. These findings suggest that formation of specific T-B conjugates results in directional release of cytokines toward the interacting B cell.

Once an effective competence signal has been generated, the B cell begins to express membrane receptors for various cytokines (see Figure 8-10c). These receptors then bind the cytokines released in a directed fashion to-

ward the B cell from the interacting T_H cell, thereby generating progression signals. Three T_H cell–derived cytokines (IL-2, IL-4, and IL-5) have been shown to provide progression signals leading to B-cell proliferation. As activated B cells proliferate, three differentiation events can occur: formation of plasma cells and memory B cells, class switching, and affinity maturation. The mechanisms of these events are discussed in a later section.

Negative Selection of Mature, Self-Reactive B Cells

Because some self-antigens do not have access to the bone marrow, B cells expressing mIgM specific for such antigens cannot be eliminated by the negative-selection process in the bone marrow described earlier. To avoid autoimmune responses from such mature self-reactive B cells, some process for deleting them or rendering them inactive must occur in peripheral lymphoid tissue.

A transgenic system developed by C. Goodnow and his coworkers has served to clarify the process of negative selection of mature B cells in the periphery. Goodnow's experimental system included two groups of transgenic mice (Figure 8-13a). One group carried a hen egg-white lysozyme (HEL) transgene linked to a metallothionine promoter, which placed transcription of the HEL gene under the control of zinc levels. The other group of transgenic mice carried rearranged immunoglobulin heavy-

and light-chain transgenes encoding anti-HEL antibody. In normal mice the frequency of HEL-specific B cells is on the order of 1 in 10^3, but in these transgenic mice the rearranged anti-HEL transgene is expressed by 60%–90% of the mature peripheral B cells. Goodnow mated the two groups of transgenics to produce "double-transgenic" offspring carrying both the HEL and anti-HEL transgenes. The question Goodnow then asked was what effect HEL, which is expressed in the periphery but not in the bone marrow, would have upon the development of B cells expressing the anti-HEL transgene.

The Goodnow double-transgenic system has yielded several interesting findings concerning negative selection of B cells (Table 8-3). He found that double-transgenic mice expressing high levels of HEL (10^{-9} M) continued to have mature, peripheral B cells bearing anti-HEL membrane antibody, but these B cells were functionally nonresponsive; that is, they were **anergic**. When these mice were given an immunizing dose of HEL, few anti-HEL plasma cells were induced and the serum anti-HEL titer was low. The endogenous concentration of HEL in these double-transgenic mice before immunization was estimated to be sufficient to occupy 45% of the anti-HEL antibodies on the B cells. A second group of double transgenics, expressing ten times lower levels of HEL (10^{-10} M) was also obtained from the matings. In this case HEL occupied less than 5% of the anti-HEL antibodies on the B cells; under these conditions the B cells were shown to be functionally active. Thus the concentration of HEL and mIg occupancy appeared to determine whether the peripheral HEL-reactive B cells became anergic or not. To determine whether the mature HEL-reactive B cells in the low-HEL double transgenics could later be rendered anergic, Goodnow fed the mice zinc water to elevate the serum HEL concentration. Within 4 days, the previously responsive mature anti-HEL B cells became functionally anergic. Thus clonal anergy could be restored in low-HEL animals by elevating the level of HEL.

Analysis of B cells from the double transgenics showed that the anergic anti-HEL cells expressed about twenty-fold lower levels of membrane IgM than reactive cells but about the same levels of membrane IgD (see Figure 8-13b). Goodnow has suggested that reduction in

(a)

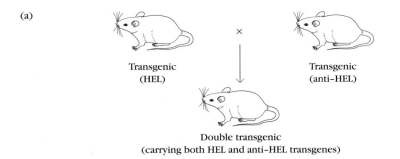

(b)

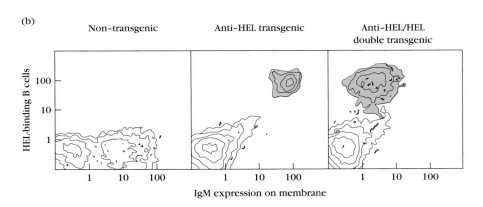

FIGURE 8-13

Goodnow's experimental system for demonstrating clonal anergy in mature peripheral B cells. (a) Production of double-transgenic mice carrying transgenes encoding HEL (hen egg-white lysozyme) and anti-HEL antibody. (b) FACS analysis of peripheral B cells that bind HEL compared with membrane IgM levels. Nontransgenics had no B cells that bound HEL (*left*). Both anti-HEL transgenics (*middle*) and anti-HEL/HEL double transgenics (*right*) had B cells that bound HEL (blue), although the level of membrane IgM was about twentyfold lower in the double transgenics. The data in Table 8-3 indicate that the B cells expressing anti-HEL in the double transgenics cannot mount a humoral response.

(a)

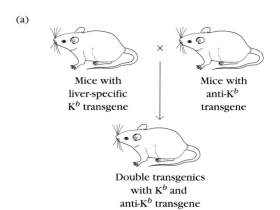

Mice with
liver-specific
K^b transgene

×

Mice with
anti-K^b
transgene

Double transgenics
with K^b and
anti-K^b transgene

(b)

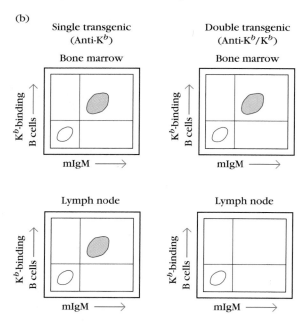

Single transgenic
(Anti-K^b)

Bone marrow

K^b-binding B cells

mIgM

Double transgenic
(Anti-K^b/K^b)

Bone marrow

K^b-binding B cells

mIgM

Lymph node

K^b-binding B cells

mIgM

Lymph node

K^b-binding B cells

mIgM

FIGURE 8-14

Experimental demonstration of clonal deletion of self-reactive mature peripheral B cells by Nemazee and Burki. (a) Production of double-transgenic mice expressing the class I K^b molecule and anti-K^b antibody. Because the K^b transgene contained a liver-specific promoter, K^b was not expressed in the bone marrow in the transgenics. (b) FACS analysis of bone marrow and peripheral (lymph node) B cells for K^b binding versus membrane IgM (mIgM). In the double transgenics, B cells expressing anti-K^b (blue) were present in the bone marrow but were absent in the lymph nodes, indicating that mature self-reactive B cells were deleted in the periphery.

the mIgM level might cause quantitative differences in signal transduction, leading to the anergic state. The observation that the anergic B cells in this system express both IgM and IgD indicates that anergy is being induced in mature B cells rather than in immature B cells.

To study what would happen if a class I MHC self-antigen were expressed only in the periphery, Nemazee and Burki modified the transgenic system used in the experiments on negative selection in the bone marrow discussed previously. To achieve this, they produced a transgene consisting of the class I K^b gene linked to a liver-specific promoter, so that the class I K^b molecule could be expressed only in the liver. Transgenic mice expressing an anti-K^b antibody on their B cells also were produced, and the two groups of transgenic mice were then mated (Figure 8-14a). In the resulting double-transgenic mice, the immature B cells expressing anti-K^b mIgM would not encounter class I K^b molecules in the bone marrow. FACS analysis of the B cells in the double transgenics showed that immature B cells expressing the transgene-encoded anti-K^b were present in the bone

TABLE 8 - 3

EXPRESSION OF ANTI-HEL TRANSGENE BY MATURE PERIPHERAL B CELLS IN SINGLE AND DOUBLE-TRANSGENIC MICE

EXPERIMENTAL GROUP	HEL LEVEL	MEMBRANE ANTI-HEL	ANTI-HEL PFC/SPLEEN*	ANTI-HEL SERUM TITER*
Anti-HEL single transgenics	None	+	High	High
Anti-HEL/HEL double transgenics				
Group 1	High (10^{-9} M)	+	Low	Low
Group 2	Low (10^{-10} M)	+	High	High
Group 2 + Zn^{2+}	High (>10^{-9} M)	+	Low	Low

* Experimental animals were immunized with hen egg-white lysozyme (HEL). Several days later, hemolytic plaque assays for the number of plasma cells secreting anti-HEL antibody were performed and the serum anti-HEL titers were determined.

SOURCE: Adapted from C. C. Goodnow, 1992, *Annu. Rev. Immunol.* **10**:489.

marrow but not in the peripheral lymphoid organs (Figure 8-14b). In the previous experiments of Nemazee and Burki, the class I MHC self-antigen (H-2^k) was expressed on all nucleated cells; in this system, immature B cells expressing the transgene-encoded antibody to this class I molecule were selected and deleted in the bone marrow (see Figure 8-5a). In their second system, however, the class I self-antigen (K^b) was expressed only in the liver, so that negative selection and deletion occurred at the mature B-cell stage in the periphery.

IN VIVO SITES FOR INDUCTION OF HUMORAL RESPONSE

In vivo activation and differentiation of B cells occurs in defined anatomic sites whose structure places certain restrictions on the kinds of cellular interactions that can take place. When an antigen is introduced into the body, it becomes concentrated in various peripheral lymphoid organs. Blood-borne antigen is filtered by the spleen, whereas tissue antigen is filtered by regional lymph nodes or lymph nodules. This discussion focuses on the generation of the humoral response in lymph nodes.

A lymph node is an extremely efficient filter capable of trapping more than 90% of any antigen carried into the node by the afferent lymphatics (see Figure 3-21). As antigen percolates through the cellular architecture of a node, it will encounter one of three types of antigen-presenting cells: interdigitating dendritic cells in the paracortex, macrophages scattered throughout the node, or specialized follicular dendritic cells in the follicles and germinal centers. Antigenic challenge leading to a humoral immune response involves a complex series of events, which take place in distinct microenvironments within a lymph node (Figure 8-15). Slightly different pathways may operate during a primary and secondary response because much of the tissue antigen is complexed with circulating antibody during a secondary response.

Antigen or antigen-antibody complexes enter the lymph nodes via afferent lymphatics, either alone or associated with antigen-transporting cells (e.g., Langerhans cells or dendritic cells) and macrophages. Lymphocytes enter the lymph nodes either through the afferent lymphatic vessels or from the blood by extravasation through high-endothelial cells in the postcapillary venules (see Figure 3-21). The initial activation of both B and T cells is thought to take place in the **paracortex**. This region is heavily populated with T cells, macrophages, and interdigitating dendritic cells. The interdigitating dendritic cells in the paracortex express high levels of class II MHC molecules and have long processes that have been shown to contact upwards of 200 T$_H$ cells.

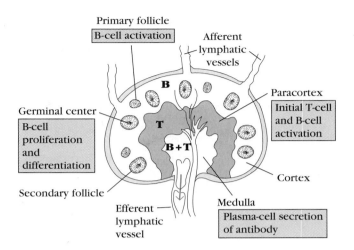

FIGURE 8-15

Schematic diagram of a peripheral lymph node showing anatomic sites at which various steps in B-cell activation, proliferation, and differentiation occur. The cortex is rich in B cells, and the paracortex in T cells; both B and T cells are present in the large numbers in the medulla. A secondary follicle comprises the follicular mantle and germinal center, which contains three distinct zones.

Within 1–2 days of antigenic challenge, the antigen is presented by macrophages and interdigitating dendritic cells to naive T cells resulting in extensive T$_H$-cell activation and proliferation within the paracortex. In addition, naive B cells from the B-cell rich cortex migrate to the T cell–rich zone of the lymph node. B cells that have bound antigen by mIg will internalize the antigen and present it in association with class II MHC molecules. On entering the T-cell zone, a B cell that is presenting antigen will seek out and interact with an activated T$_H$ cell specific for the displayed antigenic peptide, forming a T-B conjugate and inducing initial B-cell activation as described in the previous section. Once B-cell activation takes place, small foci of proliferating B cells form at the edges of the T cell–rich zone and reach a maximum size within 3–4 days of antigen challenge. The B cells within these foci differentiate into plasma cells secreting IgM and IgG isotypes. Most of the antibody produced during a primary response comes from plasma cells in these foci. (A similar sequence of events takes place in the spleen with initial B-cell activation occurring in the T cell–rich periarterial lymphatic sheath, PALS).

A few days after the formation of foci within lymph nodes, a few activated B cells, together with a few T$_H$ cells, are thought to migrate from the foci to primary follicles. These follicles then develop into secondary follicles, which provide a specialized microenvironment favorable for interactions between B cells, activated T$_H$ cells, and follicular dendritic cells. Follicular dendritic cells have long processes, along which are arrayed Fc

Visualizing Concepts

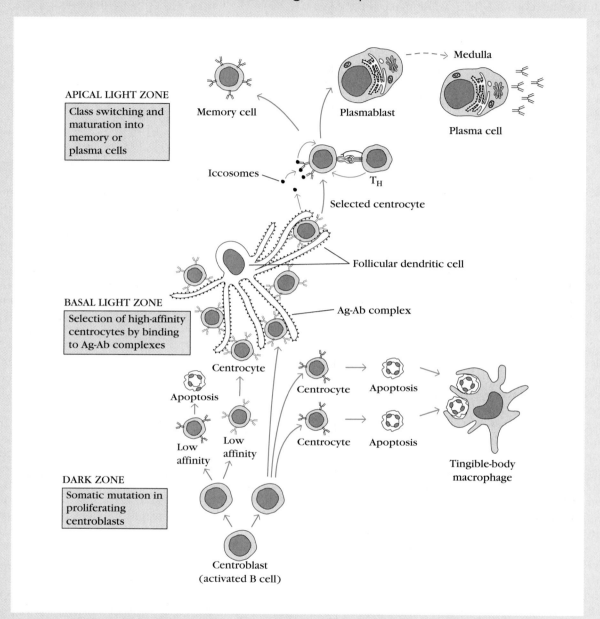

FIGURE 8-16

Overview of cellular events within secondary follicles of peripheral lymph nodes. Follicular dendritic cells bind antigen-antibody complexes along their long processes. Small B cells (centrocytes) bearing high-affinity membrane immunoglobulin (mIg antibodies shown in blue) are thought to interact with antigen presented on the follicular dendritic cells; unselected centrocytes bearing low-affinity mIg die by apoptosis and the debris is phagocytosed by tingible-body macrophages. Selected centrocytes, which may undergo class switching, then mature into memory B cells or plasmablasts; the latter migrate to the medulla where they develop into plasma cells.

receptors that bind antigen-antibody complexes effectively and retain the complexes for months to years on the cell membrane (see Figure 3-15). Because follicular dendritic cells bind antigen that has been complexed to antibody, they are thought to be particularly important in the secondary response, when circulating antibody levels are significant. The periodicity of these immune complexes along the long dendritic processes of these cells is thought to provide an optimal cross-linking matrix favoring B-cell activation. In addition, follicular dendritic cells express CD23, a cell-membrane molecule that interacts with the CR2 component of the B-cell coreceptor complex. This interaction is thought to contribute to the activating signal, facilitating further B-cell activation.

Follicular dendritic cells release small membrane-derived particles, 0.3–0.4 μm in diameter, which appear to originate from the beaded structures of the dendritic processes. These particles, which are heavily coated with immune complexes, are called **iccosomes,** for **immune-complex coating**. Especially during a secondary response, iccosomes released from follicular dendritic cells bind to mIg on B cells and are endocytosed. The endocytosed antigen is then processed and presented together with class II MHC molecules, allowing the B cells to function as effective antigen-presenting cells for activated T_H cells. Formation of T-B conjugates may follow, resulting in B-cell activation and proliferation. As cell proliferation continues, the activated B cells (together with some activated T_H cells) migrate towards the center of the follicle, forming the **germinal center**. Development of germinal centers is dependent upon the previous interaction of B cells in the foci with activated T_H cells and requires the CD40/CD40L interaction. If the CD40/CD40L interaction is blocked, then germinal centers fail to develop. Germinal centers characteristically arise within 1–3 weeks following exposure to a thymus–dependent antigen.

During the first stage of germinal-center formation, activated B cells undergo intense proliferation within the secondary follicle, filling the spaces between the network of follicular dendritic cells. The proliferating activated B cells, known as **centroblasts,** then move to one edge of the follicle, forming the **dark zone** (Figure 8-16). Centroblasts are distinguished morphologically by their large size, expanded cytoplasm, diffuse chromatin, and lack of membrane Ig. The centroblasts become densely packed within the dark zone and divide to give rise to progeny called **centrocytes,** which are small, nondividing cells that now express membrane Ig. As the number of centrocytes increases, they move from the dark zone into a region containing numerous follicular dendritic cells called the **basal light zone**. Centrocytes make close contact with antigen displayed on the long processes of follicular dendritic cells within this zone of the germinal center.

Centrocytes bearing IgM that binds to antigen presented by the follicular dendritic cells in the basal light zone undergo differentiation within the **apical light zone**, forming two types of progeny: small memory B cells and large plasmablasts. The plasmablasts leave the germinal center and migrate to the medulla of the node, where they develop into plasma cells and begin to secrete antibody molecules. Some memory B cells remain in the **follicular mantle**, while others leave the lymph node through the efferent lymphatic vessel and recirculate to other parts of the body.

The majority of centrocytes, however, cannot bind the antigen presented by the follicular dendritic cells. These cells die by apoptosis within the basal light zone of germinal centers and are phagocytosed by an unusual type of macrophage, the **tingible-body macrophage**, that specializes in phagocytosis of lymphoid cells (see Figure 8-16). The high rate of cell death by apoptosis is thought to be a means of eliminating those B cells that bear low-affinity mIg or fail to recognize the antigen that is bound by the follicular dendritic cells. This process accounts for affinity maturation in the humoral response.

B-CELL DIFFERENTIATION

Now that we've reviewed where in the body B cells are activated and differentiate, we examine in more detail the primary events in B-cell differentiation. As indicated in Figure 8-16, three important B-cell differentiation events take place in germinal centers: affinity maturation, class switching, and formation of plasma cells and memory B cells. These events require signals provided by T_H cells or follicular dendritic cells.

Affinity Maturation

In the course of a humoral immune response, the average affinity of the antibodies produced in response to an antigen increases as much as 100- to 10,000-fold. This **affinity maturation** is the result of two processes: somatic hypermutation and antigen selection of high-affinity clones.

ROLE OF SOMATIC HYPERMUTATION

When antigen-activated centroblasts proliferate in the dark zone of the germinal center, they undergo extensive **somatic hypermutation** of the heavy- and light-chain variable regions. As discussed in Chapter 7, somatic hypermutation introduces point mutations, deletions, and insertions into the V, D, and J segments of rearranged immunoglobulin genes. The majority of these mutations occur within the three complementarity-determining regions (CDRs). It is not known whether targeting to CDRs occurs because the enzymes involved in somatic hypermutation preferentially recognize the CDRs or whether mutations within the CDRs are selected over other mutations because of their impact on antigen-binding affinity.

Somatic hypermutation does not appear to occur until well into the primary response, peaking late in the second week following primary antigen challenge (see Figure 7-16). The finding that somatic mutations are located predominantly in secondary antibodies and in isotypes resulting from class switching may indicate that the mutation process is influenced by events in B-cell differentiation. Some workers have suggested that the observed increase in somatic mutations during a secondary response may result from an error-prone DNA-repair process, which would be heightened during the additional cell divisions required to generate a secondary response. The molecular mechanisms responsible for somatic hypermutation are completely unknown, but both activated T_H cells and germinal centers are required for this process to take place.

It has been estimated that the mutation rate during somatic mutation is approximately 10^{-3}/base pair/division, which is a millionfold greater than the normal mutation rate for cells. At this rate, nearly every dividing centroblast will acquire a mutation in either the heavy- or light-chain variable regions. Because somatic mutation occurs randomly, it will generate a few cells with receptors of higher affinity and many cells with receptors of lower or no affinity for antigen. Those cells with high-affinity receptors for antigen are then thought to be subjected to **positive selection**. This selection process takes place among the nondividing centrocyte population in the apical light zone of the germinal center. Binding of centrocytes with high-affinity mIg to the antigen on follicular dendritic cells is thought to deliver a positive stimulus that protects these centrocytes from apoptosis (see Figure 8-16).

A recent mathematical model developed by A. Perelson and T. Kepler suggests that affinity maturation may involve a cyclical process of rapid proliferation and somatic hypermutation followed by a period of cellular rest during which selection occurs. According to their model, once a centrocyte has been selected in the basal light zone, it re-enters the dark zone to begin another round of proliferation and mutation; the resulting progeny again move to the apical light zone for selection. This model suggests that several rounds of this cycle would be necessary to generate the 10–20 beneficial mutations needed to form a high-affinity antibody.

For affinity maturation to occur, not only must B cells bearing high-affinity mIg be generated, but cells with low-affinity mIg must be eliminated. Indeed, one of the

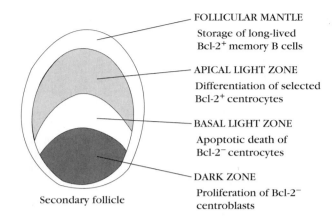

FOLLICULAR MANTLE
Storage of long-lived Bcl-2$^+$ memory B cells

APICAL LIGHT ZONE
Differentiation of selected Bcl-2$^+$ centrocytes

BASAL LIGHT ZONE
Apoptotic death of Bcl-2$^-$ centrocytes

DARK ZONE
Proliferation of Bcl-2$^-$ centroblasts

Secondary follicle

FIGURE 8-17

Schematic diagram of a secondary follicle within a peripheral lymph node. The follicular mantle surrounds the germinal center, which contains three distinguishable zones. Binding of centrocytes bearing mIg with high affinity for antigen on follicular dendritic cells in the basal light zone induces expression of Bcl-2. This oncogene product inhibits apoptosis.

striking characteristics of the germinal center is the extensive cell death by apoptosis that takes place there. This is seen most readily by the appearance of condensed chromatin fragments, indicative of apoptosis, in tingible-body macrophages. We saw in Chapter 3 that Bcl-2, which is encoded by the cellular oncogene *bcl-2*, functions to regulate apoptosis: High levels of Bcl-2 inhibit apoptosis, whereas low levels permit apoptosis to proceed. Moreover, interaction of mature B cells with antigen induces up-regulation of Bcl-2. It thus seems likely that binding of the relatively few centrocytes expressing high-affinity mIg to antigen displayed on follicular dendritic cells delivers a signal that induces expression of Bcl-2 by these centrocytes, thereby protecting them from apoptotic death. Because somatic hypermutation causes the majority of centrocytes to have diminished affinity for antigen, these cells fail to be selected by antigen captured by follicular dendritic cells. Consequently, the majority of centrocytes within the germinal center fail to express Bcl-2 and subsequently die by apoptosis (Figure 8-17). The selected high-affinity, Bcl-2$^+$ centrocytes undergo further differentiation in the apical light zone.

ANTIGEN SELECTION OF HIGH-AFFINITY CENTROCYTES

The role played by antigen in the selection of high-affinity B-cell clones was clarified in an early experiment by H. N. Eisen and G. W. Siskind, who immunized two groups of rabbits with two different doses of the hapten-carrier complex DNP-BGG. Group I was immunized with 5 mg, and group II with 250 mg of DNP-BGG. The affinity of the serum anti-DNP antibodies produced in response to the antigen was then measured at 2 weeks, 5 weeks, and 8 weeks following immunization.

As the data in Table 8-4 show, the average affinity of the group I anti-DNP antibodies increased about 140-fold from 2 weeks to 8 weeks, whereas the affinity of the group II antibodies was initially lower and did not increase. The nearly fivefold lower average affinity of the group II antibodies at 2 weeks suggests that at high immunizing doses, B cells expressing both high-affinity and low-affinity membrane antibody are activated and clonally expanded. In contrast, when the immunizing dose is low, only B cells with high-affinity membrane antibody are activated and clonally expanded (Figure 8-18). As antigen levels decline over time following immunization, competition for the available antigen increases. Now only those B cells possessing high-affinity membrane antibody are able to bind sufficient antigen to be activated and clonally expanded. Thus, with time, the average affinity of the secreted antibody increases. In the experimental system of Eisen and Siskind, antigen concentration was never limited in group II; therefore, low-affinity B cells never had to compete with the high-affinity cells for available antigen, and the response never showed an increase in antibody affinity.

Class Switching

Antibodies perform two important activities: the specific binding to an antigen, which is determined by the V_H and V_L domains; and participation in various biological effector functions, which is determined by the isotype of

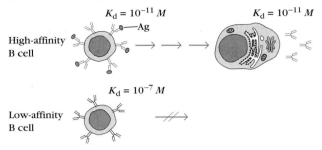

(a) Low immunizing dose

High-affinity B cell $K_d = 10^{-11} M$ — Ag $K_d = 10^{-11} M$

Low-affinity B cell $K_d = 10^{-7} M$

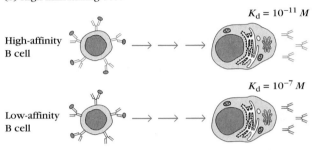

(b) High immunizing dose

High-affinity B cell $K_d = 10^{-11} M$

Low-affinity B cell $K_d = 10^{-7} M$

FIGURE 8-18

Effect of immunizing dose on affinity maturation. At low doses, only B cells bearing high-affinity membrane antibody (blue) bind antigen and are activated, leading to an increase in the average affinity of the secreted antibodies. At high doses, both high- and low-affinity cells bind antigen, so no significant change in the average affinity of the secreted antibodies occurs.

the heavy-chain constant domain. As discussed in Chapter 7, class switching allows any given V_H domain to associate with the constant region of any isotype. This enables antibody specificity to remain constant while the biological effector activities of the molecule vary.

As noted earlier, the humoral response to thymus-dependent antigens is marked by extensive class switching to isotypes other than IgM, whereas the antibody response to thymus-independent antigens is dominated by IgM. In the case of thymus-dependent antigens, membrane interaction between CD40 on the B cell and CD40L on the T_H cell appears to be necessary to induce class switching. The requirement for this interaction is highlighted by **X-linked hyper-IgM syndrome**, an immunodeficiency disorder in which T_H cells fail to express CD40L. Patients with this disorder produce IgM but not other isotypes, suggesting that class switching is dependent on the CD40/CD40L interaction. In addition, these patients do not develop germinal centers, suggesting that the CD40/CD40L interaction also is necessary for B cells to migrate to follicles and give rise to germinal centers.

The isotypes of the antibodies secreted by plasma cells following differentiation of activated B cells is dependent

TABLE 8-4

EFFECT OF IMMUNIZING DOSE AND TIME ON AVERAGE AFFINITY OF INDUCED ANTI-DNP ANTIBODIES IN RABBITS

GROUP	DNP-BGG IMMUNIZING DOSE (MG PER ANIMAL)	K OF ANTI-DNP ANTIBODIES* (L/MOL × 10⁶)		
		2 WEEKS	5 WEEKS	8 WEEKS
I	5	0.86	14	120
II	250	0.18	0.13	0.15

* Values are averages for five animals per group and are based on binding of DNP-L-lysine with serum antibody samples obtained at indicated times after immunization.

SOURCE: Adapted from H. N. Eisen and G. W. Siskind, 1964, *Biochemistry* **3**:966.

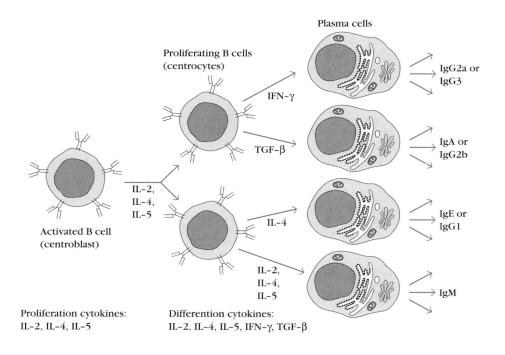

Plasma cells

Proliferating B cells
(centrocytes)

IFN-γ   IgG2a or
IgG3

TGF-β   IgA or
IgG2b

IL-2,
IL-4,
IL-5

Activated B cell
(centroblast)

IL-4   IgE or
IgG1

IL-2,
IL-4,
IL-5   IgM

Proliferation cytokines:
IL-2, IL-4, IL-5

Differention cytokines:
IL-2, IL-4, IL-5, IFN-γ, TGF-β

FIGURE 8-19

Numerous cytokines participate in B-cell proliferation and class switching during differentiation into plasma cells. Binding of the proliferation cytokines, which are released by activated T_H cells, provide the progression signal needed for proliferation of activated B cells. The indicated cytokine effects have been demonstrated; however, similar or identical effects may be mediated by other cytokines. Class switching in the response to thymus-dependent antigens also requires the CD40/CD40L interaction, which is not indicated here.

on the action of specific cytokines (Figure 8-19). Cytokines induce class switching by making the switch sites that lie 5′ to each C_H gene accessible, so that switch recombinase enzymes can bind to the site (see Figure 7-12). Exposure of activated B cells to IL-4, for example, results in DNA transcription upstream from the switch regions for $C_\gamma 1$ or C_ε, indicating that the chromatin at these switch sites is now accessible.

In the humoral response to type 1 thymus-independent (TI-1) antigens, class switching does not occur. In the response to TI-2 antigens, class switching to other isotypes can occur, although IgM is the predominant isotype produced. Several cytokines, notably IL-4, IFN-γ, and TGF-β have been shown to be required for class switching in the response to TI-2 antigens. These cytokines are produced by T_H cells, but they can also be produced by other cells enabling class switching during the response to TI-2 antigens even in the absence of T_H cells. Natural killer cells, for example, secrete both IL-4 and IFN-γ, and macrophages and B cells secrete TGF-β.

Class switching is also influenced by the microenvironment of the plasma cell. Plasma cells leaving the follicles of Peyer's patches or mesenteric lymph nodes are almost all committed to IgA production. In contrast, plasma cells originating in the tonsils, spleen, or peripheral lymph nodes are mainly committed to IgG production.

Generation of Plasma Cells and Memory B Cells

Following selection of centrocytes bearing high-affinity mIg for antigen displayed on follicular dendritic cells, the centrocytes differentiate into plasma cells and memory B cells in the apical light zone (see Figure 8-16). It appears that different membrane signals may determine whether a plasma cell or a memory cell is formed, as depicted in Figure 8-20.

Formation of plasma cells is thought to be induced by IL-1 and CD23, which are produced by follicular dendritic cells. CD23 is expressed in a membrane form and is also released in a soluble form, which acts in a paracrine fashion on nearby centrocytes. As noted earlier, CD23 is a ligand for the CR2 component of the co-receptor complex on the B cell. The interaction of either membrane or soluble CD23 with CR2 on the B cell, together with an IL-1 signal, induces the centrocyte to differentiate into a plasma cell.

Plasma cells generally lack detectable membrane-bound immunoglobulin and instead synthesize high levels of secreted antibody. Differentiation of mature B cells into plasma cells must involve a change in RNA processing so that the secreted form of the heavy chain rather than the membrane form is synthesized (see

Figure 7-18). In addition, the rate of transcription of heavy- and light-chain genes is significantly greater in plasma cells than in B cells. Several authors have suggested that the increased transcription by plasma cells might be explained by their synthesis of higher levels of transcription factors that bind to immunoglobulin enhancers compared with less-differentiated B-lineage cells. Some mechanism also must coordinate the increase in transcription of heavy-chain and light-chain genes, even though these genes are on different chromosomes.

Memory cells also are generated from selected high-affinity centrocytes in the apical light zone of germinal centers. In this case, the centrocyte is thought to bind and internalize antigen released as iccosomes from follicular dendritic cells (see Figure 8-20). The internalized antigen is processed and presented with class II MHC molecules to T_H cells scattered within the apical light zone. These T_H cells thus are activated and thereby stimulated to express CD40L, which then binds to CD40 on the centrocyte. This interaction provides a signal that is necessary for formation of a memory B cell.

Some properties of naive and memory B cells are summarized in Table 8-5. Except for membrane-bound immunoglobulins, few membrane molecules have been identified that distinguish naive B cells from memory B cells. While naive B cells only express IgM and IgD, memory B cells express additional isotypes, including IgG, IgA, and IgE. In addition, the level of IgD often appears to be reduced on memory B cells. Another membrane marker that appears to distinguish naive and memory B cells is an antigen designated J11d. Naive B cells express high levels of J11d, whereas memory B cells express little or no J11d. In addition, memory B cells express higher levels of various adhesion molecules (e.g., ICAM-1) than do naive B cells.

Some memory B cells express a single isotype, whereas others express two isotypes (IgM + IgG, IgM + IgA, or IgM + IgE). It is not known how a memory B cell can express both IgM and another isotype whose constant-region gene is 50–100 kb away. Possibly, the μ-chain mRNA is long lived, so that μ heavy chains continue to be expressed after class switching to another isotype occurs. Another possibility is that molecular mechanisms other than class switching are responsible for coexpression of IgM with IgG, IgA, or IgE. For example, some very long primary transcripts containing $V_H D_H J_H$ and multiple C_H gene segments have been detected in memory B cells. Differential processing of such long transcripts might generate different isotypes within a given memory cell; this would be analogous to the coexpression of IgM and IgD in a mature B cell (see Figure 7-19). At a later stage, class switching by the mechanism described in Chapter 7 would lead to the irreversible deletion of intervening C_H segments, so that only a single isotype is expressed.

Three models have been proposed to explain the formation of plasma cells and memory cells. The most widespread model is that memory B cells and plasma

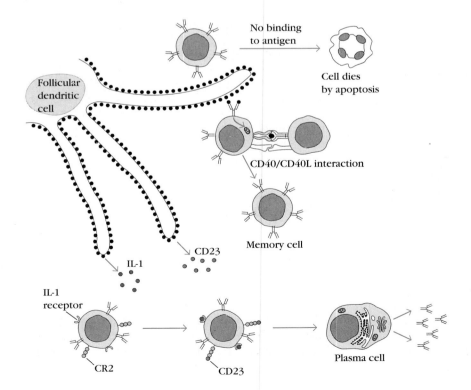

FIGURE 8-20

Different membrane signals determine whether centrocytes differentiate into plasma cells or memory cells within the apical light zone of germinal centers. Formation of plasma cells is induced by binding of IL-1 and CD23 to receptors on centrocytes. Both of these molecules are products of follicular dendritic cells. Memory B cells are generated following a T_H-derived signal triggered by interaction of CD40 on centrocytes with CD40L on activated T_H cells. Class switching may occur during formation of both plasma and memory B cells.

COMPARISON OF NAIVE AND MEMORY B CELLS

PROPERTIES	NAIVE B CELL	MEMORY B CELL
Membrane markers		
Immunoglobulin	IgM, IgD	IgM, IgD(?), IgG, IgA, IgE
Jlld	High	Low
Complement receptor	Low	High
Anatomic location	Spleen	Bone marrow, lymph node, spleen
Life span	Short-lived	May be long-lived
Recirculation	Yes	Yes
Receptor affinity	Lower average affinity	Higher average affinity due to affinity maturation*
Adhesion molecules	Low ICAM-1	High ICAM-1

* Affinity maturation results from somatic mutation during proliferation of centroblasts and subsequent antigen selection of centrocytes bearing high-affinity mIg.

cells develop from "unequal" division of a common precursor cell. A second model is that cytokines or other signals mediated by T_H cells or various accessory cells may influence the differentiation of a common precursor cell into a memory cell or a plasma cell. A third model, which is gaining support, is that memory cells and plasma cells arise from different lineages, each of which clonally expands following primary antigen exposure. Support for this last model comes from analysis of the primary and secondary antibodies induced by certain antigens. Phosphorylcholine, for example, induces antibodies characterized by a single idiotype in the primary response, whereas the antibodies produced in the secondary response, which involves stimulation and differentiation of memory B cells, completely lack this idiotype. This finding suggests that the memory cells generated in the primary response arose from a different lineage than did the plasma cells.

REGULATION OF B-CELL DEVELOPMENT

A number of transcription factors that regulate expression of various gene products at different stages of B-cell development have been identified. Among these are NF-κB, Ets-1, c-Jun, Ikaros, Oct-2, Pu.1, EBF, BCF, and E2A. Like all transcription factors, these DNA-binding proteins interact with promoter or enhancer sequences, thereby either stimulating or inhibiting transcription of the associated gene. Analyses of the effects of knocking out the gene encoding a particular transcription factor have provided clues about the role of some factors in the

B-cell development process. For example, in knockout mice carrying a disrupted *Ikaros* gene, pro-B cells fail to develop in the bone marrow. This finding suggests that Ikaros is a transcription factor that plays a role very early in B-cell development.

One of the most critical B-cell transcription factors, **B cell–specific activator protein** (BSAP), appears to function as a master B-cell regulator. It is expressed only by B-lineage cells and influences all the cell stages during B-cell maturation. Moreover, recent evidence indicates that BSAP also influences the final differentiation events leading to the formation of memory B cells and plasma cells. The latter are the only B-lineage cells that do not express BSAP. BSAP binds to promoter or enhancer sequences of various B cell–specific genes, including the λ5 and Vpre-B genes of the surrogate light chain, the J-chain gene of polymeric IgM, and the $3'\alpha$ heavy-chain enhancer region, one of the two enhancers present in heavy-chain germ-line DNA. In addition, BSAP binds to various immunoglobulin heavy-chain switch sites and to several genes involved in B-cell activation.

The heavy-chain $3'\alpha$ enhancer ($E_{3'\alpha}$) contains binding sites for several transcription factors in addition to BSAP (Figure 8-21). Binding of BSAP to $E_{3'\alpha}$ appears to influence B-cell development by preventing the binding of other transcription factors. For example, when BSAP levels are high, this factor appears to block binding of NF-αP to the $3'\alpha$ enhancer, thereby blocking transcription of the heavy-chain gene and promoting formation of memory B-cells. When BSAP levels are low, NF-αP can bind to $E_{3'\alpha}$. As a result, transcription of the immunoglobulin heavy-chain gene is increased, leading to formation of plasma cells.

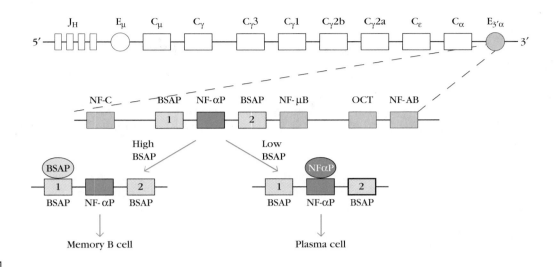

FIGURE 8-21

A portion of the immunoglobulin heavy-chain DNA showing the transcription-factor binding sites within the $3'\alpha$ enhancer region ($E_{3'\alpha}$). BSAP and NF-αP, as well as several other transcription factors, bind to specific sequences within $E_{3'\alpha}$ indicated by shaded blocks. BSAP binding, which prevents NF-αP binding, results in formation of memory B cells. When BSAP levels are low, the BSAP sites are unoccupied and NF-αP can bind to its site, leading to the formation of plasma cells. [Adapted from M. F. Neurath, E. R. Stuber, and W. Strober, 1995, *Immunol. Today* **16**:564.]

SUMMARY

1. Development of B cells involves antigen-independent maturation in the bone marrow and antigen-dependent activation and differentiation of mature B cells in the periphery, resulting in antibody-secreting plasma cells and memory B cells (see Figure 8-1).

2. During B-cell maturation, sequential Ig-gene rearrangement transforms the pro-B cell, the earliest distinctly B-lineage cell, into an immature B cell, which expresses mIgM with a single antigenic specificity (see Figure 8-3). Proliferation and development of pro-B cells into pre-B cells depends on the microenvironment provided by bone-marrow stromal cells (Figure 8-2). Pre-B cells express the heavy chain and a surrogate light chain associated with the Ig-α/Ig-β heterodimer (see Figure 8-4). Although the function of this pre-B cell receptor is not entirely clear, it is required for maturation to continue to the immature B-cell stage. Further development, including changes in RNA processing, yields mature B cells, expressing both IgM and IgD.

3. The antigen-induced activation and differentiation of mature B cells occur in the periphery, generating the humoral response. The B-cell response to soluble protein antigens requires involvement of T_H cells; in contrast, the response to certain bacterial cell-wall products (e.g., LPS) and highly polymeric molecules does not require T_H cells. The nature of the response to thymus-dependent and thymus-independent antigens differs considerably (see Table 8-2).

4. Activation of mature B cells involves signals generated by membrane events and in some cases cytokines. These signals are transduced via intracellular pathways, ultimately leading to changes in the expression of specific genes. Cross-linkage of mIg molecules by thymus-independent antigens is sufficient to trigger several signal-transduction pathways (see Figure 8-8). The recently discovered B-cell coreceptor can intensify the activating signal resulting from cross-linkage of mIg (see Figure 8-9). This may be particularly important during the primary response to low concentrations of antigen because many naive B cells express mIg with relatively low affinity for antigen. Activation induced by thymus-dependent antigens requires contact-dependent help, mediated by interaction between CD40 on B cells and CD40L on activated T_H cells, as well as cytokines released from T_H cells in a directed fashion (see Figure 8-10).

5. Generation of a humoral response to tissue antigens in vivo occurs primarily in peripheral lymph nodes (see Figures 8-16 and 8-17). Within 1–3 weeks after exposure to a thymus-dependent antigen, secondary follicles composed of a medulla surrounding a germinal center form. Intense proliferation of activated B cells (centroblasts) occurs in the dark zone of germinal centers. About 90% of the resulting centrocytes undergo death by apoptosis in the basal light zone. The remaining centrocytes, which express high-affinity mIg, inter-

act with antigen bound to follicular dendritic cells and undergo differentiation in the apical light zone, generating memory B cells and plasmablasts. The latter migrate to the medulla and develop into antibody-secreting plasma cells.

6. Affinity maturation, class switching, and formation of plasma and memory B cells all take place during B-cell proliferation and differentiation within germinal centers. Somatic hypermutation during proliferation of centroblasts and antigen selection of high-affinity centrocytes lead to affinity maturation, so that the average affinity of the induced serum antibodies increases during the course of a humoral response. Class switching depends on various cytokines (see Figure 8-19). Different membrane signals and the CD40/CD40L interaction appear to determine whether a selected centrocyte expressing high-affinity mIg develops into a memory B cell or plasma cell (see Figure 8-20).

7. Numerous transcription factors regulating various stages in B-cell development have been identified. BSAP, which appears to function as a master regulator, is expressed by and influences all B-cell stages except fully differentiated plasma cells. Binding of BSAP to the $3'\alpha$ enhancer in immunoglobulin heavy-chain genes appears to block binding of other transcription factors to this enhancer, thereby down-regulating expression of heavy chains (see Figure 8-21).

8. Induction of immune responses by self-antigens can have serious, even fatal, consequences. When a self-antigen is expressed in the bone marrow, negative selection of self-reactive immature B cells occurs. The selected cells are deleted by apoptosis or undergo further light-chain gene rearrangement resulting in production of an edited mIg that is nonreactive with the self-antigen (see Figure 8-5). In contrast, when a self-antigen is only expressed in the periphery, negative selection of the self-reactive B cells occurs at the mature B-cell stage in the periphery; the selected cells are either deleted or rendered anergic. These processes assure that an individual does not mount autoimmune responses.

REFERENCES

ARMITAGE, R. J., AND M. R. ALDERSON. 1995. B-cell stimulation. *Curr. Opin. Immunol.* **7**:243.

BOLEN, J. B. 1995. Protein tyrosine kinases in the initiation of antigen receptor signaling. *Curr. Opin. Immunol.* **7**:306.

CAMBIER, J. C., C. M. PLEIMAN, AND M. R. CLARK. 1994. Signal transduction by the B cell antigen receptor and coreceptors. *Annu. Rev. Immunol.* **12**:457.

DEFRANCO, A. L. 1993. Signaling pathways activated by protein tyrosine phosphorylation in lymphocytes. *Curr. Opin. Immunol.* **6**:364.

DESIDERIO, S. 1994. The B cell antigen receptor in B-cell development. *Curr. Opin. Immunol.* **6**:248.

FEARON, D. T., AND R. H. CARTER. 1995. The CD19/CR2/TAPA-1 complex of B lymphocytes: linking natural to acquired immunity. *Annu. Rev. Immunol.* **13**:127.

GOLD, M. R., AND A. L. DEFRANCO. 1994. Biochemistry of B lymphocyte activation. *Adv. Immunol.* **55**:221.

HAGMAN, J., AND R. GROSSCHEDL. 1994. Regulation of gene expression at early stages of B-cell differentiation. *Curr. Opin. Immunol.* **6**:222.

HODGKIN, P. D., AND A. BASTEN. 1995. B cell activation, tolerance, and antigen-presenting funtion. *Curr. Opin. Immunol.* **7**:121.

KLEINMAN, N. R. 1994. Selection in the expression of functionally distinct B-cell subsets. *Curr. Opin. Immunol.* **6**:420.

LASSOUED, K., ET AL. 1993. Expression of surrogate light chain receptors is restricted to a late stage in pre-B cell differentiation. *Cell.* **73**:73.

MACLENNAN, I. C. M. 1994. Germinal centers. *Annu. Rev. Immunol.* **12**:117.

MACLENNAN, I. C. M. 1995. Deletion of autoreactive B cells. *Curr. Biol.* **5**:103.

MELCHERS, F., ET AL. 1993. The surrogate light chain in B-cell development. *Immunol. Today.* **14**:60.

NEUBERGER, M. S., AND C. MILSTEIN. 1995. Somatic hypermutation. *Curr. Opin. Immunol.* **7**:248.

NEURATH, M. F., E. R. STUBER, AND W. STROBER. 1995. BSAP: a key regulator of B-cell development and differentiation. *Immunol. Today.* **16**:564.

NOSSEL, G. J. V. 1994. Negative selection of lymphocytes. *Cell* **76**:229.

NUÑEZ, G., ET AL. 1994. Bcl-2 and Bcl-x: regulatory switches for lymphoid death and survival. *Immunol. Today* **15**:582.

RETH, M. 1994. B cell antigen receptors. *Curr. Opin. Immunol.* **6**:3.

ROLINK, A., AND F. MELCHERS. 1993. B lymphopoiesis in the mouse. *Adv. Immunol.* **53**:123.

SEFTON, B. M., AND J. A. TADDIE. 1994. Role of tyrosine kinases in lymphocyte activation. *Curr. Opin. Immunol.* **6**:372.

VON BOEHMER, H. 1994. Positive selection of lymphocytes. *Cell* **76**:219.

STUDY QUESTIONS

1. Indicate whether each of the following statements concerning B-cell maturation is true or false. If you think a statement is false, explain why.

a. Heavy chain V_H-D_H-J_H rearrangement begins in the pre-B cell stage.

b. Immature B cells express membrane IgM and IgD.

c. The enzyme terminal deoxyribonucleotidyl transferase (TdT) is active in the pre-B cell stage.

d. The surrogate light chain is expressed by pre-B cells.

e. Self-reactive B cells can be rescued from negative selection by the expression of a different light chain.

f. In order to develop into immature B cells, pre-B cells must interact directly with bone-marrow stromal cells.

g. Most of the B cells generated every day never leave the bone marrow as mature B cells.

2. You have fluorescein (Fl)-labeled antibody to the μ heavy chain and a rhodamine (Rh)-labeled antibody to the δ heavy chain. Describe the fluorescent-antibody staining pattern of the following B-cell maturational stages assuming that you can visualize both membrane and cytoplasmic staining: (a) progenitor B cell (pro-B cell); (b) precursor B cell (pre-B cell); (c) immature B cell; (d) mature B cell; and (e) plasma cell before any class switching has occurred.

3. Describe the general structure and probable function of the B-cell coreceptor complex.

4. In the Goodnow experiment demonstrating clonal anergy of B cells, two types of transgenic mice were compared: single transgenics carrying a transgene-encoded antibody against hen egg-white lysozyme (HEL) and double transgenics carrying the anti-HEL transgene and a HEL transgene linked to the zinc-activated metallothionine promoter.

a. In both the single and double transgenics, 60%–90% of the B cells expressed anti-HEL membrane-bound antibody. Explain why.

b. How could you show that the membrane antibody on these B cells is specific for HEL and how could you determine its isotype?

c. Why was the metallothionine promoter used in constructing the HEL transgene?

d. Design an experiment to prove that the B cells, not the T_H cells, from the double transgenics were anergic.

5. Discuss the origin of the competence and progression signals required for activation and proliferation of B cells induced by (a) soluble protein antigens and (b) bacterial lipopolysaccharide (LPS).

6. DNA was isolated from three sources: liver cells, pre-B lymphoma cells, and IgM-secreting myeloma cells. Each DNA sample was digested separately with BamHI and EcoRI, which cleave germ-line heavy-chain and κ light-chain DNA as indicated in part (a) of the accompanying figure. The digested samples were analyzed by Southern blotting using a radiolabeled $C_\mu 1$ probe with the BamHI digests (blot #1) and a radiolabeled C_κ probe with the EcoRI digests (blot #2). The blot patterns are illustrated in part (b) of the figure. Based on this information, which DNA sample (designated A, B, or C) was isolated from the (a) liver cells, (b) pre-B lymphoma cells, and (c) IgM-secreting plasma cells? Explain your assignments.

For use with Question 6.

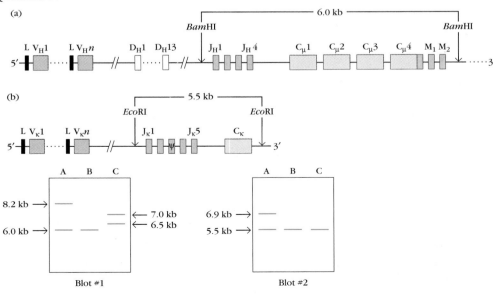

7. Fill in the blank(s) in each statement below (a–i) with the most appropriate term(s) from the following list. Terms may be used more than once or not at all.

dark zone	centroblasts
apical light zone	centrocytes
basal light zone	follicular dendritic cells
medulla	memory B cells
paracortex	plasmablasts
cortex	T_H cells

a.   Most centrocytes die by apoptosis in the _____.

b.   Initial activation of naive B cells induced by thymus-dependent antigens occurs within the _____ of lymph nodes.

c.   _____ are rapidly dividing B cells located in the _____ of germinal centers.

d.   _____ expressing high-affinity mIg interact with antigen captured by _____ in the basal light zone.

e.   Class switching occurs in the _____ and requires direct contact between B cells and _____.

f.   Centrocytes expressing mIg specific for a self-antigen present in the bone marrow are subjected to negative selection in the _____.

g.   Within lymph nodes, plasma cells are found primarily in the _____ of secondary follicles.

h.   Generation of _____ in the _____ of germinal centers is induced by interaction of centrocytes with IL-1 and CD3.

i.   Somatic hypermutation, which occurs in proliferating _____, is critical to affinity maturation.

8.   Activation and differentiation of B cells in response to thymus-dependent (TD) antigens requires T_H cells, whereas the B-cell response to thymus-independent (TI) antigens does not.

a.   Discuss the differences in the structure of TD, TI-1, and TI-2 antigens, and the characteristics of the humoral responses induced by them.

b.   Binding of which classes of antigen to mIg provides an effective competence signal for B-cell activation?

9.   B-cell activating signals must be transduced to the cell interior to influence developmental processes. Yet the cytoplasmic tails of all isotypes of mIg on B cells are too short to function in signal transduction.

a.   How do naive B cells transduce the signal induced by cross-linkage of mIg by antigen?

b.   Describe the general result of signal transduction in B cells during antigen-induced activation and differentiation.

10. In some of their experiments, Nemazee and Burki mated mice carrying a transgene encoding K^b, a class I MHC molecule, linked to a liver-specific promoter with mice carrying a transgene encoding antibody against K^b. In the resulting double transgenics, K^b-binding B cells were found in the bone marrow but not in lymph nodes. In contrast, the anti-K^b single transgenics had K^b-binding B cells in both the bone marrow and lymph nodes.

a.   Were the transgenes introduced into mice with the H-2^b haplotype or some other haplotype?

b.   Why was the K^b transgene linked to a liver-specific promoter in these experiments?

c.   What do these results suggest about the induction of B-cell tolerance to self-antigens?

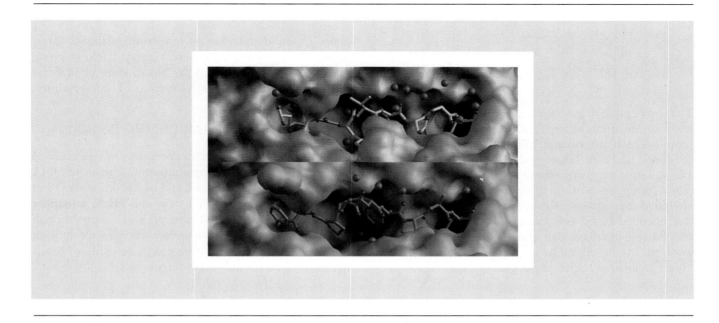

MAJOR HISTOCOMPATIBILITY COMPLEX

Every mammalian species studied to date possesses a tightly linked cluster of genes, the **major histocompatibility complex** (MHC), whose products are associated with intercellular recognition and with self/nonself discrimination. The MHC complex is a region of multiple loci that play major roles in determining whether transplanted tissue will be accepted as self (**histocompatible**) or rejected as foreign (**histoincompatible**).

The MHC plays a central role in the development of both humoral and cell-mediated immune responses. As discussed in previous chapters, T cells only recognize antigen when it is associated with an MHC molecule; thus MHC molecules play a critical role in antigen recognition by T cells. Because MHC molecules function as antigen-presenting structures, the particular set of MHC molecules expressed by an individual influences the repertoire of antigens to which that individual's T_H cells and T_C cells can respond. For this reason, the MHC partly determines the response of an individual to antigens of infectious organisms and the MHC has, therefore, been implicated in the susceptibility to disease and in the development of autoimmunity. This chapter examines the organization and inheritance of MHC genes, the structure of the MHC molecules, and the central function that these molecules play in producing an immune response.

GENERAL ORGANIZATION AND INHERITANCE OF THE MHC

The concept that the rejection of foreign tissue is the result of an immune response to cell-surface molecules (now called **histocompatibility antigens**) came from the work of R. A. Gorer and G. D. Snell in the mid-1930s. Gorer was using inbred strains of mice to identify blood-group antigens. In the course of these studies, he identified four groups of genes, designated I through IV, that encoded blood-cell antigens. Later work by Gorer and Snell established that the group II antigens were involved in the rejection of transplanted tumors and other tissue. Snell called these genes "histocompatibility genes"; their designation as histocompatibility-2 (H-2) genes was in reference to Gorer's group II blood-group antigens. Snell was awarded the Nobel Prize in 1980 for this work, attesting to the significance of his observations.

Location and Function of MHC Regions

The major histocompatibility complex is a collection of genes arrayed within a long continuous stretch of DNA on chromosome 6 in humans and on chromosome 17 in mice. The MHC is referred to as the **HLA complex** in humans and as the **H-2 complex** in mice. Although the arrangement of genes is somewhat different, in both cases the MHC genes are organized into regions encoding three classes of molecules (Figure 9-1):

Visualizing Concepts

Mouse H-2 complex

Complex	H–2						Tla	
MHC class	I	II	III			I	I	I
Region	K	IA	IE	S		D	Qa	Tla
Gene products	H-2K	IA αβ	IE αβ	C′ proteins	TNF-α TNF-β	H-2D H-2L	Qa	Tla, Qa

Human HLA complex

Complex	HLA							
MHC class	II			III		I		
Region	DP	DQ	DR	C4, C2, BF		B	C	A
Gene products	DP αβ	DQ αβ	DR αβ	C′ proteins	TNF-α TNF-β	HLA-B	HLA-C	HLA-A

FIGURE 9-1

Simplified organization of the major histocompatibility complex (MHC) in the mouse and human. The MHC is referred to as the H-2 complex in mice and as the HLA complex in humans. In both species the MHC is organized into a number of regions encoding class I (pink), class II (blue), and class III (green) gene products. The class I and class II gene products shown in this figure are considered to be the classical MHC molecules. The class III gene products include complement (C′) proteins and the tumor necrosis factors (TNF-α and TNF-β). The IEβ gene is actually located in the IA region but for pedagogical reasons is shown in the IE region.

T A B L E   9 - 1

H-2 HAPLOTYPES OF SOME MOUSE STRAINS

PROTOTYPE STRAIN	OTHER STRAINS WITH THE SAME HAPLOTYPE	HAPLOTYPE	H-2 ALLELES				
			K	IA	IE	S	D
CBA	AKR, C3H, B10.BR, C57BR	*k*	*k*	*k*	*k*	*k*	*k*
DBA/2	BALB/c, NZB, SEA, YBR	*d*	*d*	*d*	*d*	*d*	*d*
C57BL/10 (B10)	C57BL/6, C57L, C3H.SW, LP, 129	*b*	*b*	*b*	*b*	*b*	*b*
A	A/He, A/Sn, A/Wy, B10.A	*a*	*k*	*k*	*k*	*d*	*d*
A.SW	B10.S, SJL	*s*	*s*	*s*	*s*	*s*	*s*
A.TL		*t1*	*s*	*k*	*k*	*k*	*d*
DBA/1	STOLI, B10.Q, BDP	*q*	*q*	*q*	*q*	*q*	*q*

- **Class I MHC genes** encode glycoproteins expressed on the surface of nearly all nucleated cells, where they present peptide antigens of altered self-cells necessary for the activation of T_C cells.
- **Class II MHC genes** encode glycoproteins expressed primarily on antigen-presenting cells (macrophages, dendritic cells, and B cells), where they present processed antigenic peptides to T_H cells.
- **Class III MHC genes** generally encode secreted proteins associated with the immune process, including soluble serum proteins, components of the complement system, and tumor necrosis factors.

Class I MHC molecules are encoded by the K and D regions in mice and by the A, B, and C regions in humans. Additional regions, designated Qa and Tla, also encode class I molecules in mice and are closely linked to the H-2 complex. Class II molecules are encoded by the IA and IE regions in mice and by the DP, DQ, and DR regions in humans. The terminology is somewhat confusing, since the D region in mice encodes class I MHC molecules, whereas the D region (DR, DP, DQ) in humans encodes class II MHC molecules! It is a relief that the class III molecules are encoded by regions with descriptive designations such as S (for soluble protein) in the mouse and C4, C2, Bf (designating some of the individual complement proteins encoded here) in humans.

MHC Haplotypes

As discussed in more detail later, the loci constituting the MHC are highly **polymorphic**; that is, many alternate forms of the gene, or **alleles**, exist at each locus. The

MHC loci are also closely linked; for example, the recombination frequency within the H-2 complex is only 0.5%. For this reason, an individual inherits the alleles encoded by these closely linked loci as two sets, one from each parent. Each set of alleles is referred to as a **haplotype**. An individual inherits one haplotype from the mother and one haplotype from the father. In an outbred population the offspring are generally heterozygous at many loci and will express both maternal and paternal MHC alleles. The alleles are therefore **codominantly expressed**; that is, both maternal and paternal gene products are expressed in the same cells. In inbred mice, however, each H-2 locus is homozygous because the maternal and paternal haplotypes are identical, and all offspring express identical haplotypes.

Certain inbred mice strains have been designated as prototype strains, and the haplotype expressed by these strains is designated by an arbitrary italic superscript (e.g., H-2^a, H-2^b, H-2^d, H-2^k). Each designation simply is a way of referring to the entire set of inherited alleles within a strain without having to refer to each allele individually (Table 9-1). If another inbred strain has inherited the same set of alleles as the prototype strain, its MHC haplotype is the same as the prototype strain, as illustrated in Figure 9-2a. For example, the CBA, C3H, and AKR strains all have the same MHC haplotype (H-2^k). The three strains differ, however, in genes outside the H-2 complex.

If two inbred strains of mice having different MHC haplotypes are bred, the F_1 generation inherits haplotypes from both parental strains and therefore expresses both parental alleles at each MHC locus. For example, if strain C57BL/10 (H-2^b) is crossed with strain CBA (H-2^k),

(a) Hypothetical allelic composition of mouse MHC haplotypes

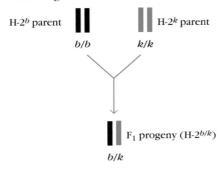

Strain	Haplotype	K	Aβ	Aα	Eβ	Eα	D
				Allele number			
CBA	k	3	22	54	11	97	13
C3H	k	3	22	54	11	97	13
C57BL/10	b	12	74	3	18	20	5

(b) Mating of inbred mouse strains with different MHC haplotypes

Homologous chromosomes with MHC loci

(c) Mating of outbred mouse strains with different MHC haplotypes

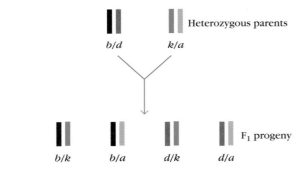

FIGURE 9-2

(a) Illustration of MHC haplotype designation. Strain CBA inherits a particular allele, indicated by an arbitrary number, at each MHC locus. The complete set of alleles is arbitrarily designated as the H-2^k haplotype. Any inbred strain (e.g., C3H) that has the same set of MHC alleles is designated as an H-2^k strain. Strains with a different set of MHC alleles (e.g., C57BL/10) are given a different haplotype designation. (b, c) Because the MHC loci are closely linked and inherited as a set, the MHC haplotype of F$_1$ progeny from mating of inbred and outbred strains can be predicted easily.

then the F$_1$ inherits both parental sets of alleles and is said to be H-2$^{b/k}$ (Figure 9-2b). Because such an F$_1$ expresses the MHC proteins of both parental strains on its cells, it is histocompatible with both strains and able to accept grafts from either parental strain. However, neither paren-

tal strain can accept a graft from the F$_1$ because half of the MHC molecules will be foreign to the parent.

As noted above, in an outbred population, each animal is generally heterozygous at each locus. Furthermore, both the maternal and paternal alleles at each MHC locus are expressed (this differs from expression of the immunoglobulin genes, which exhibit allelic exclusion, so that only one allele is expressed). The F$_1$ offspring of two heterozygous parents inherits one set of MHC alleles (i.e., one haplotype) from the father and one set from the mother (Figure 9-2c). Such an F$_1$ expresses only half of the paternal and half of the maternal class I MHC molecules on its nucleated cells. If this F$_1$ is grafted with tissue from either parent, it will recognize the foreign MHC molecules on the parental graft and reject the graft. Because the MHC loci are closely linked and are inherited as a haplotype, there is a one in four chance in outbred populations that siblings will inherit the same paternal and maternal haplotypes and therefore be histocompatible, assuming the father and mother have different haplotypes.

Congenic MHC Mouse Strains

Detailed analysis of the H-2 complex in mice was made possible by the development of congenic mouse strains. Two strains are **congenic** if they are genetically identical except at a single genetic locus or region. Any phenotypic differences that can be detected between congenic strains are related to the genetic region that distinguishes the strains. Congenic strains that are identical with each other except at the MHC can be produced by a series of crosses, backcrosses, and selections. Figure 9-3 outlines the steps by which the H-2 complex of homozygous strain B can be introduced into the background genes of homozygous strain A to generate a congenic strain, denoted A.B. The first letter in a congenic strain designation refers to the strain providing the genetic background and the second letter to the strain providing the genetically different MHC region. Thus strain A.B will be genetically identical to strain A except for the MHC locus or loci contributed by strain B.

During production of congenic mouse strains, a crossover event sometimes occurs within the H-2 complex, yielding a recombinant strain that differs from the parental strains or the congenic strain at one or a few loci within the H-2 complex. Figure 9-4 illustrates several **recombinant congenic** strains that were obtained during production of a B10.A congenic strain. Such recombinant strains have been extremely useful in analyzing the MHC because they permit comparisons of functional differences between strains that differ in only a few genes within the MHC.

FIGURE 9-3

Production of congenic mouse strain A.B, which has the genetic background of parental strain A but the H-2 complex of strain B. Crossing inbred strain A (H-2^a) with strain B (H-2b) generates F$_1$ progeny that are heterozygous (a/b) at all H-2 loci. The F$_1$ progeny are interbred to produce an F$_2$ generation, which includes a/a, a/b, and b/b individuals. The F$_2$ progeny homozygous for the B-strain H-2 complex are selected by their ability to reject a skin graft from strain A; any progeny that accept an A-strain graft are eliminated from future breeding. The selected b/b homozygous mice are then backcrossed to strain A; the resulting progeny are again interbred and their offspring are again selected for b/b homozygosity at the H-2 complex. This process of backcrossing to strain A, intercrossing, and selection for rejection of an A-strain graft is repeated for at least 12 generations. In this way A-strain homozygosity is restored at all loci except the H-2 locus, which is homozygous for the B strain.

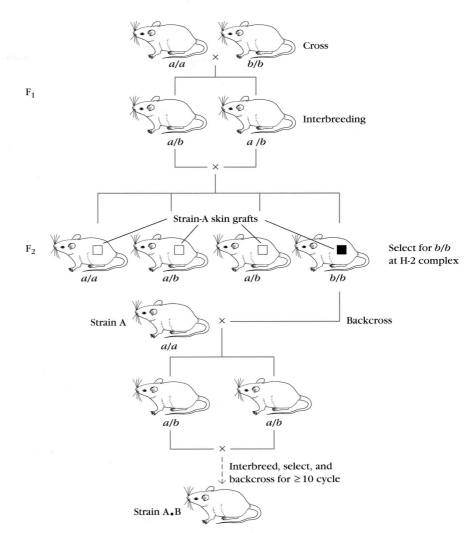

FIGURE 9-4

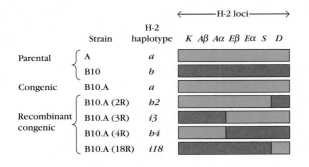

Examples of recombinant congenic mouse strains generated during production of the B10.A strain from parental strain B10 (H-2^b) and parental strain A (H-2^a). Crossover events within the H-2 complex produce recombinant strains, which have a-haplotype alleles (blue) at some H-2 loci and b-haplotype alleles (gray) at other loci.

MHC MOLECULES AND GENES

Class I and class II MHC molecules are membrane-bound glycoproteins that are closely related in both structure and function. Both types of membrane glycoproteins function as highly specialized antigen-presenting molecules that form unusually stable complexes with antigenic peptides, displaying them on the cell surface for recognition by T cells. Class III MHC molecules, in contrast, are soluble proteins and exhibit much less polymorphism than class I and II molecules.

Both class I and class II MHC molecules have been isolated and purified and the three-dimensional structures of their extracellular domains have been determined by x-ray crystallography. Figure 9-5 illustrates the considerable similarity in their structures.

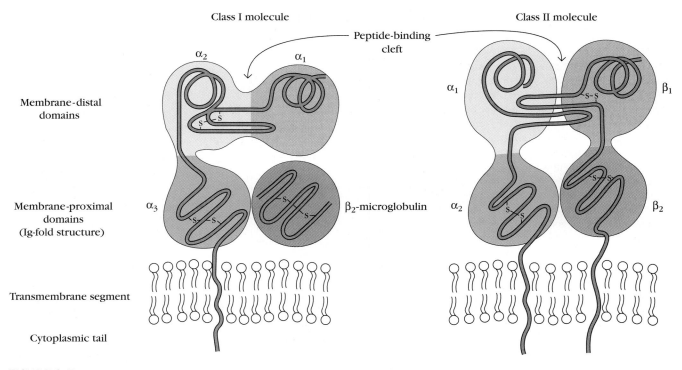

FIGURE 9-5

Schematic diagrams of a class I and class II MHC molecule showing the external domains, transmembrane segment, and cytoplasmic tail. The peptide-binding cleft is formed by the membrane-distal domains in both class I and class II molecules. The membrane-proximal domains possess the basic immunoglobulin-fold structure; thus class I and class II MHC molecules are classified as members of the immunoglobulin superfamily.

Structure of Class I Molecules

Class I MHC molecules contain a large α chain associated noncovalently with the much smaller β_2-**microglobulin** molecule (see Figure 9-5). The α chain is a polymorphic transmembrane glycoprotein of about 45 kilodaltons (kDa) encoded by genes within the A, B, and C regions of the human HLA complex and within the K and D/L regions of the mouse H–2 complex (see Figure 9-1). β_2-Microglobulin is an invariant protein of about 12 kDa encoded by a gene located on a different chromosome. Association of the α chain with β_2-microglobulin is required for expression of class I molecules on cell membranes. The α chain is anchored in the plasma membrane by its hydrophobic transmembrane segment and hydrophilic cytoplasmic tail.

Peptide mapping and amino acid sequencing have revealed that the α chain of class I MHC molecules is organized into three external domains (α_1, α_2, and α_3), each containing approximately 90 amino acids; a transmembrane domain of about 40 amino acids; and a cytoplasmic anchor segment of 30 amino acids. In size and organization β_2-microglobulin is similar to the α_3 external domain. Comparison of sequence data has shown that considerable homology exists between the α_3 domain, β_2-microglobulin, and the constant-region domains in immunoglobulins. The enzyme papain cleaves the α chain just 13 residues proximal to its transmembrane domain, releasing the extracellular portion of the molecule consisting of α_1, α_2, α_3, and β_2-microglobulin. Purification and crystallization of the extracellular portion revealed two pairs of interacting domains: a membrane-distal pair made up of the α_1 and α_2 domains and a membrane-proximal pair composed of the α_3 domain and β_2-microglobulin (Figure 9-6a).

The α_1 and α_2 domains interact to form a platform of eight antiparallel β strands spanned by two long α-helical regions. The structure forms a deep groove, or cleft, approximately 25 Å $\times$ 10 Å $\times$ 11 Å, with the long α helices as sides and the β strands of the β sheet as the bottom (Figure 9-6b). This **peptide-binding cleft** is located on the top surface of the class I MHC molecule, having a sufficient size to bind a peptide of 8–10 amino acids. The great surprise in the x-ray crystallographic analysis of class I molecules was the finding of a small peptide in the cleft that had cocrystallized with the protein. This peptide is, in fact, processed antigen bound to the α_1 and α_2 domains in this deep groove.

The α_3 domain and β_2-microglobulin are organized into two β pleated sheets each formed by antiparallel β strands of amino acids. As described in Chapter 5, this structure, known as the immunoglobulin fold, is characteristic of immunoglobulin domains. Because of this structural similarity, which is not surprising given the considerable sequence homology with the immunoglobulin constant regions, class I MHC molecules and β_2-microglobulin are classified as members of the immunoglobulin superfamily (see Figure 5-19). The α_3 domain appears to be highly conserved among class I MHC molecules and contains a sequence that is recognized by the CD8 membrane molecule present on T cells.

β_2-Microglobulin interacts extensively with the α_3 domain and also interacts with amino acids of the α_1 and α_2 domains. The interaction of β_2-microglobulin and a peptide with a class I α chain is essential for the class I molecule to reach its fully folded conformation. As discussed in detail in Chapter 10, assembly of class I molecules is believed to occur by the initial interaction of β_2-microglobulin with the folding class I α chain. This metastable "empty" dimer is then stabilized by the binding of an appropriate peptide, to form the native trimeric class I structure consisting of the class I α chain, β_2-microglobulin, and a peptide. This complete molecule is ultimately transported to the cell surface.

In the absence of β_2-microglobulin, the class I MHC α chain is not expressed on the cell membrane. This is illustrated by Daudi tumor cells, which are unable to synthesize β_2-microglobulin. These tumor cells possess class I MHC genes, which they can transcribe into mRNA. Although the mRNA is translated into protein, the cells do not express class I MHC α chains on the membrane. However, if Daudi cells are transfected with a functional gene encoding β_2-microglobulin, they will begin to express class I molecules on the membrane.

Structure of Class II Molecules

Class II MHC molecules contain two different polypeptide chains, a 33-kDa α chain and a 28-kDa β chain, which associate by noncovalent interactions (see Figure 9-5b). Like class I MHC molecules, class II MHC molecules are membrane-bound glycoproteins that contain

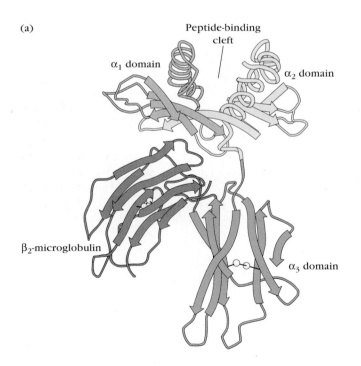

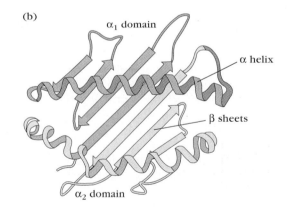

FIGURE 9-6

Representations of the three-dimensional structure of the external domains of a human class I HLA molecule based on x-ray crystallographic analysis. (a) Side view in which the β strands are depicted as thick arrows and the α helices as spiral ribbons. Disulfide bonds are shown as two interconnected spheres. The α_1 and α_2 domains interact to form the peptide-binding cleft. Note the immunoglobulin-fold structure of the α_3 domain and β_2-microglobulin. (b) The α_1 and α_2 domains as viewed from top showing the peptide-binding cleft consisting of a base of antiparallel β strands and sides of α helices. The size of this cleft in class I molecules can accommodate peptides containing 8–10 residues.

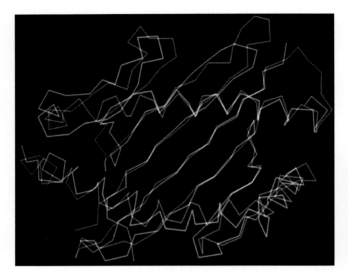

FIGURE 9-7

The membrane-distal, peptide-binding cleft of a human class II MHC molecule, HLA-DR1 (blue), superimposed over a human class I MHC molecule, HLA-A2 (red). [From J. H. Brown et al., 1993, *Nature* **364**:33.]

a dimer of the $\alpha\beta$ heterodimer, a "dimer of dimers" (Figure 9-8). The dimer is oriented so that the two peptide-binding clefts face in the opposite directions. Although it has not yet been determined whether this dimeric dimer form exists in vivo, Wiley and Strominger have speculated that it may facilitate the aggregation of two T-cell receptors (and the associated CD3 complex)

(a)

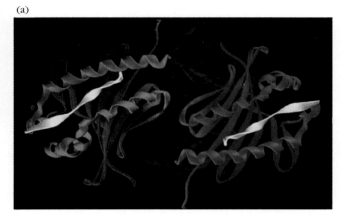

(b)

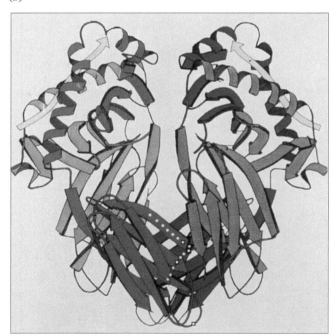

FIGURE 9-8

Antigen-binding cleft of dimeric class II DR1 molecule in (a) top view and (b) side view. This molecule crystallized as a dimer of the $\alpha\beta$ heterodimer. The crystallized dimer is shown with one DR1 molecule in red and the other DR1 molecule in blue. The bound peptides are shown in yellow. The two peptide-binding clefts in the dimeric molecule face in opposite directions. [From J. H. Brown et al., 1993, *Nature* **364**:33.]

external domains, a transmembrane segment, and a cytoplasmic anchor segment. Each chain in a class II molecule contains two external domains: α_1 and α_2 domains and β_1 and β_2 domains. The membrane-proximal α_2 and β_2 domains, like the membrane-proximal α_3/β_2-microglobulin domain of class I MHC molecules, bear sequence homology to the immunoglobulin-fold domain structure; for this reason, class II MHC molecules also are classified in the immunoglobulin superfamily. The membrane-distal domain of a class II molecule is composed of the α_1 and β_1 domains, and forms the antigen-binding cleft for processed antigen.

To date, the three-dimensional structure of only one class II MHC molecule, human HLA-DR1, has been determined by x-ray crystallographic analysis. This accomplishment, achieved in the laboratories of D. C. Wiley and J. L. Strominger in the early 1990s, was no small feat, as it took nearly ten years to obtain sufficient quantities of pure human class II DR1 for crystallographic analysis. The overall three-dimensional structure of this class II molecule is similar to that of class I molecules. The peptide-binding cleft of HLA-DR1, like that in class I molecules, is composed of a floor of eight antiparallel β strands and sides of antiparallel α helices. The similarity is so great that the class II and class I peptide-binding clefts can be superimposed (Figure 9-7).

The most striking difference between crystallized class I and class II molecules is that the latter occurs as

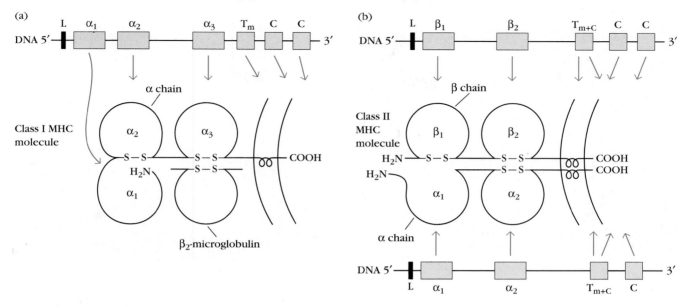

FIGURE 9-9

Schematic diagram of (a) class I and (b) class II MHC genes and molecules showing the correspondence between exons (blue) and the domains in the gene products. Each exon, with the exception of the leader (L) exon, encodes a separate domain of the MHC molecule. The gene encoding β_2-microglobulin is located on a different chromosome. Tm = transmembrane; C = cytoplasmic.

and two CD4 molecules. This aggregation may be necessary for signal transduction.

Organization of Class I and Class II Genes

A number of class I and class II MHC genes have been cloned and sequenced. Comparison of the amino acid sequence of the protein product with the DNA sequence has revealed that separate exons encode each domain (Figure 9-9).

Each of the mouse and human class I genes have a 5′ leader exon encoding a short signal peptide followed by five or six exons encoding the α chain of the class I molecule (see Figure 9-9a). The signal peptide serves to facilitate insertion of the α chain into the endoplasmic reticulum and is removed, after translation is completed, by proteolytic enzymes in the endoplasmic reticulum. The next three exons encode the extracellular α_1, α_2, and α_3 domains. The next downstream exon encodes the transmembrane (T_m) region; finally one or two 3′-terminal exons encode the cytoplasmic domains (C).

Like class I MHC genes, the class II genes are organized into a series of exons and introns mirroring the domain structure of the α and β chains (see Figure 9-9b). Both the α and the β genes encoding mouse and human class II MHC molecules have a leader exon, an

α_1 or β_1 exon, an α_2 or β_2 exon, a transmembrane exon, and one or more cytoplasmic exons.

Peptide Binding by MHC Molecules

Several hundred different allelic variants of class I and II MHC molecules have been identified in humans. Any one individual, however, expresses only a small number of these molecules—up to 6 different class I molecules and up to 12 different class II molecules. Yet this limited number of MHC molecules must be able to present an enormous array of different antigenic peptides to T cells, permitting the immune system to respond specifically to a wide variety of antigenic challenges. Thus peptide binding by class I and II molecules does not exhibit the fine specificity characteristic of antigen binding by antibodies and T-cell receptors. Instead, a given MHC molecule can bind numerous different peptides, and some peptides can bind to several different MHC molecules. Because of this broad specificity, the binding between a peptide and an MHC molecule is often referred to as "promiscuous."

Given the similarities in the structure of the peptide-binding cleft in class I and II MHC molecules it is not surprising that they exhibit some common peptide-binding features (Table 9-2). In both types of MHC

(a) **Class I MHC**

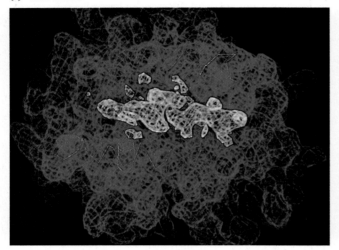

(b) **Class II MHC**

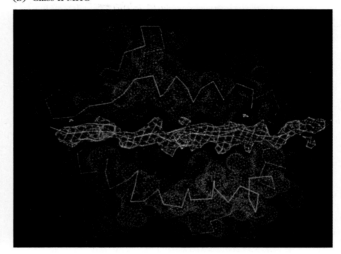

FIGURE 9-10

Models of interaction between peptides and (a) class I MHC and (b) class II MHC molecules as determined by x-ray crystallographic analysis of peptide–MHC molecule complexes. In the top models, the van der Waals surface of the MHC molecule is shown in blue and the peptide in orange/red. In the bottom models, conserved residues in the MHC molecule are shown in darker blue; polymorphic residues, in red; and other residues, in light blue. Many of the polymorphic residues are buried by the bound peptide (orange) and are not shown.

molecules, peptide ligands are held in a largely extended conformation that runs the length of the cleft. The peptide-binding cleft in class I molecules is blocked at both ends, whereas the cleft is open in class II molecules (Figure 9-10). As a result of this difference, class I molecules bind peptides that typically contain 8–10 amino acid residues, while the open groove of class II molecules accommodates slightly longer peptides of 13–18 amino acids.

The binding affinity of various peptides for MHC molecules has been determined by equilibrium dialysis (see Figure 6-2). In these experiments a labeled peptide was added to a solubilized class I or class II MHC molecule in a dialysis bag and the amount of labeled peptide bound to the MHC molecule at equilibrium was determined. Scatchard plots (see Figure 6-3) of the data revealed that the dissociation constant K_D of the peptide–MHC molecule complex is approximately 10^{-6}; the rate of association is slow, but the rate of dissociation is even slower. What this means is that the peptide–MHC molecule association is very stable under physiologic conditions; thus, most of the MHC molecules expressed

TABLE 9-2

PEPTIDE BINDING BY CLASS I AND CLASS II MHC MOLECULES

	CLASS I MOLECULES	CLASS II MOLECULES
Peptide-binding domain	$\alpha1/\alpha2$	$\alpha1/\beta1$
Nature of peptide-binding cleft	Closed at both ends	Open at both ends
General size of bound peptides	8–10 amino acids	13–18 amino acids
Peptide motifs involved in binding to MHC molecule	Anchor residues at both ends of peptide; generally hydrophobic carboxyl-terminal anchor	Anchor residues distributed along the length of the peptide
Nature of bound peptide	Extended structure in which both ends interact with MHC cleft but middle arches up away from MHC molecule	Extended structure that is held at a constant elevation above the floor of MHC cleft

on the membrane of a cell will be associated with a peptide of self or nonself origin.

CLASS I MHC–PEPTIDE INTERACTION

Class I MHC molecules bind peptides and present these peptides to CD8$^+$ T cells. In general these peptides are derived from endogenous intracellular proteins, which are digested into peptides within the cytosol. These peptides are then transported from the cytosol into the cisternae of the endoplasmic reticulum where they interact with class I MHC molecules. This process, known as the cytosolic or endogenous processing pathway, is discussed in detail in the next chapter.

Each type of class I MHC molecule (e.g., K, D, and L in mice or A, B, and C in humans) binds a unique set of peptides. In addition, each allelic variant of a class I MHC molecule (e.g., H-2K^k and H-2K^d) also binds a distinct set of peptides. Because a single nucleated cell expresses about 10^5 copies of each class I molecule, then collectively many different peptides will be expressed simultaneously on the surface of a nucleated cell by class I MHC molecules.

Various approaches have been used to obtain information about the nature of the interaction between peptide and class I MHC molecules. In one experimental approach, peptide-MHC complexes are isolated from cells, purified, and then denatured to release the bound peptide. In a healthy cell these released peptides have been shown to be various self-peptides derived from common intracellular proteins such as cytochrome c, histones, and ribosomal proteins. In an altered-self cell (e.g., a virus-infected cell), some of the self-peptides are replaced with peptides from viral proteins.

In a recent study, the peptides released from two allelic variants of a class I MHC molecule were analyzed by HPLC mass spectrometry. These two class I MHC molecules were found to bind over 2000 distinct peptides. Since there are approximately 10^5 copies of each class I allelic variant per cell, it is estimated that each of the 2000 distinct peptides is presented with a frequency of 100–4000 copies per cell. Evidence suggests that as few as 100 peptide-MHC complexes are sufficient to target a cell for recognition and lysis by a cytotoxic T lymphocyte with a receptor specific for this target structure.

The bound peptides isolated from different class I molecules have been found to have two unusual features: they generally are nonamers (nine residues), and they contain specific amino acid residues that appear to be essential for binding of the peptide to a particular MHC molecule. The finding that the peptides most frequently isolated from class I MHC molecules are nonamers suggests that this peptide length is most compatible with the size of the peptide-binding cleft in class I molecules. As noted earlier, the peptide-binding cleft in class I mole-

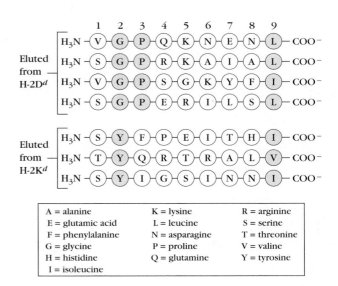

FIGURE 9-11

Examples of anchor residues in nonameric peptides eluted from two class I MHC molecules. Anchor residues (blue) tend to be hydrophobic amino acids and interact with the class I MHC molecule. [Data from V. H. Engelhard, 1994, *Curr. Opin. Immunol.* **6**:13.]

cules is closed at both ends (see Figure 9-10a); this structural feature places constraints on the size of the peptide bound, favoring nonamers. Indeed, binding studies have shown that nonameric peptides bind to class I molecules with a 100- to 1000-fold higher affinity than do peptides that are either longer or shorter.

The ability of an individual class I MHC molecule to bind to a diverse spectrum of peptides is due to the presence of the same or similar amino acid residues at several defined positions along the peptide (Figure 9-11). Because these amino acid residues anchor the peptide into the groove of the MHC molecule, they are called **anchor residues**. The side chains of the anchor residues in the peptide insert into pockets within the binding cleft of the class I MHC molecule. These pockets in the MHC molecule are lined by polymorphic amino acid residues that vary among different class I allelic variants; as a result the identity of these residues in a particular class I molecule determine the identity of the peptide anchor residues that can interact with the molecule.

All peptides examined to date that bind to class I molecules contain a carboxyl-terminal anchor. These anchors are generally hydrophobic residues (e.g., leucine, isoleucine), although a few cases of charged amino acids have been reported. Besides the anchor residue found at the carboxyl terminus, another anchor is often found at the second or second and third positions at the amino-terminal end of the peptide (see Figure 9-11). In general, any peptide of correct length that contains the same or

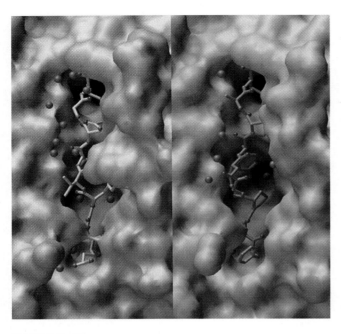

FIGURE 9-12

Model of the solvent accessible area of class I H-2K^b depicting the complex formed with a vesicular stomatitis virus (VSV-8) peptide (*left*, yellow backbone) and Sendai virus (SEV-9) nucleoprotein (*right*, blue backbone). Water molecules (blue spheres) interact with the bound peptides. The majority of the surface of both peptides is inaccessible for direct contact with T cells (VSV-8 is 83% buried; SEV-9 is 75% buried). The H-2K^b surface in the two complexes exhibits a small, but potentially significant, conformational variation, especially in the central region of the binding cleft on the right side of the peptides, which corresponds to the α helix in the α_2 domain (see Figure 9-6b). [From M. Matusumura et al., 1992, *Science* **257**:927.]

similar anchor residues will bind to the same class I MHC molecule. The discovery of conserved anchor residues in peptides that bind to various class I MHC molecules may permit prediction of which peptides in a complex antigen will bind to a particular MHC molecule based on the presence or absence of these motifs. As we discuss in Chapter 18, this may help in designing effective synthetic peptide vaccines.

X-ray crystallographic analyses of peptide–class I MHC complexes have revealed how the peptide-binding cleft in a given MHC molecule can interact stably and yet flexibly with a broad spectrum of different peptides. The anchor residues at both ends of the peptide are buried within the binding cleft, thereby holding the peptide firmly in place (Figure 9-12). As noted already, nonameric peptides are bound preferentially; the majority of contacts between class I MHC molecules and peptides involve residue 2 at the amino-terminal end and residue 9 at the carboxyl terminus of the nonameric peptide. The

bound peptide, which assumes an extended structure, interacts with the MHC cleft at both ends but arches away from the floor of the cleft in the middle (Figure 9-13). Since the middle of the peptide does not make significant contact with the cleft of the MHC molecule, peptides that are slightly longer or shorter can be accommodated by slight differences in the number of residues that bulge away from the cleft. In addition, peptides that have different middle residues but the correct anchor residues at each end can be bound to the same MHC molecule (see Figure 9-12 for examples). It is thought that the amino acids that arch away from the MHC molecule are more exposed and therefore can interact directly with the T-cell receptor.

CLASS II MHC–PEPTIDE INTERACTION

Class II MHC molecules bind peptides and present these peptides to CD4$^+$ T cells. Like class I molecules, class II molecules can bind a variety of peptides. In general these peptides are derived from exogenous proteins (either self or nonself), which are degraded within the endocytic processing pathway (see Chapter 10). Most of the peptides associated with class II MHC molecules are derived from membrane-bound proteins or proteins associated with the vesicles of the endocytic processing pathway. The membrane-bound proteins presumably are internalized by phagocytosis or by receptor-mediated endocytosis and enter the endocytic processing pathway at this point. For instance, peptides derived from digestion of membrane-bound class I MHC molecules often are bound to class II MHC molecules. Other peptides associated with class II MHC molecules are derived from digestion of the invariant chain, which is involved in the intracellular vesicular transport of class II MHC molecules from the endoplasmic reticulum to the endocytic processing pathway. When the invariant chain is digested within the endocytic pathway, the resulting peptides bind to the class II MHC cleft. Almost all class II MHC molecules investigated so far have been shown to bind the same invariant-chain peptide, a good example of promiscuous binding.

In studies similar to those done with class I molecules, peptides have been released and characterized from class II MHC–peptide complexes. The isolated peptides generally contain 13–18 amino acid residues, and thus are slightly longer than the nonameric peptides that most commonly bind to class I molecules. The peptide-binding cleft in class II molecules is open at both ends, allowing a bound peptide to extend beyond the ends, much like a long hot dog in a bun (see Figure 9-10b). This feature enables class II molecules to bind longer peptides than class I molecules. Peptides bound to class II MHC mole-

(a)

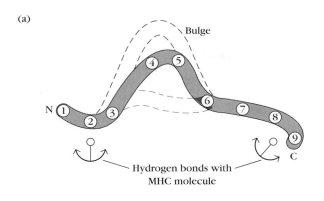

(b)

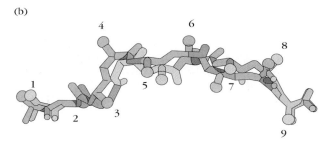

(c)

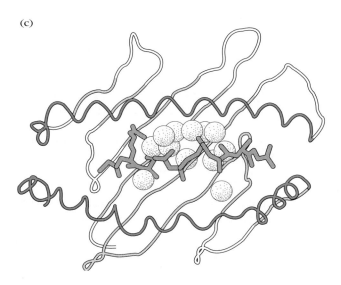

FIGURE 9-13

Conformation of peptides bound to class I MHC molecules. (a) Schematic diagram of conformational difference in bound peptides of different lengths. Longer peptides bulge in the middle, whereas shorter peptides are more extended. Contact with the MHC molecule is via hydrogen bonds involving residues 1/2 and 8/9. (b) Molecular models based on crystal structure of an influenza virus antigenic peptide (blue) and an endogenous peptide (gray) bound to a class I MHC molecule. Residues are identified by small numbers corresponding to those in part (a). (c) Representation of α_1 and α_2 domains of HLA–B27 and a bound antigenic peptide based on x-ray crystallographic analysis of the cocrystallized peptide-HLA molecule. The peptide (gray) arches up away from the β strands forming the floor of the binding cleft and interacts with twelve water molecules (white spheres). [Part (a) adapted from P. Parham, 1992, *Nature* **360**: 300; part (b) adapted from M. L. Silver et al., 1992, *Nature* **360**:367; part (c) adapted from D. R. Madden et al., 1992, *Cell* **70**:1035.]

cules maintain a roughly constant elevation on the floor of the binding cleft, another feature that distinguishes peptide binding to class I and class II molecules.

The peptides that bind to a particular class II molecule often have internal conserved "motifs," but unlike class I–binding peptides, they lack conserved anchor residues at the ends of the peptide. Instead, hydrogen bonds between the backbone of the peptide and the class II molecule are distributed throughout the binding site rather than being clustered predominantly at the ends of the site as observed for class I–bound peptides. Peptides that bind to class II MHC molecules contain a core binding sequence comprising 7–10 amino acids. Generally, this core sequence has an aromatic or hydrophobic residue at the amino terminus and three additional hydrophobic anchors in the middle portion and carboxyl-terminal end. In addition, over 30% of the peptides eluted from class II molecules contain a proline residue at position 2 and another cluster of prolines at the carboxyl-terminal end. It is thought that the prevalence and distribution of prolines may reflect the activity

of processing enzymes in the endocytic pathway, which may be specialized to cleave the protein near proline residues. Further clarification about the interaction between peptides and class II MHC molecules awaits the x-ray crystallographic analysis of more class II MHC-peptide complexes.

Polymorphism of Class I and Class II Molecules

An enormous diversity is exhibited by the MHC molecules within a species. However, the source of the diversity of MHC molecules differs from that associated with antibodies and T-cell receptors. The diversity of antibodies and T-cell receptors is generated by a continual process of random gene rearrangements and thus it changes over time within an individual. In contrast, the diversity of MHC molecules results from **polymorphism**, that is, the presence of multiple alleles at a given genetic locus within a species. Thus, the MHC molecules expressed by an individual do not change over time, but they may differ significantly from those expressed by another individual of the same species.

The MHC, one of the most polymorphic genetic complexes known in higher vertebrates, possesses an extraordinarily large number of different alleles at each locus. These alleles differ in their DNA sequences from one individual to another, and consequently the gene products expressed by different individuals have unique structural differences. The number of amino acid differences between MHC alleles can be quite significant, with up to 20 amino acid residues contributing to the uniqueness of each allele. Analysis of human HLA class I molecules has so far revealed 59 A alleles, 111 B alleles, and 37 C alleles. In mice the polymorphism is equally staggering, with more than 55 alleles now identified at the K locus and 60 alleles identified at the D locus. The current estimate of actual polymorphism in both the human and mouse MHC, suggested by serologic and functional analysis, is on the order of 100 alleles for each locus.

This enormous polymorphism results in a tremendous diversity of MHC molecules within a species. Given 100 different alleles for each class I and class II gene in the mouse H-2 complex, the theoretical diversity possible for the species is

$$100(K) \times 100(IA\alpha) \times 100(IA\beta) \times 100(IE\alpha) \times$$
$$100(IE\beta) \times 100(D) = 10^{12}!!$$

In humans the theoretical diversity is even larger, because humans have more class I and class II genes. However, because these genes are tightly linked and are inherited as a haplotype, the actual diversity within a species is less than the theoretical estimate. Still, this enormous polymorphism creates a major obstacle when it comes to matching MHC molecules for successful organ transplants.

A comparison of the amino acid sequences of several allelic MHC molecules encoded at a single locus reveals a sequence divergence of between 5% and 10%. This degree of variation is unusually high. Indeed, the sequence divergence among alleles of the MHC within a species is as great as the divergence observed for the genes encoding some enzymes (e.g., lactate dehydrogenase) across species lines. What is also unusual is that the sequence variation among MHC molecules is not randomly distributed along the entire polypeptide chain but instead is clustered in short stretches, largely within the membrane-distal α_1 and α_2 domains of class I molecules and α_1 and β_1 domains of class II molecules (Figure 9-14a).

The clustered distribution of the sequence variation in MHC molecules is thought to arise through **gene conversion**, a process whereby short donor DNA sequences base-pair with partially homologous DNA sequences in a recipient gene; excision repair or replication then inserts the donor sequence into the recipient DNA. By this process information is transferred unidirectionally from a donor DNA sequence to a partially homologous recipient DNA sequence. The molecular mechanism of gene conversion has not yet been defined, but conversion has been shown to occur in yeasts, trypanosomes, and human fetal globulin genes in addition to the class I and class II MHC genes. The large number of unexpressed pseudogenes in the MHC may serve as a pool of related gene sequences from which short, nearly homologous gene sequences can be transferred to functional class I or class II genes.

Some progress has been made in locating the polymorphic residues within the three-dimensional structure of the membrane-distal domains in class I and class II MHC molecules and in relating allelic differences to functional differences. For example, experiments described later show that different class II molecules preferentially bind various labeled peptides. In addition, studies with mutated and hybrid class II MHC molecules, as well as the recent x-ray crystallographic analysis of HLA-DR1, have located the peptide-binding cleft in the membrane-distal α_1/β_1 domain, the very region that displays localized polymorphism within class II MHC molecules. A number of researchers have suggested that such allelic differences in the class II molecules expressed by antigen-presenting cells may influence the cells' ability to recognize a particular peptide.

The polymorphic amino acids of class I MHC molecules also are clustered in the membrane-distal α_1/α_2 domain. Now that high-resolution x-ray crystallographic analyses of several class I molecules have been completed, the location of the polymorphic residues within the structure of the α_1/α_2 domain has been determined (Figure 9-14b). For example, of 17 amino acids previously shown to display significant polymorphism in the HLA-A2 molecule, 15 were shown by crystallographic analysis to be in the peptide-binding cleft of this molecule. The location of so many polymorphic amino acids within the binding site for processed antigen strongly suggests that allelic differences contribute to the observed differences in the ability of MHC molecules to interact with a given antigenic peptide.

Class III Molecules

As noted earlier, several structurally and functionally diverse proteins are encoded within the third region of the MHC (see Figure 9-1). These class III molecules include several complement components (C2, C4a, C4b, and factor B), two steroid 21-hydroxylase enzymes (21-OHA and 21-OHB), tumor necrosis factors α and β (TNF-α and TNF-β), and two heat-shock proteins.

(a)

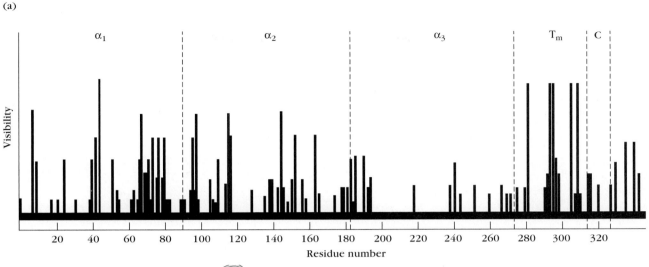

(b)

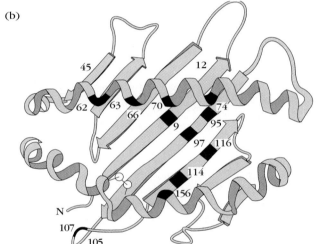

FIGURE 9-14

(a) Plots of variability in the amino acid sequence of allelic class I MHC molecules in humans versus residue position. In the external domains, most of the variable residues are in the membrane-distal α_1 and α_2 domains. (b) Location of polymorphic amino acid residues (black) in the α_1/α_2 domain of a human class I MHC molecule. [Part (a) adapted from R. Sodoyer et al., 1984, *EMBO J.* **3**:879; part (b) adapted from P. Parham, 1989, *Nature* **342**:617.]

Unlike class I and class II MHC molecules, the class III molecules are not membrane proteins and have no role in antigen presentation, although most play some role in immune responses. It is not known why the class III genes are situated within the MHC complex. Some authors have speculated that the observed genetic association of certain MHC alleles with various diseases may in some cases reflect regulatory disorders of the class III region. For example, ankylosing spondylitis is strongly associated with an allele of the B locus of the HLA complex (the *HLA-B27* allele). This disease is characterized by destruction of cartilage, and it has been suggested that because of the close linkage of the TNF-α and TNF-β genes with the *HLA-B* locus, these cytokines may be involved in cartilage destruction. Systemic lupus erythematosus is another disease associated with certain alleles of the MHC. This disease is characterized by autoanti-

body production, deposition of immune complexes, and complement-mediated damage; it is possible that regulatory defects in the expression of class III complement components may contribute to the severity of this disease.

The **heat-shock proteins** are an unusual group of highly conserved proteins that are produced by cells in response to various stresses including heat shock (for which they were named), nutrient deprivation, oxygen radicals, and viral infection. Some heat-shock proteins are thought to bind incompletely or aberrantly folded proteins and may be involved in the intracellular trafficking of proteins necessary for proper antigen presentation. These proteins have been shown to associate with ribonucleoproteins in the nucleus during heat shock. Evidence suggesting that heat-shock proteins may be linked to certain autoimmune diseases is discussed in Chapter 20.

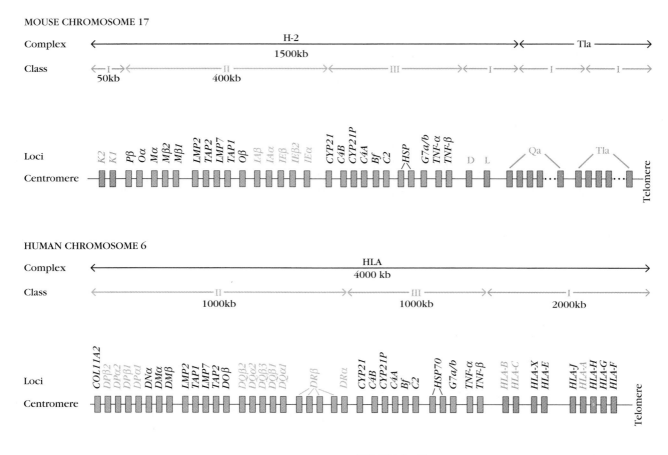

FIGURE 9-15

Detailed genomic map of the mouse and human MHC including genes encoding classical and nonclassical MHC molecules. The class I MHC genes are colored red, MHC II genes are colored blue, and genes in MHC III are colored green. Class I genes are labeled in red, class II in blue, class III in green and the nonclassical MHC genes are in black. The functions of the proteins encoded by the nonclassical class I genes are largely unknown. In the mouse, these genes are located downstream from Tla and are not shown. In contrast, several of the nonclassical class II genes encode proteins with known functions. No pseudogenes are shown in this map.

KEY

Gene	Encoded protein
C2, C4A, C4B, Bf	Complement components
COL11A2	Collagen
CYP21,CYP21P	Steroid 21-hydroxylases
G7a/b	Valyl-tRNA synthetase
HSP	Heat-shock protein
LMP2, LMP7	Proteasome-like subunits
TAP1, TAP2	Peptide-transporter subunits
TNF-α, TNF-β	Tumor necrosis factors α and β

DETAILED GENOMIC MAP OF MHC GENES

The MHC, located on chromosome 17 of mice and on chromosome 6 of humans, is now known to contain nearly 100 genes, spanning some 2000 kb of mouse DNA and some 4000 kb of human DNA. Once congenic and recombinant congenic mouse strains became available, mapping of the position and function of the individual genes within the H-2 complex began. Initially, serologic assays were used to assess the gene products encoded by the MHC genes. More recently, cloning of both mouse and human MHC genes has permitted restriction-enzyme mapping of the MHC. Detailed mapping of the MHC is progressing at a rapid pace, and additional genes are being identified within this complex each year.

Current understanding of the genomic organization of mouse and human MHC genes, based on reports through 1993, is diagrammed in Figure 9-15. Restriction-enzyme mapping has confirmed or corrected the earlier genomic maps derived from serologic analyses. In addition to the **classical** class I and class II MHC genes that had been recognized for some time (see Figure 9-1), molecular mapping has revealed a number of so-called **nonclassical** MHC genes that were not previously known.

Map of Class I MHC

In humans the class I MHC region is about 2000 kb long and contains approximately 20 genes. In mice the class I MHC consists of two regions separated by the intervening class II and class III regions. Included within the class I region are the genes encoding the well-characterized classical class I MHC molecules designated HLA-A, HLA-B, and HLA-C in humans and H-2K, H-2D, and H-2L in mice. Many nonclassical class I genes, identified by molecular mapping, also are present in both the mouse and human MHC. In mice the nonclassical class I genes are located in three regions (*H-2Q, T,* and *M*) downstream from the H-2 complex. In humans the nonclassical class I genes include the *HLA-E, HLA-F, HLA-G, HLA-H, HLA-J,* and *HLA-X* loci as well as a new family called MIC. A number of the nonclassical class I MHC genes are pseudogenes and do not encode a protein product, but others encode class I-like products.

Most of the nonclassical class I MHC gene products are categorized as **class Ib molecules**. Like the classical class I molecules, class Ib molecules generally have an α chain that associates with β_2-microglobulin. However, the class Ib molecules generally are less polymorphic and expressed at lower levels than classical class I MHC molecules. In addition, the tissue distribution of the class Ib proteins usually is more limited than that of classical class I molecules.

The functions of the nonclassical class I MHC molecules remain largely unknown, although a few studies suggest that these molecules, like the classical class I MHC molecules, may present peptides to T cells. One intriguing finding is that the class Ib molecule encoded by the *H-2M* locus is able to bind a self-peptide derived from a subunit of NADH dehydrogenase, an enzyme encoded by the mitochondrial genome. This particular self-peptide contains an amino-terminal formylated methionine. What is interesting about this finding is that peptides derived from prokaryotic organisms often have formylated amino-terminal methionine residues. One hypothesis is that this *H-2M*–encoded class I molecule may be uniquely suited to present peptides from prokaryotic organisms that are able to grow intracellularly. Such organisms include *Mycobacterium tuberculosis, Listeria monocytogenes, Brucella abortus,* and *Salmonella typhimurium.* Perhaps the limited polymorphism and unusual tissue distribution of nonclassical class I MHC molecules enables these molecules to present peptides from microorganisms that invade at specific tissue sites or infect specific types of cells.

Map of Class II MHC

The class II MHC region contains the genes encoding the α and β chains of the classical class II MHC molecules designated HLA-DR, DP, and DQ in humans and H-2IA and IE in mice. Molecular mapping of the class II MHC has revealed additional β-chain genes in both mice and humans, as well as additional α-chain genes in humans (see Figure 9-15). In the human DR region, for example, there are three or four functional β-chain genes. All of the β-chain gene products can be expressed together with the α-chain gene product in a given cell, thereby increasing the number of antigen-presenting molecules on the cell. Although the human DR region contains just one α-chain gene, the DP and DQ regions each contain two functional α-chain genes.

Genes encoding nonclassical class II MHC molecules also have been identified in both humans and mice. In mice several class II genes (*Oα, Oβ, Mα,* and *Mβ*) encode nonclassical MHC molecules that exhibit limited polymorphism and a different pattern of expression than the classical IA and IE class II molecules. In the human class II region, nonclassical genes designated *DM, DN,* and *DO* have been identified. Some of these genes are pseudogenes, and others encode proteins whose function is only beginning to be unraveled. The recently identified *DM* genes encode a class II–like molecule (HLA-DM) that facilitates the loading of antigenic peptides into the class II MHC molecules.

Mapping analysis of the class II MHC region also has revealed the presence, in both mice and humans, of two genes (*LMP2* and *LMP7*) that encode proteasome subunits and of two genes (*TAP1* and *TAP2*) that encode peptide-transporter subunits. As discussed in Chapter 10, proteasomes (containing LMP2 and LMP7) are thought to mediate cytoplasmic degradation of endogenous proteins into peptides, which then are transferred by peptide transporters (TAP1 and TAP2) into the lumen of the endoplasmic reticulum; here the peptides can interact with newly synthesized class I MHC molecules.

Map of Class III MHC

The class III region of the MHC in humans and mice contains a heterogeneous collection of more than 36 genes (see Figure 9-15). These genes encode several complement components, two steroid 21-hydroxylases, two heat-shock proteins, and two cytokines (TNF-α and TNF-β). The possible role of some of these class III MHC gene products in certain diseases was discussed previously. In addition, the genes encoding microsomal cytochrome P-450 and valyl-tRNA synthetase have been mapped to this region, as have many other genes encoding products whose functions are still unknown.

CELLULAR DISTRIBUTION OF MHC MOLECULES

In general the classical class I MHC molecules are expressed on most somatic cells, but the level of class I MHC expression varies among different cell types. The highest levels of class I molecules are expressed by lymphocytes where they constitute approximately 1% of the total plasma-membrane proteins, or some 5×10^5 molecules per cell. In contrast, fibroblasts, muscle cells, liver hepatocytes, and neural cells express very low levels of class I MHC molecules. The low level of class I MHC molecules on liver cells may reduce the likelihood of graft recognition by T cytotoxic lymphocytes of the recipient, thus contributing to the considerable success of such transplants. A few cell types (e.g., neurons, sperm cells at certain stages of differentiation, and cells of the placenta) appear to lack class I MHC molecules altogether.

As noted earlier, any particular MHC molecule can bind many different peptides. Since a single nucleated cell expresses many class I MHC molecules, each cell will display a large number of peptides in the peptide-binding clefts of its MHC molecules. If a cell is a normal healthy cell, its class I molecules will display self-peptides derived from common intracellular peptides. For example, self-peptides derived from cytochrome c, histones, and ribosomal protein have been eluted from class I MHC molecules on normal cells.

On the other hand, if a cell has been infected by a virus, then viral peptides, as well as self-peptides, will be displayed by its class I MHC molecules. A single virus-infected cell should be envisioned as having various class I molecules on its membrane, each displaying different sets of viral peptides. Because of individual allelic differences in the peptide-binding clefts of the class I MHC molecules, different individuals within a species will have the ability to bind different sets of viral peptides. Since the MHC alleles are codominantly expressed, a heterozygous individual expresses gene products encoded by both alleles at each MHC locus. An F_1 mouse, for example, expresses the K, D, and L from each parent (six different class I MHC molecules) on each of its nucleated cells (Figure 9-16). A similar situation occurs in humans; that is, a heterozygous individual expresses the A, B, and C alleles from each parent (six different class I MHC molecules) on the membrane of each nucleated cell.

Unlike class I MHC molecules, class II molecules are expressed only by antigen-presenting cells. The primary antigen-presenting cells are macrophages, dendritic cells, and B cells; thymic epithelial cells and some other cell types can function as antigen-presenting cells under cer-

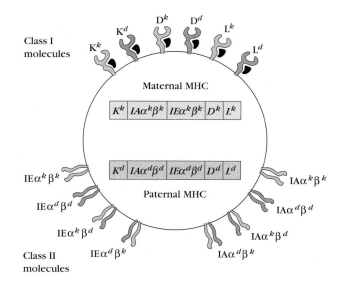

FIGURE 9-16

Diagram illustrating various MHC molecules expressed on antigen-presenting cells of a heterozygous H-2$^{k/d}$ mouse. Both the maternal and paternal MHC genes are expressed. Because the class II molecules are heterodimers, heterologous molecules containing one maternal-derived and one paternal-derived chain are produced. The α_2-microglobulin component of class I molecules (black) is encoded by a gene on a separate chromosome and may be derived from either parent.

tain conditions (see Chapter 10). Among the various cell types that express class II MHC molecules, marked differences in expression have been observed. In some cases class II expression is related to the cell's differentiation stage. For example, class II molecules cannot be detected on pre-B cells but are expressed on the membrane of mature B cells. Dendritic cells (including Langerhans cells) and mature B cells constitutively express class II MHC molecules. In contrast, monocytes and macrophages that have not interacted with antigen express only low levels of class II molecules, but these cells increase their expression significantly after they have been activated.

Because each of the classical class II MHC molecules is composed of two different polypeptide chains, which are encoded by different loci, a heterozygous individual expresses not only the parental class II molecules but also molecules containing α and β chains from different chromosomes. For example, an H-2^k mouse expresses IA^k and IE^k class II molecules; similarly, an H-2^d mouse expresses IA^d and IE^d molecules. The F_1 progeny resulting from crosses of mice with these two haplotypes express four parental class II molecules and four molecules containing one parent's α chain and the other parent's β chain (as shown in Figure 9-16). Since the human MHC contains three classical class II genes (*DP, DQ,* and *DR*), a heterozygous individual expresses six parental class II molecules and six molecules containing α and β chain combinations from either parent. The number of different class II molecules expressed by an individual is increased further by the presence of multiple β-chain genes in mice and humans, and in humans by multiple α-chain genes. The heterozygosity generated by these mechanisms presumably increases the number of different antigenic peptides that can be presented and thus is advantageous to the organism.

REGULATION OF MHC EXPRESSION

As the discussion in the previous section indicates, differential expression of the MHC genes occurs. Class II MHC genes are expressed only in a limited number of cell types, and the level of expression of both class I and class II genes varies among cell types. Research on the regulatory mechanisms that control this differential expression is still in its infancy.

Both class I and class II MHC genes are flanked by 5′ promoter sequences, which bind sequence-specific transcription factors. The promoter motifs and transcription factors that bind to these motifs are beginning to be identified. Transcriptional regulation of the MHC is mediated by both positive and negative elements. For example, an MHC II transactivator, called **CIITA**, and another transcription factor, called **RFX**, both have been shown to bind to the promoter region of class II MHC genes. Defects in these transcription factors cause one form of **bare lymphocyte syndrome**. Patients with this disorder lack class II MHC molecules on their cells and as a result suffer a severe immunodeficiency due to the central role of class II MHC molecules in T-cell maturation and activation.

The expression of MHC molecules is also regulated by various cytokines. The interferons (alpha, beta, and gamma) and tumor necrosis factor have each been shown to increase expression of class I MHC molecules on cells. Interferon gamma (IFN-γ), for example, appears to induce the formation of a specific transcription factor that binds to the promoter sequence flanking the class I MHC genes. Binding of this transcription factor to the promoter sequence appears to coordinately up-regulate transcription of the genes encoding the class I α chain, β_2-microglobulin, the proteasome subunits (LMP), and the transporter subunits (TAP). IFN-γ also has been shown to induce expression of the class II transactivator

(CIITA), thereby indirectly increasing expression of class II MHC molecules on a variety of cells including non-antigen-presenting cells (e.g., skin keratinocytes, intestinal epithelial cells, vascular endothelium, placental cells, and pancreatic beta cells). Other cytokines influence MHC expression only in certain cell types; for example, IL-4 increases expression of class II molecules by resting B cells. Expression of class II molecules by B cells is down-regulated by IFN-γ; corticosteroids and prostaglandins also decrease expression of class II molecules.

As shown in Table 9-3, MHC expression is also increased or, more commonly, decreased by a number of viruses, including human cytomegalovirus (CMV), hepatitis B virus (HBV), and adenovirus 12 (Ad12). The mechanism by which these viruses cause decreased expression of class I MHC molecules is beginning to be unraveled. In a number of cases, reduced expression of class I MHC molecules is not due to a reduction in transcription of the class I α-chain genes but rather is due to reduction in a component needed for peptide transport or MHC class I assembly. In the case of cytomegalovirus infection, a viral protein binds to β_2-microglobulin, preventing class I MHC assembly and transport to the plasma membrane. Adenovirus 12 infection causes a pronounced decrease in transcription of the transporter genes (*TAP1* and *TAP2*). As discussed in the next chapter, the TAP gene products play an important role in peptide transport from the cytoplasm into the rough endoplasmic reticulum. Blocking of TAP gene expression inhibits peptide transport; as a result, class I MHC molecules cannot assemble with β_2-microglobulin or be transported to the cell membrane. Decreased expression of class I MHC molecules, by whatever mechanism, is likely to help viruses evade the immune response by reducing the likelihood that virus-infected cells could display MHC–viral peptide complexes and become targets for CTL-mediated destruction.

MHC AND IMMUNE RESPONSIVENESS

Studies with simple synthetic antigens first showed that the ability of an animal to mount an immune response, as measured by the production of serum antibodies, is determined by its MHC haplotype. Later experiments with congenic and recombinant congenic mouse strains mapped the control of **immune responsiveness** to class II MHC genes (Table 9-4). We now know that the dependence of immune responsiveness on the class II MHC reflects the central role of class II MHC molecules in presenting antigen to T_H cells.

TABLE 9-3

EFFECT OF SOME VIRUSES ON MHC EXPRESSION

VIRUS	EFFECT ON EXPRESSION*	
	CLASS I MHC	CLASS II MHC
Adenovirus (Ad12)	↓	
Cytomegalovirus (CMV)	↓	↓
Ectromedlia virus	↓	
Hepatitis B virus (HBV)	↓	
Herpes simplex virus (HSV)	↓	
Human immunodeficiency virus (HIV)	↓	↑
Human papilloma virus 16 (HPV16)		↑
Measles virus	↑	↑
Moloney leukemia virus (MoMLV)	↑	
Rous sarcoma virus (RSV)	↓	↓
Simian immunodeficiency virus (SIV)		↑
Vaccinia virus	↓	
Vesicular stomatitis virus (VSV)	↓	
West Nile virus	↑	↑

* Increase (↑) and decrease (↓) in MHC expression are shown.

SOURCE: Adapted from D. J. Maudsley and J. D. Pound, 1991, *Immunol. Today* **12**:429.

Two explanations have been proposed to account for the variability in immune responsiveness observed among different haplotypes. According to the **determinant-selection model**, different class II MHC molecules differ in their ability to bind processed antigen.

According to the alternative **holes-in-the-repertoire model**, T cells bearing receptors that recognize foreign antigens closely resembling self-antigens may be eliminated during thymic processing. Since the T-cell response to an antigen involves a trimolecular complex of the T

TABLE 9-4

EFFECT OF H-2 HAPLOTYPE ON IMMUNE RESPONSIVENESS OF MICE TO THE SYNTHETIC COPOLYMER ANTIGENS (H, G)-A-L AND (T,G)-A-L

MOUSE STRAIN	H-2 ALLELES					RESPONSE TO (H, G)-A-L*	RESPONSE TO (T, G)-A-L*
	K	IA	IE	S	D		
A	*k*	*k*	*k*	*d*	*d*	High	Low
A.TL	*s*	*k*	*k*	*k*	*d*	High	Low
B10.A (4R)	*k*	*k*	*b*	*b*	*b*	High	Low
B10	*b*	*b*	*b*	*b*	*b*	Low	High
B10.STA62	*w27*	*b*	*w27*	*w27*	*w27*	Low	High
A.SW	*s*	*s*	*s*	*s*	*s*	Low	Low

* Indicated by production of specific serum antibodies.

cell's receptor, an antigenic peptide, and an MHC molecule (see Figure 4-9), both models may be correct. That is, the absence of an MHC molecule that can bind and present a given peptide or the absence of T-cell receptors that can recognize a given peptide–MHC molecule complex could result in the absence of immune responsiveness and so account for the observed relationship between MHC haplotype and immune responsiveness to exogenous antigens.

Determinant-Selection Model

The determinant-selection model assumes that the structure of a particular MHC molecule determines the strength of its association with any given antigen. Animals that respond, for example, to antigen A must express at least one class II MHC molecule whose structure facilitates interaction with antigen A, whereas animals that do not respond must express class II MHC molecules that do not interact effectively with antigen A. According to this model, the MHC polymorphism within a species

will generate different patterns of responsiveness and nonresponsiveness to different antigens.

If this model is correct, then class II MHC molecules from mouse strains that respond to a particular antigen and those that do not should show differential binding of that antigen. Table 9-5 presents data on the binding of various radiolabeled peptides to class II IA and IE molecules with the $H-2^d$ or $H-2^k$ haplotype. Each of the listed peptides binds significantly to only one of the class II molecules. Furthermore, as predicted, the haplotype of the class II molecule showing the highest-affinity binding for a particular peptide generally is the same as the haplotype of responder strains for that peptide.

In other experiments the nonresponder status of some strains has been linked to the deletion of a class II MHC gene. For example, $H-2^b$ and $H-2^s$ haplotype mice have undergone deletion of the *IEα* gene and therefore do not express class II IE molecules. These strains are nonresponders to a synthetic Glu-Lys-Phe peptide and to pigeon cytochrome *c*. When an *IEα* gene is introduced into a fertilized egg in these nonresponding strains, the resulting transgenic mice express the class II IE molecule

TABLE 9-5

DIFFERENTIAL BINDING OF PEPTIDES TO MOUSE CLASS II MHC MOLECULES AND CORRELATION WITH MHC RESTRICTION

LABELED PEPTIDE *	MHC RESTRICTION OF RESPONDERS[†]	PERCENTAGE OF LABELED PEPTIDE BOUND TO[‡]			
		IA^D	IE^D	IA^K	IE^K
Ovalbumin (323–339)	IA^d	**11.8**	0.1	0.2	0.1
Influenza hemagglutinin (130–142)	IA^d	**18.9**	0.6	7.1	0.3
Hen egg-white lysozyme (46–61)	IA^k	0.0	0.0	**35.2**	0.5
Hen egg-white lysozyme (74–86)	IA^k	2.0	2.3	**2.9**	1.7
Hen egg-white lysozyme (81–96)	IE^k	0.4	0.2	0.7	**1.1**
Myoglobin (132–153)	IE^d	0.8	**6.3**	0.5	0.7
Pigeon cytochrome c (88–104)	IE^k	0.6	1.2	1.7	**8.7**
λ repressor (12–26)§	IA^d + IE^k	1.6	**8.9**	0.3	2.3

* Amino acid residues included in each peptide are indicated by the numbers in parentheses.

[†] Refers to class II molecule (IA or IE) and haplotype associated with a good response to the indicated peptides as determined by studies such as that shown in Table 9-4.

[‡] Binding determined by equilibrium dialysis. Bold-faced values indicate binding was significantly greater ($p < 0.05$) than that of the other three class II molecules tested.

§ The λ repressor is an exception to the rule that high binding correlates with the MHC restriction of high-responder strains. In this case, the T_H cell specific for the λ peptide–IE^d complex has been deleted; this is an example of the hole-in-the-repertoire mechanism.

SOURCE: Adapted from S. Buus et al., 1987, *Science* **235**:1353.

and also can respond to both the synthetic Glu-Lys-Phe peptide and to pigeon cytochrome *c*.

Holes-in-the-Repertoire Model

The influence of the MHC on immune responsiveness could also be caused by an absence of functional T cells capable of recognizing a given antigen–MHC molecule complex. A good example is documented in the peptide-binding data presented in Table 9-5. The λ repressor peptide (residues 12–26) binds best in vitro to IE^d, yet the MHC restriction for this peptide is known to be associated not with IE^d but instead with IA^d and IE^k. The suggested explanation is that T cells recognizing this repressor peptide in association with IE^d may have been eliminated due to negative selection in the thymus leaving a hole in the T-cell repertoire.

An absence of functional T cells capable of recognizing a given antigen-MHC complex has been observed in several experimental systems. For example, the synthetic peptide poly Glu-Tyr induces an immune response in DBA/2 mice but not in BALB/c mice, although both strains have the $H-2^d$ haplotype and the antigen-presenting cells of both strains are capable of presenting this peptide. T cells from the responder strain were shown to respond to poly Glu-Tyr on antigen-presenting cells from both responder and nonresponder strains. In contrast, T cells from the nonresponder strain did not respond to this peptide whether it was presented by responder or nonresponder antigen-presenting cells. These results suggest that the T cells specific for poly Glu-Tyr have been functionally inactivated or clonally deleted in the nonresponder strain.

MHC AND SUSCEPTIBILITY TO INFECTIOUS DISEASES

Among the diseases associated with particular MHC alleles are a large number of autoimmune diseases, certain viral diseases, disorders of the complement system, certain neurologic disorders, and some types of allergies. In most MHC-associated diseases, however, a number of genes outside the MHC and external environmental factors also appear to play a role; therefore, unraveling the associations between specific diseases and MHC alleles has been difficult. The relation of the MHC to autoimmune diseases is discussed in Chapter 20; the discussion here is limited to the relationship of the MHC to diseases caused by pathogenic organisms.

A number of hypotheses have been offered to account for the role of the MHC in infectious diseases. Suscepti-

bility to a given pathogen may reflect the role of particular MHC alleles in responsiveness or nonresponsiveness to the pathogen. Variations in antigen presentation by different MHC alleles may determine the effectiveness of the immune response to a given pathogen. If major epitopes on a given pathogen mimic certain self-MHC molecules, it is possible that an animal may lack functional T cells specific for those epitopes. Various MHC alleles may also code for binding sites for specific viruses, bacteria, or their products.

Some evidence suggests that a reduction in MHC polymorphism within a species may predispose that species to disease. Cheetahs, for example, have been shown to be far more susceptible to viral disease than other big cats. Because the present cheetah population arose from a limited breeding stock, the species suffers from a loss of MHC diversity. The increased susceptibility of cheetahs to various viral diseases may result from a reduction in the number of different MHC molecules available to the species as a whole and a corresponding limitation on the range of processed antigens with which these MHC molecules can interact. Thus the high level of MHC polymorphism that has been observed in various species may be advantageous by providing a broad range of antigen-presenting MHC molecules. Because of this extreme polymorphism, some individuals within a species probably will not be able to develop an immune response to any given pathogen and therefore will be susceptible to infection by it. On the other hand, and perhaps of more importance, MHC polymorphism ensures that at least some members of a species will be able to respond to any one of a very large number of potential pathogens. In this way, MHC diversity appears to protect a species from a wide range of infectious diseases.

In a few cases the presence or absence of certain MHC alleles has been associated with specific diseases. For example, chickens expressing the MHC B19 allele are susceptible to the virus causing Marek's disease, whereas birds expressing the B21 allele are not susceptible. An interesting link between the MHC and disease susceptibility in humans came from a study of Dutch immigrants to South America. In 1845 a group of Dutch immigrants consisting of 367 individuals from 50 families emigrated from Europe to South America. Within two weeks of their arrival an epidemic of typhoid fever killed 50% of the immigrants, and six years later an epidemic of yellow fever killed another 20% of the population. Thereafter the annual mortality rate was relatively low, and the survivors remained and intermarried. Recently the MHC polymorphism of the "selected" descendants of the survivors was analyzed and compared with that of a similar number of Dutch families living in the Netherlands. The descendants in South America exhibited significant relative decreases in some HLA alleles, such as B7, and significant increases in other alleles, such as B13, Bw38, and Bw50. It is hypothesized that the MHC alleles carried by the descendants enabled them to respond more effectively to pathogens endemic to their South American environment.

SUMMARY

1. The major histocompatibility complex (MHC) comprises tightly linked genes that encode proteins associated with intercellular recognition and antigen presentation to T lymphocytes. The MHC, called the H-2 complex in mice and the HLA complex in humans, is organized into three regions based on the type of molecules encoded (see Figure 9-1). Class I molecules are encoded by the K and D regions in mice and the A, B, and C regions in humans. Class II molecules are encoded by the IA and IE regions in mice and the DP, DQ, and DR regions in humans. Class III molecules are encoded by the S region in mice and the C4, C2, and Bf region in humans. Many alleles exist for each class I and class II MHC gene; the entire set of MHC alleles on a chromosome is referred to as its haplotype. A given animal may be homozygous or heterozygous for MHC haplotype.

2. Class I MHC molecules consist of a large glycoprotein α chain, encoded by the class I MHC genes, and a much smaller molecule of β_2-microglobulin, encoded by a gene outside of the MHC (see Figure 9-5). The α chain contains three external domains (α_1, α_2, and α_3), a hydrophobic transmembrane segment, and a cytoplasmic tail. The latter two domains anchor the α chain to the plasma membrane, and the α_1 and α_2 domains interact to form a cleft that binds antigenic peptides. Class II MHC molecules are heterodimers composed of two noncovalently associated glycoproteins, the α and β chain, which are encoded by separate class II genes (see Figure 9-5b). Each chain contains two external domains, a transmembrane segment, and a cytoplasmic tail. The genes encoding the class I α chain and class II α and β chains are organized as a series of exons and introns, with each exon encoding a separate domain of the polypeptide chain (see Figure 9-9).

3. X-ray crystallographic analysis has been accomplished for several class I MHC molecules and one class II molecule. These analyses have revealed that the peptide-binding region in both class I and class II molecules is a deep cleft with eight antiparallel β strands forming the floor and two antiparallel α helices forming the sides (see Figure 9-6). The one class II molecule that has been crystallized did so as dimers of the $\alpha\beta$ heterodimer, suggesting that the molecule may be displayed on the membrane as a dimer (see Figure 9-8).

4. Because portions of both class I and class II MHC molecules exhibit the immunoglobulin-fold structure, these molecules are considered members of the immunoglobulin superfamily. In addition to a similarity in structure, both class I and class II MHC molecules function to present antigen to T cells. Class I molecules, which are present on nearly all nucleated cells, present processed endogenous antigen to CD8$^+$ T cells. Class II molecules, which are expressed on a limited number of antigen-presenting cells (macrophages, dendritic cells, B cells), present processed exogenous antigen to CD4$^+$ T cells.

5. The interactions between class I and II MHC molecules and peptides have been studied with several different experimental approaches. Elution experiments and binding experiments have demonstrated that peptide length and the presence or absence of certain conserved motifs in peptides influence their ability to interact with class I and class II MHC molecules (see Table 9-2). Studies with hybrid and mutated genes have demonstrated that both membrane-distal domains in class I and class II MHC molecules are necessary for antigen presentation. Direct evidence of the interaction between a peptide and the cleft formed by the two membrane distal domains in class I and class II molecules has been obtained from x-ray crystallographic analyses of peptide–MHC molecule complexes (see Figure 9-10).

6. Class III MHC molecules include a diverse group of nonmembrane proteins that play no role in antigen presentation. Disturbances in the expression of some class III molecules (e.g., certain complement components, tumor necrosis factors, and heat-shock proteins) may be associated with certain autoimmune diseases.

7. Restriction-enzyme mapping of the MHC has supplemented earlier results obtained by serologic analyses (see Figure 9-15). The detailed genomic map of the MHC developed to date includes a number of "nonclassical" class I and class II genes. Some of these are pseudogenes, but others encode protein products whose functions are under study. Genes within the class II region in both mice and humans encode proteasome subunits and peptide-transporter subunits; these proteins function in the cytosolic pathway for processing endogenous proteins.

8. Studies with congenic and recombinant congenic mouse strains have shown that MHC haplotype influences immune responsiveness and the ability to present antigen (see Tables 9-4 and 9-5). The variation in amino acid sequences (i.e., the polymorphism)

that gives rise to different haplotypes occurs primarily in the membrane-distal domains of class I and class II MHC molecules (see Figure 9-14). The polymorphic residues in class I MHC molecules have been shown to be localized primarily in the peptide-binding cleft.

REFERENCES

BJORKMAN, P. J., AND W. P. BURMEISTER. 1994. Structures of two classes of MHC molecules elucidated: crucial differences and similarities. *Curr. Opin. Struc. Biol.* **4**: 852.

BROWN, J. H., ET AL. 1993. Three-dimensional structure of the human class II histocompatibility antigen HLA-DR1. *Nature* **364**:33.

ENGELHARD, V. H. 1994. Structure of peptides associated with MHC class I molecules. *Curr. Opin. Immunol.* **6**:13.

GUO, H. C., ET AL. 1992. Different length peptides bind to HLA-Aw68 similarly at their ends but bulge out in the middle. *Nature* **360**:364.

HEDRICK, S. M. 1992. Dawn of the hunt for nonclassical MHC function. *Cell* **70**:177.

KIM, J., ET AL. 1994. Toxic shock syndrome toxin-1 complexed with a class II MHC major histocompatibility molecule HLA-DR-1. *Science* **266**:1870.

MADDEN, D. R. 1995. The three-dimensional structure of peptide-MHC complexes. *Annu. Rev. Immunol.* **13**:587.

MADDEN, D. R., ET AL. 1992. The three dimensional structure of HLA-B27 at 2.1 Å resolution suggests a general mechanism for tight peptide binding to MHC. *Cell* **70**:1035.

NEPON, G. T. 1995. Class II antigens and disease susceptibility. *Annu. Rev. Med.* **46**:17.

OGASAWARA, K., AND K. ONOE. 1993. MHC-binding motifs and the design of peptide-based vaccines. *Trends Micro.* **1**:276.

PARHAM, P. 1992. Deconstructing the MHC. *Nature* **360**:300.

PETERS, P. J., ET AL. 1991. Segregation of MHC class II molecules from MHC class I molecules in the Golgi complex for transport to lysosomal compartments. *Nature* **349**:669.

ROTZSCHKE, O. AND K. FALK. 1994. Origin, structure and motifs of naturally processed MHC class II ligands. *Curr. Opin. Immunol.* **6**:45.

SILVER, M. L., ET AL. 1992. Atomic structure of a human MHC molecule presenting an influenza virus peptide. *Nature* **360**:367.

STROYNOWSKI, I., AND J. FORMAN. 1995. Novel molecules related to MHC antigens. *Curr. Opin. Immunol.* **7**:97.

STUDY QUESTIONS

1. Indicate whether each of the following statements is true or false. If you think a statement is false, explain why.

a. A monoclonal antibody specific for β_2-microglobulin can be used to detect both class I MHC K and D molecules on the surface of cells.

b. Antigen-presenting cells express both class I and class II MHC molecules on their membrane.

c. Class III MHC genes encode membrane-bound proteins.

d. In outbred populations, an individual is more likely to be histocompatible with one of its parents than with its siblings.

e. Class II MHC molecules typically bind to slightly longer peptides than do class I molecules.

f. All cells express class I MHC molecules.

g. The majority of the peptides displayed by class I and class II MHC molecules on cells are derived from self-proteins.

2. You wish to produce a syngeneic and a congenic mouse strain. Indicate whether each of the following characteristics applies to production of syngeneic (S), congenic (C), or both (S and C) mice.

a. Requires the greatest number of generations

b. Requires backcrosses

c. Yields mice that are genetically identical

d. Requires selection for homozygosity

e. Requires sibling crosses

f. Can be started with outbred mice

g. Yields progeny that are genetically identical to the parent except for a single genetic region

3. You have generated a congenic A.B mouse strain that has been selected for the MHC. The haplotype of strain A was *a/a* and of strain B was *b/b*.

a. Which strain provides the genetic background of this mouse?

b. Which strain provides the haplotype of the MHC of this mouse?

c. To produce this congenic strain, the F_1 progeny are always backcrossed to which strain?

d. Why was backcrossing to one of the parents performed?

e. Why was interbreeding of the F_1 and F_2 progeny performed?

f. Why was selection necessary and what kind of selection was performed?

4. You cross a BALB/c (H-2^d) mouse with a CBA (H-2^k) mouse. What MHC molecules will the F_1 progeny express on (a) its liver cells and (b) its macrophages?

5. To carry out studies on the structure and function of the class I MHC molecule K^b and the class II MHC molecule IA^b, you decide to transfect the genes encoding these proteins into a mouse fibroblast cell line (L cell) derived from the C3H strain (H-2^k). L cells do not normally function as antigen-presenting cells. In the following table, indicate which of the listed MHC molecules will (+) or will not (–) be expressed on the membrane of the transfected L cells.

TRANSFECTED GENE	MHC MOLECULES EXPRESSED ON THE MEMBRANE OF THE TRANSFECTED L CELLS					
	D^K	D^B	K^K	K^B	IA^K	IA^B
None						
K^b						
IAα^b						
IAβ^b						
IAα^b and IAβ^b						

6. The SJL mouse strain, which has the H-2^s haplotype, has a deletion of the $IE\alpha$ locus.

a. List the classical MHC molecules that are expressed on the membrane of macrophages from SJL mice.

b. If the class II $IE\alpha$ and $IE\beta$ genes from an H-2^k strain are transfected into SJL macrophages, what additional classical MHC molecules would be expressed on the transfected macrophages?

7. Draw diagrams illustrating the general structure, including the domains, of class I MHC molecules, class II MHC molecules, and membrane-bound antibody on B cells. Label each chain and the domains within it, the antigen-binding regions, and regions that have the immunoglobulin-fold structure.

8. One of the characteristic features of the MHC is the large number of different alleles that occur at each locus.

a. Where are most of the polymorphic amino acid residues located in MHC molecules? What is the significance of this location?

b. How is MHC polymorphism thought to be generated?

9. As a student in an immunology laboratory class, you have been given spleen cells from a mouse immunized with the LCM virus. You determine the antigen-specific functional activity of these cells with two different assays. In assay 1, the spleen cells are incubated with macrophages that have been briefly exposed to the LCM virus; the production of interleukin 2 (IL-2) is a positive response. In assay 2, the spleen cells are incubated with LCM-infected target cells; lysis of the target cells represents a positive response in this assay. The results of the

For use with Question 9.

MOUSE STRAIN USED AS SOURCE OF MACROPHAGES AND TARGET CELLS	MHC HAPLOTYPE OF MACROPHAGES AND VIRUS-INFECTED TARGET CELLS				RESPONSE OF SPLEEN CELLS	
	K	IA	IE	D	IL-2 PRODUCTION IN RESPONSE TO LCM-PULSED MACROPHAGES (ASSAY 1)	LYSIS OF LCM-INFECTED CELLS (ASSAY 2)
C3H	k	k	k	k	+	–
BALB/c	d	d	d	d	–	+
(BALB/c × B10.A) F_1	d/k	d/k	d/k	d/d	+	+
A.TL	s	k	k	d	+	+
B10.A (3R)	b	b	b	d	–	+
B10.A (4R)	k	k	–	b	+	–

assays using macrophages and target cells of different haplotypes are presented in the accompanying table. Note that the experiment has been set up in a way to exclude alloreactive responses.

a. The activity of which cell population is detected in each of the two assays?

b. The functional activity of which MHC molecules is detected in each of the two assays?

c. From the results of this experiment, which MHC molecules are required, in addition to the LCM virus, for specific reactivity of the spleen cells in each of the two assays?

d. What additional experiments could you perform to unambiguously confirm the MHC molecules required for antigen-specific reactivity of the spleen cells?

e. Which of the mouse strains listed in the table could have been the source of the immunized spleen cells tested in the functional assays? Give your reasons.

10. A T_C-cell clone recognizes a particular measles virus peptide when it is presented by H-2D^b. Another MHC molecule has an identical peptide-binding cleft as H-2D^b but differs from H-2D^b at several other amino acids in the α_1/α_2 domain. Predict whether the second MHC molecule could present this measles virus peptide to the T_C-cell clone. Briefly explain your answer.

11. How can you determine if two different inbred mouse strains have identical MHC haplotypes?

12. Red blood cells are not nucleated and do not express any MHC molecules. Why is this property fortuitous for blood transfusions?

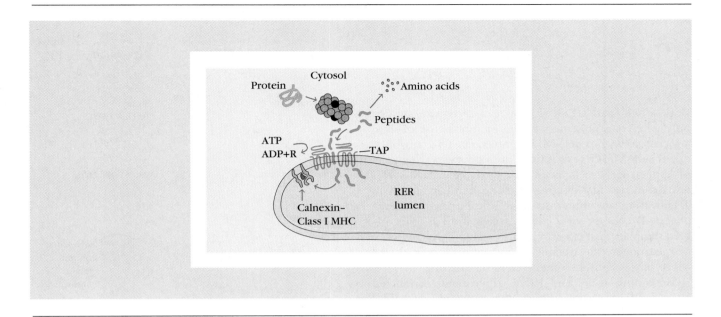

ANTIGEN PROCESSING
AND PRESENTATION

T-cell recognition of antigen requires that peptides derived from foreign antigen be displayed within the cleft of an MHC molecule on the membrane of a cell. The formation of these peptide–MHC complexes requires that a protein antigen be degraded into peptides by a sequence of events called **antigen processing**. The degraded peptides then associate with MHC molecules within the cell interior, and the peptide–MHC complexes are transported to the membrane where they are displayed (**antigen presentation**).

As discussed briefly in Chapter 1, class I and class II MHC molecules associate with peptides that have been processed in different intracellular compartments. Class I MHC molecules bind peptides derived from **endogenous antigens** that have been processed within the cytoplasm of the cell (e.g., normal cellular proteins or viral and bacterial proteins produced within infected cells). Class II MHC molecules bind peptides derived from **exogenous antigens** that are internalized by phagocytosis or endocytosis and processed within the endocytic pathway. In this chapter the mechanism of antigen processing and the means by which processed antigen and MHC molecules are combined within different intracellular compartments for presentation are examined in more detail.

SELF-MHC RESTRICTION
OF T CELLS

Both CD4$^+$ and CD8$^+$ T cells can recognize antigen only when it is presented on the membrane of a cell in association with a self-MHC molecule. This attribute, called **self-MHC restriction**, distinguishes recognition of antigen by T cells from that by B cells. Self-MHC restriction was first discovered in experiments in which T cells from one inbred strain were mixed with macrophages, B cells, or virus-infected cells from another inbred strain. In each experimental system a T-cell response to the antigen was obtained only if the T cells shared MHC alleles with the other cells in the mixture.

Beginning in the mid-1970s, experiments conducted by a number of researchers demonstrated self-MHC restriction in T-cell recognition. A. Rosenthal and E. Shevach, for example, showed that antigen-specific proliferation of T$_H$ cells occurred only in response to antigen presented by macrophages of the same MHC haplotype. In their experimental system, guinea pig macrophages from strain 2 initially were incubated with an antigen, which allowed the macrophages to process the antigen and subsequently present the antigen on their cell surface. These "antigen-pulsed" macrophages then were mixed with T cells from the same strain (strain 2), a different strain (strain 13), or (2 × 13) F$_1$ animals, and the magnitude of T-cell proliferation in response to the antigen-pulsed macrophages was measured.

The results of the Rosenthal and Shevach experiments, outlined in Figure 10-1, showed that strain 2 antigen-pulsed macrophages activated strain 2 and F$_1$ T cells but not strain 13 T cells. Similarly, strain 13 antigen-pulsed macrophages activated strain 13 and F$_1$ T cells but not strain 2 T cells. Subsequently, congenic and recombinant congenic strains of mice, which differed from each other only in selected regions of the H-2 complex, were used as the source of macrophages and T cells. These experiments confirmed that the CD4$^+$ T$_H$ cell is activated only by antigen-pulsed macrophages that share class II MHC alleles. Thus, antigen recognition by the CD4$^+$ T$_H$ cell is **class II MHC restricted**.

The self-MHC restriction of CD8$^+$ T cells was first demonstrated by R. Zinkernagel and P. Doherty in 1974. In their experimental system, mice were immunized with lymphocytic choriomeningitis (LCM) virus; several days later the animals' spleen cells, which included T$_C$ cells specific for the virus, were isolated and incubated with LCM-infected target cells of the same or different haplotype (Figure 10-2). They found that the T$_C$ cells only killed syngeneic virus-infected target cells. Later studies with congenic and recombinant congenic strains showed that the T$_C$ cell and the virus-infected tar-

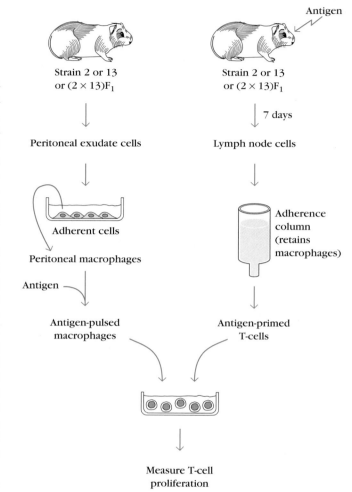

Antigen-primed T cell	Antigen-pulsed macrophages		
	Strain 2	Strain 13	(2 × 13)F$_1$
Strain 2	+	−	+
Strain 13	−	+	+
(2 × 13)F$_1$	+	+	+

FIGURE 10-1

Experimental demonstration of self-MHC restriction of T$_H$ cells. Peritoneal exudate cells from strain 2, strain 13, or (2 × 13) F$_1$ guinea pigs were incubated in plastic Petri dishes allowing enrichment of macrophages, which are adherent cells. The peritoneal macrophages were then incubated with antigen, generating "antigen-pulsed macrophages." These antigen-pulsed macrophages were incubated in vitro with antigen-primed T cells from strain 2, strain 13, or (2 × 13) F$_1$ guinea pigs and the degree of T-cell proliferation was assessed. The results indicated that T$_H$ cells could proliferate only in response to antigen presented by macrophages that shared MHC alleles. [Adapted from A. Rosenthal and E. Shevach, 1974, *J. Exp. Med.* **138**:1194 .]

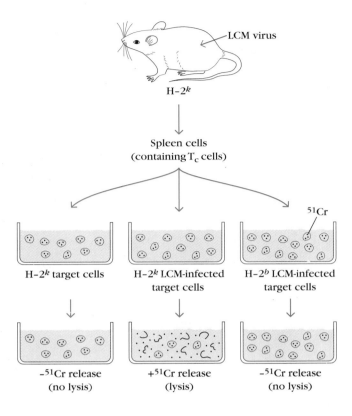

FIGURE 10-2

Classic experiment of Zinkernagel and Doherty demonstrating that antigen recognition by T_C cells exhibits MHC restriction. H-2^k mice were primed with the lymphocytic choriomeningitis (LCM) virus to induce cytotoxic T lymphocytes (CTLs) specific for the virus. Spleen cells from this LCM-primed mouse were then added to target cells of different H-2 haplotypes that were intracellularly labeled with ^{51}Cr (black dots) and either infected or not with the LCM virus. CTL-mediated killing of the target cells, as measured by the release of ^{51}Cr into the culture supernatant, occurred only if the target cells were infected and had the same MHC haplotype as the CTLs.

get cell must share class I molecules encoded by the K or D regions of the MHC. Thus, antigen recognition by CD8$^+$ T_C cells is **class I MHC restricted**. In 1996 Doherty and Zinkernagel were awarded the Nobel Prize for their major contribution to the understanding of cell-mediated immunity.

ROLE OF ANTIGEN-PRESENTING CELLS

As early as 1959, immunologists were confronted with data suggesting that T cells and B cells recognized antigen by different mechanisms. The dogma of the time, which persisted until the 1980s, was that cells of the immune system recognize the entire protein in its native conformation. However, the experiments by P. G. H. Gell and B. Benacerraf, mentioned in Chapter 4, demonstrated that when a primary antibody response and cell-mediated response were induced by a protein in its native conformation, a secondary antibody response (mediated by B cells) could be induced only by native antigen, whereas a secondary cell-mediated response could be induced by either the native or the denatured antigen (see Table 4-5). The findings of Gell and Benacerraf were viewed as an interesting enigma, but their implications were completely overlooked until the early 1980s.

Early Evidence for the Necessity of Antigen Processing

The results obtained by K. Ziegler and E. R. Unanuae were among those that contradicted the prevailing dogma that antigen recognition by B and T cells was basically similar. These researchers observed that T_H-cell activation by bacterial protein antigens was prevented by treating the antigen-presenting cells with paraformaldehyde prior to antigen exposure. However, if the antigen-presenting cells were allowed to ingest the antigen and were fixed with paraformaldehyde 1–3 h later, T_H-cell activation still occurred (Figure 10-3a,b). During that interval of 1–3 h, the antigen-presenting cells had processed the antigen and had displayed it on the membrane in a form able to activate T cells.

Subsequent experiments by R. P. Shimonkevitz showed that internalization and processing could be bypassed if antigen-presenting cells were exposed to peptide digests of an antigen instead of the native antigen (Figure 10-3c). In these experiments, antigen-presenting cells were treated with glutaraldehyde and then incubated with native ovalbumin or with ovalbumin that had been subjected to partial enzymatic digestion. The digested ovalbumin was able to interact with the glutaraldehyde-fixed antigen-presenting cells, thereby activating ovalbumin-specific T_H cells, whereas the native ovalbumin failed to do so. Taken together, the findings presented in Figure 10-3 suggest that antigen processing is a metabolic process that digests proteins into peptides, which can then be displayed on the membrane of the antigen-presenting cell together with a class II MHC molecule.

At about the same time, A. Townsend and his colleagues began to identify the proteins of influenza virus that were recognized by T_C cells. Contrary to their expectations, they found that internal proteins of the virus, such as matrix and nucleocapsid proteins, were often recognized by T_C cells better than the more exposed envelope proteins. Moreover, Townsend's work revealed that T_C cells recognized short linear peptide

Visualizing Concepts

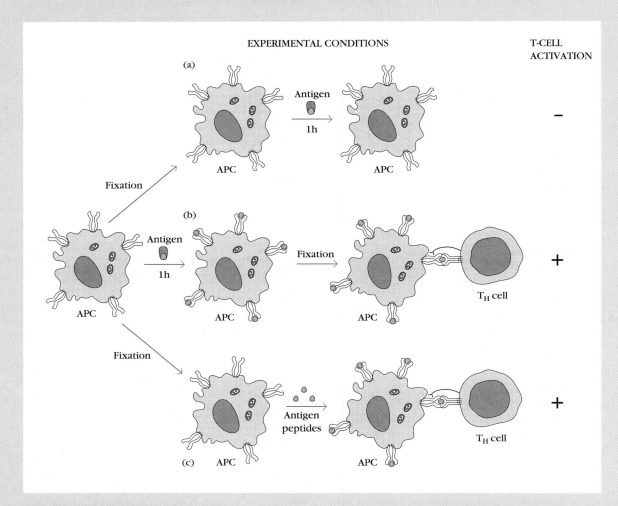

FIGURE 10-3

Experimental demonstration that antigen processing is necessary for T_H–cell activation. (a) When antigen-presenting cells (APCs) are fixed before exposure to antigen, they are unable to activate T_H cells. (b) In contrast, APCs fixed at least 1 h after antigen exposure can activate T_H cells. (c) When APCs are fixed before antigen exposure and incubated with peptide digests of the antigen (rather than native antigen), they also can activate T_H cells. T_H–cell activation is determined by measuring a specific T_H–cell response (e.g., cytokine secretion).

sequences of the influenza protein. In fact, when noninfected target cells were incubated in vitro with synthetic peptides corresponding to sequences of internal influenza proteins, these cells could be recognized by T_C cells and subsequently lysed just as well as target cells that had been infected with live influenza virus.

Cells That Function in Antigen Presentation

Since all cells expressing either class I or class II MHC molecules can present peptides to T cells, strictly speaking they all could be designated as antigen-presenting cells. However, by convention, cells that display peptides associated with class I MHC molecules to CD8$^+$ T$_C$ cells are referred to as **target cells**; cells that display peptides associated with class II MHC molecules to CD4$^+$ T$_H$ cells are called **antigen-presenting cells** (APCs). This convention is followed throughout this text.

A variety of cells can function as antigen-presenting cells. The distinguishing feature of these cells is their ability to express class II MHC molecules and to deliver a co-stimulatory signal. Three cell types are classified as **professional** antigen-presenting cells: dendritic cells, macrophages, and B lymphocytes. These cells differ in their mechanisms of antigen uptake, in whether they constitutively express class II MHC molecules, and in their co-stimulatory activity:

- Dendritic cells are the most effective of the antigen-presenting cells. Because these cells constitutively express a high level of class II MHC molecules and of co-stimulatory activity, they can activate naive T$_H$ cells.
- Macrophages must be activated by phagocytosing microorganisms before they express class II MHC molecules or the co-stimulatory B7 membrane molecule.
- B cells constitutively express class II MHC molecules but must be activated before they express the co-stimulatory B7 molecule.

Several other cell types, classified as **nonprofessional** antigen-presenting cells, can be induced to express class II MHC molecules or a co-stimulatory signal (Table 10-1).

TABLE 10-1
ANTIGEN-PRESENTING CELLS

Professional antigen-presenting cells

Dendritic cells (several types)

Macrophages

B cells

Nonprofessional antigen-presenting cells

Fibroblasts (skin)

Glial cells (brain)

Pancreatic beta cells

Thymic epithelial cells

Thyroid epithelial cells

Vascular endothelial cells

Many of these cells function in antigen presentation only for short periods of time during a sustained inflammatory response.

Because nearly all nucleated cells express class I MHC molecules, virtually any nucleated cell is able to function as a target cell presenting endogenous antigens to T$_C$ cells. Most often target cells are cells that have been infected by a virus or some other intracellular microorganism. However, target cells can also be altered self-cells such as cancer cells, aging body cells, or allogeneic cells from a graft.

EVIDENCE FOR TWO PROCESSING AND PRESENTATION PATHWAYS

Intracellular (endogenous) and extracellular (exogenous) antigens present different challenges to the immune system. Extracellular antigens are eliminated by secreted antibody, whereas intracellular antigens are most effectively eliminated by cytotoxic T lymphocytes (CTLs). To mediate these responses, the immune system uses two different antigen-presenting pathways: endogenous antigens are processed in the **cytosolic pathway** and presented on the membrane with class I MHC molecules; exogenous antigens are processed in the **endocytic pathway** and presented on the membrane with class II MHC molecules (Figure 10-4).

Early evidence suggesting that class I and class II MHC molecules present antigenic peptides derived from different processing pathways was obtained from experiments with two clones of T$_C$ cells specific for influenza virus. One clone was a typical CD8$^+$, class I–restricted T$_C$ cell, but the other was an atypical CD4$^+$, class II–restricted T$_C$ cell. As discussed in Chapter 3, the association between T-cell function and MHC restriction is not absolute. Indeed, an increasing number of reports have described cross-functional T-cell lines—that is, CD4$^+$, class II–restricted T$_C$ clones, and CD8$^+$, class I–restricted T$_H$ clones. L. A. Morrison and T. J. Braciale analyzed two T$_C$ cell lines: one a typical T$_C$ line that recognized influenza hemagglutinin (HA) associated with a class I MHC molecule and the other an atypical T$_C$ line that recognized influenza HA associated with a class II MHC molecule. These researchers sought to determine whether antigen is processed along different pathways for association with class I or class II MHC molecules. In one set of experiments, target cells that expressed both class I and class II MHC molecules were incubated with infectious influenza virus or with UV-inactivated influenza virus. (The inactivated virus retained its antigenic properties but was no longer capable of replicating

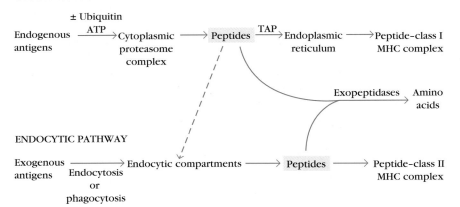

CYTOSOLIC PATHWAY

ENDOCYTIC PATHWAY

FIGURE 10-4

Overview of cytosolic and endocytic pathways for processing antigen. The resulting antigenic peptides associate with class I or class II MHC molecules, and the peptide-MHC complexes then are transported to the cell membrane. TAP = transporter of antigenic peptides.

within the target cells.) The target cells were then incubated with the class I–restricted or class II–restricted T_C cells and subsequent lysis of the target cells was determined.

The results of the Morrison and Braciale experiments, presented in Table 10-2, show that the class II–restricted T_C cells responded to target cells treated with infectious or noninfectious influenza virions, whereas the class I–restricted T_C cells responded to target cells treated with infectious virions but not to target cells treated with non-

infectious virions. Similarly, target cells that had been treated with infectious influenza virions in the presence of emetine, which inhibits viral protein synthesis, stimulated the class II–restricted T_C cells but not the class I–restricted T_C cells. Just the opposite results were obtained with target cells that had been treated with infectious virions in the presence of chloroquine, a drug that blocks the endocytic processing pathway.

These results support the distinction between exogenous and endogenous antigens and the preferential asso-

T A B L E   1 0 – 2

EFFECT OF ANTIGEN PRESENTATION
ON ACTIVATION OF CLASS I AND CLASS II MHC-RESTRICTED T_C CELLS

| | CTL ACTIVITY [†] | |
TREATMENT OF TARGET CELLS *	CLASS I RESTRICTED	CLASS II RESTRICTED
Infectious virus	+	+
UV-inactivated virus (noninfectious)	−	+
Infectious virus + emetine	−	+
Infectious virus + chloroquine	+	−
Hemagglutinin protein	−	+
Hemagglutinin gene	+	−
Synthetic hemagglutinin peptides	+	+

* Target cells, which expressed both class I and class II MHC molecules, were treated with the indicated preparations of influenza virus or other agents. Emetine inhibits viral protein synthesis, and chloroquine inhibits the endocytic processing pathway. The influenza hemagglutinin (*HA*) gene was introduced into target cells as part of a recombinant vaccinia virus vector that contained the *HA* gene but no HA polypeptide.

[†] Determined by lysis (+) and no lysis (−) of the target cells.

SOURCE: Adapted from T. J. Braciale et al., 1987, *Immunol. Rev.* **98**:95.

ciation of exogenous antigens with class II MHC molecules and of endogenous antigens with class I MHC molecules. In other words, the mode of antigen entry into cells and its subsequent processing within either the endocytic processing pathway (exogenous antigens) or cytosolic pathway (endogenous antigens) determines whether the resulting antigenic peptides will associate with class I or class II MHC molecules. In the Morrison and Braciale experiments, association of viral antigen with class II MHC molecules did not require viral replication or protein synthesis. On the other hand, association of viral antigen with class I MHC molecules required replication of the influenza virus and viral protein synthesis within the target cells. These findings provided early evidence to suggest separate routing of class I and class II MHC molecules in separate intracellular compartments. This separate routing dictates whether the class I and II MHC molecules interact with peptides derived from cytosolic degradation of endogenously synthesized proteins or with peptides derived from endocytic degradation of exogenous antigens. In the next two sections, we'll examine each of these pathways in detail.

ENDOGENOUS ANTIGENS: THE CYTOSOLIC PATHWAY

Endogenous antigens, such as those produced by a virus replicating within a cell, are degraded within the cytoplasm into peptides that can associate with class I MHC molecules. Soluble protein antigens that are experimentally delivered into the cytoplasm of a cell also have been shown to be degraded into peptides that can be presented by class I MHC molecules to T_C cells. (One way to deliver soluble protein antigens into the cytoplasm is to load them inside membrane liposomes; as these fuse with the plasma membrane, the antigen is released into the cytoplasm.) The pathway by which endogenous antigens are degraded for presentation with class I MHC molecules utilizes pathways involved in the turnover of normal intracellular proteins.

Peptide Generation by Proteasomes

In eukaryotic cells protein levels are carefully regulated. Every protein is subject to continuous turnover and is degraded at a rate that is generally expressed in terms of its half-life. Some proteins (e.g., transcription factors, cyclins, and key metabolic enzymes) appear to have very short half-lives; denatured, misfolded, or otherwise abnormal proteins also are degraded rapidly. Intracellular proteins are degraded into short peptides by a cytosolic

proteolytic system possessed by all cells. Those proteins that are targeted for proteolysis often have a small protein, called **ubiquitin**, attached to them (Figure 10-5a).

Ubiquitin-protein conjugates can be degraded by a large multifunctional protease complex called a **proteasome.** Each proteasome is a large, cylindrical particle containing four rings of protein subunits with a central channel of 10–20 Å. A proteasome, described by John Monaco as a "big ball of degradative enzymes," can cleave three or four different types of peptide bonds in an ATP-dependent process (Figure 10-5b). Degradation of ubiquitin-protein complexes is thought to occur within the central hollow of a proteasome, thus avoiding proteolysis of other proteins within the cytoplasm.

The immune system is thought to utilize this general pathway of protein degradation to produce small peptides for presentation with class I MHC molecules. The immune system appears to modify the proteasome by the addition of two subunits to the proteasome: LMP2 and LMP7. These subunits are encoded within the MHC gene cluster and are induced by increased levels of IFN-γ. The peptidase activities of proteasomes containing LMP2 and LMP7 preferentially generate peptides

(a)

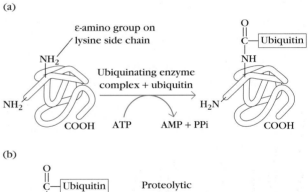

(b)

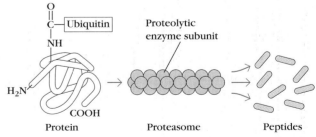

Protein   Proteasome   Peptides

FIGURE 10-5

Cytosolic proteolytic system for degradation of intracellular proteins. (a) Proteins to be degraded often are covalently linked to a small protein called ubiquitin. In this reaction, which requires ATP, a ubiquinating enzyme complex links several ubiquitin molecules to a lysine-amino group near the amino terminus of the protein. (b) Degradation of ubiquitin-protein complexes occurs within the central channel of proteasomes, generating a variety of peptides. Proteasomes are large cylindrical particles whose subunits catalyze cleavage of peptide bonds.

that bind to MHC class I molecules. Such proteasomes, for example, show increased hydrolysis of peptide bonds following basic and/or hydrophobic residues. As discussed in Chapter 9, peptides that bind to class I MHC molecules terminate almost exclusively with hydrophobic or basic residues.

Peptide Transport from the Cytosol to the RER

Insight into the role that peptide transport plays in the cytosolic processing pathway came from studies of cell lines with defects in peptide presentation by class I MHC molecules. One such mutant cell line, called RMA-S, expresses about 5% of the normal levels of class I MHC molecules on its membrane. Although RMA-S cells continue to synthesize normal levels of class I α chains and β_2-microglobulin, both molecules remain intracellular instead of appearing on the membrane. A clue to the mutation in the RMA-S cell line was the discovery by A. Townsend and his colleagues that "feeding" these cells predigested peptides restored their level of membrane-associated class I MHC molecules to normal. They suggested that peptide might be required to stabilize the interaction between the class I α chain and β_2-microglobulin. This led them to speculate that the RMA-S cell line might possibly have a defect in peptide transport. The ability to restore expression of class I MHC molecules on the membrane by feeding the cells predigested peptides would be compatible with this type of defect.

Subsequent experiments with the RMA-S cell line showed that the defect in these cells is in the protein that transports peptides from the cytoplasm to the rough endoplasmic reticulum (RER), where class I molecules are synthesized. When RMA-S cells were transfected with a functional transporter gene the cells began to express class I molecules on the membrane. The transporter protein, designated **TAP** (for **transporters associated with antigen processing**) is a membrane-spanning heterodimer consisting of two proteins: TAP1 and TAP2 (Figure 10-6a). In addition to their transmembrane segments, the TAP1 and TAP2 proteins each have one hydrophobic domain, which is thought to project through the membrane into the lumen of the RER, and one ATP-binding domain, which projects into the cytosol. Both TAP1 and TAP2 belong to the family of the ATP-binding cassette proteins found in the membranes of many cells, including bacteria; these proteins mediate ATP-dependent transport of amino acids, sugars, ions, and peptides.

Peptides generated in the cytosol by the proteasome are translocated by TAP into the RER by a process that requires the hydrolysis of ATP (Figure 10-6b). TAP has

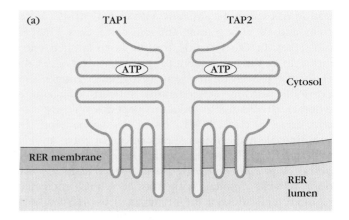

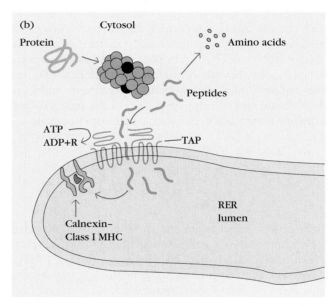

FIGURE 10-6

Generation of antigenic peptide–class I MHC complexes in cytosolic pathway. (a) Schematic diagram of TAP (transporters associated with antigen processing), a heterodimer anchored in the membrane of the rough endoplasmic reticulum (RER). The two chains are encoded by *TAP1* and *TAP2*. The cytosolic domain in each TAP subunit contains an ATP-binding site, and peptide transport is dependent on ATP hydrolysis. (b) In the cytosol, association of LMP2 and LMP7 (black spheres) with a proteasome changes its catalytic specificity to favor production of peptides that bind to class I MHC molecules. Within the RER membrane, newly synthesized class I α chain and β_2-microglobulin associate with calnexin. Physical association of this complex with TAP promotes binding of antigenic peptide by the α chain, which causes dissociation of calnexin and stabilizes the class I MHC molecule.

the highest affinity for peptides containing 8–13 amino acids, which is the optimal peptide length for class I MHC binding. In addition, TAP appears to favor peptides with hydrophobic or basic carboxyl-terminal amino acids, the preferred anchor residues for class I MHC mol-

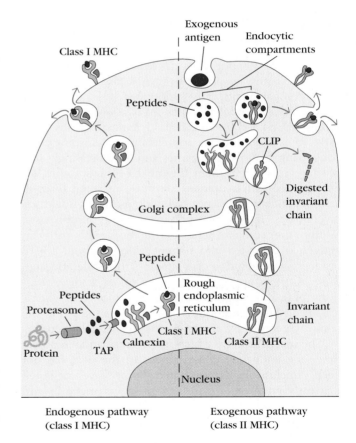

β₂ microglobulin

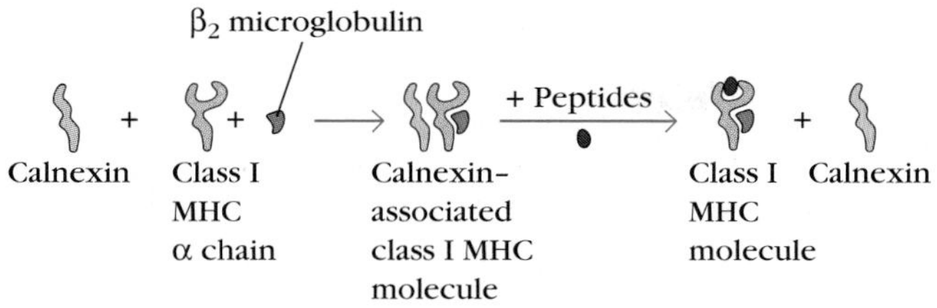

Calnexin | Class I MHC α chain | → Calnexin-associated class I MHC molecule | + Peptides → | Class I MHC molecule | + Calnexin

FIGURE 10-7

Assembly and stabilization of class I MHC molecules. Newly formed class I α chain and β_2-microglobulin associate with calnexin, a molecular chaperone, in the RER membrane. Subsequent binding of an antigenic peptide stabilizes the class I molecule and releases calnexin.

ecules. Thus, TAP seems uniquely designed to transport peptides that will interact with class I MHC molecules.

The *TAP1* and *TAP2* genes map within the class II MHC region, adjacent to the *LMP2* and *LMP7* genes (see Figure 9-16). Both the transporter genes and the *LMP* genes are polymorphic; that is, different allelic forms of these genes exist within the population. Allelic differences in LMP-mediated proteolytic cleavage of protein antigens or in the transport of different peptides from the cytosol into the RER may contribute to the observed variation among individuals in their response to different endogenous antigens.

Assembly of Peptides with Class I MHC Molecules

Like other proteins, the α chain and β_2-microglobulin components of the class I MHC molecule are synthesized on polysomes along the rough endoplasmic reticulum. Assembly of these components into a stable class I MHC molecule requires the presence of a peptide. The assembly of a stable class I MHC molecule involves the participation of **molecular chaperones**, which facilitate the folding of polypeptides. The predominant molecular chaperone involved in class I MHC assembly is **calnexin**, a resident membrane protein of the endoplasmic reticulum. Within the RER newly synthesized class I α chains rapidly associate with β_2-microglobulin and calnexin and assemble in a partially folded state. This association with calnexin appears to inhibit degradation of the α chain (Figure 10-7).

The calnexin-associated α chain–β_2-microglobulin heterodimer then physically associates with the TAP protein (see Figure 10-6b). Binding of the heterodimer to TAP is thought to promote peptide capture by the class I molecule before the peptides are exposed to the luminal environment of the RER. As a consequence of peptide binding, the class I molecule displays increased stability and dissociates from both calnexin and the TAP protein.

Overview of Class I Endogenous Pathway

The current model of the pathway by which endogenous antigens are processed and presented is shown in Figure 10-8. As mentioned earlier, endogenous antigens are thought to be degraded within the cytoplasm by the large (26S) LMP-containing proteasome complex. Peptides are then transported across the membrane of the RER by an ATP-binding transporter called TAP. The calnexin-associated class I MHC molecule then associates with the transmembrane TAP protein and captures the peptides. Binding of the peptide to the class I MHC molecule stabilizes the complex and causes its dissociation from calnexin. Finally, the class I MHC molecule–peptide complex is transported from the RER through the Golgi complex to the plasma membrane.

Endogenous pathway (class I MHC)   Exogenous pathway (class II MHC)

FIGURE 10-8

Model of separate antigen-presenting pathways for endogenous and exogenous antigens. The mode of antigen entry into cells and the site of antigen processing appear to determine whether antigenic peptides associate with class I MHC molecules in the rough endoplasmic reticulum or with class II molecules in endocytic compartments. Some elements of this model have not been experimentally demonstrated.

EXOGENOUS ANTIGENS: THE ENDOCYTIC PATHWAY

Antigen-presenting cells can internalize antigen by phagocytosis, endocytosis, or both. Macrophages internalize antigen by both processes, whereas most other APCs are not phagocytic or are poorly phagocytic and therefore internalize exogenous antigen only by endocytosis (either receptor-mediated endocytosis or pinocytosis). B cells, for example, internalize antigen very effectively by receptor-mediated endocytosis using antigen-specific membrane antibody as the receptor to capture the antigen.

Peptide Generation in Endocytic Vesicles

Once an antigen is internalized, it is degraded into peptides within compartments of the endocytic processing pathway. Internalized antigen takes 1–3 h to transverse the endocytic pathway and appear at the cell surface in the form of peptide–class II MHC complexes. The endocytic pathway appears to involve three increasingly acidic compartments: early endosomes (pH 6.0–6.5); late endosomes, or endolysosomes (pH 5.0–6.0); and lysosomes (pH 4.5–5.0). Internalized antigen moves from early to late endosomes and finally to lysosomes, encountering hydrolytic enzymes and an increasingly low pH in each compartment (Figure 10-9). Lysosomes, for example, contain a unique collection of more than 40 acid-dependent hydrolases including proteases, nucleases, glycosidases, lipases, phospholipases, and phosphatases. Within the compartments of the endocytic pathway, antigen is degraded into oligopeptides of about 13–18 residues, which bind to class II MHC molecules. Because these enzymes are optimally active under acidic conditions (pH), antigen processing can be inhibited by chemical agents (e.g., chloroquine) that increase the pH of the compartments or by protease inhibitors (e.g., leupeptin).

The mechanism by which internalized antigen moves from one endocytic compartment to the next has not been conclusively demonstrated. Some have suggested that early endosomes from the periphery move inward to become late endosomes and finally lysosomes. Others have suggested that small transport vesicles carry antigens from one compartment to the next, in a manner similar to the way in which small transport vesicles carry proteins from one compartment of the Golgi complex to the next. Eventually the endocytic compartments, or portions of them, return to the cell periphery where they fuse with the plasma membrane. In this way, the surface receptors may be recycled.

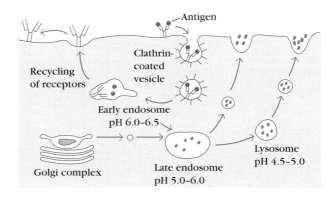

FIGURE 10-9

Generation of antigenic peptides in endocytic processing pathway. Internalized exogenous antigen (blue) moves through several acidic compartments, in which it is degraded into peptides that ultimately associate with class II MHC molecules transported in vesicles from the Golgi complex. The cell shown here is a B cell, which internalizes antigen by receptor-mediated endocytosis with the membrane-bound antibody functioning as an antigen-specific receptor.

Transport of Class II MHC Molecules to Endocytic Vesicles

Since antigen-presenting cells express both class I and class II MHC molecules, some mechanism must exist to prevent class II MHC molecules from binding to the same set of antigenic peptides as the class I molecules. Recent studies have shown that when a class II MHC molecule is synthesized within the RER, it associates with another protein called the **invariant (Ii) chain.** Three pairs of the class II $\alpha\beta$ chains associate with a pre-assembled invariant chain trimer. This trimeric protein interacts with the peptide-binding cleft of the class II molecule, preventing any endogenously derived peptides from binding to the cleft while the class II molecule is within the RER (Figure 10-10). In addition to its role in preventing peptide binding to class II MHC molecules, the invariant chain also appears to be involved in the folding of the class II α and β chains, their exit from the RER, and the subsequent routing of class II molecules to the endocytic processing pathway.

The role of the invariant chain in routing of class II molecules has been demonstrated in transfection experiments with cells that lack the genes encoding class II MHC molecules and the invariant chain. Immunofluorescent labeling of such cells transfected only with class II MHC genes revealed class II molecules localized within the Golgi complex. However, in cells transfected with both the class II MHC genes and invariant-chain gene, the class II molecules were localized in the cytoplasmic vesicular structures of the endocytic pathway. The invariant chain contains sorting signals in its cytoplasmic tail that directs the transport of the class II MHC complex from the trans-Golgi network to the endocytic compartments.

Assembly of Peptides With Class II MHC Molecules

Recent experiments indicate that most class II MHC–invariant chain complexes are transported from the RER, where they are formed, through the Golgi complex and trans-Golgi network to early endosomes. Here, within the endocytic pathway, these complexes move from early endosomes to late endosomes, and finally to lysosomes. As the proteolytic activity increases in each successive compartment, the invariant chain is gradually degraded. However, a short fragment of the invariant chain termed **CLIP** (for class II–associated invariant chain peptide) remains bound to the class II molecule after the invariant chain has been cleaved within the endosomal compartment. CLIP physically occupies the peptide-binding groove of the class II MHC molecule, presumably preventing any premature binding of antigenic peptide (see Figure 10-10).

A class II MHC–like molecule, called **HLA-DM**, is thought to play a role in the removal of CLIP and in the subsequent loading of class II molecules with antigenic peptides. Like other class II MHC molecules, HLA-DM is a heterodimer of α and β chains. However, unlike other class II molecules, HLA-DM is not expressed at the cell membrane and instead is found predominantly within the endosomal compartment. The $DM\alpha$ and $DM\beta$ genes are located near the TAP and LMP genes in the MHC complex of humans.

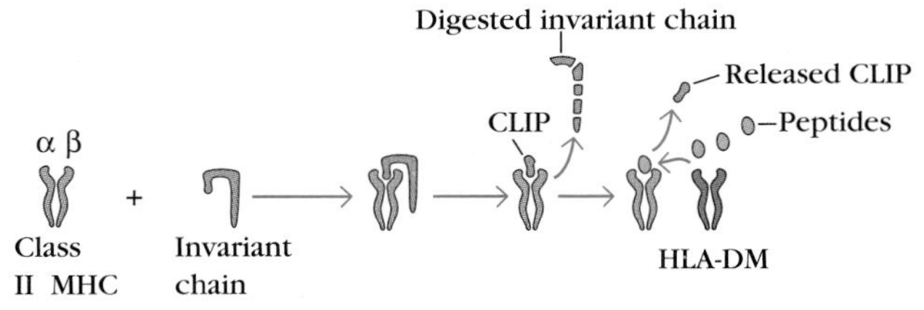

As the class II MHC molecules move through the endocytic pathway, they assume a more open conformation, called a floppy state. Experiments with so-called "falling-apart" mutants suggest that HLA-DM facilitates the exchange of CLIP associated with class II molecules in the floppy state with antigenic peptide (see Figure 10-10). In falling-apart mutants, which have a defective HLA-DM, this exchange cannot take place, and the α and β chains of the class II molecule soon dissociate.

As with class I MHC molecules, peptide binding is required to maintain the structure and stability of class II MHC molecules. Once a peptide has bound, the peptide–class II complex is transported to the plasma membrane, where the neutral pH appears to enable the complex to assume a compact, stable form. Peptide is bound so strongly in this compact form that it is very difficult to replace a class II–bound peptide on the membrane with another peptide at physiologic conditions.

Overview of Class II Exogenous Pathway

The current model of the pathway for processing and presenting exogenous antigens is summarized in Figure 10-8. As discussed previously, newly synthesized class II α and β chains associate with an invariant chain within the RER. This association precludes binding of class II MHC molecules with peptides derived from endogenous antigens or other intracellular proteins. Class II molecules, together with the associated invariant chains, are thought to be routed from the RER through the Golgi complex to the endocytic pathway. Once inside an endocytic compartment, the invariant chain is degraded by proteolytic enzymes, leaving the CLIP fragment bound to the peptide-binding cleft of the class II molecules. Within the acidic endocytic compartments, the class II molecules assume an open (floppy) conformation that facilitates replacement of CLIP with an antigenic peptide, a process mediated by HLA-DM. The resulting class II MHC–peptide complexes move to plasma membrane.

FIGURE 10-10

Assembly and classification of class II MHC molecules. Within the rough endoplasmic reticulum, a newly synthesized class II MHC molecule binds an invariant chain. The bound invariant chain prevents premature binding of peptides to the class II molecule and helps to direct the complex to endocytic compartments containing peptides derived from exogenous antigens. Digestion of the invariant chain leaves CLIP, a small fragment. HLA-DM, an MHC-like molecule expressed within endosomal compartments, mediates exchange of peptides for CLIP.

CLINICAL APPLICATIONS

The discovery that endogenous and exogenous antigens are processed in different pathways has important implications for the design of new vaccines. If a class I–restricted cell-mediated response is desired, then a vaccine must be processed within the cytosolic pathway.

This requirement is met by attenuated live vaccines capable of limited growth within the cytoplasm of infected cells and by several other types of vaccines developed in recent years. Vaccines intended to elicit a humoral antibody response, on the other hand, must possess epitopes that are recognizable by B cells (see Table 4-4). Once recognized by a B cell, the vaccine will be endocytosed and then processed within the endocytic pathway. An in-depth discussion of various approaches to designing vaccines is presented in Chapter 18.

Some evidence suggests that defects in antigen processing or presentation may contribute to certain autoimmune diseases. For example, D. Faustman and her colleagues found that expression of class I MHC molecules on cells from diabetic patients was significantly lower than that on cells from normal controls. Furthermore, nonobese diabetic (NOD) mice, which have a similar reduction in class I MHC expression, have been shown to have a genetic defect in the gene encoding the peptide-transporter protein. Faustman has speculated that a defect in transporter function may be responsible for the reduction in class I MHC expression in both the NOD mouse and human diabetics. She has suggested that autoimmune diabetes may develop in individuals who are unable to present self-peptides together with class I MHC molecules to developing thymocytes during T-cell maturation in the thymus; as a result self-reactive T cells are not eliminated as they normally are. Faustman's theory is controversial, and so far no evidence for a defect in the peptide-transporter protein in human diabetics has been reported. Indeed, some other mechanism may be responsible for the decreased expression of class I MHC molecules in NOD mice and human diabetics.

SUMMARY

1. T-cell recognition of antigen requires that antigenic peptides be displayed within the cleft of a self-MHC molecule on the membrane of a cell. This requirement is called self-MHC restriction. In general, CD4$^+$ T$_H$ cells are class II MHC restricted, whereas CD8$^+$ T$_C$ cells are class I MHC restricted.

2. Complexes between antigenic peptides and MHC molecules are formed by degradation of a protein antigen in one of two different antigen-processing pathways. Those cells that process and present peptides associated with class II MHC molecules are called antigen-presenting cells (APCs); those that process and present peptides associated with class I MHC molecules are called target cells.

3. Endogenous antigens are thought to be degraded into peptides within the cytosol by a large enzyme complex, called the proteasome, which has several types of peptidase activity. The resulting antigenic peptides are transported into the lumen of rough endoplasmic reticulum by TAP, an ATP-dependent heterodimeric protein located in the RER membrane (see Figure 10-6). Within the RER the peptides assemble with class I MHC molecules; binding of peptide stabilizes the association between the class I α chain and β_2-microglobulin. Peptide–class I complexes then are transported from the RER through the Golgi complex to the plasma membrane (see Figure 10-8, *left*).

4. Exogenous antigens, internalized by phagocytosis or endocytosis, are degraded by various hydrolytic enzymes within the acidic endocytic compartments (see Figure 10-9). Within the RER, newly formed class II MHC molecules associate with the invariant chain, which blocks binding of peptides. Class II molecules with the associated invariant chain are routed to endocytic compartments, where the invariant chain is degraded by proteolytic enzymes, leaving the CLIP fragment in the peptide-binding cleft. As the class II molecules assume a more open conformation in the low-pH compartments, antigenic peptides displace CLIP. The peptide–class II complexes are then transported to the plasma membrane (see Figure 10-8, *right*).

REFERENCES

BENHAM, A., A. TULIP, AND J. NEEFJES. 1995. Synthesis and assembly of MHC-peptide complexes. *Immunol. Today* **16**:359.

CASTELLINO, F., AND R. N. GERMAIN. 1995. Extensive trafficking of MHC class II–invariant chain complexes in the endocytic pathway and appearance of peptide-loaded class II in multiple compartments. *Immunity* **2**:73.

CIECHANOVER, A. 1994. The ubiquitin-proteasome proteolytic pathway. *Cell* **79**:13.

HARDING, C. V., AND H. J. GEUZE. 1993. Antigen processing and intracellular traffic of antigens and MHC molecules. *Curr. Opin. Cell Biol.* **5**:596.

HOWARD, J. C. 1995. Supply and transport of peptides presented by class I MHC molecules. *Curr. Opin. Immunol.* **7**:69.

MELLMAN, I., P. PIERRE, AND S. AMIGORENA. 1995. Lonely MHC molecules seeking immunogenic peptides for meaningful relationships. *Curr. Opin. Cell Biol.* **7**:564.

MOMBERG, F., J. NEEFJES, AND G. J. HAMMERLING. 1994. Peptide selection by MHC-encoded TAP transporters. *Curr. Opin. Immunol.* **6**:32.

NIEDERMANN, G., ET AL. 1995. Contribution of proteasome-mediated proteolysis to the hierarchy of epitopes presented by major histocompatibility complex class I molecules. *Immunity* **2**:289.

ROCK, K. L., AND E. R. UNANUE. 1995. Antigen recognition. *Curr. Opin. Immunol.* **7**:65.

ROMISH, K. 1994. Peptide traffic across the ER membrane: TAPs and other conduits. *Trends Cell Biol.* **4**:311.

WILLIAMS, D. B., AND T. H. WATTS. 1995. Molecular chaperones in antigen presentation. *Curr. Opin. Immunol.* **7**:77.

STUDY QUESTIONS

1. Explain the difference between the terms *antigen-presenting cell* and *target cell*, as they are commonly used in immunology.

2. Define the following terms:

a. Self-MHC restriction

b. Antigen processing

c. Endogenous antigen

d. Exogenous antigen

3. L. A. Morrison and T. J. Braciale conducted an experiment to determine whether antigens presented by class I or II MHC molecules are processed in different pathways. Their results are summarized in Table 10-2.

a. Explain why the class I–restricted T_C cells did not respond to target cells infected with UV-inactivated influenza virus?

b. Explain why chloroquine inhibited the response of the class II–restricted T_C cells to live virus.

c. Explain why emitine inhibited the response of class I–restricted but not class II–restricted T_C cells to live virus.

d. Explain why class II–restricted T_C cells responded to hemagglutinin protein but class I–restricted cells did not.

4. For each of the following cell components or processes, indicate whether it is involved in the processing and presentation of exogenous antigens (EX), endogenous antigens (EN), or both (B). Briefly explain the function of each item.

a. _____ Class I MHC molecules

b. _____ Class II MHC molecules

c. _____ Invariant (Ii) chains

d. _____ Lysosomal hydrolases

e. _____ TAP1 and TAP2 proteins

f. _____ Transport of vesicles from the RER to the Golgi complex

g. _____ Proteasomes

h. _____ Phagocytosis or endocytosis

i. _____ Calnexin

j. _____ CLIP

5. Antigen-presenting cells have been shown to present lysozyme peptide 46–61 together with the class II IA^k molecule. When CD4$^+$ T_H cells are incubated with APCs and native lysozyme or the synthetic lysozyme peptide 46–61, T_H-cell activation occurs.

a. If chloroquine is added to the incubation mixture, presentation of the native protein is inhibited, but the peptide continues to induce T_H-cell activation. Explain why this occurs.

b. If chloroquine addition is delayed for 3 h, presentation of the native protein is not inhibited. Explain why this occurs.

6. Cells that can present antigen to T_H cells have been classified into two groups—professional and nonprofessional APCs.

a. Name the three types of professional APCs. For each type indicate whether it expresses class II MHC molecules and a co-stimulatory signal constitutively or must be activated before doing so.

b. Give three examples of nonprofessional APCs. When are these cells most likely to function in antigen presentation?

7. Predict whether T_H-cell proliferation or CTL-mediated cytolysis of target cells will occur with the following mixtures of cells. The CD4$^+$ T_H cells are from lysozyme-primed mice, and the CD8$^+$ CTLs are from influenza-infected mice. Use R to indicate a response and NR to indicate no response.

a. _____ H–2^k T_H cells + lysozyme-pulsed H–2^k macrophages

b._____ H–2^k T_H cells + lysozyme-pulsed H–2$^{b/k}$ macrophages

c._____ H–2^k T_H cells + lysozyme-primed H–2^d macrophages

d._____ H–2^k CTLs + influenza-infected H–2^k macrophages

e._____ H–2^k CTLs + influenza-infected H–2^d macrophages

f._____ H–2^d CTLs + influenza-infected H–2$^{d/k}$ macrophages

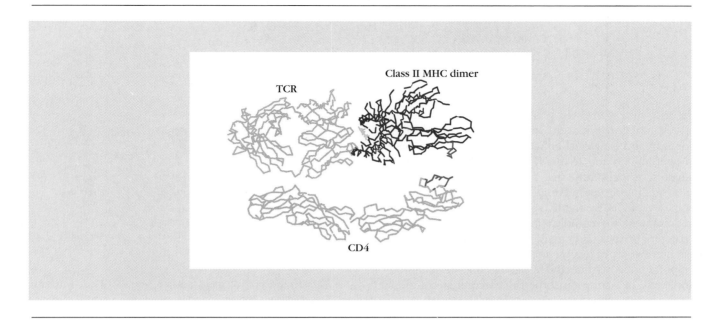

T - C E L L   R E C E P T O R

Although the antigen-specific nature of T-cell responses clearly implies that they possess an antigen-specific and clonally restricted receptor, the nature of the T-cell receptor for antigen remained unknown long after the B-cell receptor had been identified. Relevant experimental results were contradictory and difficult to conceptualize within a single model because the T-cell receptor differs from the B-cell antigen-binding receptor in two important ways. First, the T cell does not secrete its receptor as the B cell does, so that any assessment of receptor structure and specificity had to rely on complex cellular assays. Second, the T-cell receptor (TCR) is specific not for antigen alone but for antigen in association with a molecule encoded by the major histocompatibility complex (MHC). This property prevents purification of the T-cell receptor by simple antigen-binding techniques and adds complexity to any experimental system designed to investigate the receptor.

Once the T-cell receptor was finally isolated, it was found to be a heterodimer composed of either α and β or γ and δ chains. Surprisingly, the genomic organization and the mode of generation of diversity for each chain were found to be similar to that of the B-cell receptor's immunoglobulin chains. In addition, the T-cell receptor was found to be associated on the membrane with a signal-transducing complex called CD3. This signal-transducing complex has a function similar to the Ig-α/Ig-β complex of the B-cell receptor. Three-dimensional analysis of the structure of the complete T-cell receptor by x-ray crystallography continues to be hampered by difficulties in isolating and solubilizing sufficient quantities of the membrane-bound chains. Moreover, because the T-cell receptor only recognizes antigen that is complexed with self-MHC molecules, insight into antigen binding by the TCR requires three-dimensional analysis of a TCR-peptide-MHC ternary complex. Such a three-dimensional analysis has yet to be achieved.

EARLY STUDIES OF THE T-CELL RECEPTOR

In the early 1980s investigators learned much about T-cell function but were thwarted in their attempts to identify and isolate its antigen-binding receptor. Several properties, unique to the T-cell receptor, hampered its identification. Because the T cell does not secrete its antigen-binding receptor, complex cellular assays are required to assess TCR structure, specificity, and function. The requirement for complex cellular assays to assess TCR structure or specificity made it difficult to tell whether an agent that specifically stimulated or blocked T-cell responses did so directly by acting on the receptor or indirectly by acting on some other required component of the cellular function being assessed.

Self-MHC Restriction of the T-Cell Receptor

By the early 1970s, immunologists had discovered that cytotoxic T lymphocytes (CTLs) specific for virus-infected target cells could be generated. For example, when mice were infected with lymphocytic choriomenigitis (LCM) virus, they would produce CTLs that could lyse LCM-infected target cells in vitro. Yet these same CTLs failed to bind free LCM virus or viral antigens. This finding suggested that antigen recognition by T cells was fundamentally different from that of B cells. Why didn't the CTLs bind the virus or viral antigens directly? The answer began to emerge in the classical experiments of Zinkernagel and Doherty (see Figure 10-2). These studies demonstrated that antigen recognition by T cells is specific not only for viral antigen but also for an MHC molecule (Figure 11-1). T cells were shown to recognize antigen only when it is presented on the membrane of a cell by a self-MHC molecule. This attribute, called **self-MHC restriction,** distinguishes recognition of antigen by T cells from that by B cells. In 1996 Doherty and Zinkernagel were awarded the Nobel Prize for this work.

Two models were proposed to explain the MHC restriction of the T-cell receptor. The **dual-receptor model** envisioned a T cell as having two separate receptors, one for antigen and one for class I or class II MHC molecules. The **altered-self model** proposed that there was a single receptor capable of recognizing foreign antigen complexed to a self-MHC molecule. Unlike the dual-receptor model, in which an antigen and MHC molecule are recognized separately, the altered-self model predicts that a single receptor recognizes an alteration in MHC molecules induced by their association with foreign antigens.

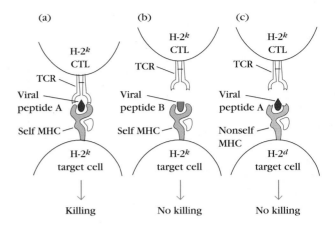

FIGURE 11-1

Self-MHC restriction of the T-cell receptor (TCR). A particular TCR is specific for both an antigenic peptide and a self-MHC molecule. In this example, the H-2^k CTL is specific for viral peptide A presented on an H-2^k target cell (a). Antigen recognition does not occur when peptide B is displayed on an H-2^k target cell (b) nor when peptide A is displayed on an H-2^d target cell (c).

The debate between proponents of these two models was waged for a number of years, until an elegant experiment by J. Kappler and P. Marrack provided a means to test each model. Two preparations of T cells with specificities for different antigen plus class II MHC complexes were used for the experiment: one preparation was a T-cell hybridoma specific for ovalbumin (OVA) in the context of an H-2^k class II MHC molecule; the other preparation was a normal T cell reactive to keyhole limpet hemocyanin (KLH) in the context of an H-2^f class II MHC molecule. The experimenters fused these two cells to produce a T-cell hybridoma expressing the receptors of both fusion partners (Figure 11-2). If the dual-receptor model were correct, then the hybrid cells should express separate receptors for each antigen and separate receptors for each class II MHC molecule; therefore, the hybrid cells should respond to both antigens presented by either H-2^k or H-2^f antigen-presenting cells. In fact, Kappler and Marrack found that the hybrid cells continued to respond only to OVA presented by H-2^k cells and to KLH presented by H-2^f cells. In other words, the original specificity for antigen and MHC haplotype appeared to segregate together in the membrane of these hybrid cells. This finding provided early support for the altered-self model.

Isolation of T-Cell Receptors

Identification and isolation of the T-cell receptor finally was accomplished by producing large numbers of monoclonal antibodies to various T-cell clones and then screening these monoclonal antibodies to find one that

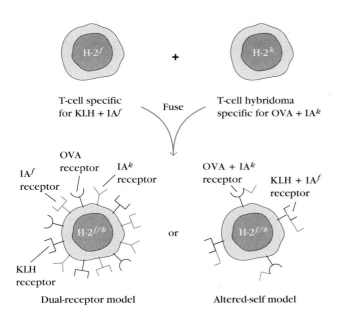

Response of fused cells				
		Expected response		
Antigen	MHC on APCs	Dual-receptor model	Altered-self model	Actual response
OVA	IA^k	+	+	+
OVA	IA^f	+	−	−
KLH	IA^k	+	−	−
KLH	IA^f	+	+	+

FIGURE 11-2

Experimental test of the dual-receptor and altered-self models of T-cell antigen recognition. T cells with two different specificities were fused, and the hybrid cells then were tested for their ability to recognize various antigen-MHC complexes. One fusion partner was specific for ovalbumin (OVA) + the class II MHC molecule IA^k on antigen-presenting cells (APCs), and the other was specific for keyhole limpet hemocyanin (KLH) + IA^f. Comparison of the expected responses of the fused cells, assuming the dual-receptor or altered-self model to be correct, with the actual responses supports the altered-self model. [Based on J. Kappler et al., 1981, *J. Exp. Med.* **153**:1198.]

was clone specific, or **clonotypic**. This approach was based on the assumption that since the T-cell receptor is specific for both an antigen and an MHC molecule, there should be significant structural differences in the receptor from clone to clone. The T-cell receptor was first identified by J. P. Allison in 1982 using this approach; other researchers soon isolated the receptor and found that it was a heterodimer consisting of α and β chains.

Using $\alpha\beta$ heterodimers isolated from membranes derived from various T-cell clones, Allison showed that some antisera bound to $\alpha\beta$ heterodimers from all the clones, whereas other antisera were clone specific. This finding suggested that the amino acid sequences of the

TCR α and β chains, like those of the immunoglobulin heavy and light chains, have constant and variable regions. Later, a second type of TCR heterodimer consisting of δ and γ chains was identified. The majority of T cells (more than 95%) express the $\alpha\beta$ heterodimer; the remaining 2%–5% of T cells express the $\gamma\delta$ heterodimer.

STRUCTURE OF T-CELL RECEPTORS

Amino acid sequencing of the $\alpha\beta$ and $\gamma\delta$ TCR heterodimers revealed a domain structure that is strikingly similar to that of the immunoglobulins; thus, they are classified as members of the immunoglobulin superfamily (see Figure 5-19). Each chain in a TCR has two domains containing an intrachain disulfide bond spanning 60–75 amino acids. The amino-terminal domain in both chains exhibits marked sequence variation, but the sequences of the remainder of each chain are conserved. Thus the TCR domains—one variable (V) and one constant (C)—are structurally homologous to the V and C domains of immunoglobulins, and the TCR molecule is thought to resemble an Fab fragment (Figure 11-3). The TCR variable domains have three hypervariable regions, which appear to be equivalent to the CDRs in immunoglobulin light and heavy chains.

In addition to the constant domain, each TCR chain contains a short connecting sequence, which has a cysteine residue involved in disulfide linking of the two chains in the TCR heterodimer. Following the connecting region is a transmembrane region of 21 or 22 amino acids, anchoring each chain in the plasma membrane. The transmembrane domains of both chains are unusual in that they contain positively charged amino acid residues. These positively charged residues enable the chains of the TCR heterodimer to interact with chains of the signal-transducing CD3 complex. Finally, each TCR chain contains a short cytoplasmic tail of 5–12 amino acids at the carboxyl-terminal end.

Because both the $\alpha\beta$ and $\gamma\delta$ T-cell receptors are transmembrane proteins, it is difficult to isolate sufficient quantities for x-ray crystallography; in addition, the chains are not soluble in the absence of detergent. To date, only the β chain and the V domain of the α chain have been analyzed by x-ray crystallography. Consequently the three-dimensional structure of the $\alpha\beta$ heterodimer can only be inferred from its homology to immunoglobulin molecules.

The crystal structure of the TCR β chain shows structural homology to immunoglobulins. The three CDRs are oriented in the V domain to form the expected antigen-binding site. It is thought that CDR1 and CDR2 form the periphery of the antigen-binding site

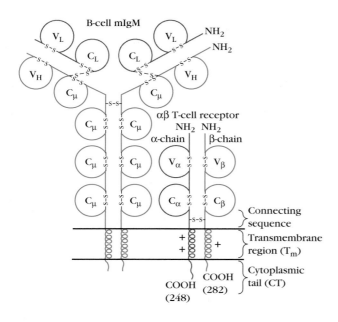

FIGURE 11-3

Schematic diagram illustrating the structural similarity between the $\alpha\beta$ T-cell receptor and membrane-bound IgM on B cells. The TCR α and β chain each contain two domains with the immunoglobulin-fold structure. The amino-terminal domains (V_α and V_β) exhibit sequence variation and contain three hypervariable regions equivalent to the CDRs in antibodies. The sequence of the constant domains (C_α and C_β) does not vary. The two chains are connected by a disulfide bond; they interact with CD3 via positive charges in their transmembrane region. The structure of the $\gamma\delta$ T-cell receptor is similar. Numbers indicate residue positions in the TCR molecule. Unlike the antibody molecule, which is bivalent, the TCR is monovalent.

and contact primarily the α-helical regions of the MHC molecule. CDR3 is located in the center of the antigen-binding site and is thought to play a more significant role in contacting the antigenic peptide held in the cleft of the MHC molecule.

ORGANIZATION AND REARRANGEMENT OF TCR GENES

The genes encoding the $\alpha\beta$ and $\gamma\delta$ T-cell receptors are expressed only in cells of the T-cell lineage. The four TCR loci (α, β, γ, and δ) have a germ-line organization that is remarkably similar to the multigene organization of the immunoglobulin (Ig) genes. As with the Ig genes, separate V, D, and J gene segments rearrange during T-cell maturation to form functional genes encoding the T-cell receptor.

Identifying and Cloning the TCR Genes

In order to identify and isolate the TCR genes, S. M. Hedrick and M. M. Davis sought to isolate mRNA encoding the α and β chains from a T_H-cell clone. This was no easy task. Because the T cell does not secrete its antigen-binding receptor, the receptor mRNA does not represent a sizable fraction of the mRNA, as it does, for example, in the plasma cell, where immunoglobulin is a major secreted cell product and mRNAs encoding the heavy and light chains are relatively easy to purify. The successful scheme of Hedrick and Davis for isolating TCR genes depended on a number of well-thought-out assumptions, which proved to be correct.

Hedrick and Davis reasoned that the TCR mRNA — like the mRNAs encoding other integral membrane proteins—would be bound to polyribosomes rather than to free cytoplasmic ribosomes. They therefore isolated the membrane-bound polyribosomal mRNA from a T_H-cell clone and used reverse transcriptase to synthesize ^{32}P-labeled cDNA probes (Figure 11-4). Because only 3% of lymphocyte mRNA is in the membrane-bound polyribosomal fraction, this step eliminated the 97% of the mRNA that did not encode any integral membrane protein.

Hedrick and Davis next used a technique called **DNA subtractive hybridization** to remove from their preparation the $[^{32}P]$cDNA that was not unique to T cells. Their rationale for this step was that since T cells and B cells are derived from a common progenitor cell, they should express many genes in common. Earlier measurements by Davis had shown that 98% of the genes expressed in lymphocytes are common to B cells and T cells. Hedrick and Davis sought to enrich for the 2% of the expressed genes that are unique to T cells, which should include the genes encoding the T-cell receptor. Therefore, by hybridizing B-cell mRNA with their T_H-cell $[^{32}P]$cDNA, they were able to remove, or subtract, all the cDNA that was common to B cells and T cells. The unhybridized $[^{32}P]$cDNA remaining after this step presumably represented the expressed polyribosomal mRNA that was unique to the T_H-cell clone, including the mRNA encoding its T-cell receptor.

Cloning of the unhybridized $[^{32}P]$cDNA generated a library from which 10 different cDNA clones were identified. To determine which of these T-cell–specific cDNA clones might represent the T-cell receptor, Hedrick and Davis used these clones as probes to look for genes on the genomic DNA that rearranged in mature T cells. This approach was based on the assumption that since the $\alpha\beta$ T-cell receptor appeared to have constant and variable regions, its genes should undergo DNA rearrangements like those observed in B cells. The two investigators isolated genomic DNA from T cells, B cells, liver cells, and macrophages, cleaved it with restriction

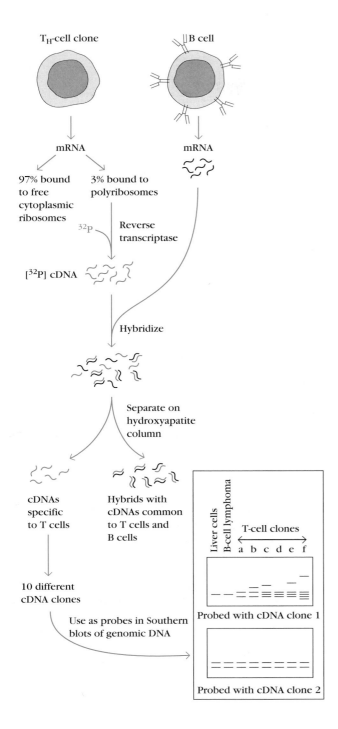

FIGURE 11-4

Production and identification of a cDNA clone encoding the T-cell receptor. The flow chart outlines the procedure used by S. Hedrick and M. Davis to obtain [^{32}P]cDNA clones corresponding to T-cell–specific mRNAs. The technique of DNA subtractive hybridization enabled them to isolate [^{32}P]cDNA unique to the T cell. The labeled T_H-cell cDNA clones were used as probes (*Inset*) in Southern-blot analyses of genomic DNA from liver cells, B-lymphoma cells, and six different T_H-cell clones (a–f). Probing with cDNA clone 1 produced a distinct blot pattern for each T-cell clone, whereas probing with cDNA clone 2 did not. Assuming that liver cells and B cells contained unrearranged germ-line DNA, and that each of the T-cell clones contained different rearranged TCR genes, the results using cDNA clone 1 as the probe identified the T-cell receptor of clone 1. The cDNA of clone 2 identified another T-cell membrane molecule encoded by DNA that does not undergo rearrangement. [Based on S. Hedrick et al., 1984, *Nature* **308**:149.]

panel). These patterns presumably represented rearranged TCR genes. Such results would be expected if rearranged TCR genes occur only in mature T cells. The observation that each of the six T-cell lines showed different Southern-blot patterns was consistent with the expected differences in TCR specificity in each T-cell line.

The cDNA clone identified by the Southern-blot analyses shown in Figure 11-4 has all the hallmarks of a putative TCR gene: it represents a gene sequence that rearranges, is expressed as a membrane-bound protein, and is expressed only in T cells. This cDNA clone was found to encode the β chain of the T-cell receptor. Later, cDNA clones were identified encoding the α chain, the γ chain, and finally the δ chain.

TCR Multigene Families

Germ-line DNA contains four TCR multigene families each encoding one of the receptor chains (Figure 11-5). As in the case of Ig genes, functional TCR genes are produced by gene rearrangements involving V and J segments in the α-chain and γ-chain families and V, D, and J segments in the β-chain and δ-chain families. In the mouse the α-, β-, and γ-chain gene segments are located on chromosomes 14, 6, and 13, respectively. The δ-chain gene segments are located on chromosome 14 between the V_α and J_α segments. This location of the δ-chain gene family is significant: A productive rearrangement of the α-chain gene segments deletes C_δ, so that in a given T cell the $\alpha\beta$ TCR receptor cannot be coexpressed with the $\gamma\delta$ receptor.

Mouse germ-line DNA contains about 100 V_α and 50 J_α gene segments and a single C_α segment. The δ-chain gene family contains about 10 V gene segments, which are largely distinct from the V_α gene segments, although some sharing of V segments has been observed

Figure labels (left panel):

T_H-cell clone

B cell

mRNA

mRNA

97% bound to free cytoplasmic ribosomes

3% bound to polyribosomes

^{32}P

Reverse transcriptase

[^{32}P] cDNA

Hybridize

Separate on hydroxyapatite column

cDNAs specific to T cells

Hybrids with cDNAs common to T cells and B cells

10 different cDNA clones

Use as probes in Southern blots of genomic DNA

Liver cells
B-cell lymphoma
T-cell clones
a b c d e f

Probed with cDNA clone 1

Probed with cDNA clone 2

endonucleases, and subjected each DNA sample to Southern-blot analysis using the 10 [^{32}P]cDNA probes to identify unique T-cell genomic DNA sequences. They looked for bands that showed DNA rearrangement in T cells but not in liver cells, B cells, or macrophages. One cDNA probe showed the same Southern-blot patterns for DNA isolated from liver cells, B cells, and macrophages but six different patterns for the DNA from six different mature T-cell lines (see Figure 11-4 inset, upper

Mouse TCR α-chain and δ-chain DNA (chromosome 14)

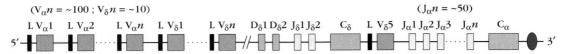

Mouse TCR β-chain DNA (chromosome 6)

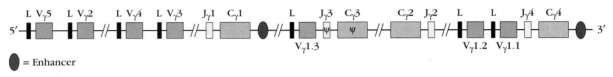

Mouse TCR γ-chain DNA (chromosome 13)

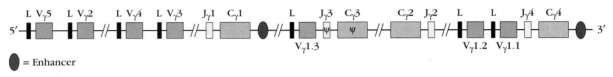

= Enhancer

ψ = pseudogene

FIGURE 11-5

Germ-line organization of the mouse TCR α-, β-, γ-, and δ-chain gene segments. Each C gene segment is composed of a series of exons and introns, which are not shown. The organization of TCR gene segments in humans is similar, although the number of the various gene segments differs in some cases (see Table 11-1). [Adapted from D. Raulet, 1989, *Annu. Rev. Immunol.* **7**:175 and M. Davis, 1990, *Annu. Rev. Biochem.* **59**:475.]

in rearranged α- and δ-chain genes. Two D_δ and two J_δ gene segments and one C_δ segment have also been identified. The β-chain gene family has 20–30 V gene segments and two repeats of D, J, and C segments, each repeat consisting of one D_β, six J_β, and one C_β. The γ-chain gene family consists of seven V_γ segments and three different functional J_γ-C_γ repeats. The organization of the TCR multigene families in humans is generally similar to that in mice, although the number of segments differs (Table 11-1).

Variable-Region Gene Rearrangements

The organization of the gene segments in the germ-line DNA encoding the α and β chains of the T-cell receptor is generally analogous to that of the immunoglobulin germ-line DNA. The α chain, like the immunoglobulin L chain, is encoded by V, J, and C gene segments. The β chain, like the immunoglobulin H chain, is encoded by V, D, J, and C gene segments. Rearrangement of the TCR α- and β-chain gene segments results in VJ joining for the α chain and VDJ joining for the β chain (Figure 11-6).

Following transcription of the rearranged TCR genes, RNA processing, and translation, the α and β chains are expressed as a disulfide-linked heterodimer on the membrane of the T cell. Unlike immunoglobulins, which can be membrane bound or secreted, the αβ heterodimer

is expressed only in a membrane-bound form; thus no differential RNA processing is required to produce membrane or secreted forms. Also, the constant-region germ-line DNA encoding the TCR α and β chains is much simpler than the immunoglobulin heavy-chain

TABLE 11-1

TCR MULTIGENE FAMILIES IN HUMANS

GENE	CHROMOSOME LOCATION	NO. OF GENE SEGMENTS			
		V	D	J	C
α Chain	14	50		70	1
δ Chain*	14	3	3	3	1
β Chain†	7	57	2	13	2
γ Chain	7	14		5	2

* The δ-chain gene segments are located between the V_α and J_α segments.

† There are two repeats, each containing 1 D_β, 6 or 7 J_β, and 1 C_β. There are two repeats, each containing 2 or 3 J_γ and 1 C_γ.

SOURCE: Data from P. A. H. Moss et al., 1992, *Annu. Rev. Immunol.* **10**:71.

Visualizing Concepts

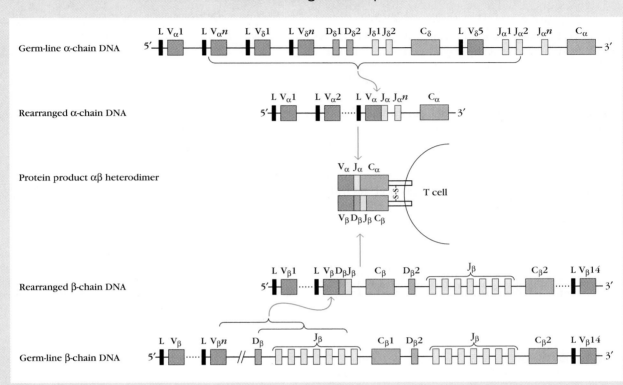

FIGURE 11-6

Example of gene rearrangements that yield a functional gene encoding the $\alpha\beta$ T-cell receptor. The α-chain DNA, analogous to immunoglobulin light-chain DNA, undergoes a variable-region V_α-J_α joining. The β-chain DNA, analogous to immunoglobulin heavy-chain DNA, undergoes two variable-region joinings: first D_β to J_β and then V_β to $D_\beta J_\beta$. Transcription of the rearranged genes yields primary transcripts, which are processed to give mRNAs encoding the α and β chains of the membrane-bound TCR. The leader sequence is cleaved from the nascent polypeptide chain and is not present in the finished protein. As no secreted TCR is produced, differential processing of the primary transcripts does not occur. Although the β-chain DNA contains two C segments, the gene products exhibit no known functional differences.

germ-line DNA, which has multiple C gene segments encoding distinct isotypes with different effector functions. TCR α-chain DNA has only a single C gene segment; the β-chain DNA has two C gene segments, but their protein products have no known functional differences.

Mechanism of TCR DNA Rearrangements

The mechanisms by which TCR germ-line DNA is rearranged to form functional receptor genes appear to be similar to the mechanisms used in Ig-gene rearrangements. For example, conserved heptamer and nonamer recognition signal sequences (RSSs), containing either 12-bp (one-turn) or 23-bp (two-turn) spacer sequences, have been identified flanking each V, D, and J gene segment in TCR germ-line DNA. The recognition signals in T cells have similar heptamer and nonamer sequences as those in B cells (see Figure 7-6). All of the TCR-gene rearrangements follow the one-turn/two-turn joining rule observed for the Ig genes.

Like the pre-B cell, the pre-T cell expresses the recombination-activating genes (*RAG-1* and *RAG-2*). The RAG1/2 recombinase enzyme recognizes the heptamer and nonamer recognition signals and catalyzes V-J and V-D-J joining during TCR-gene rearrangement by the same deletional or inversional mechanisms that occur in the Ig genes (see Figure 7-8). As described in

Chapter 7 for the immunoglobulin genes, RAG1/2 introduces a nick on one DNA strand between the coding and signal sequences. The recombinase then catalyzes a transesterification reaction resulting in hairpin formation at the coding sequence and a flush 5′ phosphorylated double-strand break at the signal sequence. Circular excision products thought to be generated by looping-out and deletion during TCR-gene rearrangement have been identified in thymocytes.

Studies with SCID mice, which lack functional T and B cells, provide evidence for the similarity in the mechanisms of Ig-gene and TCR-gene rearrangements. As discussed in Chapter 7, SCID mice have a defect in a gene required for double-stranded DNA break repair. As a result of this defect, D and J gene segments are not joined during rearrangement of both Ig and TCR DNA (see Figure 7-10). This finding suggests that the same double-stranded break-repair enzymes are involved in V-D-J rearrangements in B cells and in T cells.

Although B cells and T cells utilize very similar mechanisms for variable-region gene rearrangements, the Ig genes are not normally rearranged in T cells and the TCR genes are not rearranged in B cells. Presumably, the recombinase enzyme system is regulated in each cell lineage, so that only rearrangement of the correct receptor DNA occurs. As discussed at the end of Chapter 7, a region within the κ chain 3′ enhancer recently has been shown to suppress κ L-chain gene rearrangement in T cells. It is proposed that a protein present in T cells, but not in B cells, binds to this enhancer, thereby preventing V_κ to J_κ joining. Deletion of this region in the 3′ enhancer allows V_κ to J_κ joining to occur in T cells as well as B cells.

ALLELIC EXCLUSION OF TCR GENES

As with the Ig genes, rearrangement of the TCR β-chain genes exhibits allelic exclusion. The organization of the β-chain gene segments into two clusters means that if a nonproductive rearrangement occurs, the thymocyte can attempt a second rearrangement. This increases the likelihood that a productive rearrangement will be made for the β chain. Once a productive rearrangement occurs for one β-chain allele, the rearrangement of the other β allele is inhibited.

Allelic exclusion appears to be less stringent for the TCR α-chain genes. For example, analyses of T-cell clones expressing a functional $\alpha\beta$ T-cell receptor revealed a number of clones with productive rearrangements for both α-chain alleles. Furthermore, when an immature T-cell lymphoma expressing a particular $\alpha\beta$ T-cell receptor was subcloned, several subclones were obtained that expressed the same β-chain allele but a different α-chain allele from the original parent clone. Studies with transgenic mice also indicate that allelic ex-

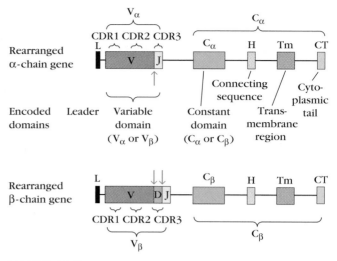

FIGURE 11-7

Schematic diagram of rearranged $\alpha\beta$-TCR genes showing the exons encoding the various domains of the $\alpha\beta$ T-cell receptor and approximate position of the CDRs. Junctional diversity (vertical arrows) generates CDR3 (see Figure 11-8). The structures of the rearranged γ- and δ-chain genes are similar although additional junctional diversity can occur in δ-chain genes.

clusion is less stringent for TCR α-chain genes than for β-chain genes. Mice carrying a productively rearranged $\alpha\beta$-TCR transgene do not rearrange and express the endogenous β-chain genes. However, the endogenous α-chain genes sometimes are expressed at varying levels in place of the already rearranged α-chain transgene.

Since allelic exclusion is not complete for the TCR α chain, more than one α chain is occasionally expressed on the membrane of a given T cell. The obvious question is how do the rare T cells that express two $\alpha\beta$ T-cell receptors maintain a single antigen-binding specificity? One possibility, suggested by some researchers, is that when a T cell expresses two different $\alpha\beta$ T-cell receptors, only one is likely to be self-MHC restricted and therefore functional.

Structure of Rearranged TCR Genes

The general structure of rearranged TCR genes is shown in Figure 11-7. The variable regions of T-cell receptors are, of course, encoded by rearranged VDJ and VJ sequences. In TCR genes, combinatorial joining of V gene segments appears to generate CDR1 and CDR2, whereas junctional flexibility and N-region nucleotide addition generate CDR3. Rearranged TCR genes also contain a short leader (L) exon upstream of the joined VJ or VDJ sequences. The amino acids encoded by the leader exon are cleaved as the nascent polypeptide enters the endoplasmic reticulum.

The constant region of each TCR chain is encoded by a C gene segment that has multiple exons corresponding to the structural domains in the protein (see Figure 11-3). The first exon in the C gene segment encodes the majority of the corresponding chain's C domain. Next is a short exon encoding the connecting sequence, followed by exons encoding the transmembrane region and cytoplasmic tail.

Generation of TCR Diversity

Although TCR germ-line DNA contains far fewer V gene segments than Ig germ-line DNA, a number of features contribute to generating more diversity among T-cell receptors than antibodies. Table 11-2 and Figure 11-8 compare the generation of diversity among antibody molecules and TCR molecules.

Combinatorial joining of variable-region gene segments generates a large number of random gene com-

binations for all the TCR chains, as it does for the Ig heavy- and light-chain genes. For example, $100 \, V_\alpha$ and $50 \, J_\alpha$ gene segments can generate 5×10^3 possible VJ combinations for the TCR α chain. Similarly, $25 \, V_\beta$, $2 \, D_\beta$, and $12 \, J_\beta$ gene segments can give 6×10^2 possible combinations. Although there are fewer TCR V_α and V_β gene segments than immunoglobulin V_H and V_κ segments, this difference is offset by the greater number of J segments in TCR germ-line DNA. Assuming that the antigen-binding specificity of a given T-cell receptor depends upon the variable region in both chains, random association of $5 \times 10^3 \, V_\alpha$ combinations with $6 \times 10^2 \, V_\beta$ combinations can generate a minimum of 3×10^6 possible combinations for the $\alpha\beta$ T-cell receptor.

As illustrated in Figure 11-8b, the location of one-turn (12-bp) and two-turn (23-bp) recognition signal sequences in TCR β- and δ-chain DNA differs from that in Ig heavy-chain DNA. Because of the arrangement of the recognition signal sequences in TCR germ-line

TABLE 11 - 2

COMPARISON OF POSSIBLE DIVERSITY IN MOUSE IMMUNOGLOBULIN AND TCR GENES

MECHANISM OF DIVERSITY	IMMUNOGLOBULINS		$\alpha\beta$ T-CELL RECEPTOR		$\gamma\delta$ T-CELL RECEPTOR	
	H CHAIN	κ CHAIN	α CHAIN	β CHAIN	γ CHAIN	δ CHAIN
ESTIMATED NUMBER OF SEGMENTS						
Multiple germ-line gene segments						
V	300	300	100	25	7	10
D	12	0	0	2	0	2
J	4	4	50	12	3	2
POSSIBLE NUMBER OF COMBINATIONS *						
Combinatorial V-J and V-D-J joining	$300 \times 12 \times 4$ $= 1.4 \times 10^4$	300×4 $= 1.2 \times 10^3$	100×50 $= 5 \times 10^3$	$25 \times 2 \times 12$ $= 6 \times 10^2$	7×3 $= 21$	$10 \times 2 \times 2$ $= 40$
Alternative joining of D gene segments	−	−	−	+ (some)	−	+ (often)
Junctional flexibility	+	+	+	+	+	+
N-region nucleotide addition [†]	+	−	+	+	+	+
P-region nucleotide addition	+	+	+	+	+	+
Somatic mutation	+	+	−	−	−	−
Total estimated diversity [‡]	$\sim 10^{11}$		$\sim 10^{15}$		$\sim 10^{18}$	

[*] A plus sign (+) indicates mechanism makes a significant contribution to diversity but to an unknown extent. A minus sign (−) indicates mechanism does not operate.

[†] See Figure 11-8d for theoretical number of combinations generated by N-region addition.

[‡] Total estimated diversity includes contribution from combinatorial association of chains.

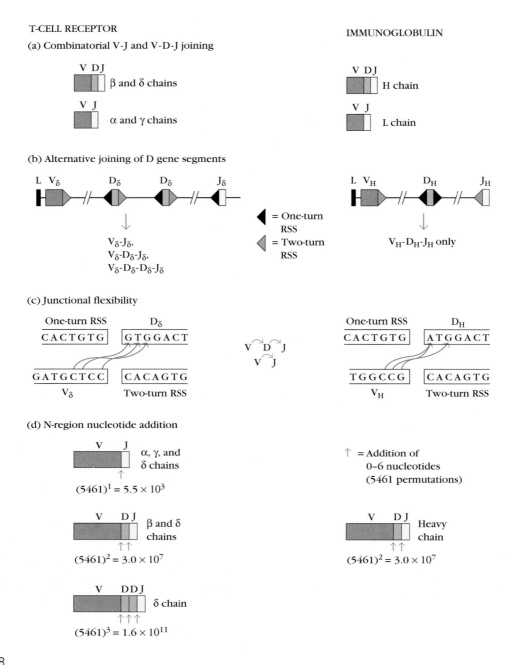

FIGURE 11-8

Comparison of mechanisms for generating diversity in TCR genes and immunoglobulin genes. In addition to the mechanisms shown, P-nucleotide addition occurs in both TCR and Ig genes, and somatic mutation occurs in Ig genes. Combinatorial association of the expressed chains generates additional diversity among TCR and Ig molecules.

DNA, **alternative joining of D gene segments** can occur while the one-turn/two-turn joining rule is observed. Thus, it is possible for a V_β gene segment to join directly with a J_β or D_β gene segment, generating a $(VJ)_\beta$ or $(VDJ)_\beta$ unit. Alternative joining of δ-chain gene segments generates similar units; in addition, one D_δ can join with another, yielding $(VDDJ)_\delta$ and in humans $(VDDDJ)_\delta$. This mechanism, which cannot occur in Ig heavy-chain DNA, generates considerable additional diversity in TCR genes.

The joining of gene segments during TCR-gene rearrangement exhibits **junctional flexibility**. As with the Ig genes, this flexibility can generate many nonproductive rearrangements, but it also increases diversity by encoding several alternative amino acids at each junction (see Figure 11-8c). In both Ig and TCR genes, nucleotides may be added at the junctions between some gene segments during rearrangement (see Figure 7-15). Variation in endonuclease cleavage of the hairpin generates additional nucleotides that are palindromic. Such **P-region nucleotide addition** can occur in the genes encoding all the TCR and Ig chains. Addition of **N-region nucleotides,** catalyzed by a terminal deoxynucleotidyl transferase, generates additional junctional diversity. Whereas N-region nucleotide addition occurs only in the Ig heavy-chain genes, it occurs in the genes encoding all the TCR chains. As many as six nucleotides can be added by this mechanism at each junction, generating up to 5461 possible combinations assuming random selection of nucleotides (see Figure 11-8d). Some of these combinations, however, lead to nonproductive rearrangements. Although each junctional region in a TCR gene encodes only 10–20 amino acids, enormous diversity can be generated in these regions. Estimates suggest that the combined effects of P- and N-region nucleotide addition and joining flexibility can generate as many as 10^{13} possible amino acid sequences in the TCR junctional regions alone.

The T-cell receptor must function to recognize both a very large number of different processed antigens and a relatively small number of self-MHC molecules. The way that diversity is generated for the TCR must allow the receptor to have the necessary variability needed for diverse peptide recognition while restricting its MHC-recognition diversity. As noted earlier, the CDR1 and CDR2 regions of the TCR, which are encoded by the V gene segments, are thought to contact the α-helices of MHC molecules. Moreover, TCR DNA has far fewer V gene segments than Ig DNA (see Table 11-2). It has been suggested that the relatively small number of V gene segments in TCR DNA have been selected to encode a limited number of CDR1 and CDR2 regions with affinity for regions of the α-helices of MHC molecules.

In contrast to the limited diversity of CDR1 and CDR2, the CDR3 of the TCR has even greater diversity than that seen in immunoglobulins. Diversity in the CDR3 region of the TCR is generated by junctional diversity in V-D-J joining, joining of multiple D gene segments, and the introduction of P and N nucleotides at the V-D-J and V-J junctions (see Figure 11-7). The CDR3 region most likely plays a major role in binding the antigenic peptide. Thus the added diversity of the CDR3 region may enable this region of the TCR to recognize a large number of different peptides.

Unlike the Ig genes, the TCR genes do not appear to undergo extensive somatic mutation. That is, the functional TCR genes generated during T-cell maturation in the thymus are generally the same as those found in the mature peripheral T-cell population. The absence of somatic mutation in T cells ensures that T-cell specificity does not change after thymic selection and therefore reduces any possibility that random mutation might generate a self-reactive T cell. Although a few experiments have provided evidence for somatic mutation of receptor genes in T cells in the germinal center, this appears to be the exception and not the rule.

T-CELL RECEPTOR COMPLEX: TCR-CD3

As discussed in Chapter 5, membrane-bound immunoglobulin on B cells associates with another membrane protein, the Ig-α/Ig-β heterodimer, to form the B-cell antigen receptor (see Figure 5-13). Similarly, the T-cell receptor associates with **CD3**, forming the TCR-CD3 membrane complex. In both cases, the accessory molecule is involved in signal transduction after interaction of a B or T cell with antigen.

The first evidence suggesting that the T-cell receptor is associated with another membrane molecule came from experiments in which fluorescent antibody to the receptor was shown to "co-cap" another membrane protein designated CD3. Later experiments by J. P. Allison and L. Lanier demonstrated that the T-cell receptor and CD3 are located quite close together in the T-cell membrane. These researchers first treated a T-cell membrane preparation with a cross-linking agent that spans 12 Å, and then precipitated the T-cell receptor with anti-TCR monoclonal antibody. Analysis of the precipitated T-cell receptors showed that they were cross-linked to CD3 molecules, indicating that the two proteins must be positioned within 12 Å of each other in the membrane.

Subsequent experiments demonstrated not only that CD3 is closely associated with the $\alpha\beta$ heterodimer but also that its expression is required for membrane expression of $\alpha\beta$ and $\gamma\delta$ T-cell receptors. Thus each heterodimer exists as a molecular complex with CD3 on the T-cell membrane. Loss of the genes encoding either CD3 or the TCR chains results in loss of the entire molecular complex from the membrane, demonstrating the obligate requirement for coexpression of both CD3 and the T-cell receptor on the membrane.

CD3 is a complex of five invariant polypeptide chains that associate to form three dimers: a heterodimer of gamma and epsilon chains ($\gamma\varepsilon$), a heterodimer of delta and epsilon chains ($\delta\varepsilon$), and a homodimer of two zeta chains ($\zeta\zeta$) or a heterodimer of zeta and eta chains ($\zeta\eta$) (Figure 11-9). The ζ and η chains, which are encoded by the same gene, differ in their carboxyl-terminal ends due to differences in RNA splicing of the primary transcript. About 90% of the CD3 complexes examined to date

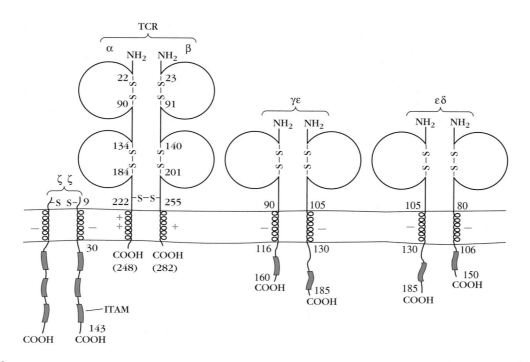

FIGURE 11-9

Schematic diagram of the TCR-CD3 complex, which constitutes the T-cell antigen-binding receptor. The figure shows the $\alpha\beta$ T-cell receptor and CD3 complex consisting of the $\zeta\zeta$ homodimer plus $\gamma\varepsilon$ and $\delta\varepsilon$ heterodimers. The external domains of the γ, δ, and ε chains of CD3 are similar to the immunoglobulin-fold structure, which may facilitate their interaction with the T-cell receptor and each other.

Ionic interactions also may occur between the oppositely charged transmembrane regions in the TCR and CD3 chains. The long cytoplasmic tails of the CD3 chains contain a common sequence, the immunoreceptor tyrosine-based activation motif (ITAM), which functions in signal transduction.

incorporate the $\zeta\zeta$ homodimer; the remainder have the $\zeta\eta$ heterodimer. The T-cell receptor complex can thus be envisioned as four dimers: The $\alpha\beta$ or $\gamma\delta$ TCR heterodimer determines the ligand-binding specificity, whereas the CD3 dimers ($\gamma\varepsilon$, $\delta\varepsilon$, and $\zeta\zeta$ or $\zeta\eta$) are required for expression of the T-cell receptor and for signal transduction.

The γ, δ, and ε chains of CD3 are members of the immunoglobulin superfamily, each containing an immunoglobulin-like extracellular domain followed by a transmembrane region and a cytoplasmic domain of more than 40 amino acids. The ζ and η chains have a distinctly different structure: Both have a very short external region of only 9 amino acids, a transmembrane region, and a long cytoplasmic tail containing 113 amino acids in ζ and 155 amino acids in η. The transmembrane region of all the CD3 polypeptide chains contains a negatively charged aspartic acid residue. These negatively charged groups may enable the CD3 complex to interact with one or two positively charged amino acids that are present in the transmembrane region of each TCR chain.

The cytoplasmic tails of the CD3 chains contain a motif called the **immunoreceptor tyrosine-based activation motif** (ITAM). This motif is found in a number of other receptors including the Ig-α/Ig-β heterodimer of the B-cell receptor complex and Fc receptors for IgE and IgG. The ITAM sites have been shown to interact with tyrosine kinases and to play an important role in signal transduction. In CD3, the γ, δ, and ε chains each contain a single copy of ITAM, whereas the ζ and η chains contain three copies (see Figure 11-9). The function of CD3 in signal transduction is discussed more fully in Chapter 12.

T-CELL ACCESSORY MEMBRANE MOLECULES

Although recognition of antigen–MHC complexes is mediated solely by the TCR–CD3 complex, a variety of other membrane molecules play an important accessory role in antigen recognition and T-cell activation (Table

11-3). Some of these accessory molecules strengthen the interaction between T cells and antigen-presenting cells or target cells; some act in signal transduction; and some exhibit both functions.

CD4 and CD8 Coreceptors

T cells can be subdivided based on their expression of CD4 or CD8 membrane molecules. As discussed in previous chapters, CD4$^+$ T cells recognize antigen in association with class II MHC molecules and largely function as helper cells, whereas CD8$^+$ T cells recognize antigen in association with class I MHC molecules and largely function as cytotoxic cells. CD4 is a 55-kDa monomeric membrane glycoprotein that contains four extracellular immunoglobulin-like domains (D_1–D_4), a hydrophobic transmembrane region, and a long cytoplasmic tail containing three serine residues, which can be phosphorylated. CD8 generally is present as a disulfide-linked $\alpha\beta$ heterodimer and less frequently as an $\alpha\alpha$ homodimer. Both the α and β chains of CD8 are small glycoproteins of approximately 30–38 kDa. Each chain consists of a single extracellular immunoglobulin-like domain, a hydrophobic transmembrane region, and a cytoplasmic tail containing 25–27 residues, several of which can be phosphorylated. The schematic diagrams of the CD4 and CD8 structures in Figure 11-10 show their various domains.

Both CD4 and CD8 possess two key properties that allow these membrane molecules to be classified as **coreceptors**: recognition of the peptide-MHC complex and signal transduction. The extracellular domains of CD4 and CD8 bind to the membrane-proximal domains of MHC molecules on APCs or target cells: CD4 binds

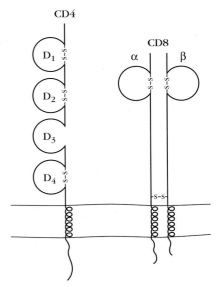

FIGURE 11-10

General structure of the CD4 and CD8 coreceptors. CD8 usually is present as an $\alpha\beta$ heterodimer, but occasionally is found as an α homodimer. The monomeric CD4 molecule contains four Ig-fold domains, whereas each chain in the CD8 molecule contains one Ig-fold domain.

to the β_2 domain of class II MHC molecules (Figure 11-11), whereas CD8 binds to the α_3 domain of MHC class I. This interaction apparently functions to increase the avidity of the interaction between a T-cell receptor and a peptide-MHC complex. The binding of T-cell receptors to peptide-MHC complexes has been shown to be augmented about 100-fold by the presence of CD4 or CD8

TABLE 11-3

SELECTED T-CELL ACCESSORY MOLECULES

NAME	LIGAND	ADHESION	SIGNAL TRANSDUCTION	MEMBER OF Ig SUPERFAMILY
CD4	Class II MHC	+	+	+
CD8	Class I MHC	+	+	+
CD2 (LFA-2)	CD58 (LFA-3)	+	+	+
LFA-1 (CD 11a/CD18)	ICAM-1 (CD54)	+	?	+/(−)
CD28	B7	?	+	+
CTLA-4	B7	?	+	−
CD45R	CD22	+	+	+
CD5	CD72	?	+	−

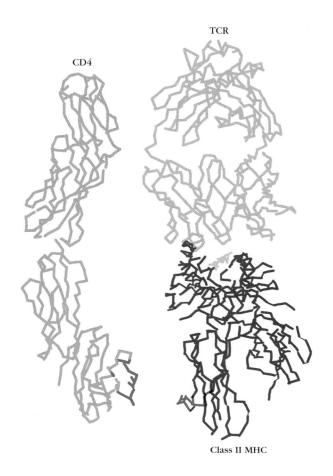

CD4

TCR

Class II MHC

FIGURE 11-11

Model of the external domains of CD4 (orange), T-cell receptor (blue), and class II MHC molecule (green) showing their orientation to each other. The top of the CD4 and TCR models in this figure would be anchored in the T-cell membrane; the bottom of the class II MHC molecule would be anchored in the membrane of an antigen-presenting cell. Interaction between CD4 and the β_2 domain in the class II molecule is mediated by the residues in red. The antigenic peptide is in pink. [From S. J. Davis and P. A. van der Merwe, 1996, *Immunol. Today* **17**(4):181.]

Recent evidence suggests that during antigen recognition by a T_H cell a TCR molecule first binds to a dimer of the class II MHC molecule. The membrane-distal domain of CD4 then binds to the β_2 domain of the class II MHC molecule, forming a ternary complex of TCR, CD4, and MHC (Figure 11-13a). Once bound to the MHC molecule, the CD4 molecule is thought to undergo a conformational change, enabling its membrane-proximal domains to interact with the membrane-proximal domains of an adjacent CD4 molecule that has complexed in a similar manner with a TCR and MHC molecule. Eventually a tetrameric structure (or even larger oligomeric structure) will be formed on the membrane (Figure 11-13b). This cross-linkage of the TCRs on a T cell, forming a lattice-type structure, may be necessary for transmembrane signaling events. It is not known whether CD8 binding to class I MHC molecules forms a similar oligomeric structure or not.

Other Accessory Membrane Molecules

In addition to CD4 and CD8, T cells possess several other accessory membrane molecules including CD2, LFA-1, CD28, and CD45R. Unlike the CD4 and CD8 coreceptors, the other accessory molecules do not interact with the peptide-MHC complex; rather, these addi-

on the membrane. The signal-transduction property of CD4 and CD8 is mediated through their cytoplasmic domains. Both CD4 and CD8 are noncovalently associated with the protein tyrosine kinase Lck. This interaction, which is essential for effective signal transduction, is similar to interaction of the B-cell coreceptor with the Lyn kinase (Figure 11-12).

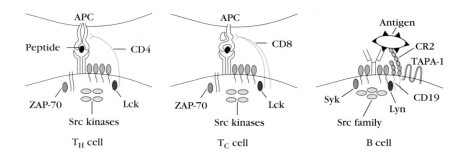

FIGURE 11-12

Comparison of interactions involving T-cell and B-cell coreceptors. The external domain of the T-cell coreceptors, CD4 and CD8, interact with MHC molecules, and the cytoplasmic tail interacts with the Lck protein tyrosine kinase. The B-cell coreceptor comprises three mole-

cules: TAPA-1; CR2, which interacts with complement on antigen; and CD19, whose cytoplasmic tail interacts with Lyn, another protein tyrosine kinase. Both T-cell and B-cell coreceptors increase the avidity of the antigen-receptor interaction and function in signal transduction.

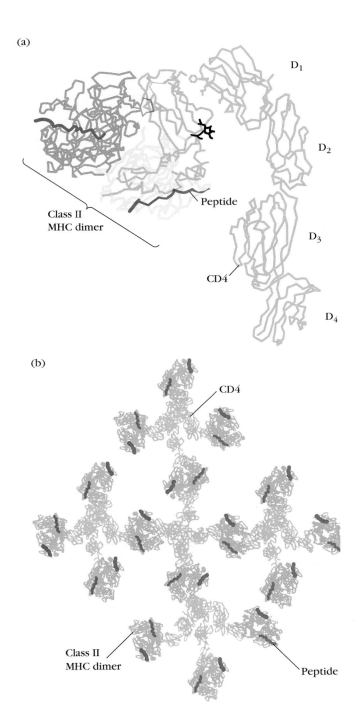

(a)

D₁

D₂

Peptide

Class II
MHC dimer

D₃

CD4

D₄

(b)

CD4

Class II
MHC dimer

Peptide

FIGURE 11-13

Models of interaction between CD4 and class II MHC molecule during antigen recognition. (a) Following binding of a T-cell receptor (not shown) to the dimer form of a class II MHC molecule (pink/blue), the membrane-distal D_1 domain of CD4 (green) interacts with the β_2 domain of the MHC molecule. (b) A lattice-type structure is formed by interaction of the membrane-proximal domains of CD4 with adjacent CD4 molecules that also are complexed to a TCR and MHC molecule. The peptide is represented by the red ribbon.

tional accessory molecules bind to other ligands present on antigen-presenting cells or target cells (see Table 11-3). These interactions strengthen the association between a T cell and an antigen-presenting cell or a target cell. As T cells are activated, the strength of adhesion between some of these accessory molecules and their respective ligands has been shown to increase, thereby prolonging the association between the interacting cells and providing time for directed secretion of various cytokines or lytic enzymes (see Chapter 16). Like CD4 and CD8, some of these other accessory molecules also function as signal-transducing molecules. The important role of these accessory molecules is demonstrated by the ability of monoclonal antibodies specific for these molecules to block T-cell activation.

Figure 11-14 schematically depicts the interactions between various T_H- and T_C-cell accessory membrane molecules and their ligands on antigen-presenting cells and target cells, respectively.

TERNARY TCR-PEPTIDE-MHC COMPLEX

Although the interaction between the T-cell receptor, an antigenic peptide, and an MHC molecule is central to development of both humoral and cell-mediated responses, the nature of this trimolecular complex is still being unraveled. As indicated earlier, the TCR recognizes complexes consisting of a peptide and MHC molecule, exhibiting specificity for both the peptide and MHC molecule. In this section, we discuss what is known about the details of this critical ternary interaction.

Evidence That TCR Alone Recognizes Peptide-MHC Complex

Discovery of CD3, CD4, and CD8 raised the possibility that these molecules associated with the TCR might be necessary for antigen recognition by T cells. The experiment of Kappler and Marrack outlined in Figure 11-2 supported the notion that a single receptor on the T cell recognizes peptide complexed to a self-MHC molecule. However, that experiment did not rule out the possibility that another membrane molecule, associated with the T-cell receptor, might contribute to recognition of either the peptide or MHC molecule.

A definitive experiment proving that the $\alpha\beta$ T-cell receptor alone recognizes both peptide and MHC molecules used an approach similar to that of the earlier Kappler and Marrack experiment but involved gene transfection instead of cell fusion. Functional TCR α- and β-chain genes from a T_C-cell clone specific for one

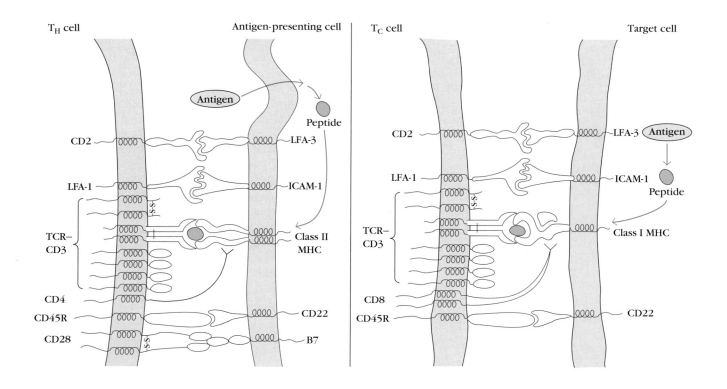

FIGURE 11-14

Schematic diagram of the interactions between the T-cell receptor and various accessory molecules with their ligands on an antigen-presenting cell (*left*) or target cell (*right*). Binding of the coreceptors, CD4 and CD8, and the other accessory molecules to their ligands strengthens the association between the interacting cells and/or aids in the signal transduction leading to T-cell activation.

hapten on H-2^d target cells were transfected into another T$_C$–cell clone specific for a different hapten on H-2^k target cells (Figure 11-15). The transfected cells expressed both their own T-cell receptor and the new transfected T-cell receptor. Cytolysis assays showed that the transfected cells recognized both hapten–MHC molecule complexes for which the original T$_C$ clones were specific; however the transfected cells did not recognize either hapten when it was presented on target cells of a different MHC haplotype. In other words, transfection of the TCR genes alone transferred reactivity to both a particular antigen and a particular MHC molecule.

Interactions Involved in Forming Ternary Complex

Both the α and β chains of the TCR heterodimer have been shown to make an equal contribution to the recognition of peptides and MHC molecules. One chain is not specific for peptide recognition and the other chain specific for MHC recognition. In addition, it is known that the same V regions of the TCR α and β chains recognize both peptide–class I MHC complexes and peptide–class II MHC complexes. That is, there do not seem to be separate V-region sequences specific for class I and class II MHC molecules. What is less clear is the relative contribution of TCR-MHC contact and TCR-peptide contact to formation of the trimolecular complex.

The high degree of TCR specificity for both antigenic peptides and MHC molecules must be achieved through the diversity of the variable region of the T-cell receptor. Although crystallographic analysis of the T-cell receptor has not been achieved as yet, the similarity between TCR and immunoglobulin genes suggests that the T-cell receptor resembles an Fab-like structure whose variable domains are folded in a β-pleated sheet structure with the CDRs facing outward. The most likely hypothesis is that the CDRs, the most diverse regions within the TCR variable domains, are involved in the TCR-peptide and TCR-MHC interactions. Various experimental results suggest that the two CDR3 loops interact with antigenic peptides, while the CDR1 and CDR2 loops are thought to interact with MHC molecules.

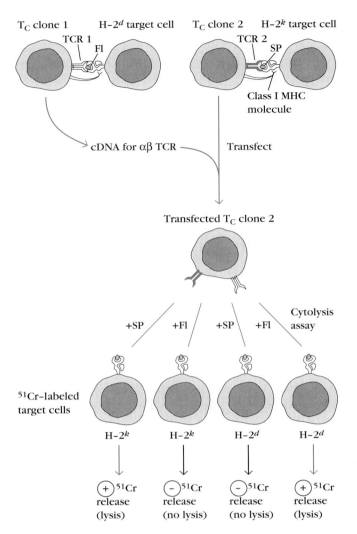

FIGURE 11-15

Experimental demonstration that the $\alpha\beta$ T-cell receptor alone recognizes both peptide and MHC molecules. cDNA corresponding to the $\alpha\beta$ T-cell receptor was prepared from T_C clone 1, which was specific for fluorescein (Fl) presented on H-2^d target cells. This cDNA was transfected into T_C clone 2, specific for 3-(p-sulphophenyldiazo)-4-hydroxy-phenylacetic acid (SP) on H-2^k target cells. The transfected cells were assayed for their ability to kill H-2^d and H-2^k target cells in the presence of Fl or SP. The target cells were labeled intracellularly with ^{51}Cr, and upon lysis ^{51}Cr was released into the media. The transfected cells could kill only those target cells presenting antigen associated with the original MHC restriction molecule.

Figure 11-16 schematically illustrates the current model of the interaction between a T-cell receptor, antigenic peptide, and MHC molecule. The peptide-binding site of the T-cell receptor appears to map to CDR3, while CDR1 and CDR2 interact with MHC molecules. As discussed in Chapter 9, the peptide-binding site

of the MHC molecule lies in a cleft between the α_1 and α_2 domains of class I molecules and between the α_1 and β_1 domains of class II molecules (see Figure 9-5). These same membrane-distal domains are involved in the interaction of MHC molecules with the T-cell receptor. The site on an antigenic peptide that interacts with a T-cell receptor is called the **epitope**, and the site that interacts with an MHC molecule is the **agretope**.

Affinity of TCR for Peptide-MHC Complexes

The affinity of T-cell receptors for peptide-MHC complexes is low, with K_d values ranging from 10^{-4} to 10^{-7} M. Thus this interaction is quite weak compared with the antigen-antibody interaction, which generally has a K_d ranging from 10^{-7} to 10^{-11} M. The low affinity of the T-cell receptor for antigenic peptide–MHC complexes means that the binding of a T cell to an antigen-presenting cell or target cell cannot depend solely on interaction of the TCR with a peptide-MHC complex. Instead, cell-adhesion molecules are thought to initiate the contact between a T cell and an antigen-presenting cell or a target cell (Figure 11-14). Once cell-to-cell contact is made, the T-cell receptor may scan the membrane for peptide-MHC complexes. During T-cell activation by a particular peptide-MHC complex, there is a transient increase in accessory membrane molecules (e.g., CD2, LFA-1), allowing close contact between the interacting cells so that cytokines or cytotoxic substances may

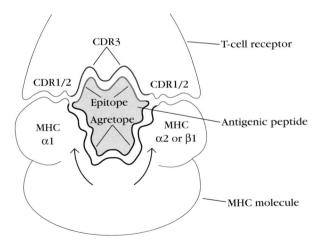

FIGURE 11-16

Schematic diagram showing the various sites in a T-cell receptor, antigenic peptide, and MHC molecule that interact in the TCR-peptide-MHC trimolecular complex. [Adapted from J. McCluskey et al., 1992, in *Antigen Processing and Recognition*, CRC Press.]

be released at the junction between the cells. Within a short time of activation, the enhanced adhesion declines and the T cell detaches from the antigen-presenting cell or target cell.

Influence of Peptide on Topology of Ternary Complex

Although CDR1 and CDR2 of the T-cell receptor interact with MHC molecules, the interaction of CDR3 with the peptide may play the most significant role in determining the final configuration of the TCR-peptide-MHC complex. E. W. Ehrlich and coworkers have obtained results suggesting that the TCR-MHC interaction is quite fluid and that different TCR-MHC interactions can be obtained depending upon which peptide is bound. In their experiments they used T cells from transgenic mice expressing an $\alpha\beta$-TCR transgene that could cross-react with two peptides of moth cytochrome c differing from each other by a single amino acid substitution. They measured the responses of the transgenic T cells to each peptide presented by 13 mutant MHC molecules that differed from each other by a single amino acid predicted to be in the a helices of the MHC molecule and to point up toward the T-cell receptor. The results showed that the T-cell response to the mutant MHC molecules depended upon which peptide was being recognized. This finding suggests that the interactions between CDR1 and CDR2 sequences and an MHC molecule vary depending upon the peptide that is carried by the MHC molecule. The final configuration of the trimolecular complex thus appears to be determined by the interaction of the peptide with CDR3 of the T-cell receptor.

ALLOREACTIVITY OF T CELLS

So far the discussion of MHC molecules has focused on their role in antigen presentation. However, as noted in Chapter 9, MHC molecules were first identified because of their role in rejection of foreign tissue. Graft-rejection reactions result from the direct response of T cells to MHC molecules, which function as **histocompatibility antigens**. Because of the extreme polymorphism of the MHC, most individuals of the same species have a unique set of histocompatibility antigens. Therefore, T cells respond even to **allogeneic** grafts (alloreactivity), and MHC molecules are considered **alloantigens**. Generally, CD4+ T cells respond to class II alloantigens, and CD8+ T cells respond to class I alloantigens.

The alloreactivity of T cells is troubling for two reasons. First, the ability of T cells to respond to allogeneic

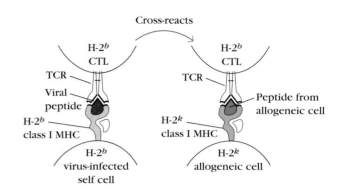

FIGURE 11-17

Possible mechanism of T-cell cross-reactivity that would explain the observed high incidence of alloreactive T cells. As schematically illustrated, a T-cell receptor specific for an H-2^b class I MHC molecule plus viral peptide (*left*) cross-reacts with an allogeneic H-2^k class I molecule plus an allogeneic peptide (*right*). According to this model, the conformation of the allogeneic peptide–MHC complex and foreign peptide–self-MHC complex is sufficiently similar that the same TCR recognizes both complexes.

histocompatibility antigens alone appears to contradict all the evidence indicating that T cells can respond only to foreign antigen plus self-MHC molecules. In responding to allogeneic grafts, however, T cells recognize a foreign MHC molecule directly, instead of responding to an antigen that has been processed and presented together with a self-MHC molecule. A second problem posed by the T-cell response to allogeneic MHC molecules is that the frequency of alloreactive T cells is quite high; it has been estimated that 1%–5% of all T cells are alloreactive, which is far higher than the frequency of T cells reactive with a particular foreign antigenic peptide plus self-MHC molecule. This finding is troubling because the high frequency of alloreactive T cells appears to contradict the basic tenet of clonal selection. If 1 T cell in 20 reacts with a given alloantigen and if one assumes there are on the order of 100 distinct H-2 haplotypes in mice, then there are not enough distinct T-cell specificities to cover all the unique H-2 alloantigens, let alone foreign antigens displayed by self-MHC molecules.

One possible biologically satisfying explanation for the high frequency of alloreactive T cells is that a particular T-cell receptor is not only specific for a foreign antigenic peptide plus a self-MHC molecule but also can cross-react with certain allogeneic MHC molecules. In other words, if an allogeneic MHC molecule plus allogeneic peptide structurally resembles a processed foreign peptide plus self-MHC molecule, the same T-cell receptor may recognize both peptide-MHC complexes (Figure 11-17). Since allogeneic cells express on the order of 10^5 class I MHC molecules per cell, T cells bearing low-affinity cross-reactive receptors might be able to bind by virtue of the high density of membrane alloantigen. Foreign antigen, on the other hand, would be sparsely displayed on the membrane of an antigen-presenting cell or altered self-cell associated with class I or class II MHC molecules, limiting responsiveness to only those T cells bearing high-affinity receptors.

Experimental evidence that antigen-specific T cells can also be alloreactive has come from studies with a number of T-cell clones. For example, after immunizing an H-2^a haplotype mouse with DNP-OVA, B. Sredni and R. H. Schwarz were able to obtain a T-cell clone that responded to DNP-OVA associated with a class II IA^a molecule. This same clone, however, also responded to allogeneic cells bearing IA^s in the absence of DNP-OVA. To determine the frequency of such antigen-specific and alloreactive T cells, Sredni and Schwarz immunized three congenic strains (B10.A, B10, and B10.S) with DNP-OVA and then isolated 20–40 antigen-specific clones from each strain. Each antigen-specific clone was then tested for alloreactivity against cells expressing different MHC haplotypes in the absence of antigen. Between 19% and 44% of the antigen-specific clones were able to respond to allogeneic cells. These findings support the hypothesis that the high percentage of alloreactive T cells reflects the existence of antigen-specific T cells whose receptor recognizes antigen plus a self-MHC molecule but can cross-react with various allogeneic MHC molecules.

SUMMARY

1. T-cell receptors, unlike antibodies, do not react with soluble antigen but rather with processed antigen associated with a self-MHC molecule on an antigen-presenting cell or a target cell. Kappler and Marrack demonstrated that a single TCR molecule interacts with both an antigenic peptide and MHC molecule (see Figure 11-2). T-cell receptors, first isolated by means of clonotypic monoclonal antibodies, are heterodimers consisting of an α and β chain or a γ and δ chain.

2. T-cell receptors are organized into variable and constant domains, which are thought to have the immunoglobulin-fold structure, similar to those in immunoglobulins (see Figure 11-3). The TCR variable region domains contain three hypervariable complementarity-determining regions (CDRs), which appear to be equivalent to those in immunoglobulins. Each chain in a TCR molecule also contains a short membrane-proximal connecting region, a hydrophobic transmembrane segment, and a short cytoplasmic tail.

3. TCR germ-line DNA is organized into multigene families corresponding to the α, β, γ, and δ chains. Each multigene family contains multiple variable-region gene segments (V and J in α- and γ-chain DNA and V, D, and J in β- and δ-chain DNA) and one or more constant-region C gene segments (see Figure 11-5). By mechanisms similar to those used by B cells to rearrange immunoglobulin germ-line DNA, T cells rearrange the variable-region TCR gene segments to form functional genes encoding either the TCR α and β chains or γ and δ chains.

4. The mechanisms generating TCR diversity are generally similar to those generating antibody diversity (see Table 11-2 and Figure 11-8). However, during rearrangement of TCR β- and δ-chain gene segments alternative joining of V, D, and J segments can occur and random N-region nucleotides can be added at the junctions between gene segments encoding all the chains. Because of these mechanisms, the potential diversity of TCR genes is significantly greater than that of immunoglobulin genes, even though somatic mutation does not occur in TCR genes, as it does in immunoglobulin genes.

5. The T-cell receptor is closely associated with CD3, a complex of five different polypeptide chains that associate to form three dimers (see Figure 11-9). Both the T-cell receptor and CD3 are coexpressed on the membrane of T cells. The cytoplasmic tail of each CD3 chain contains a common sequence known as the immunoreceptor tyrosine-based activation motif (ITAM); this motif is involved in signal transduction following interaction of a T-cell receptor and peptide-MHC complex. ITAM is also present in the Ig-α/Ig-β heterodimer on B cells and in Fc receptors for IgE and IgG.

6. T cells possess several other membrane molecules that play accessory roles in the interaction between T cells and antigen-presenting or target cells; some of these accessory molecules also function in signal transduction (see Table 11-3). The coreceptors CD4 and CD8 bind to the membrane-proximal domains of MHC molecules, thereby strengthening the relatively weak interaction between the T-cell receptor and peptide-MHC complex. CD4 and CD8 also participate in signal transduction via their long cytoplasmic tails, which are associated with a cytosolic protein kinase. The other accessory membrane molecules (e.g., CD2, LFA-1, CD28, and CD45R) each interact with their own ligand on antigen-presenting cells or target cells (see Figure 11-14).

7. Formation of the TCR-antigen-MHC complex, which is essential for an immune response, depends on several interactions (see Figure 11-16). The antigen-binding site of the T-cell receptor maps to

CDR3 and interacts with the epitope on the antigenic peptide. Sites in CDR1 and CDR2 of the T-cell receptor interact with the MHC membrane-distal domains. The peptide-binding cleft of the MHC molecule interacts with the agretope of the antigenic peptide.

8. T cells respond not only to complexes of a foreign antigenic peptide plus self-MHC molecule but also to foreign MHC molecules (histocompatibility antigens) alone. This T-cell response leads to rejection of allogeneic grafts. Some evidence suggests that this alloreactivity results from the ability of T cells specific for an antigenic peptide plus self-MHC molecule to cross-react with various allogeneic peptide–allogeneic MHC complexes (see Figure 11-17).

REFERENCES

BENTLEY, G. A., ET AL. 1995. Crystal structure of the β chain of a T cell antigen receptor. *Science* **267**:1984.

CHIEN, Y., AND M. M. DAVIS. 1993. How $\alpha\beta$ T-cell receptors "see" peptide/MHC complexes. *Immunol. Today* **14**:597.

CONSTANT, P., ET AL. 1994. Stimulation of human $\gamma\delta$ T cells by nonpeptide mycobacterial ligands. *Science* **264**:267.

DAVIS, M. M., AND Y. CHIEN. 1995. Issues concerning the nature of antigen recognition by $\alpha\beta$ and $\gamma\delta$ T-cell receptors. *Immunol. Today* **16**:316

EHRLICH, E. W., ET AL. 1993. T-cell receptor interaction with peptide/major histocompatibility complex (MHC) and superantigen/MHC ligands is dominated by antigen. *J. Exp. Med.* **178**:713.

FIELDS, B. A., ET AL. 1995. Crystal structure of the V_α domain of a T cell antigen receptor. *Science* **270**: 1821.

HEDRICK, S. M., ET AL. 1984. Isolation of cDNA clones encoding T cell–specific membrane-associated proteins. *Nature* **308**:149.

HONG, S. C., ET AL. 1992. An MHC interaction site maps to the amino-terminal half of the T-cell receptor α chain variable domain. *Cell* **69**:999.

JANEWAY, C. A. 1995. Ligands for the T-cell receptor: hard times for avidity models. *Immunol. Today* **16**:223.

JULIUS, M., C. R. MAROUN, AND L. HAUGH. 1993. Distinct roles for CD4 and CD8 as co-receptors in antigen receptor signalling. *Immunol. Today* **14**:177.

MOSS, P. A. H., W. M. C. ROSENBERG, AND J. I. BELL. 1993. The human T-cell receptor in health and disease. *Annu. Rev. Immunol.* **10**:71.

SAKIHAMA, T., A. SMOLYAR, AND E. L. REINHERZ. 1995. Molecular recognition of antigen between CD4, MHC class II and TCR molecules. *Immunol. Today* **16**:581.

TANAKA, Y., ET AL. 1994. Nonpeptide ligands for human $\gamma\delta$ T cells. *Proc. Nat'l. Acad. Sci. USA* **91**:8175.

TANAKA, Y., ET AL. 1995. Natural and synthetic nonpeptide antigens recognized by human $\gamma\delta$ T cells. *Nature* **375**:155.

YANAGI, Y., ET AL. 1984. A human T-cell specific cDNA clone encodes a protein having extensive homology to immunoglobulin chains. *Nature* **308**:145.

ZHU, C., AND D. B. ROTH. 1995. Characterization of coding ends in thymocytes of SCID mice: implications for the mechanism of V(D)J recombination. *Immunity* **2**:101.

ZINKERNAGEL, R. M., AND DOHERTY, P. C. 1974. Immunological surveillance against altered self-components by sensitized T lymphocytes in lymphocytic choriomeningitis. *Nature* **251**:547.

STUDY QUESTIONS

1. Indicate whether each of the following statements is true or false. If you think a statement is false, explain why.

a. Monoclonal antibody specific for CD4 will coprecipitate the T -cell receptor along with CD4.

b. Subtractive hybridization can be used to enrich for mRNA that is present in one cell type but absent in another cell type within the same species.

c. Clonotypic monoclonal antibody was used to isolate the T-cell receptor.

d. The T cell uses the same set of V, D, and J gene segments as the B cell but uses different C gene segments.

e. The $\alpha\beta$ TCR is bivalent and has two antigen-binding sites.

f. Each $\alpha\beta$ T cell expresses only one β-chain and one α-chain allele.

g. Even though TCR germ-line DNA contains fewer V gene segments than Ig germ-line DNA in the mouse, the potential estimated diversity of T-cell receptors is about the same as that of immunoglobulins.

h. The Ig-α/Ig-β heterodimer and CD3 serve analogous functions in the B-cell receptor and T-cell receptor, respectively.

2. Describe the critical experiment that proved that the $\alpha\beta$ T-cell receptor alone recognizes both antigen and MHC molecules.

3. Draw the basic structure of the $\alpha\beta$ T-cell receptor and compare it with the basic structure of membrane-bound immunoglobulin.

4. Several membrane molecules, in addition to the T-cell receptor, are involved in antigen recognition and T-cell activation. Describe the properties and distinct functions of the following T-cell membrane molecules: (a) CD3, (b) CD4 and CD8, and (c) CD2.

5. Indicate whether each of the properties listed below applies to the T-cell receptor (TCR), B-cell immunoglobulin (Ig), or both (TCR/Ig).

a. _____ Is associated with CD3

b. _____ Is monovalent

c. _____ Exists in membrane-bound and secreted forms

d. _____ Contains domains with the immunoglobulin-fold structure

e. _____ Is MHC restricted

f. _____ Exhibits diversity generated by imprecise joining of gene segments

g. _____ Exhibits diversity generated by somatic mutation

6. A major obstacle to identifying and cloning TCR genes is the low level of TCR mRNA in T cells.

a. To overcome this obstacle, Hedrick and Davis made three important assumptions that proved to be correct. Describe each assumption and how it facilitated identification of the genes encoding the T-cell receptor.

b. Suppose, instead, that Hedrick and Davis wanted to identify the genes encoding IL-4. What changes in the three assumptions should they make?

7. Hedrick and Davis used the technique of subtractive hybridization to isolate cDNA clones encoding the T-cell receptor. You wish to use this technique to isolate cDNA clones encoding several gene products and have available clones of various cell types to use as the source of cDNA or mRNA for hybridization. For each gene product listed in the left column of the table below, select the most appropriate cDNA and mRNA source clones from the following cell types: T_H1 cell line (A); T_H2 cell line (B); T_C cell line (C); macrophage (D); IgA-secreting myeloma cell (E); IgG-secreting myeloma cell (F); myeloid progenitor cell (G); and B-cell line (H). More than one cell type may be correct in some cases.

GENE PRODUCT	cDNA SOURCE	mRNA SOURCE
IL-2		
CD8		
J chain		
IL-1		
CD3		

8. Mice from different inbred strains listed in the *left* column of the accompanying table were infected with LCM virus. Spleen cells derived from these LCM-infected mice then were tested for their ability to lyse LCM-infected ^{51}Cr-labeled target cells from the strains *listed across the top of the table*. Indicate with (+) or (−) whether you would expect to see ^{51}Cr released from the labeled target cells.

For use with Question 8.

Source of spleen cells from LCM-infected mice	Release of ^{51}Cr from LCM-infected target cells			
	B10.D2 (H-2^d)	B10 (H-2^b)	B10.BR (H-2^k)	(BALB/c × B10) F$_1$ (H-$2^{b/d}$)
B10.D2 (H-2^d)				
B10 (H-2^b)				
BALB/c (H-2^d)				
BALB/b (H-2^b)				

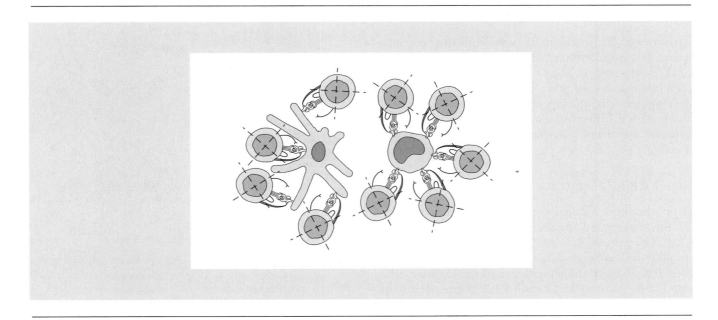

T-CELL MATURATION, ACTIVATION, AND DIFFERENTIATION

The attribute that distinguishes antigen recognition by T cells from that by B cells is MHC restriction. Both the maturation of progenitor T cells in the thymus and the activation of mature peripheral T cells are influenced by the involvement of MHC molecules. The potential antigenic diversity of T cells is reduced during maturation by a selection process that allows only MHC-restricted and nonself-reactive T cells to mature. The final stages in T-cell maturation proceed along two different developmental pathways, which generate functionally distinct CD4$^+$ and CD8$^+$ subpopulations that exhibit class II and class I MHC restriction, respectively.

Activation of mature peripheral T cells is initiated through the interaction of the T-cell receptor with an antigenic peptide displayed in the groove of an MHC molecule. The low affinity of this interaction necessitates the involvement of coreceptors and other accessory membrane molecules that function to strengthen the TCR–antigen–MHC interaction and to transduce the activating signal. Activation leads to the proliferation and differentiation of T cells into various types of effector cells and memory T cells. Because the vast majority of thymocytes and peripheral T cells express the $\alpha\beta$ T-cell receptor, all references to T cells and the T-cell receptor in this chapter denote the $\alpha\beta$ receptor unless otherwise indicated.

T-CELL MATURATION

Progenitor T cells from the bone marrow begin to migrate to the thymus at about day 11 of gestation in mice and in the eighth or ninth week of gestation in humans. The progenitor cells are attracted to the thymus by a chemotactic factor secreted by thymic epithelial cells. In a manner similar to B-cell maturation in the bone marrow, T-cell maturation is correlated with rearrangements of the germ-line TCR genes and expression of various membrane markers. However, in contrast to B-cell development thymocytes proliferate and differentiate along several different developmental pathways, which generate functionally distinct subpopulations of mature T cells.

Pre-T Cell Receptor

A novel complex called the **pre-T cell receptor** (pre TCR) is expressed on thymocytes that lack CD4 and CD8. The pre-TCR consists of the CD3 protein and a disulfide-linked heterodimer consisting of the β-chain of the TCR and a 33-kDa glycoprotein (gp33), now called pre-Tα. As illustrated in Figure 12-1, the general structure of the pre-TCR bears a striking similarity to the pre-BCR expressed by developing precursor B cells. Both pre-receptors consist of a complex of the first receptor chain to be expressed (μ heavy chain for the B cell and β chain for the T cell) complexed with a unique chain ($\lambda5$ for the B cell and pre-Tα for the T cell). The pre-BCR contains an additional noncovalently associated polypeptide, Vpre-B. Thus far, no such analogous component has been discovered for the pre-TCR, although its existence has been hypothesized.

The pre-TCR is thought to recognize some intrathymic ligand and transmit an activating signal through the CD3 complex that activates Lck, a protein tyrosine kinase. Signal transduction through the pre-TCR has several effects:

1. Recognizes that a productive TCR β-chain rearrangement has been made and selects those thymocytes expressing the β chain for further expansion and maturation
2. Suppresses further rearrangement of TCR β-chain genes so that allelic exclusion of the β chain will occur
3. Enhances rearrangement of the TCR α chain
4. Induces developmental progression to the CD4$^+$8$^+$ **double-positive** state

T-Cell Developmental Pathways

Changes in various membrane molecules and TCR-gene rearrangements during thymocyte development in the mouse have been studied with monoclonal antibodies and by restriction-endonuclease analyses of genomic DNA. The overall process is depicted in Figure 12-2. Upon entry into the thymus, progenitor T cells begin to express a membrane protein called **Thy-1,** which is a marker of all thymus-derived lymphocytes in

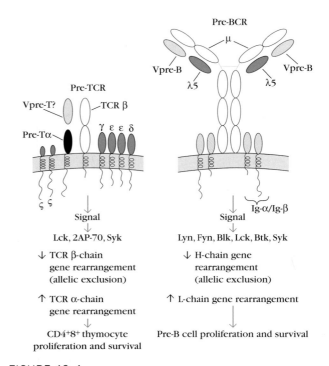

FIGURE 12-1

Comparison of the general structure of the pre-T cell receptor (pre-TCR) and pre-B cell receptor (pre-BCR) and the effects of activating them. Binding of unknown ligands to the pre-TCR and pre-BCR are thought to generate intracellular signals leading to generation of pre-T cells (CD4$^+$8$^+$ thymocytes) and pre-B cells.

the mouse. The earliest fetal thymocytes lack detectable CD4 and CD8 and are referred to as **double-negative,** or CD4$^-$8$^-$, cells. These double-negative thymocytes differentiate along one of two developmental pathways.

Those thymocytes that make productive rearrangements of both the γ- and δ-chain genes develop into double-negative, CD3$^+$ $\gamma\delta$ T cells, which account for only 0.5%–1.0% of thymocytes in adults. This thymocyte subpopulation can be detected by day 14 of gestation, reaches maximal numbers between days 17 and 18, and then declines until birth (Figure 12-3).

The majority of double-negative thymocytes progress down a different developmental pathway. They begin to rearrange the TCR β-chain genes and express the β chain with the pre-T α chain as a pre-T cell receptor. Once a signal is transmitted through the pre-TCR it halts further β-chain gene rearrangement and induces expression of both CD4 and CD8. The thymocytes at this stage are called **double-positive,** or CD4$^+$8$^+$, cells. These double-positive thymocytes begin to proliferate. During this proliferative phase, TCR α-chain gene rearrangement does not occur even though both the *RAG-1* and *RAG-2* genes are transcriptionally active.

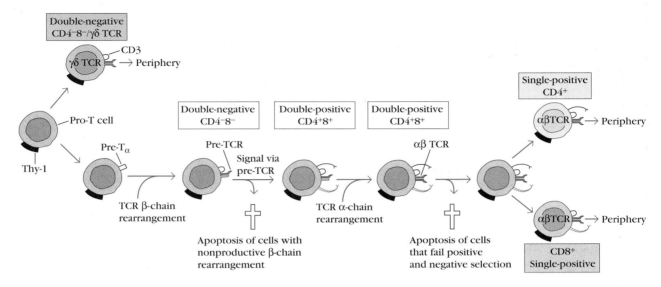

FIGURE 12-2

Proposed pathways for T-cell development in the thymus. Most of the immature thymocytes in the thymus die either because they make an unproductive TCR-gene rearrangement or because they fail positive or negative selection. Three mature T-cell populations (green, pink, blue) are produced and move to the peripheral lym-phoid organs. The vast majority of peripheral T cells express the $\alpha\beta$ TCR and either CD4 (blue) or CD8 (pink). A few T cells express the $\gamma\delta$ TCR (green); most of these lack both CD4 and CD8. [Adapted from B. J. Fowlkes and D. M. Pardoll, 1989, *Adv. Immunol.* 44:207.]

Rearrangement of the α-chain genes cannot take place at this stage because the RAG-2 protein is rapidly de-graded in proliferating cells. For this reason, α-chain gene rearrangement does not begin until the double-positive thymocytes stop proliferating and RAG-2 pro-tein levels increase. This proliferative phase contributes to T-cell diversity by generating a clone of cells with a sin-gle TCR β-chain rearrangement. Each of the cells with-in this clone can then rearrange different α-chain genes allowing for greater diversity. The TCR α-chain genes are not expressed until day 16 or 17 of gestation, and double-positive cells expressing both CD3 and the $\alpha\beta$ T-cell receptor begin to appear at day 17 and reach max-imal levels about the time of birth (see Figure 12-3).

An estimated 99% of all thymocytes do not mature and die by apoptosis within the thymus either because they fail to make a productive TCR-gene rearrangement or because they fail to survive thymic selection, which is discussed below. Double-positive thymocytes that ex-press the $\alpha\beta$ TCR-CD3 complex and survive thymic selection develop into either **single-positive CD4⁺** thymocytes, representing 10% of the total thymocyte population, or **single-positive CD8⁺** thymocytes, rep-resenting 5% of the total thymocyte population. These single-positive cells migrate to the periphery (see Figure 12-2). In addition, a small population (0.5%) of double-negative thymocytes expressing the TCR-CD3 complex can also be detected in the thymus. These cells appear late in development, usually within 5 days following birth. The origin of this population is uncertain, but it may develop from the single-positive populations through the loss of either CD4 or CD8.

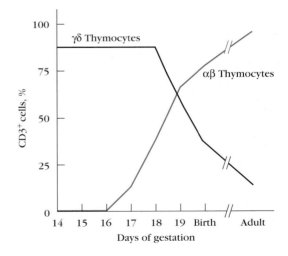

FIGURE 12-3

Time course of appearance of $\gamma\delta$ thymocytes and $\alpha\beta$ thymocytes during mouse fetal development. The graph shows the percentage of CD3⁺ cells in the thymus that are double-negative (CD4⁻8⁻) and bear the $\gamma\delta$ T-cell receptor (black) or are double-positive (CD4⁺8⁺) and bear the $\alpha\beta$ T-cell receptor (blue).

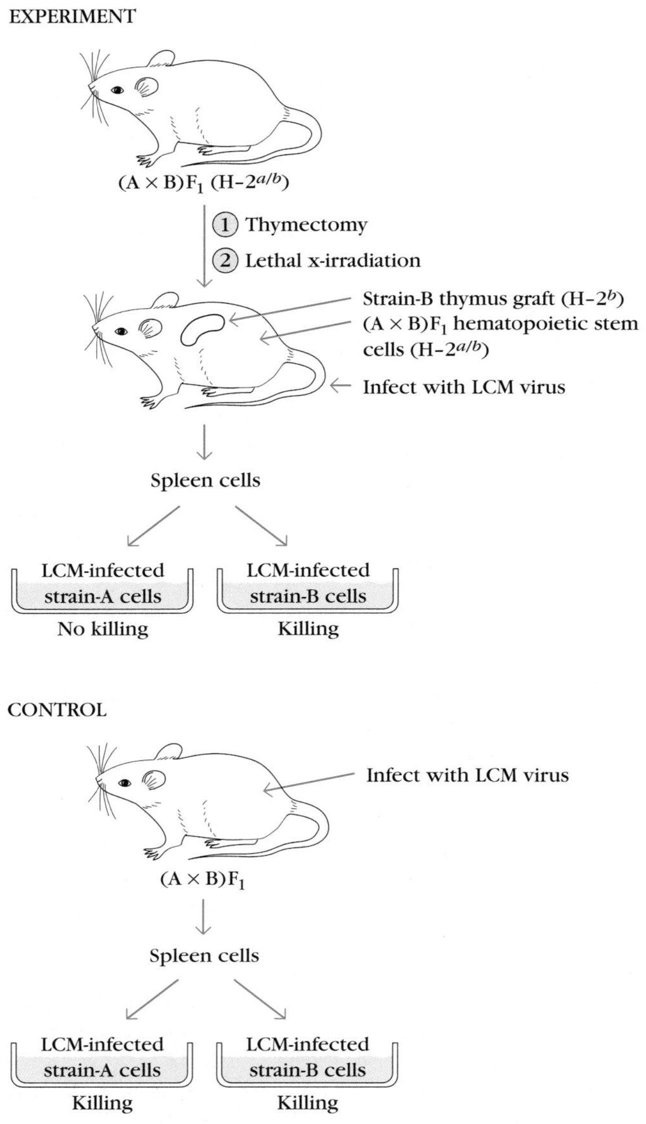

EXPERIMENT

$(A \times B)F_1$ (H-$2^{a/b}$)

① Thymectomy
② Lethal x-irradiation

Strain-B thymus graft (H-2^b)
$(A \times B)F_1$ hematopoietic stem
cells (H-$2^{a/b}$)

Infect with LCM virus

Spleen cells

LCM-infected
strain-A cells
No killing

LCM-infected
strain-B cells
Killing

CONTROL

Infect with LCM virus

$(A \times B)F_1$

Spleen cells

LCM-infected
strain-A cells
Killing

LCM-infected
strain-B cells
Killing

Thymic Selection of the T-Cell Repertoire

As discussed in the last chapter, random gene rearrangement within TCR germ-line DNA combined with
junctional diversity can potentially generate an enormous TCR repertoire with an estimated diversity ex-
ceeding 10^{15} for the $\alpha\beta$ receptor and 10^{18} for the $\gamma\delta$
receptor (see Table 11-2). The gene products encoded
by the rearranged TCR genes have no inherent affinity for foreign antigen plus a self-MHC molecule, and
theoretically should be capable of recognizing soluble
antigen (either foreign or self), self-MHC molecules,

FIGURE 12-4

Experimental demonstration that the thymus selects for maturation
only those T cells whose T-cell receptors recognize antigen presented
on target cells with the haplotype of the thymus. Thymectomized
and lethally irradiated $(A \times B)$ F_1 mice were grafted with a strain-B
thymus and reconstituted with $(A \times B)$ F_1 bone marrow cells. Following infection with the LCM virus, the CTL cells were assayed for
their ability to kill ^{51}Cr-labeled strain-A or strain-B target cells
infected with the LCM virus. Only strain-B target cells were lysed,
suggesting that the H-2^b grafted thymus had selected for maturation
only those T cells that could recognize antigen in association with
H-2^b MHC molecules.

or antigen plus a nonself-MHC molecule. Nonetheless,
the most distinctive property of mature T cells is that
they only recognize foreign antigen associated with self-
MHC molecules.

Clearly, thymocytes that undergo productive TCR-
gene rearrangement must be "selected" in some way, so
that only those thymocytes whose receptors exhibit self-
MHC restriction are permitted to mature. By processes
discussed in detail later, **positive selection** ensures that
the $\alpha\beta$ TCRs expressed in a given individual will bind
to self-MHC. Cells that fail positive selection are eliminated within the thymus by apoptosis. Also eliminated,
by **negative selection**, are thymocytes bearing a high-
affinity receptor for self-MHC molecules alone or self-
antigen plus self-MHC molecules; such thymocytes
would pose the threat of an autoimmune response if they
matured. As noted already, some 99% of all thymocyte
progeny die by apoptosis within the thymus. This high
death rate is thought to reflect the weeding out of all
thymocytes whose receptors do not specifically recognize foreign antigen plus self-MHC molecules.

Early evidence for the role of the thymus in selection
of the T-cell repertoire came from chimeric mouse experiments by R. M. Zinkernagel and his colleagues
(Figure 12-4). These researchers implanted thymectomized and lethally irradiated $(A \times B)$ F_1 mice with a B-
type thymus and then reconstituted the animal's immune
system with an intravenous infusion of F_1 bone marrow
cells. To be certain that the thymus graft did not contain
any mature T cells, it was irradiated before being transplanted. In such an experimental system, pre-T cells
from the $(A \times B)$ F_1 bone marrow mature within a thymus expressing only B-haplotype MHC molecules on
the thymic stromal cells. Would these $(A \times B)$ F_1 T cells
now be MHC-restricted for the haplotype of the thymus? To answer this question, the chimeric mice were
infected with LCM virus and the mature T cells were
then tested for their ability to kill LCM-infected target
cells from strain A or strain B mice. As shown in Figure

12-4, T_C cells from the chimeric mice could lyse only LCM-infected target cells bearing the same MHC haplotype as the implanted thymus. Apparently the implanted thymus had selected for maturation only T cells having receptors capable of recognizing antigen in association with the MHC haplotype of the thymus.

As noted above, thymocytes are thought to undergo two selection processes in the thymus (Table 12-1):

- Positive selection of thymocytes bearing receptors capable of binding self-MHC molecules, which results in **MHC restriction**
- Negative selection by elimination of thymocytes bearing high-affinity receptors for self-MHC molecules alone or self-antigen presented by self-MHC, which results in **self-tolerance**
- Both processes are necessary to generate mature T cells that are self-MHC restricted and self-tolerant.

Thymic stromal cells, including epithelial cells, macrophages, and dendritic cells, are thought to play a role in positive and negative selection. These thymic stromal cells express high levels of class I and class II MHC molecules. Immature thymocytes expressing the TCR-CD3 complex are thought to interact with these thymic stromal cells, leading to positive and negative selection by mechanisms that are not fully understood. First, we'll examine the details of each selection process and then consider some of the experimental evidence supporting the existence of these processes.

POSITIVE SELECTION

Positive selection appears to involve an interaction of immature thymocytes with epithelial cells in the cortex of the thymus (Figure 12-5). Electron micrographs reveal close contact between thymocytes and epithelial cells within the thymic cortex, and there is evidence that the T-cell receptors tend to cluster at sites of contact. Some researchers have suggested that the interaction of immature CD4$^+$8$^+$ thymocytes with thymic epithelial cells, mediated by MHC-restricted T-cell receptors, might allow the cells to receive some kind of protective signal; cells whose receptors are not MHC restricted would not interact with the thymic epithelial cells and would consequently not receive the protective signal, leading to their death by apoptosis (see Figure 12-5).

During positive selection the RAG-1, RAG-2, and Td T proteins continue to be expressed. Thus the immature thymocytes in a clone expressing a given β chain continue to rearrange TCR α-chain genes, and the resulting TCRs are then selected for self-MHC recognition. Only those cells whose $\alpha\beta$-TCR heterodimer recognizes a self-MHC molecule are selected for survival. If a cell does not express an $\alpha\beta$ TCR with affinity for a self-MHC molecule, then the cell will die within 3–4 days by apoptosis.

NEGATIVE SELECTION

The population of MHC-restricted thymocytes that survive positive selection comprises some cells with low-affinity receptors for self-antigen presented by self-MHC molecules and other cells with high-affinity receptors. The latter thymocytes undergo negative selection by an interaction with bone-marrow–derived APCs (dendritic cells and macrophages) in the medulla. During negative selection, dendritic cells and macrophages bearing class I and class II MHC molecules are thought to interact with thymocytes bearing high-affinity receptors for self-antigen plus self-MHC molecules or self-MHC molecules alone (see Figure 12-5). The nature of the interaction leading to negative selection is not known, but the selected cells are observed to undergo death by apoptosis. Tolerance to self-antigens is thereby achieved by eliminating T cells that are self-reactive and only allowing

TABLE 12-1

CHARACTERISTICS OF T-CELL SELECTION IN THE THYMUS

PROPERTY	POSITIVE SELECTION	NEGATIVE SELECTION
Site	Cortex	Medulla
Stromal cells involved	Epithelial cells	Macrophages and dendritic cells
Selection mechanism	Survival of thymocytes bearing receptors for self-MHC	Elimination of thymocytes bearing high-affinity receptors for self-MHC or self-antigen + self-MHC
Immune consequence	Self-MHC restriction	Self-tolerance

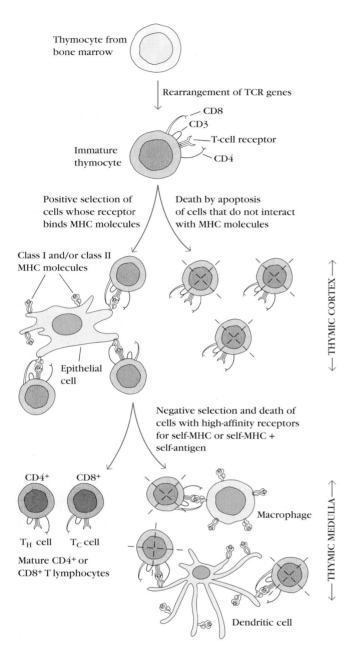

Thymocyte from bone marrow

Rearrangement of TCR genes

CD8
CD3
T-cell receptor
CD4

Immature thymocyte

Positive selection of cells whose receptor binds MHC molecules

Death by apoptosis of cells that do not interact with MHC molecules

Class I and/or class II MHC molecules

Epithelial cell

← THYMIC CORTEX →

Negative selection and death of cells with high-affinity receptors for self-MHC or self-MHC + self-antigen

CD4⁺

CD8⁺

T_H cell

T_C cell

Mature CD4⁺ or CD8⁺ T lymphocytes

Macrophage

Dendritic cell

← THYMIC MEDULLA →

FIGURE 12-5

Positive and negative selection of thymocytes in the thymus. Because of thymic selection, which involves thymic stromal cells (epithelial cells, dendritic cells, and macrophages), mature T cells are both self-MHC restricted and self-tolerant.

by the thymic cells (Figure 12-6). Analysis of the T cells from these fetal thymic organ cultures revealed the absence of CD4⁺ T cells in cultures grown with anti–class II monoclonal antibody and the absence of CD8⁺ T cells in cultures grown with anti–class I monoclonal antibody. Similarly, injection of neonatal mice with anti–class II antibody prevented the development of CD4⁺ T cells and injection of anti–class I antibody prevented the development of CD8⁺ T cells. Thus development of these two thymocyte subpopulations correlates with the ability to recognize either class I or class II MHC molecules in the thymus. The results of these experiments suggest that positive selection of the CD4⁺ or CD8⁺ cells requires interaction of thymocytes with class I or class II MHC molecules. If the class I or class II MHC molecules are blocked by antibody, developing thymocytes cannot bind to the self-MHC molecules on the thymic stromal cells and are not positively selected.

Further support that binding of thymocytes to class I or class II MHC molecules is required for positive selection in the thymus came from subsequent experimental studies with knockout mice incapable of producing functional class I or class II MHC molecules (Table 12-2). Class I–deficient mice were found to have a normal distribution of double-negative, double-positive, and CD4⁺ thymocytes but failed to produce CD8⁺ thymocytes. Class II–deficient mice had double-negative, double-positive, and CD8⁺ thymocytes but lacked CD4⁺ thymocytes. Not surprisingly, the lymph nodes of these class II–deficient mice lacked CD4⁺ T cells. Thus the absence of class I or II MHC molecules prevents positive selection of CD8⁺ or CD4⁺ T cells, respectively.

Experiments with transgenic mice provided additional evidence that interaction with MHC molecules plays a role in positive selection. In these experiments rearranged $\alpha\beta$-TCR genes derived from a CD8⁺ T-cell clone specific for influenza antigen plus H-2^k class I MHC molecules were injected into fertilized eggs from two different mouse strains, one with the H-2^k haplotype and one with the H-2^d haplotype (Figure 12-7). Since the receptor transgenes were already rearranged, other TCR-gene rearrangements were suppressed in the transgenic mice; therefore, a high percentage of the thymocytes in the transgenic mice expressed the T-cell receptor encoded by the transgene. Thymocytes expressing the TCR transgene were found to mature into CD8⁺ T cells only in the transgenic mice with the H-2^k class I

maturation of T cells specific for foreign antigen plus self-MHC molecules (**altered self**).

EXPERIMENTAL EVIDENCE FOR POSITIVE SELECTION

Ada Kruisbeek obtained experimental evidence suggesting that binding of thymocytes to class I or class II MHC molecules within the thymus leads to positive selection of MHC-restricted T cells. In her experiments, mouse fetal thymic tissue was grown in tissue-culture media containing high concentrations of monoclonal antibody to either the class I or class II MHC molecules expressed

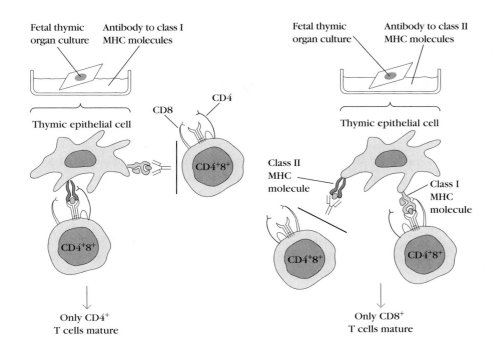

Thymic epithelial cell

CD4⁺8⁺

Only CD4⁺
T cells mature

Thymic epithelial cell

CD4⁺8⁺   CD4⁺8⁺

Only CD8⁺
T cells mature

FIGURE 12-6

Experimental demonstration that acquisition of MHC restriction depends on interaction of immature thymocytes with class I or class II MHC molecules on thymic epithelial cells. See text for discussion.

MHC haplotype (i.e., the haplotype for which the transgene receptor was restricted). In transgenic mice with a different MHC haplotype ($H-2^d$), immature, double-positive thymocytes expressing the transgene were present, but these thymocytes failed to mature into CD8⁺ T cells. These findings also suggest that interaction between T-cell receptors on immature thymocytes and self-MHC molecules is required for positive selection. In the absence of self-MHC molecules, as in the $H-2^d$ transgenic mice, positive selection and subsequent maturation do not occur.

EXPERIMENTAL EVIDENCE FOR NEGATIVE SELECTION

Evidence for deletion of thymocytes reactive with self-antigen plus MHC molecules has been accumulating in a number of diverse experimental systems. In one system thymocyte maturation was analyzed in transgenic mice bearing an $\alpha\beta$-TCR transgene specific for the H-Y antigen plus class I D^b MHC molecules. The H-Y antigen is encoded on the Y chromosome and therefore is expressed in male mice but not in female mice. In this experiment, the MHC haplotype of the transgenic mice was $H-2^b$, the same as the MHC restriction of the transgene-encoded receptor. Therefore any differences in the selection of thymocytes in male and female transgenics would be related to the presence or absence of H-Y antigen.

Analysis of thymocytes in the transgenic mice revealed that female mice contained thymocytes expressing the H-Y–specific TCR transgene, but male mice did not (Figure 12-8). In other words, H-Y–reactive thymocytes

TABLE 12-2

EFFECT OF CLASS I OR II MHC DEFICIENCY ON THYMOCYTE POPULATIONS *

| | | KNOCKOUT MICE | |
CELL TYPE	CONTROL MICE	CLASS I DEFICIENT	CLASS II DEFICIENT
CD4⁻8⁻	+	+	+
CD4⁺8⁺	+	+	+
CD4⁺	+	+	−
CD8⁺	+	−	+

* Plus sign indicates normal distribution of indicated cell types in thymus. Minus sign indicates absence of cell type.

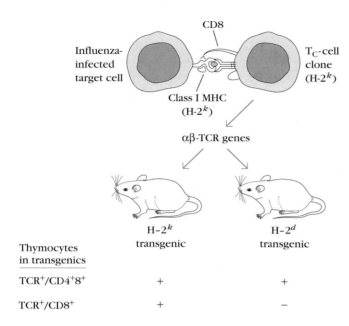

Thymocytes in transgenics

	H-2^k transgenic	H-2^d transgenic
TCR$^+$/CD4$^+$8$^+$	+	+
TCR$^+$/CD8$^+$	+	−

FIGURE 12-7

Effect of host haplotype on T-cell maturation in mice carrying transgenes encoding an H-2^k class I–restricted T-cell receptor specific for influenza virus. The presence of the rearranged TCR transgenes suppressed other gene rearrangements in the transgenics; therefore, most of the thymocytes in the transgenics expressed the $\alpha\beta$ T-cell receptor encoded by the transgene. Immature double-positive thymocytes matured into CD8$^+$ T cells only in transgenics with the haplotype (H-2^k) corresponding to the MHC restriction of the TCR transgene.

were self-reactive in the male mice and were eliminated. However, in the female transgenics, which did not express the H-Y antigen, these cells were not self-reactive and thus were not eliminated. When thymocytes from these male transgenic mice were cultured in vitro with antigen-presenting cells expressing the H-Y antigen, the thymocytes were observed to undergo apoptosis, providing a striking example of this process.

Unsolved Questions Regarding Thymic Selection

Although the general process of T-cell maturation, which generates mature CD4$^+$ and CD8$^+$ T cells, is understood, several unsolved questions regarding thymic selection remain.

What keeps positive and negative selection from eliminating the entire T-cell repertoire? If positive selection selects for thymocytes reactive with self-MHC molecules and then negative selection eliminates the self-MHC–reactive thymocytes, how do any MHC-restricted T cells survive? What keeps these two processes from eliminat-

ing the entire repertoire of MHC-restricted T cells? One hypothesis, called the **affinity model**, suggests that differences in the affinity of TCRs for self-MHC–peptide complexes determines the outcome of positive and negative selection. According to this hypothesis, all thymocytes bearing receptors that can bind to self-MHC molecules are selected during positive selection, whereas subsequently only those thymocytes bearing **high-affinity** receptors for self-MHC (or self-antigen plus self-MHC) bind during negative selection and undergo death by apoptosis. In this way, only thymocytes bearing receptors with a low affinity for self-antigen plus self-MHC molecules survive positive and negative selection, eventually leaving the thymus as mature T cells with self-MHC–restricted receptors (see Figure 12-5).

If the affinity hypothesis is to explain why all MHC-restricted thymocytes are not eliminated during negative selection, then there must be some mechanism that in-

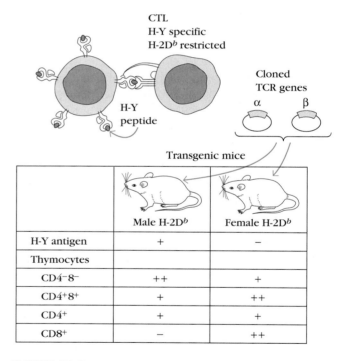

	Male H-2D^b	Female H-2D^b
H-Y antigen	+	−
Thymocytes		
CD4$^-$8$^-$	++	+
CD4$^+$8$^+$	+	++
CD4$^+$	+	+
CD8$^+$	−	++

FIGURE 12-8

Experimental demonstration that negative selection of thymocytes requires self-antigen plus self-MHC. In this experiment, H-2^b male and female transgenics were prepared carrying TCR transgenes specific for H-Y antigen plus the D^b molecule. This antigen is expressed only in males. FACS analysis of thymocytes from the transgenics showed that mature CD8$^+$ T cells expressing the transgene were absent in the male mice but present in the female mice, suggesting that thymocytes reactive with a self-antigen (in this case, H-Y antigen in the male mice) are deleted during thymic selection. [Adapted from H. von Boehmer and P. Kisielow, 1990, *Science* **248**:1370.]

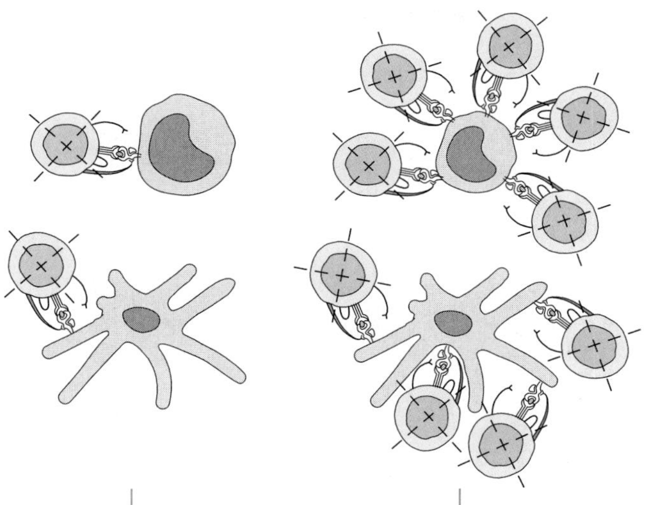

TCR single-transgenic mice
(normal CD8 level)

TCR/CD8 double-transgenie mice
(↑CD8 level)

18 × 10⁷ CD8⁺ thymocytes
(79% of transgenic thymocytes)

0.8 × 10⁷ CD8⁺ thymocytes
(6% of transgenic thymocytes)

FIGURE 12-9

Experimental demonstration that elevated levels of CD8 stimulate negative selection. Double-transgenic mice expressing elevated levels of CD8 (blue) and a class I-restricted T-cell receptor possessed many fewer thymocytes specific for the transgenic TCR than did single transgenics expressing normal CD8 levels. Presumably, the higher CD8 level on thymocytes of the double transgenics facilitates interaction of thymocytes bearing low-affinity receptors to stromal cells, leading to their elimination. [Data from E. A. Robey et al., 1992, *Cell* **69**:1089.]

creases the ability of cells bearing low-affinity receptors to bind with thymic epithelial cells during positive selection and/or that decreases their binding to dendritic cells or macrophages during negative selection. Differences in the populations of thymic stromal cells involved in positive and negative selection may influence the thymocyte–stromal cell interaction. As noted earlier, thymic cortical epithelial cells appear to be involved in positive selection, whereas most negative selection appears to involve bone-marrow–derived dendritic cells and macrophages. Some researchers have suggested that thymic cortical epithelial cells express additional membrane molecules that facilitate their interaction with thymocytes bearing low-affinity receptors for self-MHC molecules. If these membrane molecules are not expressed on thymic macrophages or dendritic cells, then thymocytes bearing low-affinity receptors for self-MHC molecules might not bind to the macrophages and dendritic cells and therefore would not be deleted during negative selection.

Another possibility is that thymocytes express different membrane molecules that influence their avidity for thymic stromal cells at different stages in thymic processing. For example, the coreceptors CD4 and CD8 are known to bind to class II and class I MHC molecules, respectively. Perhaps the expression of these or other unidentified membrane molecules sufficiently increases the avidity of thymocytes bearing low-affinity receptors so that they can bind to thymic epithelial cells during posi-

tive selection. The subsequent loss or decrease in the number of molecules expressed on the membrane during development of thymocytes may lower their avidity, so that only thymocytes with high-affinity receptors for self-MHC (or self-MHC plus self-antigen) would be able to bind to thymic stromal cells during negative selection.

To test the possibility that differential expression of CD8 affects thymic selection, E. Robey, B. J. Fowlkes, and their colleagues experimentally manipulated the level of CD8 expression in mice and then analyzed the composition of the thymocyte population. In their study, they first produced double-transgenic mice expressing a class I MHC–restricted TCR transgene and a CD8 transgene. The CD8⁺ level on the T cells in these double-transgenic mice was twice the normal level. Since the interaction of T cells with class I MHC molecules is strengthened by participation of CD8, these researchers predicted that increasing the level of CD8 expression would increase the avidity of thymocytes for class I molecules, leading to their negative selection. As predicted, FACS analyses of thymocytes from the transgenics revealed that the proportion of mature CD8⁺ thymocytes was 13-fold lower in the double transgenics, which had elevated levels of CD8, than in the single transgenics (Figure 12-9).

What is the role of peptide in thymic selection? A model system, **fetal thymic organ culture**, has been utilized to analyze thymocyte selection and the role that

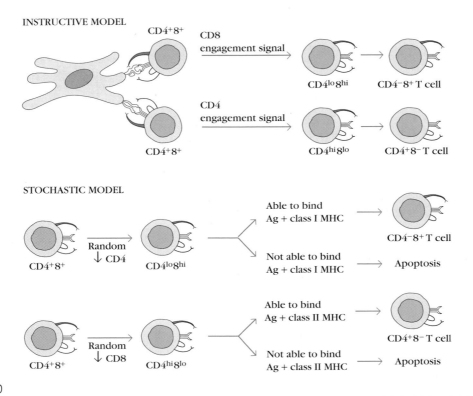

INSTRUCTIVE MODEL

CD4$^+$8$^+$

CD8 engagement signal

CD4^{lo}8^{hi} → CD4$^-$8$^+$ T cell

CD4$^+$8$^+$

CD4 engagement signal

CD4^{hi}8^{lo} → CD4$^+$8$^-$ T cell

STOCHASTIC MODEL

CD4$^+$8$^+$ → Random ↓ CD4 → CD4^{lo}8^{hi}

Able to bind Ag + class I MHC → CD4$^-$8$^+$ T cell

Not able to bind Ag + class I MHC → Apoptosis

CD4$^+$8$^+$ → Random ↓ CD8 → CD4^{hi}8^{lo}

Able to bind Ag + class II MHC → CD4$^+$8$^-$ T cell

Not able to bind Ag + class II MHC → Apoptosis

FIGURE 12-10

Proposed models of the role of the CD4 and CD8 coreceptors in thymic selection of double-positive thymocytes leading to single-positive T cells. According to the instructive model, interaction of one coreceptor with MHC molecules on stromal cells results in down-regulation of the other coreceptor. According to the stochastic model, down-regulation of CD4 or CD8 is a random process.

peptides play in this process. In this system, mouse thymic lobes are excised at a gestational age of day 16 and placed in culture. At this time the lobes consist predominantly of CD4$^-$8$^-$ thymocytes. Because these immature, double-negative, thymocytes continue to develop in the organ culture, thymic selection can be studied experimentally.

To study the role of peptides in thymic selection, the fetal thymic organ culture is modified by using mice lacking β_2-microglobulin or the peptide transporter TAP-1. In the absence of β_2-microglobulin or TAP-1, only low levels of MHC class I α chains, without bound peptide, are expressed on the stromal cells and the development of CD8$^+$ thymocytes is blocked. When exogenous peptides and β_2-microglobulin are added to these organ cultures, then class I MHC molecules bearing the peptide are expressed on the surface of the thymic stromal cells and development of CD8$^+$ T cells is restored. When a diverse peptide mixture is added, the extent of CD8$^+$ T-cell restoration is greater than when a single peptide is added. Since both single and complex peptides induce stable class I MHC assembly, this would suggest that the role of the peptide is not simply to induce stable MHC expression but that the peptide itself is recognized in the selection process.

Another modified fetal thymic organ culture has been used to analyze positive selection of a single TCR specificity. In this case, the fetal tissue was obtained by breeding mice deficient in β_2-microglobulin with transgenic mice bearing a TCR specific for an octameric peptide from ovalbumin. When the ovalbumin octameric peptide was added to the thymic organ culture, class I MHC molecules were expressed and thymocytes bearing the transgenic TCR were positively selected. Several variants of the ovalbumin peptide were able to induce positive selection. Although some of these peptide variants bind poorly to the TCR, they are still able to induce positive selection. This would suggest that even low-affinity T-cell binding is sufficient for positive selection. In addition, low doses of the peptide were shown to induce positive selection, whereas higher doses of the peptide led to elimination of the transgenic T cells by negative selection.

What is the role of CD4 and CD8 in selection? Selection of CD4$^+$8$^+$ thymocytes gives rise to class I MHC–restricted CD8$^+$ T cells and class II–restricted CD4$^+$ T cells. Two models have been proposed to explain the transition of a double-positive precursor to one of two different single-positive lineages (Figure 12-10). The **instructional model** postulates that the multiple interactions of the TCR with the $CD4^+$ or $CD8^+$ co-receptors and class I or class II MHC molecules instruct the cells to differentiate either into $CD8^+$ or $CD4^+$ single-positive cells. This model would predict that a class I MHC–specific TCR together with the CD8 coreceptor would generate a signal that is different from the signal induced by a class II MHC–specific TCR together with the CD4 coreceptor. The second model, called the **stochastic model,** suggests that CD4 or CD8 expression is switched off randomly with no relation to the specificity of the TCR. Only those thymocytes whose TCR and coreceptor recognize the same class of MHC molecule will mature. Presently, evidence exists in support of both models.

Is the signal for positive selection different from the signal for negative selection? Another unresolved question is how thymocyte recognition of self-MHC molecules is converted into a protective signal early in thymic processing (positive selection) and into a negative signal leading to apoptosis at a later stage (negative selection). One hypothesis is that the effect of TCR–mediated signal transduction may change during thymocyte maturation perhaps due to differences in coupling between the T-cell receptor and CD3. In one study, for example, cross-linking of the T-cell receptor with monoclonal antibodies induced a pronounced Ca^{2+} influx in mature single-positive thymocytes but only minimal Ca^{2+} influx in immature double-positive cells. In contrast, cross-linking of CD3 induced comparable Ca^{2+} influx in both mature and immature thymocytes. These results have led to speculation that in immature thymocytes the T-cell receptor and CD3 are not fully coupled and thus the signal generated by interaction with self-MHC molecules is incomplete; as a result such immature thymocytes undergo programmed cell death by apoptosis.

Several molecules that have been implicated in the physiologic control of apoptosis exhibit different levels of expression during thymocyte development and may contribute to the different outcomes during positive and negative selection. Among these molecules are Fas protein, a cell-surface receptor, and the *bcl-2* gene product. These proteins exhibit opposite roles in regulating apoptosis: Fas has been shown to trigger apoptosis, whereas Bcl-2 confers resistance to apoptosis. The most immature thymocytes, the double-negative ($CD4^-8^-$) cells have a high viability and exhibit a low-Fas, high–Bcl-2 phenotype, which renders them resistant to apoptosis (Table 12-3). The double-positive ($CD4^+8^+$) thymocytes, on the other hand, undergo positive and negative selection, with the majority dying by apoptosis. Interestingly, the double-positive cells exhibit a high-Fas, low–Bcl-2 phenotype, which makes them susceptible to apoptosis. Finally, mature single-positive $CD4^+$ and $CD8^+$ thymocytes, which have survived selection and are resistant to apoptosis, also exhibit the low-Fas, high–Bcl-2 phenotype.

T_H-CELL ACTIVATION

The central event in generation of both humoral and cell-mediated immune responses is the activation and clonal expansion of T_H cells. (Activation of T_C cells, which is generally similar to T_H-cell activation, is discussed in Chapter 16.) T_H-cell activation is initiated by interaction of the TCR-CD3 complex with a processed antigenic peptide bound to a class II MHC molecule on the surface of an antigen-presenting cell. This interaction and the resulting activating signals also involve a variety of accessory membrane molecules on the T_H cell and antigen-presenting cell (see Table 11-3). Interaction of a T_H cell with antigen initiates a cascade of biochemical events that induces the resting T_H cell to enter the cell cycle (G_0-to-G_1 transition) and culminates in expression of the high-affinity receptor for IL-2 and secretion of

TABLE 12-3

CORRELATION BETWEEN APOPTOSIS OF THYMOCYTES AND FAS AND BCL-2 LEVELS

CELL TYPE	FAS *	BCL-2 *	SUSCEPTIBILITY TO APOPTOSIS
$CD4^-8^-$	↓	↑	Resistant
$CD4^+8^+$	↑	↓	Susceptible
$CD4^+$	↓	↑	Resistant
$CD8^+$	↓	↑	Resistant

* ↑ indicates high expression; ↓ indicates low expression.

IL-2. In response to IL-2 (and in some cases IL-4), the activated T_H cell progresses through the cell cycle, proliferating and differentiating into memory cells or effector cells (see Figure 3-10).

Following interaction of T_H cells with antigen, numerous genes are activated. The gene products that appear can be grouped into three categories depending on how early they can be detected following antigen recognition (Table 12-4):

- **Immediate genes:** expressed within half an hour of antigen recognition; encode a number of transcription factors, including c-Fos, c-Myc, c-Jun, NF-AT, and NF-κB

T A B L E   1 2 - 4

TIME COURSE OF GENE EXPRESSION BY T_H CELLS FOLLOWING INTERACTION WITH ANTIGEN

GENE PRODUCT	FUNCTION	TIME mRNA EXPRESSION BEGINS	LOCATION	RATIO OF ACTIVATED TO NONACTIVATED CELLS
IMMEDIATE				
c-Fos	Cellular oncogene Nuclear–binding protein	15 min	Nucleus	>100
NF-AT	Nuclear–binding protein	20 min	Nucleus	50
c-Myc	Cellular oncogene	30 min	Nucleus	20
NF-κB	Nuclear–binding protein	30 min	Nucleus	>10
EARLY				
IFN-γ	Cytokine	30 min	Secreted	>100
IL-2	Cytokine	45 min	Secreted	>1000
Insulin receptor	Hormone receptor	1 h	Cell membrane	3
IL-3	Cytokine	1–2 h	Secreted	>100
TGF-β	Cytokine	<2 h	Secreted	>10
IL-2 receptor (p55)	Cytokine receptor	2 h	Cell membrane	>50
TNF-β	Cytokine	1–3 h	Secreted	>100
Cyclin	Cell cycle protein	4–6 h	Cytoplasmic	>10
IL-4	Cytokine	<6 h	Secreted	>100
IL-5	Cytokine	<6 h	Secreted	>100
IL-6	Cytokine	<6 h	Secreted	>100
c-Myb	Cellular oncogene	16 h	Nuclear	100
GM-CSF	Cytokine	20 h	Secreted	?
LATE				
HLA-DR	Class II MHC molecule	3–5 days	Cell membrane	10
VLA-4	Adhesion molecule	4 days	Cell membrane	>100
VLA-1, VLA-2, VLA-3, VLA-5	Adhesion molecules	7–14 days	Cell membrane	>100, ?, ?, ?

SOURCE: Adapted from G. Crabtree, 1989, *Science* **243**:357.

- **Early genes:** expressed within 1–2 h of antigen recognition; encode IL-2, IL-2R, IL-3, IL-6, IFN-γ, and numerous other proteins
- **Late genes:** expressed more than 2 days after antigen recognition; encode various adhesion molecules

TCR-Coupled Signaling Pathways

Although the precise molecular mechanisms that link antigen recognition by the T-cell receptor to gene activation are not fully understood, a number of signaling events common to many cells have been shown to occur in the T_H cell. These events include activation of inositol-lipid–specific phospholipase C (PLCγ_1); hydrolysis of plasma membrane inositol phospholipids; increase in intracellular Ca^{2+} levels; and activation of various protein kinases that subsequently phosphorylate a number of proteins involved in mediating the activation signal. The T-cell receptor itself has short cytoplasmic domains, which are unable to mediate signal transduction. Instead, signal transduction is mediated by the cytoplasmic domains of the CD3 complex, by the coreceptor CD4 or CD8, and by various accessory molecules including CD2 and CD45. It appears that signal transduction is accomplished by a series of protein-phosphorylation events catalyzed by protein kinases and dephosphorylation events catalyzed by protein phosphatases.

As discussed in Chapter 11, the cytoplasmic domains of each CD3 chain contain a sequence motif, called the **immunoreceptor tyrosine-based activation motif** (ITAM), that is thought to interact with protein tyrosine kinases during signal transduction (see Figure 11-9). Two protein tyrosine kinases (Fyn and ZAP-70) have been shown to be associated with the cytoplasmic domains of the ε and ζ chains of CD3. In addition, the cytoplasmic domain of CD4 and CD8 is associated with the protein tyrosine kinase Lck. It is hypothesized that TCR aggregation coupled with the coaggregation of the coreceptors, CD4 or CD8, focuses the kinases in one place, facilitating their activation (Figure 12-11). Activation of these protein tyrosine kinases appears to require the activity of CD45. This membrane molecule has a cytoplasmic tail with two protein tyrosine phosphatase domains, which are thought to catalyze dephosphorylation of a tyrosine residue of Lck and Fyn. This dephosphorylation step is thought to activate these two tyrosine kinases so that they begin to phosphorylate the ε and ζ chains of CD3, phospholipase C (PLCγ_1), and other cellular substrates.

Phosphorylation of PLCγ_1 allows it to hydrolyze phosphatidylinositol 4,5-bisphosphate (PIP$_2$), a membrane phospholipid, into two important products, inositol 1,4,5-trisphosphate (IP$_3$) and diacylglycerol (DAG). Once

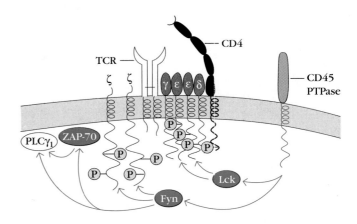

FIGURE 12-11

Initial steps in T_H-cell activation. Following antigen recognition, CD45, a protein phosphatase, activates Fyn and Lck. These protein kinases then phosphorylate tyrosine residues in the ε and ζ chains of CD3. ZAP-70, another kinase, and Fyn then phosphorylate PLCγ_1, triggering one of several signaling pathways detailed in Figure 12-12. PTPase = protein tyrosine phosphatase; PLCγ_1 = phospholipase C. [Adapted from M. Izquierdo and D. A. Cantrell, 1992, *Trends Cell Biol.* **2**:268.]

formed, IP$_3$ and DAG initiate two necessary signaling pathways (Figure 12-12). In one pathway, IP$_3$ triggers an increase in intracellular Ca^{2+} and the subsequent activation of a calmodulin–dependent phosphatase called **calcineurin**, which dephosphorylates the inactive cytosolic form of the T-cell–specific nuclear factor NF-AT. In the other pathway, DAG activates protein kinase C (PKC), which then phosphorylates various cellular substrates and mediates release of the nuclear factor NF-κB. Both nuclear factors enter the nucleus where they participate in activation of various genes, including the IL-2 gene. A third signaling pathway is generated by the CD28-B7 interaction discussed below. This pathway works together with the TCR-mediated signaling pathways to activate a protein kinase, designated JNK, that is involved in the phosphorylation of the nuclear factor c-Jun.

Of the DNA-binding proteins involved in T_H-cell activation, only NF-AT is T-cell specific; the others are found in many types of cells. Following antigen recognition by T_H cells, NF-ATc-PO$_4$, the phosphorylated cytosolic form of NF-AT, is dephosphorylated by calcineurin. NF-ATc then translocates to the nucleus where it dimerizes with AP1; the resulting complex then binds to the IL-2 enhancer (see Figure 12-12). If dephosphorylation of NF-ATc-PO$_4$ is inhibited, as it is by cyclosporin A and FK506, then T_H-cell activation is blocked and the immune response is reduced (Figure 12-13). Because of their potent immunosuppressive capabilities,

Visualizing Concepts

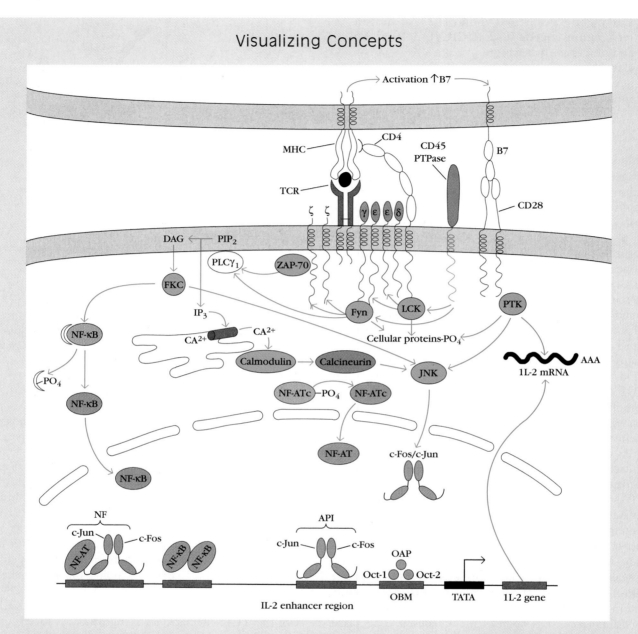

FIGURE 12-12

Overview of biochemical pathways thought to transduce the signals required for T_H–cell activation and the DNA-binding proteins that bind to the IL-2 enhancer region. The TCR-mediated signal results in production of two nuclear factors, NF-AT and NF-κB, via two separate pathways involving DAG and IP_3. In the presence of the co-stimulatory signal, generated by the CD28-B7 interaction, a third nuclear factor, c-Jun, is also produced. Binding of these and other nuclear factors to response elements in the IL-2 enhancer region (*bottom*) stimulates transcription of the IL-2 gene, leading to increased secretion of IL-2 about 45 min after antigen recognition. The co-stimulatory signal also appears to stabilize IL-2 mRNA. PTPase = protein tyrosine phosphatase; PLCγ_1 = phospholipase C; PKC = protein kinase C; PTK = protein tyrosine kinase; PIP_2 = phosphatidylinositol 4,5-bisphosphate; IP_3 = inositol 1,4,5-trisphosphate; DAG = diacylglycerol.

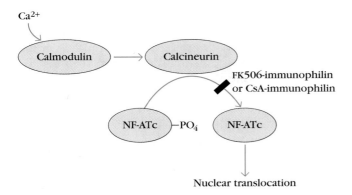

FIGURE 12-13

Mechanism of immunosuppression by cyclosporin A (CsA) and FK506, both of which bind to cytosolic proteins called immunophilins. The complex blocks the phosphatase activity of calcineurin, thereby preventing production of NF-ATc, which is necessary for T-cell activation. The immunophilins are *cis-trans* peptidyl-prolyl isomerase enzymes. CsA binds to an immunophilin called cyclophilin, and FK506 binds to one called FKBP.

cyclosporin A and FK506 have proven to be extremely effective in prolonging graft survival in transplant recipients (see Chapter 23).

The Co-stimulatory Signal

T-cell activation in response to antigen displayed on the membrane of an APC involves the dynamic interaction of multiple membrane molecules generating the necessary intracellular signals. The TCR dictates the antigen specificity of the response and plays a central role in initiating activation. However, this interaction, by itself, is not sufficient for full activation of naive T cells. It is now widely believed that naive T cells require two distinct signals for activation and subsequent proliferation into effector cells:

- The initial signal (signal 1) is generated by interaction of an antigenic peptide with the TCR-CD3 complex.
- A subsequent antigen-nonspecific co-stimulatory signal (signal 2) is provided primarily by interactions between CD28 on the T cell and B7 on the APC.

The B7 molecule is a member of the immunoglobulin superfamily, having a single V-like domain and a single C-like domain. There are two related forms of B7 (B7-1 and B7-2). Both molecules have a similar organization of extracellular domains but markedly different

cytosolic domains (Figure 12-14). Both B7 molecules are expressed on dendritic cells, activated macrophages, and activated B cells. The ligands for B7 are CD28 and CTLA-4, both of which are expressed as monomers or homodimers on the T-cell membrane; like B7 they are members of the immunoglobulin superfamily. CD28 is expressed by both resting and activated T cells and binds B7 with moderate affinity. In contrast, CTLA-4 binds B7 with a 20-fold higher affinity, but it is expressed only on activated T cells and at much lower levels (only 3% of CD28 levels).

As discussed in a later section, T cells can be activated experimentally in such a way that only the TCR-coupled signaling pathways operate. In this case, activation results in very little production of IL-2 compared with normal activation in which the CD28-B7 co-stimulatory signal also operates. The co-stimulatory signal appears to synergize with the TCR-coupled signals to augment IL-2 production and T-cell proliferation. Very little is known about how signal transduction is mediated via the CD28-B7 interaction. As shown in Figure 12-12, the co-stimulatory signal may act together with the TCR-mediated signal to activate JNK, which in turn phosphorylates c-Jun. In addition, the signal mediated through CD28 may act to increase the half-life of the mRNA encoding IL-2.

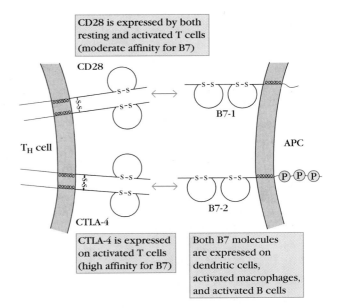

FIGURE 12-14

T_H-cell activation requires a co-stimulatory signal provided by antigen-presenting cells (APCs). One co-stimulatory signal is generated by interaction of B7 on APCs with CD28 or CTLA-4 on T_H cells. All of these membrane molecules belong to the immunoglobulin superfamily. [Adapted from P. S. Linsley and J. A. Ledbetter, 1993, *Annu. Rev. Immunol.* **11**:191.]

Altered Peptide Ligands as Antagonists or Partial Agonists

Recognition of a peptide–MHC complex by a T cell does not always result in activation. Investigations of T-cell responses to altered peptide ligands associated with MHC molecules have revealed that some peptides can induce a partial activating signal (**partial agonist peptides**) and some peptides can block the activating signal altogether (**antagonist peptides**). Such **altered peptide ligands** contain a single amino acid substitution in the epitope (i.e., the region that contacts the TCR), but have no alterations in the agretope (i.e., the region that contacts the MHC). Although these altered peptides are recognized like normal immunogenic peptides by the MHC molecule, they induce qualitatively different responses in the T cell.

Altered peptide ligands not only affect the magnitude of T-cell stimulation but may activate only some, rather than all, of the usual T-cell effector responses. For example, in one experiment altered peptide ligands stimulated a T_H2 clone to produce cytokines but did not induce proliferation. In another experiment altered peptide ligands induced a T_H1 clone to express the receptor for IL-2 but blocked secretion of IL-2. Such partial activation or antagonism by altered peptide ligands was shown to be associated with a characteristic pattern of phosphorylation of the CD3 ζ chain that is distinct from the pattern observed when T cells are exposed to an optimally activating antigenic peptide. This altered pattern of ζ-chain phosphorylation is also associated with a failure to activate ZAP-70 (see Figure 12-11).

These results with altered peptides suggest that the TCR transmits qualitatively different signals depending on how it contacts the ligand displayed by antigen-presenting cells. It is possible that some pathogens may utilize altered peptide ligands as a way to escape an immunologic attack. Certainly, the high mutation rate of the human immunodeficiency virus (HIV-1) would allow for altered peptides to arise during the course of infection, and these might act in an antagonistic or partial activating fashion, thereby increasing its virulence.

Clonal Expansion Versus Clonal Anergy

T_H-cell recognition of an antigenic peptide–MHC complex on an antigen-presenting cell results either in activation and **clonal expansion** or in a state of nonresponsiveness called **clonal anergy**. Anergy is a state of inactivation marked by the inability of cells to proliferate in response to a peptide-MHC complex. Whether clonal expansion or clonal anergy ensues is determined by the presence or absence of a co-stimulatory signal (signal 2), such as that provided by interaction of CD28 on T_H cells with B7 on antigen-presenting cells. If a resting T_H cell receives the TCR-mediated signal (signal 1) in the absence of a suitable co-stimulatory signal, then the T_H cell will become anergic.

One way of inducing clonal anergy is to incubate resting T_H cells with glutaraldehyde-fixed APCs, which do not express B7 (Figure 12-15a). The fixed APCs are able to present peptides together with class II MHC molecules, thereby providing signal 1, but they are unable to provide the necessary co-stimulatory signal 2. In the absence of a co-stimulatory signal, there is minimal production of cytokines, especially of IL-2. Anergy can also be induced by incubating T_H cells with normal APCs in the presence of the Fab portion of anti-CD28 (Figure 12-15b). That the anergic state is not simply the absence of a response, but rather an active state of unresponsiveness, can be demonstrated by incubating anergic T_H cells with normal APCs. In this case, the anergic T_H cells cannot be activated by the antigenic peptides displayed on the normal APCs (Figure 12-15c).

The systems illustrated in Figure 12-15d,e have shown that the co-stimulatory signal 2 is distinct from signal 1 provided by TCR recognition of an antigenic peptide–MHC complex. In these systems, T_H cells are incubated with fixed APCs and either normal, unfixed APCs expressing allogeneic MHC molecules or anti-CD28. IL-2 production and clonal expansion occurs in both systems because the T_H cells receive signal 1 by interacting with the fixed APCs and signal 2 by interacting with the unfixed allogeneic APCs or anti-CD28. Normally, the co-stimulatory signal is provided by the same APC that presents antigen.

The demonstration of T-cell anergy and the role of accessory membrane molecules in providing the co-stimulatory signal necessary for T_H-cell activation opens possibilities for immune intervention. For example, treatment with monoclonal antibodies to CD28 or CTLA-4 might increase the T-cell response to infectious agents or tumors. Alternatively, blocking of CD28, CTLA-4, or B7 might provide a means of inducing clonal anergy. For example, CTLA-4Ig, a soluble fusion protein consisting of the extracellular domain of CTLA-4 and the constant region of the IgG1 heavy chain, has been shown to completely block T-cell activation. In another study, this reagent was found to completely abolish graft rejection in mice transplanted with human pancreatic islet cells (see Chapter 23).

Superantigen-Induced T-Cell Activation

As mentioned in Chapter 4, superantigens are viral or bacterial proteins that bind simultaneously to the V_β

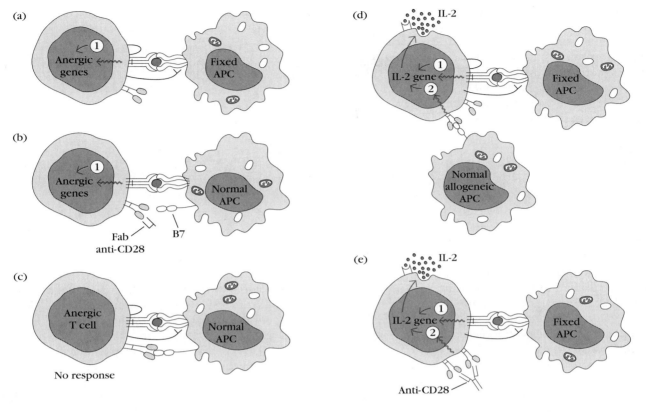

FIGURE 12-15

Experimental demonstration of clonal anergy versus clonal expansion. (a,b) Only signal 1 is generated when resting T_H cells are incubated with glutaraldehyde-fixed antigen-presenting cells (APCs) or with normal APCs in the presence of the Fab portion of anti-CD28.

(c) The resulting anergic T cells cannot respond to normal APCs. (d,e) In the presence of normal allogeneic APCs or anti-CD28, both of which produce the co-stimulatory signal 2, T cells are activated by fixed APCs.

domain of a T-cell receptor and to the α chain of a class II MHC molecule. Both exogenous and endogenous superantigens have been identified. Cross-linkage of a T-cell receptor and class II MHC molecule by either type of superantigen provides an activating signal that induces T-cell activation and proliferation (Figure 12-16).

Exogenous superantigens are soluble proteins secreted by bacteria. Included in the exogenous superantigens are a variety of **exotoxins** secreted by gram-positive bacteria, such as staphylococcal enterotoxins, toxic-shock syndrome toxin, and exfoliative dermatitis toxin; mycoplasma arthritidis supernatant; and streptococcal pyrogenic exotoxins. Each of these exogenous superantigens binds particular V_β sequences in T-cell receptors (Table 12-5) and cross-links the TCR to a class II MHC molecule.

Endogenous superantigens are cell-membrane proteins encoded by certain viruses that infect mammalian cells. One group of endogenous superantigens is encoded by mouse mammary tumor virus (MTV). This retrovirus can integrate into the DNA of certain inbred

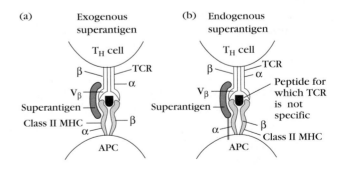

FIGURE 12-16

Superantigen-mediated cross-linkage of T-cell receptor and class II MHC molecules. Each superantigen (dark blue) binds to all TCRs bearing a particular V_β sequence regardless of their antigenic specificity. (a) Exogenous superantigens are soluble secreted bacterial proteins, including various exotoxins. (b) Endogenous superantigens are membrane-embedded proteins produced by certain viruses; they include Mls antigens encoded by mouse mammary tumor virus.

mouse strains; after integration, retroviral proteins are expressed on the membrane of the infected cells. These viral proteins, called **minor lymphocyte stimulating** (Mls) determinants, bind particular V_β sequences in T-cell receptors and cross-link the TCR to a class II MHC molecule. Four Mls superantigens, originating in different MTV strains, have been identified. These superantigens exhibit different V_β specificity, and the four *Mls* loci are located on different chromosomes (Table 12-6).

Because superantigens bind outside of the TCR antigen-binding cleft, any T cell expressing a particular V_β sequence will be activated by a particular superantigen. Mice have about 20 V_β gene segments; therefore, assuming equal frequency of expression, about 1 in 20 T cells (roughly 5%) will express a given V_β domain in their T-cell receptors and respond to a particular superantigen. The massive activation following cross-linkage by a superantigen results in overproduction of T_H-cell cytokines leading to systemic toxicity. The food poisoning induced by staphylococcal enterotoxins and the toxic shock induced by toxic-shock syndrome toxin (TSST-1) are two examples of the consequences of cytokine overproduction induced by superantigens.

In addition to inducing T-cell activation, superantigens also can influence T-cell maturation in the thymus. This occurs because a superantigen present in the thymus during thymic processing will facilitate binding of all thymocytes bearing a TCR V_β domain corresponding to the superantigen specificity to thymic stromal cells, leading to deletion of those thymocytes. Such massive deletion creates what is commonly called "holes in the repertoire," characterized by the absence of all T cells whose receptors possess a particular V_β domain.

Evidence that an exogenous superantigen can induce negative selection of a subset of thymocytes expressing receptors with a particular V_β was obtained by injecting neonatal mice with staphylococcal enterotoxin B (SEB),

TABLE 12-6

PROPERTIES OF MLS ENDOGENOUS SUPERANTIGENS

MLS ALLELE	RETROVIRAL CARRIER	CHROMOSOME LOCATION	V_β SPECIFICITY
Mls1	MTV-7	1	6, 7, 8.1, 9
Mls2	MTV-13	4	3
Mls3	MTV-6	16	3, 5
Mls4	MTV-1	7	3

TABLE 12-5

EXOGENOUS SUPERANTIGENS AND THEIR V_β SPECIFICITY

SUPERANTIGEN	DISEASE *	V_β SPECIFICITY	
		MOUSE	HUMAN
Staphylococcal products			
Enterotoxins			
SEA	Food poisoning	1, 3, 10, 11, 12, 17	nd
SEB	Food poisoning	3, 8.1, 8.2, 8.3	3, 12, 14, 15, 17, 20
SEC1	Food poisoning	7, 8.2, 8.3, 11	12
SEC2	Food poisoning	8.2, 10	12, 13, 14, 15, 17, 20
SEC3	Food poisoning	7, 8.2	5, 12
SED	Food poisoning	3, 7, 8.3, 11, 17	5, 12
SEE	Food poisoning	11, 15, 17	5.1, 6.1-6.3, 8, 18
Toxic-shock syndrome toxin (TSST1)	Toxic-shock syndrome	15, 16	2
Exfoliative dermatitis toxin (ExFT)	Scalded-skin syndrome	10, 11, 15	2
Mycoplasma arthritidis supernatant (MAS)	Arthritis, shock	6, 8.1-8.3	nd
Streptococcal pyrogenic exotoxins (SPE-A, B, C, D)	Rheumatic fever, shock	nd	nd

* Disease results from infection by bacteria producing the indicated superantigens.

TABLE 12-7

NEGATIVE SELECTION OF THYMOCYTES MEDIATED BY SEB, AN EXOGENOUS SUPERANTIGEN*

PERCENTAGE OF THYMOCYTES EXPRESSING V_β

SEB (μG)	IMMATURE THYMOCYTES DAY 15			MATURE THYMOCYTES DAY 10			MATURE THYMOCYTES DAY 1		
	$V_\beta3$	$V_\beta6$	$V_\beta8$	$V_\beta3$	$V_\beta6$	$V_\beta8$	$V_\beta3$	$V_\beta6$	$V_\beta8$
0	5.1	10.4	21.5	5.7	15.8	18.9	6.5	12.2	12.1
20	2.1	10.5	14.2	1.2	19.5	0.0	1.6	15.5	0.2
100	2.3	12.8	10.8	1.1	17.6	0.2	1.1	16.9	0.1

* Mice were injected intraperitoneally with a solution containing the indicated amounts of SEB on the day of birth and every other day thereafter. Mice given 20 μg of SEB grew and survived as well as those given none. Mice given 100 μg SEB were significantly smaller than their littermates and had higher mortality rates. SEB is specific for the $V_\beta3$ and $V_\beta8$ domains.

which binds to virtually all T cells bearing receptors with $V_\beta3$ or $V_\beta8$. Thymocytes from SEB-injected mice and noninjected controls then were stained with monoclonal antibody specific for $V_\beta3$ or $V_\beta8$. These analyses revealed a slight reduction in immature (double-positive) thymocytes and a dramatic reduction in mature (single-positive) thymocytes bearing $V_\beta3$ or $V_\beta8$ in the SEB-injected mice compared with controls (Table 12-7).

Negative selection of thymocytes mediated by endogenous Mls superantigens has also been demonstrated. The inbred AKR mouse strain, for example, has MTV-7 integrated in chromosome 1 and expresses Mls1, whereas the B10.BR strain contains no MTV strain and thus does not express any Mls superantigen. Since the Mls1

superantigen binds to the $V_\beta6$, $V_\beta7$, $V_\beta8.1$, and $V_\beta9$ domains in T-cell receptors, negative selection during thymic processing would be expected to eliminate T cells expressing receptors with these V_β domains in AKR mice but not in B10.BR mice. As shown in Table 12-8, both mouse strains have immature thymocytes expressing the V_β domains to which Mls1 binds, but only B10.BR mice contain mature thymocytes bearing T-cell receptors with these V_β domains. Thus negative selection, mediated by the Mls1 superantigen, eliminates T cells bearing the $V_\beta6$, $V_\beta7$, $V_\beta8.1$, or $V_\beta9$ domain in the AKR strain. Note in Table 12-8 that the presence of Mls1 had no effect on thymocytes bearing the $V_\beta3$ or $V_\beta5$ domain to which Mls1 does not bind.

TABLE 12-8

NEGATIVE SELECTION OF THYMOCYTES MEDIATED BY MLS1, AN ENDOGENOUS SUPERANTIGEN*

EXPRESSION OF V_β

STRAIN	MLS1	$V_\beta3$	$V_\beta5$	$V_\beta6$	$V_\beta7$	$V_\beta8.1$	$V_\beta9$
IMMATURE $\alpha\beta$ THYMOCYTES							
AKR	Present	+	+	+	+	+	+
B10.BR	Absent	+	+	+	+	+	+
MATURE PERIPHERAL $\alpha\beta$ T CELLS							
AKR	Present	+	+	−	−	−	−
B10.BR	Absent	+	+	+	+	+	+

* Chromosome 1 of the AKR strain carries the MTV-7 genome, which encodes Mls1. This superantigen is specific for $V_\beta6$, $V_\beta7$, $V_\beta8.1$, and $V_\beta9$. The B10.BR strain does not carry MTV.

T-CELL DIFFERENTIATION

An estimated 90%–95% of peripheral T cells express the $\alpha\beta$ T-cell receptor–CD3 complex. There are about twice as many CD4$^+$ T cells as CD8$^+$ T cells in the periphery. In general CD4$^+$ cells function as T helper cells and CD8$^+$ cells function as cytotoxic cells. Since both populations express the $\alpha\beta$ T-cell receptor, some researchers have proposed that T$_H$ and T$_C$ cells may express different V$_\alpha$ and V$_\beta$ gene segments. The available evidence, however, seems to suggest that both populations can use the same pool of V$_\alpha$ and V$_\beta$ gene segments. In one study, for example, the same V$_\beta$ gene product was identified on both class I MHC–restricted T$_C$ cells and class II MHC–restricted T$_H$ cells.

CD4$^+$ and CD8$^+$ T cells leave the thymus and enter the circulation as resting cells in the G$_0$ stage of the cell cycle. These naive T cells, which have not yet encountered antigen, are characterized by condensed chromatin, very little cytoplasm, and little transcriptional activity. Naive T cells continually recirculate between the blood and lymph systems. During recirculation naive T cells reside in secondary lymphoid tissues such as lymph nodes. If a naive cell does not encounter antigen in a lymph node, it exits through the efferent lymphatics, ultimately draining into the thoracic duct and rejoining the blood. It is estimated that each naive T cell recirculates from the blood to the lymph nodes and back again every 12–24 hours. Because only about 1 in 10^5 naive T cells is specific for any given antigen, this large-scale recirculation increases the chances of a naive T cell encountering appropriate antigen. Naive T cells have generally been thought to survive only about 5–7 weeks in the absence of antigen-stimulated activation, but recent evidence suggests they may have a considerably longer life span.

Generation of Effector and Memory T Cells

If a naive T cell recognizes an antigen-MHC complex on an appropriate antigen-presenting cell or target cell, it will be activated, initiating a **primary response**. About 48 hours after activation, the naive T cell enlarges into a blast cell and begins undergoing repeated rounds of cell division. As discussed earlier, activation depends on signal 1 induced by engagement of the TCR complex and the co-stimulatory signal 2 induced by the CD28-B7 interaction (see Figure 12-12). These signals trigger entry of the T cell into the G$_1$ phase of the cell cycle and, at the same time, induce transcription of the gene for IL-2 and the α chain of the high affinity IL-2 receptor. In addition, the co-stimulatory signal increases the half-life of the IL-2 mRNA. The increase in IL-2 transcription, together with stabilization of the IL-2 mRNA, increases

IL-2 production by 100-fold in the activated T cell. Secretion of IL-2 and its subsequent binding to the high affinity IL-2 receptor induces the activated naive T cell to proliferate and differentiate (Figure 12-17). T cells activated in this way divide 2–3 times per day for 4–5 days, generating a large clone of progeny cells, which differentiate into memory or effector T-cell populations.

The various **effector T cells** carry out specialized functions such as cytokine secretion and B-cell help (activated CD4$^+$ T$_H$ cells) and cytotoxic killing activity (CD8$^+$ CTLs). The generation and activity of CTLs and T$_{DTH}$ cells are described in detail in Chapter 16. Effector cells are derived from both naive and memory cells following antigen activation. Effector cells are short-lived cells with life spans ranging from a few days to a few weeks. The effector and naive populations express different cell-membrane molecules, which contribute to differences in the recirculation patterns of these two groups of cells.

As discussed in more detail in Chapters 13 and 16, CD4$^+$ effector T cells form two subpopulations charac-

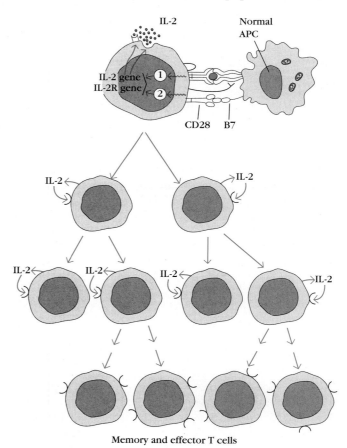

Memory and effector T cells

FIGURE 12-17

Activation of a T$_H$ cell by both signal 1 and co-stimulatory signal 2 up-regulates expression of IL-2 and the high-affinity IL-2 receptor, leading to proliferation and differentiation.

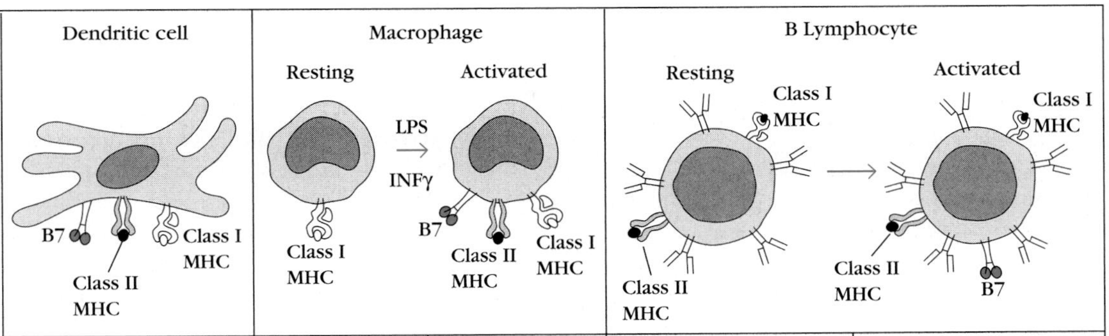

	Dendritic cell	Macrophage		B Lymphocyte	
		Resting	Activated	Resting	Activated
Antigen uptake	Endocytosis phagocytosis (by Langerhans cells)	Phagocytosis	Phagocytosis	Receptor-mediated endocytosis	Receptor-mediated endocytosis
Class II MHC expression	Constitutive (+++)	Inducible (−)	Inducible (++)	Constitutive (++)	Constitutive (+++)
Co-stimulatory activity	Constitutive B7 (+++)	Inducible B7 (−)	Inducible B7 (++)	Inducible B7 (−)	Inducible B7 (++)
T-cell activation	Naive T cells Effector T cells Memory T cells	(−)	Effector T cells Memory T cells	Effector T cells Memory T cells	Naive T cells Effector T cells Memory T cells

FIGURE 12-18

Differences in the properties of professional antigen-presenting cells affect their ability to present antigen and induce T-cell activation. Note that activation of effector and memory T cells does not require the co-stimulatory B7 molecule.

terized by the panel of cytokines that they secrete. One population, called the **T$_H$1 subset**, is distinguished by its secretion of IL-2, IFN-γ, and TNF-β. The T$_H$1 subset is responsible for classical cell-mediated functions, such as delayed-type hypersensitivity and the activation of cytotoxic T lymphocytes. The other subset, called the **T$_H$2 subset**, is distinguished by its secretion of IL-4, IL-5, IL-6, and IL-10 and functions more effectively as a helper for B-cell activation.

The **memory T-cell** population is derived from both naive T cells and from effector cells after they have encountered antigen. Memory T cells are generally thought to be long-lived, antigen-activated T cells that respond with heightened reactivity to a subsequent challenge with the same antigen, generating a **secondary response.** Recent evidence suggests, however, that some memory T cells may be relatively short-lived cells maintained in the population by continued activation by persisting antigen. An expanded population of memory T cells appears to remain long after the population of effector T cells has declined. In general, memory T cells express the same membrane molecules as effector cells.

Like naive T cells, most memory T cells are resting cells in the G_0 stage of the cell cycle, but they appear to have less stringent requirements for activation than do naive T cells. For example, naive T$_H$ cells are activated only by dendritic cells, whereas memory T$_H$ cells can be activated by macrophages, dendritic cells, and B cells. It is thought that the expression of high levels of numerous adhesion molecules by memory T$_H$ cells enables these cells to adhere to a broad spectrum of antigen–presenting cells. Memory cells also display differences in their recirculation patterns that distinguish them from naive or effector T cells.

Co-stimulatory Differences among Antigen-Presenting Cells

Only professional antigen-presenting cells (dendritic cells, macrophages, and B cells) are able to present antigen together with class II MHC molecules and deliver the co-stimulatory signal necessary for complete T-cell activation leading to proliferation and differentiation. The principal co-stimulatory molecules expressed on antigen–presenting cells are the glycoproteins B7-1 and B7-2 (see Figure 12-14). The professional antigen-presenting cells differ in their ability to display antigen and also differ in their ability to deliver the co-stimulatory signal (Figure 12-18).

Dendritic cells constitutively express high levels of class I and class II MHC molecules as well as high levels of B7-1 and B7-2. For this reason dendritic cells are very potent activators of naive, memory, and effector T cells. In contrast, resting macrophages express few, if any, class II MHC molecules or co-stimulatory B7 molecules on their membrane; consequently, resting macrophages are not able to activate naive T cells and are poor activators of memory and effector T cells. Macrophages can be activated following phagocytosis of bacteria or by bacterial products such as LPS or by IFN-γ, a T_H1-derived cytokine. Activated macrophages up-regulate their expression of class II MHC molecules and the co-stimulatory B7 molecule. Thus activated macrophages are common activators of memory and effector T cells, but their role in activating naive T cells is still questionable.

B cells also serve as antigen-presenting cells in T-cell activation. Resting B cells express class II MHC molecules but fail to express the co-stimulatory B7 molecule. Consequently, resting B cells cannot activate naive T cells, although they can activate the effector and memory T-cell populations. Upon activation, B cells up-regulate their expression of class II MHC molecules and begin expressing B7. These activated B cells can now activate naive T cells in addition to the memory and effector populations.

PERIPHERAL $\gamma\delta$ T CELLS

In 1986 a small population of peripheral-blood T cells was discovered that expressed CD3 but failed to stain with monoclonal antibody specific for the $\alpha\beta$ T-cell receptor, indicating an absence of the $\alpha\beta$ heterodimer. These cells eventually were found to express the $\gamma\delta$ receptor.

Distribution of $\gamma\delta$ T Cells

T cells bearing the $\gamma\delta$ heterodimer constitute 0.5%–10% of human peripheral blood lymphocytes and 1%–3% of the T-cell population in lymphoid organs of the mouse. But surprisingly they appear to represent a major T-cell population in the skin, intestinal epithelium, and pulmonary epithelium. Up to 1% of the epidermal cells in the skin of mice are $\gamma\delta$ T cells, called "dendritic epidermal cells" (DECs) or intraepidermal lymphocytes. These cells express Thy-1, the earliest T-cell marker, and the $\gamma\delta$ TCR–CD3 complex, but fail to express either CD4 or CD8. A second population of $\gamma\delta$ T cells has been identified in the intestinal epithelium of the mouse; these are called "intestinal epithelial lymphocytes" (IELs), or intra-epithelial lymphocytes. These cells express the $\gamma\delta$-

TCR–CD3 complex, but unlike DECs, they also express CD8. Another unusual characteristic of intestinal epithelial lymphocytes is that 25%–50% of them fail to express Thy-1. Whether these cells lose the Thy-1 marker and acquire CD8 after thymic processing or whether they differentiate at a site other than the thymus remains to be determined.

Unlike $\alpha\beta$ T cells, which recirculate extensively, $\gamma\delta$ T cells in these epithelial tissues appear not to circulate and instead remain fixed in these tissue sites. The $\gamma\delta$ T cells in different epithelial tissue sites appear to express different V_γ and V_δ gene segments. Comparison of a number of DEC clones, for example, has revealed an unusual limitation in TCR diversity. Each of the DEC clones was shown to express a restricted repertoire encoded by $V_\gamma 3J_\gamma 1$ and $V_\delta 1D_\delta 2J_\delta 2$ gene segments, with essentially no N-region diversification. In contrast, IELs were found to express $V_\delta 5J_\delta 1C_\delta 1$. This selective expression of different V gene segments in different epithelial tissues may make these T cells specialized to respond to certain types of antigens that tend to be found at these sites.

Ligands Recognized by $\gamma\delta$ T Cells

Both the nature of the antigens recognized by $\gamma\delta$ T cells and the functions of these cells have remained elusive. In 1994 several startling findings began to cause another paradigm in immunology to crumble—namely, that all T cells are self-MHC restricted and recognize only peptide antigens displayed in the cleft of the self-MHC molecule. In one study, a $\gamma\delta$ T-cell clone was found to bind directly to a herpes virus protein without requiring antigen processing and presentation together with MHC. This finding suggests that some $\gamma\delta$ T cells bind to epitopes in much the same way that antibodies do.

Also like antibodies, the $\gamma\delta$ TCR appears to have a broader specificity for antigens, binding to nonpeptide antigens as well as peptides. For example, $\gamma\delta$ T cells have been shown to bind to some mycobacterial antigens that are protease resistant; one such ligand is isopentyl pyrophosphate. Thus $\gamma\delta$ T cells may have been selected to respond to a unique type of antigen, entirely different from the type recognized by the more common $\alpha\beta$ T cells.

Function of $\gamma\delta$ T cells

The limited gene-segment repertoire and unusual ligand recognition exhibited by the $\gamma\delta$ heterodimer suggest that $\gamma\delta$ T cells may play a unique role in immunity. The nature of that role is a matter of intense speculation. The finding that $\gamma\delta$ T cells can mediate tumor-cell lysis in a non-MHC-restricted manner indicates that they may function like natural killer cells. The ability of $\gamma\delta$ T cells to respond to a mycobacterial antigen called purified protein derivative (PPD) may be an important clue regarding their function. The PPD antigen belongs to a group of highly conserved proteins, found in all organisms, called heat-shock proteins. These proteins, as their name implies, are produced by cells in response to sudden increases in temperature or other environmental stresses. But heat-shock proteins are also induced by internal stresses such as inflammatory responses, viral infections, and cancer. Mycobacterial PPD exhibits sequence homology with a mammalian heat-shock protein that is a normal component of the mitochondrial matrix. This observation has led to the proposal that $\gamma\delta$ T cells may be uniquely suited to respond to mammalian heat-shock proteins and may have evolved to eliminate damaged cells as well as microbial invaders.

C. A. Janeway has suggested that the $\gamma\delta$ T cell may represent the most primitive and earliest cell-mediated immune system, uniquely specialized to recognize epithelial-cell alterations outside the basement-membrane barrier. One proposal is that these $\gamma\delta$ T cells, which may be especially suited to combat epidermal or intestinal antigens, form a surveillance system monitoring the integrity of the external epithelial cell milieu. These cells may be able to recognize heat-shock proteins or alterations caused by ultraviolet irradiation in the outer epidermal layer. DECs may be activated by epidermal keratinocytes, which have been shown to be both effective antigen-presenting cells and secretors of IL-1. Such a system would protect the epithelial-cell surfaces, preventing the spread of infection or cancer across the basement membrane into the internal milieu.

SUMMARY

1. T-cell maturation occurs in the thymus as progenitor T cells from the bone marrow enter the thymus and rearrange the TCR genes. The earliest thymocytes lack detectable CD4 and CD8 and are referred to as double-negative cells. These double-negative thymocytes differentiate along two developmental pathways (see Figure 12-2). Those thymocytes that make a productive rearrangement of the $\gamma\delta$-TCR genes develop into CD4$^-$, CD8$^-$, CD3$^+$ $\gamma\delta$ T cells, which account for only 0.5%–1.0% of thymocytes. The majority of double-negative thymocytes rearrange the $\alpha\beta$-TCR genes and develop into CD4$^+$, CD3$^+$ $\alpha\beta$ T cells or CD8$^+$, CD3$^+$ $\alpha\beta$ T cells. Immature thymocytes in the $\alpha\beta$ pathway express a pre-T cell receptor that is analogous to the pre-B cell receptor (see Figure 12-1).

2. Rearrangement of germ-line TCR genes during T-cell maturation in the thymus appears to produce many functional genes encoding receptors that are not specific for foreign antigen plus self-MHC molecules. Thymocytes with unwanted TCR specificities are deleted in a two-step selection process (see Figure 12-5). First, positive selection of all thymocytes bearing receptors that can bind a self-MHC molecule, which confers MHC restriction. Second, negative selection and elimination of thymocytes bearing high-affinity receptors for self-MHC molecules alone or self-antigen plus self-MHC, which confers self-tolerance. As a result of this thymic selection, only thymocytes that are both self-MHC restricted and self-tolerant develop into mature T cells.

3. T_H-cell activation is initiated by interaction of the TCR-CD3 complex with a peptide-MHC complex on an antigen-presenting cell. The activating signal is not transduced solely by the TCR-CD3 complex but also is mediated and regulated by a variety of accessory molecules, including the coreceptors CD4 and CD8, as well as CD45. Signal transduction is accomplished by a series of protein phosphorylation events catalyzed by protein kinases and dephosphorylation events catalyzed by protein phosphatases (see Figures 12-11 and 12-12).

4. In addition to the signals mediated by the T-cell receptor and its associated accessory molecules (signal 1), activation of the T_H cell requires an additional co-stimulatory signal (signal 2) provided by the antigen-presenting cell. The co-stimulatory signal is commonly induced by interaction between the B7 molecule on the membrane of the APC with CD28 (or CTLA-4) on the membrane of the T_H cell (see Figure 12-14).

5. T_H-cell recognition of an antigenic peptide–MHC complex on an antigen-presenting cell results either in activation and clonal expansion or in a state of nonresponsiveness called clonal anergy. The presence or absence of the co-stimulatory signal (signal 2) determines whether activation results in clonal expansion or clonal anergy (see Figure 12-15).

6. Some 90%–99% of the peripheral T cells express the $\alpha\beta$ T-cell receptor. Those T cells that express CD4 recognize antigen associated with a class II MHC molecule and generally function as T_H cells; those T cells that express CD8 recognize antigen associated with a class I MHC molecule and generally function as T_C cells. Naive T cells are resting cells (G_0) that have not encountered antigen. Activation of naive cells initiates a primary response leading to generation of effector and memory T cells (see Figure 12-17). Memory T cells, which are more easily activated than naive cells, are responsible for the secondary response. Effector cells, which are relatively short lived, perform helper, cytotoxic, or delayed-type hypersensitivity functions. The professional antigen-presenting cells—dendritic cells, macrophages, and B cells—differ in

their ability to display antigen and activate different T-cell populations (see Figure 12-18)

7. T cells expressing the $\gamma\delta$ T-cell receptor constitute only a small percentage of the total T-cell population. The $\gamma\delta$ TCR exhibits a broader specificity for antigen than the $\alpha\beta$ TCR, and at least in some cases is not MHC restricted. The $\gamma\delta$ T cells are concentrated in several epithelial tissues and may represent a primitive cell-mediated immune system that evolved to protect the integrity of external epithelial surfaces.

REFERENCES

ABRAHAM, R. T., L. M. KARNITZ, J. PAUL SECRIST, AND P. J. LEIBSON. 1992. Signal transduction through the T-cell antigen receptor. *Trends Biol. Sci.* **17**(Oct.):434.

ALLISON, J. P. 1994. CD28-B7 interactions in T-cell activation. *Curr. Opin. Immunol.* **6**:414.

ANDERSON, S. J., AND R. M. PERLMUTTER. 1995. A signaling pathway governing early thymocyte maturation. *Immunol. Today* **16**:99.

ARNAIZ-VILLENA, A., ET AL. 1992. Human T-cell activation deficiencies. *Immunol. Today* **13**:259.

BEYERS, A. D., L. L. SPRUYT, AND A. F. WILLIAMS. 1993. Multimolecular associations of the T-cell antigen receptor. *Trends Cell Biol.* **2**:253.

BOISE, L., ET AL. 1995. CD28 costimulation can promote T cell survival by enhancing the expression of Bcl-X_L. *Immunity* **3**:87.

BRADLEY, L. M., M. CROFT, AND S. L. SWAIN. 1993. T-cell memory: new perspectives. *Immunol. Today* **14**:197.

CLIPSTONE, N. A., AND G. R. CRABTREE. 1992. Identification of calcineurin as a key signalling enzyme in T-lymphocyte activation. *Nature* **357**:695.

DORSHKIND, K. 1994. Transcriptional control points during lymphopoiesis. *Cell* **79**:751.

FOWLKES, B. J., AND E. SCHWEIGHOFFER. 1995. Positive selection of T cells. *Curr. Opin. Immunol.* **7**:188.

HATADA, M. H., ET AL. 1995. Molecular basis for interaction of the protein tyrosine kinase ZAP-70 with the T-cell receptor. *Nature* **377**:32.

HERMAN, A., J. W. KAPPLER, P. MARRACK, AND A. M. PULLEN. 1991. Superantigens: mechanism of T-cell stimulation and role in immune responses. *Annu. Rev. Immunol.* **9**:745.

JAMESON, S. C., AND M. J. BEVAN. 1995. T-cell receptor antagonists and partial agonists. *Immunity* **2**:1.

JANEWAY, C. A., AND K. BOTTOMLY. 1994. Signals and signs for lymphocyte responses. *Cell* **76**:275.

JULIUS, M., C. R. MAROUN, AND L. HAUGHN. 1993. Distinct roles for CD4 and CD8 as co-receptors in antigen receptor signalling. *Immunol. Today* **14**:177.

JUNE, C. H., J. A. BLUESTONE, L. M. NADLER, AND C. B. THOMPSON. 1994. The B7 and CD28 receptor families. *Immunol. Today* **15**:321.

KRUISBEEK, A., AND U. STORB. 1994. Lymphocyte development. *Curr. Opin. Immunol.* **6**:199.

MACDONALD, H., AND H. ACHA-ORBEA. 1994. Superantigen as suspect. *Nature* **371**:283.

NEGISHI, I., ET AL. 1995. Essential role for ZAP-70 in both positive and negative selection of thymocytes. *Nature* **376**:435.

NOSSAL, G. 1994. Negative selection of lymphocytes. *Cell* **76**:229.

O'KEEFE, S. J., ET AL. 1992. FK506-, and CsA-sensitive activation of the interleukin-2 promoter by calcineurin. *Nature* **357**:692.

OKUMURA, M., AND M. THOMAS. 1995. Regulation of immune function by protein tyrosine phosphatases. *Curr. Opin. Immunol.* **7**:312.

OWEN, J. J. T., AND N. C. MOORE. 1995. Thymocyte-stromal-cell interactions and T-cell selection. *Immunol. Today* **16**:336.

PEREIRA, P., AND S. TONEGAWA. 1993. Gamma/delta cells. *Annu. Rev. Immunol.* **11**:637.

PERLMUTTER, R. W., ET AL. 1993. Regulation of lymphocyte function by protein phosphorylation. *Annu. Rev. Immunol.* **11**:451.

RHODES, J., ET AL. 1995. Therapeutic potentiation of the immune system by costimulatory Schiff-base-forming drugs. *Nature* **377**:71.

ROBEY, E. A., ET AL. 1992. The level of CD8 expression can determine the outcome of thymic selection. *Cell* **69**:1089.

ROTH, P., AND A. DEFRANCO. 1995. Intrinsic checkpoints for lineage progression. *Curr. Bio.* **5**:349.

ROTHENBERG, E. V. 1994. Signaling mechanisms in thymocyte selection. *Curr. Opin. Immunol.* **6**:257.

SCHREIBER, S. L., AND G. R. CRABTREE. 1992. The mechanism of action of cyclosporin A and FK506. *Immunol. Today* **13**:136.

SCHWARZ, R. H. 1992. Costimulation of T lymphocytes: the role of CD28, CTLA-4 and B7/BB1 in interleukin-2 production and immunotherapy. *Cell* **72**:1066.

SEFTON, B., AND J. TADDIE. 1994. Role of tyrosine kinases in lymphocyte activation. *Curr. Opin. Immunol.* **6**:372.

SIGAL, N. H., AND F. J. DUMONT. 1992. Cyclosporin A, FK506 and rapamycin: pharmacologic probes of lymphocyte signal transduction. *Annu. Rev. Immunol.* **10**:519.

SLOAN-LANCASTER, J., AND P. M. ALLEN. 1995. Significance of T-cell stimulation by altered peptide ligands in T cell biology. *Curr. Opin. Immunol.* **7**:103.

SPRENT, J., AND S. R. WEBB. 1995. Intrathymic and extrathymic clonal deletion of T cells. *Curr. Opin. Immunol.* **7**:196.

TAKAHAMA, Y., ET. AL. 1994. Positive selection of CD4+ T cells by TCR ligation without aggregation even in the absence of MHC. *Nature* **371**:67.

VON BOEHMER, H. 1994. Positive selection of lymphocytes. *Cell* **76**:219.

WEBB, S. R., AND N. R. J. GASCOIGNE. 1994. T-cell activation by superantigens. *Curr. Opin. Immunol.* **6**:467.

WEISS, A., AND D. R. LITTMAN. 1994. Signal transduction by lymphocyte antigen receptors. *Cell* **76**:263.

STUDY QUESTIONS

1. You have a CD8+ CTL clone (from an H-2^k mouse) that has a T-cell receptor specific for the H-Y antigen. You clone the $\alpha\beta$-TCR genes from this clone and use them to prepare transgenic mice with the H-2^k or H-2^d haplotype.

a. How can you distinguish the immature thymocytes from the mature CD8+ thymocytes in the transgenic mice?

b. For each transgenic mouse listed in the table below, indicate whether the mouse would (+) or would not (−) have immature double-positive and mature CD8+ thymocytes bearing the transgenic T-cell receptor.

TRANSGENIC MOUSE	IMMATURE THYMOCYTES	MATURE CD8+ THYMOCYTES
H-2^k female		
H-2^k male		
H-2^d female		
H-2^d male		

c. Explain your answers for the H-2^k transgenics.

d. Explain your answers for the H-2^d transgenics.

2. Cyclosporin A is a powerful immunosuppressive drug that now is given to transplant recipients. Describe how this drug suppresses the immune response.

3. Antigen activation of T$_H$ cells leads to the release or induction of various nuclear factors that activate gene transcription.

a. Which two transcription factors required for proliferation of activated T$_H$ cells are present in the cytoplasm of resting T$_H$ cells in inactive forms?

b. To which enhancer do these transcription factors bind?

4. You have fluorescein-labeled anti-CD4 and rhodamine-labeled anti-CD8. You use these antibodies to stain thymocytes and lymph-node cells from normal mice and from RAG-1 knockout mice. In the diagrams below, draw the FACS plots that you would expect.

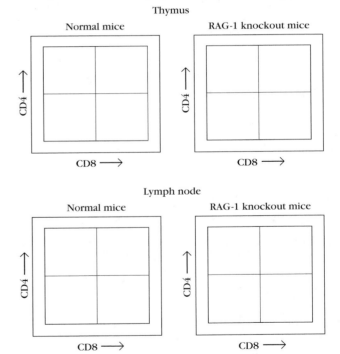

5. In order to demonstrate positive thymic selection experimentally, researchers analyzed the thymocytes from H-2^b mice, which have a deletion of the class II *IE* gene, and from H-2^b mice in which the class II *IA* gene had been knocked out.

a. What MHC molecules would you find on antigen-presenting cells from the normal H-2^b mice?

b. What MHC molecules would you find on antigen-presenting cells from the IA knockout H-2^b mice?

c.   Would you expect to find CD4$^+$ T cells, CD8$^+$ T cells, or both in each type of mouse? Why?

6.   In his classic chimeric-mouse experiments, Zinkernagel took bone marrow from mouse 1 and a thymus from mouse 2 and transplanted them into mouse 3, which was thymectomized and lethally irradiated. He then challenged the reconstituted mouse with LCM virus and removed its spleen cells. These spleen cells were then incubated with LCM-infected target cells with different MHC haplotypes, and the lysis of the target cells was monitored. The results of two such experiments using H-2^b strain C57BL/6 mice and H-2^d strain BALB/c mice is shown in the accompanying table.

a.   What was the haplotype of the thymus-donor strain in experiment A and experiment B?

b.   Why were the H-2^b target cells not lysed in experiment A but were lysed in experiment B?

c.   Why were the H-2^k target cells not lysed in either experiment?

7.   Fill in the blank(s) in each statement below (a–k) with the most appropriate term(s) from the following list. Terms may be used once, more than once, or not at all.

protein phosphatase(s)	CD8
protein kinase(s)	CD4
phospholipase(s)	CD28
class I MHC	CD45
class II MHC	B7
IL-2	IL-6

a.   Fyn and ZAP-70 are _____ associated with the cytoplasmic domains of _____.

b.   _____ is a T-cell membrane protein that has cytosolic domains with phosphatase activity.

c.   Dendritic cells express _____ constitutively, whereas B cells must be activated before they express this membrane molecule.

d.   Calcineurin, a _____, is involved in generating the active form of the transcription factor NF-AT.

e.   Activation of T$_H$ cells results in secretion of _____ and expression of its receptor, leading to proliferation and differentiation.

f.   The co-stimulatory signal needed for complete T$_H$-cell activation is triggered by interaction of _____ on the T cell and _____ on the APC.

g.   Knockout mice lacking class I MHC molecules fail to produce thymocytes bearing _____.

h.   Macrophages must be activated before they express _____ molecules and _____ molecules.

i.   T cells bearing _____ are absent from the lymph nodes of knockout mice lacking class II MHC molecules.

j.   PIP$_2$ is split by a _____ to yield DAG and IP$_3$.

k.   In activated T$_H$ cells, DAG activates a _____, which acts to generate the transcription factor NF-κB.

8.   You wish to determine the percentage of various types of thymocytes in a sample of cells from mouse thymus using the indirect immunofluorescence method.

a.   You first stain the sample with goat anti-CD3 (primary antibody) and then with rabbit FITC-labeled anti-goat Ig (secondary antibody), which emits a green color. Analysis of the stained sample by flow cytometry indicates that 70% of the cells are stained. Based on this result, how many of the thymus cells in your sample are expressing antigen-binding receptors on their surface? Explain your answer. What are the remaining unstained cells likely to be?

b.   You then separate the CD3$^+$ cells with the fluorescent-activated cell sorter (FACS) and restain them. In this case, the primary antibody is hamster anti-CD4 and the secondary antibody is rabbit PE-labeled anti-hamster-Ig, which emits a red color. Analysis of the stained CD3$^+$ cells shows that 80% of them are stained. Based on this result, can you determine how many T$_C$ cells are present in this sample? If you can, then how many T$_C$ cells are there? If you cannot, what additional experiment would you perform in order to determine the number of T$_C$ cells that are present?

For use with Question 6.

EXPERIMENT	BONE MARROW DONOR	THYMECTOMIZED, x-IRRADIATED RECIPIENT	LYSIS OF LCM-INFECTED TARGET CELLS		
			H-2^d	H-2^k	H-2^b
A	C57BL/6 × BALB/c	C57BL/6 × BALB/c	+	−	−
B	C57BL/6 × BALB/c	C57BL/6 × BALB/c	−	−	+

PART III

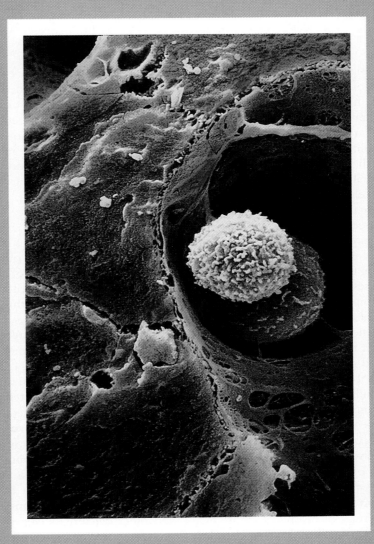

Two leukocytes travel within a capillary of the liver.
[© P. M. Motta and T. Fujita]

IMMUNE EFFECTOR
MECHANISMS

Recognition of antigen by the immune system induces a variety of effector mechanisms associated with the humoral and cell-mediated responses. Part III concentrates on these effector mechanisms. Secreted antibodies and complement components are effectors of humoral immunity, whereas both specific and nonspecific cells are the key effectors of cell-mediated immunity. The humoral branch of the immune system functions primarily to eliminate extracellular bacteria and bacterial products, whereas the cell-mediated branch functions to eliminate altered self-cells (infected cells and tumor cells) and foreign grafts.

The cytokines discussed in Chapter 13 are small proteins that assist in regulating the development of immune effector cells and/or possess direct effector functions. Secreted by activated lymphocytes, macrophages, and certain other cells, cytokines are critical components of both humoral and cell-mediated immune responses. Many cytokines exert their biological effects by binding to specific receptors found on the membrane of target cells. These receptors can be grouped into five structurally diverse protein families. When a cytokine binds to its receptor, it triggers intracellular signals which lead to specific changes in gene expression. Some cytokines chemotactically attract certain cell types, while others have direct cytotoxic or antiviral effects.

In vitro, the interaction of antibody and antigen leads to precipitation or agglutination of the antigen-antibody (immune) complexes. In vivo, however, activation of the complement system, consisting of nearly 30 serum and membrane proteins, is the primary effector mechanism of the humoral immune response. In Chapter 14 we see how complement activation generates numerous products that function in clearance of immune complexes, lysis of invading microorganisms, and neutralization of viral infectivity. Some complement products also facilitate phagocytosis and play major roles in an inflammatory response.

In Chapter 15 we learn about the movement of immune-system cells throughout the body and the cell-adhesion molecules that direct their movement to specific sites. This trafficking delivers lymphocytes to lymphoid tissues where they can encounter antigen and undergo proliferation and differentiation, as discussed in earlier chapters. Phagocytic cells directed to sites of tissue injury or local infection mediate inflammation, a localized nonspecific response that acts to contain infection or harmful substances within a confined site. Neutrophils, macrophages, and numerous mediators play critical roles in the inflammatory response. Under certain circumstances, the inflammatory response can be prolonged or excessive, with deleterious effects.

Chapter 16 describes the two major types of effector mechanisms involved in cell-mediated immunity—direct cytotoxic processes and delayed-type hypersensitivity (DTH) reactions. Antigen-specific cytotoxic T lymphocytes (CTLs) and several nonspecific cell types carry out the destruction of altered self-cells. At least in some cases, target-cell destruction results from the stimulation of intracellular pathways leading to apoptosis. Intracellular bacteria and various contact antigens can induce a type of localized inflammatory response called a DTH reaction, which is mediated primarily by $CD4^+$ T_H1 cells, activated macrophages, and various cytokines. The common assays for measuring cell-mediated cytotoxicity and the humoral response are described in this chapter, as well as the differences between the primary and secondary antibody responses. The chapter ends with a discussion of the various mechanisms which regulate immune effector responses.

In some cases, normal immune effector mechanisms for removing antigen can have exaggerated effects or occur inappropriately, leading to extensive tissue damage and other deleterious consequences. The four types of such hypersensitive reactions are covered in Chapter 17. Individuals who are allergic to pollens, mold spores, certain foods, or some drugs can blame type I hypersensitivity. A recipient who receives a blood transfusion that is not matched to their ABO blood group will develop a type II reaction, leading to destruction of the transfused blood cells. Some autoimmune diseases and infectious diseases are associated with type III reactions, which are triggered by antigen-antibody complexes. The manifestations of these three types of hypersensitivity occur within a few hours. The DTH response (type IV hypersensitivity) to intracellular pathogens and contact antigens (e.g., poison oak, poison ivy, certain organic compounds) typically takes 2 to 3 days to develop.

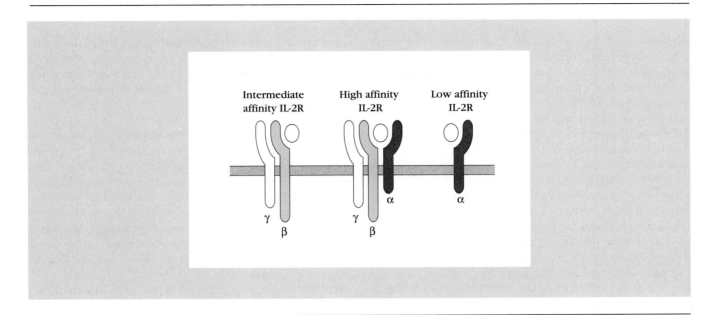

Intermediate
affinity IL-2R

High affinity
IL-2R

Low affinity
IL-2R

γ

β

γ

β

α

α

C Y T O K I N E S

The development of an effective immune response involves lymphoid cells, inflammatory cells, and hematopoietic cells. The complex interactions among these cells are mediated by a group of secreted low-molecular-weight proteins that are collectively designated **cytokines** to denote their role in cell-to-cell communication. Cytokines assist in regulating the development of immune effector cells, and some cytokines possess direct effector functions of their own. Just as hormones serve as messengers of the endocrine system, so cytokines serve as messengers of the immune system; however, unlike endocrine hormones, which exert their effects over large distances, cytokines generally act locally.

This chapter focuses on the biological activity and structure of cytokines, the structure of and signal trans-duction by cytokine receptors, the role of cytokine abnormalities in the pathogenesis of certain diseases, and possible therapeutic uses of cytokines or their receptors. The important role of cytokines in the inflammatory response is discussed in Chapter 15.

PROPERTIES OF CYTOKINES

Cytokines are a group of low-molecular-weight regulatory proteins secreted by white blood cells and a variety of other cells in the body in response to a number of inducing stimuli. Cytokines bind to specific receptors on the membrane of target cells, triggering signal-transduction pathways that ultimately alter gene expression in the target cells (Figure 13-1a). The nature of the target cell for a particular cytokine is determined by the presence of specific membrane receptors. In general, the cytokines and their receptors exhibit very high affinity for each other with dissociation constants ranging from 10^{-10} to 10^{-12} M. Because of this high affinity, pico-molar concentrations of cytokines can mediate a biological effect.

A particular cytokine may bind to receptors on the membrane of the same cell that secreted it, exerting

autocrine action; it may bind to receptors on a target cell in close proximity to the producer cell, exerting **paracrine** action; in a few cases it may bind to target cells in distant parts of the body, exerting **endocrine** action (Figure 13-1b). Cytokines regulate the intensity and duration of the immune response by stimulating or inhibiting the activation, proliferation, and/or differentiation of various cells and by regulating the secretion of antibodies or other cytokines. As discussed later, binding of a given cytokine to responsive target cells generally stimulates expression of cytokine receptors as well as of other cytokines, which in turn affect other target cells. Thus, the cytokines secreted by a single lymphocyte following antigen-specific activation can influence the activity of various cells involved in the immune response. For example, cytokines produced by activated T_H cells can influence the activity of B cells, T_C cells, natural killer cells, macrophages, granulocytes, and hematopoietic stem cells, thereby activating an entire network of interacting cells.

Cytokines exhibit the attributes of pleiotropy, redundancy, synergy, and antagonism, which permit them to regulate cellular activity in a coordinated interactive way (Figure 13-2). A given cytokine that has different biological effects on different target cells has a **pleiotropic** action. Two or more cytokines that mediate similar functions are said to be **redundant**; this property makes it difficult to ascribe a particular activity to a single cytokine. Cytokine **synergism** occurs when the combined effect of two cytokines on cellular activity is greater than the additive effects of the individual cytokines. In some cases cytokines exhibit **antagonism**; that is, the effects of one cytokine inhibit or offset the effects of another cytokine.

The term *cytokine* encompasses those cytokines secreted by lymphocytes, formerly known as **lymphokines**, and those cytokines secreted by monocytes and macrophages, formerly known as **monokines**. Although these two terms continue to be used in the literature, they are misleading because many lymphokines and monokines are secreted by a broad spectrum of cells and not simply by lymphocytes and monocytes as their name would imply. For this reason the more inclusive term cytokine is preferred.

Many of the cytokines are referred to as **interleukins**, a name indicating that they are secreted by some leukocytes and act upon other leukocytes. Presently interleukins 1–17 have been identified. Other cytokines are known by common names; these include the interferons and tumor necrosis factors. A group of low-molecular-weight cytokines, including interleukin 8, is classified in the **chemokine** family. These molecules play an important role in the inflammatory response and are discussed in Chapter 15.

Because cytokines share many properties with hormones and growth factors, the distinction between these

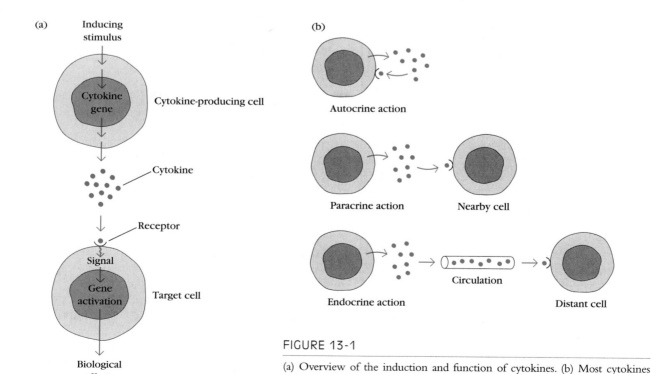

FIGURE 13-1

(a) Overview of the induction and function of cytokines. (b) Most cytokines exhibit autocrine and/or paracrine action; fewer exhibit endocrine action.

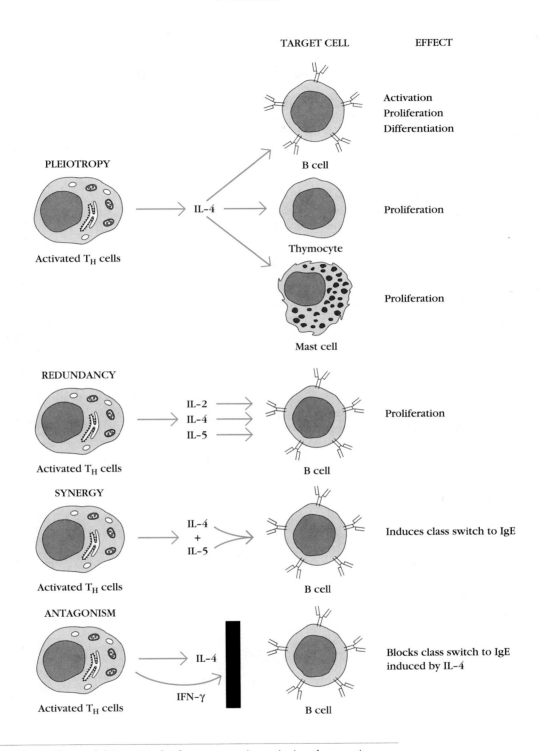

TARGET CELL   EFFECT

PLEIOTROPY

Activated T$_H$ cells

IL–4

B cell — Activation / Proliferation / Differentiation

Thymocyte — Proliferation

Mast cell — Proliferation

REDUNDANCY

Activated T$_H$ cells

IL–2
IL–4
IL–5

B cell — Proliferation

SYNERGY

Activated T$_H$ cells

IL–4
+
IL–5

B cell — Induces class switch to IgE

ANTAGONISM

Activated T$_H$ cells

IL–4

IFN–γ

B cell — Blocks class switch to IgE induced by IL–4

FIGURE 13-2

Examples of the cytokine attributes of pleiotropy, redundancy, synergy (synergism), and antagonism.

three classes of mediators is often blurred. All three classes of mediators are secreted soluble factors that elicit their biological effects at picomolar concentrations by binding to receptors on target cells. Growth factors tend to be produced constitutively, whereas cytokine production is carefully regulated. Cytokines generally are secreted following activation of a particular cell and secretion is short-lived, generally ranging from a few hours to a few days. Unlike hormones, which generally act long range in an endocrine fashion, most cytokines act over a short distance in an autocrine or paracrine fashion. In addition, most hormones are produced by specialized glands and tend to have a unique action on one or a few target cells. In contrast, cytokines are often produced by a variety of cells and bind to receptors present on numerous types of cells.

The activity of cytokines was first recognized in the mid-1960s, when culture supernatants derived from in vitro cultures of lymphocytes were found to contain factors that could regulate proliferation, differentiation, and maturation of allogeneic immune-system cells. Soon after, it was discovered that production of these factors by cultured lymphocytes was induced by activation with antigen or with nonspecific mitogens. Biochemical isolation and purification of cytokines was hampered because of their low concentration in culture supernatants and the absence of well-defined assay systems for individual cytokines. The development of gene cloning techniques during the 1970s and 1980s overcame the first problem, and discovery of cell lines whose growth depended on the presence of a particular cytokine provided researchers with simple assay systems.

General Structure of Cytokines

Once the genes encoding various cytokines had been cloned, sufficient quantities of purified preparations became available for detailed studies on the structure and function of these important proteins. Cytokines are proteins or glycoproteins that generally have a molecular mass of less than 30 kDa. Structural predictions based on sequence analyses, in some cases confirmed by x-ray crystallographic analysis, suggest that many cytokines belong to a family of structurally related proteins, called the **hematopoietins**. Included in the hematopoietin family are many interleukins (2–7, 9, 11–13, and 15), GM-CSF, G-CSF, oncostatin M (OSM), leukemia-inhibitory factor (LIF), and ciliary neurotrophic factor (CNTF).

Although the amino acid sequences of the various hematopoietins differ considerably, all of them have a high degree of α-helical structure and little or no β-sheet structure. The molecules share a similar polypeptide fold with four α-helical regions (A–D) in which the first and second helices and the third and fourth helices run roughly parallel to one another and are connected by loops. The structure of two hematopoietins, IL-2 and IL-4, are depicted in Figure 13-3.

Function of Cytokines

Cytokines generally function as intercellular messenger molecules that evoke particular biological activities after binding to a receptor on a responsive target cell. Although a variety of cells can secrete cytokines, the two principal producers are the T_H cell and the macrophage. Cytokines released from these two cells activate an entire network of interacting cells (Figure 13-4). Among the numerous physiologic responses that require cytokine involvement are development of cellular and humoral immune responses, induction of the inflammatory response, regulation of hematopoiesis, control of cellular proliferation and differentiation, and induction of wound healing.

Table 13-1 summarizes the main biological activities of a number of cytokines. It should be kept in mind that most of the listed functions have been identified from analysis of the effects of recombinant cytokines in in vitro systems and often at nonphysiologic concentrations.

(a) Interleukin 2

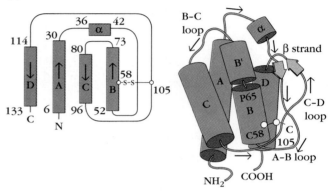

(b) Interleukin 4

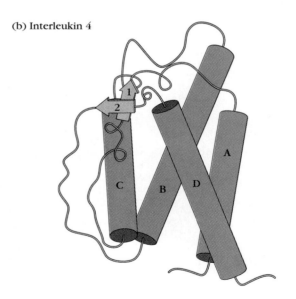

FIGURE 13-3

Several representations of the hematopoietin structure. (a) *Left:* Topographical representation of the primary structure of IL-2 showing α-helical regions (A–D) and connecting chains of the molecule. *Right:* Proposed three-dimensional model of IL-2. (b) Ribbon model of IL-4 deduced from x-ray crystallographic analysis of the molecule. The four α helices are shown in red and the two β sheets in blue. The structure of other cytokines belonging to the hematopoietin family are thought to be generally similar. [Part (b) from J. L. Boulay and W. E. Paul, 1993, *Curr. Biol.* **3**:573.]

Visualizing Concepts

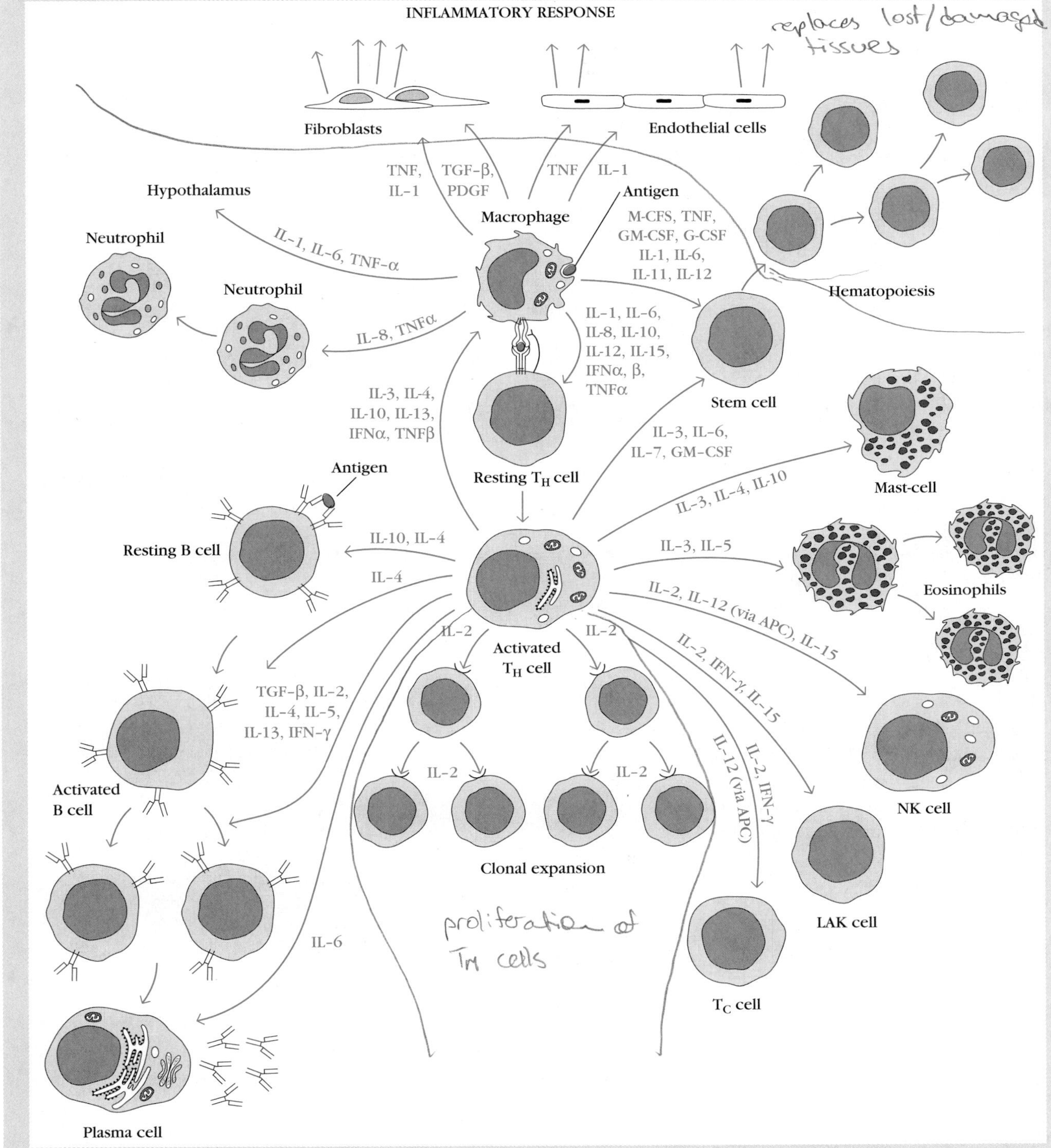

FIGURE 13-4

Interaction of antigen (blue) with macrophages and the subsequent activation of resting T_H cells leads to release of numerous cytokines, generating a complex network of interacting cells in the immune response.

T A B L E   1 3 – 1

SELECTED FUNCTIONS OF SOME CYTOKINES

CYTOKINE	SECRETED BY*	MAJOR BIOLOGICAL FUNCTIONS	
		TARGET CELLS/TISSUES	ACTIVITY
Interleukin 1 (IL-1α, IL-1β)	Monocytes, macrophages, B cells, dendritic cells, endothelial cells, other cell types	T_H cells	Co-stimulates activation
		B cells	Promotes maturation and clonal expansion
		NK cells	Enhances activity
		Vascular endothelial cells	Increases expression of ICAMs
		Macrophages and neutrophils	Chemotactically attracts
		Hepatocytes	Induces synthesis of acute-phase proteins
		Hypothalamus	Induces fever
Interleukin 2 (IL-2)	T_H1 cells	Antigen-primted T_H and T_C cells	Induces proliferation
		Antigen-specific T-cell clones	Supports long-term growth
		NK cells (some) and T_C cells	Enhances activity
Interleukin 3 (IL-3)	T_H cells, NK cells, mast cells	Hematopoietic cells	Supports growth and differentiation
		Mast cells	Stimulates growth and histamine secretion
Interleukin 4 (IL-4)	T_H2 cells, mast cells, NK cells	Antigen-primed B cells	Co-stimulates activation
		Activated B cells	Stimulates proliferation and differentiation; induces class switch to IgG1 and IgE
		Resting B cells	Up-regulates class II MHC expression
		Thymocytes and T cells	Induces proliferation
		Macrophages	Up-regulates class II MHC expression; increases phagocytic activity
		Mast cells	Stimulates growth
Interleukin 5	T_H2 cells, mast cells	Activated B cells	Stimualtes proliferation and differentation; induces class switch to IgA
		Eosinophils	Promotes growth and differentiation
Interleukin 6	Monocytes, macrophages, T_H2 cells, bone-marrow stromal cells	Proliferating B cells	Promotes terminal differentiation into plasma cells
		Plasma cells	Stimulates antibody secretion
		Myeloid stem cells	Helps promote differentiation
		Hepatocytes	Induces synthesis of acute-phase proteins

(continued on the following page)

TABLE 13 - 1 (continued)

SELECTED FUNCTIONS OF SOME CYTOKINES

CYTOKINE	SECRETED BY*	MAJOR BIOLOGICAL FUNCTIONS	
		TARGET CELLS/TISSUES	ACTIVITY
Interleukin 7 (IL-7)	Bone-marrow, thymic stromal cells	Lymphoid stem cells	Induces differentiation into progenitor B and T cells
		Resting T cells	Increases expression of IL-2 and its receptor
Interleukin 8 (IL-8)	Macrophages, endothelial cells	Neutrophils	Chemokine; chemotactically attracts; induces adherence to vascular endothelium and extravasation into tissues
Interleukin 9 (IL-9)	T_H cells	Some T_H cells	Acts as mitogen, supporting proliferation in absence of antigen
Interleukin 10 (IL-10)	T_H2 cells	Macrophages	Suppresses cytokine production and thus indirectly reduces cytokine production by T_H1 cells
		Antigen-presenting cells	Down-regulates class II MHC expression
Interleukin 11 (IL-11)	Bone-marrow stromal cells	Plasmacytomas	Supports growth
		Progenitor B cells	Promotes differentiation
		Megakaryocytes	Promotes differentiation
		Hepatocytes	Induces synthesis of acute-phase proteins
Interleukin 12 (IL-12)	Macrophages, B cells	Activated T_C cells	Acts synergistically with IL-2 to induce differentation into CTLs
		NK and LAK cells and activated T_H1 cells	Stimulates proliferation
Interleukin 13 (IL-13)	T_H cells	Macrophages	Inhibits activation and release of inflammatory cytokines; important regulator of inflammatory response
Interleukin 15 (IL-15)	T cells	T cells, intestinal epithelium	Stimulates growth of intestinal epithelium, T cell proliferation
		NK	Supports proliferation
		Activated B cells	Co-mitogen for proliferation and differentiation
Interleukin 16 (IL-16)	T cells (primarily $CD8^+$) Eosinophils	$CD4^+$ T cells	Chemotaxis; induces expression of class II MHC; induces synthesis of cytokines; suppresses antigen-induced proliferation

(continued on the following page)

T A B L E   1 3 - 1   (c o n t i n u e d)

SELECTED FUNCTIONS OF SOME CYTOKINES

CYTOKINE	SECRETED BY*	MAJOR BIOLOGICAL FUNCTIONS	
		TARGET CELLS/TISSUES	ACTIVITY
Interleukin 16 (IL-16)		Monocytes	Chemotaxis; induces class II MHC
		Eosinophils	Chemotaxis; induces cell adhesion
Interferon alpha (IFN-α)	Leukocytes	Uninfected cells	Inhibits viral replication
Interferon beta (IFN-β)	Fibroblasts	Uninfected cells	Inhibits viral replication
Interferon gamma (IFN-γ)	T_H1, T_C, NK cells	Uninfected cells	Inhibits viral replication
		Macrophages	Enhances activity
		Many cell types	Increases expression of class I and class II MHC molecules
		Proliferating B cells	Induces class switch to IgG2a; blocks IL-4–induced class switch to IgE and IgG1
		T_H2 cells	Inhibits proliferation
		Inflammatory cells	Mediates various effects important in delayed-type hypersensitivity
Leukemia-inhibitory factor (LIF)	Thymic epithelial cells, bone-marrow stromal cells	Hepatocytes	Induces synthesis of acute-phase proteins
		Embryonic stem (ES) cells	Supports proliferation and differentiation
Oncostatin M (OSM)	Macrophages, T cells	Tumor cells	Inhibits growth
		Hepatocytes	Induces synthesis of acute-phase proteins
		Kaposi's sarcoma	Stimulates growth
Transforming growth factor β (TGF-β)	Platelets, macrophages, lymphocytes, mast cells	Monocytes and macrophages	Chemotactically attracts
		Activated macrophages	Induces increased IL-1 production
		Epithelial, endothelial, lymphoid, and hematopoietic cells	Inhibits proliferation, thus limiting inflammatory response and promoting wound healing
		Proliferating B cells	Induces class switch to IgA
Tumor necrosis factor α (TNF-α)	Macrophages, mast cells	Tumor cells	Has cytotoxic effect
		Inflammatory cells	Induces cytokine secretion and is responsible for extensive weight loss (cachexia) associated with chronic inflammation
Tumor necrosis factor β (TNF-β)	T_H1 and T_C cells	Tumor cells	Has cytotoxic and other effects similar to TNF-α
		Macrophages and neutrophils	Enhances phagocytic activity

* Activated cells generally exhibit greater cytokine secretion than unactivated cells.

However, cytokines rarely, if ever, act alone in vivo. Instead, a target cell is exposed to a milieu containing a mixture of cytokines, whose combined synergistic or antagonistic effects can have very different consequences. In addition, cytokines often induce the synthesis of other cytokines, resulting in cascades of cytokine activity in which later cytokines may influence the activity of earlier cytokines.

It is difficult to reconcile the nonspecificity of cytokines with the established specificity of the immune system. What keeps the nonspecific cytokines from activating cells in a nonspecific fashion during the immune response? Clearly mechanisms must operate to ensure that the specificity of the immune response is maintained. One way in which specificity is maintained is by careful regulation of the expression of cytokine receptors on cells. Often cytokine receptors are expressed on a cell only after that cell has interacted with antigen. In this way nonspecific cytokine activation is limited to antigen-activated lymphocytes. Another means of maintaining specificity may be a requirement for cell-to-cell interaction to generate effective concentrations of a cytokine at the juncture of interacting cells. In the case of the T_H cell, a major producer of cytokines, close cellular interaction occurs when the T-cell receptor recognizes an antigen-MHC complex on an appropriate antigen-presenting cell, such as a macrophage, dendritic cell, or B lymphocyte. Cytokines secreted at the junction of these interacting cells reach concentrations high enough to affect the target cell. In addition, the half-life of cytokines in the bloodstream or other extracellular fluids into which they are secreted is usually very short, ensuring that they act for only a limited period of time.

CYTOKINE RECEPTORS

As noted already, to exert their biological effects, cytokines must first bind to specific receptors expressed on the membrane of responsive target cells. Because these receptors are expressed by many types of cells, the cytokines can affect a diverse array of cells. Biochemical characterization of cytokine receptors initially progressed at a very slow pace because their levels on the membrane of responsive cells is quite low. As in the case of the cytokines themselves, cloning of the genes encoding cytokine receptors has led to rapid advances in the identification and characterization of these receptors.

General Structure of Cytokine Receptors

Receptors for the various cytokines are quite diverse structurally, belonging to five families of receptor proteins (Figure 13-5):

- Immunoglobulin superfamily receptors
- Class I cytokine receptor family (also known as the hematopoietin receptor family)
- Class II cytokine receptor family (also known as the interferon receptor family
- TNF receptor family
- Chemokine receptor family

Most of the cytokine-binding receptors that function in the immune and hematopoietic systems belong to the class I cytokine receptor family. The members of this receptor family have conserved amino acid sequence motifs in the extracellular domain consisting of four positionally conserved cysteine residues (CCCC) and a conserved sequence of Trp-Ser-X-Trp-Ser (WSXWS), where X is a nonconserved amino acid. The receptors for all the cytokines classified as hematopoietins belong to the class I cytokine receptor family, which also is called the hematopoietin receptor family. The known ligands for class II cytokine receptors are the three interferons α, β, and γ. These receptors possess the conserved CCCC motifs, but lack the WSXWS motif present in class I cytokine receptors.

Another common feature of the hematopoietin (class I cytokine) receptor family is that most of these receptors are composed of two types of polypeptide chains: a **cytokine-specific subunit** and a **signal-transducing subunit**, which often is not specific for the cytokine. Most of these receptors are dimers, comprising one cytokine-specific and one signal-transducing subunit, but a few are trimers. The signal-transducing subunit is required for high-affinity binding of a cytokine as well as for transduction of an activating signal across the membrane. The signal-transducing subunits of all the class I and class II cytokine receptors studied to date have been shown to induce tyrosine phosphorylation, although none has tyrosine kinase activity in itself. This finding suggests that the cytosolic domain of the signal-transducing subunit is closely associated with a cytosolic protein kinase.

Subfamilies of Class I Cytokine Receptors

One of the most significant findings to emerge in the last couple of years regarding class I cytokine receptors is that they often share common signal-transducing subunits with other members of the same family. For example, several class I cytokine receptor subfamilies have been identified, with all the receptors in one subfamily having an identical signal-transducing subunit. Figure 13-6 schematically illustrates the members of three receptor subfamilies: the GM-CSF subfamily, the IL-2 subfamily, and the IL-6 subfamily.

RECEPTOR FAMILY

LIGANDS

(a) Immunoglobulin superfamily
    receptors

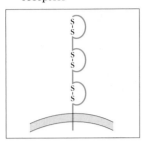

IL-1
M-CSF
C-Kit

(b) Class I cytokine receptors
    (hematopoietin)

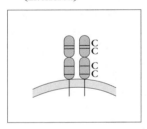

Conserved
cysteines

WSXWS

IL-2	IL-13
IL-3	IL-15
IL-4	GM-CSF
IL-5	G-CSF
IL-6	OSM
IL-7	LIF
IL-9	CNTF
IL-11	Growth hormone
IL-12	Prolactin

(c) Class II cytokine receptors
    (interferon)

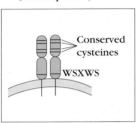

C
C
C
C

IFN α
IFN β
IFN γ

(d) TNF receptors

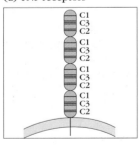

C1
C3
C2
C1
C3
C2
C1
C3
C2
C1
C3
C2

TNF α
TNF β
CD40
Nerve growth factor (NGF)
FAS

(e) Chemokine receptors

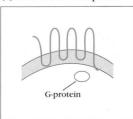

G-protein

IL-8
RANTES
MIP-1
PF4
MCAF
NAP-2

FIGURE 13-5

Schematic diagrams showing the structural features that define the five types of cytokine-binding receptor proteins. The receptors for most of the interleukins belong to the class I cytokine recpetor family.

The sharing of signal-transducing subunits among receptors explains the redundancy and antagonism exhibited by some cytokines. Consider the GM-CSF receptor subfamily, which includes the receptors for IL-3, IL-5, and GM-CSF (see Figure 13-6a). Each of these cytokines binds to a unique low-affinity, cytokine-specific receptor consisting of an α subunit only. All three low-affinity α subunits can associate noncovalently with a common signal-transducing β subunit. The resulting dimeric receptor not only exhibits increased affinity for the cytokine but also can transduce a signal across the membrane following cytokine binding (Figure 13-7). Interestingly, IL-3, IL-5, and GM-CSF exhibit considerable redundancy. Both IL-3 and GM-CSF act upon hematopoietic stem cells and progenitor cells, activate monocytes, and induce megakaryocyte differentiation. All three of these cytokines induce eosinophil proliferation and basophil degranulation with release of histamine.

Since the receptors for IL-3, IL-5, and GM-CSF share a common signal-transducing β subunit, each of these cytokines would be expected to transduce a similar activation signal, accounting for the redundancy among their biological effects. In fact, all three cytokines induce the same patterns of protein phosphorylation and phosphorylate the protein kinase Raf. Furthermore, IL-3 and GM-CSF exhibit antagonism; IL-3 binding has been shown to be inhibited by GM-CSF, and conversely, the binding of GM-CSF has been shown to be inhibited by IL-3. Since the signal-transducing β subunit is shared between these two cytokines, their antagonism is due to competition for a limited number of β subunits by the cytokine-specific α subunits.

A similar situation is found among the IL-6 receptor subfamily, which includes the receptors for IL-6, IL-11, IL-12, leukemia-inhibitory factor (LIF), oncostatin M (OSM), and ciliary neurotrophic factor (CNTF)(see Figure 13-6b). In this case, a common signal-transducing subunit, called gp130, associates with one or two different cytokine-specific subunits. LIF and OSM, which must share certain structural features, both bind to the same α subunit. As expected, the cytokines that bind to receptors in this subfamily display overlapping biological activities: IL-6, OSM, and LIF induce synthesis of acute-phase proteins by liver hepatocytes; IL-6, OSM, and LIF induce differentiation of myeloid leukemia cells into macrophages; IL-6, LIF, and CNTF affect neuronal development; IL-6, IL-11, and OSM stimulate megakaryocyte maturation and platelet production; and IL-6

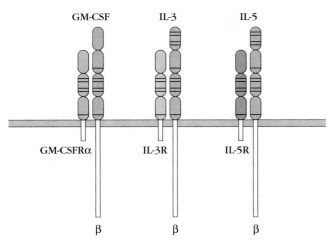

(a) GM-CSF receptor subfamily (common β subunit)

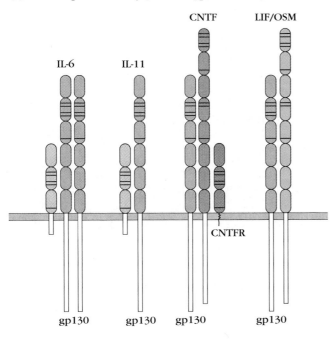

(b) IL-6 Receptor subfamily (common gp/30 subunit)

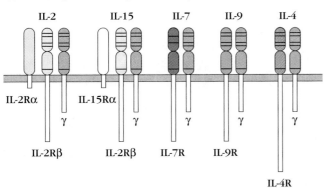

(c) IL-2 receptor subfamily (common γ subunit)

FIGURE 13-6

Schematic diagrams of the three subfamilies of class I cytokine receptors. All members of a subfamily have a common signal-transducing subunit, but a unique cytokine-specific subunit. In addition to the conserved cysteines and WSXWS motifs that characterize class I cytokine receptors, fibronectin-like and immunoglobulin-like domains are present in some of these receptors. To date, two receptors of the IL-6 subfamily (IL-6 and CNTF) and two of the IL-2 subfamily (IL-2 and IL-15) have been shown to be trimeric proteins. (Adapted from K. Sugamura et al. 1996, *Annu. Rev. Immunol.* **14**:179.)

and OSM stimulate proliferation of Kaposi's sarcoma cells. The presence of gp130 in all receptors of the IL-6 subfamily explains their common signaling pathways as well as the binding competition for limited gp130 molecules that is observed among these cytokines.

A third signal-transducing subunit defines the IL-2 receptor subfamily, which includes receptors for IL-2, IL-4, IL-7, IL-9, and IL-15 (see Figure 13-6c). Unlike the other members of the class I cytokine receptor family, the IL-2 and the IL-15 receptors are trimers, consisting of a cytokine-specific α chain and two chains—β and γ—responsible for signal transduction. The IL-2 receptor γ chain functions as the signal-transducing subunit in the other receptors in this subfamily, which are all dimers. Recently, it has been shown that **X-linked severe combined immunodeficiency** (XSCID) results from a defect in the γ-chain gene, which maps to the X chromosome. The immunodeficiencies observed in this disorder are due to the loss of all the cytokine functions mediated by the IL-2 subfamily receptors.

IL-2 Receptor

Because of the central role of IL-2 and its receptor in the clonal proliferation of T cells, the IL-2 receptor is the most studied of the cytokine receptors. As noted in the previous section, the complete trimeric receptor comprises three distinct subunits—the α, β, and γ chains. The β and γ chains belong to the class I cytokine receptor family, containing the characteristic C-C-C-C and W-S-X-W-S motifs, whereas the α chain has a quite different structure and is not a member of this receptor family (see Figure 13-6c).

The IL-2 receptor occurs in three forms that exhibit different affinities for IL-2: the low-affinity monomeric IL-2Rα, the intermediate-affinity dimeric IL-2Rβγ, and the high-affinity trimeric IL-2Rαβγ (Figure 13-8). Because the α chain is expressed by activated but not resting T cells, it is often referred to as the TAC (T-cell activation) antigen. A monoclonal antibody, designated **anti-TAC**, which binds to the 55-kDa α chain, is often used to identify IL-2Rα on cells. Signal transduction by the IL-2 receptor requires both the β and γ chains, but

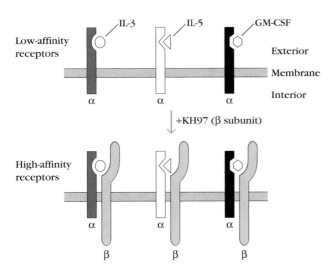

FIGURE 13-7

Schematic diagram of the low-affinity and high-affinity receptors for IL-3, IL-5, and GM-CSF. The cytokine-specific subunits exhibit low-affinity binding and cannot transduce an activation signal. Noncovalent association of each subunit with a common β subunit (KH97) yields a high-affinity dimeric receptor that can transduce a signal across the membrane. [Adapted from T. Kishimoto et al., 1992, *Science* **258**:593.]

only the trimeric receptor containing the α chain as well binds IL-2 with high affinity. Although the γ chain appears to be constitutively expressed on most lymphoid cells, expression of the α and β chains is more restricted and is markedly enhanced following antigen activation of resting lymphocytes. This phenomenon ensures that only antigen-activated CD4+ and CD8+ T cells will express the high-affinity IL-2 receptor and proliferate in response to physiologic levels of IL-2. Activated T cells express approximately 5×10^3 high-affinity receptors and ten times as many low-affinity receptors. NK cells express the β and γ subunits constitutively, accounting for their ability to bind IL-2 with an intermediate affinity and to be activated by IL-2.

Signal Transduction Mediated by Cytokine Receptors

As mentioned previously, class I and class II cytokine receptors lack signaling motifs (e.g., an intrinsic tyrosine kinase domain). Yet one of the first events that occurs following the interaction of a cytokine with one of these receptors is a series of protein tyrosine phosphorylations. Recent findings suggest a unifying model for signaling by cytokine receptors. It now appears that signal transduction through most, if not all, class I and class II cytokine receptors begins with cytokine-induced dimerization of receptor subunits. This dimerization of receptor subunits juxtaposes their cytosolic domains, allowing

the dimeric receptor to engage the intracellular signaling machinery.

Figure 13-9 outlines the model of signal transduction that is thought to apply generally to class I and class II cytokine receptors. The **JAK kinases**, a recently discovered family of cytosolic protein tyrosine kinases, become activated by interacting with the cytosolic domains of the dimerized receptor. Depending on the cytokine/receptor system, one or more of the four known JAK kinases are involved. The activated JAK kinases then begin to phosphorylate each other, the cytosolic domain of the receptor, and a family of transcription factors known as **STATs** (**signal transducers and activators of transcription**). Following their phosphorylation, the STAT proteins dimerize in the cytoplasm and subsequently translocate to the nucleus where they bind to sequence-specific DNA regulatory elements, thereby activating gene transcription.

These exciting advances have demonstrated a direct pathway whereby cytokine binding leads to changes in gene transcription. An important property of the cytokine-STAT pathway is its specificity. That is, each particular cytokine (or group of redundant cytokines) induces transcription of a specific subset of genes; the resulting gene products then mediate the various effects typical of that cytokine. As additional receptor-associated kinases, STAT proteins, and DNA regulatory elements are identified, the molecular basis of this specificity will be defined more precisely.

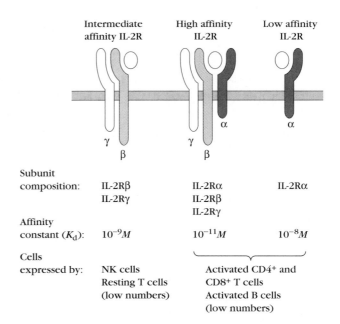

	Intermediate affinity IL-2R	High affinity IL-2R	Low affinity IL-2R
Subunit composition:	IL-2Rβ IL-2Rγ	IL-2Rα IL-2Rβ IL-2Rγ	IL-2Rα
Affinity constant (K_d):	$10^{-9}M$	$10^{-11}M$	$10^{-8}M$
Cells expressed by:	NK cells Resting T cells (low numbers)	Activated CD4+ and CD8+ T cells Activated B cells (low numbers)	

FIGURE 13-8

Comparison of the three forms of the IL-2 receptor. Signal transduction is mediated by the β and γ chains, but all three chains are required for high-affinity binding of IL-2.

Visualizing Concepts

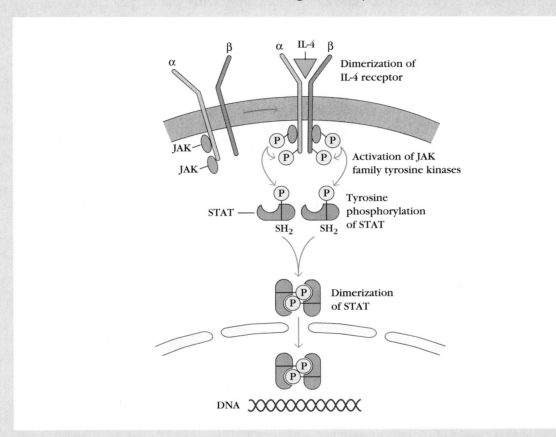

FIGURE 13-9

Model of signal transduction mediated by most class I and class II cytokine receptors. Cytokine binding induces dimerization of the receptor subunits. Association of JAK tyrosine kinases with the dimeric receptor activates the kinases, which then phosphorylate various tyrosine residues, including one or more in STAT transcription factors. After the phosphorylated STATs dimerize, they translocate to the nucleus where they activate transcription of specific genes.

CYTOKINE ANTAGONISTS

A number of proteins that inhibit the biological activity of cytokines have been reported. These proteins act in one of two ways: either they bind directly to a cytokine receptor but fail to activate the cell, or they bind directly to a cytokine inhibiting its activity. The best-characterized inhibitor is the IL-1 receptor antagonist (IL-1Ra), which binds to the IL-1 receptor but has no activity. Binding of IL-1Ra to the IL-1 receptor blocks binding of both IL-1α and IL-1β, thus accounting for the antagonistic properties of IL-1Ra. Production of IL-1Ra appears to play a role in regulating the intensity of the inflammatory response. IL-1Ra has been cloned and is currently being investigated as a potential treatment for chronic inflammatory diseases.

Cytokine inhibitors are a second group of soluble cytokine receptors, which are found in the bloodstream and extracellular fluid. These soluble receptors result from enzymatic cleavage of the extracellular domain of cytokine receptors. The released soluble fragments can bind cytokines, thereby neutralizing their activity. Among the soluble cytokine receptors that have been detected are those for IL-2, IL-4, IL-6, IL-7, IFN-γ, TNF-α, TNF-β, and LIF. Of these, the soluble IL-2 receptor, which is released following chronic T-cell activation, is the best characterized. The amino-terminal 192 amino acids of the α subunit is released by proteolytic cleavage, forming a 45-kDa soluble IL-2 receptor (sIL-2R). The shed receptor can bind IL-2 and prevent its interaction with the membrane-bound IL-2R. The presence of sIL-2R has been used as a clinical marker of chronic T-cell activation and is observed in a number of diseases including auto-immunity, transplant rejection, and AIDS.

In addition, some viruses produce cytokine-binding proteins. The poxviruses, for example, have been shown to encode a soluble TNF-binding protein and a soluble IL-1–binding protein. Since both TNF and IL-1 exhibit a broad spectrum of activities in the inflammatory response, these soluble cytokine-binding proteins may prohibit or diminish the inflammatory effects of the cytokine, thereby conferring upon the virus a selective advantage.

CYTOKINE SECRETION BY T$_H$1 AND T$_H$2 SUBSETS

The immune response to a specific antigen must induce an appropriate set of effector functions that can eliminate the particular pathogen involved in the infection. For example, the neutralization of a soluble bacterial toxin requires antibodies, whereas the response to an intracellular virus or bacterial cell requires cell-mediated cytotoxicity or delayed-type hypersensitivity. In the last few years a large body of evidence has accumulated suggesting that differences in cytokine-secretion patterns among T$_H$-cell subsets play a major role in regulating the choice of immune functional modality.

CD4$^+$ T$_H$ cells exert most of their helper functions through secreted cytokines, which either act on the cells that produce them in an autocrine fashion or modulate the responses of other cells through paracrine pathways. Although CD8$^+$ CTLs also secrete cytokines, their array of cytokines generally is more restricted than that of CD4$^+$ T$_H$ cells. As discussed in previous chapters, two mouse CD4$^+$ T$_H$-cell subpopulations can be distinguished in vitro by the cytokines they secrete. As shown in Table 13-2, these two subsets, designated T$_H$1 and T$_H$2, both secrete IL-3 and GM-CSF, but otherwise they differ in the cytokines they secrete.

The differences in the cytokines secreted by T$_H$1 and T$_H$2 cells are thought to reflect different biological functions of these two subsets:

- The T$_H$1 subset is responsible for classical cell-mediated functions (e.g., delayed-type hypersensitivity and activation of T$_C$ cells).
- The T$_H$2 subset functions primarily as a helper for B-cell activation.

The T$_H$1 subset may be particularly suited to respond to viral infections and intracellular pathogens because it secretes IL-2 and IFN-γ, which activate T$_C$ cells and macrophages. The T$_H$2 subset may be more suited to respond to freeliving bacteria and helminthic parasites and may mediate allergic reactions, since IL-4 and IL-5 are known to induce IgE production and eosinophil activation, respectively. In humans, there is now considerable evidence for T$_H$1-like and T$_H$2-like subsets, although the expression of a few cytokines such as IL-2 and IL-10 does not show such a clear segregation as seen in the mouse.

TABLE 13-2

CYTOKINE SECRETION AND PRINCIPAL FUNCTIONS OF MOUSE T$_H$1 AND T$_H$2 SUBSETS

CYTOKINE/FUNCTION	T$_H$1	T$_H$2
CYTOKINE SECRETION		
IL-2	+	–
IFN-γ	++	–
TNF-β	++	–
GM-CSF	++	+
IL-3	++	++
IL-4	–	++
IL-5	–	++
IL-10	–	++
IL-13	–	++
FUNCTIONS		
Help for total antibody production	+	++
Help for IgE production	–	++
Help for IgG2a production	++	+
Eosinophil and mast-cell production	–	++
Macrophage activation	++	–
Delayed-type hypersensitivity	++	–
T$_C$-cell activation	++	–

SOURCE: Adapted from F. Powrie and R. L. Coffman, 1993, *Immunol. Today* **14**:270.

Because the T_H1 and T_H2 subsets were originally identified in long-term in vitro cultures, some researchers have doubted that they represent true in vivo subpopulations and have suggested instead that they represent different maturational stages of a single lineage. Nevertheless, numerous reports in both mice and humans suggest that the in vivo outcome of the immune response depends on the relative levels of T_H1-like or T_H2-like activity: T_H1 cytokines are generally elevated in responses to intracellular pathogens, and T_H2 cytokines are elevated in allergic diseases and helminthic infections.

Development of T_H1 and T_H2 Subsets

The cytokine environment that is present as antigen-primed T_H cells differentiate is thought to determine the subset that develops. Two cytokines in particular, IL-4 and IL-12, play decisive roles in determining whether a T_H1 or T_H2 response develops. For example, when T_H cells are activated in vitro by an antigen together with IL-4, they develop into the T_H2 subset; in contrast, activation with the same antigen in the presence of IL-12 results in the development of the T_H1 subset. The cytokine environment has also been shown to regulate T_H-cell subset development in vivo. When transgenic mice expressing a T-cell receptor specific for ovalbumin were challenged with the ovalbumin antigen in the presence of IL-12, they produced a T_H1 response; in contrast, immunization with ovalbumin in the presence of IL-4 produced a T_H2 response.

Based on recent studies some researchers have proposed that $CD4^+$ T cells develop into polarized T_H1 or T_H2 subsets via a T_H0 precursor (Figure 13-10). These T_H0 precursors secrete IL-2, IL-4, and IFN-γ and have the potential of differentiating into either T_H1 or T_H2 subsets. Evidence for such a T_H0 precursor comes from experiments using transgenic mice in which IL-4—secreting cells were eliminated with the drug gancyclovir. This treatment also eliminated IFN-γ production, even though IL-4 and IFN-γ are secreted by different fully differentiated subsets (see Table 13-2). This finding suggests the existence of a common precursor T_H0 cell, capable of secreting both cytokines.

Cytokine Cross-Regulation

The cytokines produced by the T_H1 and T_H2 subsets exhibit **cross-regulation**; that is, the cytokines secreted by one subset can block the production and/or activity of the cytokines secreted by the other subset (Figure 13-11). For instance, IFN-γ (secreted by the T_H1 subset) preferentially inhibits proliferation of the T_H2 subset, and IL-10 (secreted by the T_H2 subset) down-regulates secretion of IFN-γ and IL-2 by the T_H1 subset. Similarly,

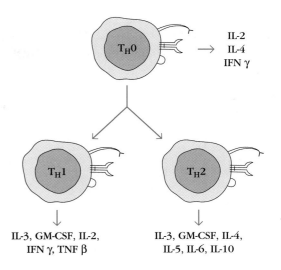

FIGURE 13-10

$CD4^+$ T cells develop into T_H1 or T_H2 subsets via a T_H0 precursor. Each of the T_H subsets secretes distinct cytokines.

IFN-γ and IL-2 (secreted by the T_H1 subset) promote IgG2a production by B cells but inhibit IgG1 and IgE production. On the other hand, IL-4 (secreted by the T_H2 subset) promotes production of IgG1 and IgE and suppresses production of IgG2a. The phenomenon of cross-regulation provides an explanation for the observation that there is an inverse relationship between antibody production and delayed-type hypersensitivity; that is, when antibody production is high, delayed-type hypersensitivity is low and vice versa.

Interleukin 10 does not inhibit T_H1 cells directly; instead, it acts on monocytes and macrophages and interferes with their ability to activate the T_H1 subset. This interference is thought to result from the demonstrated ability of IL-10 to dramatically down-regulate the expression of class II MHC molecules on these antigen-presenting cells. IL-10 has other potent immunosuppressant effects on the monocyte-macrophage lineage: it suppresses the production of nitrogen oxides and other bactericidal metabolites involved in the destruction of pathogens and the production of various inflammatory mediators (e.g., IL-1, IL-6, IL-8, GM-CSF, G-CSF, and TNF-α). These suppressive effects on the macrophage serve to further diminish the biologic consequences of T_H1 activation.

Role of T_H1/T_H2 Balance in Determining Disease Outcomes

The progression of some diseases may depend on the balance between the T_H1 and T_H2 subsets. A well-studied example of this phenomenon is leprosy, which is caused by *Mycobacterium leprae*, an intracellular pathogen

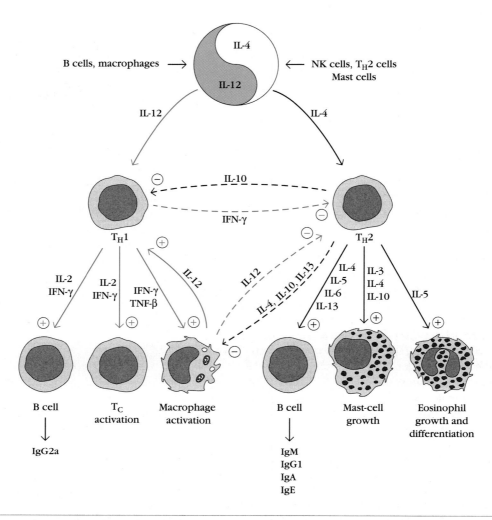

FIGURE 13-11

Cross-regulation by cytokines secreted from T_H1 and T_H2 subsets. Solid arrows indicate stimulatory effects; dashed arrows indicate inhibitory effects. IL-12 and IL-4 preferentially stimulate formation of the T_H1 and T_H2 subsets, respectively.

that is able to survive within the phagosomes of macrophages. Leprosy is not a single clinical entity; rather the disease presents as a spectrum of clinical responses, with two major forms of disease, tuberculoid and lepromatous, at each end of the spectrum. In **tuberculoid leprosy**, a cell-mediated immune response develops with the formation of granulomas, resulting in the destruction of most of the organisms so that only a few organisms remain in the tissues. Although skin and peripheral nerves are damaged, tuberculoid leprosy progresses slowly and patients usually survive. In **lepromatous leprosy**, the cell-mediated response is depressed and instead humoral antibodies are formed, sometimes resulting in hypergammaglobulinemia. The organisms are widely disseminated in macrophages, often reaching numbers as high as 10^{10} per gram of tissue. Lepromatous leprosy progresses into disseminated infection of the bone and cartilage with extensive nerve damage.

The development of lepromatous or tuberculoid leprosy depends on the balance of T_H1 and T_H2 cells (Figure 13-12). In tuberculoid leprosy the immune response is characterized by a T_H1-type response with T_{DTH} activity and a cytokine profile consisting of high levels of IL-2, IFN-γ, and TNF-α. In lepromatous leprosy there is a T_H2-type immune response with high levels of IL-4, IL-5, and IL-10. This cytokine profile explains the diminished cell-mediated immunity and increased serum antibody production in lepromatous leprosy.

There is also evidence for changes in T_H-subset activity in AIDS. Early in the disease T_H1 activity is high, but as AIDS progresses, there is a shift from a T_H1-like to a T_H2-like response that correlates with disease progres-

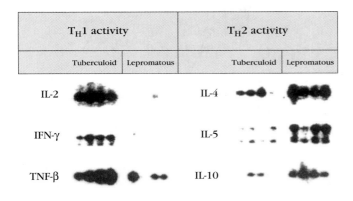

T$_H$1 activity		T$_H$2 activity	
Tuberculoid	Lepromatous	Tuberculoid	Lepromatous

IL-2	IL-4
IFN-γ	IL-5
TNF-β	IL-10

FIGURE 13-12

Correlation between type of leprosy and relative T$_H$1 or T$_H$2 activity. mRNA isolated from lesions from tuberculoid and lepromatous leprosy patients was analyzed by Southern blotting using the cytokine probes indicated. Cytokines produced by T$_H$1 cells predominate in the tuberculoid patients, while cytokines produced by T$_H$2 cells predominate in the lepromatous patients. [From P. A. Sieling and R. L. Modlin, 1994, *Immunobiology* **191**:378.]

sion (see Chapter 22). In addition, some pathogens may influence the activity of the T$_H$ subsets. The Epstein-Barr virus, for instance, produces a protein that has been shown to have sequence homology with IL-10. This viral protein, designated vIL-10 in reference to this homology, has IL-10–like activity and tends to suppress T$_H$1 activity via cross-regulation. Some researchers have speculated that vIL-10 may reduce the cell-mediated response to the virus, thus conferring a survival advantage to the Epstein-Barr virus.

CYTOKINE-RELATED DISEASES

Defects in the complex regulatory networks governing the expression of cytokines and cytokine receptors have been implicated in a number of diseases. In this section, we discuss several diseases resulting from overexpression or underexpression of cytokines or cytokine receptors.

Bacterial Septic Shock

The role of cytokine overproduction in pathogenesis can be illustrated by bacterial septic shock. This condition may develop within a few hours following infection by certain gram-negative bacteria including *E. coli, Klebsiella pneumoniae, Pseudomonas aeruginosa, Enterobacter aerogenes,* and *Neisseria meningitidis.* The symptoms of bacterial septic shock, which often is fatal, include a drop in blood pressure, fever, diarrhea, and widespread blood clotting

in various organs. This condition afflicts about 500,000 Americans annually and causes more than 70,000 deaths. The annual cost for treating bacterial septic shock is an estimated $5–10 billion.

Bacterial septic shock appears to develop when bacterial cell-wall **endotoxins** stimulate macrophages to overproduce IL-1 and TNF-α. It is the increased levels of IL-1 and TNF-α that cause septic shock. In one study, for example, higher levels of TNF-α were found in patients who died of meningitis than in those who recovered. Furthermore, a condition resembling bacterial septic shock can be produced by injection of recombinant TNF-α in the absence of gram-negative bacterial infection. Several studies offer some hope that neutralization of TNF-α or IL-1 activity with monoclonal antibodies or antagonists may prevent this fatal shock from developing in these bacterial infections. In one study, monoclonal antibody to TNF-α was shown to prevent an otherwise fatal endotoxin-induced shock in animal models. And another study has shown that injection of a recombinant IL-1 receptor antagonist (IL-1Ra), which prevents binding of IL-1 to the IL-1 receptor, reduced the mortality due to septic shock in humans from 45% to 16%. It is hoped that these experimental results will have therapeutic benefit for the treatment of bacterial septic shock in humans.

Bacterial Toxic Shock and Similar Diseases

A variety of microorganisms produce toxins that act as **superantigens**. As discussed in previous chapters, superantigens bind simultaneously to a class II MHC molecule and to the V$_β$ domain of the T-cell receptor, activating all T cells bearing a particular V$_β$ domain. Unlike conventional antigens, superantigens are not internalized, processed, and presented by antigen-presenting cells. Instead they bind directly to class II MHC molecules, apparently outside of the antigen-binding cleft. Likewise, superantigens are thought to bind to an exposed region of the β pleated sheet on the side of the T-cell receptor, well away from the sites that bind normal antigenic peptides (see Figure 4-14). Because of their unique binding ability, superantigens can activate large numbers of T cells irrespective of their antigenic specificity.

Although less than 0.01% of T cells respond to a given conventional antigen, between 5% and 25% of T cells can respond to a given superantigen. The large proportion of T cells responsive to a particular superantigen results from the limited number of TCR V$_β$ genes carried in the germ line. Mice, for example, have about 20 V$_β$ genes. Assuming that each V$_β$ gene is expressed with equal frequency, then each superantigen would be expected to interact with 1 in 20 T cells, or 5% of the total T-cell population.

A number of bacterial superantigens have been implicated as the causative agent of several diseases such as bacterial toxic shock and food poisoning (see Table 12-5). Included among these bacterial superantigens are several enterotoxins, exfoliating toxins, and toxic-shock syndrome toxin (TSST1) from *Staphylococcus aureus*; pyrogenic exotoxins from *Streptococcus pyrogenes*; and *Mycoplasma arthritidis* supernatant (MAS). The large number of T cells activated by these superantigens results in excessive production of cytokines. The toxic-shock syndrome toxin, for example, has been shown to induce extremely high levels of TNF and IL-1. As in the case of bacterial septic shock, these cytokines can induce systemic reactions including fever, widespread blood clotting, and shock.

Lymphoid and Myeloid Cancers

Abnormalities in the production of cytokines or their receptors have been associated with some types of cancer. For example, abnormally high levels of IL-6 are secreted by cardiac myxoma (a benign heart tumor) cells, myeloma and plasmacytoma cells, and cervical and bladder cancer cells. In the case of myeloma cells, IL-6 appears to operate in an autocrine manner to stimulate cell proliferation. When monoclonal antibodies to IL-6 are added to in vitro cultures of myeloma cells, their growth is inhibited. In addition, transgenic mice that express high levels of IL-6 have been found to exhibit a massive, fatal plasma-cell proliferation, called **plasmacytosis**. Although these plasma cells are not malignant, the high rate of plasma-cell proliferation possibly contributes to the development of cancer.

Perhaps the strongest case for an association between malignancy and inappropriate expression of a cytokine and/or its receptor comes from the often-fatal **adult T-cell leukemia** associated with the HTLV-1 retrovirus. The leukemic T cells express IL-2 and the high-affinity trimeric IL-2 receptor in the absence of activation by antigen or mitogen. An HTLV protein called Tax-1 has been shown to induce expression of a cellular transcription factor (or factors) that binds to the promoter regions of the genes encoding IL-2 and IL-2R, thus activating these genes (Figure 13-13). As a result, a T cell infected with HTLV-1 expresses IL-2 and its receptor constitutively, rendering the cell responsive to IL-2–induced proliferation in the absence of antigen activation. The role of other cytokine abnormalities in the pathogenesis of various cancers is examined in Chapter 24.

Chagas' Disease

The protozoan *Trypanosoma cruzi* is the causative agent of Chagas' disease, which is characterized by severe immune

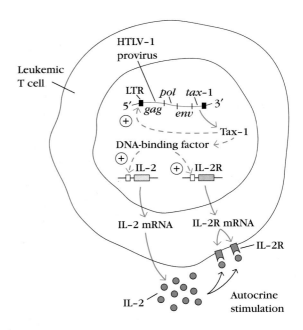

FIGURE 13-13

In adult T-cell leukemia, infection of T cells with HTLV-1 leads to constitutive expression of IL-2 and the IL-2 receptor (IL-2R). The resulting autostimulation causes T-cell proliferation in the absence of antigen. The virus-encoded protein Tax-1 promotes transcription of the provirus genome by binding to the 5′ LTR. It also stimulates expression of an unknown DNA-binding factor(s) that binds to the promoters (open boxes) of the IL-2 and IL-2R genes, stimulating transcription of these genes.

suppression. The ability of *T. cruzi* to mediate immune suppression can be observed by culturing peripheral-blood T cells in the presence and in the absence of *T. cruzi* and then evaluating their immune reactivity. Antigen, mitogen, or anti-CD3 monoclonal antibody normally can activate peripheral T cells, but in the presence of *T. cruzi* T cells are not activated by any of these agents. The defect in these lymphocytes has been traced to a dramatic reduction in the expression of the 55-kDa α subunit of the IL-2 receptor. Co-culturing of T cells with *T. cruzi* and subsequent staining with fluorescein-labeled anti-TAC, which binds to the α subunit, revealed a 90% decrease in the level of the α subunit.

As noted earlier, the high-affinity IL-2 receptor contains the α, β, and γ subunits (see Figure 13-8). Although the mechanism by which *T. cruzi* suppresses expression of the subunit is still unknown, the suppression can be induced across a filter that prevents contact between the lymphocytes and protozoa. This finding suggests that a diffusible factor mediates suppression. Such a factor, once isolated, might have numerous clinical applications for regulating the level of activated T cells in leukemias and autoimmune diseases.

(a) Suppression of T$_H$-cell activation

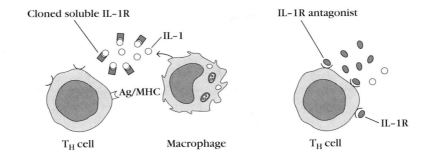

(b) Suppression of T$_H$-cell proliferation and T$_C$-cell activation

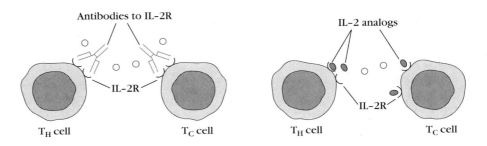

(c) Destruction of activated T$_H$ cells

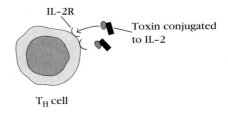

FIGURE 13-14

Experimental cytokine-related therapeutic agents offer the prospect of selectively modulating the immune response. (a,b) The agents (blue) bind either to the cytokine (open circles) or to the cytokine receptor on the cell surface, thereby preventing interaction of the cytokine with its receptor. (c) Conjugation of a toxin with a cytokine results in destruction of cells expressing the cytokine receptor.

THERAPEUTIC USES OF CYTOKINES AND THEIR RECEPTORS

The availability of purified cloned cytokines and soluble cytokine receptors offers the prospect of specific clinical therapies to modulate the immune response selectively. Because activation and proliferation of T$_H$ cells in response to alloantigens on organ transplants initiates activation of T$_C$ cells and subsequent graft rejection, various cytokine-related approaches have been tried experimentally to prolong graft survival.

For example, a cloned soluble form of the IL-1 receptor, which lacks the transmembrane and cytoplasmic domains, blocks activation of T$_H$ cells in response to alloantigens and has been shown to prolong heart transplants in animal models (Figure 13-14a). Binding of IL-1, which is a co-stimulator of T$_H$–cell activation, also can be inhibited with the recombinant IL-1 receptor antagonist; this agent binds to the IL-1 receptor but does not induce activation. Proliferation of activated T$_H$ cells and activation of T$_C$ cells can be blocked by anti-TAC, which binds to the α subunit of the high-affinity IL-2 receptor (Figure 13-14b). Administration of anti-TAC, for instance, has prolonged the survival of heart transplants in rats. Similar results have been obtained with IL-2 analogs that retain their binding ability but have lost their biological activity. Such analogs have been produced by site-directed mutagenesis of cloned IL-2 genes. Finally, cytokines conjugated to various toxins (e.g., the β chain of diphtheria toxin) have been shown to diminish rejection of kidney and heart transplants in animals. Such conjugates containing IL-2 selectively bind to and kill activated T_H cells (Figure 13-14c).

In immunodeficiency diseases and in cancer, enhanced—rather than diminished—T-cell activation is desirable. Intervention with cloned IL-2, IFN-γ, and TNF-α have each had some degree of clinical success. Culturing of various populations of NK cells or T_C cells in the presence of high concentrations of IL-2 has been shown to generate cells with effective antitumor properties. The role of such cells, referred to as **lymphokine-activated killer (LAK) cells**, in tumor therapy is examined in Chapter 24.

Cytokine therapy may also prove to be effective in the treatment of allergies. Given the opposing effects of IL-12 and IL-4 on isotype production, it may be possible to enhance production of a desired isotype selectively. Selective inhibition of IgE may benefit patients with allergies. In animal models, for example, monoclonal antibody to IL-4 has been used to decrease IgE production. Clearly these approaches have enormous clinical applications for the millions of people who suffer from allergies.

Cytokine-related therapy does have limitations, however. During an immune response, cytokines produced locally by interacting cells may reach relatively high local concentrations that cannot be mimicked by clinical administration. In addition, cytokines often have a very short half-life, so that repeated administration may be required in order to maintain effective levels. For example, recombinant human IL-2 has a half-life of only 7–10 min when administered intravenously. Finally, the pleiotropic effects of many cytokines can cause unpredictable and undesirable side effects. The side effects from administration of recombinant IL-2, for instance, range from mild ones (e.g., fever, chills, diarrhea, and weight gain) to anemia, thrombocytopenia, shock, respiratory distress, and coma.

SUMMARY

1. The complex cellular interactions involving cells of the immune, inflammatory, and hematopoietic systems are mediated by a group of secreted, low-molecular-weight proteins, collectively called cytokines. Most cytokines act on nearby target cells, although in some cases a cytokine can act on the cell that secretes it or on a distant cell. The biological activities of cytokines exhibit pleiotropy, redundancy, synergy, and antagonism, which contribute to the complexity of cytokine networks (see Figure 13-2).

2. Studies on the structure and function of cytokines advanced greatly with cloning of cytokine genes. Cytokines are proteins or glycoproteins, usually with a molecular mass of less than 30 kDa. Most of the cytokines involved in immune responses share certain structural features that define the hematopoietin family of proteins (see Figure 13-3). The cytokines characterized to date include the interferons α, β, and γ; interleukins 1–16; tumor necrosis factor α and β; and transforming growth factor β (see Table 13-1).

3. A particular cytokine can act on any target cell that expresses receptors for that cytokine. An important way in which the activity of cytokines is directed toward specific cells is by regulation of the expression of their receptors. For example, only activated T_H cells express the high-affinity IL-2 receptor (see Figure 13-8). As long as the antigen-MHC-TCR interaction continues, the high-affinity IL-2 receptor is expressed, but once this interaction ceases, expression of the IL-2 receptor stops as well.

4. The cell-surface proteins that bind cytokines can be classified into five types based on their structures (see Figure 13-5). Most of the cytokines critical in immune and inflammatory responses bind to class I or class II cytokine receptors, which possess certain conserved motifs in their extracellular domains. Most of these receptors are heterodimers, containing a cytokine-specific subunit and signal-transducing subunit. Some class I cytokine receptors share a common signal-transducing subunit, accounting for the redundancy among the biological effects of these cytokines (see Figure 13-6).

5. Cytokine-induced dimerization of the subunits of class I and class II cytokine receptors permits association of cytosolic JAK kinases with the receptor cytoplasmic domain. This association activates the kinases, which then phosphorylate tyrosine residues in STAT proteins, a family of transcription factors. The phosphorylated STATs dimerize and move to the nucleus where they activate transcription of specific genes (see Figure 13-9). The resulting gene products mediate the biological effects associated with various cytokines.

6. Antigen-stimulated T_H cells in the presence of certain cytokines are thought to develop preferentially into T_H1 and T_H2 subsets, with characteristic patterns of cytokine secretion (see Figure 13-10, Table 13-2). The cytokines secreted by the T_H1 subset act primarily in cell-mediated responses, whereas those secreted by the T_H2 subset function mostly in B-cell activation and humoral response.

7. Abnormalities in the expression of either cytokines or their receptors may result in various diseases including bacterial toxic shock, certain lymphoid and myeloid cancers, and Chagas' disease. Cytokine-related therapies that either increase or decrease the immune response offer promise of reducing graft rejection, treating certain cancers and immunodeficiency diseases, and reducing allergic reactions.

REFERENCES

AKIRA, S., AND T. KISHIMOTO. 1992. IL-6 and NF-IL6 in acute-phase response and viral infection. *Immunol. Rev.* **127**:25.

ARAI, K., ET AL. 1990. Cytokines: coordinators of immune and inflammatory responses. *Annu. Rev. Biochem.* **59**:783.

BARON, S., ET AL. 1991. The interferons: mechanism of action and clinical applications. *JAMA* **266**:1375.

BAZAN, J. F. 1992. Unraveling the structure of IL-2. *Science* **257**:410.

BEUTLER, B. 1990. The tumor necrosis factors: cachectin and lymphotoxin. *Hosp. Prac.* (Feb. 15):45.

BOULAY, J. L., AND W. E. PAUL. 1993. Hematopoietin subfamily classification based on size, gene organization and sequence homology. *Curr. Biol.* **3**:573.

CENTER, D. M., ET AL. 1996. Interleukin 16 and its function as a CD4 ligand. *Immunol. Today* **17**:476.

DALTON, D. K., et al. 1993. Multiple defects of immune cell function in mice with disrupted interferon-γ genes. *Science* **259**:1739.

DEBETS, R., AND H. F. J. SAVELKOUL. 1994. Cytokine antagonists and their potential therapeutic use. *Immunol. Today* **15**:455.

HERMAN, A., et al. 1991. Superantigens: mechanism of T-cell stimulation and role in immune responses. *Annu. Rev. Immunol.* **9**:745.

HOU, J., ET AL. 1994. An interleukin-4–induced transcription factor: IL-4 STAT. *Science* **265**:1701.

HUANG, S., ET AL. 1993. Immune response in mice that lack the interferon-γ receptor. *Science* **259**:1742.

IHLE, J. N., ET AL. 1995. Signaling through the hematopoietic cytokine receptors. *Annu. Rev. Immunol* **13**:369.

IHLE, J. N., AND I. M. KERR. 1995. JAKS and Stats in signaling by the cytokine receptor superfamily. *Trends Genet.* **11**:69.

IVASHKIV, L. B., 1995. Cytokines and STATS: how can signals achieve specificity? *Immunity* **3**:1.

KARNITZ, L. M., AND R. T. ABRAHAM. 1995. Cytokine receptor signaling mechanisms. *Curr. Opin. Immunol.* **7**:320.

KISHIMOTO, T., T. TAGA, AND S. AKIRA. 1994. Cytokine signal transduction. *Cell* **76**:253.

MOORE, K. W., ET AL. 1993. Interleukin-10. *Annu. Rev. Immunol.* **11**:165.

POWRIE, F., AND R. L. COFFMAN. 1993. Cytokine regulation of T-cell function: potential for therapeutic intervention. *Immunol. Today* **14**:270.

SCHOENHAUT, D. S., ET AL. 1992. Cloning and expression of murine IL-12. *J. Immunol.* **148**:3433.

SMITH, K. 1990. Interleukin-2. *Sci. Am.* **262**:50.

SUGAMURA, K., ET AL. 1996. The interleukin-2 receptor γ chain: Its role in the multiple cytokine receptor complexes and T cell development in XSCID. *Annu. Rev. Immunol.* **14**:179.

TAGA, T., AND T. KISHIMOTO. 1995. Signaling mechanisms through cytokine receptors that share signal transducing receptor components. *Curr. Opin. Immunol.* **7**:17.

TRINCHIERI, G. 1995. Interleukin-12: a proinflammatory cytokine with immunoregulatory functions that bridge innate resistance and antigen-specific adaptive immunity. *Annu. Rev. Immunol.* **13**:251.

VASSALLI, P. 1992. The pathophysiology of tumor necrosis factors. *Annu. Rev. Immunol.* **10**:411.

WALDMANN, T. A. 1993. The IL-2/IL-2 receptor system: a target for rational immune intervention. *Immunol. Today* **14**:264.

WALTER, M. R., ET AL. 1995. Crystal structure of a complex between interferon-γ and its soluble high-affinity receptor. *Nature* **376**:230.

STUDY QUESTIONS

1. Indicate whether each of the following statements is true or false. If you think a statement is false, explain why.

   a. The high-affinity IL-2 receptor consists of two transmembrane proteins.

   b. The anti-TAC monoclonal antibody recognizes the IL-1 receptor on T cells.

   c. All cytokine-binding receptors contain two or three subunits.

   d. Expression of the β subunit of the IL-2 receptor is indicative of T-cell activation.

e. Some cytokine receptors possess domains with tyrosine kinase activity that function in signal transduction.

f. All members of each subfamily of the class I cytokine (erythropoietin) receptors share a common signal-transducing subunit.

2. When IL-2 is secreted by one T cell in a peripheral lymphoid organ, do all the T cells in the vicinity proliferate in response to the IL-2 or only some of them? Explain.

3. Briefly describe the similarities and differences among cytokines, growth factors, and hormones.

4. Indicate which subunit(s) of the IL-2 receptor are expressed by the following types of cells:

a. _____ Resting T_H cells

b. _____ Activated T_H cells

c. _____ Activated T_H cells + cyclosporin A

d. _____ Resting T_C cells

e. _____ CTLs

f. _____ NK cells

5. Superantigens have been implicated in several diseases and have been useful as research tools.

a. What properties of superantigens distinguish them from conventional antigens?

b. By what mechanism are bacterial superantigens thought to cause symptoms associated with food poisoning and toxic-shock syndrome?

c. Does the activity of superantigens exhibit MHC restriction?

6. IL-3, IL-5, and GM-CSF exhibit considerable redundancy in their effects. What structural feature of the receptors for these cytokines might explain this redundancy?

7. Adult T-cell leukemia is associated with infection by HTLV-1. What is the likely mechanism by which HTLV-1 infection leads to uncontrolled proliferation of T cells in the absence of antigen activation?

8. Considerable evidence indicates the existence of two T_H-cell subsets, differing in the pattern of cytokines they secrete.

a. What type of immune response is mediated by the T_H1 subset? What type of antigen challenge is likely to induce a T_H1-mediated response?

b. What type of immune response is mediated by the T_H2 subset? What type of antigen challenge is likely to induce a T_H2-mediated response?

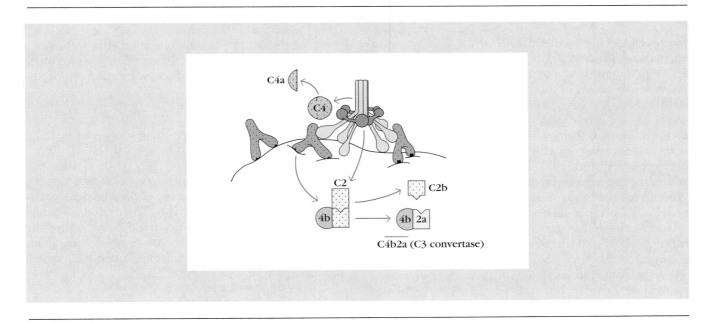

C4a

C4

C2

C2b

4b

4b 2a

C4b2a (C3 convertase)

THE COMPLEMENT SYSTEM

The complement system, the major effector of the humoral branch of the immune system, consists of nearly 30 serum and membrane proteins. Following initial activation, the various complement components interact, in a highly regulated enzymatic cascade, to generate reaction products that facilitate antigen clearance and generation of an inflammatory response. There are two pathways of complement activation: the classical pathway and the alternative pathway. The two pathways share a common terminal reaction sequence that generates a macromolecular membrane-attack complex (MAC), which lyses a variety of cells, bacteria, and viruses.

The complement reaction products amplify the initial antigen-antibody reaction and convert that reaction into a more effective defense mechanism. A variety of small, diffusible reaction products that are released during complement activation induce localized vasodilation and attract phagocytic cells chemotactically, leading to an inflammatory reaction. As antigen becomes coated with complement reaction products, it is more readily phagocytosed by phagocytic cells that bear receptors for these complement products. In addition, some of the complement products have been shown to play a role in the activation of B lymphocytes. Finally, the terminal components of the complement system generate the membrane-attack complex.

This chapter describes the similarities and differences in the two pathways, the regulation of the complement system, the effector functions of various complement components, and the consequences of hereditary deficiencies in some components.

THE COMPLEMENT COMPONENTS

The proteins and glycoproteins composing the complement system are synthesized largely by liver hepatocytes, although significant amounts of complement components are also produced by blood monocytes, tissue macrophages, and epithelial cells of the gastrointestinal and genitourinary tracts. These components constitute 15% (by weight) of the serum globulin fraction and circulate in the serum in functionally inactive forms, many of them as proenzymes in which the enzymatically active site is masked. Each proenzyme is activated by cleavage of the molecule, thereby removing an inhibitory fragment and exposing the active site. Activation of the complement system involves a sequential enzyme cascade in which the proenzyme product of one step becomes the enzyme catalyst of the next step. Each activated component has a short half-life before being inactivated.

Each complement component is designated by numerals (C1–C9), by letter symbols (e.g., factor D), or by trivial names (e.g., homologous restriction factor). The peptide fragments formed by activation of a component are denoted by small letters, with the smaller fragment designated "a" and the larger fragment designated "b" (e.g., C3a, C3b). The larger "b" fragments bind to the target near the site of activation, and the smaller "a" fragments diffuse from the site and play a role in initiating a localized inflammatory response. The comple-

ment fragments interact with one another to form functional complexes. Those complexes that have enzymatic activity are designated by a bar over the number or symbol (e.g., $\overline{C4b2a}$, $\overline{C3bBb}$).

COMPLEMENT ACTIVATION

The early steps in complement activation, culminating in formation of C5b, can occur via the **classical pathway** or the **alternative pathway**. The final steps leading to formation of a membrane-attack complex are the same in both pathways. The complement components involved in each pathway, and the sequence in which they take part, are outlined in Figure 14-1.

Classical Pathway

Complement activation via the classical pathway is commonly initiated by the formation of soluble antigen-antibody complexes (**immune complexes**) or by the

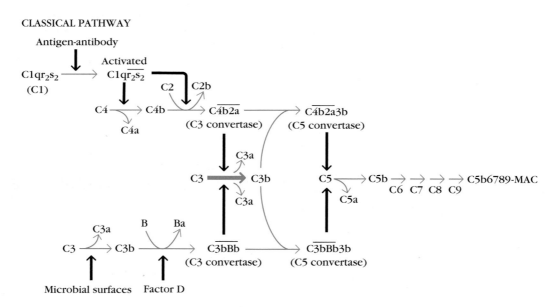

FIGURE 14-1

Overview of the complement activation pathways. The classical pathway is initiated by binding of C1 to antigen-antibody complexes. The alternative pathway is initiated by binding of C3b to activating surfaces such as microbial cell walls. Both pathways generate C3 and C5 convertases and bound C5b, which is converted into a membrane-attack complex (MAC) by a common sequence of terminal reactions.

Hydrolysis of C3 is the major amplification step in both pathways, generating large amounts of C3b, which forms part of C5 convertase. C3b also can diffuse away from the activating surface and bind to immune complexes or cell surfaces, where it functions as an opsonin. Blue arrows indicate reaction steps; black arrows indicate enzymatic or activating activity.

binding of antibody to antigen on a suitable target, such as a bacterial cell. IgM and certain subclasses of IgG (IgG1, IgG2, and IgG3) can activate the classical complement pathway, as can certain nonimmunologic activators. The initial stage of activation involves **C1, C2, C3,** and **C4,** which are present in plasma in functionally inactive forms (Table 14-1). The components were named in order of their discovery and before their functional roles had been determined, so that their names do not reflect the sequence in which they react.

The complexing of antibody with antigen induces conformational changes in the Fc portion of the antibody molecule that exposes a binding site for the C1 component of the complement system. C1 exists in serum as a macromolecular complex consisting of C1q and two molecules each of C1r and C1s, held together in a complex (C1qr$_2$s$_2$) stabilized by Ca^{2+} ions. The C1q molecule is composed of 18 polypeptide chains that associate to form six collagen-like triple helical arms, the tips of which bind to exposed C1q-binding sites in the C$_H$2 domain of the antibody molecule (Figure 14-2a,b). The C1r$_2$s$_2$ complex can exist in two configurations. When it is free and not bound to C1q, it assumes an S-shaped form; on binding to C1q, C1r$_2$s$_2$ assumes a shape similar to a figure 8 (Figure 14-2c,d,e). Each C1r and C1s monomer contains a catalytic domain and an interaction domain; the latter facilitates interaction with C1q or with each other.

Each C1 molecule must bind, via its C1q globular heads, to at least two Fc sites for a stable C1-antibody interaction to occur. When pentameric IgM is bound to antigen on a target surface, at least three binding sites for C1q are exposed. Circulating IgM, however, assumes a planar configuration in which the C1q-binding sites are not exposed (Figure 14-3). For this reason, circulating IgM cannot activate the complement cascade by itself. An IgG molecule, on the other hand, contains only a single C1q-binding site in the C$_H$2 domain of the Fc, so that firm C1q binding is achieved only when two IgG molecules are within 30–40 nm of each other on a target surface or in a complex, providing two attachment sites for C1q. This difference in the structure of IgM and IgG accounts for the observation that a single molecule of IgM bound to a red blood cell is enough to activate the classical complement pathway and lyse the red blood cell, whereas some 1000 molecules of IgG are required if two molecules, randomly distributed, are to end up close enough to each other to initiate C1q binding.

The intermediates in the classical activation pathway are depicted schematically in Figure 14-4. Binding of C1q to Fc binding sites induces a conformational change in C1r that autocatalytically converts C1r to an active serine protease enzyme, C$\overline{\text{1r}}$, which then cleaves C1s to a similar active enzyme, C$\overline{\text{1r}}$. C$\overline{\text{1s}}$ has two substrates, C4 and C2 (see Figure 14-1). The C4 component is a glycoprotein containing three polypeptide chains (α, β, and γ). C4 is activated when C$\overline{\text{1s}}$ hydrolyzes a small fragment (C4a) from the amino terminus of the chain, exposing a binding site on the larger fragment (C4b). The C4b fragment attaches to the target surface in the vicinity of C1,

T A B L E   1 4 - 1

CLASSICAL COMPLEMENT PATHWAY:
PROTEINS THAT PARTICIPATE IN FORMATION OF C5 CONVERTASE

COMPONENT	ACTIVE PROTEIN/ SPLIT PRODUCT	IMMUNOLOGIC FUNCTION
C1	C1q	Binds to Fc region of IgM and IgG
	C1r	Serine protease: enzymatically activates C1s
	C1s	Serine protease: enzymatically activates C4 and C2
C4	C4a	Peptide mediator of inflammation (anaphylatoxin)
	C4b	Binds C2 forming complex that is cleaved by C1s to yield C$\overline{\text{4b2a}}$
C2	C2a	Serine protease: C$\overline{\text{4b2a}}$ acts as C3 convertase
	C2b	Unknown function
C3	C3a	Peptide mediator of inflammation (anaphylatoxin)
	C3b	Binds to C$\overline{\text{4b2a}}$ to form C5 convertase; major opsonin

(a)

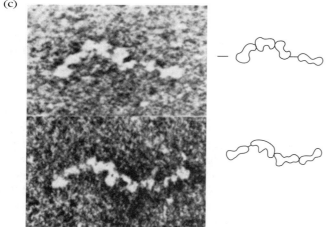

(b)

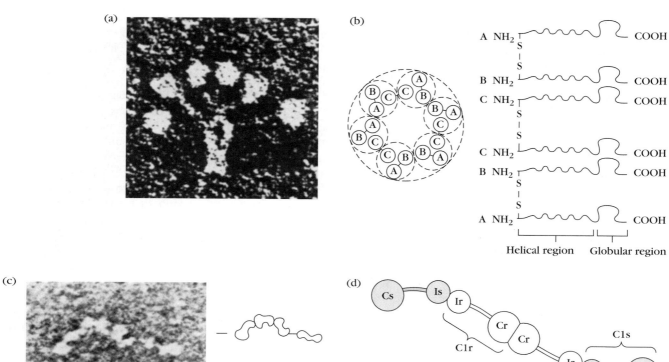

Helical region   Globular region

(c)

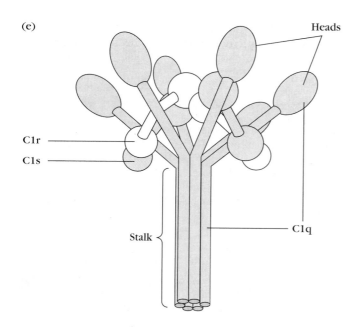

(d)

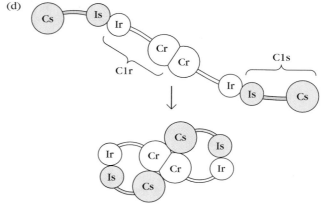

(e)

FIGURE 14-2

Structure of C1q, C1r₂s₂, and the C1 macromolecular complex. (a) Electron micrograph of C1q molecule showing stalk and six globular heads. (b) Cross-section of stalk of C1q (*left*) and schematic diagram of chain structure of two triplets (*right*). A C1q molecule consists of 18 polypeptide chains arranged into six triplets, each of which contains one A, one B, and one C chain. The stalk of the molecule corresponds to helical domains in the chains, and the heads correspond to globular regions. (c) Electron micrograph of free $C1\overline{r_2s_2}$ complexes showing characteristic S shape. (d) Diagram of $C1r_2s_2$ complex in S-shaped form (*top*) and figure-8 form (*bottom*), which it assumes on binding with C1q. Each C1r and C1s monomer contains a catalytic domain (C) with enzymatic activity and an interaction domain (I), which facilitates binding with C1q or with each other. (e) Diagram of $C1q\overline{r_2s_2}$ complex. [Part (a) from H. R. Knobel et al., 1975, *Eur. J. Immunol.* **5**:78; part (c) from J. Tschopp et al., 1980, *Proc. Nat'l. Acad. Sci. USA* **77**:7014.]

(a) (b)

(c) (d)

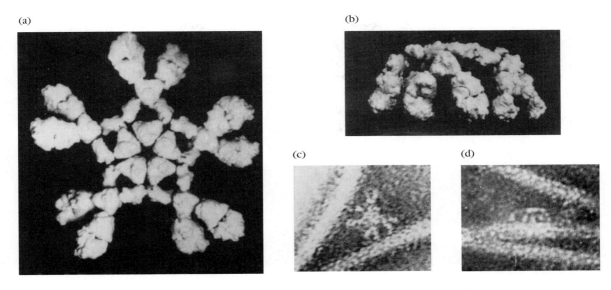

FIGURE 14-3

Models of pentameric IgM in planar form (a) and "staple" form (b). Several C1q-binding sites in the Fc region are accessible in the staple form, whereas none are exposed in the planar form. Electron micro- graphs of IgM antiflagellum antibody bound to flagella, showing the planar form (c) and stable form (d). [From A. Feinstein et al., 1981, *Monogr. Allergy* **17**:28 and, 1981, *Ann. N.Y. Acad. Sci.* **190**:1104.]

and the C2 proenzyme then attaches to the exposed binding site on C4b, where the C2 is then cleaved by the neighboring $\overline{C1s}$; the smaller fragment (C2b) diffuses away.* The resulting $\overline{C4b2a}$ complex is called **C3 con-vertase**, referring to its role in converting the C3 proen-zyme into an enzymatically active form.

The native C3 component consists of two polypep-tide chains, α and β. Hydrolysis of a short fragment (C3a) from the amino terminus of the α chain by the C3 con-vertase generates C3b (Figure 14-5). A single C3 conver-tase molecule can generate over 200 molecules of C3b, resulting in tremendous **amplification** at this step of the sequence. Some of the C3b binds to $\overline{C4b2a}$ to form a trimolecular complex ($\overline{C4b2a3b}$) called **C5 conver-tase**. The C3b component of this complex binds C5 and alters its conformation, so that the $\overline{C4b2a}$ component can cleave C5 into C5a, which diffuses away, and C5b, which attaches to the antigenic surface. The **bound**

C5b initiates formation of the membrane-attack com-plex in a sequence described later. Some of the C3b gen-erated by C3 convertase activity does not associate with $\overline{C4b2a}$; instead it diffuses away and then coats immune complexes and particulate antigens, functioning as an opsonin as discussed in a later section.

Alternative Pathway

Bound C5b can also be generated by the second major pathway of complement activation, the alternative path-way (see Figure 14-1). This pathway involves four serum proteins: **C3, factor B, factor D**, and **properdin** (Table 14-2). Unlike the classical pathway, which generally requires antibody to be initiated, the alternative pathway is initiated in most cases by various cell-surface con-stituents that are foreign to the host (Table 14-3). For example, both gram-negative and gram-positive bacteria have cell-wall constituents that can activate the alterna-tive pathway. The intermediates in the alternative path-way for generating C5b are depicted schematically in Figure 14-6.

Serum C3, which contains an unstable thioester bond, is subject to slow spontaneous hydrolysis to yield C3a and C3b. The C3b component can bind to foreign surface antigens (such as those on bacterial cells or viral particles) or even to the host's own cells (see Figure 14-5c). The membranes of most mammalian cells have high levels of

---

* Contrary to the usual convention, the larger C2 fragment is des-ignated C2a and the smaller fragment, C2b. Several years ago, a pro-posal was made to reverse the C2 fragment designation, so it would be similar to the other components; the first edition of this text adopted this proposal. However, this change in nomenclature ulti-mately was not approved, and subsequent editions of this text use the original nomenclature.

Visualizing Concepts

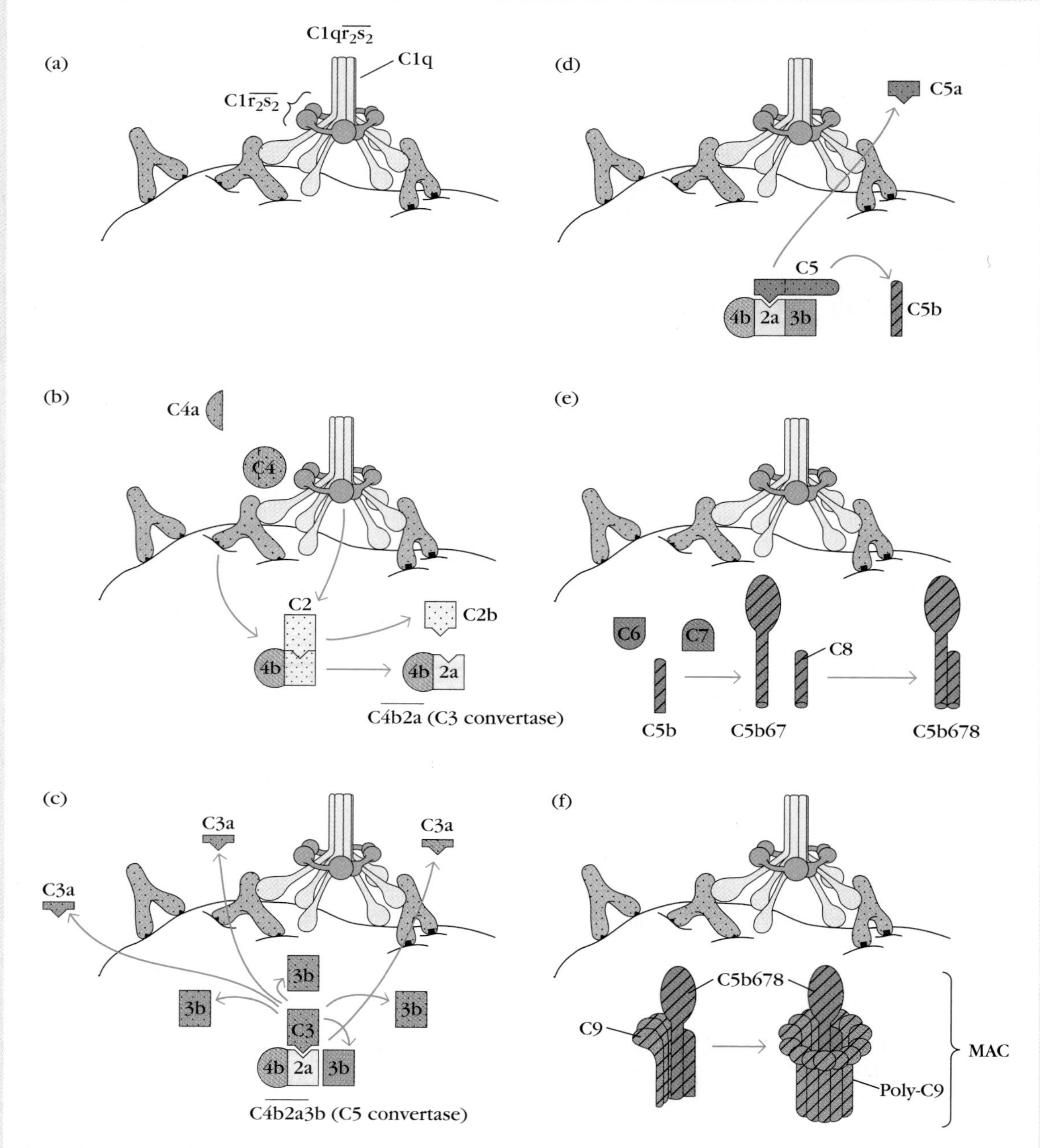

FIGURE 14-4

Schematic diagram of intermediates in the classical pathway of complement activation. Complement components, shown in solid colors, are bound to the antigenic surface but do not penetrate it; components that can insert into the cell membrane are marked with diagonal lines; and the freely diffusible components are stippled. The completed membrane-attack complex (MAC) forms a large pore in the membrane. See text for details.

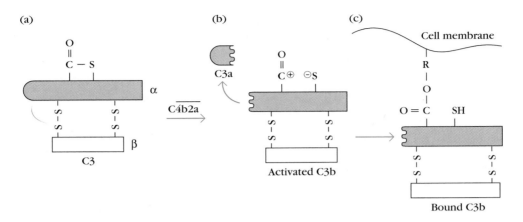

FIGURE 14-5

Hydrolysis of C3 by C3 convertase $\overline{C4b2a}$. (a) Native C3. (b) Activated C3 showing site of cleavage by $\overline{C4b2a}$, resulting in production of the C3a and C3b fragments. (c) A labile internal thioester bond in C3 is activated as C3b is formed, allowing the C3b fragment to bind to free hydroxyl or amino groups (R) on a cell membrane. Bound C3b exhibits various biological activities, including binding of C5 and binding to C3b receptors on phagocytic cells.

sialic acid, which contributes to the rapid inactivation of bound C3b molecules on host cells. Because many foreign antigenic surfaces (e.g., bacterial cell walls, yeast cell walls, and certain viral envelopes) have only low levels of sialic acid, C3b bound to these surfaces remains active for a longer time. Bound C3b can bind another serum protein called factor B by way of an Mg^{2+}-dependent bond. Binding to C3b exposes a site on factor B that serves as the substrate for an enzymatically active serum protein called factor D. Factor D cleaves the C3b-bound factor B, releasing a small fragment (Ba), which diffuses away, and generating $\overline{C3bBb}$. The $\overline{C3bBb}$ complex has C3 convertase activity and thus is analogous to the $\overline{C4b2a}$ complex in the classical pathway (Table 14-4). The C3 convertase activity of $\overline{C3bBb}$ has a half-life of only 5 min unless the serum protein properdin binds to it, stabilizing it and extending the half-life of this convertase activity to 30 min.

The $\overline{C3bBb}$ generated in the alternative pathway can activate unhydrolyzed C3 to generate more C3b auto-

TABLE 14 - 2

ALTERNATIVE COMPLEMENT PATHWAY: PROTEINS THAT PARTICIPATE IN FORMATION OF C5 CONVERTASE

COMPONENT	ACTIVE PROTEIN/ SPLIT PRODUCT	IMMUNOLOGIC FUNCTION
C3	C3a	Peptide mediator of inflammation (anaphylatoxin)
	C3b	Binds factor B, forming complex that is cleaved by factor D to yield $\overline{C3bBb}$
Factor B	Ba	Unknown function
	Bb	Serine protease: $\overline{C3bBb}$ acts as C3 convertase, which generates $\overline{C3bBb3b}$ (C5 convertase)
Factor D	D	Serine protease: cleaves factor B that is bound to C3b to form C3 convertase
Properdin		Binds to and stabilizes $\overline{C3bBb}$

INITIATORS OF THE ALTERNATIVE PATHWAY OF COMPLEMENT ACTIVATION

PATHOGENS AND PARTICLES OF MICROBIAL ORIGIN	NONPATHOGENS
Many strains of gram-negative bacteria	Human IgG, IgA, and IgE in complexes
Lipopolysaccharides from gram-negative bacateria	Rabbit and guinea pig IgG in complexes
Many strains of gram-positive bacteria	Cobra venom factor
Teichoic acid from gram-positive cell walls	Heterologous erythrocytes (rabbit, mouse, chicken)
Fungal and yeast cell walls (zymosan)	Anionic polymers (dextran sulfate)
Some viruses and virus-infected cells	Pure carboyhydrates (agarose, inulin)
Some tumor cells (Raji)	
Parasites (trypanosomes)	

SOURCE: Adapted from M. K. Pangburn, 1986, in *Immunobiology of the Complement System,* Academic Press.

catalytically. As a result, the initial steps are repeated and amplified, so that more than 2×10^6 molecules of C3b can be deposited on an antigenic surface in less than 5 min. The C3 convertase activity of $C\overline{3bBb}$ generates the $C\overline{3bBb3b}$ complex, which exhibits **C5 convertase** activity, analogous to the $C\overline{4b2a3b}$ complex in the classical pathway. The nonenzymatic C3b component binds C5, and the $C\overline{3bBb}$ component subsequently hydrolyzes the bound C5 to generate C5a and C5b; the latter binds to the antigenic surface (see Figure 14-6).

Terminal Sequence: Formation of Membrane-Attack Complex

The terminal sequence of complement activation involves C5b, C6, C7, C8, and C9, which interact sequentially to form a macromolecular structure called the **membrane-attack complex,** or MAC (Table 14-5). This complex displaces the membrane phospholipids, forming a large transmembrane channel that disrupts the

membrane and enables ions and small molecules to diffuse through it freely.

As noted previously, in both the classical and alternative pathways, a C5 convertase cleaves C5, which contains two protein chains (α and β). Following binding of C5 to the nonenzymatic C3b component of the convertase, the amino terminus of the α chain is cleaved, generating the small C5a fragment, which diffuses away, and the large C5b fragment, which provides a binding site for the subsequent components of the membrane-attack complex (see Figure 14-4d). The C5b component is extremely labile and is inactivated within 2 min unless C6 binds to it and stabilizes its activity.

Up to this point all the complement reactions take place on the hydrophilic surface of membranes or on immune complexes in the fluid phase. As C5b6 binds to C7, the resulting complex undergoes a hydrophilic-amphiphilic structural transition that exposes hydrophobic regions, which serve as binding sites for membrane phospholipids. If the reaction occurs on a target-cell membrane, the hydrophobic binding sites enable the C5b67 complex to insert into the phospholipid bilayer (see Figure 14-4e). If, however, the reaction occurs on an immune complex or other noncellular activating surface, then the hydrophobic binding sites cannot anchor the complex and it is released. Released C5b67 complexes can bind to nearby cells and mediate **"innocent-bystander"** lysis. In a number of diseases in which immune complexes are produced, tissue damage results from such innocent-bystander lysis. This autoimmune process will be discussed in Chapter 20.

Binding of C8 to membrane-bound C5b67 induces a conformational change in C8, so that it too undergoes a hydrophilic-amphiphilic structural transition exposing a

COMPLEMENT COMPONENTS IN THE FORMATION OF C3 AND C5 CONVERTASES

	CLASSICAL PATHWAY	ALTERNATIVE PATHWAY
Precursor proteins	C4 + C2	C3 + factor B
Activating protease	$C\overline{1s}$	Factor D
C3 convertase	$C\overline{4b2a}$	$C\overline{3bBb}$
C5 convertase	$C\overline{4b2a3b}$	$C\overline{3bBb3b}$
C5-binding component	C3b	C3b

Visualizing Concepts

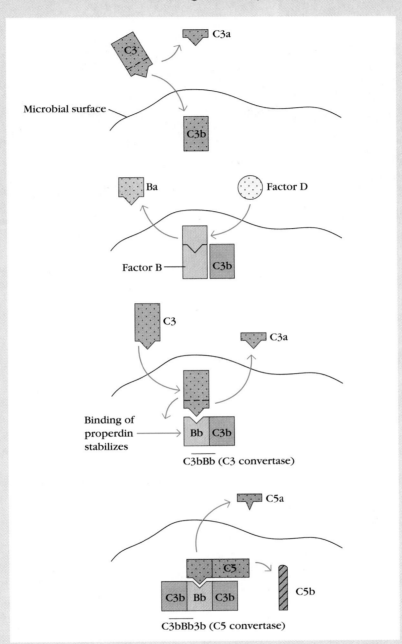

FIGURE 14-6

Schematic diagram of intermediates in formation of bound C5b by alternative pathway of complement activation. The C3bBb complex is stabilized by binding of properdin. Membrane-bound intermediates are shown in solid colors; components that can penetrate the cell membrane are marked with diagonal lines; freely diffusible components are stippled. Conversion of bound C5b to the membrane-attack complex occurs by the same sequence of reactions as in the classical pathway (see Figure 14-4e,f). See text for details.

(a)   (b)

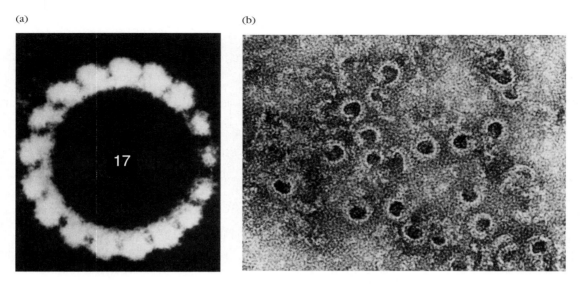

FIGURE 14-7

(a) Photomicrograph of poly-C9 complex formed by in vitro polymerization of C9. (b) Photomicrograph of complement-induced lesions on the membrane of a red blood cell. These lesions result from formation of membrane-attack complexes. [Part (a) from E. R. Podack, 1986, in *Immunobiology of the Complement System*, Academic Press; part (b) from J. Humphrey and R. Dourmashkin, 1969, *Adv. Immunol.* **11**:75.]

hydrophobic region, which interacts with the plasma membrane. The C5b678 complex creates a small pore 10 Å in diameter; formation of this pore can lead to lysis of red blood cells but not of nucleated cells. The final step in formation of the MAC is the binding and polymerization of C9, a perforin-like molecule, to the C5b678 complex. As many as 10–16 molecules of C9 can be bound and polymerized by a single C5b678 complex. During polymerization the C9 molecules undergo a hydrophilic-amphiphilic transition, so that they also can insert into the membrane (see Figure 14-4f). The completed MAC, which has a tubular form and functional pore size of 70–100 Å, consists of a C5b678 complex surrounded by a **poly-C9 complex** (Figure 14-7). Since ions and small molecules can diffuse freely through the central channel of the MAC, the cell cannot maintain its osmotic stability and is lysed by an influx of water and loss of electrolytes.

TABLE 14-5

TERMINAL COMPLEMENT PATHWAY: PROTEINS INVOLVED IN THE FORMATION OF THE MEMBRANE-ATTACK COMPLEX (MAC)

COMPONENT	ACTIVE PROTEIN/ SPLIT PRODUCT	IMMUNOLOGIC FUNCTION
C5	C5a	Peptide mediator of inflammation (anaphylatoxin)
	C5b	Binds C6 to initiate formation of MAC
C6	C6	C5b6 binds C7
C7	C7	C5b67 binds C8; after an amphiphilic transition, the resulting complex inserts into the lipid bilayer
C8	C8	C5b678 binds multiple C9 molecules, initiating their polymerization
C9	C9	Polymerizes to complete formation of MAC pore

REGULATION OF THE COMPLEMENT SYSTEM

Because the complement system is nonspecific and thus capable of attacking host cells as well as microorganisms, elaborate regulatory mechanisms are required to confine the complement activation to designated targets. Both the classical and alternative pathways include a number of extremely labile components, which undergo spontaneous inactivation as they diffuse away from target cells. For example, the target-binding site on C3b undergoes spontaneous hydrolysis by the time it has diffused 40 nm away from the $\overline{\text{C4b2a}}$ or $\overline{\text{C3bBb}}$ convertase enzymes. This rapid hydrolysis limits binding of C3b to nearby host cells. In addition, both pathways include a series of regulatory proteins that inactivate various complement components (Table 14-6). For example, a glycoprotein called **C1 inhibitor** (C1Inh) can form a complex with $C1r_2s_2$, causing it to dissociate from C1q and preventing further activation of C4 or C2 (Figure 14-8a).

The reaction catalyzed by the C3 convertase enzymes of the classical and alternative pathways is the major amplification step in complement activation, generating hundreds of molecules of C3b. The C3b generated by these enzymes can bind to nearby cells, mediating damage to the healthy cells by opsonization to phagocytic

TABLE 14-6

PROTEINS THAT REGULATE COMPLEMENT SYSTEM

PROTEIN	TYPE OF PROTEIN	PATHWAY AFFECTED	IMMUNOLOGIC FUNCTION
C1 inhibitor (C1Inh)	Soluble	Classical	Serine protease inhibitor: causes $C1r_2s_2$ to dissociate from C1q
C4b-binding protein (C4bBP)*	Soluble	Classical	Blocks formation of C3 convertase by binding C4b; cofactor for cleavage of C4b by factor I
Factor H *	Soluble	Alternative	Blocks formation of C3 convertase by binding C3b; cofactor for cleavage of C3b by factor I
Complement-receptor type 1 (CR1) * Membrane-cofactor protein (MCB) *	Membrane bound	Classical & alternative	Block formation of C3 convertase by binding C4b or C3b; cofactor for factor I–catalyzed cleavage of C4b or C3b
Decay-accelerating factor (DAF) *	Membrane bound	Classical & alternative	Accelerates dissociation of $\overline{\text{C4b2a}}$ and $\overline{\text{C3bBb}}$ (C3 convertases)
Factor I	Soluble	Classical & alternative	Serine protease: Cleaves C4b or C3b using C4bBP, CR1, factor H, DAF, or MCP as cofactor
S protein	Soluble	Terminal	Binds soluble C5b67 and prevents its insertion into cell membrane
Homologous restriction factor (HRF) Membrane inhibitor of reactive lysis (MIRL)	Membrane bound	Terminal	Bind to C5b678 on autologous cells, blocking binding of C9
Anaphylatoxin inactivator	Soluble	Effector	Blocks anaphylatoxin activity of C3a, C4a, and C5a

* An RCA (regulator of complement activation) protein. In humans, all RCA proteins are encoded on chromosome 1 and contain short consensus repeats.

Visualizing Concepts

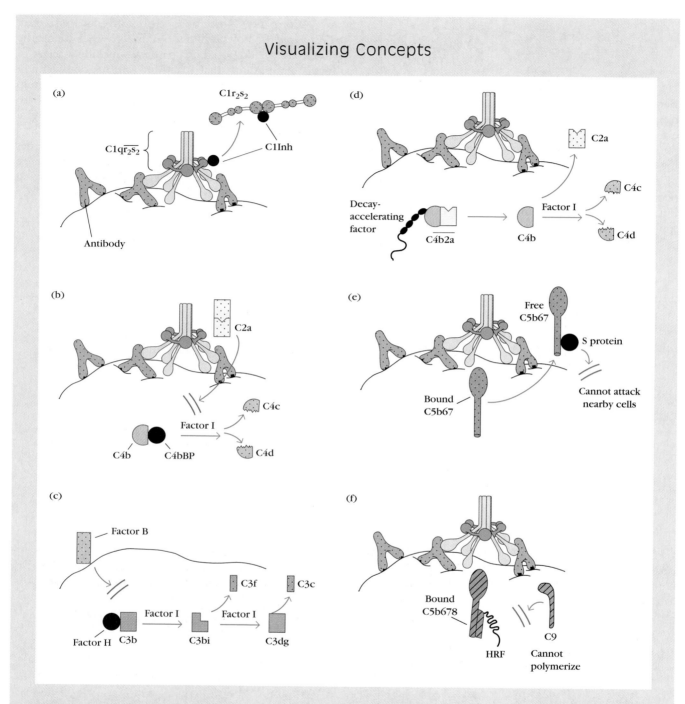

FIGURE 14-8

Schematic diagram of regulation of complement system by regulatory proteins (black), which either cause dissociation of various intermediates or block their formation. Membrane-bound intermediates are shown in solid colors; components that can penetrate the cell membrane are marked with diagonal lines; freely diffusible components are stippled. C1Inh = C1 inhibitor; C4bBP = C4b-binding protein; HRF = homologous restriction factor. See text and Table 14-6 for details.

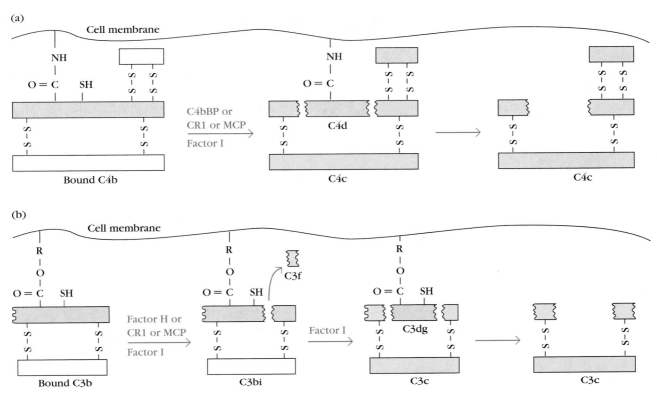

FIGURE 14-9

Inactivation of bound C4b and C3b by regulatory proteins of the complement system. (a) In the classical pathway, C4bBP (C4b-binding protein), CR1 (complement receptor type 1), or MCP (membrane cofactor protein) bind to C4b and act as cofactors for factor I–mediated cleavage of C4b. (b) In the alternative pathway, factor H, CR1, or MCP bind to C3b and act as cofactors for factor I–mediated cleavage of C3b. Free diffusible fragments are blue. See text for details.

cells bearing C3b receptors or by induction of the membrane-attack complex. It is estimated that circulating red blood cells are exposed to thousands of C3b molecules each day. C3b-mediated damage to healthy cells is prevented by a family of related proteins that regulate C3 convertase activity in the classical and alternative pathways. These C3 convertase regulatory proteins all contain repeating amino acid sequences (or motifs), containing about 60 residues, termed **short consensus repeats** (SCRs). All these proteins are encoded at a single chromosomal location on chromosome 1 in humans, known as the **regulators of complement activation** (RCA) gene cluster.

In the classical pathway three structurally different RCA proteins act similarly to prevent assembly of C3 convertase (Figure 14-8b). These regulatory proteins include soluble **C4b-binding protein** (C4bBP) and two membrane-bound proteins, **complement receptor type 1** (CR1) and **membrane cofactor protein**

(MCP). Each of these regulatory proteins binds to C4b and prevents its association with C2a. Once C4bBP, CR1, or MCP is bound to C4b, another regulatory protein, **factor I**, cleaves the C4b into bound C4d and soluble C4c (Figure 14-9a). A similar regulatory sequence occurs in the alternative pathway. In this case CR1, MCP, or a regulatory component called **factor H** binds to C3b and prevents its association with factor B (Figure 14-8c). Once CR1, MCP, or factor H is bound to C3b, factor I cleaves the C3b into a bound C3bi fragment and a soluble C3f fragment. Further cleavage of C3bi by factor I releases C3c and leaves C3dg bound to the membrane (Figure 14-9b).

RCA proteins also act on the assembled C3 convertase, causing it to dissociate. Included among these regulatory proteins are the previously mentioned C4bBP, CR1, and factor H, as well as an additional protein, **decay-accelerating factor** (DAF). DAF, a glycoprotein, is anchored covalently to a glycophospholipid membrane protein. Each of these RCA proteins accelerates decay (dissociation) of C3 convertase, releasing the component with enzymatic activity (C2a or Bb) from the cell-bound component (C4b or C3b). Once dissociation of the C3 convertase occurs, then factor I cleaves the remaining membrane-bound C4b or C3b component to irreversibly inactivate the convertase (Figure 14-8d).

Regulatory proteins also operate at the level of the membrane-attack complex. The ability of the C5b67 complex to be released and then bind to nearby cells poses a threat of innocent-bystander lysis of healthy cells. A number of serum proteins can counter this threat by binding to released C5b67 and preventing its insertion into the membrane of nearby cells. A serum protein called **S protein** can bind to C5b67, inducing a hydrophilic transition and thereby preventing insertion of C5b67 into the membrane of nearby cells (Figure 14-8e). The binding of the S protein to C5b67 also keeps C9

from binding to the soluble C5b67 and polymerizing, and thereby prevents the futile consumption of C9.

Complement-mediated lysis of cells is more effective if the complement is from a different species than the cells being lysed. This unusual phenomenon, which remained unexplained for several years, is now known to depend on two membrane proteins that block MAC formation. These two proteins, present on the membrane of many cell types, are **homologous restriction factor (HRF)** and **membrane inhibitor of reactive lysis (MIRL)**. Both HRF and MIRL protect cells from nonspecific complement-mediated lysis by binding to C8, preventing assembly of poly-C9 and its insertion into the plasma membrane (Figure 14-8f). However, this inhibition occurs only if the complement components are from the same species as the target cells. For this reason, MIRL and HRF are said to display homologous restriction, for which the latter was named.

TABLE 14-7

SUMMARY OF BIOLOGICAL EFFECTS MEDIATED BY COMPLEMENT PRODUCTS

EFFECT	COMPLEMENT PRODUCT MEDIATING *
Cell lysis	C5b–9, the membrane-attack complex (MAC)
Inflammatory Response:	
Degranulation of mast cells and basophils[†]	C3a, C4a, and C5a (anaphylatoxins)
Degranulation of eosinophils	C3a, C5a
Extravasation and chemotaxis of leukocytes at inflammatory site	C3a, **C5a**, C5b67
Aggregation of platelets	C3a, C5a
Inhibition of monocyte/macrophage migration and induction of their spreading	Bb
Release of neutrophils from bone marrow	C3c
Release of hydrolytic enzymes from neutrophils	C5a
Increased expression of complement receptors type 1 and 3 (CR1 and CR3) on neutrophils	C5a
Opsonization of particulate antigens, increasing their phagocytosis	**C3b**, C4b, C3bi
Viral neutralization	C3b, C5b–9 (MAC)
Solubilization and clearance of immune complexes	C3b

* Boldfaced component is most important in mediating indicated effect.
[†] Degranulation leads to release of histamine and other mediators that induce contraction of smooth muscle and increased permeability of vessels.

BIOLOGICAL CONSEQUENCES OF COMPLEMENT ACTIVATION

Complement serves as an important mediator of the humoral response by amplifying the response and converting it into an effective defense mechanism to destroy invading microorganisms and viruses. The MAC mediates cell lysis, while other complement components or split products participate in the inflammatory response, opsonization of antigen, viral neutralization, and clearance of immune complexes (Table 14-7).

Many of the biological activities of the complement system depend on the binding of complement fragments to complement receptors, which are expressed by various cells. In addition, some complement receptors play an important role in regulating complement activity by binding biologically active complement components and degrading them into inactive products. The complement receptors and their primary ligands, which include various complement components and their proteolytic breakdown products, are listed in Table 14-8.

Cell Lysis

The **membrane-attack complex** formed by complement activation is capable of lysing a broad spectrum of microorganisms, viruses, erythrocytes, and nucleated cells. Because the alternative pathway of activation generally occurs without an initial antigen-antibody interaction, this pathway serves as an important innate system of nonspecific defense against infectious microorganisms. The requirement for an initial antigen-antibody reaction in the classical pathway supplements the nonspecific innate defense of the alternative pathway with a more specific defense mechanism.

The importance of cell-mediated immunity in host defense against viral infections has been emphasized in previous chapters. Nevertheless antibody and complement do play a role in host defense against viruses and are often crucial in containing viral spread during acute

TABLE 14-8

COMPLEMENT-BINDING RECEPTORS

RECEPTOR	MAJOR LIGANDS	ACTIVITY	CELLULAR DISTRIBUTION
CR1 (CD35)	C3b, C4b	Blocks formation of C3 convertase; binds immune complexes to cells	Erythrocytes, neutrophils, monocytes, macrophages, eosinophils, follicular dendritic cells, B cells, some T cells
CR2 (CD21)	C3d, C3dg,* C3bi	Part of B-cell coreceptor; binds Epstein-Barr virus	B cells, some T cells
CR3 (CD11b/18) CR4 (CD11c/18)	C3bi	Bind cell-adhesion molecules on neutrophils, facilitating their extravasation; bind immune complexes, enhancing their phagocytosis	Monocytes, macrophages, neutrophils, natural killer cells, some T cells
C3a/C4a receptor	C3a, C4a	Induces degranulation of mast cells and basophils	Mast cells, basophils, granulocytes
C5a receptor	C5a	Induces degranulation of mast cells and basophils	Mast cells, basophils, granulocytes, monocytes, macrophages, platelets, endothelial cells

* Cleavage of C3dg by serum proteases generates C3d and C3g.

(a)

(b)

(c)

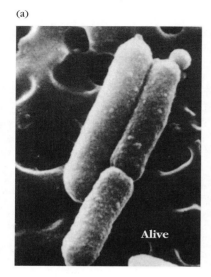
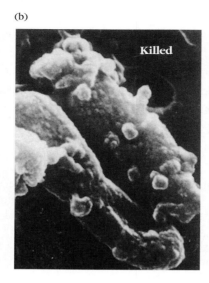
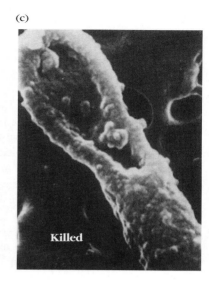

FIGURE 14-10

Scanning electron micrographs of *E. coli* showing (a) intact cells and (b, c) cells killed by complement-mediated lysis. Note membrane blebbing on lysed cells. [From R. D. Schreiber et al., 1979, *J. Exp. Med.* **149**:870.]

infection and in protecting against reinfection. Most—perhaps all—enveloped viruses are susceptible to complement-mediated lysis. The viral envelope is largely derived from the plasma membrane of the infected host cell and is therefore susceptible to pore formation via the membrane-attack complex. Among the pathogenic viruses shown to be lysed by complement-mediated lysis are herpes virus, myxoviruses, paramyxoviruses, and retroviruses.

The complement system is generally quite effective in lysing gram-negative bacteria (Figure 14-10). However, some gram-negative bacteria and most gram-positive bacteria have mechanisms for evading complement-mediated damage (Table 14-9). For example, a few gram-negative bacteria can develop resistance to complement-mediated lysis that correlates with the virulence of the organism. In *Escherichia coli* and *Salmonella*, resistance to complement is associated with the smooth bacterial phenotype, which is characterized by the presence of long polysaccharide side chains in the cell-wall lipopolysaccharide (LPS) component. It has been proposed that the increased LPS in the wall of resistant strains may prevent insertion of the MAC into the bacterial membrane, so that the complex is released from the bacterial cell rather than forming a pore. Strains of *Neisseria gonorrhoeae* resistant to complement-mediated killing have been associated with disseminated gonococcal infections in humans. Some evidence suggests that the membrane proteins of resistant *Neisseria* strains undergo noncovalent interactions with the MAC that

prevent its insertion into the outer membrane of the bacterial cells. These examples of resistant gram-negative bacteria are the exception; most gram-negative bacteria are susceptible to complement-mediated lysis.

In contrast, gram-positive bacteria are generally resistant to complement-mediated lysis because the thick peptidoglycan layer in their cell wall prevents insertion of the MAC into the inner membrane. Although complement activation can occur on the cell membrane of encapsulated bacteria such as *Streptococcus pneumoniae*, the capsule prevents interaction between C3b deposited on the membrane and the CR1 on phagocytic cells. Some bacteria possess an elastase that inactivates C3a and C5a, preventing these split products from inducing an inflammatory response. In addition to these mechanisms of evasion, various bacteria, viruses, fungi, and protozoans contain proteins that can interrupt the complement cascade on their surfaces, thus mimicking the effects of the normal complement regulatory proteins C4bBP, CR1, and DAF.

Nucleated cells tend to be more resistant to complement-mediated lysis than red blood cells. Lysis of nucleated cells requires formation of multiple membrane-attack complexes, whereas a single MAC can lyse a red blood cell. Many nucleated cells, including the majority of cancer cells, can endocytose the MAC. If the complex is removed soon enough, the cell can repair any membrane damage and restore its osmotic stability. This is the reason why complement-mediated lysis by monoclonal antibody specific for tumor-cell antigens is often not effective; rather, such monoclonal antibodies must be conjugated with toxins or radioactive isotopes to be effective tumor-killing agents.

Inflammatory Response

The complement cascade is often viewed in terms of the final outcome of cell lysis, but various peptides generated during formation of the MAC play a decisive role in the development of an effective inflammatory response (see Table 14-7). As noted already, the complement "split products" C3a, C4a, and C5a, called **anaphylatoxins**, bind to receptors on mast cells and blood basophils and induce degranulation with release of histamine and other pharmacologically active mediators. These mediators induce smooth-muscle contraction and increased vascular permeability. A serum protein called **anaphylatoxin inactivator** can bind C3a, C4a, and C5a, blocking their anaphylatoxin activity.

C3a, C5a, and C5b67 act together to induce monocytes and neutrophils to adhere to vascular endothelial cells, extravasate through the endothelial lining of the capillary, and migrate toward the site of complement activation in the tissues. C5a is most potent in mediating these processes, with picomolar quantities being effective. Activation of the complement system thus results in influxes of fluid that carries antibody and phagocytic cells to the site of antigen entry. The role of complement in the inflammatory response is discussed more fully in Chapter 15.

T A B L E   1 4 - 9

MICROBIAL EVASION OF COMPLEMENT-MEDIATED DAMAGE

MICROBIAL COMPONENT	MECHANISM OF EVASION	EXAMPLES
GRAM-NEGATIVE BACTERIA		
Long polysaccharide chains in cell-wall LPS	Side chains prevent insertion of MAC in bacterial membrane	Resistant strains of *E. coli* and *Salmonella* sp.
Outer membrane protein	MAC interacts with membrane protein and fails to insert into bacterial membrane	Resistant strains of *Neisseria gonorrhoeae*
Elastase	Anaphylotoxins C3a and C5a are inactivated by microbial elastase	*Pseudomonas aeruginosa*
GRAM-POSITIVE BACTERIA		
Peptidoglycan layer of cell wall	Insertion of MAC into bacterial membrane is prevented by thick layer of peptidoglycan	*Streptococcus* sp.
Bacterial capsule	Capsule provides physical barrier between C3b deposited on bacterial membrane and CR 1 on phagocytic cells	*Streptococcus pneumoniae*
OTHER MICROBES		
Proteins that mimic complement regulatory proteins	Proteins present in various bacteria, viruses, fungi, and protozoans inhibit the complement cascade	Vaccinia virus, herpes simplex, Epstein-Barr virus, *Trypanosoma cruzi, Candida albicans*

KEY: CR 1 = type 1 complement receptor; LPS = lipopolysaccharide; MAC = membrane-attack complex (C5b–9).

Opsonization of Antigen

C3b is the major **opsonin** of the complement system, although C4b and C3bi also have opsonizing activity. The amplification that occurs with C3 activation results in a coating of C3b on immune complexes and particulate antigens. Each of the phagocytic cells expresses complement receptors (CR1, CR3, and CR4) that bind C3b, C4b, or C3bi (see Table 14-8). When antigen has been coated with C3b during complement activation by either pathway, the coated antigen binds to cells bearing CR1. If the cell is a phagocyte (e.g., a neutrophil, monocyte, or macrophage), phagocytosis will be enhanced (Figure 14-11).

Activation of phagocytic cells by various agents, including C5a anaphylatoxin, has been shown to increase the number of CR1s from 5000 on resting phagocytes to 50,000 on activated cells, greatly facilitating their phagocytosis of C3b-coated antigen. Once C3b-coated antigen has bound to CR1, some of the C3b is degraded into C3bi and C3f. This enables the antigen to bind to CR3, which triggers phagocytosis more effectively than CR1.

Viral Neutralization

The complement system plays an important role in host defense by neutralizing viral infectivity. Some viruses (e.g., retroviruses, Epstein-Barr virus, Newcastle disease virus, and rubella virus) can activate the alternative or even the classical pathway in the absence of antibody. For most viruses, the binding of serum antibody to the repeating subunits of the viral structural proteins creates particulate immune complexes ideally suited for complement activation by the classical pathway.

The complement system mediates viral neutralization by a number of mechanisms. Some degree of neutralization is achieved through the formation of larger viral aggregates, simply because these aggregates reduce the net number of infectious viral particles. Although antibody does play a role in the formation of viral aggregates, in vitro studies show that the C3b component facilitates aggregate formation in the presence of as little as two molecules of antibody per virion. For example, polyoma virus coated with antibody is neutralized when serum containing activated C3 is added.

The binding of antibody and/or complement to the surface of a viral particle creates a thick protein coating that can be visualized by electron microscopy (Figure 14-12). This coating neutralizes viral infectivity by blocking attachment to susceptible host cells. The deposits of antibody and complement on viral particles also facilitate binding of the viral particle to cells possessing Fc or type 1 complement receptors (CR1). In the case of phagocytic cells, such binding can be followed by phagocytosis and intracellular destruction of the ingested viral particle. Finally, complement is effective in lysing most, if not all, enveloped viruses, resulting in fragmentation of the envelope and disintegration of the nucleocapsid.

(a)

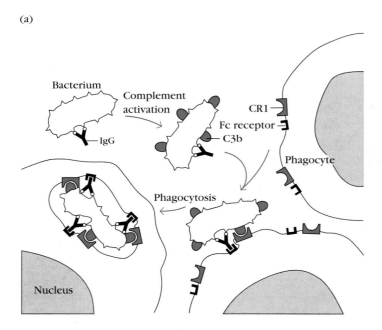

(b)

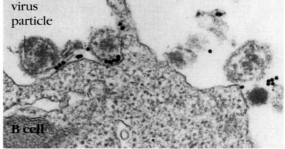

FIGURE 14-11

(a) Schematic representation of the role of C3b in opsonization. (b) Electron micrograph of Epstein-Barr virus coated with antibody and C3b and bound to the C3b receptors (CR1) on a B lymphocyte. [From N. R. Cooper and G. R. Nemerow, 1986, in *Immunobiology of the Complement System*, Academic Press.]

(a)   (b)   (c)

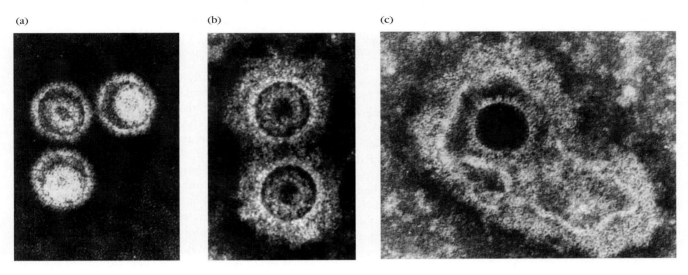

FIGURE 14-12

Electron micrographs of negatively stained preparations of Epstein-Barr virus. (a) Control without antibody. (b) Antibody-coated particles. (c) Particles coated with antibody and complement. [From N. R. Cooper and G. R. Nemerow, 1986, in *Immunobiology of the Complement System,* Academic Press.]

Solubilization of Immune Complexes

The role of the complement system in clearing immune complexes can be seen in patients with the autoimmune disease **systemic lupus erythematosus** (SLE). These individuals produce large quantities of immune complexes and suffer tissue damage as a result of complement-mediated lysis and the induction of type II or type III hypersensitivity (see Chapter 17). Although complement plays a significant role in the development of tissue damage in SLE, the paradoxical finding is that deficiencies in C1, C2, C4, and CR1 predispose an individual to SLE; indeed, 90% of individuals who completely lack C4 develop SLE. The complement deficiencies are thought to interfere with effective solubilization and clearance of immune complexes; the result is the persistence of these complexes and subsequent tissue damage by the very system whose deficiency was to blame.

The coating of soluble immune complexes with C3b is thought to facilitate their binding to CR1 on erythrocytes. Although red blood cells express lower levels of CR1 ($\sim 5 \times 10^2$ per cell) than granulocytes ($\sim 5 \times 10^4$ per cell), there are about 10^3 red blood cells for every white blood cell; therefore, erythrocytes account for about 90% of the CR1 in the blood. For this reason, erythrocytes play an important role in binding C3b-coated immune complexes and carrying these complexes to the liver and spleen. In these organs, immune complexes are stripped from the red blood cells and are phagocytosed, thereby preventing their deposition in tissues. In SLE patients, deficiencies in C1, C2, and C4 each contribute to reduced levels of C3b on immune complexes and hence inhibit their clearance. The lower levels of CR1 expressed on the erythrocytes of SLE patients also may interfere with the proper binding and clearance of immune complexes.

COMPLEMENT DEFICIENCIES

Genetic deficiencies have been described for each of the complement components with the exception of factor B. Homozygous deficiencies in any of the early components of the classical pathway (C1q, C1r, C1s, C4, and C2) manifest similar clinical presentations, notably a marked increase in **immune-complex diseases** such as systemic lupus erythematosus, glomerulonephritis, and vasculitis. These deficiencies highlight the important role of the early complement reactions in generating C3b, which is critical for solubilization and clearance of immune complexes. In addition to immune-complex diseases, individuals with such complement deficiencies may suffer from recurrent infections by pyogenic bacteria such as streptococci and staphylococci. These organisms are gram-positive and therefore resistant in any case to the lytic effects of the MAC. Nonetheless, the early complement components ordinarily prevent recurrent infection by mediating a localized inflammatory response and opsonizing the bacteria. Deficiencies in factor D and properdin—early components of the alternative pathway—appear to be associated with *Neisseria* infections but not with immune-complex disease.

C3 deficiencies have the most severe clinical manifestations, reflecting the central role of C3 in activation of C5 and formation of the MAC. The first patient identified with a C3 deficiency was a child who suffered from frequent severe bacterial infections and was erroneously thought to have agammaglobulinemia. When tests revealed normal immunoglobulin levels, a deficiency in C3 was discovered. This case highlights the critical function of the complement system in converting a humoral antibody response into an effective host-defense mechanism. The majority of patients with C3 deficiency have recurrent bacterial infections and manifest immune-complex diseases.

Individuals with homozygous deficiencies in the components involved in the MAC develop recurrent meningococcal and gonococcal infections caused by *Neisseria* species. In normal individuals these gram-negative bacteria are generally susceptible to complement-mediated lysis or are cleared by the opsonizing activity of C3b. Few of these individuals manifest immune-complex disease, so generally they must produce enough C3b to clear immune complexes. Interestingly, a deficiency in C9 results in no clinical symptoms, suggesting that in some cases the entire MAC is not necessary for complement-mediated lysis to occur.

Congenital deficiencies of complement regulatory proteins have also been reported. The C1 inhibitor (C1Inh) regulates activation of the classical pathway by preventing excessive C4 and C2 activation by C1. Deficiency of C1Inh is an autosomal dominant condition with a frequency of 1 in 1000. The deficiency gives rise to a disease called **hereditary angioedema**, which manifests clinically as localized edema of the tissue, often following trauma but sometimes with no known cause. The edema can be in subcutaneous tissues or within the bowel or upper respiratory tract, where it causes abdominal pain or obstruction of the airway.

A number of the membrane-bound regulatory components including decay-accelerating factor (DAF) and homologous restriction factor (HRF) are anchored to the plasma membrane by glycosyl phosphatidylinositol membrane anchors. In individuals with **paroxysmal nocturnal hemoglobinuria** the glycosyl phosphatidylinositol membrane anchor is defective, resulting in an absence of DAF and HRF from the cell membrane. As a consequence of this defect, much lower levels of complement are able to lyse the red blood cells, and the individual suffers from chronic hemolytic anemia.

SUMMARY

1. The complement system comprises a group of serum proteins, many of which exist in inactive and active forms. Complement activation involves an enzymatic cascade that generates various complement proteins, which play an important role in antigen clearance. The two pathways of complement activation, the classical pathway and the alternative pathway, involve different complement proteins and are initiated differently (see Figure 14-1). The two pathways converge in a common terminal reaction sequence that generates a membrane-attack complex (MAC) responsible for cell lysis.

2. The classical pathway, which involves in order the C1, C4, C2, and C3 components, is initiated by binding of IgM and certain subclasses of IgG to soluble antigen or cell-surface antigens. The reaction sequence generates the enzymatically active $\overline{C4b2a3b}$ complex (C3 convertase), which can split C3 into C3a and C3b, and the $\overline{C4b2a3b}$ complex (C5 convertase), which can split C5 into C5a and C5b. The alternative pathway is most commonly initiated by surface constituents of a variety of microorganisms (bacteria, fungi, some viruses, and some parasites); however, this pathway also can be initiated by IgG-, IgA-, and IgE-antigen complexes (see Table 14-3). This pathway involves C3, factor B, factor D, and properdin. The reaction sequence generates $C3b\overline{Bb}$ (C3 convertase) and $C3b\overline{Bb3b}$ (C5 convertase) analogous to the convertases in the classical pathway. Both the classical and alternative pathways generate bound C5b. This component reacts sequentially with C6, C7, C8, and C9 to produce the membrane-attack complex, which mediates cell lysis by forming a large pore in the cell membrane (see Figures 14-4 and 14-6).

3. Because of its nonspecific nature, the complement system requires elaborate regulatory mechanisms to prevent damage to normal tissues. Both pathways have a number of extremely labile components that lose their activity as they diffuse from the site of activation. In addition, both pathways have a number of regulatory components that function to inactivate complement products and prevent excessive buildup of enzymatically active components (see Figure 14-8 and Table 14-6).

4. The complement system serves as an important effector of the humoral immune response with various components mediating specific effects (see Table 14-7). It destroys foreign cells through the process of MAC-mediated lysis. The complement system also induces a localized inflammatory response with a buildup of fluid and inflammatory cells, and it facili-

tates phagocytosis of antigen through its effect as an opsonin. Complement also acts to neutralize viral infectivity by several mechanisms and aids in solubilizing immune complexes.

5. Inherited deficiencies of most of the complement components have been described. The consequences of these conditions depend on which complement component is deficient. C3 deficiencies, which are clinically the most severe, are often associated with immune-complex disease and susceptibility to recurrent bacterial infections. These effects reflect the central role of C3 in both the classical and alternative pathways of complement activation. Deficiency of the regulatory protein C1 inhibitor (C1Inh) is fairly common and is associated with a localized edema called hereditary angioedema.

REFERENCES

AHEARN, J. M., AND D. T. FEARON. 1989. Structure and function of the complement receptors, CR1 (CD35) and CR2 (CD21). *Adv. Immunol.* **46**:183.

BREKKE, O. H., T. E. MICHAELSEN, AND I. SANDLIE. 1995. The structural requirements for complement activation by IgG: does it hinge on the hinge? *Immunol. Today* **16**:85.

COOPER, N. R. 1991. Complement evasion strategies of microorganisms. *Immunol. Today* **12**:327.

DAVIS, A. E. 1988. C1 inhibitor and hereditary angioneurotic edema. *Annu. Rev. Immunol.* **6**:595.

ERDEI, A., G. FUST, AND J. GERGELY. 1991. The role of C3 in the immune response. *Immunol. Today* **12**:332.

FRANK, M. M., AND L. F. FRIES. 1991. The role of complement in inflammation and phagocytosis. *Immunol. Today* **12**:322.

HOURCADE, D., M. HOLERS, AND J. P. ATKINSON. 1989. The regulators of complement activation (RCA) gene cluster. *Adv. Immunol.* **45**:381.

KINOSHITA, T. 1991. Biology of complement: the overture. *Immunol. Today* **12**:291.

LISZEWSKI, M. K., T. W. POST, AND J. P. ATKINSON. 1991. Membrane cofactor protein (MCP or CD46): newest member of the regulators of complement activation gene cluster. *Annu. Rev. Immunol.* **9**:431.

MORGAN, B. P., AND M. J. WALPORT. 1991. Complement deficiency and disease. *Immunol. Today* **12**:301.

MULLER-EBERHARD, H. J. 1986. The membrane attack complex of complement. *Annu. Rev. Immunol.* **4**:503.

MULLER-EBERHARD, H. J. 1988. Molecular organization and function of the complement system. *Annu. Rev. Biochem.* **57**:321.

PASCUAL, M., AND L. E. FRENCH. 1995. Complement in human disease: looking towards the 21st century. *Immunol. Today* **16**:58.

PERLMUTTER, D. H., AND H. R. COLTEN. 1986. Molecular immunobiology of complement biosynthesis. *Annu. Rev. Immunol.* **4**:231.

REID, K. B. M., AND A. J. DAY. 1989. Structure-function relationships of the complement components. *Immunol. Today* **10**:177.

WILSON, J. G., ET AL. 1987. Deficiency of the C3b/C4b receptor (CR1) of erythrocytes in systemic lupus erythematosus. *J. Immunol.* **138**:2706.

STUDY QUESTIONS

1. Indicate whether each of the following statements is true or false. If you think a statement is false, explain why.

a. A single molecule of bound IgM can activate the C1q component of the classical complement pathway.

b. C3a and C3b are fragments of C3.

c. The C4 and C2 complement components are present in the serum in a functionally inactive proenzyme form.

d. Nucleated cells tend to be more resistant to complement-mediated lysis than red blood cells.

e. Enveloped viruses cannot be lysed by complement because their outer envelope is resistant to pore formation by the membrane-attack complex.

f. C4-deficient individuals have difficulty eliminating immune complexes.

2. Explain why serum IgM cannot activate complement by itself.

3. Would you expect a C1 or C3 complement deficiency to be more serious clinically? Why?

4. Some microorganisms produce enzymes that can degrade the Fc portion of antibody molecules. Why would such enzymes be advantageous for the survival of microorganisms that possess them?

5. Complement activation can occur via the classical or alternative pathway.

a. How do the two pathways differ in the substances that can initiate activation?

b. Which portion of the overall activation sequence differs in the two pathways? Which portion is similar?

c. How do the biological consequences of complement activation via the classical and the alternate pathways differ?

6. Enucleated cells, such as red blood cells, are more susceptible to complement-mediated lysis than nucleated cells.

a. Explain why the red blood cells of an individual are not normally destroyed as the result of innocent-bystander lysis by complement.

b. Under what conditions might complement cause lysis of an individual's own red blood cells?

7. Briefly explain the mechanism of action of the following complement regulatory proteins. Indicate which pathway(s) each protein regulates.

a. C1 inhibitor (C1Inh)

b. C4b-binding protein (C4bBP)

c. Homologous restriction factor (HRF)

d. Decay-accelerating factor

e. Factor H

f. Membrane cofactor protein (MCP)

8. For each complement component(s) or reaction (a–l), select the most appropriate description listed below (1–13). Each description may be used once, more than once, or not at all.

Complement Component(s)/Reactions:

a. C3b

b. C1, C4, C2, and C3

c. C9

d. C3, factor B, and factor D

e. C1q

f. $\overline{C4b2a3b}$

g. C5b, C6, C7, C8, and C9

h. C3 → C3a + C3b

i. C3a, C5a, and C5b67

j. C3a, C4a, and C5a

k. $\overline{C4b2a}$

l. C3b + B → $\overline{C3bBb}$ + Ba

Descriptions:

1) Reaction that produces major amplification during activation

2) Are early components of alternative pathway

3) Compose the membrane-attack complex

4) Mediates opsonization

5) Are early components of classical pathway

6) Has perforin-like activity

7) Binds to Fc region of antibodies

8) Have chemotactic activity

9) Has C3 convertase activity

10) Induce degranulation of mast cells (are anaphylatoxins)

11) Has C5 convertase activity

12) Reaction catalyzed by factor D

13) Reaction catalyzed by $\overline{C1q\overline{r_2s_2}}$

9. You have prepared knockout mice with mutations in the genes that encode various complement components. Each knockout strain cannot express one of the complement components listed across the top of the table below. Predict the effect of each mutation on the steps in complement activation and on the complement effector functions indicated in the table below using the following symbols: NE = no effect; D = process/ function decreased but not abolished; A = process/ function abolished.

	Component knocked out						
	C1q	C4	C3	C5	C6	C9	Factor B
Complement Activation Formation of C3 convertase in classical pathway							
Formation of C3 convertase in alternative pathway							
Formation of C5 convertase in classical pathway							
Formation of C5 convertase in alternative pathway							
Effector Functions C3b-mediated opsonization							
Neutrophil chemotaxis							
Cell lysis							

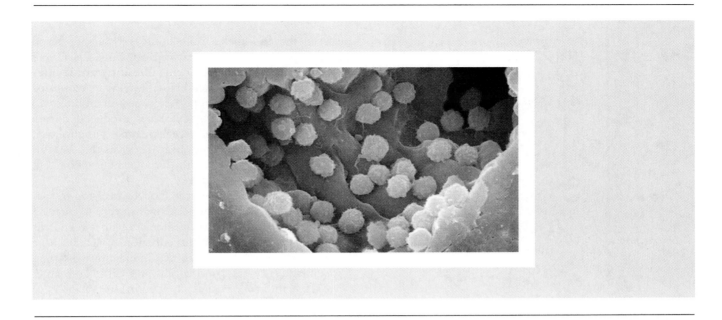

LEUKOCYTE MIGRATION
AND INFLAMMATION

Lymphocytes circulate continually in the blood and lymph and also migrate into the tissues at sites of infection or tissue injury. This recirculation not only increases the chances that lymphocytes specific for a particular antigen will encounter that antigen but also is critical to development of an inflammatory response. **Inflammation** is a complex response to localized injury or other trauma, which involves various immune-system cells and numerous mediators. This chapter covers the molecules and processes that play a role in leukocyte migration, various molecules that mediate inflammation, and the characteristic physiologic changes that accompany inflammatory responses.

LYMPHOCYTE RECIRCULATION

Lymphocytes are capable of a remarkable level of recirculation, continuously moving through the blood and lymph to the various lymphoid organs (Figure 15-1). Following a brief transit time of approximately 30 min in the bloodstream, nearly 45% of all lymphocytes are carried from the blood directly to the spleen where they reside for approximately 5 h. Almost equal numbers (42%) of lymphocytes exit from the blood into various peripheral lymph nodes where they reside for about 12 h. A smaller number of lymphocytes (10%) migrate to **tertiary extralymphoid tissues** by crossing endothelial cells lining the capillaries. These tissues normally have few, if any, lymphoid cells but can import lymphoid cells during an inflammatory response. The most immunologically active tertiary extralymphoid tissues are those that interface with the external environment such as the skin and various mucosal epithelia of the gastrointestinal, pulmonary, and genitourinary tracts.

The process of continual lymphocyte recirculation allows maximal numbers of antigenically committed lymphocytes to encounter and interact with antigen. An

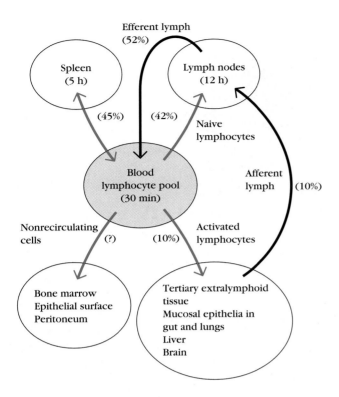

FIGURE 15-1

Lymphocyte recirculation routes. The percentage of the lymphocyte pool that circulates to various sites and the average transit times in the major sites are indicated. Lymphocytes migrate from the blood into lymph nodes via specialized postcapillary venules called high-endothelial venules (HEVs). [Adapted from A. Ager, 1994, *Trends Cell Biol.* **4**:326.]

individual lymphocyte may make a complete circuit from the blood to the tissues and lymph and back again as often as 1–2 times per day. Since only about one in 10^5 lymphocytes recognizes a particular antigen, it would appear that a large number of antigen-committed T or B cells must contact antigen on a given antigen-presenting cell within a relatively short period of time in order to generate a specific immune response. The odds of the small percentage of lymphocytes committed to a given antigen actually making contact with that antigen when it is present are greatly increased by the extensive recirculation of lymphocytes.

CELL-ADHESION MOLECULES

The vascular endothelium serves as an important "gate-keeper," regulating the movement of blood-borne molecules and leukocytes into the tissues. In order for circulating leukocytes to enter inflamed tissue or peripheral lymphoid organs, the cells must adhere to and pass between the endothelial cells lining the walls of blood vessels, a process called **extravasation**. Endothelial cells express leukocyte-specific **cell-adhesion molecules** (CAMs). Some of these membrane proteins are expressed constitutively; others are only expressed in response to localized concentrations of cytokines produced during an inflammatory response. Recirculating lymphocytes, monocytes, and granulocytes bear receptors that bind to CAMs on the vascular endothelium, enabling these cells to extravasate into the tissues.

In addition to their role in leukocyte adhesion to vascular endothelial cells, many CAMs also serve to increase the strength of the functional interactions between cells of the immune system. Various adhesion molecules have been shown to contribute to the interactions between T_H cells and APCs, T_H and B cells, and CTLs and target cells. These interactions are examined in later chapters.

A number of endothelial and leukocyte CAMs have been cloned and characterized, providing new details about the extravasation process. Most of these CAMs belong to four families of proteins: the selectin family, the mucin-like family, the integrin family, and the immunoglobulin (Ig) superfamily (Figure 15-2).

Selectin Family

The **selectin** family of membrane glycoproteins has a distal lectin-like domain that enables these molecules to bind to specific carbohydrate groups. Selectins interact primarily with sialylated carbohydrate moieties often linked to mucin-like molecules. The selectin family includes three molecules designated L, E, and P. Most circulating leukocytes express L-selectin, whereas E-selectin and P-selectin are expressed on vascular endothelial cells. Selectin molecules are responsible for the initial stickiness of leukocytes to vascular endothelium.

Mucin-like Family

Mucins are a group of serine and threonine-rich proteins that are heavily glycosylated. Their extended structure allows them to present sialylated carbohydrate ligands to selectins. For example, L-selectin on leukocytes recognizes sialylated carbohydrates on two mucin-like molecules (CD34 and GlyCAM-1) expressed on certain endothelial cells of lymph nodes. Another mucin-like molecule (PSGL-1) found on neutrophils interacts with E- and P-selectin expressed on inflamed endothelium.

Integrin Family

The **integrins** are heterodimeric proteins (consisting of an α and $\alpha\beta$ chain) that are expressed by leukocytes and facilitate adherence to the vascular endothelium or other

(a) General structure of CAM families

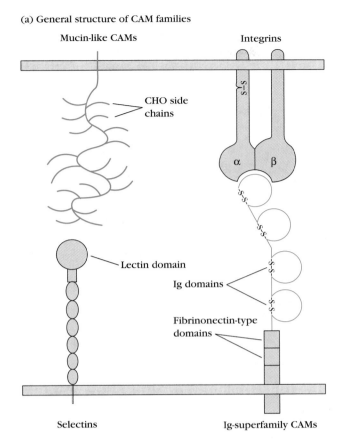

(b) Selected CAMs belonging to each family

Mucin-like CAMs:	Selectins:
GlyCAM-1	L-selectin
CD34	P-selectin
PSGL-1	E-selectin
MAdCAM-1	

Ig-superfamily CAMs:	Integrins:
ICAM-1, -2, -3	α4β1 (VLA-4, LPAM-2)
VCAM-1	α4β7 (LPAM-1)
LFA-2 (CD-2)	α6β1 (VLA-6)
LFA-3 (CD58)	αLβ2 (LFA-1)
MAdCAM-1	αMβ2 (Mac-1)
	αXβ2 (CR4, p150/95)

FIGURE 15-2

Schematic diagrams depicting the general structure of the four families of cell-adhesion molecules (a) and representative molecules in each family (b). The lectin domain in selectins interacts primarily with carbohydrate (CHO) moieties on mucin-like molecules. Both chains in integrin molecules contribute to the binding site, which interacts with an Ig domain in CAMs belonging to the Ig superfamily. MAdCAM-1 contains both mucin-like and Ig-like domains and thus can bind to both selectins and integrins.

cell-to-cell interactions. The integrins are grouped into categories depending upon which β subunit they contain. Different integrins are expressed by different populations of leukocytes, allowing these cells to bind to different CAMs belonging to the immunoglobulin superfamily expressed along the vascular endothelium. As discussed later, some integrins must be activated before they can bind with high affinity to their ligands.

The importance of integrin molecules in leukocyte extravasation is demonstrated by **leukocyte-adhesion deficiency** (LAD), an autosomal recessive disease characterized by recurrent bacterial infections and impaired healing of wounds. This disorder stems from abnormal synthesis of the β chain of the integrin heterodimer. The leukocytes of an affected individual lack functional integrin molecules and thus cannot extravasate from the blood vessels to the tissues. As a result, an inflammatory response cannot develop in the tissues, and affected individuals have more frequent and more severe bacterial infections than normal individuals.

Immunoglobulin Superfamily

Several adhesion molecules contain a variable number of immunoglobulin-like domains and thus are classified in the **immunoglobulin superfamily** (see Figure 5-19). Included in this group are ICAM-1, ICAM-2, ICAM-3, and VCAM, which are expressed on vascular endothelial cells and bind to various integrin molecules. A more recently discovered cell-adhesion molecule, called MAdCAM-1, has both Ig-like domains and mucin-like domains. This molecule is expressed on mucosal endothelium and directs lymphocyte entry into mucosa. It binds to integrins via its immunoglobulin-like domain and to selectins via its mucin-like domain.

NEUTROPHIL EXTRAVASATION

As an inflammatory response develops, a variety of cytokines and other inflammatory mediators acts upon the local blood vessels inducing increased expression of endothelial CAMs. The vascular endothelium is then said to be **activated**, or **inflamed**. Neutrophils are generally the first cell type to bind to inflamed endothelium and extravasate into the tissues. To accomplish this, neutrophils must recognize the inflamed endothelium and adhere strongly enough so that they are not swept away by the flowing blood. The bound neutrophils must then

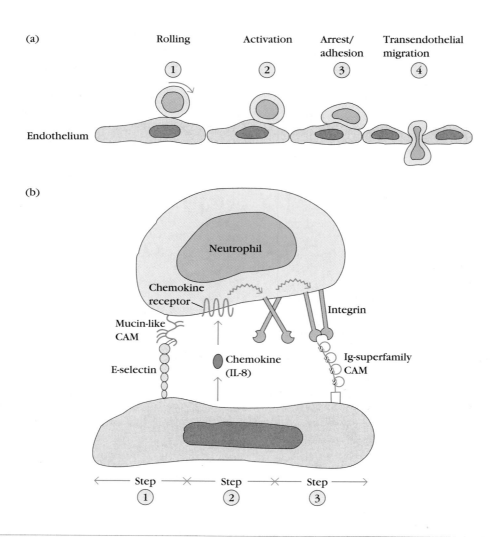

FIGURE 15-3

(a) The four sequential, but overlapping, steps in neutrophil extravasation. (b) Cell-adhesion molecules and chemokines involved in the first three steps of neutrophil extravasation. Initial rolling is mediated by binding of E-selectin molecule on the vascular endothelium to sialylated carbohydrate moieties on mucin-like CAMs. A chemokine such as IL-8 then binds to a G-protein–linked receptor on the neutrophil, triggering an activating signal. This signal induces a conformational change in the integrin molecules enabling them to adhere firmly to Ig-superfamily molecules on the endothelium.

penetrate the endothelial layer and migrate into the underlying tissue. Monocytes and eosinophils extravasate using a similar process, but since the steps have been best established for neutrophils we will focus on this cell.

The process of neutrophil extravasation can be divided into four sequential steps: (1) rolling, (2) chemoattractant activating stimulus, (3) arrest and adhesion, and (4) transendothelial migration (Figure 15-3a). In the first step, neutrophils attach loosely to the endothelium by a low-affinity selectin-carbohydrate interaction. During an inflammatory response cytokines and other inflammatory mediators act upon the local endothelium inducing expression of adhesion molecules of the selectin family on

the inflamed endothelium. These E- and P-selectin molecules bind to mucin-like cell-adhesion molecules on the neutrophil membrane or with a sialylated lactosaminoglycan, called sialyl Lewis^x (Figure 15-3b). This interaction tethers the neutrophil briefly to the endothelial cell, but the sheer force of the circulating blood soon detaches the neutrophil. Selectin molecules on another endothelial cell again tether the neutrophil; this process is repeated so that the neutrophil tumbles end-over-end along the endothelium, a type of binding referred to as **rolling**.

As the neutrophil rolls, it is activated by various **chemoattractants;** these are either localized on the endothelial cell surface or secreted locally by cells involved in the inflammatory response. Among the chemoattractants are members of a more recently described family of chemoattractive cytokines called **chemokines**. Two chemokines involved in this process are interleukin 8 (IL-8) and macrophage inflammatory protein (MIP-1b). Other chemoattractants are platelet-activating factor (PAF), the complement split product C5a, and various N-formyl peptides produced by bacteria during an infection. Binding of these chemoattractants to receptors on the neutrophil membrane triggers an activating signal mediated by **G proteins** associated with the receptor. This signal induces a conformational change in the integrin molecules in the neutrophil membrane, increasing their affinity for the Ig-superfamily adhesion molecules on the endothelium. Subsequent interaction between integrins and Ig-superfamily CAMs stabilizes adhesion of the neutrophil to the endothelial cell, enabling the cell to adhere firmly to the endothelial cell.

The subsequent transendothelial migration of the neutrophil into the tissues involves the directed migration of the neutrophil through interendothelial junctions and across the reticular cells that make up the vessel wall. The steps in transendothelial migration, still largely unknown, are thought to be mediated by further chemoattractant activation and subsequent integrin-Ig superfamily interactions or by a separate migration stimulus.

LYMPHOCYTE EXTRAVASATION

Various subsets of lymphocytes exhibit directed extravasation at inflammatory sites and secondary lymphoid organs. The recirculation of lymphocytes thus is carefully controlled to ensure that appropriate populations of B and T cells are recruited into different tissues. As with neutrophils, extravasation of lymphocytes involves interactions among a number of cell-adhesion molecules (Table 15-1).

High-Endothelial Venules

Some regions of vascular endothelium found in postcapillary venules of various lymphoid organs are composed of specialized cells with a plump, cuboidal ("high") shape; such regions are called **high-endothelial venules**, or HEVs (Figure 15-4a,b). These regions contrast sharply with the flattened appearance of endothelial cells lining the rest of the capillary. Each of the secondary lymphoid organs, with the exception of the spleen, contains HEVs. When frozen sections of lymph nodes, Peyer's patches, or tonsils are incubated with lymphocytes and washed to remove unbound cells, over 85% of the bound cells are found adhering to HEVs, even though HEVs account for only 1%–2% of the total area of the frozen section (Figure 15-4c).

It has been estimated that as many as 1.4×10^4 lymphocytes extravasate every second through HEVs into a single lymph node. The development and maintenance of HEVs in lymphoid organs is influenced by cytokines produced in response to antigen capture. For example, HEVs fail to develop in animals raised in a germ-free environment. The role of antigenic activation of lymphocytes in the maintenance of HEVs has been demonstrated by surgically blocking the afferent lymphatic vasculature to a node, so that antigen entry to the node is blocked. Within a short period of time, the HEVs show impaired function and eventually revert to a more flattened morphology.

High-endothelial venules express a variety of cell-adhesion molecules. Like other vascular endothelial cells, HEVs express CAMs of the selectin family (E- and P-selectin), the mucin-like family (GlyCAM-1 and CD34), and the immunoglobulin superfamily (ICAM-1, ICAM-2, ICAM-3, VCAM-1, and MAdCAM-1). Some of these adhesion molecules are distributed in a tissue-specific manner. These tissue-specific adhesion molecules have been called **vascular addressins** (VAs) because they serve to direct the extravasation of different populations of recirculating lymphocytes to particular lymphoid organs.

Homing of Lymphocytes

The general process of lymphocyte extravasation is similar to neutrophil extravasation. An important feature distinguishing the two processes is that different subsets of lymphocytes migrate differentially into different tissues. This process is called **trafficking**, or **homing**. The different trafficking patterns of lymphocyte subsets is mediated by receptors on the surface of recirculating lymphocytes that recognize particular vascular addressins on the HEVs of different secondary lymphoid tissues and endothelium at sites of inflammation. Because these receptors direct the circulation of various populations of lymphocytes to particular lymphoid and inflammatory tissues, they have been called **homing receptors**. Researchers have identified a number of lymphocyte and endothelial cell-adhesion molecules that participate in the interaction of lymphocytes with HEVs and with endothelium at tertiary sites or sites of inflammation (see Table 15-1).

Also contributing to trafficking differences among different lymphocyte subsets are the chemokines. Macrophage inflammatory protein (MIP-1b) preferentially attracts naive T cells, whereas monocyte chemoattractant

(a)

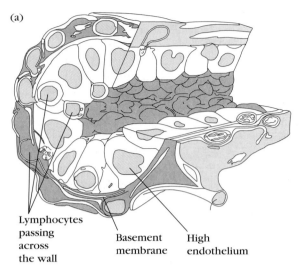

Lymphocytes
passing
across
the wall

Basement
membrane

High
endothelium

(b)

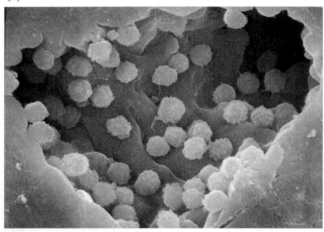

(c)

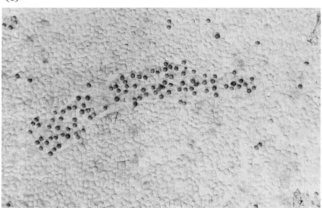

FIGURE 15-4

(a) Schematic cross-sectional diagram of a lymph node postcapillary venule with high endothelium. Lymphocytes are shown in various stages of attachment to the HEV and in migration across the wall into the cortex of the node. (b) Scanning electron micrograph showing numerous lymphocytes bound to the surface of a high-endothelial venule. (c) Micrograph of frozen sections of lymphoid tissue. Some 85% of the lymphocytes (darkly stained) are bound to HEVs (in cross section), which comprise only 1%–2% of the total area of the tissue section. [Part (a) adapted from A. O. Anderson and N. D. Anderson, 1981, in *Cellular Functions in Immunity and Inflammation*, J. J. Oppenheim et al. (eds.), Elsevier, North-Holland; part (b) from S. D. Rosen and L. M. Stoolman, 1987, *Vertebrate Lectins,* Van Nostrand Reinhold; part (c) from S. D. Rosen, 1989, *Curr. Opin. Cell Biol.* **1**:913.]

Naive Lymphocytes

Naive lymphocytes are not able to mount an immune response until they have been activated to become an effector cell. The site of activation of a naive cell occurs exclusively in specialized microenvironments within secondary lymphoid tissue (e.g., peripheral lymph nodes, Peyer's patches, tonsils, and spleen). Within these specialized microenvironments, dendritic cells capture antigen and present it to the naive lymphocyte resulting in its activation (see Figures 3-21 and 3-22). Naive cells do not exhibit a preference for a particular type of secondary lymphoid tissue but instead are disseminated to secondary lymphoid tissue throughout the body by recognizing adhesion molecules on HEVs.

The initial attachment of naive lymphocytes to HEVs is generally mediated by the binding of the homing receptor L-selectin to vascular addressins such as GlyCAM-1 and CD34 on HEVs (Figure 15-5a). The trafficking pattern of naive cells is designed to keep these cells constantly recirculating through secondary lymphoid tissue, whose primary function is to trap blood-borne or tissue-borne antigen. Since only about 1 in 10^5 lymphocytes is specific for a particular antigen, this type of trafficking ensures that maximal numbers of naive cells will encounter the trapped antigen.

Once naive lymphocytes encounter antigen trapped in a secondary lymphoid tissue, they become activated and enlarge into lymphoblasts. Activation takes about 48 h, and during this time the blast cells are retained in the paracortical region of the secondary lymphoid tissue. During this phase, called the **shut-down phase**, antigen-specific lymphocytes cannot be detected in the circulation (Figure 15-6). Rapid proliferation and differentiation of naive cells occurs during the shut-down phase. The effector and memory cells that are generated by this process then leave the lymphoid tissue and begin to recirculate.

protein (MCP-1) and RANTES preferentially attract memory T cells. Thus differences in vascular addressins, homing receptors, and chemokines and their receptors determine the recirculation pattern of particular lymphocyte subsets.

EFFECTOR AND MEMORY LYMPHOCYTES

The trafficking patterns of effector and memory lymphocytes differ from those of naive lymphocytes. Effector cells tend to home to regions of infection by recognizing inflamed vascular endothelium and chemoattractant molecules that are generated during the inflammatory response. Interestingly, memory lymphocytes exhibit selective homing to the type of tissue in which they first encountered antigen. Presumably this ensures that a particular memory cell will return to the tissue where it is most likely to re-encounter a subsequent antigenic threat.

Effector and memory cells express increased levels of certain cell-adhesion molecules, allowing these cells to enter tertiary extralymphoid tissue (such as skin and mucosal epithelia) and sites of inflammation in addition to secondary lymphoid organs. Inflamed endothelium expresses a number of adhesion molecules, including E- and P-selectin and the Ig-superfamily molecules VCAM-1 and ICAM-1, that bind to the receptors expressed at high levels on memory/effector cells.

Unlike naive lymphocytes, which do not exhibit a preference for a particular type of secondary lymphoid tissue, the memory and effector populations have subsets

TABLE 15-1

SOME INTERACTIONS BETWEEN CELL-ADHESION MOLECULES IMPLICATED IN LEUKOCYTE EXTRAVASATION*

RECEPTOR ON CELLS	EXPRESSION	LIGANDS ON ENDOTHELIUM	STEP INVOLVING INTERACTION [†]	MAIN FUNCTION
CLA or ESL-1	Effector T cells	E-selectin	Tethering/rolling	Homing to skin and migration into inflamed tissue
L-selectin	All leukocytes	GlyCAM-1, CD34, MAdCAM-1	Tethering/rolling	Lymphocyte recirculation via HEVs to peripheral lymph nodes and migration into inflamed tertiary sites
LFA-1 ($\alpha L\beta 2$)	Leukocyte subsets	ICAM-1, 2, 3	Adhesion/arrest	General role in lymphocyte extravasation via HEVs and leukocyte migration into inflamed tissue
LPAM-1 ($\alpha 4\beta 7$)	Effector T cells, monocytes	MAdCAM-1, VCAM-1	Rolling/adhesion	Homing of T cells to gut via mucosal HEV; migration into inflamed tissue
Mac-1 ($\alpha M\beta 2$)	Monocytes	VCAM-1	—	Monocyte migration into inflamed tissue
PSGL-1	Neutrophils	E- and P-selectin	Tethering/rolling	Neutrophil migration into inflamed tissue
VLA-4 ($\alpha 4\beta 1$)	Neutrophils, T cells, monocytes	VCAM-1, MAdCAM-1, fibronectin	Rolling/adhesion	General role in leukocyte migration into inflamed tissue
VLA-6 ($\alpha 6\beta 1$)	T cells	Lamanin	—	Homing of progenitor T cells to thymus; possible role in T-cell homing to nonmucosal sites

* Most endothelial and leukocyte CAMs belong to four groups of proteins as shown in Figure 15-2. In general, molecules in the integrin family bind to Ig-superfamily CAMs, and molecules in the selectin family bind to mucin-like CAMs. Members of the selectin and mucin-like families can be expressed on both leukocytes and endothelial cells, whereas integrins are expressed only on leukocytes, and Ig-superfamily CAMs are expressed only on endothelium.

[†] See Figures 15-3a and 15-7 for an illustration of steps in the extravasation process.

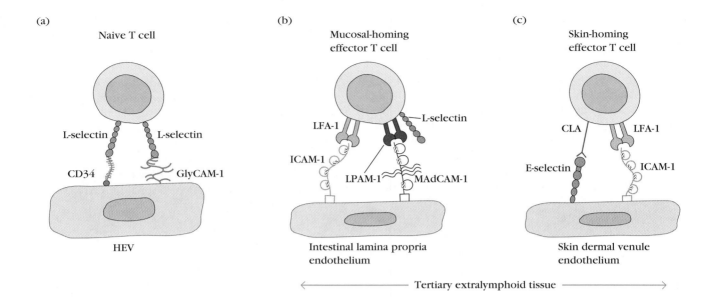

(a) Naive T cell

L-selectin   L-selectin

CD34   GlyCAM-1

HEV

(b) Mucosal-homing
effector T cell

LFA-1   L-selectin

ICAM-1

LPAM-1   MAdCAM-1

Intestinal lamina propria
endothelium

(c) Skin-homing
effector T cell

CLA   LFA-1

E-selectin   ICAM-1

Skin dermal venule
endothelium

←——————— Tertiary extralymphoid tissue ———————→

FIGURE 15-5

Examples of homing receptors and vascular addressins involved in selective trafficking of naive and effector T cells. (a) Naive T cells tend to home to secondary lymphoid tissue through regions of HEVs. The initial interaction involves the homing receptor L-selectin and mucin-like cell-adhesion molecules such as CD34 or GlyCAM-1 expressed on HEVs. (b, c) Various subsets of effector T cells express high levels of particular homing receptors that allow them to home to endothelium in various tertiary extralymphoid tissues. The initial interactions in homing of effector T cells to mucosal and skin sites are illustrated.

that exhibit tissue-selective homing behavior. Such tissue **tropism** is imparted not by a single adhesion receptor but by different combinations of adhesion molecules that enable different subsets of effector cells to preferentially home to different sites. For example, a mucosal homing subset of memory/effector cells has high levels of the integrins LPAM-1 ($\alpha 4\beta 7$) and LFA-1 ($\alpha L\beta 2$) and high levels of L-selectin, which bind to MAdCAM and various ICAMs on intestinal lamina propria venules (Figure 15-5b). A second subset of memory/effector cells displays preferential homing to the skin. This subset expresses high levels of cutaneous lymphocyte antigen (CLA) and LFA-1, which bind to E-selectin and ICAMs on dermal venules of the skin (Figure 15-5c).

Some effector and memory cells express reduced levels of L-selectin and therefore do not tend to home through HEVs into peripheral lymph nodes. Instead, these effector and memory populations enter peripheral lymph nodes via the afferent lymphatic vessels.

Adhesion-Molecule Interactions

The extravasation of lymphocytes into secondary lymphoid tissue or regions of inflammation is a multistep process involving a cascade of adhesion-molecule interac-

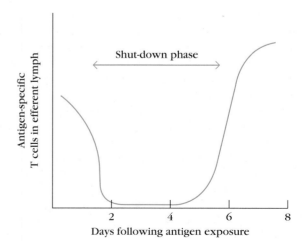

Shut-down phase

Antigen-specific
T cells in efferent lymph

2   4   6   8

Days following antigen exposure

FIGURE 15-6

T-cell activation in the paracortical region of a lymph node results in the brief loss of lymphocyte recirculation. During this shut-down phase, antigen-specific T cells cannot be detected leaving the node in the efferent lymph.

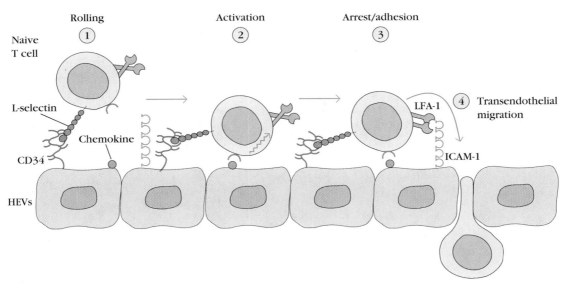

FIGURE 15-7

Steps in extravasation of a naive T cell through a high-endothelial venule into a lymph node. Extravasation of lymphocytes involves the same basic steps as neutrophil extravasation but some of the cell-adhesion molecules differ. Activation of the integrin LFA-1, induced by chemokine binding to the lymphocyte, leads to firm adhesion followed by migration between the endothelial cells into the tissue.

tions similar to those involved in neutrophil emigration from the bloodstream. Figure 15-7 depicts the typical interactions involved in extravasation of naive T cells across HEVs into lymph nodes. The first step usually involves a selectin–carbohydrate interaction similar to that seen with neutrophil adhesion. Naive lymphocytes initially bind to HEVs by L-selectin, which serves as a homing receptor directing the lymphocytes to particular tissues expressing a corresponding mucin-like vascular addressin such as CD34 or GlyCAM-1. Lymphocyte rolling is less pronounced than that of neutrophils. Although the initial selectin–carbohydrate interaction is quite weak, the slow rate of blood flow in postcapillary venules, particularly in regions of HEVs, reduces the likelihood that the sheer force of the flowing blood will dislodge the tethered lymphocyte.

In the second step, an integrin-activating stimulus is mediated by chemokines that are either localized on the endothelial surface or secreted locally. The thick glycocalyx covering of the HEVs may function to retain these soluble chemoattractant factors on the HEVs. It is thought that HEVs secrete lymphocyte-specific chemoattractants, which may explain why neutrophils do not extravasate into lymph nodes at the HEVs even though they express L-selectin. Chemokine binding to G protein–coupled receptors on the lymphocyte leads to activation of integrin molecules on the membrane, as occurs in neutrophil extravasation. Once activated, the integrin

molecules interact with Ig-superfamily adhesion molecules (e.g., ICAM-1), so the lymphocyte adheres firmly to the endothelium. The molecular mechanisms involved in the final step, transendothelial migration, are poorly understood.

MEDIATORS OF INFLAMMATION

A variety of inflammatory mediators are released by cells of innate or acquired immunity during an inflammatory response. These mediators serve to trigger or enhance specific aspects of the inflammatory response. Inflammatory mediators are released by tissue mast cells, blood platelets, and a variety of leukocytes, including neutrophils, monocytes/macrophages, eosinophils, basophils, and lymphocytes.

Chemokines

Chemokines are a group of small polypeptides, containing 70–80 residues, that chemotactically attract different types of leukocytes and regulate the expression and conformation of integrins in leukocyte membranes. The chemokines possess four conserved cysteine residues and can be separated into two distinctive subgroups based on the position of two of the four invariant cysteine residues (Table 15-2):

- **C-C subgroup** chemokines, in which the conserved cysteines are contiguous, include macrophage chemotactic and activating factor (MCAF), RANTES, and macrophage inflammatory protein 1a and 1b (MIP-1a and MIP-1b).
- **C-X-C subgroup** chemokines, in which the conserved cysteines are separated by another amino acid, include IL-8, neutrophil-activating protein 2 (NAP-2), platelet factor 4 (PF-4), melanoma growth stimulatory activity (MGSA), and β-thromboglobulin (βTG).

The chemokines induce the adherence of various leukocytes to the vascular endothelium. Following migration of leukocytes into tissues, the cells are attracted toward high localized concentrations of chemokines. In humans, most C-X-C chemokines attract neutrophils but not monocytes, whereas C-C chemokines attract monocytes but not neutrophils.

One of the best characterized chemokines is IL-8. This chemokine is produced by a variety of cells including monocytes/macrophages, neutrophils, and endothelial cells. IL-8 is retained on inflamed endothelium,

T A B L E   1 5 - 2

SELECTED CHEMOKINES

CHEMOKINE	SECRETED BY	CHEMOTACTIC FOR
C-C SUBGROUP		
Macrophage chemotactic and activating factor (MCAF)	Monocytes Macrophages Fibroblasts	Monocytes Macrophages T cells
Macrophage inflammatory protein-1a (MIP-1a)	Monocytes Macrophages Neutrophils Endothelium	Monocytes Macrophages T cells B cells Basophil Eosinophil
Macrophage inflammatory protein-1b (MIP-1b)	Monocytes Macrophages Neutrophils Endothelium	Monocytes Macrophages Naive T cells B cells
RANTES	T cells Platelets	Monocytes Memory T cells Eosinophils Basophils
C-X-C SUBGROUP		
Interleukin 8 (IL-8)	Monocytes Macrophages Endothelium Fibroblasts Neutrophils	Neutrophils Basophils T cells
Neutrophil-activating protein (NAP-2)	Platelets	Neutrophils Basophils
Platelet factor 4 (PF-4)	Platelets	Neutrophils Fibroblasts

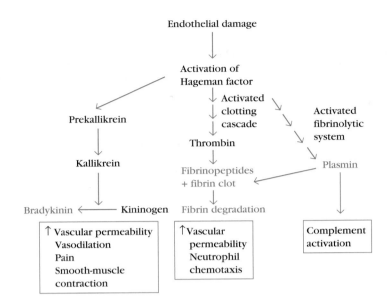

FIGURE 15-8

Tissue damage induces formation of plasma enzyme mediators by the kinin system, the clotting system, and the fibrinolytic system. These mediators cause vascular changes, among the earliest signs of inflammation, and various other effects. Plasmin not only degrades fibrin clots but also activates the classical complement pathway.

probably by binding to proteoglycan molecules on the inflamed endothelium or in the underlying extracellular matrix. As described earlier, binding of IL-8 to IL-8 receptors on neutrophils activates the integrin molecules on the neutrophil surface, allowing firm adhesion of neutrophils to the inflamed endothelium. Only after firm adhesion will neutrophils migrate between the endothelial cells, entering the tissue to participate in an inflammatory response (see Figure 15-3b).

Plasma Enzyme Mediators

Plasma contains four interconnected mediator-producing systems: the kinin system, the clotting system, the fibrinolytic system, and the complement system. With the exception of the complement system, these systems share a common intermediate as illustrated in Figure 15-8. When tissue damage occurs these four systems are activated to form a web of interacting systems that generate a number of mediators of inflammation.

KININ SYSTEM

The kinin system is an enzymatic cascade that begins when a plasma clotting factor, called Hageman factor, is activated following tissue injury. The activated Hageman factor then activates prekallikrein to form kallikrein, which cleaves kininogen to produce **bradykinin** (Figure 15-8). This inflammatory mediator is a potent vasoactive basic peptide that increases vascular permeability, causes vasodilation, induces pain, and induces contraction of smooth muscle. Kallikrein also acts directly on the complement system by cleaving C5 into C5a and C5b. The C5a complement component is an anaphylatoxin that

induces mast cell degranulation, resulting in the release of a number of inflammatory mediators from the mast cell.

CLOTTING SYSTEM

Another enzymatic cascade that is triggered following damage to blood vessel walls results in formation of large quantities of thrombin. Thrombin acts on soluble fibrinogen in tissue fluid or plasma to produce insoluble strands of **fibrin** and **fibrinopeptides**. The insoluble fibrin strands crisscross one another forming a **clot,** which serves as a barrier to the spread of infection. The clotting system is triggered very rapidly following tissue injury to prevent bleeding and limit spread of invading pathogens into the bloodstream. The fibrinopeptides act as inflammatory mediators inducing increased vascular permeability and neutrophil chemotaxis.

FIBRINOLYTIC SYSTEM

Removal of the fibrin clot from the injured tissue is achieved by the fibrinolytic system. The end product of this pathway is the enzyme **plasmin,** which is formed by the conversion of plasminogen into plasmin. Plasmin, a potent proteolytic enzyme, breaks down fibrin clots into degradation products that are chemotactic for neutrophils. Plasmin also contributes to the inflammatory response by activating the classical complement pathway.

COMPLEMENT SYSTEM

Activation of the complement system by both classical and alternative pathways results in the formation of a number of complement split products that serve as important mediators of inflammation. Binding of the **anaphylatoxins** (C3a, C4a, and C5a) to receptors on the membrane of tissue mast cells induces degranulation with release of histamine and other pharmacologically active mediators. These mediators induce smooth-muscle contraction and increases in vascular permeability. C3a, C5a, and C5b67 act together to induce monocytes and neutrophils to adhere to vascular endothelial cells, extravasate through the endothelial lining of the capillary, and migrate toward the site of complement activation in the tissues. Activation of the complement system thus results in influxes of fluid that carries antibody and phagocytic cells to the site of antigen entry. Other roles of complement products in the inflammatory response are listed in Table 14-7.

Lipid Inflammatory Mediators

Following membrane perturbations, phospholipids in the membrane of several cell types (e.g., macrophages, monocytes, neutrophils, and mast cells) are degraded into **arachidonic acid** and lyso–platelet-activating factor (Figure 15-9). The latter is subsequently converted into **platelet-activating factor** (PAF). This factor causes platelet activation and has many inflammatory effects, including eosinophil chemotaxis and the activation and degranulation of neutrophils and eosinophils.

Metabolism of arachidonic acid via the cyclooxygenase pathway produces **prostaglandins** and **thromboxanes**. Different prostaglandins are produced by different cells: monocytes and macrophages produce large quantities of PGE2 and PGF2; neutrophils produce moderate amounts of PGE2; mast cells produce PGD2. Prostaglandins have diverse biological activities, including increased vascular permeability, increased vascular dilation, and induction of neutrophil chemotaxis. The thromboxanes cause platelet aggregation and constriction of blood vessels.

Arachidonic acid is also metabolized via the lipoxygenase pathway to yield **leukotrienes**. There are four leukotrienes: LTB4, LTC4, LTD4, and LTE4. Three of these leukotrienes (LTC4, LTD4 and LTE4) together make up what was called **slow-reacting substance of anaphylaxis** (SRS-A); these mediators induce smooth muscle contraction. LTB4 is a potent chemoattractant of neutrophils. The leukotrienes are produced by a variety of cells including monocytes, macrophages, and mast cells.

Cytokine Inflammatory Mediators

A number of cytokines play a significant role in the development of an acute or chronic inflammatory response. IL-1, IL-6, and TNF-α exhibit a number of redundant and pleiotropic effects that together contribute to the inflammatory response. A number of these effects are listed in Table 15-3. In addition, IFN-γ contributes to the inflammatory response, acting later in the acute response and contributing in a major way to chronic inflammation by attracting and activating macrophages. The role of these inflammatory cytokines in the development of acute and chronic inflammation will be discussed more fully in the next section.

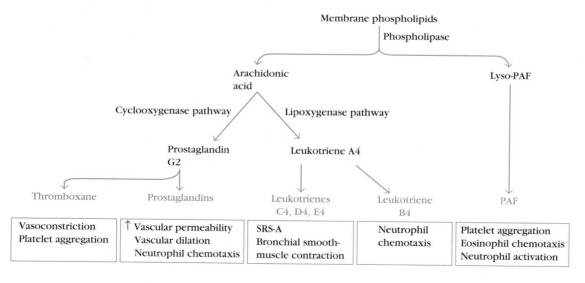

FIGURE 15-9

The breakdown of membrane phospholipids generates important mediators of inflammation, including thromboxane, prostaglandins, leukotrienes, and platelet-activating factor (PAF).

TABLE 15-3

REDUNDANT AND PLEIOTROPIC EFFECTS OF IL-1, TNF-α, AND IL-6

EFFECT	IL-1	TNF-α	IL-6
Endogenous pyrogen fever	+	+	+
Synthesis of acute-phase proteins by liver	+	+	+
Increased vascular permeability	+	+	+
Increased adhesion molecules on vascular endothelium	+	+	−
Fibroblast proliferation	+	+	−
Platelet production	+	−	+
Induction of IL-8	+	+	−
Induction of IL-6	+	+	−
T-cell activation	+	+	+
B-cell activation	+	+	+
Proliferation of Kaposi's sarcoma	+	−	+
Increased immunoglobulin synthesis	−	−	+

THE INFLAMMATORY PROCESS

Inflammation is a physiologic response to a variety of stimuli such as infections and tissue injury. In general, an acute inflammatory response exhibits rapid onset and is of short duration. Acute inflammation is generally accompanied by a systemic response, known as the acute-phase response, which is characterized by a rapid alteration in the levels of several plasma proteins. In some diseases persistent immune activation can result in chronic inflammation resulting in pathologic consequences.

Central Role of Neutrophils in Inflammation

In the early stages of an inflammatory response the predominant cell type infiltrating the tissue is the neutrophil. Neutrophil infiltration into the tissue peaks within the first 6 h of an inflammatory response. Neutrophil production in the bone marrow increases to meet this need. A normal adult produces 10^{11} neutrophils per day, but during a period of acute inflammation, neutrophil production increases tenfold.

The neutrophils leave the bone marrow and circulate within the blood. In response to mediators of acute inflammation, vascular endothelial cells increase their expression of E- and P-selectin. Thrombin and histamine induce increased expression of P-selectin; cytokines such as IL-1 or TNF-α induce increased expression of E-selectin. The circulating neutrophils express mucins such as PSGL-1 or the tetrasaccharides sialyl Lewis^a or sialyl Lewis^x, which bind to E- and P-selectin.

As described earlier, this binding mediates the attachment or tethering of neutrophils to the vascular endothelium, allowing the cells to roll in the direction of the blood flow. During this time chemoattractants, such as IL-8 or platelet-activating factor (PAF), act upon the neutrophils triggering a G-protein–mediated activating signal that leads to a conformational change in the integrin adhesion molecules, resulting in neutrophil adhesion and subsequent transendothelial migration (see Figure 15-3).

Once in tissues, the activated neutrophils also express increased levels of receptors for chemoattractants and therefore exhibit **chemotaxis**, migrating towards a gradient of the chemoattractant. Among the inflammatory mediators that are chemotactic for neutrophils are the chemokines (IL-8 and NAP-2), complement split products (C3a, C5a, and C5b67), fibrinopeptides, prostaglandins, and leukotrienes. In addition, molecules released by microorganisms, such as formyl methionyl peptides, are also chemotactic for neutrophils. In addition, activated neutrophils express increased levels of Fc receptors for antibody and receptors for complement. These receptors enable activated neutrophils to bind more effectively to antibody or complement-coated pathogens; this process, known as **opsonization,** increases phagocytic uptake by neutrophils.

The activating signal also stimulates metabolic pathways resulting in a respiratory burst, which leads to the production of **reactive oxygen intermediates** and **reactive nitrogen intermediates**. Release of some of these reactive intermediates and the release of mediators from neutrophil primary and secondary granules (proteases, phospholipases, elastases, and collagenases) play an important role in killing various pathogens. These substances also contribute to the tissue damage that can occur during an inflammatory response. The accumulation of dead cells and microorganisms, together with accumulated fluid and various proteins, makes up what is known as **pus.**

Acute Inflammatory Response

Infection or tissue injury induces a complex cascade of nonspecific events, known as the inflammatory response, that provides early protection by restricting the tissue damage to the site of infection or tissue injury. The acute inflammatory response involves both localized and systemic responses.

LOCALIZED RESPONSE

The hallmark signs of a localized acute inflammatory response, first described almost 2000 years ago, are swelling (*tumor*), redness (*rubor*), heat (*calor*), pain (*dolor*), and loss of function. Within minutes after tissue injury, there is an increase in vascular diameter (**vasodilation**), resulting in an increase in the volume of blood to the area and a reduction in the flow of blood. The increased blood volume causes heat and tissue redness. Vascular permeability also increases, leading to leakage of fluid from the blood vessels, particularly at postcapillary venules. This results in tissue **edema** and in some instances **extravasation** of leukocytes, contributing to the swelling and redness in the area. When fluid exudes from the bloodstream, the kinin, clotting, and fibrinolytic systems are activated (see Figure 15-8). Many of the vascular changes that occur early in a local response are due to the direct effects of plasma enzyme mediators like bradykinin and fibrinopeptides, which induce vasodilation and increased vascular permeability. Some of the vascular changes are due to the indirect effects of the complement anaphylatoxins (C3a, C4a and C5a), which induce local mast cell degranulation with release of histamine. Histamine is a potent mediator of inflammation, causing vasodilation and smooth-muscle contraction. The prostaglandins can also contribute to the vasodilation and increased vascular permeability associated with the acute inflammatory response.

Within a few hours of the onset of these vascular changes, neutrophils adhere to the endothelial cells, migrating out of the blood into the tissue spaces (Figure 15-10). These neutrophils phagocytose invading pathogens and release mediators that contribute to the inflammatory response. Among the mediators is macrophage inflammatory protein (MIP-1a and MIP-1b), a chemokine that attracts macrophages to the site of inflammation. Macrophages arrive about 5–6 hours after an inflammatory response begins. These macrophages are activated cells that exhibit increased phagocytosis and an increase in release of mediators and cytokines that contribute to the inflammatory response.

Activated tissue macrophages secrete three cytokines (IL-1, IL-6, and TNF-α) that induce many of the localized and systemic changes observed in the acute inflammatory response (see Table 15-3). All three cytokines act locally inducing coagulation and an increase in vascular permeability. Both TNF-α and IL-1 induce increased expression of adhesion molecules on vascular endothelial cells. For instance, TNF-α stimulates expression of E-selectin, an endothelial adhesion molecule that selectively binds neutrophils. IL-1 induces increased expression of ICAM-1 and VCAM-1, which bind to integrins on lymphocytes and monocytes. Circulating neutrophils, monocytes, and lymphocytes adhere to the wall of a blood vessel by recognizing these adhesion molecules and then move through the vessel wall into the tissue spaces. IL-1 and TNF-α also act on macrophages and endothelial cells inducing production of the chemokine IL-8. IL-8 contributes to the influx of neutrophils by increasing their adhesion to vascular endothelial cells and by acting as a potent chemotactic factor. Other cytokines also serve as chemotactic factors for various leukocyte populations. For instance, IFN-γ has been shown to chemotactically attract macrophages, bringing increased numbers of phagocytic cells to a site where antigen is localized. In addition, IFN-γ and TNF-α activate macrophages and neutrophils, promoting increased phagocytic activity and increased release of lytic enzymes into the tissue spaces.

A local acute inflammatory response can occur without the overt involvement of the immune system. Often, however, cytokines released at the site of inflammation facilitate both the adherence of immune-system cells to vascular endothelial cells and their migration through the vessel into the tissue spaces. The result is an influx of lymphocytes, neutrophils, monocytes, eosinophils, basophils, and mast cells to the site of tissue damage, where these cells participate in clearance of the antigen and healing of the tissue.

The duration and intensity of the local acute inflammatory response must be carefully regulated to control tissue damage and facilitate the tissue-repair mechanisms that are necessary for wound healing. TGF-β has been shown to play an important role in limiting the inflammatory response. It also promotes accumulation and proliferation of fibroblasts and the deposition of an extracellular matrix that is required for proper tissue repair.

SYSTEMIC ACUTE-PHASE RESPONSE

The local inflammatory response is accompanied by a systemic response known as the **acute-phase response** (Figure 15-11). This response is marked by the induction of fever, increased synthesis of hormones such as ACTH and hydrocortisone, increased production of white blood cells (leukocytosis), and production of a large number of

Visualizing Concepts

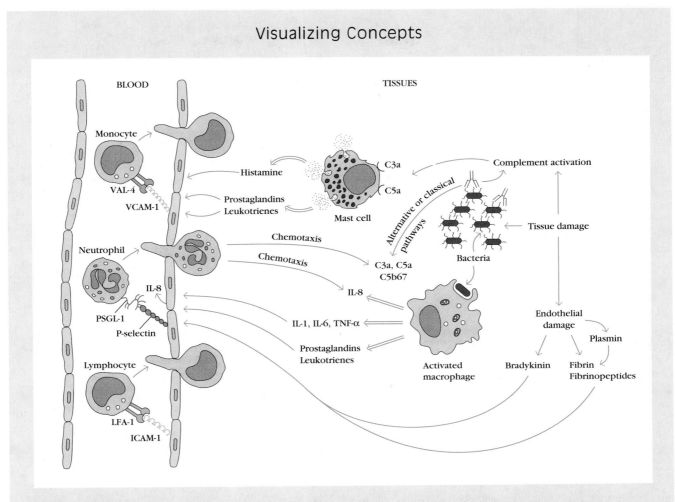

FIGURE 15-10

Overview of the cells and mediators involved in a local acute inflammatory response. Tissue damage leads to the formation of complement products that act as opsonins, anaphylatoxins, and chemotactic agents. Bradykinin and fibrinopeptides induced by endothelial damage mediate vascular changes. Neutrophils generally are the first leukocytes to migrate into the tissue, followed by monocytes and lymphocytes. Only some of the interactions involved in the extravasation of leukocytes are depicted.

acute-phase proteins in the liver. The increase in body temperature inhibits the growth of a number of pathogens and appears to enhance the immune response to the pathogen.

C-reactive protein is a prototype acute-phase protein whose serum level increases by 1000-fold during an acute-phase response. It is composed of five identical polypeptides held together by noncovalent interactions. C-reactive protein binds to a wide variety of microorganisms and activates complement, resulting in deposition of

the opsonin C3b on the surface of microorganisms. Phagocytic cells, which express C3b receptors, can then readily phagocytose the C3b-coated microorganisms (see Figure 14–11a).

Many systemic acute-phase effects are due to the combined action of IL-1, TNF-α, and IL-6 (see Figure 15-11). Each of these cytokines acts on the hypothalamus to induce a fever response. Within 12–24 h of the onset of an acute-phase inflammatory response, increased levels of IL-1, TNF-α, and IL-6 (as well as LIF and OSM)

Visualizing Concepts

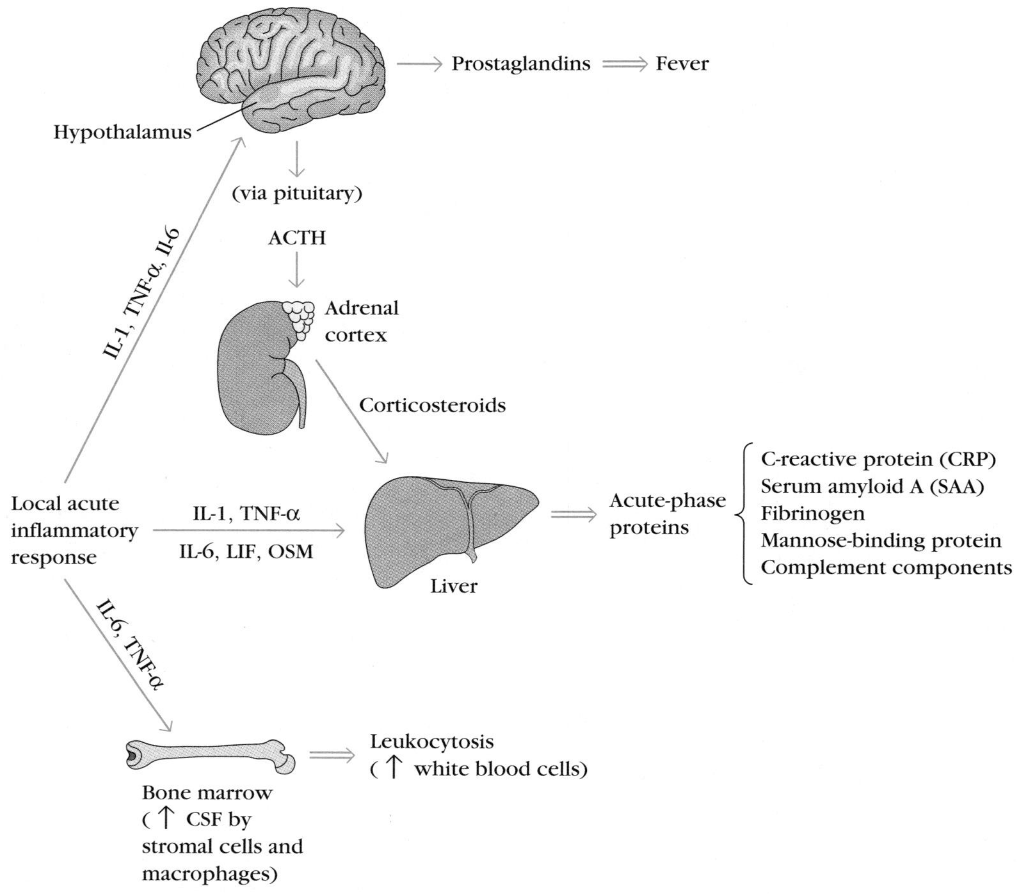

FIGURE 15-11

Overview of the organs and mediators involved in a systemic acute-phase response. IL-1, IL-6, and TNF-α, which are produced by activated macrophages at the site of inflammation, are particularly important in mediating acute-phase effects. LIF = leukemia inhibitory factor; OSM = oncostatin M.

induce production of acute-phase proteins by hepatocytes. TNF-α also acts on vascular endothelial cells and macrophages to induce secretion of colony-stimulating factors (M-CSF, G-CSF, and GM-CSF). These CSFs stimulate hematopoiesis, resulting in transient increases in the necessary white blood cells to fight the infection.

The redundancy in the ability of at least five cytokines (TNF-α, IL-1, IL-6, LIF, and OSM) to induce produc-

tion of acute-phase proteins by the liver results from the induction of a common transcription factor, NF-IL6, following interaction of each of these cytokines with its receptor. Amino acid sequencing of cloned NF-IL6 revealed that it has a high degree of sequence homology with C/EBP, a liver-specific transcription faction (Figure 15-12a). Both NF-IL6 and C/EBP contain a leucine-zipper domain and a basic DNA-binding domain, and

(a)

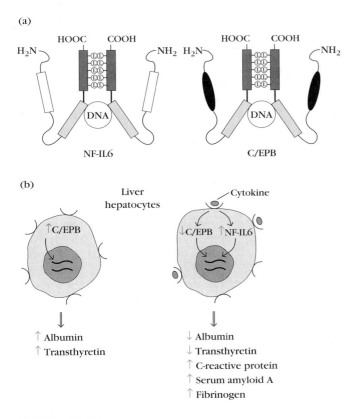

(b)

FIGURE 15-12

Comparison of the structure and function of C/EBP and NF-IL6. (a) Both transcription factors are dimeric proteins containing a leucine-zipper domain (dark gray) and a basic DNA-binding domain (blue). (b) C/EBP is expressed constitutively in liver hepatocytes and promotes transcription of albumin and transthyretin genes. During an inflammatory response, binding of IL-1, IL-6, TNF-α, LIF, or OSM to receptors on liver hepatocytes induces production of NF-IL6, which promotes transcription of the genes encoding various acute-phase proteins. Concurrently, C/EBP levels decrease and in turn the levels of albumin and transthyretin also decrease.

both proteins bind to the same nucleotide sequence in the promoter or enhancer of the genes encoding various liver proteins. C/EBP, which stimulates production of albumin and transthyretin, is expressed constitutively by liver hepatocytes. As an inflammatory response develops and the cytokines interact with their respective receptors on liver hepatocytes, expression of NF-IL6 increases and that of C/EBP decreases (Figure 15-12b). The inverse relationship between these two transcription factors accounts for the observation that serum levels of proteins such as albumin and transthyretin decline while those of acute-phase proteins increase during an inflammatory response.

Chronic Inflammatory Response

Chronic inflammation develops during persistence of an antigen. Some microorganisms, for example, have cell-wall components that enable them to resist phagocytosis. Such organisms often induce a chronic inflammatory response, resulting in significant tissue damage. Chronic inflammation also occurs in a number of autoimmune diseases in which self-antigens continually activate T cells. Finally, chronic inflammation also contributes to the tissue damage and wasting associated with many types of cancer.

The accumulation and activation of macrophages is the hallmark of chronic inflammation. Cytokines released by the chronically activated macrophages also stimulate fibroblast proliferation and collagen production. A type of scar tissue develops at sites of chronic inflammation, a process called **fibrosis**. Although fibrosis is a wound-healing reaction, it can interfere with normal tissue function. Chronic inflammation often leads to formation of a **granuloma**. This is a tumor-like mass consisting of a central area of activated macrophages surrounded by activated lymphocytes. The center of the granuloma often contains **multinucleated giant cells** formed by the fusion of activated macrophages. These giant cells typically are surrounded by large modified macrophages that resemble epithelial cells and therefore are called **epitheloid cells**. The development of a granuloma in delayed-type hypersensitivity is discussed more fully in Chapter 16.

ROLE OF IFN-γ AND TNF-α

Two cytokines in particular, IFN-γ and TNF-α, play a central role in the development of chronic inflammation. T_H1 cells, NK cells, and T_C cells release IFN-γ, while activated macrophages secrete TNF-α.

All three members of the interferon family of glycoproteins (IFN-α, IFN-β, and IFN-γ) are released from virus-infected cells and confer antiviral protection on neighboring cells. However, IFN-γ has a number of pleiotropic activities that distinguish it from IFN-α and IFN-β and contribute to the inflammatory response (Figure 15-13). One of the most striking effects of IFN-γ is its ability to activate macrophages. Activated macrophages exhibit increased expression of class II MHC molecules, increased cytokine production, and increased microbicidal activity, compared with nonactivated macrophages, and thus are more effective in antigen presentation and killing of intracellular microbial pathogens. In a chronic inflammatory response, the accumulation of large numbers of activated macrophages is responsible for much of the tissue damage. These cells release various

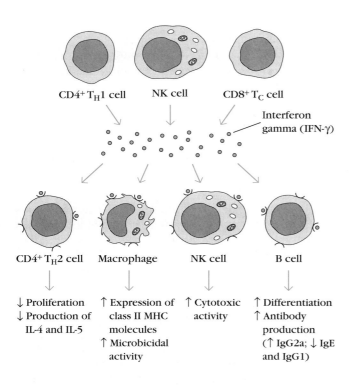

FIGURE 15-13

Summary of pleiotropic activity of interferon gamma (IFN-γ). The activation of macrophages induced by IFN-γ plays a critical role in chronic inflammation. This cytokine is secreted by T_H1 cells, NK cells, and T_C cells and acts on numerous cell types. [Adapted from Research News, 1993, *Science* **259**:1693.]

hydrolytic enzymes and reactive oxygen and nitrogen intermediates, resulting in damage to the surrounding tissue (see Tables 3-5 and 3-6).

One of the principal cytokines secreted by activated macrophages is TNF-α. The activity of this cytokine was first observed around the turn of the century by a surgeon, William Coley. He noted that when cancer patients developed certain bacterial infections, the tumors would become necrotic. In the hope of providing a cure for cancer, Coley began to inject cancer patients with supernatants derived from various bacterial cultures. These culture supernatants, called "Coley's toxins," induced hemorrhagic necrosis in the tumor but had numerous undesirable side-effects, making them unsuitable for cancer therapy. Decades later the active component of Coley's toxin was shown to be a lipopolysaccharide (endotoxin) component of the bacterial cell wall. This endotoxin does not itself induce tumor necrosis but instead induces macrophages to produce TNF-α. This cytokine has a direct cytotoxic effect on tumor cells but not on normal cells (Figure 15-14a). Potential immunotherapeutic approaches using TNF-α for the treatment of cancer are examined in Chapter 24.

Several lines of evidence indicate that TNF-α also contributes to much of the tissue wasting that characterizes chronic inflammation. For example, mice carrying a TNF-α transgene become severely wasted (Figure 15-14b). In studies by A. Cerami and coworkers rabbits were found to lose nearly half of their body mass within 2 months after being infected with trypanosomes. They

---

(a)   Treated   Untreated

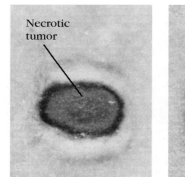
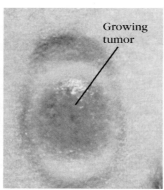

(b)

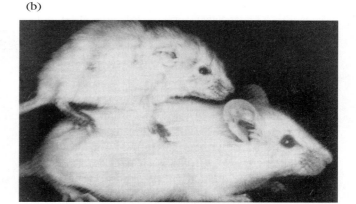

FIGURE 15-14

Biological activities of TNF-α. (a) A cancerous tumor in a mouse injected with endotoxin (*left*) shows hemorrhagic necrosis compared with a tumor in an untreated mouse (*right*). Endotoxin induces the production of TNF-α, which then acts to destroy the tumor.

(b) Transgenic mouse (*top*) bearing a TNF-α transgene becomes anorectic and severely wasted. Normal mouse is shown on the bottom. [Part (a) from L. J. Old, 1988, *Sci. Am.* **258**:59; part (b) from B. Beutler, 1993, *Hosp. Prac.* (April 15):45.]

subsequently discovered that a macrophage-derived factor was responsible for the profound wasting and called the factor **cachetin**. Cloning of the genes for TNF-α and cachetin revealed that they were the same protein.

Activation of macrophages by IFN-γ promotes increased transcription of the TNF-α gene and increases the stability of TNF-α mRNA. Both effects result in increased TNF-α production. TNF-α acts synergistically with IFN-γ to initiate a chronic inflammatory response. Both cytokines together induce much greater increases in ICAM-1, E-selectin, and class I MHC molecules than either cytokine alone. The increase in intercellular adhesion molecules facilitates the recruitment of large numbers of cells in a chronic inflammatory response.

CHRONIC INFLAMMATORY DISEASES

Recent studies suggest that regions of plump endothelial cells resembling HEVs appear along the vasculature in tertiary extralymphoid sites of chronic infection. These HEV-like regions, which appear to be sites of lymphocyte extravasation into the inflamed tissue, express several mucins (e.g., GlyCAM-1, MAdCAM-1, and CD34) that are often displayed on normal HEVs. Several cytokines, notably IFN-γ and TNF-α, that are associated with chronic inflammation may play a role in the induction of HEV-like regions along the vasculature.

These HEV-like regions have been observed in a number of chronic inflammatory diseases in humans, including rheumatoid arthritis, Crohn's disease, ulcerative colitis, Graves' disease, Hashimoto's thyroiditis, and diabetes mellitus (Table 15-4). Development of this HEV-like vasculature is likely to facilitate a large-scale influx of leukocytes contributing to chronic inflammation. These observations suggest that a potentially effective approach for treating chronic inflammatory diseases may be to try to control the development of these HEV-like regions.

ANTI-INFLAMMATORY AGENTS

Although development of an effective inflammatory response can play an important role in the body's defense, the response can sometimes be detrimental. Allergies, autoimmune diseases, microbial infections, transplants, and burns may be accompanied by a chronic inflammatory response. Various therapeutic approaches are available for reducing long-term inflammatory responses and thus the complications associated with them.

Agents That Reduce Leukocyte Extravasation

Because leukocyte extravasation is an integral part of the inflammatory response, one approach for reducing inflammation is to impede this process. Theoretically, one way to reduce leukocyte extravasation is to block the activity of various adhesion molecules with antibodies. In animal models, for example, antibodies to the integrin LFA-1 have been used to reduce neutrophil buildup in inflammatory tissue. Antibodies to ICAM-1 have also been used, with some success, in preventing the tissue necrosis associated with burns and in reducing the likelihood of kidney-graft rejection in animal models. The results with antibodies specific for ICAM-1 have been so

TABLE 15-4

CHRONIC INFLAMMATORY DISEASES ASSOCIATED WITH HEV-LIKE VASCULATURE

DISEASE	AFFECTED ORGAN	PLUMP ENDOTHELIUM	MUCIN-LIKE CAMS ON ENDOTHELIUM*
Crohn's disease	Gut	+	+
Diabetes mellitus	Pancreas	+	+
Graves' disease	Thyroid	+	+
Hashimoto's thyroiditis	Thyroid	+	+
Rheumatoid arthritis	Synovium	+	+
Ulcerative colitis	Gut	+	+

* Includes GlyCAM-1, MAdCAM-1, and CD34.

SOURCE: Adapted from J. P. Girard and T. A. Springer, 1995, *Immunol. Today* **16**:449.

encouraging that this antibody is now being tested in clinical trials on human kidney-transplant patients.

Corticosteroids

The corticosteroids, which are cholesterol derivatives, include prednisone, prednisolone, and methylprednisolone. These potent anti-inflammatory agents exert various effects that result in a reduction in the numbers and activity of immune-system cells.

Corticosteroid treatment causes a decrease in the number of circulating lymphocytes as the result either of steroid-induced lysis of lymphocytes (lympholysis) or of alterations in lymphocyte-circulation patterns. Some species (e.g., hamster, mouse, rat, and rabbit) are particularly sensitive to corticosteroid-induced lympholysis. In these animals corticosteroid treatment at dosages as low as 10^{-7} M causes such widespread lympholysis that the weight of the thymus is reduced by 90%; the spleen and lymph nodes also shrink visibly (see Figure 3-19 for structure of lymphatic vessels). Immature thymocytes in these species appear to be particularly sensitive to corticosteroid-mediated killing. In rodents, corticosteroids induce programmed cell death in immature thymocytes, whereas mature thymocytes are resistant to this activity. Within 2 h following in vitro incubation with corticosteroids, immature thymocytes begin to show the characteristic morphology of apoptosis, and 90% of the chromatin is degraded into the characteristic nucleosome ladder by 24 h after treatment. The steps involved in the induction of apoptosis by corticosteroids remain to be determined. In humans, guinea pigs, and monkeys, corticosteroids do not induce apoptosis but instead affect lymphocyte-circulation patterns, causing a decrease in thymic weight and a marked decrease in the number of circulating lymphocytes.

Like other steroid hormones, the corticosteroids are lipophilic and thus can cross the plasma membrane and bind to receptors in the cytosol. The resulting receptor-hormone complexes are subsequently transported to the nucleus where they bind to specific regulatory DNA sequences, either up-regulating or down-regulating transcription. The corticosteroids have been shown to induce increased transcription of the NF-κB inhibitor (IκB). Binding of this inhibitor to NF-κB in the cytosol prevents the translocation of NF-κB into the nucleus and consequently prevents NF-κB activation of a number of genes, including genes involved in T-cell activation and cytokine production (see Figure 12-12).

Corticosteroids also reduce both the phagocytic and killing ability of macrophages and neutrophils, and this effect may contribute to their anti-inflammatory action. In addition, they reduce chemotaxis, so that fewer inflammatory cells are attracted to the site of T_H-cell activation. In the presence of corticosteroids, expression of class II MHC molecules and IL-1 production by macrophages is dramatically reduced; such reductions would be expected to lead to corresponding reductions in T_H-cell activation. Corticosteroids also stabilize the lysosomal membrane, so that decreased levels of lysosomal enzymes are released at the site of inflammation.

Nonsteroidal Anti-Inflammatory Drugs

Since the time of Hippocrates extracts of willow bark have been used for relief of pain. The active ingredient, salicylate, which is found in aspirin, is just one of many nonsteroidal anti-inflammatory drugs (NSAIDs). NSAIDs are the most frequently used medication for treating pain and inflammation. One mechanism by which these drugs exert anti-inflammatory effects is by inhibiting the cyclooxygenase pathway by which prostaglandins and thromboxanes are produced from arachidonic acid (see Figure 15-9). The reduction in prostaglandin production limits the increase in vascular permeability and neutrophil chemotaxis in the inflammatory response. Clinically, NSAIDs have been shown to be effective for treatment of many acute and chronic inflammatory reactions.

SUMMARY

1. Lymphocytes undergo constant recirculation between the blood, lymph, lymphoid organs, and tertiary extralymphoid tissues (see Figure 15-1). This extensive recirculation greatly increases the chances of the small number of lymphocytes specific for a given antigen (about 1 in 10^5 cells) actually encountering that antigen when it is present in the body. Although the tertiary extralymphoid tissues normally contain few lymphoid cells, migration of lymphoid cells into these sites occurs during the inflammatory response.

2. Migration of leukocytes into inflamed tissue or lymphoid organs requires interaction between cell-adhesion molecules (CAMs) on the vascular endothelium and those on the circulating cells. Most of these CAMs fall into one of four protein families: the selectins, mucin-like family, integrins, or Ig superfamily (see Figure 15-2). Selectins and mucin-like CAMs interact with each other, and members of each family are expressed on both leukocytes and endothelial cells. Integrins, expressed on leukocytes, interact with Ig-superfamily CAMs, expressed on endothelial cells.

3. Neutrophils are generally the first cell type to move from the bloodstream into inflammatory sites. Extravasation of both neutrophils and lymphocytes involves four steps: rolling, chemoattractant-activating signal,

arrest and adhesion, and transendothelial migration (see Figures 15-3 and 15-7). Unlike neutrophils, various lymphocyte populations exhibit differential extravasation into various tissues. Homing receptors on lymphocytes interact with tissue-specific adhesion molecules, called vascular addressins, on high-endothelial venules (HEVs) in lymphoid organs and on the endothelum in tertiary extralymphoid tissues (see Table 15-1). Naive lymphocytes home to secondary lymphoid organs, extravasating across HEVs, whereas effector lymphocytes selectively home to inflamed vascular endothelium (see Figure 15-5).

4. Several types of mediators play a role in the inflammatory response. Chemokines are a group of small polypeptides that act as chemoattractant and activating molecules during leukocyte extravasation (see Table 15-2). Plasma enzyme mediators include bradykinin and fibrinopeptides, which increase vascular permeability; plasmin, a proteolytic enzyme that degrades fibrin clots into chemotactic products and activates complement; and various complement products that act as anaphylatoxins, opsonins, and chemotactic molecules for neutrophils and monocytes (see Figure 15-8). Lipid inflammatory mediators, derived from membrane phospholipids, include thromboxanes, prostaglandins, leukotrienes, and platelet-activating factor (see Figure 15-9). Three cytokines, IL-1, IL-6, and TNF-α, mediate many of the local and systemic features of the acute inflammatory response (see Table 15-3).

5. Inflammation is a physiologic response to a variety of stimuli such as tissue injury and infection. An acute inflammatory response involves both localized and systemic effects. The localized response begins when tissue and endothelial damage induces formation of plasma enzyme mediators that lead to vasodilation and increased vascular permeability (see Figure 15-10). Neutrophils and then monocytes extravasate into the site. Activation of tissue macrophages and degranulation of mast cells lead to release of numerous inflammatory mediators, some of which induce systemic acute-phase effects. The systemic response includes induction of fever, leukocytosis, and production of corticosteroids and acute-phase proteins, including C-reactive protein (see Figure 15-11).

6. Chronic inflammation results from persistence of antigen due to infection with certain resistant microorganisms or various pathologic conditions. Two cytokines, IFN-γ and TNF-α, are central to the chronic inflammatory response, which often involves granuloma formation and tissue wasting. Several human chronic inflammatory diseases are marked by the presence of an HEV-like vasculature in particular organs (see Table 15-4).

7. A chronic inflammatory response may accompany allergies, autoimmune diseases, microbial infections, transplants, and burns. Antibodies to cell-adhesion molecules involved in leukocyte extravasation have shown promise in reducing chronic inflammation associated with burns and graft rejection. Corticosteroids have numerous effects that contribute to their anti-inflammatory action. A variety of nonsteroidal anti-inflammatory drugs (NSAIDs) are available and are the most commonly used medications for pain and inflammation.

REFERENCES

AGREE, A. 1994. Lymphocyte recirculation and homing: roles of adhesion molecules and chemoattractants. *Trends Cell Biol.* **4**:326.

AHUJA, S. K., J. L. GAO, AND P. M. MURPHY. 1994. Chemokine receptors and molecular mimicry. *Immunol. Today* **15**:281.

BARGATZE, R. F., M. A. JUTILA, AND E. C. BUTCHER. 1995. Distinct roles of L-selectin and integrins $\alpha 4\beta 7$ and LFA-1 in lymphocyte homing to Peyer's patch-HEV in situ: the multistep model confirmed and refined. *Immunity* **3**:99.

BAUMANN, H., AND J. GAULDIE. 1994. The acute response. *Immunol. Today* **15**:74.

BRADLEY, L. M., AND S. R. WATSON. 1996. Lymphocyte migration into tissue: the paradigm derived from CD4 subsets. *Curr. Opin. Immunol.* **8**:312.

DIANZANI, U., AND F. MALAVASI. 1995. Lymphocyte adhesion to endothelium. *Crit. Rev. Immunol.* **15**:167.

GIRARD, J. P., AND T. A. SPRINGER. 1995. High endothelial venules (HEVs): specialized endothelium for lymphocyte migration. *Immunol. Today* **16**:449.

HOGG, N., AND C. BERLIN. 1995. Structure and function of adhesion receptors in leukocyte trafficking. *Immunol. Today* **16**.

HYNES, R. O. 1994. The impact of molecular biology on models for cell adhesion. *Bioessays* **16**:663.

HYNES, R. O., AND A. D. LANDER. 1992. Contact and adhesive specificities in the associations, migrations, and targeting of cells and axons. *Cell* **68**:303.

MARX, J. 1995. How the glucocorticoids suppress immunity. *Science* **270**:232.

PICKER, L. J. 1994. Control of lymphocyte homing. *Curr. Opin. Immunol.* **6**:394.

PICKER, L. J., AND E. C. BUTCHER. 1992. Physiological and molecular mechanisms of lymphocyte homing. *Annu. Rev. Immunol.* **10**:561.

SPRINGER, T. A. 1994. Traffic signals for lymphocyte recirculation and leukocyte emigration: the multi-step paradigm. *Cell* **76**:301.

STEEL, D. M., AND A. S. WHITEHEAD. 1994. The major acute phase reactants: C-reactive protein, serum amyloid P component and serum amyloid A protein. *Immunol. Today* **15**:81.

STUDY QUESTIONS

1. Indicate whether each of the following statements is true or false. If you think a statement is false, explain why.

a. Chemokines are chemoattractants for lymphocytes but not other leukocytes.

b. Integrins are expressed on both leukocytes and endothelial cells.

c. Leukocyte extravasation involves multiple interactions between cell-adhesion molecules.

d. Most secondary lymphoid organs contain high-endothelial venules (HEVs).

e. Mucin-like CAMs interact with selectins.

f. An acute inflammatory response only involves localized effects in the region of tissue injury or infection.

g. MAdCAM-1 is an endothelial adhesion molecule that binds to L-selectin and to several integrins.

h. Granuloma formation is a common symptom of local inflammation.

2. Various inflammatory mediators induce expression of ICAMs on a wide variety of tissues. What effect might this induction have on the localization of immune cells?

3. Extravasation of neutrophils and lymphocytes occur by generally similar mechanisms, although some differences distinguish the two processes.

a. List in order the four basic steps in leukocyte extravasation.

b. At what sites are neutrophils most likely to extravasate? Why?

c. Different lymphocyte subpopulations preferentially migrate into different tissues, a process called homing (or trafficking). Discuss the roles of the three types of molecules that permit homing of lymphocytes.

4. Which three cytokines secreted by activated macrophages play a major role in mediating the localized and systemic effects associated with an acute inflammatory response?

5. An effective inflammatory response requires differentiation and proliferation of various nonlymphoid white blood cells. Explain how hematopoiesis in the bone marrow is induced by tissue injury or local infection.

6. For each pair of molecules listed below, indicate whether the molecules interact during the 1st, 2nd, 3rd, or 4th step in neutrophil extravasation at an inflammatory site. Use N to indicate any molecules that do not interact.

a. _____ Chemokine and L-selectin
b. _____ E-selectin and mucin-like CAM
c. _____ IL-8 and E-selectin
d. _____ Ig-superfamily CAM and integrin
e. _____ ICAM and chemokine
f. _____ Chemokine and G-protein–coupled receptor
g. _____ ICAM and integrin

7. Discuss the main effects of IFN-γ and TNF-α during a chronic inflammatory response.

8. Five cytokines (IL-1, IL-6, TNF-α, LIF, and OSM) induce production of C-reactive protein and other acute-phase proteins by hepatocytes. Briefly explain how these different cytokines can exert the same effect on hepatocytes.

9. For each inflammation-related term (a–h), select the descriptions listed below (1–11) that apply. Each description may be used once, more than once, or not at all; more than one description may apply to some terms.

Terms:

a. _____ Tertiary extralymphoid tissue
b. _____ P- and E-selectin
c. _____ Prostaglandins
d. _____ Nonsteroidal anti-inflammatory drugs
e. _____ ICAM-1, -2, -3
f. _____ MAdCAM
g. _____ Bradykinin
h. _____ Inflamed endothelium

Descriptions:

1) Bind to sialylated carbohydrate moieties
2) Inhibit cyclooxygenase pathway
3) Induce expression of NK-$\kappa\beta$ inhibitor
4) Has both Ig domains and mucin-like domains
5) Region of vascular endothelium found in postcapillary venules
6) Expressed by inflamed endothelium
7) Exhibits HEV-like vasculature in chronic inflammation
8) Belong to Ig-superfamily of CAMs
9) Exhibits increased expression of CAMs
10) Increase vascular permeability and induce fever
11) Induce fever

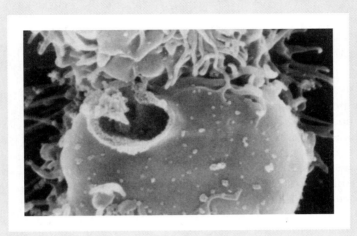

CELL-MEDIATED AND
HUMORAL EFFECTOR RESPONSES

The cell-mediated and humoral branches of the immune system serve different functions and involve different effector mechanisms for generating immunity. The effectors of the humoral branch are secreted antibodies, which can neutralize soluble antigens. Binding of antibodies to surface antigens on microorganisms also can activate the complement system, leading to lysis of the invaders, opsonization, and viral neutralization. The primary effectors in the cell–mediated branch are various effector cells, although antibody sometimes plays a secondary role. Both antigen-specific and nonspecific cells contribute to the cell-mediated immune response. Specific cells include cytokine-secreting CD4$^+$ T$_H$1 and T$_H$2 cells and CD8$^+$ T cytotoxic lymphocytes (CTLs); nonspecific cells include macrophages, neutrophils, eosinophils, and natural killer cells. The activity of both specific and nonspecific components is dependent on high localized concentrations of various cytokines. Unlike the humoral branch of the immune system, which serves mainly to eliminate extracellular bacteria and bacterial products, the cell-mediated branch is responsible for the clearance of intracellular pathogens, virus-infected cells, tumor cells, and foreign grafts. The system is adapted to recognizing altered self-cells and eliminating them from the body.

In previous chapters various aspects of the humoral and cell-mediated effector responses have been discussed: antigen–antibody interactions (Chapter 5); the complement system (Chapter 14); functions of cytokine-secreting CD4$^+$ T$_H$1 and T$_H$2 cells (Chapter 13); and the inflammatory response (Chapter 15). This chapter focuses on specific and nonspecific cytotoxic effector mechanisms, the delayed-type hypersensitivity (DTH) response mediated by effector T$_H$ cells, the characteristics of the primary and secondary humoral response, experimental assays of cytotoxic and humoral responses, and regulation of immune effector responses.

EFFECTOR RESPONSES IN THE CELL-MEDIATED BRANCH

The importance of cell-mediated immunity becomes evident when the system is defective. Children with Di-George syndrome, who are born without a thymus and therefore lack the T-cell component of the cell-mediated immune system, generally are able to cope with infections of extracellular bacteria, but they cannot effectively eliminate intracellular pathogens. Their lack of functional cell-mediated immunity results in repeated infections with viruses, intracellular bacteria, and fungi. The severity of the cell-mediated immunodeficiency in these children is such that even attenuated vaccines, capable of only limited growth in normal individuals, can produce life-threatening infections.

Cell-mediated immune responses can be divided into two major categories involving different effector populations. One group involves effector cells having direct cytotoxic activity. The second group involves a subpopulation of effector $CD4^+$ T cells that mediate delayed-type hypersensitivity reactions. Before the details of these responses are described, the general properties of effector T cells and their differences from naive T cells are reviewed.

General Properties of Effector T Cells

The three types of effector T cells—$CD4^+$ T_H1 and T_H2 cells and $CD8^+$ CTLs—exhibit several properties that set them apart from naive T_H and T_C cells (Table 16-1). In particular, effector cells are characterized by their less stringent activation requirements, increased expression of cell-adhesion molecules, and production of both membrane-bound and soluble effector molecules.

ACTIVATION REQUIREMENTS

T cells at different stages of differentiation may respond with different efficiencies to signal 1 mediated by the T-cell receptor and may consequently require different levels of the co-stimulatory signal 2. As discussed in Chapter 12, activation of naive T cells and their subsequent proliferation and differentiation into effector T cells requires both signal 1, delivered by interaction of the TCR complex and CD4 or CD8 coreceptor with a foreign peptide–MHC molecule complex, and the co-stimulatory signal 2, delivered by the antigen-presenting cell (see Figure 12-17). In contrast, antigen-experienced effector cells (as well as memory cells) are able to respond to signal 1 with little, if any, signal 2.

One reason for this difference in the activation requirements is that naive and effector T cells express different isoforms of CD45, designated CD45RA and CD45RO. This membrane molecule has phosphatase activity and is involved in signal 1 transduction by catalyzing dephosphorylation of a tyrosine residue on the protein tyrosine kinases Lck and Fyn (see Figure 12-11). The different isoforms of CD45 are produced by alternative splicing of the RNA transcript of the CD45 gene. The CD45RO isoform, expressed on effector T cells, associates better with the CD4 and CD8 coreceptors than does the CD45RA isoform, expressed by naive T cells. As a result, effector T cells are more sensitive to signal 1 activation by a peptide-MHC complex. They also have less stringent requirements for the co-stimulatory signal 2 and therefore are able to respond to peptide-MHC complexes displayed on target cells or antigen-presenting cells that lack the co-stimulatory B7 molecule (see Figure 12-18).

CELL-ADHESION MOLECULES

Compared with naive T cells, effector T cells also express higher densities of several cell-adhesion molecules,

---

T A B L E   1 6 - 1

COMPARISON OF NAIVE AND EFFECTOR T CELLS

PROPERTY	NAIVE T CELLS	EFFECTOR T CELLS
Co-stimulatory signal (CD28-B7 interaction)	Required for activation	Not required for activation
CD45 isoform	CD45RA	CD45RO
Cell-adhesion molecules (CD2 and LFA-1)	Low	High
Trafficking patterns	HEVs in secondary lymphoid tissue	Tertiary lymphoid tissues; inflammatory sites

including CD2 and the integrin LFA-1, which bind, respectively, to LFA-3 and ICAMs, on antigen-presenting cells and various target cells. The level of LFA-1 and CD2 is twofold to fourfold higher on effector T cells than on naive T cells, enabling the effector T cells to bind more effectively to antigen-presenting cells and to various target cells that express low levels of ICAMs or LFA-3.

The initial interaction of an effector T cell with an antigen-presenting cell or target cell is weak, allowing the TCR to scan the membrane for specific peptides presented by self-MHC molecules. If no peptide–MHC molecule complex recognized by the effector cell is present, then the effector cell will disengage from the APC or target cell. Recognition of a peptide-MHC complex by the TCR, however, provides a signal that increases the affinity of LFA-1 for ICAMs on the APC or target-cell membrane, prolonging the interaction between the cells. For example, T_H1 effector cells will remain bound to macrophages displaying peptide–class II MHC complexes; T_H2 effector cells will remain bound to specific B cells displaying peptide–class II MHC complexes; CTL effector cells will remain bound to virus-infected target cells displaying peptide–class I MHC complexes.

As discussed in Chapter 15, effector T cells display different trafficking patterns from naive T cells. Naive T cells express high levels of the homing receptor L-selectin, which binds to the vascular addressins GlyCAM-1 and CD34 present on high-endothelial venules (HEVs) of secondary lymphoid tissue. Effector T cells express increased levels of homing receptors CLA, LPAM-1, and LFA-1, allowing the effector cells to enter tertiary lymphoid tissue (such as skin and mucosal epithelia) and sites of inflammation in addition to secondary lymphoid tissue (see Table 15-1).

EFFECTOR MOLECULES

Unlike naive T cells, effector T cells express certain effector molecules, which may be membrane bound or soluble (Table 16-2). The membrane-bound molecules belong to the tumor necrosis factor (TNF) family of membrane proteins and include the Fas ligand (FAS) on $CD8^+$ CTLs, TNF-β on T_H1 cells, and the CD40 ligand on T_H2 cells. Each of the effector T-cell populations also secretes distinct panels of effector molecules. CTLs secrete cytotoxins (perforins and granzymes) as well as two cytokines, IFN-γ and TNF-β. As discussed in Chapter 13, the T_H1 and T_H2 subsets secrete largely nonoverlapping sets of cytokines.

Each of these membrane-bound and secreted molecules plays an important role in various T-cell effector functions. The Fas ligand, perforins, and granzymes, for example, mediate target-cell destruction by the CTL; membrane-bound TNF-β and soluble IFN-γ and GM-CSF promote macrophage activation by the T_H1 cell; and the membrane-bound CD40 ligand and soluble IL-4, IL-5, and IL-6 all play a role in B-cell activation by the T_H2 cell.

Direct Cytotoxic Responses

One way the immune system eliminates foreign cells and altered self-cells is to mount a cytotoxic reaction that results in lysis of target cells. The various cell-mediated cytotoxic effector mechanisms can be subdivided into two general categories: those involving antigen-specific cytotoxic T lymphocytes (CTLs) and those involving nonspecific cells, such as natural killer (NK) cells and macrophages. The target cells to which these effector mechanisms are directed include allogeneic cells, malignant cells, virus-infected cells, and chemically conjugated cells.

CTL-MEDIATED CYTOTOXICITY

Cytotoxic T lymphocytes, or CTLs, are generated by immune activation of T cytotoxic (T_C) cells. These effector cells have lytic capability and play critical roles in the recognition and elimination of altered self-cells (e.g., virus-infected cells and tumor cells) and in graft-rejection

TABLE 16-2

EFFECTOR MOLECULES PRODUCED BY EFFECTOR T CELLS

CELL TYPE	SOLUBLE EFFECTORS	MEMBRANE-BOUND EFFECTORS
CTL	Cytotoxins (perforins and granzymes), IFN-γ, TNF-β	Fas ligand (FAS)
T_H1	IL-2, IL-3, TNF-β, IFN-γ, GM-CSF (high)	Tumor necrosis factor β (TNF-β)
T_H2	IL-3, IL-4, IL-5, IL-6, IL-10, IL-13, GM-CSF (low)	CD40 ligand

reactions. In general, CTLs are $CD8^+$ and are therefore class I MHC restricted, although in rare instances $CD4^+$ class II–restricted T cells have been shown to function as CTLs. Since virtually all nucleated cells in the body express class I MHC molecules, CTLs can recognize and eliminate almost any altered body cell.

The CTL-mediated immune response can be divided into two phases, reflecting different aspects of the cytotoxic T-cell response. The first phase involves the activation and differentiation of naive T_C cells into functional effector CTLs. In the second phase, effector CTLs recognize antigen–class I MHC complexes on specific target cells, initiating a sequence of events that culminates in target-cell destruction.

Phase 1: Generation of CTLs Naive T_C cells are incapable of killing target cells and are therefore referred to as **CTL precursors** (CTL-Ps) to denote their functionally immature state. Only after a CTL-P has been activated will the cell differentiate into a functional CTL possessing cytotoxic activity. Generation of CTLs from CTL-Ps appears to require at least three sequential signals:

- An antigen-specific signal 1 transmitted by the TCR complex upon recognition of a peptide–MHC molecule complex
- A co-stimulatory signal transmitted by the CD28-B7 interaction
- A signal induced by the interaction of IL-2 with the high-affinity IL-2 receptor, resulting in proliferation and differentiation of the antigen-activated CTL-P into an effector CTL

Unactivated CTL-Ps do not express IL-2 or IL-2 receptors, do not proliferate, and do not display cytotoxic activity (Figure 16-1). Antigen activation induces a CTL-P to begin expressing the IL-2 receptor and to a lesser extent IL-2, the principal cytokine required for proliferation and differentiation of activated CTL-Ps into effector CTLs. In some cases, the amount of IL-2 secreted by an antigen-activated CTL-P may be sufficient to induce its own proliferation and differentiation; this is particularly true of memory CTL-Ps, which have lower activation requirements than naive cells (Figure 16-2a). In general, though, most activated CTL-Ps require additional IL-2 produced by proliferating T_H1 cells to proliferate and differentiate into effector CTLs. The fact that the IL-2 receptor is not expressed until after a CTL-P has been activated by antigen plus a class I MHC molecule ensures that only antigen-specific CTL-Ps are clonally expanded by IL-2 and acquire cytotoxicity.

The proliferation and differentiation of both antigen-activated T_H cells and CTL-Ps are dependent on IL-2.

In IL-2 knockout mice the absence of IL-2 has been shown to abolish CTL-mediated cytotoxicity. Following antigen clearance, the levels of IL-2 decline. This decline in IL-2 induces T_H1 cells and CTLs to undergo programmed cell death by apoptosis. In this way the immune response is rapidly terminated, lessening the likelihood of nonspecific tissue damage from the inflammatory response.

The role of T_H1 cells in the generation of CTLs from naive CTL-Ps is not completely understood. It is unlikely that a T_H1 cell and CTL-P interact directly. Some have suggested that activation and differentiation of both T_H and CTL-P populations occur at sites of organized lymphoid tissue such as regional lymph nodes. In a primary response to a virus, for example, naive T cells are unable to respond to the virus except in organized lymphoid tissues. Within organized lymphoid tissues, T_H1 cells and CTL-Ps may interact with common antigen-presenting cells (e.g., interdigitating dendritic cells) that have internalized and processed the virus in the endocytic pathway (Figure 16-2b). Such APCs would present antigenic viral peptides associated with both class I and class II MHC molecules and thus would be recognized by both $CD4^+$ and $CD8^+$ T cells. Another possibility is that organized lymphoid tissue forms an anatomic niche rich in cytokines, providing an ideal milieu for CTL-P activation.

Phase 2: Destruction of Target Cells The effector phase of a CTL-mediated response involves a carefully orchestrated sequence of events culminating in target-cell destruction by CTLs (Figure 16-3). Long-term cultures of CTL clones have been used to identify many of the membrane molecules and membrane events involved in this process. These studies have revealed that two major pathways are responsible for CTL-mediated destruction of target cells:

- Directional delivery of cytotoxic proteins (including perforin and granzymes) released from CTLs and taken up by target cells
- Interaction of the membrane-bound Fas ligand on CTLs with the Fas receptor on the surface of target cells

Recent evidence suggests that apoptosis is the primary mechanism of target-cell destruction in both pathways.

The primary events in the pathway involving the release of cytotoxic proteins are conjugate formation, membrane attack, CTL dissociation, and target-cell destruction (Figure 16-4). When antigen-specific CTLs are incubated with appropriate target cells, the two cell types interact and undergo conjugate formation.

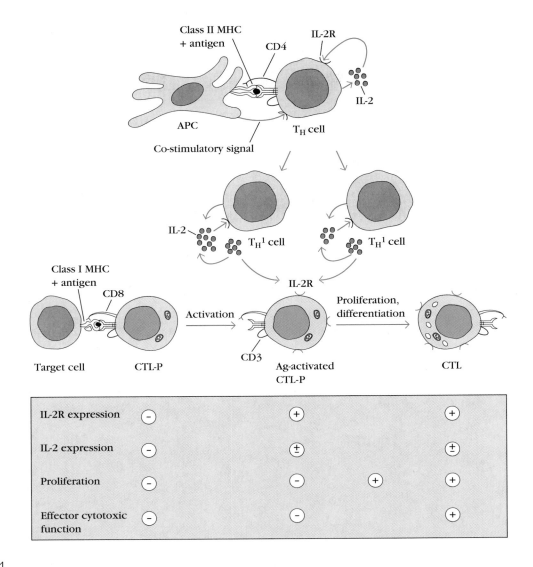

FIGURE 16-1

Generation of effector CTLs. Upon interaction with antigen–class I MHC complexes on appropriate target cells, CTL-Ps begin to express IL-2 receptors (IL-2R) and lesser amounts of IL-2. Proliferation and differentiation of antigen-activated CTL-Ps generally require additional IL-2 secreted by T_H1 cells resulting from antigen activation and proliferation of CD4+ T_H cells. In the subsequent effector phase, CTLs destroy specific target cells.

Formation of a CTL–target cell conjugate is followed within several minutes by a Ca^{2+}-dependent, energy-requiring step in which the CTL inflicts membrane damage on the target cell. Following this step the CTL dissociates from the target cell and goes on to bind to another target cell. Within a variable period of time (from 15 min to 3 h) after CTL dissociation, the target cell is destroyed. Each of the steps involved in this process have been studied in more detail with cloned CTLs.

The TCR–CD3 membrane complex on a CTL recognizes antigen in association with class I MHC molecules on a target cell. Following this antigen-specific recognition, the integrin receptor LFA-1 on the CTL membrane binds to intercellular cell-adhesion molecules (ICAMs) on the target-cell membrane allowing conjugate formation between the two cells. M. L. Dustin and T. A. Springer found that antigen-mediated CTL activation converts LFA-1 from a low-avidity state to a high-avidity state (Figure 16-5). Because of this phenomenon, CTLs adhere to and form conjugates only with appropriate target cells that display antigenic peptides associated with class I MHC molecules. LFA-1 persists in

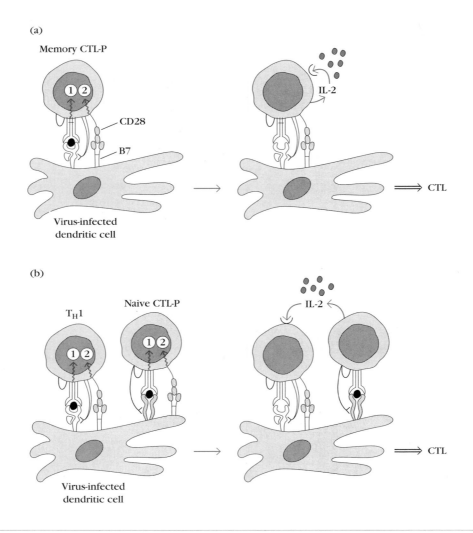

FIGURE 16-2

Proliferation of memory CTL-Ps may not require help from T_H cells. (a) Antigen-activated memory CTL-Ps appear to secrete sufficient IL-2 to autostimulate their own proliferation and differentiation into effector CTLs. They also may not require the CD28–B7 co-stimulatory signal for activation. (b) A T_H1 cell may provide the IL-2 necessary for proliferation of an antigen-activated naive CTL-P when it binds to the same APC as the CTL-P.

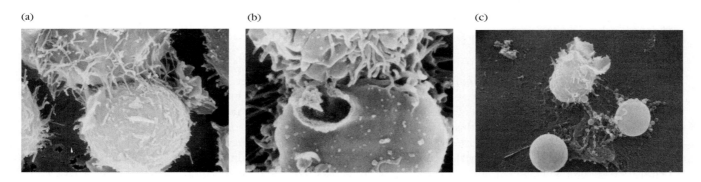

FIGURE 16-3

Scanning electron micrographs of tumor-cell destruction by a CTL. (a) A CTL (top left) makes contact with a smaller tumor cell. (b) Membrane damage to the tumor cell results in a visible cavity and allows an influx of water, resulting in cell swelling. (c) Lysis of the tumor cell has occurred leaving only cell debris and the nucleus (right). [From J. D. E. Young and Z. A. Cohn, 1988, *Sci. Am.* **258**(1):38.]

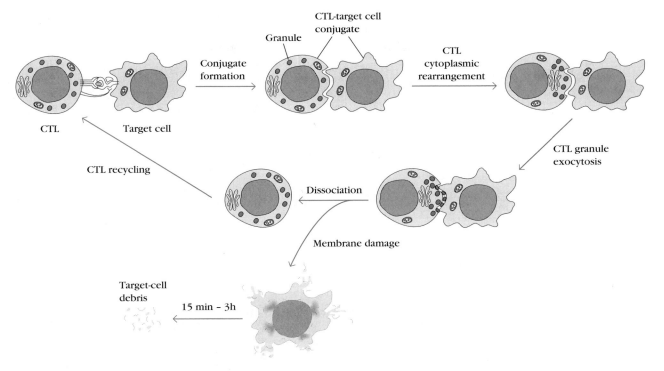

FIGURE 16-4

Stages in CTL-mediated killing of target cells. T-cell receptors on a CTL interact with processed antigen–class I MHC complexes on an appropriate target cell, leading to formation of a CTL/target-cell conjugate. The Golgi stacks and granules in the CTL reorient towards the point of contact with the target cell, and the granules' contents are released by exocytosis. Following dissociation of the conjugate, the CTL is recycled and the target cell is destroyed in time as the result of damage to its membrane and/or the action of cytotoxic mediators. [Adapted from P. A. Henkart, 1985, *Annu. Rev. Immunol.* **3**:31.]

the high-avidity state for only 5–10 min after antigen-mediated activation, and then it returns to the low-avidity state. This downshift in LFA-1 avidity is thought to facilitate CTL dissociation from the target cell.

Electron microscopy of cultured CTL clones reveals the presence of intracellular electron-dense storage granules. These granules have been isolated by fractionation and shown to mediate target-cell damage by themselves. Analysis of isolated CTL storage granules has shown that they contain some high-molecular-weight proteoglycans, various toxic cytokines (e.g., TNF-β), a pore-forming protein called **perforin**, and several proteases called **granzymes** (or **fragmentins**) with serine esterase activity. Although CTL-Ps lack cytoplasmic granules and perforin, CTL-P activation results in the appearance of these cytoplasmic granules and expression of 65-kDa perforin monomers within them.

Immediately following formation of a CTL–target cell conjugate, the Golgi stacks and storage granules reorient within the cytoplasm of the CTL, becoming concentrated near the junction with the target cell (Figure 16-6). Perforin monomers then are released from the granules

by exocytosis into the junctional space between the two cells. As the perforin monomers contact the target-cell membrane, they undergo a conformational change, exposing an amphipathic domain that inserts into the target-cell membrane; the monomers then polymerize (in the presence of Ca2$^+$) to form a cylindrical pore with an internal diameter of 5–20 nm (Figure 16-7a). A large number of perforin pores are visible on the target-cell membrane in the region of conjugate formation (Figure 16-7b). Interestingly, perforin exhibits some sequence homology with the terminal C9 component of the complement system, and the membrane pores formed by perforin are similar to those observed in complement-mediated lysis (see Figure 14-7). The importance of perforin to CTL-mediated killing is demonstrated by perforin-deficient knockout mice, which are unable to eliminate lymphocytic choriomeningitis virus (LCMV) even though they mount a significant CD8$^+$ immune response to the virus.

In addition to perforin, granzymes and other lytic substances are released from CTL granules. The pores are thought to facilitate entry of these substances into the

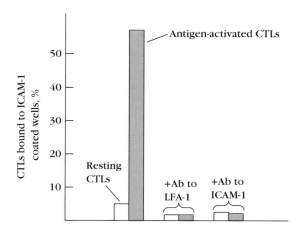

FIGURE 16-5

Effect of antigen activation on ability of CTLs to bind to the intercellular cell-adhesion molecule ICAM-1. Resting mouse CTLs were first incubated with anti-CD3 antibodies. Cross-linkage of CD3 molecules on the CTL membrane by anti-CD3 has the same activating effect as interaction with antigen–class I MHC complexes on a target cell. Adhesion was assayed by binding of radiolabeled CTLs to microwells coated with ICAM-1. Antigen activation increased CTL binding to ICAM-1 more than 10-fold. The presence of excess monoclonal antibody to LFA-1 or ICAM-1 in the microwells abolished binding, demonstrating that both molecules are necessary for adhesion to occur. [Based on M. L. Dustin and T. A. Springer, 1989, *Nature* **341**:619.]

target cell. Granzymes have been implicated in fragmentation of the target-cell DNA into oligomers of 200 bp; this type of DNA fragmentation is typical of apoptosis. Since granzymes are proteases, they cannot mediate directly DNA fragmentation. Rather, they may activate an endogenous apoptotic pathway within the target cell. This apoptotic process does not require mRNA or protein synthesis in either the CTL or target cell. Within 5 min following CTL contact, target cells begin to exhibit DNA fragmentation. Interestingly, viral DNA within infected target cells has also been shown to be fragmented during this process. This observation has led to speculation that the rapid onset of DNA fragmentation following CTL contact may prevent continued viral replication and assembly during the time prior to target-cell destruction.

Granzyme B has been shown to have protease activity closely related to interleukin 1β converting enzyme (ICE); both ICE and granzyme B have an unusual proteolytic specificity, cleaving substrates adjacent to aspartic residues. ICE is an endogenous protease that plays a central role in the endogenous apoptotic pathway. A number of external stimuli—including certain viruses, growth-factor withdrawal, and DNA damage—activate this en-

dogenous apoptotic pathway by converting ICE from an inactive to an active form (Figure 16-8). Once activated, ICE is thought to cleave an unidentified substrate leading to DNA degradation. It is hypothesized that granzyme B may either activate ICE or act in its place to trigger this endogenous apoptotic pathway.

Some CTL lines that are potent killers have been shown to lack perforin and granzymes. In these cases cytotoxicity is mediated by the action of a transmembrane death-signaling receptor called Fas present on the target-cell membrane. Fas (also known as APO-1) was originally identified as a cell-membrane protein that induced apoptosis when activated by antibodies. Fas is a member of the TNF family of cytokine receptors (see

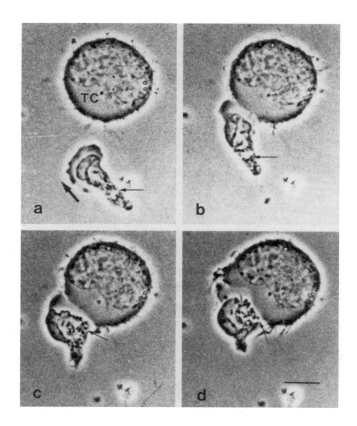

FIGURE 16-6

Formation of a conjugate between a CTL and target cell and reorientation of CTL cytoplasmic granules as recorded by time-lapse cinematography. (a) A motile mouse CTL (thin arrow) approaches an appropriate target cell (TC). Thick arrow indicates direction of movement. (b) Initial contact of the CTL and target cell has occurred. (c) Within 2 min of initial contact, the membrane-contact region has broadened and the rearrangement of dark cytoplasmic granules within the CTL (thin arrow) is under way. (d) Further movement of dark granules towards the target cell is evident 10 min after initial contact. [From J. R. Yanelli et al., 1986, *J. Immunol.* **136**:377.]

(a)

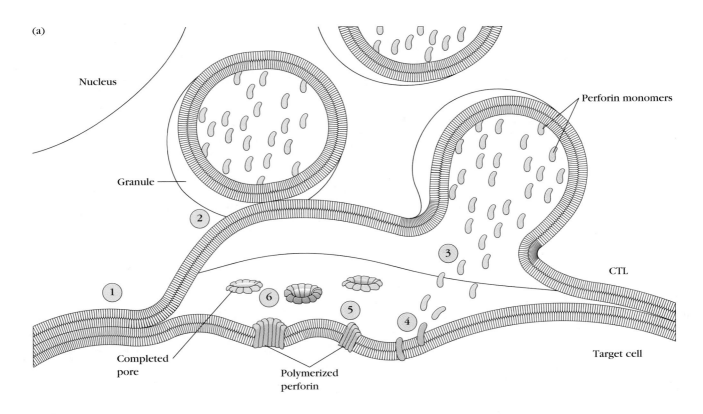

Nucleus

Granule

Perforin monomers

CTL

Completed pore

Polymerized perforin

Target cell

FIGURE 16-7

CTL-mediated pore formation in target-cell membrane. (a) In this model, a rise in intracellular $Ca2^+$ triggered by CTL–target cell interaction (1) induces exocytosis, in which the granules fuse with the CTL cell membrane (2) and release monomeric perforin into the small intracellular space between the two cells (3). The released perforin monomers undergo a $Ca2^+$-induced conformational change that allows it to insert into the target-cell membrane (4). In the presence of $Ca2^+$, the monomers polymerize within the membrane (5), forming cylindrical pores (6). (b) Electron micrograph of perforin pores on the surface of a rabbit erythrocyte target cell. [Part (a) adapted from J. D. E. Young and Z. A. Cohn, 1988, *Sci. Am.* **258**(1):38; part (b) from E. R. Podack and G. Dennert, 1983, *Nature* **301**:442.]

(b)

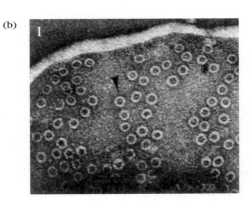

Figure 13-5d). CTLs express a cell-surface protein, with sequence homology to tumor necrosis factor, that binds to Fas. Interaction of this Fas ligand on a CTL with Fas on a target cell induces a signal in the target cell that activates the endogenous apoptotic pathway. Fas-induced apoptosis is also thought to involve ICE activation resulting in DNA degradation (see Figure 16-8).

The Fas ligand is expressed on effector T cells but not on naive T cells; CTLs express higher levels than T_H1 or T_H2 cells. The presence of the Fas ligand on T_H1 and T_H2 cells may account for reports that some $CD4^+$ T cells display cytotoxic activity in the absence of perforin or granzymes.

NK CELL–MEDIATED CYTOTOXICITY

Natural killer (NK) cells were discovered quite by accident when immunologists were measuring tumor-specific CTL activity in mice with tumors. Normal unimmunized mice and mice with unrelated tumors served as negative controls. Much to the consternation of the researchers, the controls showed significant tumor lysis. Characterization of the cells responsible for this nonspecific tumor-cell killing revealed that a population of large, granular lymphocytes was responsible. The cells, which were named natural killer (NK) cells for their nonspecific cytotoxicity, make up 5%–10% of the

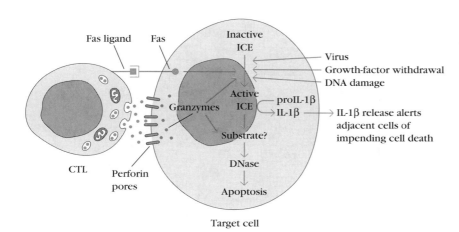

Target cell

FIGURE 16-8

Proposed model of target-cell apoptosis stimulated by CTLs. Activation of interleukin 1β converting enzyme (ICE) leads to apoptosis. Granzymes released from some CTLs may activate ICE or act directly in the apoptotic pathway. In some cases, a signal induced by interaction of the Fas ligand and Fas, a TNF-type cytokine receptor on the target cell, also is thought to activate ICE. [Adapted from M. J. Smyth and J. A. Trapani, 1995, *Immunol. Today* **16**(4):202.]

recirculating lymphocyte population. These cells have been implicated in viral immunity and in defense against tumors.

NK cells are involved in the early response to infection with certain viruses and intracellular bacteria. NK activity is stimulated by IFN-α, IFN-β, and IL-12. In the course of a viral infection, these cytokines rapidly rise, followed closely by a wave of NK cells that peaks in about 3 days (Figure 16-9). NK cells provide the first line of defense to virus infection, controlling viral replication during the time required for activation, proliferation, and differentiation of T_C cells into functional CTLs at about day 7. The importance of NK cells in defense against viral infections is illustrated by the case report of a young woman who completely lacked these cells. Even though this patient had normal T- and B-cell counts, she suffered severe varicella virus infections and a life-threatening cytomegalovirus infection.

NK-Cell Lineage The lineage of NK cells remains uncertain, as they express some membrane markers of T lymphocytes and some markers of monocytes and granulocytes. Moreover, different NK cells express different sets of membrane molecules. It is not known whether this heterogeneity reflects subpopulations of NK cells or different stages in their activation or maturation. Among the membrane molecules expressed by NK cells are Thy-1, CD2, the 75-kDa β subunit of the IL-2 receptor, and CD16 (or FcγRIII), which is a receptor for the Fc region of IgG. Monoclonal antibody to CD16 has been shown to remove almost all NK-cell activity from peripheral blood, and this reagent can be used to separate NK cells from other cell types.

A population of CD16$^+$ cells has been identified in the bone marrow and fetal thymus with anti-CD16. At day 14.5 of gestation, a major fetal thymocyte population bears the phenotype CD16$^+$, CD4$^-$, CD8$^-$, and TCR$^-$.

Interestingly, if these fetal thymocytes are isolated and injected into the thymus of an irradiated adult mouse, they differentiate into double-positive TCR$^+$, CD4$^+$, CD8$^+$, CD16$^-$ cells and later mature into the single-positive CD4$^+$ or CD8$^+$ subpopulations, expressing the T-cell receptor. However, if the CD16$^+$, CD4$^-$, CD8$^-$ fetal thymocytes are grown in tissue culture in the presence of exogenous IL-2, the cells maintain their CD16$^+$ phenotype and acquire the functional cytotoxic properties of

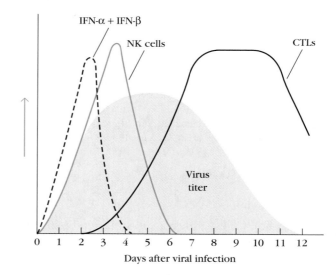

FIGURE 16-9

Time course of viral infection. IFN-α and IFN-β (dashed curve) are released from virus-infected cells soon after infection. These cytokines stimulate the NK cells, quickly leading to a rise in the NK-cell population (blue curve). NK cells help contain the infection during the period required for generation of CTLs (solid black curve). Once the CTL population reaches a peak, the virus titer (blue area) rapidly decreases.

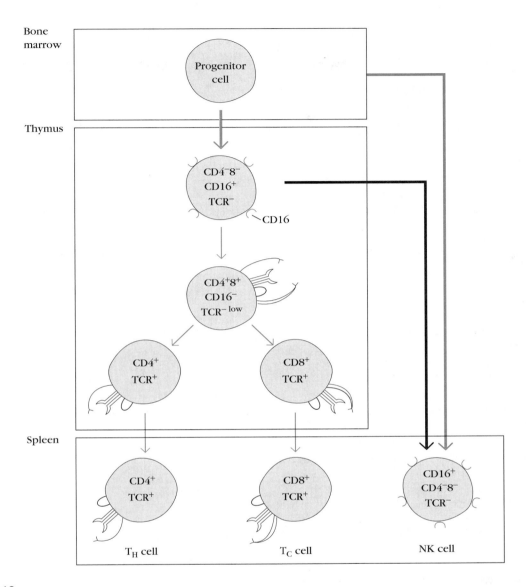

FIGURE 16-10

Model of thymocyte development involving a CD16+, NK-like in-termediate. CD16 has been identified on hematopoietic cells in the bone marrow and fetal thymus. This membrane molecule is present on mature NK cells but is absent from CD8+ and CD4+ T cells. According to this model, bone marrow progenitor cells that bypass the thymus (thick blue arrow) or fail to undergo thymic induction (thick black arrow) give rise to peripheral NK cells. NK-cell development clearly can bypass the thymus, since NK cells are found in athymic mice. [Adapted from H. R. Rodewald et al., 1992, *Cell* **69**:139.]

NK cells. This has led to the suggestion that both CD4+ and CD8+ T cells and NK cells may be derived from a common lineage (Figure 16-10). However, the observation that NK cells can develop in SCID mice suggests that either NK cells develop from a lineage distinct from T cells or else that they develop from a common early progenitor cell prior to the rearrangement of the TCR genes.

Mechanism of NK-Cell Killing Natural killer cells appear to kill tumor cells and virus-infected cells by a process similar to that employed by CTLs. The cytoplasm of NK cells contains numerous granules containing per-forin and granzymes. Unlike CTLs, which need to be activated before granules appear, NK cells are constitutively cytotoxic, always having large granules in their cytoplasm. After an NK cell adheres to a target cell, degranulation occurs with release of perforin and granzymes at the junction of the interacting cells. The released perforin forms pores in the same way described for the CTL (see Figure 16-7). NK cells have also been shown to mediate target-cell destruction by apoptosis. In addition to granzymes, a number of toxic molecules (e.g., TNF-α) may contribute to target-cell apoptosis mediated by NK cells.

Despite these similarities, NK cells differ from CTLs in several significant ways. First, NK cells do not express antigen-specific T-cell receptors or CD3. In addition, target-cell recognition by NK cells is not MHC restricted; that is, the same levels of NK-cell activity are observed with syngeneic and allogeneic tumor cells. Moreover, although prior priming enhances CTL activity, no increase in NK-cell activity occurs after a second injection with the same tumor cells. In other words, the NK-cell response generates no immunologic memory.

NK-Cell Receptors Given that NK cells do not express antigen-specific receptors, the mechanism by which NK cells recognize altered self-cells and distinguish them from normal body cells has baffled immunologists for years. One clue to this puzzle is the observation that virus-infected cells and tumor cells express lower levels of class I MHC molecules than do normal cells. One model, called the **two-receptor model**, suggests that NK cells receive signals from two receptors enabling these cells to distinguish healthy cells from infected or cancerous cells.

According to this model, a receptor called **NKR-P1** binds to oligosaccharides that are expressed on the surface of tumor and virus-infected cells, which often have abnormal patterns of glycosylation. Interaction of the NKR-P1 receptor with its oligosaccharide ligand signals to the NK cell to kill. This killing signal can be prevented by a signal from a second receptor, called Ly49, present on the NK-cell surface (Figure 16-11, *top*). This receptor binds to certain alleles of class I MHC molecules. Binding of the **Ly49** receptor to a class I MHC molecule transmits a negative signal that overrides the NKR-P1 signal. Thus when MHC expression is reduced, as it is on virus-infected or cancerous cells, the Ly49 signal is also reduced, allowing the NKR-P1 signal to induce killing of the target cell (Figure 16-11, *bottom*).

ANTIBODY-DEPENDENT CELL-MEDIATED CYTOTOXICITY

A number of cells that have cytotoxic potential express membrane receptors for the Fc region of the antibody molecule. When antibody is specifically bound to a target cell, these receptor-bearing cells can bind to the antibody Fc region, and thus to the target cells, and subsequently cause lysis of the target cell. Although the cytotoxic cells involved are nonspecific, the specificity of the antibody directs them to specific target cells. This type of cyto-

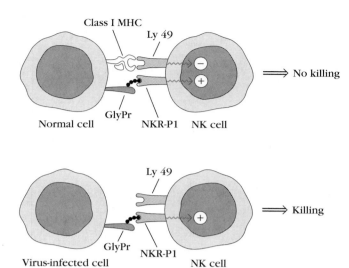

FIGURE 16-11

Two-receptor model of how cytotoxic activity of NK cells is restricted to altered self-cells. The NKR-P1 receptor on NK cells interacts with carbohydrate moieties (black circles) on membrane glycoproteins (GlyPr) of normal and altered self-cells, inducing a killing signal (+). Engagement of a second NK receptor called Ly49 with class I MHC molecules delivers another signal (−) that counteracts the killing signal. Expression of class I molecules on normal cells thus prevents their destruction by NK cells. Because class I expression is decreased on altered self-cells, the killing signal predominates, leading to their destruction.

toxicity is referred to as **antibody-dependent cell-mediated cytotoxicity** (ADCC).

Among the cells that can mediate ADCC are NK cells, macrophages, monocytes, neutrophils, and eosinophils. Antibody-dependent cell-mediated killing of cells infected with the measles virus can be observed in vitro by adding antimeasles antibody together with macrophages to a culture of measles-infected cells. Similarly, cell-mediated killing of helminths, such as schistosomes or blood flukes, can be observed in vitro by incubating newly infected larvae (schistosomules) with antibody to the schistosomules together with eosinophils.

Target-cell killing by ADCC, which does not involve complement-mediated lysis, appears to involve a number of different cytotoxic mechanisms (Figure 16-12). When macrophages, neutrophils, or eosinophils bind to a target cell by way of the Fc receptor, they become more active metabolically; as a result, the lytic components in their cytoplasmic lysosomes or granules increase. Release of these lytic components at the site of the Fc-mediated contact may result in damage to the target cell. In addition, activated monocytes, macrophages, and NK cells have been shown to secrete tumor necrosis factor (TNF), which may have a cytotoxic effect on the bound target cell. Since both NK cells and eosinophils contain perforin in cytoplasmic granules, their target-cell killing also may involve perforin-mediated membrane damage similar to the mechanism described for CTL-mediated cytotoxicity.

EXPERIMENTAL ASSESSMENT OF CELL-MEDIATED CYTOTOXICITY

Three experimental systems have been particularly useful for measuring the activation and effector phases of cell-mediated cytotoxic responses. The **mixed-lymphocyte reaction** (MLR) is an in vitro system for assaying T_H-cell proliferation in a cell-mediated response; **cell-mediated lympholysis** (CML) is an in vitro assay of effector cytotoxic function; and the **graft-versus-host reaction** in experimental animals provides an in vivo system for studying cell-mediated cytotoxicity.

Mixed-Lymphocyte Reaction (MLR) In 1965, X. Ginsburg and D. H. Sachs observed that when rat lymphocytes were cultured on a monolayer of mouse fibroblast cells, the rat lymphocytes proliferated and destroyed the mouse fibroblasts. In 1970 it was discovered that functional CTLs could also be generated by co-culturing

allogeneic spleen cells in a system termed the mixed-lymphocyte reaction (MLR). The T lymphocytes in an MLR undergo extensive blast transformation and cell proliferation. The degree of proliferation can be assessed by adding [^{3}H]thymidine to the culture medium and monitoring uptake of label into DNA in the course of repeated cell divisions.

Both populations of allogeneic T lymphocytes proliferate in an MLR unless one population is rendered unresponsive by treatment with mitomycin C or lethal x-irradiation (Figure 16-13). In the latter system, called a **one-way MLR**, the unresponsive population provides stimulator cells that express alloantigens foreign to the responder T cells. Within 24–48 h the responder T cells begin dividing in response to the alloantigens of the stimulator cells, and by 72–96 h a population of functional CTLs is generated. With this experimental system functional CTLs can be generated entirely in vitro, after which their activity can be assessed with various effector assays.

The significant role of T_H cells in the one-way MLR can be demonstrated by use of antibodies to the T_H-cell membrane marker CD4. In a one-way MLR, responder T_H cells recognize allogeneic class II MHC molecules on the stimulator cells and proliferate in response to these differences. Removal of the CD4$^+$ T_H cells from the responder population with anti-CD4 plus complement abolishes the MLR and prevents generation of CTLs. In addition to T_H cells, accessory cells such as macrophages also are necessary for the MLR to proceed. When adherent cells (largely macrophages) are removed from the stimulator population, the proliferative response in the MLR is abolished and functional CTLs are no longer generated. It is now known that the function of these macrophages is to activate class II MHC–restricted T_H cells whose proliferation is measured in the MLR. In the absence of T_H-cell activation, there is no proliferation.

Cell-Mediated Lympholysis (CML) Development of the cell-mediated lympholysis (CML) assay was a major experimental advance that contributed to understanding of the mechanism of target-cell killing by CTLs. In this assay suitable target cells are labeled intracellularly with chromium-51 (^{51}Cr) by incubating the target cells with Na$_2$^{51}CrO$_4$. After the ^{51}Cr diffuses into a cell, it binds to cytoplasmic proteins, reducing passive diffusion of the label out of the cell. When specifically activated CTLs are incubated for 1–4 h with such labeled target cells, the cells lyse and the ^{51}Cr is released. The amount of ^{51}Cr released is directly related to the number of target cells lysed by the CTLs. By means of this assay the specificity of CTLs for allogeneic cells, tumor cells, virus-infected cells, and chemically modified cells has been demonstrated (Figure 16-14).

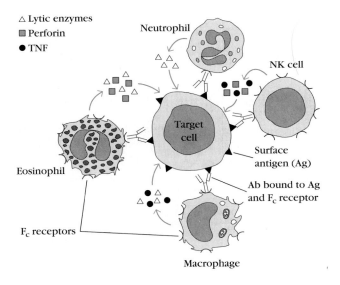

△ Lytic enzymes
■ Perforin
● TNF

Neutrophil

NK cell

Target cell

Surface antigen (Ag)

Ab bound to Ag and F_c receptor

Eosinophil

F_c receptors

Macrophage

FIGURE 16-12

Antibody-dependent cell-mediated cytotoxicity (ADCC). Nonspecific cytotoxic cells are directed to specific target cells by binding to the Fc region of antibody bound to surface antigens on the target cells. Various substances (e.g., lytic enzymes, TNF, perforin) secreted by the nonspecific cytotoxic cells then mediate target-cell destruction.

(a)

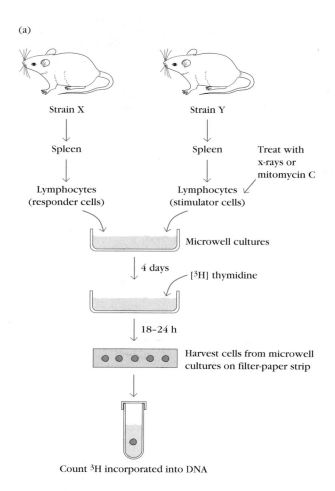

(b)

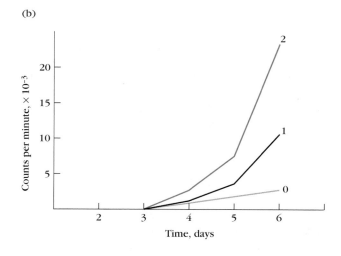

FIGURE 16-13

One-way mixed-lymphocyte reaction (MLR). (a) This assay measures the proliferation of lymphocytes from one strain (responder cells) in response to allogeneic cells that have been x-irradiated or treated with mitomycin C to prevent proliferation (stimulator cells). The amount of [³H]thymidine incorporated into the DNA is directly proportional to the extent of responder-cell proliferation. (b) The amount of [³H]thymidine uptake in a one-way MLR depends on the degree of differences in class II MHC molecules between the stimulator and responder cells. Curve 0 = no class II MHC differences; curve 1 = one class II MHC difference; curve 2 = two class II MHC differences. These results demonstrate that the greater the class II MHC differences, the greater the proliferation of responder cells.

The T cells responsible for CML were identified by selectively depleting different T-cell subpopulations by means of antibody-plus-complement lysis. In general, the activity of CTLs exhibits class I MHC restriction. That is, CTLs can only kill target cells that present antigen associated with syngeneic class I MHC molecules. Occasionally, however, CD4⁺, class II–restricted T cells have been shown to function as CTLs.

Graft-versus-Host Reaction

The graft-versus-host (GVH) reaction is an in vivo indication of cell-mediated cytotoxicity. The reaction develops when immunocomponent lymphocytes are injected into an allogeneic recipient whose immune system is compromised. The grafted lymphocytes begin to attack the host, and the host's compromised state prevents an immune response against the graft. In humans, GVH reactions often develop following transplantation of bone marrow into patients who have had radiation exposure or who have leukemia, immunodeficiency diseases, or autoimmune anemias. The clinical manifestations of the GVH reaction include diarrhea, skin lesions, jaundice, spleen enlargement, and death. Epi-

thelial cells of the skin and gastrointestinal tract often become necrotic, causing the skin and intestinal lining to be sloughed.

Experimentally, GVH reactions develop when immunocompetent lymphocytes are transferred into a neonatal or an x-irradiated animal. The recipients, especially neonatal ones, often exhibit weight loss. The grafted lymphocytes generally are carried to a number of organs, including the spleen, where they begin to proliferate in response to the allogeneic MHC antigens of the host. This proliferation induces an influx of host cells, which in turn undergo intense proliferation that results in visible spleen enlargement, or splenomegaly. The intensity of a GVH reaction can be assessed by calculating the spleen index as follows:

$$\text{Spleen index} = \frac{\text{Weight of exp. spleen/Total body weight}}{\text{Weight of control spleen/Total body weight}}$$

A spleen index of 1.3 or greater is considered to be indicative of a positive GVH reaction. Spleen enlargement results from proliferation of both CD4⁺ and CD8⁺ T-cell populations. NK cells also have been shown to

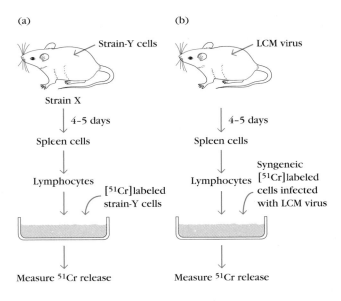

(a)   (b)

Strain-Y cells   LCM virus

Strain X

4–5 days   4–5 days

Spleen cells   Spleen cells

Lymphocytes   Lymphocytes

[51Cr]labeled   Syngeneic
strain-Y cells   [51Cr]labeled
                             cells infected
                             with LCM virus

Measure 51Cr release   Measure 51Cr release

FIGURE 16-14

In vitro cell-mediated lympholysis (CML) assay. This assay can measure the activity of cytotoxic T lymphocytes (CTLs) against allogeneic cells (a) or virus-infected cells (b). In both cases the release of ^{51}Cr into the supernatant indicates the presence of CTLs that can lyse the target cells.

play a role in the GVH reaction, and these cells may contribute to some of the skin lesions and intestinal wall damage observed.

Delayed-Type Hypersensitivity

When some subpopulations of activated T_H cells encounter certain types of antigens, they secrete cytokines that induce a localized inflammatory reaction called **delayed-type hypersensitivity** (DTH). The reaction is characterized by large influxes of nonspecific inflammatory cells, in which the macrophage is a major participant. Historically, this type of reaction was first described in 1890 by Robert Koch, who observed that individuals infected with *Mycobacterium tuberculosis* developed a localized inflammatory response when injected intradermally with a filtrate derived from a mycobacterial culture. He called this localized skin reaction a "tuberculin reaction."

Later, as it became apparent that a variety of other antigens could induce this response, its name was changed to delayed-type hypersensitivity in reference to the delayed onset of the reaction and to the extensive tissue damage (hypersensitivity) that is often associated with the reaction. The term **hypersensitivity** is somewhat misleading for it suggests that a DTH response is always detrimental. Although in some cases a DTH response does cause extensive tissue damage and is in itself patho-

logic, in many cases tissue damage is limited, and the response plays an important role in defense against intracellular pathogens and contact antigens.

PHASES OF THE DTH RESPONSE

The development of the DTH response requires an initial **sensitization phase** of 1–2 weeks following primary contact with the antigen. During this period T_H cells are activated and clonally expanded by antigen presented together with the requisite class II MHC molecule on an appropriate antigen-presenting cell (Figure 16-15a). A variety of antigen-presenting cells have been shown to be involved in the activation of a DTH response, including Langerhans cells and macrophages. Langerhans cells are dendritic cells found in the epidermis. These cells are thought to pick up antigen that enters through the skin and transport the antigen to regional lymph nodes where T cells are activated by the antigen. In some species, including humans, the vascular endothelial cells express class II MHC molecules and also function as antigen-presenting cells in the development of the DTH response. Generally, the T cells activated during the sensitization phase are CD4$^+$, primarily of the T_H1 subtype, but in a few cases CD8$^+$ cells have also been shown to induce a DTH response. The activated T cells are often designated as T_{DTH} cells to denote their function in the DTH response, although in reality they are simply a subset of T_H cells (or in some cases T_C cells).

A secondary contact with antigen induces the **effector phase** of the DTH response (Figure 16-15b). In the effector phase, T_{DTH} secrete a variety of cytokines that are responsible for the recruitment and activation of macrophages and other nonspecific inflammatory cells. A DTH response normally does not become apparent until an average of 24 h following secondary contact with the antigen; the response generally peaks 48–72 h after secondary contact. The delayed onset of this response reflects the time required for the cytokines to induce localized influxes of macrophages and activation of these cells. Once a DTH response begins, a complex interplay of nonspecific cells and mediators is set in motion that can result in tremendous amplification. By the time the DTH response is fully developed, only about 5% of the participating cells are antigen-specific T_{DTH} cells; the remainder are macrophages and other nonspecific cells.

Macrophages function as the principal effector cells of the DTH response. Cytokines elaborated by T_{DTH} cells induce blood monocytes to adhere to vascular endothelial cells and migrate from the blood into the surrounding tissues. During this process the monocytes differentiate into activated macrophages. As discussed in Chapter 3, **activated macrophages** exhibit increased levels of phagocytosis and an increased ability to kill

Visualizing Concepts

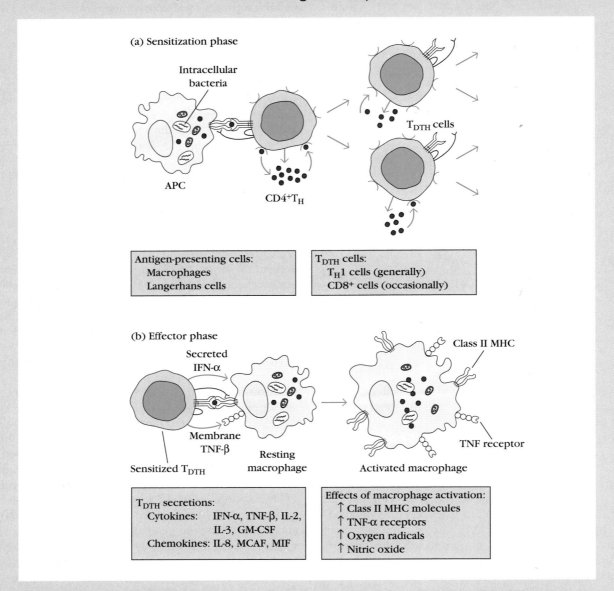

FIGURE 16-15

Overview of the DTH response. (a) In the sensitization phase following initial contact with antigen (e.g., peptides derived from intracellular bacteria), T_H cells proliferate and differentiate into T_{DTH} cells. (b) In the effector phase following subsequent exposure of sensitized T_{DTH} cells to antigen, the T_{DTH} cells secrete a variety of cytokines and chemokines. These factors attract and activate macrophages and other nonspecific inflammatory cells. Activated macrophages are more effective in presenting antigen, thus perpetuating the DTH response, and function as the primary effector cells in this reaction. MCAF = macrophage chemotactic and activating factor; MIF = macrophage-inhibition factor.

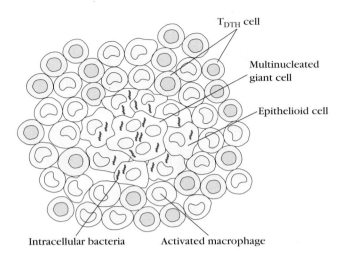

Labels: T_{DTH} cell, Multinucleated giant cell, Epithelioid cell, Intracellular bacteria, Activated macrophage

FIGURE 16-16

A prolonged DTH response can lead to formation of a granuloma, a nodule-like mass. Lytic enzymes released from activated macrophages in a granuloma can cause extensive tissue damage.

microorganisms via various cytotoxic mediators (see Table 3-5). In addition, activated macrophages express increased levels of class II MHC molecules and cell-adhesion molecules and therefore function as more effective antigen-presenting cells.

The influx and activation of macrophages in the DTH response provide an effective host defense against intracellular pathogens. Generally the pathogen is rapidly cleared with little tissue damage. However, in some cases, especially if the antigen is not easily cleared, a prolonged DTH response can itself become destructive to the host as the intense inflammatory response develops into a visible granulomatous reaction. A **granuloma** develops when continuous activation of macrophages induces the macrophages to adhere closely to one another, assuming an epithelioid shape and sometimes fusing to form mult-inucleated giant cells (Figure 16-16). These giant cells displace the normal tissue cells, forming palpable nodules, and release high concentrations of lytic enzymes, which destroy the surrounding tissue. In these cases the response can lead to blood-vessel damage and extensive tissue necrosis.

CYTOKINES INVOLVED IN THE DTH REACTION

Numerous cytokines play a role in generating a DTH reaction. The pattern of cytokines implicated in a DTH response suggest that T_{DTH} cells may be primarily of the T_H1 subset (see Table 16-2). IL-2 functions in an autocrine manner to amplify the population of cytokine-producing T cells. Among the cytokines produced by T_{DTH} cells are a number that serve to activate and attract macrophages to the site of activation. IL-3 and GM-CSF induce localized hematopoiesis of the granulocyte-monocyte lineage. IFN-γ and TNF-β (together with macrophage-derived TNF-α and IL-1) act on nearby endothelial cells, inducing a number of changes that facilitate extravasation of monocytes and other nonspecific inflammatory cells. Circulating neutrophils and monocytes adhere to the adhesion molecules displayed on the vascular endothelial cells and extravasate into the tissue spaces. Neutrophils appear early in the reaction, peaking by about 6 h and then declining in numbers. The monocyte infiltration occurs between 24 and 48 h after antigen exposure.

As the monocytes enter the tissues to become macrophages, they are chemotactically drawn to the site of the DTH response by factors such as monocyte chemotactic and activating factor (MCAF) and IFN-γ. Another chemokine, called **migration-inhibition factor** (MIF), inhibits further macrophage migration and thus prevents the macrophages from migrating beyond the site of a DTH reaction. As macrophages accumulate at the site of a DTH reaction, they are activated by cytokines, particularly IFN-γ and membrane-bound TNF-β produced by T_{DTH} cells. As noted earlier, activated macrophages are more effective antigen-presenting cells than unactivated macrophages. Thus the activated macrophages can efficiently mediate activation of more T_{DTH} cells, which in turn secrete more cytokines that recruit and activate even more macrophages. This self-perpetuating response, however, is a double-edged sword, with a fine line existing between a beneficial, protective response and a detrimental response characterized by extensive tissue damage.

A 1993 report of experiments with knockout mice that could not produce IFN-γ demonstrated the importance of this cytokine in the DTH response. When these knockout mice were infected with an attenuated (non-pathogenic) strain of *Mycobacterium bovis* (BCG), nearly all the animals died within 60 days, whereas wild-type mice survived (Figure 16-17). Macrophages from the IFN-γ knockout mice were shown to have reduced levels of class II MHC molecules and of bactericidal metabolites such as nitric oxide and superoxide anion.

PROTECTIVE ROLE OF THE DTH RESPONSE

A variety of intracellular pathogens and contact antigens can induce a DTH response (Table 16-3). Cells harboring intracellular pathogens are rapidly destroyed by lytic enzymes released by activated macrophages that accumulate at the site of a DTH reaction (Figure 16-18). The initial response, however, is nonspecific and often results in

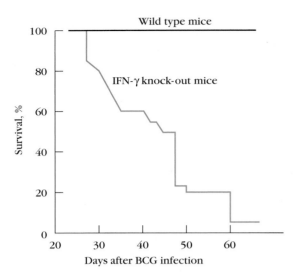

FIGURE 16-17

Experimental demonstration of role of IFN-γ in host defense against intracellular pathogens. Knockout mice were produced by introducing a targeted mutation in the gene encoding IFN-γ. The mice were then infected with 10^7 colony-forming units of attenuated *Mycobacterium bovis* (BCG) and their survival monitored. [Adapted from D. K. Dalton et al., 1993, *Science* **259**:1739.]

significant damage to healthy tissue. Generally this is the price the body pays for successful elimination of cells harboring intracellular and fungal pathogens. The response to *Mycobacterium tuberculosis* illustrates the double-edged

nature of the DTH response. Immunity to this intracellular bacterium involves a DTH response in which activated macrophages wall-off the organism and contain it within a granuloma-type lesion called a **tubercle.** Often, however, the concentrated release of lytic enzymes from the activated macrophages within tubercles leads to tissue damage within the lung.

The vitally important role of the DTH response in protecting the host against various intracellular pathogens is illustrated by AIDS. In this disease, CD4+ T cells are severely depleted, resulting in a loss of the DTH response. Often patients suffering with AIDS develop life-threatening infections from intracellular bacteria, fungi, or protozoans that would not threaten an individual whose DTH response was intact. The immune response in AIDS patients is discussed in more depth in Chapter 22.

DETECTION OF THE DTH REACTION

The presence of a DTH reaction can be measured experimentally by injecting antigen intradermally into an animal and observing whether a characteristic skin lesion develops at the injection site. A positive skin-test reaction indicates that the individual has a population of sensitized T_{DTH} cells specific for the test antigen. For example, to determine whether an individual has been exposed to *M. tuberculosis,* a protein derived from the cell wall of this mycobacterium (PPD) is injected intradermally. Development of a red, slightly swollen, firm lesion at the site between 48 and 72 h later indicates that the individual

TABLE 16-3
INTRACELLULAR PATHOGENS AND CONTACT ANTIGENS THAT INDUCE DELAYED-TYPE HYPERSENSITIVITY

Intracellular bacteria	Intracellular viruses
Mycobacterium tuberculosis	Herpes simplex virus
Mycobacterium leprae	Variola (smallpox)
Listeria monocytogenes	Measles virus
Brucella abortus	
	Contact antigens
Intracellular fungi	Poison oak and ivy
Pneumocystis carinii	Picrylchloride
Candida albicans	Hair dyes
Histoplasma capsulatum	Nickel salts
Cryptococcus neoformans	
Intracellular parasites	
Leishmania sp.	

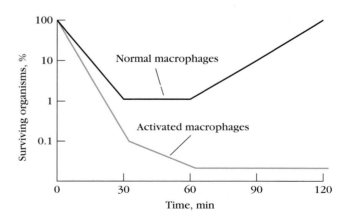

FIGURE 16-18

Survival of the intracellular pathogen *Listeria monocytogenes* when mixed with normal macrophages (not activated by IFN-γ) or activated macrophages in vitro. Note the logarithmic scale. The much greater ability of activated macrophages to destroy intracellular pathogens is evident.

has been exposed to *M. tuberculosis* antigens, either through direct exposure to the organism or through immunization, which is performed in some parts of the world. Development of a skin lesion in a previously sensitized individual results from the intense infiltration of cells to the site of injection during a DTH reaction; 80%–90% of these cells are macrophages.

PATHOLOGIC DTH RESPONSES

In some cases the DTH response to an intracellular pathogen can cause such extensive tissue damage that the response itself is pathologic and constitutes a truly hypersensitive condition. Much of the tissue damage in tuberculosis results from the accumulation of activated macrophages whose lysosomal enzymes destroy healthy lung tissue. Delayed-type hypersensitive reactions can also develop to inappropriate antigens such as poison oak and skin-contact sensitizers. Such examples, of truly hypersensitive conditions, in which tissue damage far outweighs any beneficial effects, are discussed in Chapter 18.

EFFECTOR RESPONSES IN THE HUMORAL BRANCH

The humoral immune response, which is uniquely adapted to the elimination of extracellular pathogens, is characterized by the production of large numbers of antibody molecules specific for antigenic determinants (epitopes) on a foreign pathogen. The potential diversity generated by this branch of the immune system can provide 10^8–10^{11} different antigen-binding specificities (see Table 7-2). This enormous antigen-binding diversity is coupled with conservation of constant-region sequences, which confer biological effector functions on antibody molecules.

Humoral effector functions facilitate effective elimination of foreign pathogens from a host animal in a variety of ways discussed in other chapters. Antibodies perform this function by the following mechanisms:

- Activating the complement system, resulting in lysis of microorganisms
- Acting as opsonins, enhancing phagocytosis of microorganisms
- Binding to and neutralizing bacterial toxins
- Binding to viruses and inhibiting their ability to infect host cells
- Binding to potential pathogens at mucous membrane surfaces, thereby preventing colonization
- Binding to Fc receptors on NK cells or macrophages in ADCC, conferring specificity for antigen on these otherwise nonspecific cells (see Figure 16-12)

In this section, we consider the differences between the primary and secondary humoral response, the experimental assay of antibody-secreting plasma cells, and the use of hapten-carrier conjugates in studying the humoral response.

Primary and Secondary Responses

The kinetics and other characteristics of the humoral response differ considerably depending on whether they result from activation of naive lymphocytes (primary response) or memory lymphocytes (secondary response). In both cases, activation leads to production of secreted antibodies of various isotypes, which vary in their ability to mediate specific effector functions (see Table 5-4).

The first contact of an individual with an exogenous antigen generates a **primary humoral response,** characterized by the production of antibody-secreting plasma cells and memory B cells. The kinetics of the primary response, as measured by serum antibody level, vary depending on the nature of the antigen, the route of antigen administration, the presence or absence of adjuvants, and the species or strain being immunized (see Chapter 4).

In all cases, however, a primary response is characterized by a **lag phase,** during which naive B cells undergo clonal selection in response to the antigen and differentiate into plasma cells and memory cells (Figure 16-19). The lag phase is followed by a logarithmic increase in serum antibody level, which reaches a peak, plateaus for a variable time, and then declines. In the case of an antigen such as sheep red blood cells (SRBCs), the lag phase lasts 3–4 days; peak plasma-cell levels are attained within 4–5 days; and peak serum antibody levels are attained by 5–7 days. Eight or nine successive cell divisions occur within the 4- to 5-day period, generating plasma and memory cells. For soluble protein antigens the lag phase is a little longer, often lasting about a week, and peak plasma-cell levels are attained by 9–10 days. During a primary humoral response, IgM is secreted initially, often followed by IgG. Depending on the persistence of the antigen, a primary response can last for varying periods, sometimes only a few days and sometimes several weeks.

The memory B cells formed during a primary response stop dividing and enter the G_0 phase of the cell cycle. These cells have variable life spans, and some persist for the life of the individual. The existence of long-lived memory B cells accounts for a phenomenon called **"original antigenic sin,"** which was first observed when the antibody response to influenza vaccines was monitored. Monitoring revealed that immunization with an influenza vaccine of one strain elicited an antibody response to that strain but, paradoxically, also elicited an antibody response of greater magnitude to another influenza strain that the individual had been exposed to

Visualizing Concepts

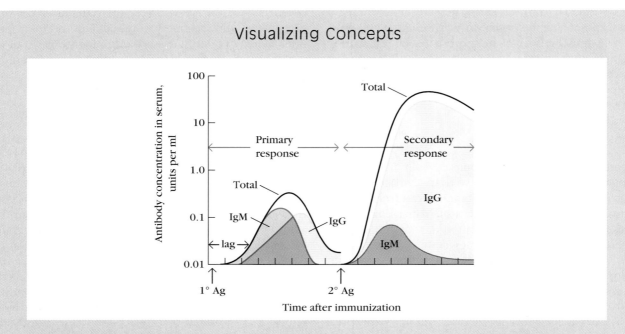

FIGURE 16-19

Concentration and isotype of serum antibody following primary (1°) and secondary (2°) immunization with antigen. The antibody concentrations are plotted on a logarithmic scale. The time units are not specified because the kinetics differ somewhat with type of antigen, administration route, presence or absence of adjuvant, and the species or strain of animal.

during childhood. It was as if the memory of the first antigen exposure had left a life-long imprint on the immune system. This phenomenon can be explained by the presence of a memory-cell population, elicited by the influenza strain encountered in childhood, that is activated by cross-reacting epitopes on the vaccine strain. This process then generates a secondary response, characterized by antibodies with higher affinity for the earlier viral strain.

The capacity to develop a **secondary humoral response** depends on the existence of a population of memory B cells and memory T cells. Antigen activation of these memory cells results in a secondary antibody response that can be distinguished from the primary response in several ways (Table 16-4). The secondary response has a shorter lag period and thus occurs more rapidly, reaches a greater magnitude, and lasts for a longer duration. In addition, the secondary response is characterized by secretion of antibody with a higher affinity for the antigen and isotypes other than IgM predominate (see Figure 16-19).

The population of memory B cells specific for a given antigen is considerably larger than the population of corresponding naive B cells, accounting in part for some of

the differences between the primary and secondary response. Furthermore, memory B cells are more easily activated than naive B cells. The processes of affinity maturation and class switching discussed in Chapter 8 are responsible for the higher affinity and different isotypes exhibited in a secondary response. The higher levels of antibody coupled with the overall higher affinity provide an effective host defense against reinfection. The change in isotype that occurs in the secondary response provides antibodies whose biological effector functions are particularly suited to eliminate a given pathogen.

Experimental Assessment of Humoral Immunity

For many years the humoral immune response could be monitored only by quantifying antibody production by various assays based on the antigen-antibody interaction (see Chapter 6). This changed with development of the hemolytic plaque assay, which permits determination of the number of plasma cells. Originally developed by N. K. Jerne, A. A. Nordin, and C. Henry, and later modified by other researchers, this assay has played a significant role in studies of the humoral response.

HEMOLYTIC PLAQUE ASSAYS

The original **direct hemolytic plaque assay,** which is similar in principle to a viral plaque assay, is used to measure the number of plasma cells in mice primed with SRBCs. Spleen cells from primed mice are mixed in warm, melted agar with an excess of SRBCs (Figure 16-20a). The agar containing the cell suspension is poured into a Petri dish, whose bottom is covered with a layer of hard agar, and allowed to cool and solidify. The splenic lymphocytes are thus immobilized in the agar, surrounded by a sea of SRBCs. The Petri dish is incubated for 1 h at 37°C, during which time antibody secreted by plasma cells diffuses into the agar matrix and binds to the SRBCs in the vicinity of each antibody-secreting plasma cell. Guinea pig serum containing complement is then added. The complement reacts with the antibody bound to the SRBCs and mediates their lysis, leaving each plasma cell surrounded by a clear plaque devoid of red blood cells. The plaques are counted, and their number is the number of antibody-producing plasma cells specific for the SRBC antigen. This assay, referred to as the **direct plaque-forming cells** (PFC), identifies primarily IgM-producing plasma cells.

The hemolytic plaque assay can be adapted to determine not only the number of IgM-secreting plasma cells and IgG-secreting plasma cells. In the case of IgM, complement-mediated lysis is triggered by the binding of a single pentameric IgM molecule to an SRBC. However, in the case of IgG, which exists as a monomer, complement-mediated lysis does not occur unless the Fc regions from two IgG molecules are located within 30–40 nm of each other on the membrane of an SRBC. Such close proximity of two IgG molecules does not normally result from the random binding of IgG secreted by a single plasma cell. Therefore an anti-isotype antibody that reacts with the bound IgG is added to the Petri dish after the first hour of incubation. The dishes are incubated for an additional hour, at which time the complement is added, and the dishes are incubated for another hour (Figure 16-20b). This procedure, called the **indirect hemolytic plaque assay,** results in lysis of SRBCs to which IgM or IgG are bound. Subtraction of the number of plaques formed in the direct assay from the number formed in the indirect assay gives the number of IgG-secreting plasma cells, or **indirect PFC.** Since most of the antibody secreted during a primary response is IgM, the direct PFC is high and the indirect PFC is low. In contrast, a secondary response leads to a low direct PFC and a high indirect PFC, reflecting the switch from IgM to IgG secretion.

The hemolytic plaque assay also can be modified to quantitate plasma cells secreting antibodies directed against specific proteins, polysaccharides, or small haptens. In this case, the animal is immunized with the desired antigen, but before the SRBCs are mixed with the isolated spleen cells, they are coated with the immunizing antigen. The induced antibody binds to these antigen-coated SRBCs, which are lysed after the complement is added (Figure 16-20c). Uncoated SRBCs can serve as a control, since they do not lyse in response to antibody secreted from the antigen-specific plasma cells.

ELISPOT ASSAY

In another modification of the Jerne plaque-forming assay, called the **"Elispot assay,"** plasma cells can be quantitated without use of SRBCs. In this assay, the

TABLE 16-4

COMPARISON OF PRIMARY AND SECONDARY ANTIBODY RESPONSES

PROPERTY	PRIMARY RESPONSE	SECONDARY RESPONSE
Responding B cell	Naive (virgin) B cell	Memory B cell
Lag period following antigen administration	Generally 4–7 days	Generally 1–3 days
Time of peak response	7–10 days	3–5 day
Magnitude of peak antibody response	Varies depending on antigen	Generally 100–1000 times higher than primary response
Isotype produced	IgM predominates early in the response	IgG predominates
Antigens	Thymus-dependent and thymus-independent	Thymus-dependent
Antibody affinity	Lower	Higher

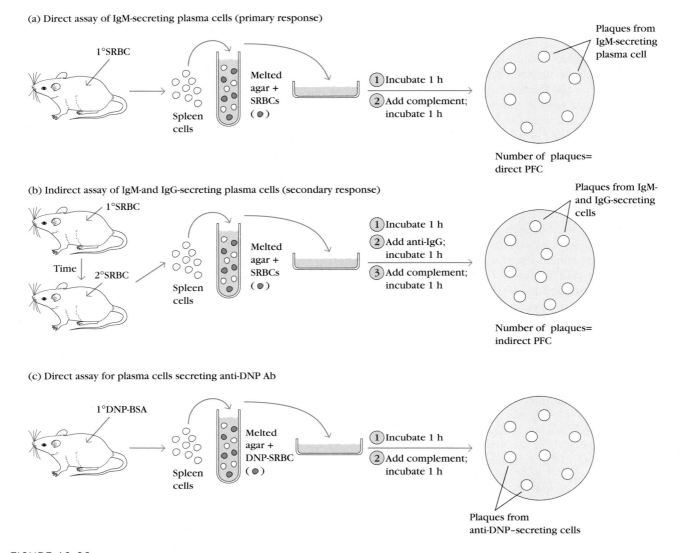

FIGURE 16-20

Hemolytic plaque assays. (a) A direct assay detects IgM-secreting plasma cells, which are predominant in a primary response. (b) In an indirect assay, which detects both IgM- and IgG-secreting plasma cells, antibodies against mouse IgG are added so that complement-mediated lysis of IgG-SRBC complexes will occur. By subtracting the direct PFC from the indirect PFC, the number of IgG-secreting plasma cells can be determined. In a secondary response, the indirect PFC is high and the direct PFC is low. (c) The response to immunization with antigens other than SRBCs can be determined with the hemolytic plaque assay if the immunizing protein or hapten is coupled to SRBCs.

antigen-primed lymphocytes are incubated in a Petri dish to which antigen has been bound. As the plasma cells secrete antibody, it binds to antigen in the vicinity of the plasma cell. After removal of the cells, the bound antibody is visualized by an ELISA assay in which the dish is first incubated with enzyme-labeled anti-Ig followed by an appropriate substrate. The enzyme-substrate reaction produces a colored spot, allowing enumeration of the plasma cells (see Figure 6-14a).

Humoral Response to Hapten-Carrier Conjugates

As discussed in Chapter 4, when animals are immunized with small organic compounds (**haptens**) conjugated to large proteins (**carriers**), the conjugate induces a humoral immune response with antibodies formed both to hapten epitopes and to unaltered epitopes on the carrier protein. Since the chemical conjugation allows multiple

TABLE 16-5

COMMON HAPTEN-CARRIER CONJUGATES USED IN IMMUNOLOGIC RESEARCH

HAPTEN-CARRIER ACRONYM	HAPTEN	CARRIER PROTEIN
DNP-BGG	Dinitrophenol	Bovine gamma-globulin
TNP-BSA	Trinitrophenyl	Bovine serum albumin
NIP-KLH	5-Nitrophenyl acetic acid	Keyhole limpet hemocyanin
ARS-OVA	Azophenylarsonate	Ovalbumin
LAC-HGG	Phenyllactoside	Human gamma-globulin

molecules of a single hapten to be coupled to the carrier protein and since the position of the hapten is easily accessible to the B cell's membrane-bound antibody, the hapten functions as the immunodominant B-cell epitope (see Figure 4-12).

Hapten-carrier conjugates provided immunologists with an ideal system for studying cellular interactions involved in the humoral response. Unlike complex proteins, whose B-cell epitopes are often conformational sequences dependent on the tertiary structure of the protein, a hapten constitutes a defined B-cell epitope that can be presented to B cells on different protein carriers. Studies with hapten-carrier conjugates demonstrated that the generation of a humoral antibody response requires associative recognition by T_H cells and B cells, each recognizing different epitopes on the same antigen.

A variety of different hapten-carrier conjugates have been used in immunologic research (Table 16-5). After an animal has been immunized with a hapten-carrier conjugate, the humoral response to the hapten is assessed with a modified hemolytic plaque assay, with hapten-conjugated SRBCs as the indicator cells (see Figure 16-20c). A direct hemolytic plaque assay is used to quantitate plasma cells secreting IgM antihapten antibody, and an indirect assay is used to quantitate plasma cells secreting IgG antihapten antibody, an indicator of a secondary response.

One of the earliest findings with hapten-carrier conjugates was that a hapten had to be chemically coupled to a larger carrier molecule to induce a humoral response to the hapten. If an animal was immunized with both hap-

ten and carrier separately, no plasma cells specific for the hapten were generated. A second important observation was that in order to generate a secondary antibody response to a hapten, the animal had to be immunized with the same hapten-carrier conjugate used for the primary immunization. If the secondary immunization was with the same hapten but conjugated to a different, unrelated carrier, no secondary antihapten response occurred. This phenomenon, called the **carrier effect,** could be circumvented by priming the animal separately with the unrelated carrier (Table 16-6).

Similar experiments conducted with an adoptive-transfer system showed that hapten-primed cells and carrier-primed cells were distinct populations. In these studies one mouse was primed with the DNP-BSA conjugate and another was primed with the unrelated carrier BGG, which was not conjugated to the hapten. In one experiment, spleen cells from both mice were mixed and injected into a lethally irradiated syngeneic recipient. When this mouse was challenged with DNP conjugated to the unrelated carrier BGG, there was a secondary antihapten response, as indicated by a positive hemolytic plaque assay to DNP (Figure 16-21a). In a second experiment, spleen cells from the BGG-immunized mice were treated with anti-T-cell antiserum (anti-Thy-1) and complement to remove the T cells. When this T-cell–depleted sample was mixed with the DNP-BSA–primed spleen cells and injected into an irradiated mouse, no secondary antihapten response was observed upon immunizing with DNP-BGG (Figure 16-21b). However, similar treatment

TABLE 16-6

SECONDARY HUMORAL RESPONSE TO DNP IN MICE IMMUNIZED WITH VARIOUS COMBINATIONS OF DNP AND CARRIER PROTEIN*

PRIMARY IMMUNIZATION	SECONDARY IMMUNIZATION	SECONDARY ANTI-DNP PFC
DNP-BSA	DNP-BSA	+
DNP + BSA	DNP + BSA	−
DNP-BSA	DNP + BSA	−
DNP-BSA	DNP-BGG	−
DNP-BSA + BGG	DNP-BGG	+

* Following the secondary immunization, spleen cells were isolated and an indirect hemolytic plaque assay was performed to determine the secondary anti-DNP PFC, using DNP-SRBCs as the indicator cells.

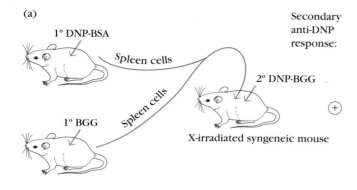

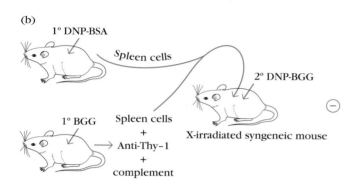

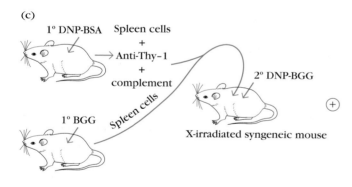

FIGURE 16-21

Adoptive-transfer experiments demonstrating that hapten-primed and carrier-primed cells are separate populations. (a) X-irradiated syngeneic mice reconstituted with spleen cells from both DNP-BSA–primed mice and BGG-primed mice and challenged with DNP-BGG generated a secondary anti-DNP response. (b) Removal of T cells from the BGG-primed spleen cells, by treatment with anti-Thy-1 antiserum, abolished the secondary anti-DNP response. (c) Removal of T cells from the DNP-BSA–primed spleen cells had no effect on the secondary response to DNP. These experiments show that carrier-primed cells are T cells and hapten-primed cells are B cells. The secondary anti-DNP response was measured with an indirect hemolytic plaque assay.

of the DNP-BSA–primed spleen cells did not abolish the secondary antihapten response to DNP-BGG (Figure 16-21c). Later experiments, in which antisera were used to specifically deplete CD4$^+$ or CD8$^+$ T cells, showed that the removal of the CD4$^+$ T-cell subpopulation primed with the second carrier abolished the carrier effect. These experiments demonstrate that the response of hapten-primed B cells to the hapten-carrier conjugate requires the presence of carrier-primed CD4$^+$ T$_H$ cells specific for carrier epitopes. (It is important to keep in mind that the B-cell response is not limited to the hapten determinant; in fact some B cells do react to epitopes on the carrier, but because the assay system uses hapten-conjugated SRBCs, it measures only the antihapten response.)

The experiments with hapten-carrier conjugates revealed that both T$_H$ cells and B cells must recognize antigenic determinants on the same molecule for B-cell activation to occur. This feature of the T- and B-cell interaction in the humoral response is called **associative, or linked, recognition.** The conclusions drawn from hapten-carrier experiments apply generally to the humoral response and support the requirement for T-cell help in B-cell activation discussed in Chapter 8. In the case of a protein such as BSA, for example, the B cell binds to B-cell epitopes on the protein via its membrane-bound antibody. After binding, the BSA is internalized, processed in the endocytic processing pathway, and presented as a processed peptide together with a class II MHC molecule on the membrane of the B cell. An activated T$_H$ cell then recognizes the processed peptide together with the class II MHC molecule, leading to activation and proliferation of the B cell (see Figure 8-10).

The hapten-carrier systems also highlight the important differences in epitope recognition by B and T cells, which were discussed in Chapter 4. B cells recognize the hapten determinant because it is accessible and hydrophilic, of a size comparable to that of the antigen-binding sites on B cells, and present in multiple copies, making it the immunodominant B-cell epitope. T cells, in contrast, recognize certain internal, hydrophobic residues of the carrier that are displayed following antigen processing (together with class II MHC molecules) on the membrane of an antigen-presenting cell (see Table 4-4).

REGULATION OF THE IMMUNE EFFECTOR RESPONSE

Upon encountering an antigen, the immune system can either develop an immune response or enter a state of unresponsiveness called **tolerance.** The development of immunity or tolerance, both of which involve specific recognition of antigen by antigen-reactive T or B cells, needs to be carefully regulated since an inappropriate response—whether it be immunity to self-antigens or tolerance to a potential pathogen—can have serious and possibly life-threatening consequences.

Regulation of the immune response takes place in both the humoral and the cell-mediated branch. Every time an antigen is introduced, important regulatory decisions determine the branch of the immune system to be activated, the intensity of the response, and its duration. In previous chapters, we've seen that T_H1-like and T_H2-like cytokines help regulate which branch of the immune system is activated; cytokines also are critical in determining which antibody isotypes are produced. In the remainder of this chapter, other immune regulatory mechanisms are discussed. Greater knowledge about these regulatory events, which are still not well understood, may allow selective up-regulation or down-regulation of immune reactivity, when such fine-tuning would be desirable.

Antigen-Mediated Regulation

The immunologic history of an animal influences the quality and quantity of its immune response. A naive animal responds very differently than a previously primed animal to antigen challenge. Previous antigen encounter may have rendered the animal tolerant to the antigen or may have resulted in the formation of memory cells. In some cases the presence of a competing antigen can regulate the immune response to an unrelated antigen. This **antigenic competition** is illustrated by injecting mice with a competing antigen a day or two before immunization with a test antigen. As Table 16-7 reveals, the

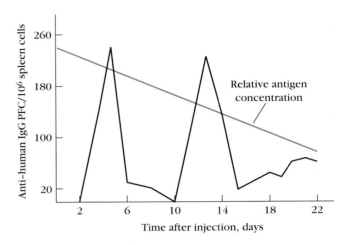

FIGURE 16-22

Following a single primary immunization of rabbits with human IgG, the number of splenic plasma cells secreting anti-human IgG antibodies showed a cyclical pattern despite the linear decrease in serum antigen concentration. This finding indicates that the immune response is not regulated solely by antigen concentration. [Adapted from C. G. Romball and W. O. Weigle, 1973, *J. Exp. Med.* **138**:1426.]

response to horse red blood cells (HRBCs) is severely reduced by prior immunization with sheep red blood cells (SRBCs) and vice versa. At the cellular level, a competing antigen may interfere with antigen presentation to and activation of T_H cells; alternatively, the immune response to the competing antigen may generate various cytokines that down-regulate a subsequent response.

Although antigen concentration is the primary regulator of the intensity of an immune response, other regulators operate at a coarse or fine level to contribute to the intensity and duration of the response. An early finding suggesting that a decline in antigen level is not solely responsible for immune regulation came from experiments of C. G. Romball and W. O. Weigle. They injected rabbits with a single dose of human IgG and then determined the number of plaque-forming plasma cells at various times. Although antigen concentrations declined in a linear fashion, the number of plasma cells generated in response to the antigen showed a cyclical response, peaking, declining, and peaking again several times (Figure 16-22). This cyclical response indicates that something other than antigen concentration must be regulating the response.

Antibody-Mediated Suppression

As in so many biochemical reactions subject to feedback inhibition by the end product, antibody exerts feedback

TABLE 16-7
ANTIGENIC COMPETITION BETWEEN SRBCS AND HRBCS

IMMUNIZING ANTIGEN		HEMOLYTIC PLAQUE ASSAY (DAY 8)*	
AG1 (DAY 0)	AG2 (DAY 3)	TEST AG	PFC/10^6 SPLEEN CELLS
None	HRBC	HRBC	205
SRBC	HRBC	HRBC	13
None	SRBC	SRBC	626
HRBC	SRBC	SRBC	78

* See Figure 16-20 for assay details.

inhibition on its own further production. If an animal is immunized with a specific antigen and is injected with preformed antibody to that same antigen just before or within 5 days after antigen priming, the immune response to the antigen is reduced as much as 100-fold.

One explanation for antibody-mediated suppression is that the passively administered antibody competes with antigen-reactive B cells for antigen, so that the B cells do not clonally expand. Evidence for such competition between passively administered antibody and antigen-reactive B cells comes from studies in which it took over 10 times more low-affinity anti-DNP antibody than high-affinity anti-DNP antibody to induce comparable suppression. Furthermore, the competition for antigen between passively administered antibody and antigen-reactive B cells drives the response toward higher affinity. Only the high-affinity antigen-reactive cells can compete successfully with the passively administered antibody for the available antigen. This process is similar to affinity maturation, which occurs in the course of an immune response as the antibody formed early in the response begins to bind to the antigen, decreasing its concentration so that only the high-affinity antigen-reactive cells are stimulated later in the response (see Table 8-4).

Because of antibody-mediated suppression, certain vaccines (e.g., those for measles and mumps) are not administered to infants before the age of 1 year. The level of naturally acquired maternal IgG that the fetus acquires by transplacental transfer remains high for about 6 months after birth. If an infant is immunized with the measles or mumps vaccine while this maternal antibody is still present, the humoral response is low and the production of memory cells is inadequate to confer long-lasting immunity.

Immune Complexes as Regulators

Preformed antigen-antibody complexes have been shown in some experiments to enhance and in others to suppress the immune response. These immune complexes may exert their effect by binding to Fc receptors on various cells. It has not yet been possible to predict the effect of immune-complex size on immune responsiveness. There is evidence suggesting that patients with malignant tumors often develop circulating immune complexes in which antibody is complexed with tumor antigens. These complexes have been shown to suppress the immune response in these patients.

Idiotype Regulation: The Network Theory

The enormous diversity of antibody and T-cell receptor (TCR) specificities that can be generated by the immune system is mind-boggling. Current estimates sug-

gest that the immune system is capable of generating on the order of 10^{11} distinct antibody specificities and 10^{15}–10^{18} distinct TCR specificities. Since a mouse produces only 10^8 lymphocytes per day, only a fraction of the potential repertoire is expressed during the lifetime of a mouse. Because antigen-specific antibodies and T-cell receptors are not expressed during fetal development of the immune system, their variable-region sequences can be recognized as nonself by the immune system.

In 1973 Niels Jerne proposed a conceptual theory, called the **network theory,** that predicted the consequences of immune-system recognition of self-antibody; for this work, Jerne was awarded a Nobel Prize in 1984. According to the network theory, as antibody is produced in response to an antigen, it in turn induces the formation of antibodies to its unique variable-region sequences. Jerne referred to each individual antigenic determinant of the variable region as an **idiotope.** Each antibody contains multiple idiotopes, and the sum of the individual idiotopes is called the **idiotype** of the antibody. In some cases, a particular idiotope and the actual antigen-combining site, which Jerne called the **paratope,** are identical; in other cases the idiotopes consist of variable-region sequences outside the antigen-binding site (Figure 16-23a).

The network theory proposes that during a humoral response the antibodies formed in response to the antigen in turn induce the formation of secondary antibodies to the individual idiotopes of the first (primary) antibody. The idiotype of the primary antibody (Ab-1) activates a network of B cells whose receptors recognize the individual idiotopes of Ab-1. These B cells then differentiate into plasma cells that secrete anti-idiotype antibody (Ab-2). The individual idiotopes of Ab-2 can then further extend the network by inducing production of an anti-anti-idiotype, or Ab-3 (Figure 16-23b). This antibody often resembles idiotopes of Ab-1, and the network begins to limit itself as decreased levels of antibody are produced in each successive activation.

Anti-idiotype regulation can also function within the T-cell branch of the immune system, since the $\alpha\beta$ and $\gamma\delta$ T-cell receptors have variable regions and are therefore capable of expressing idiotopes that can be recognized by other T or B cells. The idiotype network involving B and T cells represents a complex circuitry of interacting cells that functions either to enhance or to suppress immune activation. The complexity of the idiotype network has made it difficult to predict whether administration of anti-idiotype antibodies or T cells bearing anti-idiotype receptors will up-regulate or down-regulate immune responsiveness.

A central principle of the network theory is that some anti-idiotype antibody will be directed against the paratope and therefore will appear as the **internal image** of

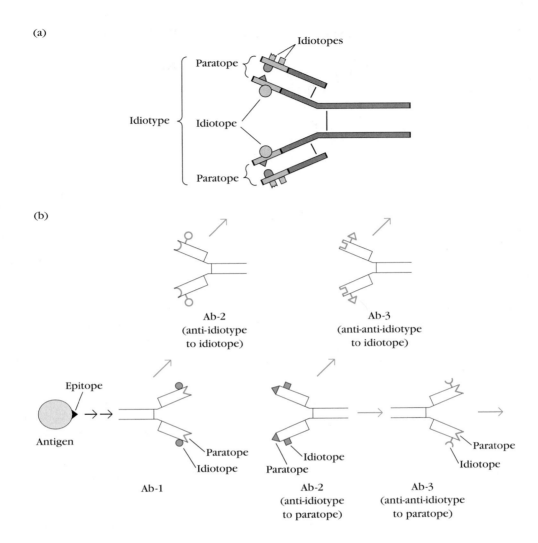

FIGURE 16-23

Network theory proposed by Niels Jerne. (a) Each antibody molecule expresses unique variable-region epitopes called idiotopes; the sum of the idiotopes is its idiotype. Idiotopes may coincide with the antigen-binding site, or paratope. (b) According to the network theory, the immune response to an antigen results in the formation of anti-idiotype antibodies specific for the individual idiotopes of the primary antibody (Ab-1). These anti-idiotype antibodies (Ab-2) in turn induce the formation of anti-anti-idiotype antibodies (Ab-3). A network of interacting antibodies is thus formed that serves to regulate the immune response. Note that the anti-idiotype antibody to the paratope of Ab-1 is an internal image of the original epitope on the antigen.

the original epitope on the antigen. For example, if mice are immunized with anti-insulin antibody (Ab-1), they produce anti-idiotype antibody (Ab-2) to Ab-1. Some of this anti-idiotype antibody will bind to the insulin-binding paratope of Ab-1. This anti-paratope antibody thus mimics the original insulin ligand; indeed this molecular mimicry is evidenced by the ability of the anti-paratope antibody to bind to the insulin receptor and induce glycolysis, just as insulin would. By re-expressing the image of the original epitope in the form of anti-paratope antibody, the immune system will continue to be activated even after the original antigen has been cleared; this may

ensure that sufficient clonal proliferation and memory-cell production occurs in response to the original epitope.

The regulatory activity of anti-idiotype antibody was first observed in vivo with a system involving a myeloma protein from BALB/c mice. Designated TEPC-15, this myeloma was found to be an IgA antibody specific for phosphorylcholine (PC). (Before techniques producing monoclonal antibodies were developed, immunologists depended on spontaneously occurring myelomas as sources of homogeneous antibodies.) Since phosphorylcholine is the major component of the pneumococcal cell-wall C polysaccharide, TEPC-15 could serve as an

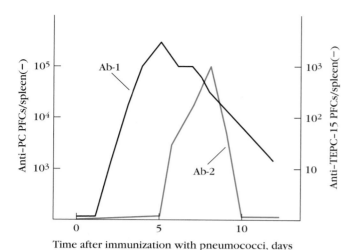

FIGURE 16-24

Production of anti-idiotype antibodies following immunization of BALB/c mice with pneumococci. Splenic plasma cells secreting antibody to the phosphorylcholine (PC) component of the pneumococcal cell wall (Ab-1 curve) were detected in a hemolytic plaque assay using PC-coated SRBCs. Splenic plasma cells secreting anti-idiotype antibody (Ab-2 curve) were detected using SRBCs coated with the myeloma protein TEPC-15, which is specific for PC. [Adapted from H. Cozenza, 1976, *Eur. J. Immunol.* **6**:114.]

antigen to assess anti-idiotype antibody production in mice that had been immunized with pneumococci. When BALB/c mice were immunized with pneumococci, the number of plaque-forming plasma cells was determined in two hemolytic plaque assays (see Figure 16-20). The first assay detected plasma cells secreting antibody to PC by use of sheep red blood cells coated with PC as the test antigen; the second assay detected plasma cells secreting anti-idiotype antibody by use of SRBCs coated with TEPC-15. As Figure 16-24 reveals, a peak anti-PC PFC was reached about 4 days after immunization followed by a peak anti-idiotype PFC 4 days later. Note that the plots in Figure 16-24 are similar to the cyclical pattern of IgG production shown in Figure 16-22.

In addition to their possible role in immune regulation, anti-idiotype antibodies offer possibilities as vaccines. Immunization with anti-idiotype antibody theoretically provides a way for exposing an individual to an epitope, and thus inducing immunity, without risking exposure to a pathogen (see Chapter 18).

Neuroendocrine Regulation (Neuroimmunomodulation)

For centuries clinical observations have implicated psychosocial factors in susceptibility to disease. Reports abound suggesting a relationship between stress and immune function. Large numbers of popular books have appeared suggesting that psychoneuroimmune interactions could provide a biological mechanism for resistance or susceptibility to disease. Research in this area has been hampered by several limitations: The interdisciplinary nature of this area requires a breadth of expertise in immunology, neurobiology, and endocrinology that few people have, and the quantification of stress in general is fraught with numerous methodological difficulties. Nevertheless the past decade has witnessed a virtual explosion of interdisciplinary research that has documented the effects of the neural and endocrine systems on the activity of the immune system. The interaction appears to be two directional; that is, neuroendocrine mechanisms regulate the immune response, and an active immune response induces changes in both neural and endocrine functions (Figure 16-25).

The central nervous system interacts with the immune system through autonomic innervation of lymphoid organs and through neuroendocrine mediators. The autonomic nervous system consists of motor neurons that conduct nerve impulses from the brain stem or spinal cord to heart muscle tissue and to various smooth muscles and glandular epithelial tissue. Composed of the sympathetic and parasympathetic systems, the autonomic nervous system serves to regulate the body's involuntary functions. Often both parasympathetic and sympathetic systems innervate an organ, exerting opposite effects on the organ. For example, the parasympathetic system slows down the heartbeat, whereas the sympathetic system accelerates the heartbeat; the ratio between sympathetic and parasympathetic impulses therefore determines the rate of heartbeat. During periods of stress (when strong

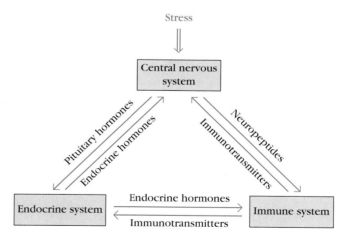

FIGURE 16-25

Schematic overview of the relationships between the neuroendocrine system and the immune system. See text for discussion. [Adapted from D. N. Khansari et al., 1990, *Immunol. Today* **11**:170.]

emotions such as anger or fear are elicited), the sympathetic nervous system predominates. The sympathetic system releases two **neurotransmitters:** acetylcholine from cholinergic fibers and norepinephrine from adrenergic fibers.

Both primary and secondary lymphoid organs are innervated by the autonomic nervous system, particularly by adrenergic sympathetic nerve fibers, which often end in regions where lymphocytes are clustered. For example, adrenergic fibers crisscross the stromal-cell matrix of the bone marrow and are scattered throughout the cortex and medulla of the thymus. Similarly, a variety of compartments within lymph nodes and spleen are innervated by adrenergic fibers. In some regions, such as the periarteriolar lymphatic sheath (PALS), these nerve fibers have been shown to form intimate anatomic associations with T lymphocytes and interdigitating dendritic cells.

During periods of stress the close functional relation between the nervous system and the endocrine system is highlighted. For example, a number of neuroendocrine responses are commonly observed during periods of stress, regardless of the nature of the stress. During a stress response the hypothalamus acts on the anterior pituitary gland to secrete adrenocorticotropin (ACTH), which then acts upon the adrenal cortex inducing secretion of glucocorticoids (including hydrocortisone). In addition, the sympathetic nervous system and adrenal medulla are stimulated, resulting in production of the neurotransmitters acetylcholine and norepinephrine, and release of epinephrine from the adrenal medulla. Other neuroendocrine mediators (e.g., growth hormones, prolactin, melatonin, endorphins, and enkephalins) also are associated with the stress response.

Many of the neuroendocrine and neurotransmitter substances that are released during a stress response have been shown to either enhance or suppress the immune response (Table 16-8). Lymphocytes have receptors for a variety of neuroendocrine substances including ACTH,

TABLE 16-8

NEUROENDOCRINE FACTORS WITH IMMUNOMODULATORY PROPERTIES

FACTOR	ACTION*	IMMUNE RESPONSE AFFECTED
Glucocorticoids (hydrocortisone)	S	Antibody production, NK-cell activity, cytokine production
Catecholamines (epinephrine)	S	Lymphocyte proliferation in response to mitogens
Acetylcholine	E	Number of lymphocytes and macrophages in bone marrow
β-Endorphin	E/S	Antibody production, activation of macrophages and T cells
Enkephalin	E/S	T-cell activation (enhanced at low dose; suppressed at high dose)
Prolactin	E	Macrophage activation, IL-2 production
Growth hormone	E	Antibody production, macrophage activation, IL-2 modulation
VIP	S/E	Cytokine production
Melatonin	E	Mixed-lymphocyte reaction (MLR), antibody production
ACTH	E/S	Cytokine production, NK-cell activity, antibody production, macrophage activation
Somatostatin	S/E	Plaque-forming count, response to mitogens
Sex hormones	S/E	Lymphocyte transformation, mixed-lymphocyte reaction

* E = enhancement; S = suppression
SOURCE: Adapted from D. N. Khansari et al., 1990, *Immunol. Today* **11**:170.

acetylcholine, epinephrine, vasoactive intestinal peptide (VIP), substance P, prolactin, growth hormone, somatostatin, β-endorphin, and enkephalin. Perhaps the best-studied neuroendocrine substance is the glucocorticoid hydrocortisone, which has been shown to exhibit pronounced immunosuppressive effects on the immune response. Other neuroendocrine substances have been shown to have various effects on the immune system ranging from marked immunosuppression to immunopotentiation.

Conversely, the immune system is able to modulate the neural and endocrine systems. A number of thymic hormones, including thymosin and thymopoietin, have been shown to induce increased production of ACTH by the pituitary. Furthermore, a number of cytokines have been shown to modulate neural or endocrine responses. IL-1, for example, induces a constellation of effects that modulate the hypothalamus fever response, ACTH production by the pituitary, and glucocorticoid production by the adrenal cortex. In addition, some evidence indicates that cells of the immune system can produce a variety of neuropeptides and neuroendocrine hormones. Thus an interacting network exists between the nervous system, endocrine system, and immune system and changes in any one system can modulate the activity of the other systems.

The evidence that the neural and endocrine systems regulate the immune system raises the possibility that psychologic factors may also impact on immune function. A number of studies have suggested that a positive mental state is associated with a longer survival time for both cancer and AIDS patients. In contrast, patients hospitalized for major depression have been found to have significantly reduced immune responses to various mitogens. Perhaps the most provocative experiments indicating a relation between psychologic factors and immune function comes from the work indicating that behavioral conditioning can modify the immune response.

For instance, in these studies by R. Ader and N. Cohen, rats were injected with the immunosuppressive drug cyclophosphamide and at the same time were fed saccharin-flavored water (a conditioning stimulus). The rats were subsequently immunized with sheep red blood cells and antibody titers were later measured. As expected, the antibody response was suppressed by the cyclophosphamide. However, when the animals were later fed saccharin-flavored water (the conditioning stimulus) and were then reimmunized with SRBC, the immune response was suppressed compared with that of control animals that had received the initial treatment but had not been re-exposed to the conditioning stimulus at the time of the secondary injection.

A few studies suggest that conditioning also may be able to modify the immune response in humans. D. H. Bovbjerg and colleagues studied the immune function of 20 ovarian cancer patients undergoing chemotherapy. A blood sample was drawn from each patient at home several days before each chemotherapy visit and a second sample was drawn at the hospital just prior to chemotherapy. Cell counts were the same in both blood samples, but the proliferative response to mitogen stimulation in the sample taken just prior to chemotherapy was significantly reduced. Thus, anticipation of chemotherapy in the hospital setting appears to have reduced the immune function in these women.

In another study healthy volunteers received the tuberculin skin test once a month for 6 months. The test was administered by injecting PPD from a green vial into one arm and saline from a red vial into the other arm. Each volunteer was skin-test positive, developing a positive skin test only in the arm receiving the PPD. After 6 months the colored vials were switched, so that the PPD was now in the red vial and the saline was in the green vial; neither the experimenter nor the subject was aware of the switch. The results revealed a significant reduction in swelling and redness elicited by the PPD compared with the six previous times.

SUMMARY

1. The cell-mediated branch of the immune system involves three types of antigen-specific effector cells: $CD4^+$ T_H1 and T_H2 and cytotoxic T lymphocytes (CTLs). Compared with naive T_H and T_C cells, the effector cells are more easily activated, express higher levels of cell-adhesion molecules, exhibit different trafficking patterns, and produce both soluble and membrane effector molecules (see Tables 16-1 and 16-2).

2. Phase I of the CTL-mediated immune response involves the activation and differentiation of T_C cells, called CTL precursors (CTL-Ps). Interaction of a CTL-P with an antigen–class I MHC complex leads to expression of IL-2 receptors and of IL-2 on the activated CTL-P. IL-2 produced by the CTL-P itself and/or by proliferating T_H cells than binds to the IL-2 receptors, inducing proliferation and differentiation of the CTL-P into an effector CTL (see Figure 16-1).

3. Phase II of the CTL-mediated response involves several steps: recognition of specific target cells bearing antigen and class I MHC molecules, formation of CTL/target-cell conjugates, reorientation of cytoplasmic granules within the CTL towards the region of close membrane interaction with the target cell, release of the granular contents within the zone of cel-

lular adhesion, formation of pores in the target-cell membrane, dissociation of the CTL from the target cell, and the subsequent destruction of the target cell (see Figure 16-4). Perforin monomers released from the CTL granules insert into target-cell membrane and polymerize, forming pores (see Figure 16-7). Target-cell killing by some CTLs appears to occur via apoptosis induced by soluble granzymes released from the CTL or the membrane-bound Fas ligand (see Figure 16-8).

4. Various nonspecific cytotoxic cells also can kill target cells without having to interact with antigen-MHC complexes. NK cells, for example, mediate lysis of tumor cells and virus-infected cells by perforin-induced pore formation similar to the mechanism employed by CTLs. The presence of relatively high levels of class I MHC molecules on normal cells appears to protect them against NK cell–mediated killing (see Figure 16-11). NK cells and several other types of nonspecific cytotoxic cells can bind to the Fc region of antibody on target cells and subsequently release lytic enzymes, perforin, or TNF, which damage the target-cell membrane (see Figure 16-12). This process, called antibody-dependent cell-mediated cytotoxicity (ADCC), thus directs nonspecific cytotoxic cells to specific target cells.

5. Cell-mediated immunity involving delayed-type hypersensitivity plays an important role in host defense against intracellular pathogens. T_{DTH} cells, which differentiate from activated T_H cells, secrete a number of T_H1-like cytokines that cause macrophages to accumulate and to become activated. The activated macrophages, which are more effective killers of intracellular pathogens, are the primary effector cells in the DTH response (see Figure 16-15).

6. The kinetics of antibody formation and other properties of primary and secondary humoral responses differ (see Figure 16-19 and Table 16-4). The primary response is marked by a long lag period, a logarithmic rise in antibody formation, a short plateau, and then a relatively rapid decline. IgM is the first antibody class to be secreted, followed by IgG later in the primary response. The secondary response has a shorter lag period, a more rapid logarithmic phase, a longer plateau, and a slower decline than the primary response. Little IgM is produced in the secondary response, which is characterized by production of IgG or other isotypes and a higher average antibody affinity for antigen.

7. Cytokines, antigen, antibody, and immune complexes all play a role in regulating the immune response. Despite a linear decline in the antigen level following antigen exposure, plasma cells and antibody specific for a given antigen appear cyclically following antigen exposure (see Figure 16-22), indicating that antigen concentration is not the only regulating factor. Antibody may suppress the immune response by binding to antigen and preventing further B-cell activation. Immune complexes have been shown to both increase and decrease the immune response to an antigen.

8. The unique variable-region amino acid sequences of antibodies and T-cell receptors are recognized as antigenic determinants by the immune system. Thus the secreted antibodies and clonally expanded T-cell receptors generated in an immune response can in turn elicit anti-idiotype antibodies. According to the network theory, a series (or network) of anti-idiotype antibodies are induced during an immune response; these anti-idiotype antibodies act to up-regulate or down-regulate the response (see Figure 16-23).

9. Several of the in vitro assays of cell-mediated and humoral immune responses have critical roles in immunologic research. The one-way mixed-lymphocyte reaction (MLR) measures the proliferation of T_H cells in response to allogeneic stimulator cells that have been x-irradiated or treated with mitomycin (see Figure 16-13). The activity of CTLs can be assessed with the cell-mediated lympholysis (CML) assay (see Figure 16-14). The hemolytic plaque assay is used to determine the number of antibody-secreting plasma cells; it can be modified to detect only plasma cells secreting a particular antigen (see Figure 16-20).

REFERENCES

AKBAR, A. N., AND M. SALMON. 1995. Selection and survival of activated lymphocytes. *Sci. Am. Sci Med.* (March/April):48.

ARMITAGE, R. J., W. C. FANSLOW, L. STROCKBINE, ET AL. 1992. Molecular and biological characterization of a murine ligand for CD40. *Nature* **357**:80.

ATKINSON, E. A., AND R. C. BLEACKLEY. 1995. Mechanisms of lysis by cytotoxic T cells. *Crit. Rev. Immunol.* **15**:359.

BERKE, G. 1995. Unlocking the secrets of CTL and NK cells. *Immunol. Today* **16**:343.

BOVBJERG, D. H., ET AL. 1990. Anticipatory imune suppression and nausea in women receiving cyclin chemotherapy for ovarian cancer. *J. Consult. Clin. Psych.* **58**:153–157.

CLARK, E. A., AND P. J. L. LANE. 1991. Regulation of human B-cell activation and adhesion. *Annu. Rev. Immunol.* **9**:97.

Correa, I., and D. H. Raulet. 1995. Binding of diverse peptides to MHC class I molecules inhibits target cell lysis by activated natural killer cells. *Immunity* **2**:61.

Croft, M. 1994. Activation of naive, memory and effector T cells. *Curr. Opin. Immunol.* **6**:431.

Gray, D. 1993. Immunological memory. *Annu. Rev. Immunol.* **11**:49.

Gray, D. 1994. Regulation of immunological memory. *Curr. Opin. Immunol.* **6**:425.

Griffiths, G. M. 1995. The cell biology of CTL killing. *Curr. Opin. Immunol.* **7**:343

Henkart, P.A., and M.V. Sitkovsky. 1994. Two ways to kill target cells. *Curr. Biol.* **4**:923.

Kupfer, A., and S. J. Singer. 1991. The specific interaction of helper T cells and antigen-presenting B cells. IV. Membrane and cytoskeleton reorganizations in the bound T cell as a function of antigen dose. *J. Exp. Med.* **170**:1697.

Parker, D. C. 1993. T cell–dependent B-cell activation. *Annu. Rev. Immunol.* **11**:331.

Peter, P. J., et al. 1989. Molecules relevant for T cell–target cell interaction are present in cytolytic granules of human T lymphocytes. *Eur. J. Immunol.* **19**:1469.

Pober, J. S., and R. S. Cotran. 1990. Cytokines and endothelial cell biology. *Physiol. Rev.* **70**:427.

Rahemtulla, A., et al. 1991. Normal development and function of CD8+ cells but markedly decreased helper cell activity in mice lacking CD4. *Nature* **353**:180.

Reth, M., et al. 1991. The B-cell antigen receptor complex. *Immunol. Today* **12**:196.

Rodewald, H. R., et al. 1992. A population of early fetal thymocytes expressing FcγRII/III contains precursors of T lymphocytes and natural killer cells. *Cell* **69**:139.

Rousset, F., E. Barcia, and J. Banchereau. 1991. Cytokine-induced proliferation and immunoglobulin production of human B lymphocytes triggered through their CD40 antigen. *J. Exp. Med.* **173**:705.

Sher, A., and R. L. Coffman. 1992. Regulation of immunity to parasites by T cells and T cell-derived cytokines. *Annu. Rev. Immunol.* **10**:385.

Smyth, M. J., and J. A. Trapani. 1995. Granzymes: exogenous proteinases that induce target cell apoptosis. *Immunol. Today* **16**(4):202.

Snapper, C. M., and J. J. Mond. 1993. Towards a comprehensive view of immunoglobulin class switching. *Immunol. Today* **14**:15.

Sprent, J. 1994. T and B memory cells. *Cell* **76**:315.

Squier, M. K. T., and J. J. Cohen. 1994. Cell-mediated cytotoxic mechanisms. *Curr. Opin. Immunol.* **6**:447.

Szakal, A. K., M. H. Kosco, and J. G. Tew. 1989. Microanatomy of lymphoid tissue during humoral immune responses: structure-function relationships. *Annu. Rev. Immunol.* **7**:91.

Tartaglia, L. A., et al. 1993. Tumor necrosis factor's cytotoxic activity is signaled by the p55 TNF receptor. *Cell* **73**:213.

Taub, D. D., et al. 1993. Preferential migration of activated CD4+ and CD8+ T cells in response to MIP-1a and MIP-1b. *Science* **260**:355.

Tschopp, J., and M. Nabholz. 1990. Perforin-mediated target-cell lysis by cytolytic T lymphocytes. *Annu. Rev. Immunol.* **8**:279.

Versteeg, R. 1992. NK cells and T cells: mirror images? *Immunol. Today* **13**:244.

Vitetta, E. S., et al. 1991. Memory B and T cells. *Annu. Rev. Immunol.* **9**:193.

Yokoyama, W. M. 1995. Natural killer cell receptors. *Curr. Opin. Immunol.* **7**:110.

STUDY QUESTIONS

1. Indicate whether each of the following statements is true or false. If you believe a statement is false, explain why.

a. The indirect hemolytic plaque assay detects only IgG-secreting plasma cells.

b. Cytokines can regulate which branch of the immune system is activated.

c. Immunization with a hapten-carrier conjugate results in production of antibodies to both hapten and carrier epitopes.

d. All the antibodies secreted by a single plasma cell have the same idiotype and isotype.

e. If mice are immunized with HRBCs and then are immunized a day later with SRBCs, the antibody response to the SRBCs will be much higher than that achieved in control mice immunized only with SRBCs.

f. Anti-idiotype antibody appears as the internal image of the original antigen.

g. Both CTLs and NK cells release perforin after interacting with target cells.

h. The idiotype of an antibody molecule is composed of multiple idiotopes.

i. Antigen activation of naive CTL-Ps requires a co-stimulatory signal delivered by interaction of CD28 and B7.

j. TEPC-15 is an anti-idiotype antibody induced in the immune response to the phosphorylcholine determinant of pneumococcal polysaccharide.

2. You have a monoclonal antibody specific for LFA-1. You perform CML assays of a CTL clone, using target cells for which the clone is specific, in the presence and absence of this antibody. Predict the relative amounts of ^{51}Cr released in the two assays. Explain your answer.

3. You decide to co-culture lymphocytes from the strains listed in the table below in order to observe the mixed-lymphocyte reaction (MLR). In each case, indicate which lymphocyte population(s) you would expect to proliferate.

POPULATION 1	POPULATION 2	PROLIFERATION
C57BL/6 (H-2^b)	CBA (H-2^k)	
C57BL/6 (H-2^b)	CBA (H-2^k) mitomycin C-treated	
C57BL/6 (H-2^b)	(CBA × C57BL/6) F$_1$ (H-2$^{k/b}$)	
C57BL/6 (H-2^b)	C57L (H-2^b)	

4. Four mice are immunized with antigen under the conditions listed below (a–d). In each case, indicate whether the induced serum antibodies will have high affinity or low affinity and be largely IgM or IgG.

a. A primary response to a low antigen dose

b. A secondary response to a low antigen dose

c. A primary response to a high antigen dose

d. A secondary response to a high antigen dose

5. In the mixed-lymphocyte reaction (MLR), the uptake of [^{3}H]thymidine often is used to assess cell proliferation.

a. Which cell type proliferates in the MLR?

b. How could you prove the identity of the proliferating cell?

c. Explain why production of IL-2 also can be used to assess cell proliferation in the MLR.

6. Three groups of mice were immunized according to the schedule shown in the accompanying table. Spleen cells were isolated from the immunized mice, and the number of plaque-forming cells was determined; the direct and indirect PFC for each group are listed below.

IMMUNIZATION SCHEDULE	DIRECT PFC/10^6 SPLEEN CELLS	INDIRECT PFC/10^6 SPLE\EN CELLS
(A) 1° DNP-BSA	310	343
(B) 1° DNP-BSA 2° DNP-BSA	62	4060
(C) 1° DNP-BSA 2° DNP-BGG	366	386

a. Which assays are used to measure a primary (1°) and secondary (2°) plaque-forming response? Describe each assay.

b. Calculate the number of IgM-secreting and IgG-secreting plasma cells/10^6 spleen cells for each group of mice.

c. Why is the indirect PFC so much higher than the direct PFC for group B but not for group A or C?

7. Indicate whether each of the properties listed below is exhibited by T$_H$ cells, CTLs, both T$_H$ cells and CTLs, or neither cell type.

a. _____ Can make IL-1

b. _____ Can make IL-2

c. _____ Is class I MHC restricted

d. _____ Expresses CD8

e. _____ Is required for B-cell activation

f. _____ Is cytotoxic for target cells

g. _____ Is the main proliferating cell in an MLR

h. _____ Is the effector cell in a CML assay

i. _____ Is class II MHC restricted

j. _____ Expresses CD4

k. _____ Is the primary effector cell in a DTH response

l. _____ Expresses CD3

m. _____ Adheres to target cells via LFA-1

n. _____ Can express the IL-2 receptor

o. _____ Expresses the ab T-cell receptor

p. _____ Is the principal target of HIV

q. _____ Responds to soluble antigens alone

r. _____ Produces perforin

s. _____ Expresses the CD40 ligand on its surface

8. Mice from several different inbred strains were infected with LCM virus, and several days later their spleen cells were isolated. The ability of the primed spleen cells to lyse LCM-infected, ^{51}Cr-labeled target cells from various strains was determined. In the accompanying table, indicate with a (+) or (−) whether the spleen cells listed in the left column would cause ^{51}Cr release from the target cells listed in the headings across the top of the table.

9. A mouse is infected with influenza virus. How could you assess whether the mouse has T_H and T_C cells specific for influenza?

For use with Question 8.

SOURCE OF PRIMED SPLEEN CELLS	^{51}Cr RELEASE FROM LCM-INFECTED TARGET CELLS			
	B10.D2 (H-2^d)	B10 (H-2^b)	B10.BR (H-2^k)	(BALB/C × B10) F$_1$ (H-2$^{b/d}$)
B10D2 (H-2^d)				
B10 (H-2^b)				
BALB/c (H-2^d)				
(BALB/c × B10) (H-2$^{b/d}$)				

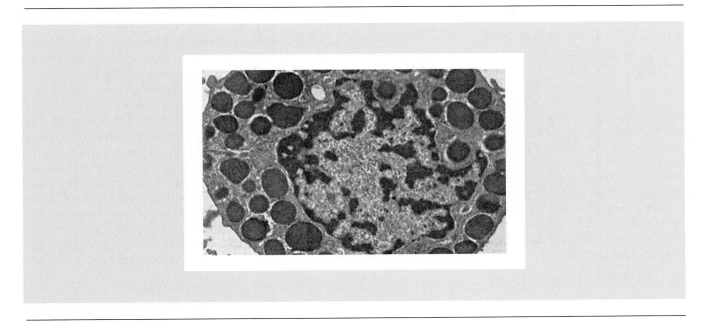

HYPERSENSITIVE REACTIONS

An immune response evokes a battery of effector molecules that act to remove antigen by various mechanisms discussed in previous chapters. Generally, these effector molecules induce a subclinical, localized inflammatory response that eliminates antigen without extensive tissue damage to the host. Under certain circumstances, however, this inflammatory response can have deleterious effects, resulting in significant tissue damage or even death. Such an immune response is termed **hypersensitivity** or **allergy**. Although hypersensitivity denotes an increased response, the response is not always heightened but may, instead, reflect an inappropriate immune response to an antigen. Hypersensitive reactions may develop in the course of either humoral or cell-mediated responses.

Reactions within the humoral branch are initiated by antibody or antigen-antibody complexes and are termed **immediate hypersensitivity** because the symptoms manifest within minutes or hours following an encounter with antigen by a sensitized recipient. Three types of such reactions are commonly recognized. Reactions within the cell-mediated branch are initiated by T$_{DTH}$ cells and are referred to as **delayed-type hypersensitivity** (DTH) in reference to the delay of symptoms for days following antigen exposure. Although DTH reactions, as discussed in Chapter 16, provide an important line of defense against intracellular pathogens, they sometimes cause extensive tissue damage that is pathologic and truly hypersensitive. This chapter examines the mechanisms and consequences of the four primary types of hypersensitive reactions.

GELL AND COOMBS CLASSIFICATION

Several types of hypersensitive reactions can be distinguished, reflecting differences in the effector molecules generated in the course of the reaction. In immediate hypersensitive reactions, different antibody isotypes induce different immune effector molecules. IgE antibodies, for example, induce mast cell degranulation with release of histamine and other biologically active molecules. IgG and IgM antibodies, on the other hand, induce hypersensitive reactions by activating complement. The effector molecules in these reactions are the membrane-attack complex and such complement split products as C3a, C4a, and C5a. In delayed-type hypersensitivity reactions, the effector molecules are various cytokines secreted by T_{DTH} cells.

As it became clear that different immune mechanisms can give rise to hypersensitive reactions, P. G. H. Gell and R. R. A. Coombs proposed a classification scheme in which hypersensitive reactions are divided into four types (I, II, III, and IV), each involving distinct mechanisms, cells, and mediator molecules. These are summarized in Table 17-1. This classification scheme has served an important function in identifying the mechanistic differences among various hypersensitive reactions. But it is important to point out that a great deal more complexity exists due to a vast array of secondary effects that blur the boundaries of the classification scheme.

TABLE 17-1

GELL AND COOMBS CLASSIFICATION OF HYPERSENSITIVE REACTIONS

TYPE	DESCRIPTIVE NAME	INITIATION TIME	MECHANISM	TYPICAL MANIFESTATIONS
IMMEDIATE REACTIONS				
Type 1	IgE-mediated hypersensitivity	2–30 min	Ag induces cross-linkage of IgE bound to mast cells and basophils with release of vasoactive mediators	Systemic anaphylaxis Localized anaphylaxis: Hay fever Asthma Hives Food allergies Eczema
Type II	Antibody-mediated cytotoxic hypersensitivity	5–8 h	Ab directed against cell-surface antigens mediates cell destruction via complement activation or ADCC	Blood-transfusion reactions Erythroblastosis fetalis Autoimmune hemolytic anemia
Type III	Immune complex–mediated hypersensitivity	2–8 h	Ag-Ab complexes deposited in various tissues induce complement activation and an ensuing inflammatory response	Localized Arthus reaction Generalized reactions: Serum sickness Glomerulonephritis Rheumatoid arthritis Systemic lupus erythematosus
DELAYED REACTIONS				
Type IV	Cell-mediated hypersensitivity	24–72 h	Sensitized T_{DTH} cells release cytokines that activate macrophages or T_C cells, which mediate direct cellular damage	Contact dermatitis Tubercular lesions Graft rejection

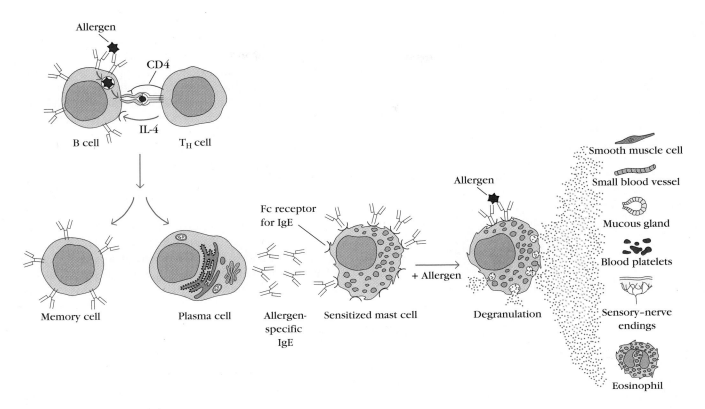

FIGURE 17-1

General mechanism underlying a type I hypersensitive reaction. Exposure to an allergen activates B cells to form IgE-secreting plasma cells. The secreted IgE molecules bind to IgE-specific Fc receptors on mast cells and blood basophils. Second exposure to the allergen leads to cross-linking of the bound IgE, triggering the release of pharmacologically active mediators from mast cells and basophils. The mediators cause smooth-muscle contraction, increased vascular permeability, and vasodilation.

IgE-MEDIATED (TYPE I) HYPERSENSITIVITY

A type I hypersensitive reaction is induced by certain types of antigens, referred to as **allergens**, and has all the hallmarks of a normal humoral response. That is, an allergen induces a humoral antibody response by the same mechanisms as described in Chapter 8 for other soluble antigens, resulting in generation of antibody-secreting plasma cells and memory cells. What distinguishes a type I hypersensitive response from a normal humoral response is that the plasma cells secrete IgE. This class of antibody binds with high affinity to **Fc receptors** on the surface of tissue mast cells and blood basophils. Such IgE-coated mast cells and basophils are said to be **sensitized**. A later exposure to the same allergen cross-links the membrane-bound IgE on sensitized mast cells and basophils, causing **degranulation** of these cells (Figure 17-1). The pharmacologically active mediators released from the granules exert biological effects on the surrounding tissues. The principal effects—vasodilation and smooth-muscle contraction—may be either systemic or localized, depending on the extent of mediator release.

Components of Type I Reactions

As depicted in Figure 17-1, several components are critical to development of type I hypersensitive reactions. We'll consider these components first and then describe the mechanism of degranulation.

ALLERGENS

The vast majority of humans mount significant IgE responses only as a defense against parasitic infections. After an individual is exposed to a parasite, serum IgE levels increase and remain high until the parasite is successfully cleared from the body. **Atopic** persons, however, may have a genetic defect affecting regulation of the IgE response. These regulatory defects allow nonparasitic

TABLE 17-2

COMMON ANTIGENS ASSOCIATED WITH TYPE I HYPERSENSITIVITY

Proteins	*Foods*
Foreign serum	Nuts
Vaccines	Seafood
	Eggs
Plant pollens	Peas, beans
Rye grass	
Ragweed	*Insect products*
Timothy grass	Bee venom
Birch trees	Wasp venom
	Ant venom
Drugs	Cockroach calyx
Penicillin	
Sulfonamides	*Mold spores*
Local anesthetics	
Salicylates	*Animal hair and dander*

antigens to stimulate inappropriate IgE production, leading to tissue-damaging type I hypersensitivity. The term *allergen* refers specifically to nonparasitic antigens capable of stimulating type I hypersensitive responses in allergic individuals.

Most allergic IgE responses occur on mucous membrane surfaces in response to allergens that enter the body either by inhalation or ingestion. Of the common allergens listed in Table 17-2, relatively few have been purified and characterized. Those that have include the allergens from rye grass pollen, ragweed pollen, codfish, birch pollen, timothy grass pollen, and bee venom. Each of these allergens has been shown to be a multiallergen system containing a number of allergenic components. Ragweed pollen, a major pollen allergen in the United States, is a case in point. It has been reported that a square mile of ragweed yields 16 tons of pollen in a single season. The pollen particles are inhaled, and their tough outer wall is dissolved by enzymes in the mucous secretions, releasing the allergenic substances. Chemical fractionation of ragweed has revealed a variety of substances, most of which are not allergenic but are capable of eliciting an IgM or IgG response. Of the five fractions that are allergenic (i.e., able to induce an IgE response), two evoke allergenic reactions in about 95% of ragweed-sensitive individuals and are called major allergens; these are designated the E and K fractions. The other three, called Ra3, Ra4, and Ra5, are minor allergens that induce an allergic response in only 20%–30% of sensitive subjects.

What makes these agents allergens? Why are some pollens (e.g., ragweed) highly allergenic, whereas other equally abundant pollens (e.g., nettle) are rarely allergenic? No single physicochemical property seems to distinguish the highly allergenic E and K fractions of ragweed from the less allergenic Ra3, Ra4, and Ra5 fractions and from the nonallergenic fractions. Rather, allergens as a group appear to possess diverse properties. Some allergens, including foreign serum and egg albumin, are potent antigens; others, such as plant pollens, are weak antigens. Although most allergens are small proteins or protein-bound substances having a molecular weight between 15,000 and 40,000, attempts to identify some common chemical property of these antigens, one that would render them all allergenic, have failed. It appears that allergenicity is a consequence of a complex series of interactions involving not only the allergen but also the dose, the sensitizing route, sometimes an adjuvant, and—most importantly—the genetic constitution of the recipient.

REAGINIC ANTIBODY (IgE)

As discussed in Chapter 5, the existence of a human serum factor that reacted with allergens was first demonstrated by K. Prausnitz and H. Kustner in 1921. The local wheal and flare response that occurs when an allergen is injected into a sensitized individual is referred to as the **P-K reaction**. Because the serum components responsible for the P-K reaction displayed specificity for allergen, they were assumed to be antibodies, but the nature of these P-K antibodies, or **reagin**, was not demonstrated for many years.

Experiments conducted by K. and T. Ishizaka in the mid-1960s showed that the biological activity of reaginic antibody in a P-K test could be neutralized by rabbit antiserum against whole atopic human sera but not by rabbit antiserum specific for the four known human immunoglobulin classes (IgA, IgG, IgM, and IgD) (Table 17-3). And when rabbits were immunized with sera from ragweed-sensitive individuals, the rabbit antiserum could inhibit (neutralize) a positive ragweed P-K test even after precipitation of the rabbit antibodies specific for the known human IgG, IgA, IgM, and IgD isotypes. The Ishizakas called this new isotype IgE in reference to the E antigen of ragweed that they used to characterize it.

Serum IgE levels in normal individuals fall within the range of 0.1–0.4 μg/ml; even the most severely allergic individuals rarely have IgE levels greater than 1 μg/ml. These low levels made physiochemical studies of IgE difficult, and it was not until the discovery of an IgE myeloma by S. G. O. Johansson and H. Bennich in 1967 that extensive chemical analysis of IgE could be undertaken. IgE was found to be composed of two heavy (ε) and two light chains with a combined molecular weight of 190,000. The higher molecular weight compared to IgG (150,000) is due to the presence of an additional constant-region domain (see Figure 5-15). This additional domain (C_H4) contributes to an altered conformation of the Fc portion of the molecule that enables it to bind to glycoprotein receptors on the surface of basophils and mast cells. Although the half-life of IgE in the serum is only 2–3 days, once IgE is bound to its receptor on mast cells and basophils, it is stable in the bound state for a number of weeks.

Mast Cells and Basophils

The cells that bind IgE were identified by incubating human leukocytes and tissue cells with either ^{125}I-labeled IgE myeloma protein or ^{125}I-labeled anti-IgE. In both cases autoradiography revealed that the labeled probe bound to blood basophils and tissue mast cells. Basophils are granulocytes that circulate in the blood of most vertebrates; in humans they account for 0.5%–1.0% of the circulating white blood cells. Their granulated cytoplasm stains with basic dyes, hence the name basophil. Electron microscopy reveals a multilobed nucleus, few mitochondria, numerous glycogen granules, and electron-dense membrane-bound granules scattered throughout the cytoplasm (see Figure 3-13c).

Mast cell precursors are formed in the bone marrow during hematopoiesis and are carried to virtually all vascularized peripheral tissues where they differentiate into mature cells. Mast cells are found throughout connective tissue, particularly near blood and lymphatic vessels. Some tissues, including the skin and mucous membrane surfaces of the respiratory and gastrointestinal tract, contain high concentrations of mast cells; skin, for example, contains 10,000 mast cells per mm^3. Electron micrographs of mast cells reveal numerous membrane-bound granules, which contain pharmacologically active mediators, distributed throughout the cytoplasm (Figure 17-2). After activation, these mediators are released from the granules, resulting in the clinical manifestations of the type I hypersensitive reaction.

Mast cell populations in different anatomic sites exhibit significant variation in the types and amounts of allergic mediators they contain and in their sensitivity to activating stimuli and cytokines. Mast cells also secrete a variety of cytokines including IL-1, IL-3, IL-4, IL-5, IL-6, GM-CSF, TGF-β, and TNF-α. Because these cytokines exert diverse biological effects (see Table 13-1), mast cells contribute to a broad spectrum of physiologic, immunologic, and pathologic processes.

IgE-Binding Fc Receptors

The reaginic activity of IgE depends on its ability to bind to a receptor specific for the Fc region of the ε

T A B L E   1 7 - 3

IDENTIFICATION OF IgE BASED ON REACTIVITY OF ATOPIC SERUM IN P-K TEST

SERUM	TREATMENT	ALLERGEN ADDED	P-K REACTION AT SKIN SITE
Atopic	None	−	−
Atopic	None	+	+
Nonatopic	None	+	−
Atopic	Rabbit antiserum to human atopic serum *	+	−
Atopic	Rabbit antiserum to human IgM, IgG, IgA, and IgD†	+	+

* Serum from an atopic individual was injected into rabbits to produce antiserum against human atopic serum. When this antiserum was reacted with human atopic serum, it neutralized the P-K reaction.

† Serum from an atopic individual was reacted with rabbit antiserum to the known classes of human antibody (IgM, IgA, IgG, and IgD) to remove these isotypes from the atopic serum. The treated atopic serum continued to give a positive P-K reaction, indicating that a new immunoglobulin isotype was responsible for this reactivity.

SOURCE: Based on K. Ishizaka and T. Ishizaka, 1967, *J. Immunol.* **99**:1187.

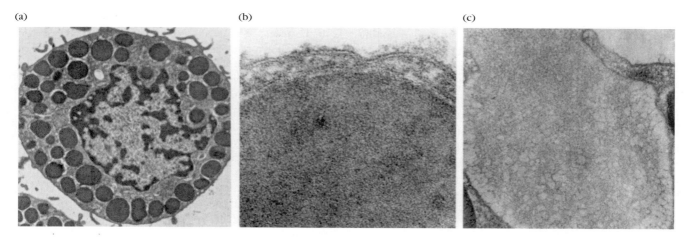

FIGURE 17-2

(a) Electron micrograph of a typical mast cell reveals numerous elec-tron-dense membrane-bounded granules prior to degranulation. (b) Close-up of intact granule underlying the plasma membrane of a mast cell. (c) Granule releasing its contents during degranulation. [From S. Burwen and B. Satir, 1977, *J. Cell Biol.* **73**:662.]

heavy chain. Two classes of FcεR have been identified, designated FcεRI and FcεRII, which are expressed by different cell types and differ by 1000-fold in their affin-ity for IgE.

High-Affinity Receptor (FcεRI) Mast cells and baso-phils express FcεRI, which binds IgE with a high affinity ($K_D = 1–2 \times 10^{-9}$ M). The high affinity of this receptor enables it to bind IgE despite the low serum concentra-tion of IgE (1×10^{-7} M). Between 40,000 and 90,000 FcεRI molecules have been shown to be present on a human basophil.

The FcεRI receptor contains four polypeptide chains: an α and a β chain and two identical disulfide-linked γ chains (Figure 17-3a). The external region of the α chain contains two 90-aa domains that exhibit homology with the immunoglobulin-fold structure, placing the molecule in the immunoglobulin superfamily (see Figure 5-19). FcεRI interacts with the C_H3/C_H3 and C_H4/C_H4 do-mains of the IgE molecule via the two Ig-like domains of the α chain. The β chain spans the plasma membrane four times and is thought to link the α chain to the γ homodimer. The two γ chains are disulfide-linked and extend a considerable distance into the cytoplasm. Each γ chain has a conserved sequence in its cytosolic domain known as an **immunoreceptor tyrosine activation motif** (ITAM). Two other membrane receptors that have this motif are the ζ chains of CD3 associated with the T-cell receptor and the Ig-α/Ig-β chains associated with membrane immunoglobulin on B cells. The ITAM motif on these three receptors is thought to interact with

protein tyrosine kinases to transduce an activating signal to the cell. Allergen-mediated cross-linkage of the bound IgE results in aggregation of the FcεRI receptors and rapid tyrosine phosphorylation, which initiates the process of mast-cell degranulation.

Low-Affinity Receptor (FcεRII) The other IgE receptor, designated FcεRII (or CD23), is specific for the C_H3/C_H3 domain of IgE and has a lower affinity for IgE ($K_D = 1 \times 10^{-6}$ M) than does FcεRI (Figure 17-3b). The FcεRII receptor appears to play a variety of roles in regulating the intensity of the IgE response. Allergen cross-linkage of IgE bound to FcεRII has been shown to activate B cells, alveolar macrophages, and eosinophils. When this receptor is blocked with monoclonal anti-bodies, IgE secretion by B cells is diminished. A soluble form of FcεRII (or sCD23), which is generated by auto-proteolysis of the membrane receptor, has been shown to enhance IgE production by B cells. Interestingly, atopic individuals have higher levels of CD23 on their lympho-cytes and macrophages and higher levels of sCD23 in their serum than nonatopic individuals.

Mechanism of IgE-Mediated Degranulation

The biochemical events mediating degranulation of mast cells and blood basophils have many features in com-mon. For simplicity this section presents a general over-view of mast cell degranulation mechanisms without calling attention to the slight differences between mast

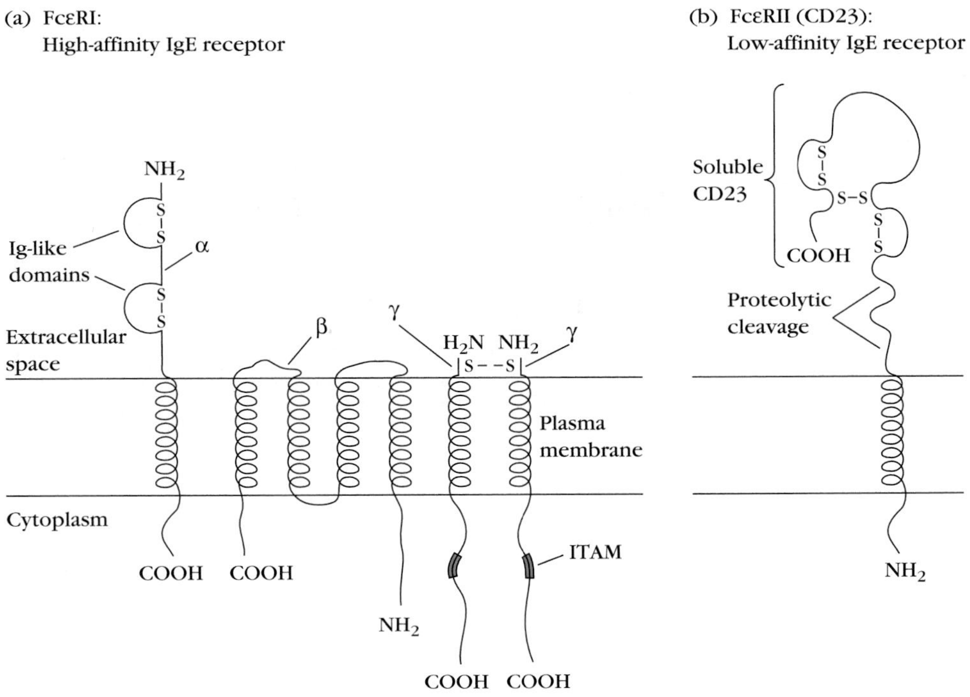

(a) FcεRI:
High-affinity IgE receptor

(b) FcεRII (CD23):
Low-affinity IgE receptor

FIGURE 17-3

Schematic diagrams of the high-affinity (FcεRI) and low-affinity (FcεRII) receptors that bind the Fc region of IgE. (a) Each γ chain of the high-affinity receptor contains an ITAM, a motif also present in the Ig-α/Ig-β heterodimer of the B-cell receptor and in the CD3 complex of the T-cell receptor. (b) The low-affinity receptor is unusual because it is oriented in the membrane with its NH₂-terminus directed toward the cell interior and its COOH-terminus directed toward the extracellular space.

cells and basophils. Although mast cell degranulation generally is initiated by allergen cross-linkage of bound IgE, a number of other stimuli can also initiate the process, including the anaphylatoxins (C3a, C4a, and C5a); various drugs such as synthetic ACTH, codeine, and morphine; and compounds such as the calcium ionophore. This section focuses on the biochemical events following allergen cross-linkage of bound IgE.

RECEPTOR CROSS-LINKAGE

IgE-mediated degranulation begins when an allergen cross-links receptor-bound (fixed) IgE on the surface of a mast cell or basophil. In itself, the binding of IgE to FcRI apparently has no effect on a target cell. It is only after cross-linkage by allergen of the fixed IgE-receptor complex that degranulation proceeds. The importance of cross-linkage is indicated by the inability of monovalent allergens, which cannot cross-link the fixed IgE, to trigger degranulation. Experimental studies with preformed IgE-allergen complexes, in which the ratio of IgE to allergen was carefully monitored, revealed that only complexes having IgE:allergen ratios of 2:1 or

greater could induce degranulation. Complexes in antigen excess (having an IgE:allergen ratio of 1:2) failed to induce degranulation because the requisite cross-linkage of receptors did not occur.

Other experiments have revealed that it is actually the cross-linkage of two or more FcRI molecules—with or without IgE—that is essential for degranulation. Although cross-linkage is normally effected by the interaction of fixed IgE with divalent or multivalent allergen, it also can be effected by a variety of experimental means that bypass the need for allergen and in some cases even for IgE (Figure 17-4).

INTRACELLULAR EVENTS LEADING TO MAST CELL DEGRANULATION

The cytoplasmic domains of the β and γ chains of FcεRI are associated with protein tyrosine kinases (PTKs). Cross-linkage of the FcεRI receptors activates the associated PTKs resulting in the phosphorylation of tyrosines within the ITAMs of the γ subunit as well as phosphorylation of residues on the β subunit and on phospholipase C. These phosphorylation events induce the production

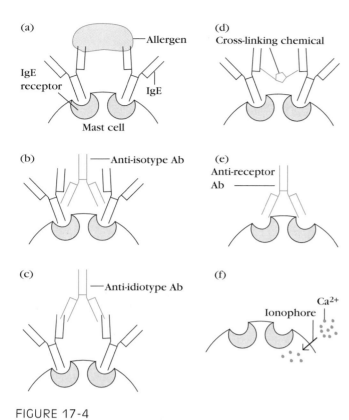

FIGURE 17-4

Schematic diagrams of mechanisms that can trigger degranulation of mast cells. (a) Allergen cross-linkage of cell-bound IgE molecules. (b, c) Antibody cross-linkage of IgE. (d) Chemical cross-linkage of IgE. (e) Cross-linkage of IgE receptors by antireceptor antibody. (f) Enhanced Ca^{2+} influx stimulated by an ionophore that increases membrane permeability to Ca^{2+} ions. Note that mechanisms (b), (c), and (d) do not require allergen; mechanisms (e) and (f) require neither allergen nor IgE; and mechanism (f) does not even require receptor cross-linkage.

of a number of second messengers that mediate the process of degranulation (Figure 17-5).

Within 15 s after cross-linkage of FcεRI, methylation of various membrane phospholipids is observed, resulting in an increase in membrane fluidity and the formation of Ca^{2+} channels. The influx of Ca^{2+} reaches a peak within 2 min of FcεRI cross-linkage (Figure 17-6). The Ca^{2+} increase is due to both a release of Ca^{2+} from intracellular stores in the endoplasmic reticulum and from the uptake of extracellular Ca^{2+}. The Ca^{2+} influx eventually leads to the formation of arachidonic acid, which is converted into two classes of potent mediators: the **prostaglandins** and the **leukotrienes**. The influx of Ca^{2+} also promotes the assembly of microtubules and the contraction of microfilaments, both of which are necessary for the movement of granules to the plasma membrane. The importance of the Ca^{2+} influx in mast cell degran-

ulation is highlighted by the use of drugs, such as cromolyn sodium, to block this influx as a treatment for allergies.

Concomitant with phospholipid methylation and Ca^{2+} influx, there is a transient increase in membrane-bound adenylate cyclase activity, with a rapid peak of cAMP reached at about 1 min after cross-linkage of FcεRI. The effects of cAMP are exerted through the activation of cAMP-dependent protein kinases, which phosphorylate the granule-membrane proteins, thereby changing the granules' permeability to water and Ca^{2+} (see Figure 17-5). The consequent swelling of the granules facilitates their fusion with the plasma membrane, releasing their contents. The increase in cAMP is transient and is followed by a drop in cAMP to levels below baseline (see Figure 17-6). This drop in cAMP appears to be necessary for degranulation to proceed. When cAMP levels are increased by certain drugs, the degranulation process is blocked. Several of these drugs (including theophylline and epinephrine) are often given to treat allergic disorders and are discussed later in the chapter.

Mediators of Type I Reactions

The clinical manifestations of type I hypersensitive reactions are related to the biological effects of the mediators released during mast cell or basophil degranulation. These mediators are pharmacologically active agents that act on local tissues as well as on populations of secondary effector cells, including eosinophils, neutrophils, T lymphocytes, monocytes, and platelets. The mediators thus serve as an amplifying terminal effector mechanism, much as the complement system serves as an amplifier and effector of an antigen-antibody interaction. When generated in response to parasitic infection, these mediators initiate a beneficial defense process. Localized smooth-muscle contraction and the consequent vasodilation and increased vascular permeability bring an influx of plasma and inflammatory cells to attack the pathogen. On the other hand, mediator release induced by inappropriate antigens, such as allergens, results in unnecessary increases in vascular permeability and inflammation whose detrimental effects far outweigh any beneficial effect.

The mediators can be classified as either primary or secondary (Table 17-4). The **primary mediators** are produced before degranulation and are stored in the granules. The most significant primary mediators are histamine, proteases, eosinophil chemotactic factor, neutrophil chemotactic factor, and heparin. The **secondary mediators** either are synthesized after target-cell activation or are released by the breakdown of membrane phospholipids during the degranulation process. The

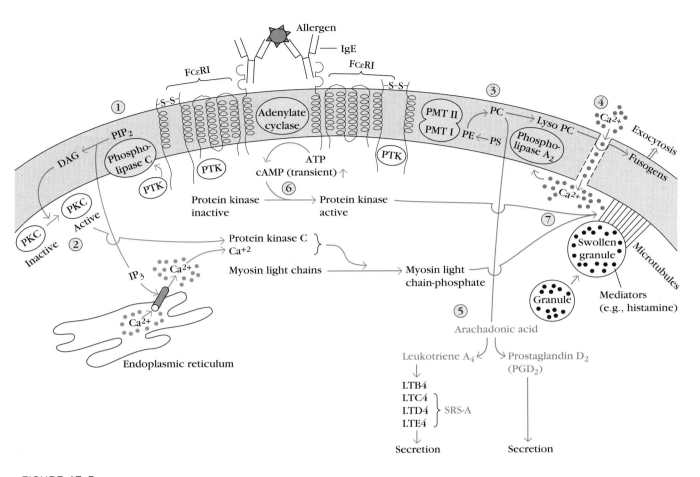

FIGURE 17-5

Diagrammatic overview of biochemical events in mast cell activation and degranulation. Allergen cross-linkage of bound IgE results in FcεRI aggregation and activation of protein tyrosine kinase (PTK). (1) PTK then phosphorylates phospholipase C, which converts phosphatidylinositol-4,5 bisphosphate (PIP$_2$) into diacylglycerol (DAG) and inositol triphosphate (IP$_3$). (2) DAG activates protein kinase C (PKC), which phosphorylates myosin light chains necessary for microtubular assembly and the fusion of the granules with the plasma membrane. IP$_3$ is a potent mobilizer of intracellular Ca^{2+} stores. Cross-linkage of FcεRI also activates an enzyme that converts phosphatidylserine (PS) into phosphatidylethanolamine (PE). (3) Eventually PE is methylated to form phosphatidylcholine (PC) by two phospholipid methyl transferase enzymes I and II (PMT I and II). (4) The accumulation of PC on the exterior surface of the plasma membrane causes an increase in membrane fluidity and facilitates the formation of Ca^{2+} channels. The resulting influx of Ca^{2+} activates phospholipase A$_2$, which promotes the breakdown of PC to form lysophosphatidylcholine (lyso PC) and arachidonic acid. (5) Arachidonic acid is converted into potent mediators: the leukotrienes and prostaglandin D$_2$. (6) FcεRI cross-linkage also activates the membrane adenylate cyclase leading to a transient increase of cAMP within 15 s. A later drop in cAMP levels is mediated by protein kinase and is required for degranulation to proceed. (7) cAMP-dependent protein kinases are thought to phosphorylate the granule-membrane proteins, thereby changing the granules' permeability to water and Ca^{2+}. The consequent swelling of the granules facilitates fusion with the plasma membrane and release of the mediators.

secondary mediators include platelet-activating factor, leukotrienes, prostaglandins, bradykinin, and various cytokines. The differing manifestations of type I hypersensitivity in different species or different tissues partly reflect variations in the primary and secondary mediators present. The main biological effects of several of these mediators are discussed briefly in the following sections.

HISTAMINE

Histamine, which is formed by decarboxylation of the amino acid histidine, is a major component of mast cell granules, accounting for about 10% of granule weight. Because it is stored—preformed—in the granules, its biological effects are observed within minutes of mast

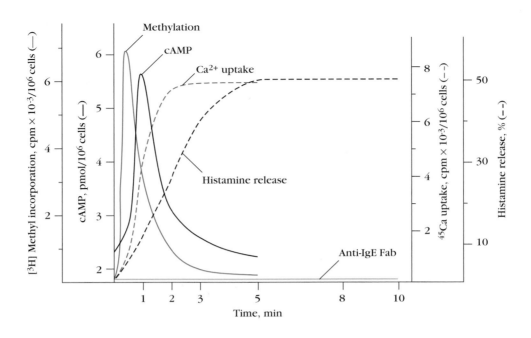

FIGURE 17-6

Kinetics of major biochemical events following cross-linkage of bound IgE on cultured human basophils with F(ab′)$_2$ fragments of anti-IgE. Curves are shown for phospholipid methylation (solid blue), cAMP production (solid black), Ca^{2+} influx (dashed blue), and histamine release (dashed black). In control experiments with anti-IgE Fab fragments, no significant changes were observed. [Adapted from T. Ishizaka et al., 1985, *Int. Arch. Allergy Appl. Immunol.* **77**:137.]

cell activation. Once released from mast cells, histamine initially binds to specific receptors on various target cells. Three types of histamine receptors—designated H$_1$, H$_2$, and H$_3$—have been identified; these receptors have different tissue distributions and mediate different effects when they bind histamine.

Most of the biologic effects of histamine in allergic reactions are mediated by the binding of histamine to H$_1$ receptors. This binding induces contraction of intestinal and bronchial smooth muscles, increased permeability of venules, and increased mucus secretion by goblet cells. Interaction of histamine with H$_2$ receptors increases vasopermeability and dilation and stimulates exocrine glands. Binding of histamine to H$_2$ receptors on mast cells and basophils suppresses degranulation; thus histamine exerts negative-feedback control on mediator release. The function of the most recently discovered histamine receptor, H$_3$, is under investigation.

LEUKOTRIENES AND PROSTAGLANDINS

As secondary mediators, the leukotrienes and prostaglandins are not formed until the mast cell undergoes degranulation and its plasma membrane is broken down. An ensuing enzymatic cascade generates the prostaglandins and the leukotrienes (see Figure 17-5). It therefore takes a longer time for the biological effects of these mediators to become apparent. Their effects are more pronounced and longer-lasting, however, than those of histamine. The leukotrienes mediate bronchoconstriction, increased vascular permeability, and mucus production. Prostaglandin D$_2$ causes bronchoconstriction.

The contraction of human bronchial and tracheal smooth muscles appears at first to be mediated by histamine, but within 30–60 s further contraction is mediated by the leukotrienes and prostaglandins. Being active at nanomole levels, the leukotrienes are as much as 1000 times more potent as bronchoconstrictors than histamine, and they are also more potent stimulators of vascular permeability and mucus secretion. In humans the leukotrienes are thought to contribute to the prolonged bronchospasm and buildup of mucus seen in asthmatics.

CYTOKINES

Adding to the complexity of the type I reaction is the variety of cytokines released from mast cells and eosinophils. Some of these may contribute to the clinical manifestations of type I hypersensitivity. Human mast cells secrete IL-4, IL-5, IL-6, and TNF-α. These cytokines alter the local microenvironment, eventually leading to the recruitment of inflammatory cells such as neutrophils and eosinophils. IL-4 increases IgE production by B cells. IL-5 is especially important in the recruitment and activation of eosinophils. The high concentrations of TNF-α secreted by mast cells may contribute to shock in systemic anaphylaxis. (This effect may parallel the role of TNF-α in bacterial septic shock and toxic-shock syndrome discussed in Chapter 13.)

Consequences of Type I Reactions

The clinical manifestations of type I reactions can range from serious life-threatening conditions, such as systemic anaphylaxis and asthma, to hay fever and eczema, which are merely annoying.

SYSTEMIC ANAPHYLAXIS

Systemic anaphylaxis is a shock-like and often fatal state whose onset occurs within minutes of a type I hypersensitive reaction. This type of response was first reported in 1839 by Magendie, who noted the sudden death of dogs following repeated injections of egg albumin. This report went unnoticed until 1902 when two French physicians, Paul J. Portier and Charles R. Richet, observed a similar phenomenon. The two physicians were trying to develop an antitoxin to protect swimmers from the painful stings of the Portuguese man-of-war jellyfish and sea anemones. While attempting to immunize dogs with a sublethal extract of sea anemone tentacles, they observed that a secondary challenge several weeks later with the same sublethal extract brought on a rapid sequence of symptoms including vomiting, bloody diarrhea, asphyxia, unconsciousness, and death. They called the response **anaphylaxis** (from Greek *ana*, against, and *phylaxis*, protection) to denote that this was an inappropriate response, counter to host protective mechanisms. For his work on anaphylaxis, Richet was awarded a Nobel Prize in medicine in 1913.

TABLE 17-4

PRINCIPAL MEDIATORS INVOLVED IN TYPE I HYPERSENSITIVITY

MEDIATOR	EFFECTS
PRIMARY	
Histamine	Increased vascular permeability; smooth-muscle contraction
Serotonin	Increased vascular permeability; smooth-muscle contraction
Eosinophil chemotactic factor (ECF-A)	Eosinophil chemotaxis
Neutrophil chemotactic factor (NCF-A)	Neutrophil chemotaxis
Proteases	Bronchial mucus secretion; degradation of blood-vessel basement membrane; generation of complement split products
SECONDARY	
Platelet-activating factor	Platelet aggregation and degranulation; contraction of pulmonary smooth muscles
Leukotrienes (slow reactive substance of anaphylaxis, SRS-A)	Increased vascular permeability; contraction of pulmonary smooth muscles
Prostaglandins	Vasodilation; contraction of pulmonary smooth muscles; platelet aggregation
Bradykinin	Increased vascular permeability; smooth-muscle contraction
Cytokines IL-1 and TNF-α	Systemic anaphylaxis; increased expression of CAMs on venular endothelial cells
IL-2, IL-3, IL-4, IL-5, IL-6, TGF-β, and GM-CSF	Various effects (see Table 13-1)

Systemic anaphylaxis can be induced in a variety of experimental animals and is seen occasionally in humans. Each species exhibits characteristic symptoms of anaphylaxis, which reflect differences in the distribution of mast cells and in the biologically active contents of their mast cell granules. The animal model of choice for studying systemic anaphylaxis has been the guinea pig. Anaphylaxis can be induced in guinea pigs with relative ease, and its symptoms closely parallel those observed in humans.

Active **sensitization** in guinea pigs is induced by a single injection of a foreign protein such as egg albumin. After an incubation period of about 2 weeks, the animal is usually challenged with an intravenous injection of the same protein. Within 1 min the animal becomes restless, its respiration becomes labored, and its blood pressure drops. As the smooth muscles of the gastrointestinal tract and bladder contract, the guinea pig defecates and urinates. Finally bronchiole constriction results in death by asphyxiation within 2–4 min of the injection. These events all stem from the systemic vasodilation and smooth-muscle contraction brought on by mediators released during the course of the reaction. Postmortem examination reveals that massive edema, shock, and bronchiole constriction are the major causes of death.

Systemic anaphylaxis in humans is characterized by a similar sequence of events. A wide range of antigens have been shown to trigger this reaction in susceptible humans, including bee, wasp, hornet, and ant stings; drugs, such as penicillin, insulin, and antitoxins; and seafood and nuts. If not treated quickly, these reactions can be fatal. **Epinephrine** is the drug of choice used to treat systemic anaphylactic reactions. Epinephrine counteracts the effects of mediators like histamine and the leukotrienes by relaxing the smooth muscles and reducing vascular permeability. Epinephrine also improves cardiac output, which is necessary to prevent vascular collapse during an anaphylactic reaction. In addition, epinephrine increases cAMP levels in the mast cell, thereby blocking further degranulation.

LOCALIZED ANAPHYLAXIS (ATOPY)

In localized anaphylaxis the reaction is limited to a specific target tissue or organ, often involving epithelial surfaces at the site of allergen entry. The tendency to manifest localized anaphylactic reactions is inherited and is referred to as **atopy**. Atopic allergies, which afflict at least 20% of the population in developed countries, include a wide range of IgE-mediated disorders including allergic rhinitis (hayfever), asthma, atopic dermatitis (eczema), and food allergies.

Allergic Rhinitis The most common atopic disorder, affecting 10% of the U. S. population, is allergic rhinitis, commonly known as **hay fever**. This results from air-borne allergens reacting with sensitized mast cells in the conjunctivae and nasal mucosa to induce the release of pharmacologically active mediators from mast cells; these mediators then cause localized vasodilation and increased capillary permeability. The symptoms include watery exudation of the conjunctivae, nasal mucosa, and upper respiratory tract, as well as sneezing and coughing.

Asthma Another common manifestation of localized anaphylaxis is asthma. For reasons that are still unclear, the incidence of asthma has increased dramatically in developed countries. What is even more alarming, is that the severity of the disease also appears to be increasing. The increase in asthma mortality is highest among children, and in the United States the mortality is highest among African-American children of the inner city. Epidemiologic studies have so far failed to explain the increased incidence of asthma in this population. A clue to the increase in asthma in inner-city children may be the finding that cockroach calyx is a major allergen associated with asthma. During 1990, the cost for the treatment of asthma in the United States was $6.4 billion.

In some cases airborne or blood-borne allergens, such as pollens, dust, fumes, insect products, or viral antigens, trigger an asthmatic attack (**allergic asthma**); in other cases an asthmatic attack can be induced by exercise or cold, apparently independent of allergen stimulation (**intrinsic asthma**). Like hay fever, asthma is triggered by degranulation of mast cells with release of mediators, but instead of occurring in the nasal mucosa, the reaction develops in the lower respiratory tract. The resulting contraction of the bronchial smooth muscles leads to bronchoconstriction. Airway edema, mucus secretion, and inflammation contribute to the bronchial constriction and to airway obstruction. Asthmatic patients may have abnormal levels of receptors for neuropeptides. For example, asthmatic patients have been reported to have increased expression of receptors for substance P, a peptide that contracts smooth muscles, and decreased expression of receptors for vasoactive intestinal peptide, a peptide that relaxes smooth muscles.

Most clinicians view asthma as primarily an inflammatory disease. The asthmatic response can be divided into early and late responses (Figure 17-7). The **early response** occurs within minutes of allergen exposure and involves primarily histamine, leukotrienes (LTC_4), and prostaglandin D_2 (PGD_2). The effects of these mediators lead to bronchoconstriction, vasodilation, and some buildup of mucus. The **late response** occurs hours later and involves additional mediators including IL-4, IL-5, IL-16, TNF-α, eosinophil chemotactic factor (ECF), and platelet-activating factor (PAF). The overall effects of these mediators is to recruit inflammatory cells, including eosinophils and neutrophils, into the bronchial tissue.

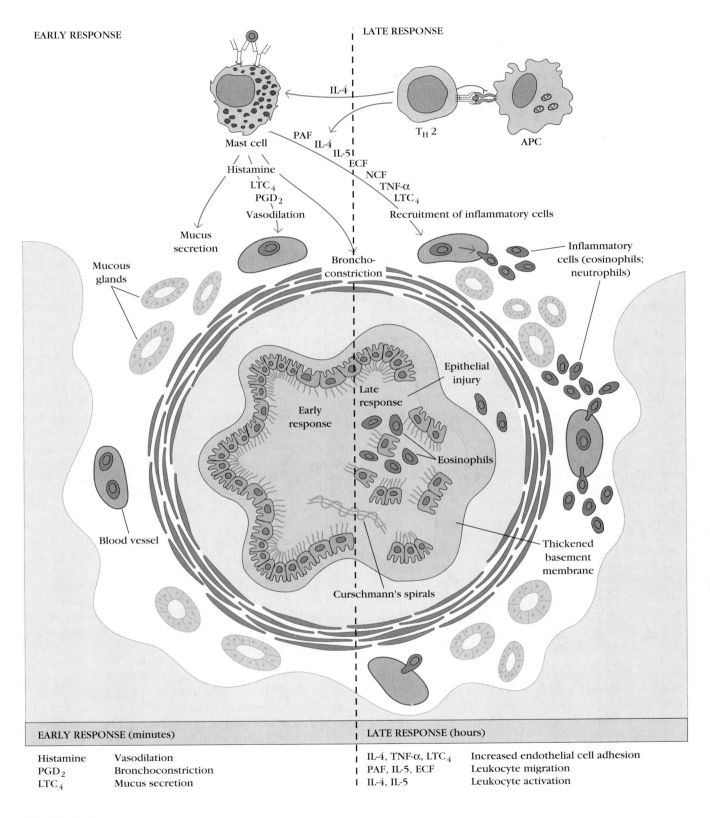

EARLY RESPONSE

LATE RESPONSE

IL-4

Mast cell

T$_H$2

APC

PAF
IL-4
IL-5
ECF
NCF
TNF-α
LTC$_4$

Histamine
LTC$_4$
PGD$_2$
Vasodilation

Recruitment of inflammatory cells

Mucus
secretion

Broncho-
constriction

Mucous
glands

Inflammatory
cells (eosinophils;
neutrophils)

Epithelial
injury

Late
response

Early
response

Eosinophils

Blood vessel

Thickened
basement
membrane

Curschmann's spirals

EARLY RESPONSE (minutes)		LATE RESPONSE (hours)	
Histamine	Vasodilation	IL-4, TNF-α, LTC$_4$	Increased endothelial cell adhesion
PGD$_2$	Bronchoconstriction	PAF, IL-5, ECF	Leukocyte migration
LTC$_4$	Mucus secretion	IL-4, IL-5	Leukocyte activation

FIGURE 17-7

The early and late inflammatory response in asthma. The immune cells involved in the early and late response are represented at the top. The effects of various mediators on an airway, represented in cross-section, are illustrated in the center. See text for explanation.

The neutrophils and eosinophils are capable of causing significant tissue injury by releasing toxic enzymes, oxygen radicals, and cytokines. These events lead to occlusion of the bronchial lumen with mucus, proteins, and cellular debris; sloughing of the epithelium; thickening of the basement membrane; fluid buildup (edema); and hypertrophy of the bronchial smooth muscles. A mucus plug often forms and adheres to the bronchial wall. The mucus plug contains clusters of detached epithelial-cell fragments, eosinophils, some neutrophils, and spirals of bronchial tissue known as Curschmann's spirals.

Food Allergies   Various foods also can induce localized anaphylaxis in allergic individuals. Allergen cross-linking of IgE on mast cells along the upper or lower gastrointestinal tract can induce localized smooth-muscle contraction and vasodilation and thus such symptoms as vomiting or diarrhea. Mast cell degranulation along the gut can increase the permeability of mucous membranes, so that the allergen enters the bloodstream. Various symptoms can ensue, depending on where the allergen is deposited. For example, some individuals develop asthmatic attacks after ingesting certain foods. Others develop **atopic urticaria**, commonly known as **hives**, when a food allergen is carried to sensitized mast cells in the skin causing swollen (edematous), red (erythematous) eruptions; this response is known as a **wheal and flare reaction**.

Atopic Dermatitis   Atopic dermatitis (**allergic eczema**) is an inflammatory disease of skin that is frequently associated with a family history of atopy. The disease is observed most frequently in young children, often developing during infancy. Serum IgE levels are often elevated. The allergic individual develops skin eruptions that are erythematous and filled with pus. Unlike a delayed-type hypersensitive reaction, which involves T_H1 cells, the skin lesions in atopic dermatitis have T_H2 cells and an increased number of eosinophils.

LATE-PHASE REACTION

As a type I hypersensitive reaction begins to subside, mediators released during the course of the reaction often induce a localized inflammatory reaction, called the **late-phase reaction**. The late-phase reaction begins to develop 4–6 h following the initial type I reaction and persists for 1–2 days. The reaction is characterized by infiltration of neutrophils, eosinophils, macrophages, lymphocytes, and basophils. The localized late-phase response also may be partly mediated by cytokines released from mast cells. Both TNF-α and IL-1 increase the expression of cell-adhesion molecules on venular endothelial cells, thus facilitating the buildup of neutrophils, eosinophils, and monocytes that characterizes the late-phase response.

Eosinophils play a principal role during the late-phase reaction, accounting for some 30% of the cells that accumulate. Eosinophil chemotactic factor, released by mast cells during the initial reaction, attracts large numbers of eosinophils to the affected site. Various cytokines released at the site, including IL-3, IL-5, and GM-CSF, contribute to the growth and differentiation of the eosinophils. Eosinophils express Fc receptors for IgG and IgE isotypes and bind directly to antibody-coated allergen. Much like mast cell degranulation, binding of antibody-coated antigen activates eosinophils, leading to their degranulation and release of inflammatory mediators, including leukotrienes, major basic protein, platelet-activation factor, cationic protein, and eosinophil-derived neurotoxin. The release of these eosinophil-derived mediators may play a protective role in parasitic infections. However, in response to allergens, these mediators contribute to extensive tissue damage in the late-phase reaction. The influx of eosinophils in the late-phase response has been shown to contribute to the chronic inflammation of the bronchial mucosa that characterizes persistent asthma.

Neutrophils are another major participant in late-phase reactions, also accounting for 30% of the inflammatory cells. Neutrophils are attracted to the area of a type I reaction by neutrophil chemotactic factor, released from degranulating mast cells. In addition, a variety of cytokines released at the site, including IL-8, have been shown to activate neutrophils resulting in release of their granule contents, including lytic enzymes, platelet-activating factor, and leukotrienes.

Regulation of the Type I Response

As noted earlier, the genetic constitution of an animal, the antigen dose, and the mode of antigen presentation influence the level of the IgE response induced by an antigen (i.e., its allergenicity). For example, inbred strains of mice have been shown to differ in their tendency to mount an IgE response. Some strains (e.g., SJL) fail to produce an IgE response to allergens, whereas other strains (e.g., BDF1) have an increased propensity for IgE production. Breeding experiments have shown that this genetic variation is not linked to the MHC. A genetic component also has been shown to influence susceptibility to type I hypersensitive reactions in humans. When both parents are allergic, there is a 50% chance that a child will also be allergic; when only one parent is allergic, there is a 30% chance that a child will manifest some kind of type I reaction.

The effect of antigen dosage on the IgE response is illustrated by immunization of BDF1 mice. Repeated low doses of an appropriate antigen induce a persistent IgE response in these mice, but higher antigen doses result in transient IgE production and a shift toward IgG. The mode of antigen presentation also influences the development of the IgE response. For example, immunization of Lewis-strain rats with keyhole limpet hemocyanin (KLH) plus aluminum hydroxide gel or *Bordetella pertussis* as an adjuvant induces a strong IgE response, whereas injection of KLH with complete Freund's adjuvant produces a largely IgG response. Similar experimental findings have been reported in mice. Infection with the nematode *Nippostrongylus brasiliensis* (Nb), like certain adjuvants, preferentially induces an IgE response. For example, Nb-infected mice develop higher levels of IgE specific for an unrelated antigen than do uninfected control mice.

The relative levels of the T_H1 and T_H2 subsets also are key to regulating type I hypersensitive responses. T_H1 cells reduce the response, whereas T_H2 cells enhance the response. Cytokines secreted by T_H2 cells—namely, IL-3, IL-4, IL-5, and IL-10—stimulate the type I response in several ways. IL-4 enhances class switching to IgE and regulates the clonal expansion of IgE-committed B cells; IL-3, IL-4, and IL-10 enhance mast cell production; and IL-3 and IL-5 enhance eosinophil maturation, activation, and accumulation. In contrast, T_H1 cells produce IFN-γ, which inhibits the type I response.

The pivotal role of IL-4 in regulating the type I response was demonstrated in experiments by W. E. Paul and coworkers. When these researchers activated normal, unprimed B cells in vitro with LPS, only 2% of the cells expressed membrane IgG1 and only 0.05% expressed membrane IgE. However, when unprimed B cells were incubated with LPS plus IL-4, the percentage of cells expressing IgG1 increased to 40%–50% and the percentage expressing IgE increased to 15%–25%. In an attempt to determine whether IL-4 plays a role in vivo in regulating IgE production, Paul primed Nb-infected mice with TNP-KLH in the presence or in the absence of monoclonal antibody to IL-4. The antibody to IL-4 inhibited the production of IgE specific for TNP-KLH by 99% in these Nb-infected mice compared with controls.

Further support for the role of IL-4 in the IgE response comes from the experiments of K. Rajewski and coworkers with IL-4 knockout mice. These IL-4–deficient mice were unable to mount an IgE response to helminthic antigens. Increased levels of CD4$^+$ T_H2 cells and increased levels of IL-4 have also been detected in atopic individuals. When allergen-specific CD4$^+$ T cells from atopic individuals are cloned and added to an autologous B-cell culture, the B cells synthesize IgE, whereas allergen-specific CD4$^+$ T cells from nonatopic individuals do not support IgE production.

In contrast to IL-4, IFN-γ decreases IgE production, suggesting that the balance of IL-4 and IFN-γ may determine the amount of IgE produced (Figure 17-8). Since IFN-γ is secreted by the T_H1 subset and IL-4 by the T_H2 subset, the relative activity of these subsets may influence an individual's response to allergens. According to this proposal, atopic and nonatopic individuals would exhibit qualitatively different type I responses to an allergen: the response in atopic individuals would involve the T_H2 subset and result in production of IgE; the response in nonatopic individuals would involve the T_H1 subset and result in production of IgM or IgG. To test this hypothesis, allergen-specific T cells were cloned from atopic and nonatopic individuals. The cloned T cells from the atopic individuals were predominantly of the T_H2 phenotype (IL-4 secreting), whereas the cloned T cells from nonatopic individuals were predominantly of the T_H1 phenotype (IFN-γ secreting). Needless to say, there is keen interest in down-regulating IL-4 as a possible treatment for allergic individuals.

Detection of Type I Hypersensitivity

Type I hypersensitivity is commonly identified and assessed by **skin testing**. Small amounts of potential allergens are introduced at specific skin sites by either

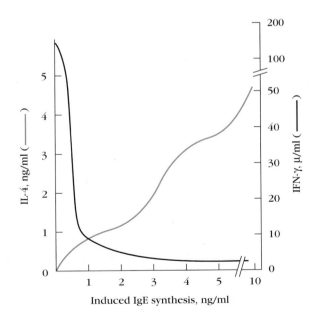

FIGURE 17-8

Effect of IL-4 and IFN-γ on in vitro production of IgE. These plots show the amount of IgE produced by plasma cells cultured in the presence of various concentrations of IL-4 (blue curve) or IFN-γ (black curve). [Adapted from G. Del Prete, 1988, *J. Immunol.* **140**: 4193.]

intradermal injection or superficial scratching. A number of tests can be applied to sites on the forearm or back of an individual at one time. If a person is allergic to the allergen, local mast cells will degranulate and the release of histamine and other mediators produces a wheal and flare within 30 min (Figure 17-9). The advantage of skin testing is that it is relatively inexpensive to perform and allows screening of a large number of allergens in a single sitting. The disadvantage of skin testing is that it sometimes sensitizes the allergic individual to new allergens and in some rare cases may induce systemic anaphylactic shock. A few individuals also manifest a late-phase reaction, which comes 4–6 h after testing and sometimes lasts for up to 24 h. As noted already, eosinophils accumulate during a late-phase reaction and release of eosinophil-granule contents contributes to the tissue damage in a late-phase reaction site.

Another method of assessing type I hypersensitivity is to determine the serum level of total IgE antibody by the **radioimmunosorbent test** (RIST). This highly sensitive technique, based on the radioimmunoassay, can determine nanogram levels of total IgE. The patient's serum is reacted with agarose beads or paper disks coated with rabbit anti-IgE. After the beads or disks are washed, ^{125}I-labeled rabbit anti-IgE is added. The beads or disks are counted in a gamma counter. The radioactivity count is proportional to the level of IgE in the patient's serum (Figure 17-10a).

The similar **radioallergosorbent test** (RAST) detects the serum level of IgE specific for a given allergen. The allergen is coupled to beads or disks, the patient's serum is added, and unbound antibody is washed away. The amount of specific IgE bound to the solid-phase allergen is then measured by adding ^{125}I-labeled rabbit anti-IgE, washing the beads, and counting the bound radioactivity (Figure 17-10b).

Therapy for Type I Hypersensitivities

Clearly the obvious first step in controlling type I hypersensitivities is to identify the offending allergen and avoid contact if possible. Often the removal of house pets, dust-control measures, or avoidance of offending foods can eliminate a type I response. Elimination of inhalant allergens (such as pollens) is a physical impossibility, however, and other means of intervention must be pursued.

Immunotherapy involving repeated injections of increasing doses of allergens (**hyposensitization**) has been known for some time to reduce the severity of type I reactions, or even eliminate them completely, in a significant number of individuals suffering from allergic rhinitis. Such repeated introduction of allergen by subcutaneous injections appears to cause a shift toward IgG

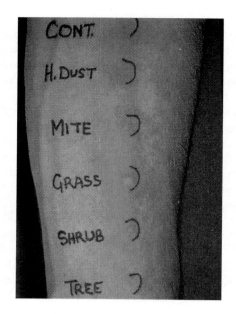

FIGURE 17-9

Skin testing by intradermal injection of allergens into the forearm of an individual. In this individual, a wheal and flare response developed within a few minutes at the site where grass was injected, indicating that the individual is allergic to grass. [From L. M. Lichtenstein, 1993, *Sci. Am.* **269**(2):117. Used with permission.]

production or to induce T-cell–mediated suppression (possibly via a shift to the T_H1 subset and IFN-γ production) that turns off the IgE response (Figure 17-11). In this situation, the IgG antibody is referred to as **blocking antibody** because it competes for the allergen, binds to it, and forms a complex that can be removed by phagocytosis; as a result, the allergen is not available to cross-link the fixed IgE on the mast cell membrane and allergic symptoms decrease.

Another approach for treating allergies stems from the finding that soluble antigens tend to induce a state of anergy by activating T cells in the absence of the necessary co-stimulatory signal (see Figure 12-15). Presumably a soluble antigen is internalized by endocytosis, processed, and presented with class II MHC molecules, but fails to induce expression of the requisite co-stimulatory ligand (B7) on antigen-presenting cells. Immunologic Pharmaceuticals has reported the identification of T-cell epitopes of ragweed pollen, cat hair, and house dust mites. When animals were injected with soluble antigens containing these T-cell epitopes, the animals became anergic to the corresponding allergen. Phase I clinical trials in humans are under way to determine if the soluble antigens will induce a similar allergen-specific state of nonresponsiveness in atopic individuals.

(a)

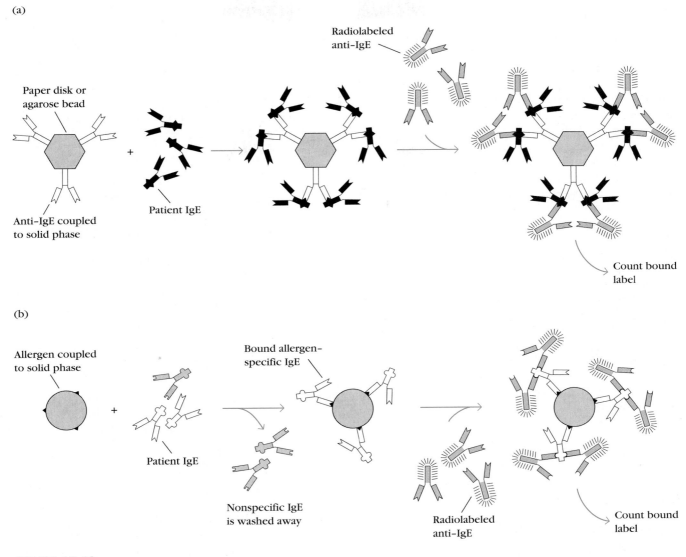

(b)

FIGURE 17-10

Procedures for assessing type I hypersensitivity. (a) Radioimmuno-sorbent test (RIST) can quantify nanogram amounts of total serum IgE. (b) Radioallergosorbent test (RAST) can quantify nanogram amounts of serum IgE specific for a particular allergen.

Knowledge of the mechanism of mast cell degranulation and the mediators involved in type I reactions opened the way to drug therapy for allergies. **Antihistamines** have been the most useful drugs in alleviating allergic rhinitis symptoms. These drugs act by binding to the histamine receptors on target cells and blocking the binding of histamine. The H_1 receptors are blocked by the classical antihistamines, and the H_2 receptors by a newer class of antihistamines.

Several drugs block release of allergic mediators by interfering with various biochemical steps in mast cell activation and degranulation (Table 17-5). Disodium cromoglycate (cromolyn sodium) prevents Ca^{2+} influx into mast cells. Theophylline, which is commonly administered orally or through inhalers to asthmatics, blocks phosphodiesterase, which catalyzes conversion of cAMP to 5′-AMP. The resulting prolonged increase in cAMP levels blocks degranulation. A number of drugs stimulate the β-adrenergic system by stimulating β receptors. As mentioned earlier, epinephrine (also known as adrenaline) is commonly administered during anaphylactic shock. It acts by binding to β receptors on

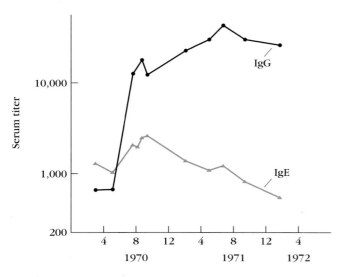

FIGURE 17-11

Hyposensitization treatment of type I allergy. Injection of ragweed anti-gen periodically for 2 years into a ragweed-sensitive individual induced a gradual decrease in IgE levels and a dramatic increase in IgG. Both antibodies were measured by a radioimmunoassay. [Adapted from K. Ishizaka and T. Ishisaka, 1973, in *Asthma Physiology, Immunopharmacology and Treatment*, K. F. Austen and L. M. Lichtenstein (eds.), Academic Press.]

T A B L E   1 7 - 5

MECHANISM OF ACTION OF SOME DRUGS USED TO TREAT TYPE I HYPERSENSITIVITY

DRUG	ACTION
Antihistamines	Block H1 and H2 receptors on target cells
Cromolyn sodium	Blocks Ca^{2+} influx into mast cells
Theophylline	Prolongs high cAMP levels in mast cells by inhibiting phosphodiesterase, which cleaves cAMP to 5′-AMP*
Epinephrine (adrenalin)	Stimulates cAMP production by binding to β-adrenergic receptors on mast cells*
Cortisone	Reduces histamine levels by blocking conversion of histidine to histamine and stimulates mast-cell production of cAMP*

* Although cAMP rises transiently during mast cell activation, degranulation is prevented if cAMP levels remain high.

bronchial smooth muscles and mast cells, elevating the cAMP levels within these cells. The increased levels of cAMP lead to relaxation of the bronchial muscles and decreased mast cell degranulation. A number of epineph-rine analogs have been developed that bind to select β receptors and induce cAMP increases with fewer side effects than epinephrine. Cortisone and various other anti-inflammatory drugs also have been used to reduce type I reactions.

ANTIBODY-MEDIATED CYTOTOXIC (TYPE II) HYPERSENSITIVITY

Type II hypersensitive reactions involve antibody-medi-ated destruction of cells. This type of reaction is best exemplified by blood-transfusion reactions in which host antibodies react with foreign antigens present on the incompatible transfused blood cells and mediate destruc-tion of these cells. Antibody can mediate cell destruction by activating the complement system to create pores in the membrane of the foreign cell (see Figure 14-1). Antibody can also mediate cell destruction by antibody-dependent cell-mediated cytotoxicity (ADCC). In this process, cytotoxic cells with Fc receptors bind to the Fc region of antibodies on target cells and promote killing of the cells (see Figure 16-12). Antibody bound to a foreign cell also can serve as an opsonin, enabling pha-gocytic cells with Fc or C3b receptors to bind and phagocytose the antibody-coated cell (see Figure 14-11).

In this section, we examine three examples of type II hypersensitive reactions. Certain autoimmune diseases also involve autoantibody-mediated cellular destruction via type II mechanisms. These diseases are discussed in Chapter 20.

Transfusion Reactions

A large number of proteins and glycoproteins on the membrane of red blood cells are encoded by different genes, each of which has a number of alternative alleles. An individual possessing one allelic form of a blood-group antigen can recognize other allelic forms on trans-fused blood as foreign and mount an antibody response. In some cases the antibodies are acquired by natural exposure to similar antigenic determinants on a variety of microorganisms thought to be normal flora of the gut. This is the case with the ABO blood-group antigens (Figure 17-12a).

Antibodies to the A, B, and O antigens, called **iso-hemagglutinins**, are usually of the IgM class. An indi-vidual with blood type A, for example, recognizes B-like epitopes on intestinal microorganisms and produces iso-

(a)

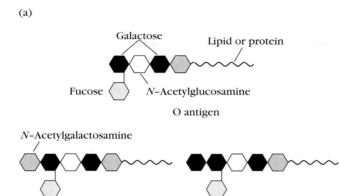

(b)

Genotype	Blood-group phenotype	Antigens on erythrocytes (*agglutinins*)	Serum antibodies (*isohemagglutinins*)
AA or AO	A	A	Anti-B
BB or BO	B	B	Anti-A
AB	AB	A and B	None
OO	O	None	Anti-A and anti-B

FIGURE 17-12

ABO blood group. (a) Structure of terminal sugars, which constitute the distinguishing epitopes, in the A, B, and O blood antigens. (b) ABO genotypes and corresponding phenotypes, agglutinins, and iso-hemagglutinins.

hemagglutinins to the B-like epitopes. This same individual does not respond to A-like epitopes on the same intestinal microorganisms because these A-like epitopes are too similar to self and a state of self-tolerance to these epitopes should exist (Figure 17-12b). If a type A individual is accidentally transfused with blood containing type B cells, the anti-B isohemagglutinins will bind to the B blood cells and mediate their destruction by means of complement-mediated lysis. Antibodies to other blood-group antigens are acquired through repeated blood transfusions because minor allelic differences in these antigens can stimulate antibody production. These antibodies are usually of the IgG class.

Transfusion of blood into a recipient possessing antibodies to one of the blood-group antigens can result in a **transfusion reaction**. The clinical manifestations of transfusion reactions result from massive intravascular hemolysis of the transfused red blood cells by antibody plus complement. The clinical manifestations may have immediate or delayed onset. Reactions having immediate onset are most commonly associated with ABO blood-group incompatibilities, which lead to complement-mediated lysis triggered by the IgM isohemagglutinins. Within hours free hemoglobin can be detected in the plasma; it is filtered through the kidneys, resulting in hemoglobinuria. Some of the hemoglobin gets con-

verted to bilirubin, which at high levels is toxic. Typical symptoms include fever, chills, nausea, clotting within blood vessels, pain in the lower back, and hemoglobin in the urine. Treatment involves prompt termination of the transfusion and maintenance of urine flow with a diuretic because the accumulation of hemoglobin in the kidney can cause acute tubular necrosis.

Delayed hemolytic transfusion reactions generally occur in individuals who have received repeated transfusions of ABO-compatible blood that is incompatible for other blood-group antigens. The reactions develop between 2 and 6 days following transfusion and reflect the secondary nature of these reactions. The transfused blood induces clonal selection and production of IgG against a variety of blood-group membrane antigens. The most common blood-group antigens inducing delayed transfusion reactions are ABO, Rh, Kidd, Kell, and Duffy. The predominant isotype involved in these reactions is IgG, which is less effective than IgM in activating complement. For this reason, complement-mediated lysis of the transfused red blood cells is incomplete, and many of the transfused cells are destroyed at extravascular sites by agglutination, opsonization, and subsequent phagocytosis by macrophages. Symptoms include fever, low hemoglobin, increased bilirubin, mild jaundice, and anemia. Free hemoglobin is usually not detected in the plasma or urine in these reactions because RBC destruction occurs in extravascular sites.

Transfusion reactions can be prevented by proper cross-matching between the donor's and the recipient's blood. Cross-matching can reveal the presence of the antibodies in donor or recipient sera that can cause these reactions.

Hemolytic Disease of the Newborn

Hemolytic disease of the newborn develops when maternal IgG antibodies specific for fetal blood-group antigens cross the placenta and destroy fetal red blood cells. The consequences of such transfer can be minor, serious, or lethal. Severe hemolytic disease of the newborn, called **erythroblastosis fetalis**, most commonly develops when an Rh+ fetus expresses an **Rh antigen** on its blood cells that the Rh− mother does not express.

During pregnancy, fetal red blood cells are separated from the mother's circulation by a layer of cells in the placenta called the trophoblast. During her first pregnancy with an Rh+ fetus, an Rh− woman is usually not exposed to enough of fetal red blood cells to activate her Rh-specific B cells. At the time of delivery, however, separation of the placenta from the uterine wall allows larger amounts of fetal umbilical-cord blood to enter the mother's circulation. These fetal red blood cells activate Rh-specific B cells, resulting in production of Rh-specific plasma cells and memory B cells in the mother. The secreted IgM antibody clears the Rh+ fetal red cells from the mother's circulation, but the memory cells remain, a threat to any subsequent pregnancy with an Rh+ fetus. Activation of these memory cells in a subsequent pregnancy results in the formation of IgG anti-Rh antibodies, which cross the placenta and damage the fetal red blood cells (Figure 17-13). Mild to severe anemia

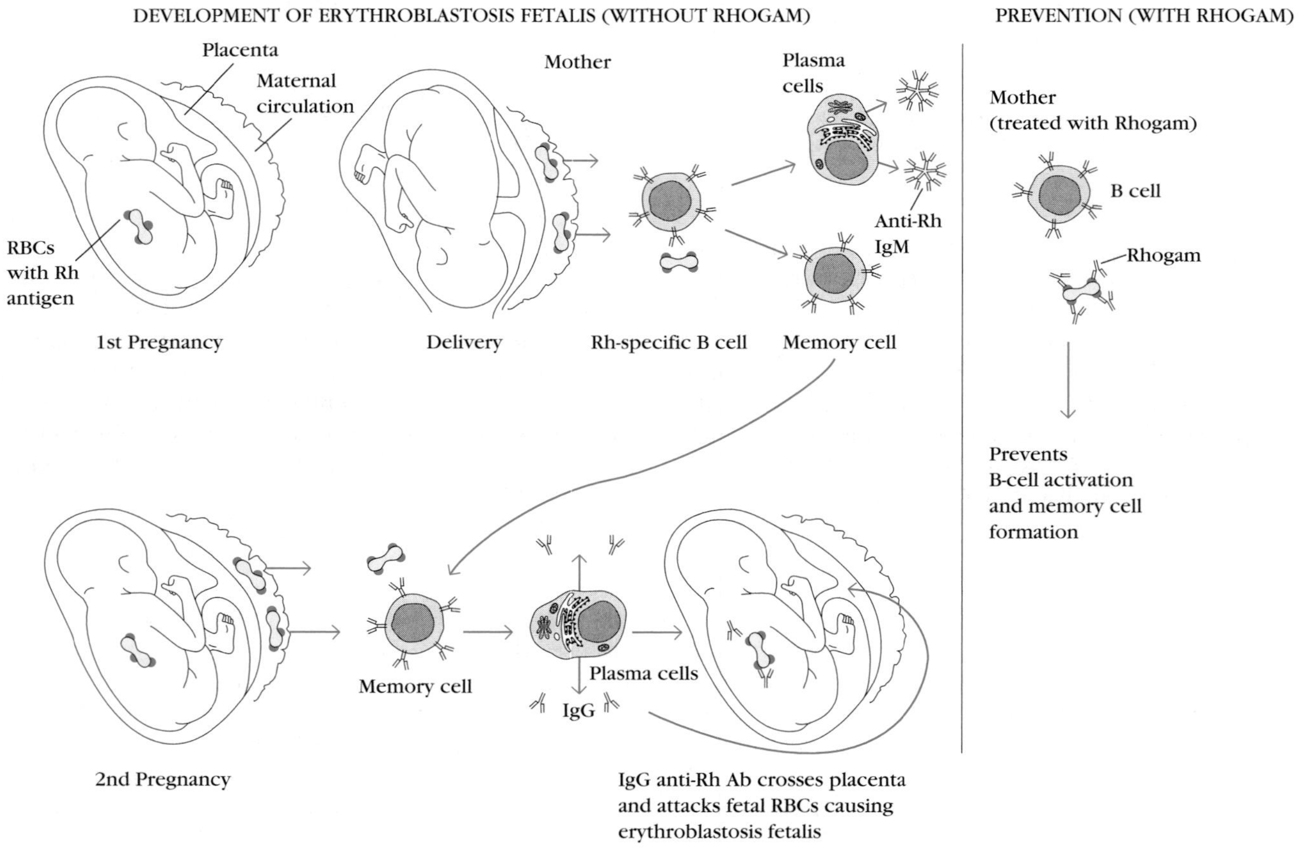

FIGURE 17-13

Development of erythroblastosis fetalis (hemolytic disease of the newborn) caused by an Rh− mother carrying an Rh+ fetus (*left*) and effect of treatment with anti–Rh antibody, or Rhogam (*right*). See text for details.

can develop, sometimes with fatal consequences. In addition, conversion of hemoglobin to bilirubin can present an additional threat to the newborn because the lipid-soluble bilirubin may accumulate in the brain and cause brain damage.

Hemolytic disease of the newborn caused by Rh incompatibility can be almost entirely prevented by the administration of antibodies to the Rh antigen within 24–48 h after delivery. These antibodies, called **Rhogam**, bind to any fetal red blood cells that enter the mother's circulation at the time of delivery and facilitate their clearance before B-cell activation and ensuing memory-cell production can take place. In a subsequent pregnancy with an Rh$^+$ fetus, a Rhogam-treated mother is unlikely to produce IgG anti-Rh antibodies; thus the fetus is protected from the damage that occurs when these antibodies cross the placenta.

The development of hemolytic disease of the newborn caused by Rh incompatibility can be detected by testing maternal serum at intervals during pregnancy for antibodies to the Rh antigen. A rise in the titer of these antibodies as pregnancy progresses indicates that the mother has been exposed to Rh antigens and is producing increasing amounts of antibody. The presence of maternal IgG on the surface of fetal red blood cells can be detected by a **Coombs test**. Isolated fetal red blood cells are incubated with goat antibody to human IgG antibody (the Coombs reagent). If maternal IgG is bound to the fetal red blood cells, the cells agglutinate with the Coombs reagent.

Treatment of hemolytic disease caused by Rh incompatibility depends on the severity of the reaction. If the reaction is severe, the fetus can be given an intrauterine blood-exchange transfusion with Rh$^-$ red blood cells. These transfusions are given every 10–21 days until delivery. In less severe cases, a blood-exchange transfusion is not given until after birth, primarily to remove bilirubin; the infant is also exposed to low levels of UV light to break down the bilirubin and prevent any cerebral damage. The mother can also be treated during the pregnancy by **plasmapheresis**. In this procedure a cell-separation machine is used to separate the mother's blood into two fractions, cells and plasma. The plasma containing the anti-Rh antibody is discarded, and the cells are reinfused into the mother in an albumin or fresh plasma solution.

The majority of cases (65%) of hemolytic disease of the newborn have relatively minor consequences and are caused by ABO blood-group incompatibility between the mother and fetus. Type A or B fetuses carried by type O mothers most commonly develop these reactions. A type O mother is most likely to develop IgG antibody to the A or B blood-group antigens either through natural exposure or through exposure to fetal blood-group A or B antigens in successive pregnancies. Usually the fetal anemia resulting from this incompatibility is mild; the major clinical manifestation is a slight elevation of bilirubin, with jaundice. Depending on the severity of the anemia and jaundice, a blood-exchange transfusion may be required in these infants. In general the reaction is mild, however, and exposure of the infant to low levels of UV light is enough to break down the bilirubin and avoid any cerebral damage.

Drug-Induced Hemolytic Anemia

Certain antibiotics (e.g., penicillin, cephalosporin, and streptomycin) can adsorb nonspecifically to proteins on RBC membranes, forming a complex similar to a hapten-carrier complex. In some patients, such drug-protein complexes induce formation of antibodies, which then bind to the adsorbed drug on red blood cells, inducing complement-mediated lysis and thus progressive anemia. When the drug is withdrawn, the hemolytic anemia disappears. Penicillin is notable in that it can induce all four types of hypersensitivity with various clinical manifestations (Table 17-6).

TABLE 17 - 6

PENICILLIN-INDUCED HYPERSENSITIVE REACTIONS

TYPE OF HYPERSENSITIVE REACTION	ANTIBODY OR LYMPHOCYTES INDUCED	CLINICAL MANIFESTATIONS
I	IgE	Urticaria, systemic anaphylaxis
II	IgM, IgG	Hemolytic anemia
III	IgG	Serum sickness, glomerulonephritis
IV	T$_{DTH}$ cells	Contact dermatitis

IMMUNE COMPLEX–MEDIATED (TYPE III) HYPERSENSITIVITY

The reaction of antibody with antigen generates immune complexes. Generally this complexing of antigen with antibody facilitates the clearance of antigen by phagocytic cells. In some cases, however, large amounts of immune complexes can lead to tissue-damaging type III hypersensitive reactions. The magnitude of the reaction depends on the quantity of immune complexes as well as their distribution within the body. Depending on where these complexes are carried, different tissue-damaging reactions can be observed. When the complexes are deposited in tissue very near the site of antigen entry, a localized reaction develops. When the complexes are formed in the blood, a reaction can develop wherever the complexes are deposited (e.g., on blood-vessel walls, in the synovial membrane of joints, on the glomerular basement membrane of the kidney, on the choroid plexus of the brain). In any case, tissue is damaged at the site of deposition.

Type III hypersensitive reactions develop when immune complexes activate the complement system's array of immune effector molecules (see Figure 14-1). As discussed in Chapter 14, the C3a, C4a, and C5a complement split products are anaphylatoxins that cause localized mast cell degranulation and consequent increase in local vascular permeability. C3a, C5a, and C5b67 are also chemotactic factors for neutrophils, which can accumulate in large numbers at the site of immune-complex deposition. Larger immune complexes are deposited on the basement membrane of blood-vessel walls or kidney glomeruli, whereas smaller complexes may pass through the basement membrane and be deposited in the subepithelium. The type of lesion that results depends on the site of deposition of the complexes.

Much of the tissue damage in type III reactions stems from release of lytic enzymes by neutrophils as they attempt to phagocytose immune complexes. The C3b complement component acts as an opsonin, coating immune complexes. A neutrophil binds to a C3b-coated immune complex by means of the type I complement receptor, which is specific for C3b. Because the complex is attached to the basement-membrane surface, phagocytosis is impeded, allowing lytic enzymes to be released during the unsuccessful attempts of the neutrophil to ingest the adhering immune complex. Further activation of the membrane-attack mechanism of the complement system can also contribute to the tissue destruction. In addition, the activation of complement can induce aggregation of platelets, and the resulting release of clotting factors can lead to formation of microthrombi.

Localized Type III Reactions

Injection of an antigen intradermally or subcutaneously into an animal that has high levels of circulating antibody specific for that antigen leads to formation of localized immune complexes, which mediate an acute **Arthus reaction** within 4–8 h (Figure 17-14). Microscopic examination of the tissue reveals neutrophils adhering to the vascular endothelium and then migrating into the tissues at the site of immune-complex deposition. As the reaction develops, localized tissue and vascular damage results in an accumulation of fluid (edema) and red blood cells (erythema) at the site. The severity of the reaction can vary from mild swelling and redness to tissue necrosis.

Following an insect bite, a sensitive individual may have a rapid, localized type I reaction at the site. Often, some 4–8 h later, a typical Arthus reaction also develops at the site with pronounced erythema and edema. Intrapulmonary Arthus-type reactions induced by bacterial spores, fungi, or dried fecal proteins can also cause pneumonitis or alveolitis. These reactions are known by a variety of common names reflecting the source of the antigen. For example, "farmer's lung" develops after inhalation of thermophilic actinomycetes from moldy hay, and "pigeon fancier's disease" results from inhalation of a serum protein in dust derived from dried pigeon feces.

Generalized Type III Reactions

When large amounts of antigen enter the bloodstream and bind to antibody, circulating immune complexes can form. If antigen is in excess, small complexes form; because these are not easily cleared by the phagocytic cells, they can cause tissue-damaging type III reactions at various sites. Historically, generalized type III reactions were often observed after the administration of antitoxins containing foreign serum, such as horse antitetanus or antidiphtheria serum. In such cases, the recipient of a foreign antiserum develops antibodies specific for the foreign serum proteins; these antibodies then form circulating immune complexes with the foreign serum antigens. Typically, within days or weeks after exposure to foreign serum antigens, an individual begins to manifest a combination of symptoms that are called **serum sickness** (Figure 17-15). These symptoms include fever, weakness, generalized vasculitis (rashes) with edema and erythema, lymphadenopathy, arthritis, and sometimes glomerulonephritis. The precise manifestations of serum sickness depend on the quantity of immune complexes formed as well as the overall size of the complexes, which determine the site of tissue deposition.

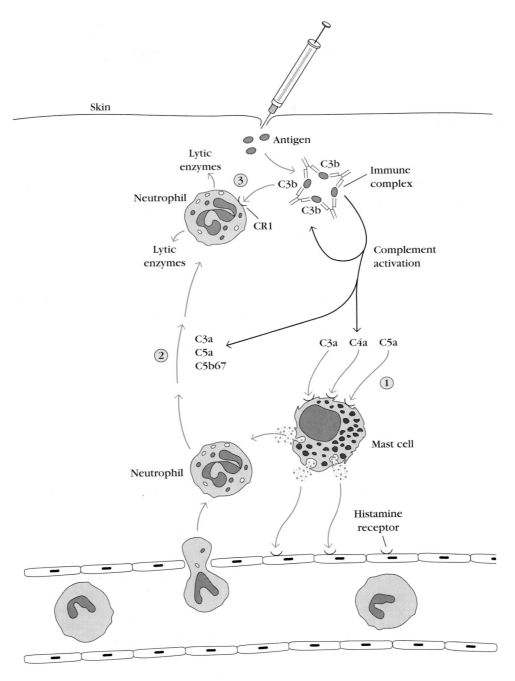

FIGURE 17-14

Development of a localized Arthus reaction (type III hypersensitive reaction). Complement activation initiated by immune complexes (classical pathway) produces complement intermediates that (1) mediate mast cell degranulation, (2) chemotactically attract neutrophils, and (3) stimulate release of lytic enzymes from neutrophils trying to phagocytose C3b-coated immune complexes. See text for further discussion.

Formation of circulating immune complexes contributes to the pathogenesis of a number of conditions other than serum sickness. These include the following:

Autoimmune Diseases
   Systemic lupus erythematosus
   Rheumatoid arthritis
   Goodpasture's syndrome

Drug Reactions
    Allergies to penicillin and sulfonamides

Infectious Diseases
    Poststreptococcal glomerulonephritis
    Meningitis
    Hepatitis
    Mononucleosis
    Malaria
    Trypanosomiasis

Complexes of antibody with various bacterial, viral, and parasitic antigens have been shown to induce a variety of type III hypersensitive reactions, including skin rashes, arthritic symptoms, and glomerulonephritis. Poststreptococcal glomerulonephritis, for example, develops when circulating complexes of antibody and streptococcal antigens are deposited in the kidney and damage the glomeruli. A number of autoimmune diseases stem from circulating complexes of antibody and self-proteins, glycoproteins, or even DNA. In systemic lupus erythematosus, complexes of DNA and anti-DNA antibodies accumulate in synovial membranes, causing arthritic symptoms, or accumulate on the basement membrane of the kidney, causing progressive kidney damage.

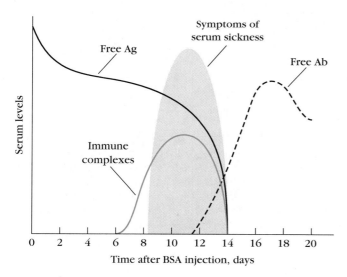

FIGURE 17-15

Correlation between immune-complex formation and development of symptoms of serum sickness. A large dose of antigen (BSA) was injected into a rabbit at day 0. As antibody formed, it complexed with the antigen and was deposited in the kidneys, joints, and capillaries. The symptoms of serum sickness (light blue curve) corresponded to the peak in immune-complex formation. As the immune complexes were cleared, free circulating antibody (dashed black curve) was detected and the symptoms of serum sickness subsided. [Based on F. G. Germuth, Jr., 1953, *J. Exp. Med.* **97**:257.]

T$_{DTH}$-MEDIATED (TYPE IV) HYPERSENSITIVITY

Type IV hypersensitive reactions develop when antigen activates sensitized T$_{DTH}$ cells; these cells generally appear to be a T$_H$1 subpopulation although sometimes T$_C$ cells are involved. As illustrated in Figure 16-15, activation of T$_{DTH}$ cells by antigen on appropriate antigen-presenting cells results in the secretion of various cytokines, including interleukin 2 (IL-2), interferon gamma (IFN-γ), macrophage-inhibition factor (MIF), and tumor necrosis factor β (TNF-β). The overall effect of these cytokines is to draw macrophages into the area and activate them, promoting increased phagocytic activity and increased concentrations of lytic enzymes for more effective killing. As lytic enzymes leak out of the activated macrophages into the surrounding tissue, localized tissue destruction can ensue. These reactions typically take 48–72 h to develop, the time required for initial T$_{DTH}$-cell activation and cytokine secretion to mediate accumulation of macrophages and the subsequent release of their lytic enzymes.

As discussed in Chapter 16, several lines of evidence suggest that the type IV (or DTH) reaction is important in host defense against parasites and bacteria that can live intracellularly. Because these organisms are inside the host's cells, circulating antibodies cannot reach them. However, the heightened phagocytic activity and the buildup of lytic enzymes from macrophages in the area lead to nonspecific destruction of cells, and thus of the intracellular pathogen. When this defense process is not entirely effective, the continued presence of the pathogen's antigens can provoke a chronic DTH reaction, which is characterized by excessive numbers of macrophages, continual release of lytic enzymes, and consequent tissue destruction. The granulomatous skin lesions seen with *Mycobacterium leprae* and the lung cavitation seen with *Mycobacterium tuberculosis* are both examples of the tissue damage that can result when chronic delayed-type hypersensitive reactions develop (see Figures 16-16 and 19-9).

The reaction to an intradermal injection of an antigen can serve as a test for the presence of T$_{DTH}$ cells previously sensitized by that antigen. The use of the PPD antigen to detect previous exposure to *M. tuberculosis* was described in Chapter 16. Similar skin tests to detect previous exposure to the bacterium causing leprosy and the fungus causing coccidiomycosis utilize **lepromin** and **coccidiodin**, respectively, as test antigens. In these tests, the appearance of swelling and redness at the injection site within 48–72 h constitutes a positive reaction. The depletion in CD4$^+$ T cells associated with AIDS can be monitored by repeated skin testing with any of the various antigens that induce a type IV DTH response in most normal individuals. As AIDS progresses, the decline in T_{DTH} cells is reflected in decreased skin reactivity to such antigens.

Many contact-dermatitis reactions, including the response to formaldehyde, trinitrophenol, nickel, turpentine, various cosmetics and hair dyes, poison oak, and poison ivy, are mediated by T_{DTH} cells. Most of these substances are small molecules that can complex with skin proteins. This complex is internalized by antigen-presenting cells in the skin (e.g., Langerhans cells), then processed and presented together with class II MHC molecules, causing activation of sensitized T_{DTH} cells. In the reaction to poison oak, for example, a pentadeca-catechol compound from the leaves of the plant complexes with skin proteins. When T_H cells react with this compound appropriately displayed by local antigen-presenting cells, they differentiate into sensitized T_{DTH} cells. A subsequent exposure to pentadecacatechol will elicit activation of T_{DTH} cells and induce cytokine production (Figure 17-16). Approximately 48–72 h after this secondary exposure, the secreted cytokines cause macrophages to accumulate at the site. Activation of these macrophages and release of their lytic enzymes result in the redness and pustules that characterize a reaction to poison oak.

SUMMARY

1. Hypersensitive reactions are inflammatory reactions within the humoral or cell-mediated branches of the immune system that lead to extensive tissue damage or even death. These reactions are classified into four main types based on the mechanism that induces them (see Table 17-1). Each type generates characteristic effector molecules and clinical manifestations.

2. A type I hypersensitive reaction is mediated by IgE antibodies, whose Fc region binds to receptors on mast cells or blood basophils (see Figure 17-1). Cross-linkage by allergen of the fixed IgE initiates a sequence of intracellular events leading to mast cell or basophil degranulation with release of pharmacologically active mediators (see Table 17-4). The mediators are the immune effector molecules in this reaction. The principal effects of these mediators are smooth-muscle contraction and vasodilation. Clinical manifestations of type I reactions include potentially life-threatening systemic anaphylaxis and localized responses such as hay fever and asthma (see Figure 17-7).

3. A type II hypersensitive reaction occurs when antibody reacts with antigenic determinants present on the surface of cells, leading to cell damage or death through complement-mediated lysis or antibody-

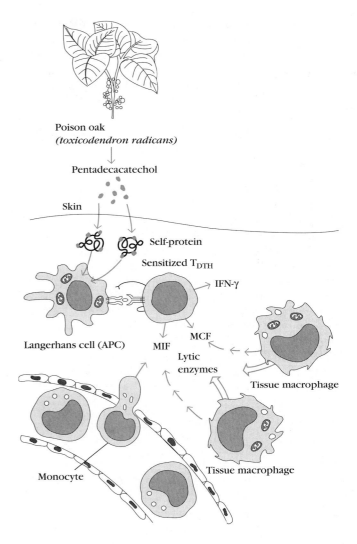

FIGURE 17-16

Development of delayed-type hypersensitivity reaction following second exposure to poison oak. Cytokines such as IFN-γ, MCF, and MIF released from sensitized T_{DTH} cells mediate this reaction. Tissue damage results from lytic enzymes released from activated macrophages. MCF = macrophage-chemotactic factor; MIF = migration-inhibition factor. See also Figure 16-15.

dependent cell-mediated cytotoxicity (ADCC). Transfusion reactions, resulting from mismatching of donor and recipient blood, and hemolytic disease of the newborn are two clinical conditions caused by type II reactions. The latter is most likely when an Rh^- mother carries an Rh^+ fetus (see Figure 17-13).

4. A type III hypersensitive reaction is mediated by the formation of immune complexes and the ensuing activation of complement. Complement split products serve as immune effector molecules that cause

localized vasodilation and chemotactically attract neutrophils. Deposition of immune complexes near the site of antigen entry can induce an Arthus reaction in which lytic enzymes released by the accumulated neutrophils and the complement membrane-attack complex cause localized tissue damage (see Figure 17-14). Generalized type III reactions occur when circulating immune complexes are deposited at various sites; the manifestations of these reactions vary depending on the site of tissue deposition.

5. A type IV hypersensitive reaction involves the cell-mediated branch of the immune system. Antigen activation of sensitized T_{DTH} cells induces release of various cytokines, which serve as the immune effector molecules in this reaction (see Figure 17-16). The net effect of these cytokines is to cause an accumulation and activation of macrophages, which release lytic enzymes that cause localized tissue damage.

REFERENCES

ANSARI, A. A., ET AL. 1989. Human immune responsiveness to Lolium perenne pollen allergen Lol p III (rye III) is associated with HLA-DR3 and DR5. *Hum. Immunol.* **25**:59.

AUBRY, J. P., ET AL. 1992. CD21 is a ligand for CD23 and regulates IgE production. *Nature* **358**:505.

BONNEFOY, J. Y., ET AL. 1993. A new pair of surface molecules involved in human IgE regulation. *Immunol. Today* **14**:1.

DASER, A., ET AL. 1995. Role and modulation of T-cell cytokines in allergy. *Curr. Opin. Immunol.* **7**:762.

FINKELMAN, F. D., ET AL. 1988. IL-4 is required to generate and sustain in vivo IgE response. *J. Immunol.* **141**:2335.

GORDON, J. R., P. R. BURD, AND S. J. GALI. 1990. Mast cells as a source of multifunctional cytokines. *Immunol. Today* **11**:457.

HOLT, P. G. 1994. Immunoprophylaxis of atopy: light at the end of the tunnel? *Immunol. Today* **15**:484.

HOYNE, G. F., ET AL. 1995. Peptide modulation of allergen-specific immune responses. *Curr. Opin. Immunol.* **7**:757.

KAWAKAMI, T., ET AL. 1992. Tyrosine phosphorylation is required for mast cell activation by FcεRI cross-linking. *J. Immunol.* **148**:3513.

KUHN, R., K. RAJEWSKI, AND W. MULLER. 1991. Generation and analysis of interleukin-4 deficient mice. *Science* **254**:707.

KUMAR, A., AND W. W. BUSSE. 1995. Airway inflammation in asthma. *Sci. Am. Sci. Med.* (March/April):38.

MARSH, D. G., ET AL. 1994. Linkage analysis of IL-4 and other chromosome 5q31.1 markers and total serum immunoglobulin E concentrations. *Science* **264**:1152.

PAUL-EUGÈNE, N., ET AL. 1993. Functional interaction between β_2-adrenoceptor agonists and interleukin-4 in the regulation of CD23 expression and release and IgE production in human. *Molec. Immunol.* **30**:157.

RAZIN, E., I. PECHT, AND J. RIVERA. 1995. Signal transduction in the activation of mast cells and basophils. *Immunol. Today* **16**:370.

TEIXEIRA, M. M., T. J. WILLIAMS, AND P. G. HELLEWELL. 1995. Mechanisms and pharmacological manipulation of eosinophil accumulation. *Trends Pharmacol. Sci.* **16**:418.

THOMAS, P., ET AL. 1992. Glycosylation-inhibiting factor from human T cell hybridomas constructed from peripheral blood lymphocytes of a bee venom-sensitive allergic patient. *J. Immunol.* **148**:729.

WILLIAMS, J., ET AL. 1992. Regulation of low-affinity IgE receptor (CD23) expression on mononuclear phagocytes in normal and asthmatic subjects. *J. Immunol.* **149**:2823.

STUDY QUESTIONS

1. Indicate whether each of the following statements is true or false. If you think a statement is false, explain why.

a. Mice infected with *Nippostrongylus brasiliensis* exhibit decreased production of IgE.

b. IL-4 decreases IgE production by B cells.

c. The initial step in the process of mast cell degranulation is cross-linking of Fc receptors.

d. Antihistamines are effective for the treatment of type III hypersensitivity.

e. Most pollen allergens contain a single allergenic component.

f. Babies can acquire IgE-mediated allergies by passive transfer of maternal antibody.

g. Transfusion reactions are a manifestation of type II hypersensitivity.

h. Most T_{DTH} cells belong to the T_H1 subset.

2. In an immunology laboratory exercise, you are studying the response of mice injected intradermally

with complete antibodies to the IgE Fc receptor (FcεRI) or with Fab fragments of such antibodies.

a. Predict the response expected with each type of antibody.

b. Would the responses observed depend on whether or not the mice were allergic? Explain.

3. Serum sickness can result when an individual is given a large dose of antiserum such as a mouse antitoxin to snake venom. How could you take advantage of recent technological advances to produce an antitoxin that would not produce serum sickness in patients who receive it?

4. What immunologic mechanisms most likely account for a person developing each of the following reactions following an insect bite?

a. Within 1–2 min after being bitten, swelling and redness appear at the site and then disappear by 1 h.

b. 6–8 h later swelling and redness again appear and persist for 24 h.

c. 72 h later the tissue becomes inflamed, and tissue necrosis follows.

5. Indicate which type(s) of hypersensitive reaction (I–IV) apply to the following characteristics. Each characteristic can apply to one, or more than one, type.

a. Is an important defense against intracellular pathogens.

b. Can be induced by penicillin.

c. Involves histamine as an important mediator.

d. Can be induced by poison oak in sensitive individuals.

e. Can lead to symptoms of asthma.

f. Occurs as result of mismatched blood transfusion.

g. Systemic form of reaction is treated with epinephrine.

h. Can be induced by pollens and certain foods in sensitive individuals.

i. May involve cell destruction via antibody-dependent cell-mediated cytotoxicity.

j. One form of clinical manifestation is prevented by Rhogam.

k. Localized form characterized by wheal and flare reaction.

6. In the table below, indicate whether each immunologic event listed does (+) or does not (–) occur in each type of hypersensitive response.

For use with Question 6.

IMMUNOLOGIC EVENT	TYPE I HYPERSENSITIVITY	TYPE II HYPERSENSITIVITY	TYPE III HYPERSENSITIVITY	TYPE IV HYPERSENSITIVITY
IgE-mediated degranulation of mast cells				
Lysis of antibody-coated blood cells by complement				
Tissue destruction in response to poison oak				
C3a- and C5a-mediated mast-cell degranulation				
Chemotaxis of neutrophils				
Chemotaxis of eosinophils				
Activation of macrophages by IFN-γ				
Deposition of antigen-antibody complexes on basement membranes of capillaries				
Sudden death due to vascular collapse (shock) shortly after injection or ingestion of antigen				

PART IV

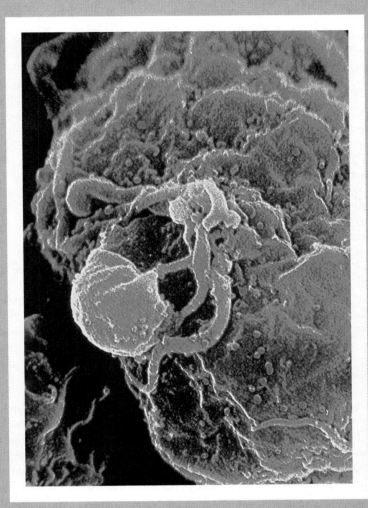

AIDS viruses infect a T-lymphocyte. [© S. Camazine/NIH]

THE IMMUNE SYSTEM
IN HEALTH AND DISEASE

Immunology provides many clues for understanding the pathogenesis of numerous diseases and for developing various measures to either prevent or treat disease. The chapters in Part IV deal with these direct medical applications.

Since Pasteur's public demonstration of the technique of vaccination a little more than 100 years ago, immunologists have developed vaccines against many of the most devastating infectious diseases. The routine immunization of children in many countries has dramatically reduced the toll taken by common childhood illnesses during the past 50 years. In Chapter 18, we first discuss the common types of vaccines, and then see how modern advances in immunology are being applied in designing new vaccines that pose less risk to recipients.

If the human immune system were 100% effective, we would never suffer serious infectious diseases. However, each year millions of people become infected with pathogens, and, especially in less-developed countries, many die from such infections. Chapter 19 reviews the response of the immune system to the four major types of pathogens—viruses, bacteria, protozoans, and parasitic worms—focusing on specific diseases as examples. We also discuss the strategies used by various pathogens to evade immune destruction, so that they can become established within a host. By knowing in detail how the immune system responds to a particular pathogen and how that pathogen escapes, researchers are better able to devise preventive and therapeutic measures.

Lymphocytes that recognize self-antigen normally are either eliminated during B-cell and T-cell maturation or are rendered nonfunctional by various processes. The sometimes devastating consequences of a breakdown in the mechanisms for generating self-tolerance are discussed in Chapter 20. Autoimmune reactions are the cause of several fairly common, chronic disorders including insulin-dependent diabetes mellitus, myasthenia gravis, multiple sclerosis, and rheumatoid arthritis. Most current therapies for autoimmune diseases nonspecifically reduce the immune response; although these may alleviate the autoimmune symptoms, they compromise the patient's ability to ward off infections. Researchers are devising more specific therapies based on knowledge about the molecular mechanisms involved in the immune response.

In Chapter 21 we examine the causes and devastating consequences of immunodeficiency diseases. Those afflicted with such disorders suffer from frequent, prolonged, severe infections, often caused by pathogens that a normal immune system can effectively combat. A wide array of congenital defects give rise to various immunodeficiency diseases. Some disorders are marked by defects in phagocytic cells; others lead to abnormalities in antibody production or in functioning of the complement system. Those afflicted with combined immunodeficiencies, the most serious of these disorders, are unable to mount effective humoral or cell-mediated immune responses. These patients often die in infancy, although bone marrow transplants and in some cases gene therapy offer therapeutic possibilities.

In addition to congenital defects, secondary causes (e.g., infection, malnutrition, and certain drugs) can compromise the immune system. The most significant of the acquired immunodeficiencies—AIDS—renders its victims susceptible to numerous opportunistic infections and rare forms of cancer, which usually are the immediate causes of death. The rapid worldwide spread of AIDS that began in the early 1980s led to an explosion of research about its cause, its effects on the immune system, and approaches for treating or preventing it. This vast body of research is summarized in Chapter 22. The causative agent, human immunodeficiency virus (HIV), is a retrovirus that infects CD4$^+$ T cells, as well as certain other cell types. HIV infection is typically followed by an asymptomatic latent period, which may last up to 10 years. Eventually, the CD4$^+$ T-cell count falls dramatically and a variety of other immunologic abnormalities develop.

In the past several decades great strides have been made in transplantation of tissues and organs. The major obstacle to successful transplantation is rejection of the graft by the recipient's immune system. Chapter 23 is devoted to the analysis of the immunologic basis for graft rejection and to the methods for promoting acceptance. Graft rejection results primarily from a cell-mediated response to histocompatibility antigens (primarily but not exclusively MHC molecules) present on the graft cells that differ from those of the recipient. Tissue typing to minimize the differences in histocompatibility antigens between donor and recipient greatly increases the chances of graft acceptance. Drugs that suppress the immune system are helpful, but they increase the recipient's risk of infection. Promising efforts are under way to develop more specific techniques for promoting graft acceptance, including the use of various monoclonal antibodies.

Under certain conditions, normal cells undergo transformation into tumor (cancer) cells, which are characterized by unregulated cell growth. As we see in Chapter 24, tumor cells can be viewed as altered self-cells, which express cell-membrane antigens that may induce a cell-mediated immune response. Although the immune response to tumor cells is often ineffective, promotion or supplementation of these natural defense mechanisms is the basis for some cancer treatments. This chapter concludes with a discussion of various cancer immunotherapies.

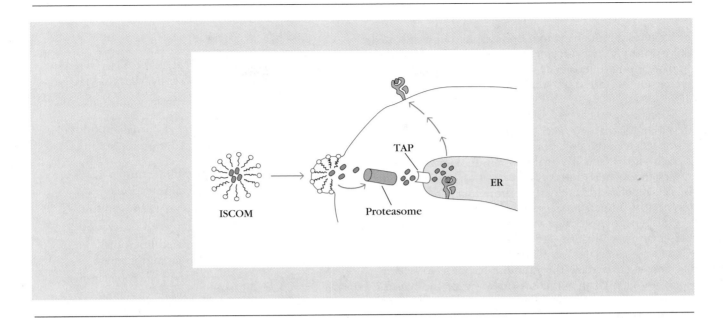

VACCINES

The discipline of immunology has its roots in the early vaccination trials of Edward Jenner and Louis Pasteur. Since these early efforts, vaccines have been developed for many diseases that were once major afflictions of mankind. The incidence of diseases such as diphtheria, measles, mumps, pertussis (whooping cough), rubella (German measles), poliomyelitis, and tetanus has declined dramatically as vaccination has become more common. According to the World Health Organization,

immunization of children in Third World countries increased from 5% to 60% between 1974 and the late 1980s. Despite this progress, more than 5 million infants worldwide continue to die every year from diseases that could be avoided by existing vaccines. Among them are an estimated 2 million deaths from measles and 800,000 from neonatal tetanus, both of which can be completely avoided by immunization. Clearly, vaccination is a cost-effective weapon for disease prevention. Perhaps in no other case have the benefits of vaccination been as dramatically evident as in the eradication of smallpox, one of mankind's long-standing and most terrible scourges. Since October 1977, not a single naturally acquired smallpox case has been reported anywhere in the world.

Unfortunately, because of economic or scientific obstacles, vaccines are either nonexistent or not readily available for several diseases associated with significant rates of morbidity or mortality. For example, more than 250 million people are chronically infected with hepatitis B virus (HBV); malaria causes 1–2 million deaths each year; diarrheal diseases (e.g., infections caused by rotavirus, *Shigella* sp., *Vibrio cholerae*, and toxin-producing *Escherichia coli*) annually kill an estimated 4–5 million people; the common cold and influenza continue to infect untold millions yearly. And despite unprecedented efforts, no effective vaccine has been developed against human immunodeficiency virus (HIV), which had infected an estimated 20 million people worldwide by 1995.

Recent advances in immunology have led to the development of new and promising vaccine strategies. Knowledge of the differences in epitopes recognized by T cells and B cells has enabled immunologists to begin to design vaccines to maximize activation of the humoral or cell-mediated branch of the immune system. As differences in antigen-processing pathways became evident, scientists began to design vaccines to maximize antigen presentation with class I or class II MHC molecules. Genetic engineering techniques can be used to develop vaccines to maximize the immune response to selected epitopes. This chapter focuses on some of the existing vaccine strategies as well as on some experimental designs that may become the vaccines of the future.

ACTIVE AND PASSIVE IMMUNIZATION

Immunity to infectious microorganisms can be achieved by active or passive **immunization**. In each case, immunity can be acquired by natural processes or by artificial means involving injection of antibodies or vaccines (Table 18-1).

Passive Immunization

Passive immunization, in which **preformed antibodies** are transferred to a recipient, can occur naturally by transplacental transfer of maternal antibodies to the developing fetus. Maternal antibodies to diphtheria, tetanus, streptococci, rubeola, rubella, mumps, and poliovirus all afford passively acquired protection to the developing fetus. Maternal antibodies present in colostrum also provide passive immunity to the infant.

Passive immunization can also be achieved by injecting a recipient with preformed antibodies. Passive immunization is used to provide immediate protection to individuals who have been exposed to an infectious organism and are suspected of lacking active immunity to that organism. As an example, if individuals who have not received up-to-date active immunization against tetanus suffer a puncture wound, they are given an injection of horse antiserum to tetanus toxin. The preformed horse antibody neutralizes any tetanus toxin produced by *Clostridium tetani* in the wound. Passive immunization is

TABLE 18-1	
AQUISITION OF IMMUNITY THROUGH PASSIVE AND ACTIVE IMMUNIZATION	
TYPE	ACQUIRED THROUGH
Passive immunization	Natural maternal antibody
	Artificial immune serum
Active immunization	Natural infection
	Artificial infection:
	Attenuated organisms
	Inactivated organisms
	Purified microbial macromolecules
	Cloned microbial antigens (alone or in vectors)
	Synthetic peptides
	Anti-idiotype antibodies
	Multivalent complexes

routinely administered to individuals exposed to botulism, tetanus, diphtheria, hepatitis, measles, and rabies (Table 18-2). Passively administered antiserum is also administered to provide protection from snake bites and black widow spider bites. Because passive immunization does not activate the immune system, it generates no memory response.

Passive immunization should only be given when necessary because certain risks are associated with the injection of preformed antibody. If the antibody was produced in another species, such as a horse, the recipient can mount a strong response to the isotypic determinants of the foreign antibody. This anti-isotype response can lead to certain complications. Some individuals, for example, produce IgE antibody specific for a passive antibody. Immune complexes of this IgE bound to the passively administered antibody can mediate systemic mast cell degranulation, leading to systemic anaphylaxis. Other individuals produce IgG or IgM antibodies specific for the foreign antibody, which form complement-activating immune complexes. The deposition of these complexes in the tissues can lead to type III hypersensitive reactions. Even when human gamma globulin is administered passively, the recipient can generate an anti-allotype response to the human immunoglobulin, although its level is usually much lower than that of an anti-isotype response.

T A B L E   1 8 - 2

COMMON AGENTS USED
FOR PASSIVE IMMUNIZATION

DISEASE	AGENT
Black widow spider bite	Horse antivenin
Botulism	Horse antitoxin
Diphtheria	Horse antitoxin
Hepatitis A and B	Pooled human immune gamma globulin
Measles	Pooled human immune gamma globulin
Rabies	Pooled human immune gamma globulin
Snake bite	Horse antivenin
Tetanus	Pooled human immune gamma globulin or horse antitoxin

Active Immunization

The goal of active immunization is to elicit **protective immunity** and **immunologic memory** so that a subsequent exposure to the pathogenic agent will elicit a heightened immune response with successful elimination of the pathogen. Active immunization can be achieved through natural infection with a microorganism, or it can be acquired artificially through administration of a **vaccine**. In active immunization, as the name implies, the immune system plays an active role, with proliferation of antigen-reactive T and B cells resulting in formation of memory cells. Active immunization with various types of vaccines has played an important role in the reduction of deaths from infectious diseases, especially among children.

Vaccination of children is begun at about 2 months of age. The recommended program of childhood immunizations in this country, updated in 1995 by the Centers for Disease Control (CDC), is outlined in Table 18-3. The program includes the following vaccines:

- Hepatitis B vaccine (new)
- Diphtheria-pertussis-tetanus (DPT) combined vaccine
- Trivalent (Sabin) oral polio vaccine (OPV)
- Measles-mumps-rubella (MMR) combined vaccine

- *Haemophilus influenzae* (Hib) vaccine
- Varicella zoster vaccine for chickenpox (new)

The introduction and spreading use of various vaccines for childhood immunization led to a dramatic decrease in the incidence of common childhood diseases in the United States (Figure 18-1). As long as widespread, effective immunization programs are maintained, the incidence of these childhood diseases should remain low.

As indicated in Table 18-3, childhood immunization often requires multiple **boosters** at appropriately timed intervals to achieve effective immunity. One reason for this is the persistence of maternal antibodies in the young infant. For example, passively acquired maternal antibodies bind to epitopes on the DPT vaccine and block adequate immune-system activation; therefore, this vaccine must be given several times after the maternal antibody has been catabolized to achieve adequate immunity. Passively acquired maternal antibody also interferes with the effectiveness of the measles vaccine; for this reason, the MMR vaccine is not given before 12–15 months of age. In Third World countries, however, the measles vaccine is administered at 9 months, even though maternal antibodies are still present, because 30%–50% of young children in these countries contract the disease

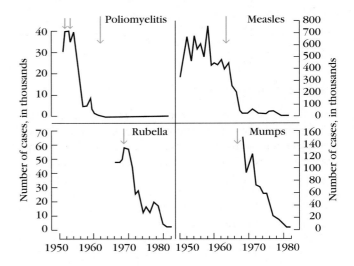

FIGURE 18-1

Reported annual number of cases of poliomyelitis, measles, rubella (German measles), and mumps in the United States (1950–1980) as reported by the Centers for Disease Control. The effect of introduction of vaccines (indicated by blue arrows) on the incidence of these diseases is obvious. [Data from Centers for Disease Control; adapted from C. A. Mims and D. O. White, 1984, *Viral Pathogenesis and Immunology,* Blackwell Scientific.]

T A B L E   1 8 - 3

RECOMMENDED VACCINATION SCHEDULE FOR INFANTS AND CHILDREN

AGE	VACCINE
Birth–2 months	Hepatitis B
2 months	Diphtheria-pertussis-tetanus (DPT) Poliomyelitis (OPV)* *Haemophilus influenzae* type b (Hib)
4 months	Diphtheria-pertussis-tetanus (DPT) Poliomyelitis (OPV)* *Haemophilus influenzae* type b (Hib)
6–18 months	Hepatitis B Poliomyelitis (OPV)*
12–15 months	Diphtheria-pertussis-tetanus (DPT) Varicella zoster (VZV)* Measles, mumps, rubella (MMR)
4–6 years	Diphtheria-pertussis-tetanus (DPT) Poliomyelitis (OPV) Measles, mumps, rubella (MMR)[†]
11–12 years	Diphtheria-tetanus Varicella zoster (VZV)[‡]

* Sabin vaccine consisting of three attenuated strains of poliovirus.

[‡] Varicella zoster virus (VZV) causes chickenpox

[†] Final dose of MMR may be given instead at 11–12 years.

SOURCE: Centers for Disease Control, 1995 Guidelines.

before 15 months of age. Multiple immunizations with the oral polio vaccine are required to ensure that an adequate immune response is generated to each of the three strains of poliovirus that make up the vaccine.

Recommendations for vaccination of adults vary depending on the risk group. Vaccines for meningitis, pneumonia, and influenza are often given to groups living in close quarters (e.g., military recruits) or to individuals with reduced immunity (e.g., the elderly). International travelers are also routinely immunized against such endemic diseases as cholera, yellow fever, plague, typhoid, hepatitis, typhus, and polio.

Vaccination is not 100% effective. Instead, with any vaccine a small percentage of recipients will respond poorly and therefore will not be adequately protected. This is not a serious problem if the majority of the population is immune to an infectious agent. In this case the probability of a susceptible individual contacting an infected individual is so low that the susceptible individual is not likely to become infected. This phenomenon is known as **herd immunity**. The appearance of measles epidemics among college students and unvaccinated preschool-age children in the United States during the mid- to late-1980s resulted partly from an overall decrease in vaccinations among the population that had lowered the herd immunity of the population (Figure 18-2). Among preschool-age children, 88% of those who developed measles were unvaccinated. Most of the college students who contracted measles had been vaccinated as children; the failure of the vaccine to protect them may have resulted from the presence of passively acquired maternal antibodies that reduced their overall response to the vaccine. This increase in the incidence of measles prompted the Immunization Practices Advisory Committee of the Centers for Disease Control to recommend that children receive two immunizations with the combined measles-mumps-rubella vaccine, one at 12–15 months of age and one at entry to kindergarten.

The CDC has called attention to the decline in vaccination rates and herd immunity among American children. For example, a 1995 publication reports that in California nearly one third of all infants are unvaccinated and that about half of all children under the age of 2 are behind schedule on their vaccinations. Such a decrease in herd immunity portends serious consequences, as illustrated by recent events in the new independent states of the former Soviet Union. By the mid-1990s, a diphtheria epidemic was raging in many regions of these new countries, linked to a decrease in herd immunity resulting from decreased vaccination rates following breakup of the Soviet Union. The World Health Organization estimated that 100,000–200,000 individuals in the affected areas would contract diphtheria in 1995.

DESIGNING VACCINES FOR ACTIVE IMMUNIZATION

Several factors must be kept in mind in developing a successful vaccine. First and foremost, the development of an immune response does not necessarily mean that a state of immunity has been achieved. Often the branch of the immune system that is activated is critical, and therefore vaccine designers must recognize the impor-

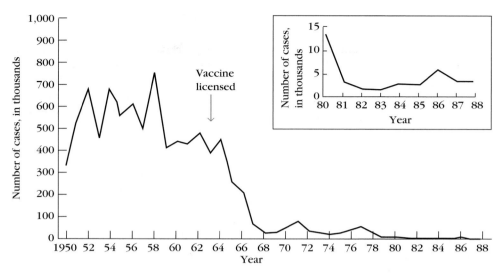

FIGURE 18-2

Introduction of the measles vaccine in 1962 led to a dramatic decrease in the annual incidence of this disease in the United States. Occasional outbreaks of measles in the 1980s *(inset)* occurred mainly among unvaccinated young children and among college students; most of the latter had been vaccinated, but only once, when they were young. [Data from Centers for Disease Control.]

tant differences between activation of the humoral and cell-mediated branches. A second factor is the development of immunologic memory. For example, a vaccine that induces a protective primary response may fail to induce memory-cell formation, leaving the host unprotected after the primary response to the vaccine subsides.

The role of memory cells in immunity depends, in part, on the incubation period of the pathogen. In the case of influenza virus, which has a very short incubation period (<3 days), disease symptoms are already under way by the time memory cells are activated. Effective protection against influenza therefore depends on maintaining high levels of neutralizing antibody by repeated reimmunizations. For pathogens with a longer incubation period, demonstrable neutralizing antibody at the time of infection is not necessary. The poliovirus, for example, requires more than 3 days to begin to infect the central nervous system. An incubation period of this length provides the necessary time for memory B cells to respond with production of high levels of serum antibody. Thus the vaccine for polio is designed to induce high levels of immunologic memory. Following immunization with the Salk vaccine, serum antibody levels peak within 2 weeks and then decline, but the memory response continues to climb, reaching maximal levels at 6 months and persisting for years (Figure 18-3). If an immunized individual is later exposed to the poliovirus, these memory cells will respond by differentiating into plasma cells that produce high levels of serum antibody, which protect the individual from infection.

In the remainder of this chapter, various approaches to the design of vaccines—both currently used vaccines and experimental ones—are described and examined in terms of their ability to induce humoral and cell-mediated immunity and memory-cell production.

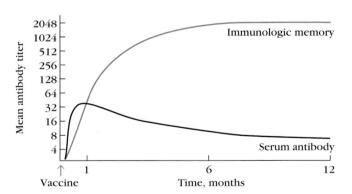

FIGURE 18-3

Immunization with a single dose of the Salk polio vaccine induces a rapid increase in serum antibody levels, which peak by 2 weeks and then decline. Induction of immunologic memory follows a slower time course, reaching maximal levels 6 months after vaccination. The persistence of the memory response for years following primary vaccination is responsible for immunity to poliomyelitis. [From M. Zanetti et al., 1987, *Immunol. Today* **8**:18.]

WHOLE-ORGANISM VACCINES

As Table 18-4 indicates, many of the common vaccines currently in use consist of **inactivated** (killed) or live but **attenuated** (avirulent) bacterial cells or viral particles. The primary characteristics of these two types of vaccines are compared in Table 18-5.

Attenuated Viral or Bacterial Vaccines

In some cases microorganisms can be attenuated so that they lose their ability to cause significant disease (pathogenicity) but retain their capacity for transient growth within an inoculated host. Attenuation can often be achieved by growing a pathogenic bacterium or virus for prolonged periods under abnormal culture conditions. This procedure selects mutants that are better suited to growth in the abnormal culture conditions and are therefore less capable of growth in the original host. For example, an attenuated strain of *Mycobacterium bovis* called **Bacillus Calmette-Guerin** (BCG) was developed by growing *M. bovis* on a medium containing increased concentrations of bile. After 13 years this strain had adapted to growth with increased bile and had become sufficiently attenuated that it was suitable as a vaccine for tuberculosis. The Sabin polio vaccine and the measles vaccine consist of viral strains that have been successfully attenuated and now serve as successful vaccines. The poliovirus used in the Sabin vaccine was attenuated by growth in monkey kidney epithelial cells. The measles vaccine contains a strain of rubella virus that was grown in duck embryo cells and later in human cell lines.

Attenuated vaccines have some advantages and some disadvantages. Because of their capacity for transient growth, such vaccines provide prolonged immune-system exposure to the individual epitopes on the attenuated organisms, resulting in increased immunogenicity and memory-cell production. As a consequence, these vaccines often require only a single immunization, eliminating the need for repeated boosters. This property is a major advantage in Third World countries where epidemiologic studies have shown that roughly 20% of individuals fail to return for each subsequent booster. The ability of many attenuated vaccines to replicate within host cells makes them particularly suitable for inducing a cell-mediated response.

The Sabin polio vaccine, consisting of three attenuated strains of poliovirus, is administered orally to children on a sugar cube or in sugar liquid. The attenuated viruses colonize the intestine and induce protective immunity to all three strains of virulent poliovirus. The ability of the attenuated Sabin vaccine to colonize the intestines enables it to induce production of secretory IgA, which serves as an important defense against naturally acquired poliovirus. The vaccine also induces IgM and IgG classes of antibody. Unlike most other attenuated vaccines, which require a single immunizing dose, the Sabin polio vaccine requires boosters because the three strains of attenuated poliovirus in the vaccine in-

T A B L E   1 8 - 4

CLASSIFICATION OF COMMON VACCINES FOR HUMANS

DISEASE OR PATHOGEN	TYPE OF VACCINE
WHOLE ORGANISMS	
Bacterial cells:	
Cholera	Inactivated
Pertussis	Inactivated
Plague	Inactivated
Tuberculosis	Attenuated BCG*
Viral particles:	
Influenza	Inactivated
Measles	Attenuated
Mumps	Attenuated
Polio (Sabin)	Attenuated
Polio (Salk)	Inactivated
Rubella	Inactivated
Varicella zoster (chickenpox)	Attenuated
Yellow fever	Attenuated
PURIFIED MACROMOLECULES	
Toxoids:	
Diphtheria	Inactivated exotoxin
Tetanus	Inactivated exotoxin
Capsular polysaccaharide:	
Haemophilus influenzae type b	Polysaccharide + protein carrier
Neisseria meningitidis	Polysaccharide
Streptococcus pneumoniae	23 distinct capsular polysaccharides
Surface antigen:	
Hepatitis B	Recombinant surface antigen (HbsAg)

* Bacillus Calmette–Guerin (BCG) is an avirulent strain of *Mycobacterium bovis*.

terfere with each other's replication in the intestine. With the first immunization, one strain will predominate in its growth, inducing immunity to that strain. With the second immunization, the immunity generated by the previous immunization will limit the growth of the previously predominant strain, enabling one of the two remaining strains to predominate and induce immunity. Finally with the third immunization, immunity to all three strains is achieved.

The major disadvantage of attenuated vaccines is the possibility of their **reversion** to a virulent form. The rate of reversion of the Sabin polio vaccine leading to subsequent paralytic disease is about one case in four million doses of vaccine. Another concern with attenuated vaccines is the presence of other viruses as contaminants. In 1960 it was discovered that the oncogenic virus SV40 had contaminated some monkey kidney cultures used in production of the Sabin vaccine; as a result more stringent vaccine testing was required to eliminate this contaminant. Attenuated vaccines also may be associated with complications similar to those seen in the natural disease. A small percentage of recipients of the measles vaccine, for example, develop postvaccine encephalitis. Although these complications are undesirable, the risk of such complications is far less than that observed in a naturally acquired measles infection.

In some cases, however, postvaccine complications may render a potential vaccine unacceptable. This situation is illustrated by trials conducted several years ago with an experimental measles vaccine. This vaccine—an attenuated strain of the virus called the Edmonston-Zagreb strain—is immunogenic in infants as young as 4–6 months old. As noted earlier, maternal antibodies render the standard measles vaccine ineffective when it is given before 9 months of age. The new vaccine was developed for use in Third World countries where many infants are infected with the measles virus at a very early age. Unfortunately, trials of the Edmonston-Zagreb vaccine in Guinea-Bissau, Senegal, and Haiti had to be halted when many vaccinated children began dying from common endemic disorders such as diarrhea, pneumonia, and parasitic diseases. Mortality rates were higher in girls than boys, an unexplained finding. The high rate of postvaccine complications with the Edmonston-Zagreb strain may result from vaccine-mediated immunosuppression, since the measles virus is known to cause transient immunosuppression. Some have speculated that the potent immunogenicity of the Edmonston-Zagreb strain, even in the presence of maternal antibodies, may be associated with potent immunosuppressive effects, placing vaccinated infants at risk for infections with other endemic pathogens that unvaccinated infants can resist.

Genetic engineering techniques provide a way to attenuate a virus irreversibly by selectively removing genes that are necessary for virulence. This has been done with a herpes virus vaccine for pigs, in which the thymidine kinase gene was removed. Because thymidine kinase is required for the virus to grow in certain types of cells

---

TABLE 18 - 5

COMPARISON OF ATTENUATED (LIVE) AND INACTIVATED (KILLED) VACCINES

CHARACTERISTIC	ATTENUATED VACCINE	INACTIVATED VACCINE
Production	Selection for avirulent organisms: virulent pathogen is grown under adverse culture conditions or prolonged passage of a virulent human pathogen in different hosts	Virulent pathogen is inactivated by chemicals or irradiation with γ-rays
Booster requirement	Generally requires only a single booster	Requires multiple boosters
Relative stability	Less stable	More stable (advantageous for Third World countries where refrigeration is limited)
Type of immunity induced	Produces humoral and cell-mediated immunity	Produces mainly humoral immunity
Reversion tendency	May revert to virulent form	Cannot revert to virulent form

(e.g., neurons), removal of this gene rendered the virus incapable of causing disease. It is possible that similar genetic engineering techniques could eliminate the risk of reversion of the attenuated polio vaccine. One strategy for developing an AIDS vaccine involves research on HIV variants in the hope of developing an irreversibly attenuated strain.

Inactivated Viral or Bacterial Vaccines

Another common approach in vaccine production is to inactivate the pathogen by heat or by chemical means so that the pathogen is no longer capable of replication in the host. It is critically important to maintain the structure of epitopes on surface antigens during inactivation. Heat inactivation is generally unsatisfactory because it causes extensive protein denaturation; thus any epitopes that depend on higher orders of protein structure are likely to be altered. Chemical inactivation with formaldehyde or various alkylating agents has had success. The Salk polio vaccine and the pertussis (whooping cough) vaccine are produced by formaldehyde inactivation.

Unlike immunization with attenuated vaccines, which generally requires only one dose to induce long-lasting immunity, repeated boosters of killed vaccines are often needed to maintain the immune status of the host. In addition, killed vaccines induce a predominantly humoral antibody response; they are less effective than attenuated vaccines in inducing cell-mediated immunity and in eliciting a secretory IgA response.

Even though they contain killed pathogens, inactivated whole-organism vaccines are still associated with certain risks. A serious complication with the first Salk vaccines was inadequate formaldehyde killing of the virus in two vaccine lots, which caused paralytic polio in a high percentage of recipients. The pertussis vaccine highlights another problem that can arise with a complex whole-organism vaccine. Encephalitis-type reactions occur in a small percentage of infants receiving this vaccine (Table 18-6). The components of the vaccine responsible for these reactions have not been determined.

Purified Macromolecules as Vaccines

Some of the risks associated with attenuated or killed whole-organism vaccines can be avoided with vaccines that consist of specific, purified macromolecules derived from pathogens. Three general forms of such vaccines are in current use: inactivated exotoxins, capsular polysaccharide, and recombinant surface antigens (see Table 18-4).

POLYSACCHARIDE VACCINES

The virulence of some pathogenic bacteria depends primarily on the antiphagocytic properties of their hydrophilic polysaccharide capsule. Coating of the capsule with antibodies and/or complement greatly increases the ability of macrophages and neutrophils to phagocytose such pathogens. These findings provide the rationale for vaccines consisting of purified capsular polysaccharides.

The current vaccine for *Streptococcus pneumoniae*, which causes pneumococcal pneumonia, consists of 23 antigenically different capsular polysaccharides. It is marketed as Pneumovax 23 by Merck and as Pnu-Immune 23 by Lederle Laboratories. The vaccine induces formation of opsonizing antibodies and is administered to high-risk groups such as infants, splenectomized patients, other immune-suppressed individuals, and the elderly. The vaccine for *Neisseria meningitidis*, a common cause of bacterial meningitis, also consists of purified capsular polysaccharides.

One limitation of polysaccharide vaccines is their inability to activate T_H cells. They activate B cells in a thymus-independent type 2 (TI-2) manner, resulting in IgM production but little class switching, no affinity maturation, and little, if any, development of memory cells. Several investigators have reported the induction of IgA-secreting plasma cells in humans receiving subcutaneous immunization with the pneumococcal polysaccharide vaccine. In this case, since T_H cells are not involved in the response, the vaccine may activate IgA-specific memory B cells previously generated by naturally occurring bacterial antigens at mucosal surfaces. Because these bacteria have both polysaccharide and protein epitopes, they would activate T_H cells, which in turn could mediate class switching and memory-cell formation.

T A B L E   1 8 - 6

RISKS VERSUS BENEFITS OF THE PERTUSSIS VACCINE FOR WHOOPING COUGH

PROBLEM	RISK OF OCCURRENCE AFTER	
	VACCINATION	DISEASE
Seizures	1:1750	1:25–1:50
Encephalitis	1:110,000	1:1000–1:4000
Severe brain damage	1:310,000	1:2000–1:8000
Death	1:1,000,000	1:200–1:1000

SOURCE: I. Tizard, *Immunology: An Introduction*, 2d ed., Saunders.

One way to involve T_H cells directly in the response to a polysaccharide antigen is to conjugate the antigen to some sort of protein carrier. For example, the vaccine for *Haemophilus influenzae* type b (Hib), the major cause of bacterial meningitis in children under 5 years of age, consists of type b capsular polysaccharide covalently linked to a protein carrier, tetanus toxoid. The polysaccharide-protein conjugate is considerably more immunogenic than the polysaccharide alone, and because it activates T_H cells, it enables class switching from IgM to IgG. Although this type of vaccine can induce memory B cells, it cannot induce memory T cells specific for the pathogen. In the case of the Hib vaccine, it appears that the memory B cells can be activated to some degree in the absence of a population of memory T_H cells, thus accounting for the efficacy of this vaccine.

TOXOID VACCINES

Some bacterial pathogens, including those causing diphtheria and tetanus, produce exotoxins. These exotoxins produce many of the disease symptoms resulting from infection. Diphtheria and tetanus vaccines, for example, can be made by purifying the bacterial exotoxin and then inactivating the toxin with formaldehyde to form a **toxoid**. Vaccination with the toxoid induces antitoxoid antibodies, which are also capable of binding to the toxin and neutralizing its toxic effects. In production of toxoid vaccines the conditions must be closely controlled to achieve detoxification without excessive modification of the epitope structure.

One of the problems encountered with vaccines consisting of purified macromolecules is the difficulty of obtaining sufficient quantities of the purified components. In the case of the diphtheria and tetanus toxoid vaccines, this limitation has been overcome by cloning the exotoxin genes and then expressing them in easily grown host cells. In this way, large quantities of the exotoxin can be produced, purified, and subsequently inactivated.

RECOMBINANT ANTIGEN VACCINES

Theoretically the gene encoding any immunogenic protein can be isolated and cloned in bacterial, yeast, or mammalian cells using recombinant DNA technology (see Chapter 2). A number of genes encoding surface antigens from viral, bacterial, and protozoan pathogens have been successfully cloned in bacterial, yeast, insect, or mammalian expression systems, and the expressed antigens used for vaccine development. The first such recombinant antigen vaccine approved for human use was the hepatitis B vaccine. This vaccine was developed by

cloning the gene for the major surface antigen of hepatitis B virus (HBsAg) in yeast cells. The recombinant yeast cells are grown in large fermenters and HBsAg accumulates intracellularly in the cells. The yeast cells are harvested and disrupted by high pressure, releasing the recombinant HBsAg, which is then purified by conventional biochemical techniques. The recombinant hepatitis B vaccine has been shown to induce the production of protective antibodies. This vaccine holds much promise for the 250 million carriers of chronic hepatitis B worldwide!

Several recombinant vaccines for human immunodeficiency virus, presently being assessed in volunteers as potential vaccines for AIDS, are discussed in Chapter 22. Other recombinant vaccines that are being evaluated in animal models include the β subunit of cholera toxin, the enterotoxin of *E. coli*, the circumsporozoite protein of the malaria parasite, and a glycoprotein membrane antigen from Epstein-Barr virus. Animals immunized with these recombinant vaccines have in some cases mounted a protective immune response to a subsequent challenge with the live pathogen. One disadvantage of recombinant protein or glycoprotein vaccines is that they are processed as exogenous antigens and therefore do not tend to induce much activation of class I MHC–restricted T_C cells. In other words, they primarily induce humoral immunity.

RECOMBINANT VECTOR VACCINES

It is possible to introduce genes encoding major antigens of especially virulent pathogens into attenuated viruses or bacteria. The attenuated organism serves as a **vector**, replicating within the host and expressing the gene product of the pathogen. A number of organisms have been used for vector vaccines, including vaccinia virus, the canarypox virus, attenuated poliovirus, adenoviruses, attenuated strains of *Salmonella*, and the BCG strain of *Mycobacterium bovis*.

Vaccinia virus, the attenuated vaccine used to eradicate smallpox, has been widely employed as a vector vaccine. This large, complex virus, with a genome of about 200 genes, can be engineered to carry several dozen foreign genes without impairing its capacity to infect host cells and replicate. The procedure for producing a vaccinia vector carrying a foreign gene from a pathogen is outlined in Figure 18-4. The genetically engineered vaccinia expresses high levels of the inserted gene product, which can then serve as a potent immunogen in an inoculated host. E. Paoletti has inserted genes from

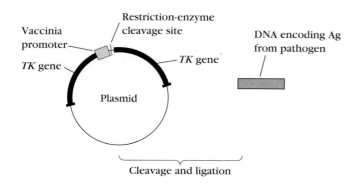

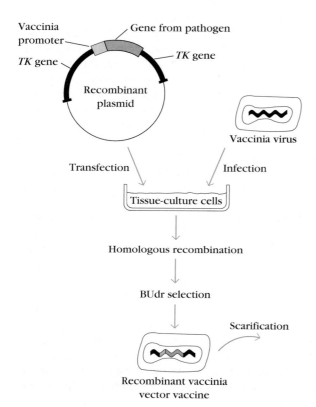

FIGURE 18-4

Production of vaccinia vector vaccine. The gene encoding the desired antigen (blue) is inserted into a plasmid vector adjacent to a vaccinia promoter (gray) and flanked on either side by the vaccinia thymidine kinase (*TK*) gene (black). When tissue-culture cells are incubated simultaneously with vaccinia virus and the recombinant plasmid, the antigen gene and promoter are inserted into the vaccinia virus genome by homologous recombination at the site of the nonessential *TK* gene, resulting in a *TK⁻* recombinant virus. Cells containing the recombinant vaccinia virus are selected by addition of bromodeoxyuridine (BUdr), which kills TK⁺ cells. [Adapted from B. Moss, 1985, *Immunol. Today* **6**:243.]

Other attenuated vector vaccines may prove to be safer than the vaccinia vaccine. The canarypox virus has recently been tried as a vector vaccine. Like its relative, vaccinia, the canarypox virus is a large virus that can easily be engineered to carry multiple genes. Unlike vaccinia, the canarypox virus does not appear to be virulent even in individuals with severe immune suppression. Another possible vector is an attenuated strain of *Salmonella typhimurium*, which has been engineered with genes from the bacterium that causes cholera. The advantage of this vector vaccine is that *Salmonella* infects cells of the mucosal lining of the gut and therefore will induce secretory IgA production. Effective immunity against a number of diseases, including cholera and gonorrhea, depends on increased production of secretory IgA at mucous membrane surfaces. One of the poliovirus strains used in the Sabin vaccine is another candidate for a safe and effective vector vaccine. In this case the poliovirus vector is genetically engineered so that a portion of the gene encoding the outer capsid protein of poliovirus is replaced by DNA encoding the epitope of choice. The resulting poliovirus chimera will express the desired epitope in a highly accessible presentation protruding from the poliovirus nucleocapsid.

DNA VACCINES

In a recently developed vaccination strategy, plasmid DNA encoding a viral antigen is injected directly into the muscle of the recipient. The DNA is taken up by muscle cells and the encoded protein antigen is expressed, leading to both a humoral antibody response and cell-mediated response to the viral antigen. What is most surprising about this finding is that the injected DNA is taken up and expressed by the muscle cells with much greater efficiency than seen with transfection experiments in tissue culture. The DNA appears either to inte-

hepatitis B virus, herpes simplex, and influenza into vaccinia virus. Vaccine trials in the laboratory have shown that this engineered vaccinia induces antibodies and cell-mediated immunity to all three engineered gene products. Like the smallpox vaccine, genetically engineered vaccinia vector vaccines can be administered simply by dermal scratching, causing a limited localized infection in host cells. If the foreign gene product expressed by the vaccinia is a viral envelope protein, it is inserted into the membrane of the infected host cell, inducing development of cell-mediated immunity as well as antibody-mediated immunity.

grate into the chromosomal DNA or to be maintained for long periods in an episomal form. It is unclear whether the viral antigen is expressed only by the muscle cells or whether dendritic cells in the area also take up the plasmid DNA and express the viral antigen. The fact that muscle cells express only low levels of class I MHC molecules and fail to express co-stimulatory molecules suggests that dendritic cells in the area also may be involved.

DNA vaccines offer several advantages over many of the existing vaccines. Their ability to induce both humoral and cell-mediated immunity without requiring a live attenuated vaccine is a major benefit. In addition, because DNA vaccines allow prolonged expression of the antigen, significant immunological memory should be generated. An improved method for administering these vaccines involves coating microscopic gold beads with the plasmid DNA and then delivering the coated particles through the skin into the underlying muscle with an air gun (called a **gene gun**). A number of companies, including Vical and Merck, have begun testing DNA vaccines in animal models. So far, the results are encouraging and have shown that these vaccines are able to induce protective immunity against a number of pathogens, including the influenza virus.

Enthusiasm for the potential of DNA vaccines must, however, be tempered by several unknowns. It is not known exactly which cells take up the DNA. Neither is it known what the consequences of long-term antigen expression will be. Chronic persistent expression of the antigen by the muscle cells, for example, may eventually lead to a state of immunologic nonresponsiveness to the antigen or to a state of autoimmunity. Finally, the safety of introducing foreign DNA molecules at high copy number remains unknown.

SYNTHETIC PEPTIDE VACCINES

Among the synthetic peptide vaccines currently being evaluated are those for hepatitis B virus, the malaria parasite, diphtheria toxin, influenza (see Chapter 19), and HIV (see Chapter 22). Construction of synthetic peptides for use as vaccines to induce either humoral or cell-mediated immunity requires an understanding of the nature of T-cell and B-cell epitopes.

Although the amino acid sequence of many important antigens from pathogens is known, few have been subjected to x-ray crystallographic analysis, so their three-dimensional structure is unknown. However, because B-cell epitopes must constitute accessible surface regions, vaccine designers commonly analyze the primary structure of an antigen to identify strongly hydrophilic sequences, which most likely correspond to such surface regions. Synthetic peptides corresponding to these potential B-cell epitopes are then prepared. Ideally, vaccines for inducing humoral immunity should include peptides composing immunodominant B-cell epitopes. Such epitopes can be identified by determining the dominant antibody in the sera of individuals who are recovering from a disease and then testing various synthetic peptides for their ability to react with that antibody with a high affinity. In one such experiment, two linear synthetic peptides representing potential B-cell epitopes of HBsAg were tested for their binding affinity to pooled antisera from individuals who had recovered from hepatitis B. It was found that a synthetic peptide consisting of cyclical repeats of amino acids 139–147 had a tenfold higher affinity than cyclical repeats of amino acids 124–137. The cyclical peptide 139–147 was therefore chosen as a potential candidate for a synthetic hepatitis B vaccine.

An effective memory response for both humoral and cell-mediated immunity requires generation of a population of memory T_H cells. A successful vaccine must therefore include immunodominant T-cell epitopes. With synthetic peptide vaccines it is difficult to identify those epitopes owing to the role, unpredictable as yet, of the MHC in influencing immunodominance for the T-cell system. T cells recognize processed peptides that, in the majority of cases, appear to represent internal peptides. As illustrated in Figure 4-9, these peptides must have a site (the **agretope**) that enables them to interact with MHC molecules as well as a site (the **epitope**) that enables them to interact with the T-cell receptor. Since MHC molecules differ in their ability to present peptides to T cells, MHC polymorphism within a species influences the level of T-cell responsiveness by different individuals to different peptides.

Moreover, different subpopulations of T cells probably recognize different epitopes. Experiments by E. Sercarz have identified some peptides that induce a strong helper response and other peptides that induce immunologic suppression. These helper and suppressor peptides generally represent different, nonoverlapping amino acid sequences within an antigen. For example, immunization with the amino-terminal residues (1–17) of hen egg-white lysozyme suppressed the response to native lysozyme. By identifying suppressing peptides and eliminating them from synthetic vaccines, it might be possible to generate enhanced immunity. These suppressing peptides may also be valuable in situations where it is desirable to decrease the immune response, as in treating autoimmune diseases.

MULTIVALENT SUBUNIT VACCINES

One of the limitations with synthetic peptide vaccines and recombinant protein vaccines is that these vaccines tend to be poorly immunogenic; in addition, they tend to induce a humoral antibody response but are less likely to induce a cell-mediated response. What is needed is some method of structuring a synthetic peptide vaccine to contain both immunodominant B-cell and T-cell epitopes. Furthermore, if a CTL response is desired, the vaccine must be delivered intracellularly so that the peptides can be processed and presented together with class I MHC molecules. A number of innovative techniques

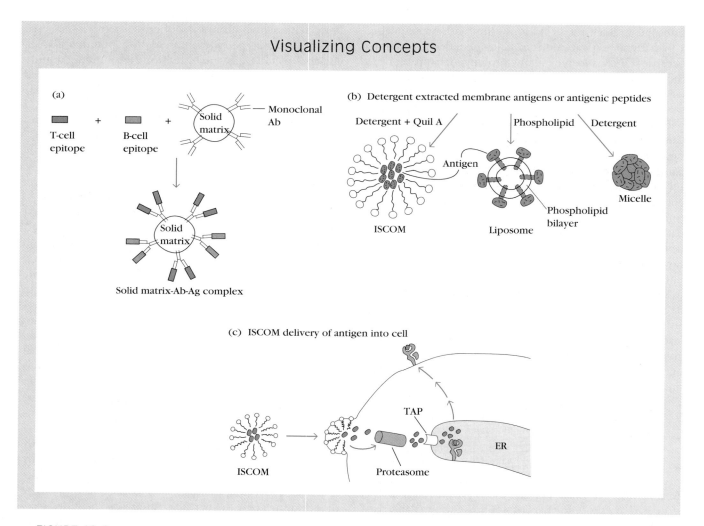

Visualizing Concepts

FIGURE 18-5

Multivalent subunit vaccines. (a) Solid matrix–antibody–antigen complexes can be designed to contain synthetic peptides representing both T-cell epitopes (blue) and B-cell epitopes (gray). (b) Protein micelles, liposomes, and immunostimulating complexes (ISCOMs) can all be prepared with extracted antigens or antigenic peptides (blue). In micelles and liposomes, the hydrophilic residues of the antigen molecules are oriented outward. In ISCOMs, the long fatty-acid tails of the external detergent layer are adjacent to the hydrophobic residues of the centrally located antigen molecules. (c) ISCOMs and liposomes can deliver antigens inside cells, so they mimic endogenous antigens. Subsequent processing by the cytosolic pathway and presentation with class I MHC molecules induces a cell-mediated response.

are currently being employed to develop multivalent vaccines that can present multiple copies of a given peptide or a mixture of peptides to the immune system.

One approach is to prepare **solid matrix–antibody-antigen** (SMAA) complexes by attaching monoclonal antibodies to particulate solid matrices and then saturating the antibody with the desired antigen. The resulting complexes are then used as vaccines. By attaching different monoclonal antibodies to the solid matrix, it is possible to bind a mixture of peptides or proteins, composing immunodominant epitopes for both T cells and B cells, to the solid matrix (Figure 18-5a). These multivalent complexes have been shown to induce vigorous humoral and cell-mediated responses. Their particulate nature contributes to their increased immunogenicity by facilitating phagocytosis by phagocytic cells.

Another means of obtaining a multivalent vaccine is to utilize detergent to incorporate protein antigens or synthetic antigenic peptides into protein micelles, into lipid vesicles (called liposomes), or into immunostimulating complexes (Figure 18-5b). **Micelles** are formed by mixing proteins in detergent and then removing the detergent. The individual proteins will orient themselves with the hydrophilic residues oriented toward the aqueous environment and the hydrophobic residues at the center so as to exclude their interaction with the aqueous environment. **Liposomes** containing protein antigens are prepared by mixing the proteins with a suspension of phospholipids under conditions that form vesicles bounded by a bilayer. The proteins are incorporated into the bilayer with the hydrophilic residues exposed. **Immunostimulating complexes** (ISCOMs) are lipid carriers prepared by mixing protein or peptide antigens with detergent and a glycoside called Quil A.

Membrane proteins from different pathogens including influenza virus, measles virus, hepatitis B virus, and HIV have been incorporated into micelles, liposomes, and ISCOMs and are currently being assessed as potential vaccines. In addition to their increased immunogenicity, liposomes and ISCOMs appear to fuse with the plasma membrane delivering the antigen intracellularly where it can be processed by the cytosolic pathway and thus induce a cell-mediated response (Figure 18-5c).

ANTI-IDIOTYPE VACCINES

As discussed in Chapter 16, an anti-idiotype antibody can in effect serve as the internal image of an antigen. This discovery opened the door to the potential introduction of anti-idiotype antibodies as vaccines. What they promise, of course, is the generation of an effective

immune response to a dangerous pathogen without exposure of the vaccinated individual to any form of the pathogen (Figure 18-6).

Anti-idiotype vaccines have been shown to induce protective immunity in mice against hepatitis B virus and

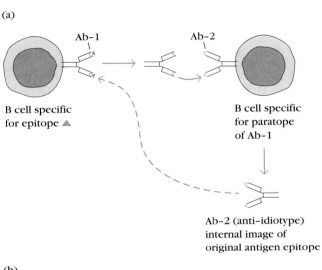

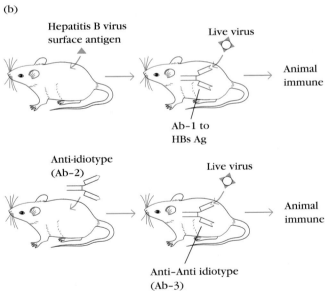

FIGURE 18-6

Use of anti-idiotype antibody as a vaccine. (a) The binding site on some anti-idiotype antibodies (Ab-2) resembles the structure of the epitope on the original antigen. Such anti-paratope antibody can interact with B cells specific for the original antigen, thus inducing production of more antibody against the antigen. (b) Immunization with anti-idiotype antibody has been shown experimentally to protect mice against hepatitis B virus without exposing the animal to the virus. HBsAg = hepatitis B surface antigen.

TABLE 18-7

EVALUATION OF SOME ANTI-IDIOTYPE VACCINES

INFECTIOUS AGENTS	NATURE OF ANTI-IDIOTYPE VACCINE	SPECIES TESTED	ADJUVANT	PROTECTION
VIRUSES				
Hepatitis	P/M	Mice	+	+
Rabies	P	Mice	+	ND
Tobacco mosaic	P	Mice	+	ND
Polio type II	M	Mice	−	−
Reovirus	M	Mice	−	ND
Sendai	M	Mice	−	+
BACTERIA				
Streptococcus pneumoniae	M	Mice	−	+
Escherichia coli	M	Mice	+	+
Listeria monocytogenes	M	Mice	+	+
PARASITES				
Trypanosoma rhodesiense	M	Mice	−	+
Schistosoma mansoni	M	Rats	−	+
Trypanosoma cruzi	P	Mice	+	ND

KEY: P = polyclonal antibody; M = monoclonal antibody; ND = not determined.
SOURCE: M. Zanetti et al., 1987, *Immunol. Today* **8**:18.

several other pathogens (Table 18-7). One anti-idiotype vaccine currently being developed for protection against HIV is designed to bind to a conserved region on the gp120 envelope glycoprotein that is required for binding of the virus to CD4 molecules on the host-cell membrane. The development of anti-idiotype vaccines for humans holds much promise, particularly when immunization with a killed or attenuated vaccine would pose an unacceptable risk to the patient.

SUMMARY

1. A state of immunity can be induced by passive or active immunization (Table 18-1). Passive immunization involves transfer of preformed antibodies and provides short-term protection without the requirement for an active immune response. Active immunization induces clonal selection of lymphocytes and results in memory-cell formation.

2. In developing a vaccine, the branch of the immune system to be activated must be considered. To induce humoral immunity, epitopes must be accessible to B-cell immunoglobulin receptors and should represent immunodominant epitopes of the infectious agent. To induce cell-mediated immunity, a vaccine capable of transient intracellular growth is desirable to maximize the presentation of antigens with class I MHC molecules.

3. Three types of vaccines are currently used in humans: attenuated (avirulent) microorganisms, inactivated (killed) microorganisms, or purified macromolecules (see Table 18-4). Attenuated vaccines undergo transient growth in the recipient and therefore stimulate a more pronounced immune response and memory-cell production without the requirement for addi-

tional boosters. They do, however, pose a risk for reversion to a pathogenic state. Inactivated vaccines require repeated boosters but pose no risk of reversion to a pathogenic state. The use of purified macromolecules, which are less complex than whole-organism vaccines, avoids certain complications due to unknown side effects. By applying recombinant DNA techniques, it is possible to produce large quantities of a defined antigen for immunization.

4. Recombinant vectors, including vaccinia virus, canarypox virus, and attenuated *S. typhimurium*, can be engineered to carry multiple genes from infectious microorganisms (see Figure 18-4). An advantage of recombinant vector vaccines is that the engineered vector replicates in host cells, which serves to maximize cell-mediated immunity to the expressed antigens.

5. Plasmid DNA encoding a protein antigen from a pathogen has been shown to serve as an effective vaccine. When the DNA is injected directly into muscle, it either integrates into the muscle cell genome or is maintained in an episomal form for a prolonged time. Subsequent expression of the antigen induces both humoral and cell mediated immunity.

6. Synthetic peptides that represent immunodominant T-or B-cell epitopes are being evaluated as vaccines for several diseases. This approach enables immunologists to produce defined vaccines that may permit selective activation of the humoral or cell-mediated branches of the immune system. Various types of multivalent vaccines have been devised to induce both humoral and cell-mediated immunity (see Figure 18-5).

7. Anti-idiotype vaccines offer the possibility of achieving a state of immunity without having to expose the recipient to the uncertainties of vaccines derived from whole organisms or purified macromolecules (see Figure 18-6).

REFERENCES

BLOOM, B. 1989. Vaccines for the third world. *Nature* **342**:115.

BRACIALE, T. J. 1993. Naked DNA and vaccine design. *Trends Microbiol.* **1**:323.

DONNELLY, J. J., ET AL. 1995. Preclinical efficacy of a prototype DNA vaccine: enhanced protection against antigenic drift in influenza virus. *Nature Med.* **1**:583.

ETLINGER, H. M. 1992. Carrier sequence selection—one key to successful vaccines. *Immunol. Today* **13**:52.

EVANS, D. J., ET AL. 1989. An engineered poliovirus chimera elicits broadly reactive HIV-1 neutralizing antibodies. *Nature* **339**:385.

HENDERSON, D. A. 1976. The eradication of smallpox. *Sci. Am.* **235**:25

MILCH, D. R. 1989. Synthetic T and B cell recognition sites: implications for vaccine development. *Adv. Immunol.* **45**:195.

PARDOLL, D. M., AND A. M. BECKERLEG. 1995. Exposing the immunology of naked DNA vaccines. *Immunity* **3**:165.

STEWARD, M. W., AND C. R. HOWARD. 1987. Synthetic peptides: a next generation of vaccines? *Immunol. Today* **8**:51.

STOVER, C. K., V. FDELA CRUG, AND T. R. FUERST, ET AL. 1991. New use of BCG for recombinant vaccines. *Nature* **351**:456.

TAKAHSHI, H., ET AL. 1990. Induction of CD8$^+$ cytotoxic T cells by immunization with purified HIV-1 envelope protein in Iscoms. *Nature* **344**:873.

TASTEMAIN, C. 1995. Diphtheria disaster relief. *Nature Med.* **1**:503.

VAN DEN DOBBELSTEEN, G. P., AND E. P. VAN REES. 1995. Mucosal immune responses to pneumococcal polysaccharides: implications for vaccination. *Trends Microbiol.* **3**:155.

WEISS, R. 1992. Measles battle loses potent weapon. *Science* **258**:546.

STUDY QUESTIONS

1. Indicate whether each of the following statements is true or false. If you think a statement is false, explain why.

a. Transplacental transfer of maternal IgG antibodies against measles confers short-term immunity on the fetus.

b. Attenuated vaccines are more likely to induce cell-mediated immunity than killed vaccines are.

c. Multivalent subunit vaccines generally induce a greater response than synthetic peptide vaccines.

d. One disadvantage of DNA vaccines is that they don't generate significant immunologic memory.

e. Macromolecules generally contain a large number of potential epitopes.

f. A DNA vaccine only induces a response to a single epitope.

2. What are the advantages and disadvantages of using attenuated organisms as vaccines?

3.   A young girl who had never been immunized to tetanus stepped on a rusty nail and got a deep puncture wound. The doctor cleaned out the wound and gave the child an injection of tetanus antitoxin.

a.   Why was antitoxin given instead of a booster shot of tetanus toxoid?

b.   If the girl receives no further treatment and steps on a rusty nail again 3 years later, will she be immune to tetanus?

4.   What are the advantages of the Sabin polio vaccine compared with the Salk vaccine?

5.   In an attempt to develop a synthetic peptide vaccine, you have analyzed the amino acid sequence of a protein antigen for (a) hydrophobic peptides and (b) strongly hydrophilic peptides. How might peptides of each type be used as a vaccine to induce different immune responses?

6.   Explain the phenomenon of herd immunity. How does this phenomenon relate to the appearance of certain epidemics?

7.   You have developed a synthetic peptide vaccine representing an immunodominant T-cell epitope for strain A mice. When the vaccine is tested in strain B mice, no T-cell response occurs. What is the most likely explanation for this finding? How could you test this hypothesis?

8.   Explain the relationship between the incubation period of a pathogen and the approach needed to achieve effective active immunization.

9.   List the three types of purified macromolecules that are currently used as vaccines.

10. The Salk polio vaccine has been recommended for use by HIV-infected children instead of the Sabin polio vaccine. Why do you think this recommendation was made?

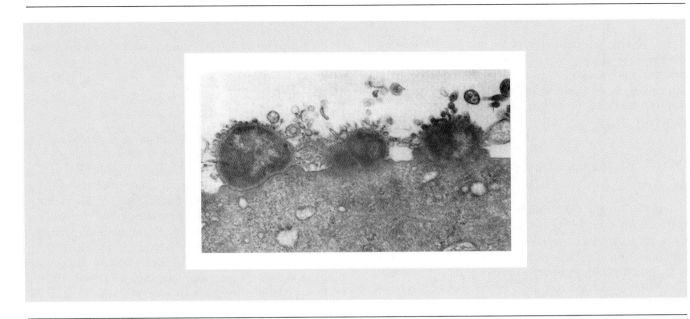

IMMUNE RESPONSE
TO INFECTIOUS DISEASES

VIRAL INFECTIONS

BACTERIAL INFECTIONS

PROTOZOAN DISEASES

DISEASES CAUSED BY PARASITIC WORMS
(HELMINTHS)

In order for a pathogen to establish an infection in a susceptible host, a series of coordinated events is required to circumvent the specific and nonspecific host defenses. Generally, pathogens use a variety of strategies to escape immune destruction. Many pathogens reduce their own antigenicity either by growing within host cells, where they are sequestered from immune attack, or by shedding their membrane antigens. Other pathogens mimic host-cell membrane molecules, either by expressing molecules with similar sequences or by acquiring a covering of host membrane molecules. In some cases pathogens are able to selectively suppress the immune response or regulate the response to generate a branch of immune activation that is ineffective. Continual variation in surface antigens is another strategy that enables a pathogen

to elude the immune system. This antigenic variation may occur by the gradual accumulation of mutations, or it may involve an abrupt change in surface antigens.

Infectious diseases, which have plagued human populations throughout history, still cause the death of millions each year. Although widespread use of vaccines and drug therapy has dramatically reduced mortality from infectious diseases in developed countries, infectious diseases continue to be the leading cause of death in the Third World. It is estimated that over 600 million people are infected with tropical diseases, resulting in some 20 million deaths each year (Table 19-1). Despite these alarming numbers, estimated expenditures for research on infectious diseases prevalent in the Third World are less than 5% of total health-research expenditures worldwide. Not only is this a tragedy for these countries, but some of these diseases are beginning to emerge or re-emerge in developed countries. For example, some U. S. troops returned from the Persian Gulf with schistosomiasis; cholera cases have recently increased worldwide with more than 30 cases reported in the United States in 1992; and a new drug-resistant strain of *Mycobacterium tuberculosis* is spreading at an alarming rate within the United States.

In this chapter the concepts discussed in earlier chapters, such as antigenicity (Chapter 4), immune effector mechanisms (Part III), and vaccine development (Chapter 18), are applied to selected infectious diseases caused by viruses, bacteria, protozoa, and helminths—the four major types of pathogens.

VIRAL INFECTIONS

A number of specific immune effector mechanisms, together with nonspecific defense mechanisms, are called into play to eliminate an infecting virus (Table 19-2). At the same time the virus acts to subvert one or more of these mechanisms in order to prolong its own survival. The outcome of the infection will depend on how ef-

T A B L E   1 9 - 1

INFECTIOUS DISEASES: THE LEADING KILLERS IN 1990

CAUSE OF DEATH	ESTIMATED NUMBER
Acute respiratory infections	6,900,000
Diarrheal diseases	4,200,000
Tuberculosis	3,300,000
Malaria	1,000,000–2,000,000
Hepatitis	1,000,000–2,000,000
Measles alone	220,000
Meningitis, bacterial	200,000
Schistosomiasis (parastic tropical disease)	200,000
Pertussis alone (whooping cough)	100,000
Amoebiasis (parasitic infection)	40,000–60,000
Hookworm (parasitic infection)	50,000–60,000
Rabies	35,000
Yellow fever (epidemic)	30,000
African trypanosomiasis (sleeping sickness)	20,000 or more

SOURCE: World Health Organization, 1992, *Global Health Situation and Projections*: cited in A. Gibbons, 1992, *Science* **256**:1135.

fectively the host's defensive mechanisms resist the offensive tactics of the virus.

Viral Neutralization by Humoral Antibody

Antibodies specific for viral surface antigens are often crucial in containing the spread of a virus during acute infection and in protecting against re-infection. Most viruses express surface receptor molecules that enable them to initiate infection by binding specifically to host-cell membrane molecules. For example, influenza virus binds to sialic acid residues in cell-membrane glycoproteins and glycolipids; rhinovirus binds to intercellular adhesion molecules (ICAMs); and Epstein-Barr virus binds to type 2 complement receptors on B cells. If antibody is produced to the viral receptor, it can block infection altogether by preventing binding of viral particles to host cells. Secretory IgA in mucous secretions plays an important role in host defense against viruses by blocking viral attachment to mucosal epithelial cells. The advantage of the attenuated oral polio vaccine, discussed in Chapter 18, is that it induces production of secretory IgA, which effectively blocks attachment of poliovirus along the gastrointestinal tract.

Viral neutralization by antibody sometimes involves mechanisms that operate following viral attachment to host cells. In some cases antibodies may block viral penetration by binding to epitopes that are necessary to mediate fusion of the viral envelope with the plasma membrane. If the induced antibody is of a complement-activating isotype, lysis of enveloped virions can ensue. Antibody or complement can also agglutinate viral particles and function as an opsonizing agent to facilitate Fc or C3b receptor-mediated phagocytosis of the viral particles.

Cell-Mediated Antiviral Mechanisms

Although antibodies have an important role in containing the spread of a virus in the acute phases of infection, they are not usually able to eliminate the virus once infection has occurred—particularly if the virus is capable of entering a latent state in which its DNA is integrated into host chromosomal DNA. Once an infection is established, cell-mediated immune mechanisms are most important in host defense. In general $CD8^+$ T_C cells and $CD4^+$ T_H1 cells are the main components of cell-mediated antiviral defense, although in some cases $CD4^+$ T_C cells have also been implicated. Activated T_H1 cells produce a number of cytokines, including IL-2, IFN-γ, and TNF, that serve, either directly or indirectly, to defend against viruses. IFN-γ acts directly by inducing an antiviral state in cells. IL-2 acts indirectly by assisting in the activation of CTL precursors into an effector population. Both IL-2 and IFN-γ activate NK cells, which play an important role in host defense during the first days of many viral infections until a specific CTL response develops.

In most viral infections specific CTL activity arises within 3–4 days after infection, peaks by 7–10 days, and then declines. Within 7–10 days of primary infection most virions are eliminated, paralleling the development of CTLs. CTLs specific for the virus eliminate virus-infected self-cells and thus eliminate potential sources of new viral production. The role of CTLs in defense against viruses is demonstrated by the ability of virus-specific CTLs to confer protection for the specific virus on nonimmune recipients. The viral specificity of the CTL can be demonstrated using adoptive transfer. Adoptive transfer of a CTL clone specific for influenza virus strain X will protect mice against influenza virus X but not against influenza virus strain Y.

Viral Evasion of Host-Defense Mechanisms

Despite their restricted genome size, a number of viruses have been found to encode proteins that interfere at various levels with specific or nonspecific host defenses. Presumably the advantage of such proteins is that they enable viruses to replicate more effectively amidst antiviral host defenses. A major nonspecific defense against viruses are **interferon** α and **interferon** β, which are produced by various cells in response to a viral infection. These cytokines induce an antiviral protein called DAI in nearby uninfected cells. However, a number of viruses, including adenoviruses and Epstein-Barr virus, have been shown to overcome the antiviral effect of the interferons by blocking or inhibiting the action of DAI.

Antibody-mediated destruction of viruses requires complement activation resulting either in direct lysis of the viral particle or opsonization and elimination of the virus via phagocytic cells. A number of viruses have strategies to evade complement-mediated destruction. Vaccinia virus, for example, secretes a protein that binds to the C4b complement component, inhibiting the classical complement pathway; and herpes simplex viruses have a glycoprotein component that binds to the C3b complement component, inhibiting both the classical and alternative pathways.

A number of viruses escape immune attack by constantly changing their antigens. In the case of the influenza virus, which is discussed more fully later, continual antigenic variation results in the frequent

TABLE 19-2

MECHANISMS OF HUMORAL AND CELL-MEDIATED IMMUNE RESPONSES TO VIRUSES

RESPONSE TYPE	EFFECTOR MOLECULE OR CELL	ACTIVITY
Humoral	Antibody (especially secretory IgA)	Blocks binding of virus to host cells, thus preventing infection or reinfection
	IgG, IgM, and IgA antibody	Blocks fusion of viral envelope with host-cell plasma membrane
	IgG and IgM antibody	Enhances phagocytosis of viral particles (opsonization)
	IgM antibody	Agglutinates viral particles
	Complement activated by IgG or IgM antibody	Mediates opsonization by C3b and lysis of enveloped viral particles by membrane-attack complex
Cell-mediated	IFN-γ secreted by T_H or T_C cells	Has direct antiviral activity
	Cytotoxic T lymphocytes (CTLs)	Kill virus-infected self-cells
	NK cells and macrophages	Kill virus-infected cells by antibody-dependent cell-mediated cytotoxicity (ADCC)

emergence of new infectious strains of the virus. The absence of protective immunity to these newly emerging strains leads to repeated epidemics of influenza. Antigenic variation among rhinoviruses, the causative agent of the common cold, is responsible for the inability to produce an effective vaccine for colds. Nowhere is antigenic variation greater than in the human immunodeficiency virus (HIV), the causative agent of AIDS. Estimates suggest that HIV accumulates mutations at a rate 65 times faster than influenza virus. Because of the importance of AIDS, Chapter 22 is devoted in its entirety to this disease.

A large number of viruses evade the immune response by causing generalized immunosuppression. Among these are the paramyxoviruses causing mumps, the measles virus, Epstein-Barr virus (EBV), cytomegalovirus, and HIV. In some cases immunosuppression is caused by direct viral infection of lymphocytes or macrophages. The virus can then directly destroy the immune cells by cytolytic mechanisms or alter the function of these cells. In other cases immunosuppression occurs as a result of a cytokine imbalance. For example, EBV produces a protein, called BCRF1, that is homologous to IL-10; like IL-10, BCRF1 suppresses cytokine production by the T_H1 subset, resulting in decreased levels of IL-2, TNF, and IFN-γ. Other viruses suppress the immune response by suppressing class I MHC expression: cytomegaloviruses produce a protein that binds to β_2-microglobulin, blocking class I MHC expression on the membrane; and adenoviruses synthesize an integral membrane protein that binds to class I MHC molecules within the endoplasmic reticulum preventing their translocation to the cell membrane. The immunosuppression that is often observed in retrovirus infections may be due to a retroviral envelope protein, called p15E, that inhibits signal transduction by protein kinase C during T-cell activation (see Figure 12-12).

Influenza

The influenza virus infects the upper respiratory tract and major central airways in humans, horses, birds, pigs, and even seals. It has been responsible for some of the worst **pandemics** (worldwide epidemics) in human history, one of which killed more than 20 million people in 1918–1919, a toll surpassing the number of casualties in World War I. Some areas, such as Alaska and the Pacific Islands, lost more than half of their population during that pandemic.

Properties of the Influenza Virus

Influenza viral particles, or virions, are roughly spherical or ovoid in shape, with an average diameter of 90–100 nm. The virions are surrounded by an outer envelope—a lipid bilayer acquired from the plasma membrane of the in-

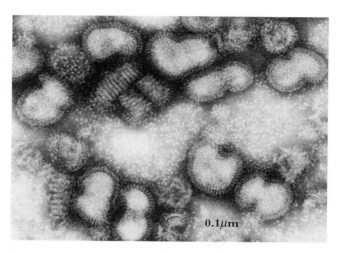

0.1 μm

FIGURE 19-1

Electron micrograph of influenza virus reveals roughly spherical viral particles enclosed in a lipid bilayer with protruding hemagglutinin (HA) and neuraminidase (NA) glycoprotein spikes. [Courtesy of G. Murti, Department of Virology, St. Jude Children's Research Hospital, Memphis, Tenn.]

fected host cell during the process of budding. Inserted into the envelope are two glycoproteins, **hemagglutinin** (HA) and **neuraminidase** (NA), which form radiating projections that are visible in electron micrographs (Figure 19-1). The hemagglutinin projections, in the form of trimers, are responsible for the attachment of the virus to host cells. There are approximately 1000 hemagglutinin projections per influenza virion. The hemagglutinin trimer binds to sialic acid groups on host-cell glycoproteins and glycolipids by way of a conserved amino acid sequence that forms a small groove in the hemagglutinin molecule. Neuraminidase, as its name indicates, cleaves N-acetylneuraminic (sialic) acid from nascent viral glycoproteins and host-cell membrane glycoproteins, an activity that presumably facilitates viral budding from the infected host cell. Within the envelope an inner layer of matrix protein surrounds the nucleocapsid, which consists of eight different strands of ssRNA associated with protein and RNA polymerase (Figure 19-2). Each RNA strand encodes a different influenza protein.

Three basic types of influenza (A, B, and C) can be distinguished by differences in their nucleoprotein and matrix proteins. Type A is the most common and is responsible for the major human pandemics. Antigenic variation in hemagglutinin and neuraminidase has allowed type A influenza virus to be subtyped. According to the nomenclature of the World Health Organization, each virus strain is defined by its animal host of origin (specified, if other than human), geographical origin,

Visualizing Concepts

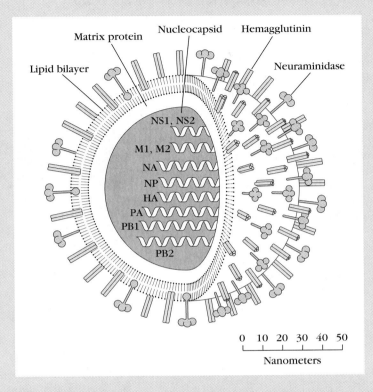

FIGURE 19-2

Schematic representation of influenza structure. The envelope is covered with neuraminidase and hemagglutinin spikes. Inside is an inner layer of matrix protein surrounding the nucleocapsid, which consists of eight ssRNA strands associated with nucleoprotein. The eight RNA strands encode ten proteins: PB1, PB2, PA, HA (hemagglutinin), NP (nucleoprotein), NA (neuraminidase), M1, M2, NS1, and NS2.

strain number, year of isolation, and antigenic description of HA and NA (Table 19-3). For example, A/SW/Iowa/15/30 (H1N1) designates strain-A isolate 15 that arose in swine in Iowa in 1930, and A/Hong Kong/1/68 (H3N2) denotes strain-A isolate 1 that arose in humans in Hong Kong in 1968; the H and N spikes are antigenically distinct in these two strains. There are 13 different hemagglutinins and 9 neuraminidases among the type A influenza viruses.

The distinguishing feature of influenza virus is its variability. The virus can change its surface antigens so completely that the immune response to one viral epidemic gives little or no protection against a subsequent epidemic. The antigenic variation results primarily from changes in the hemagglutinin and neuraminidase spikes protruding from the viral envelope (Figure 19-3). Two

different mechanisms generate antigenic variation in HA and NA: antigenic drift and antigenic shift. **Antigenic drift** involves a series of spontaneous point mutations that occur gradually, resulting in minor changes in HA and NA. **Antigenic shift** results in the sudden emergence of a new subtype of influenza bearing an HA and possibly NA dramatically different from that of the preceding virus.

The first human influenza virus was isolated in 1934 and was given the subtype designation H0N1. This subtype persisted until 1947 when a major antigenic shift generated a new subtype, H1N1. This subtype supplanted the previous subtype and became prevalent worldwide until 1957 when H2N2 emerged. The H2N2 subtype prevailed for the next decade and was replaced in 1968 by H3N2. Antigenic shift in 1977 saw the re-emergence of H1N1. The last antigenic shift in 1989 brought the re-emergence of H3N2 which remained dominant throughout the next several years. However, an H1N1 strain re-emerged in Texas in 1995, and current influenza vaccines contain both H3N2 and H1N1 strains (see Table 19-3). With each antigenic shift, hemagglutinin and neuraminidase undergo major sequence changes, resulting in major antigenic variations for which the immune system lacks memory. Thus each antigenic shift finds the population immunologically unprepared, resulting in major outbreaks of influenza, which sometimes reach pandemic proportions.

Between pandemic-causing antigenic shifts, the influenza virus undergoes antigenic drift, generating minor antigenic variations, which account for strain differences. The immune response contributes to the emergence of these different influenza strains. As an individual infected

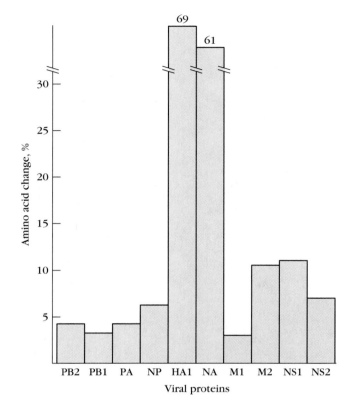

FIGURE 19-3

Amino acid sequence variation in 10 influenza viral proteins from two H3N2 strains and one H1N1 strain. The surface glycoproteins hemagglutinin (HA1) and neuraminidase (NA) show significant sequence variation; in contrast, the sequences of internal viral proteins, such as matrix proteins (M1 and M2) and nucleoprotein (NP), are largely conserved. [Adapted from G. G. Brownlee, 1986, in *Options for the Control of Influenza*, Alan R. Liss.]

TABLE 19-3

SOME INFLUENZA A STRAINS AND THEIR HEMAGGLUTININ (H) AND NEURAMINIDASE (N) SUBTYPE

SPECIES	VIRUS STRAIN DESIGNATION	ANTIGENIC SUBTYPE
Human	A/Puerto Rico/8/34	H0N1
	A/Fort Monmouth/1/47	H1N1
	A/Singapore/1/57	H2N2
	A/Hong Kong/1/68	H3N2
	A/USSR/80/77	H1N1
	A/Brazil/11/78	H1N1
	A/Bangkok/1/79	H3N2
	A/Taiwan/1/86	H1N1
	A/Shanghai/16/89	H3N2
	A/Johannesburg/33/95	H3N2
	A/Wuhan/359/95	H3N2
	A/Texas/36/95	H1N1
Swine	A/Sw/Iowa/15/30	H1N1
	A/Sw/Taiwan/70	H3N2
Horse (Equine)	A/Eq/Prague/1/56	H7N7
	A/Eq/Miami/1/63	H3N8
Birds	A/Fowl/Dutch/27	H7N7
	A/Tern/South America/61	H5N3
	A/Turkey/Ontario/68	H8N4

with a given influenza strain mounts an effective immune response, the strain is eliminated. However, the accumulation of point mutations sufficiently alters the antigenicity of some variants so that they are able to escape immune elimination (Figure 19-4a). These variants become a new strain of influenza, causing another local epidemic cycle. The role of antibody in such immunologic selection can be demonstrated in the laboratory by mixing an influenza strain with monoclonal antibody specific for that strain and then culturing the virus in cells. The antibody will neutralize all unaltered viral particles and only those viral particles with mutations resulting in altered antigenicity will escape. Within a short period in culture, a new influenza strain can be shown to emerge.

Antigenic shift is thought to occur through genetic reassortment between influenza virions from humans

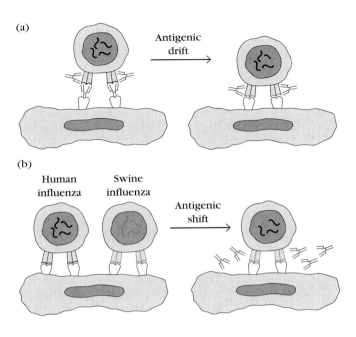

(a)

Antigenic drift

(b)

Human influenza   Swine influenza

Antigenic shift

FIGURE 19-4

Two mechanisms generate variations in influenza surface antigens. (a) In antigenic drift, the accumulation of point mutations eventually yields a variant protein that is no longer recognized by antibody to the original antigen. (b) Antigenic shift may occur via reassortment of an entire ssRNA between human and animal virions coinfecting the same cell. Only four of the eight RNA strands are depicted.

and from various animals, including horses, pigs, and ducks (Figure 19-4b). The fact that influenza contains eight separate strands of ssRNA makes possible the reassortment of the RNA strands of human and animal virions within a single cell coinfected with both viruses. Evidence for in vivo genetic reassortment between influenza A viruses from human and domestic pigs was obtained by R. G. Webster and C. H. Campbell in 1971. After infecting a pig simultaneously with human Hong Kong influenza (H3N2) and with swine influenza (H1N1), they were able to recover virions expressing H3N1. In some cases, an apparent antigenic shift may represent the re-emergence of a previous strain that has remained hidden for several decades. For example, in May of 1977 a strain of influenza, A/USSR/77 (H1N1), appeared that proved to be identical to a strain that had caused an epidemic 27 years earlier. The virus could have been preserved over the years in a frozen state or in an animal reservoir. When such a re-emergence occurs, the HA and NA antigens expressed are not really new; however, they will be seen by the immune system as if they were new because no memory cells specific for these an-

tigenic subtypes will exist in the population. Thus from an immunologic point of view, the re-emergence of a previous influenza A strain can have the same effect as an antigenic shift that generates a new subtype.

HOST RESPONSE TO INFLUENZA INFECTION

Humoral antibody specific for the HA molecule is produced during an influenza infection. This antibody protects against influenza infection, but its specificity is strain-specific and is readily bypassed by antigenic drift in the HA and NA glycoproteins. Antigenic drift in the HA molecule results in amino acid substitutions in several antigenic domains at the molecule's distal end (Figure 19-5). Two of these domains are on either side of the conserved sialic acid-binding cleft, which is necessary for binding of virions to target cells. Serum antibodies to these regions, which are important in blocking initial viral infectivity, peak within a few days of infection and then decrease over the next 6 months; the titers then plateau and remain relatively stable for the next several years. This antibody does not appear to be required for recovery from influenza, as patients with agammaglobulinemia recover from the disease. Instead the serum antibody appears to play a significant role in resistance to reinfection by the same strain. When serum antibody levels are high for a particular HA molecule, both mice and humans are resistant to infection by virions expressing that particular HA molecule. If mice are infected with influenza virus and antibody production is experimentally suppressed, the mice recover from the infection only to become reinfected with the same viral strain.

Cell-mediated immunity involving CTLs specific for influenza-infected host cells develops 3–4 days after infection, reaches a peak by day 8, and then disappears by about day 20. In mice, transfer of influenza-specific T_C clones has been shown to confer immunity to a lethal dose of influenza virus on syngeneic adoptive-transfer recipients. Unlike the humoral response, which is specific for each influenza subtype, CTL activity can be cross-reactive; that is, CTLs sometimes recognize and kill syngeneic cells infected with any type A influenza subtype (Table 19-4). This cross-reactivity is important for the development of a better vaccine for influenza, since current vaccines—which are designed to induce antibodies to HA and NA—yield poor protection owing to the continual changes in these glycoproteins. If a vaccine could induce CTL memory that is cross-reactive for all three human pandemic viral subtypes (H1N1, H2N2, and H3N2), then the vaccine might be more protective. It is therefore important to determine which influenza antigens induce cross-reactive CTLs and to characterize the cross-reactive epitopes on these antigens. As discussed

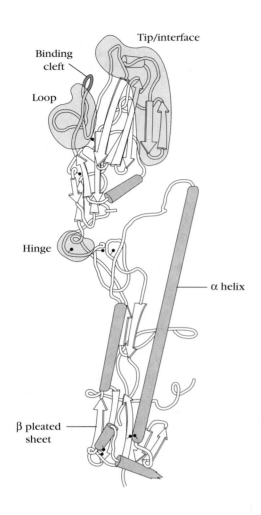

Binding cleft

Tip/interface

Loop

Hinge

α helix

β pleated sheet

FIGURE 19-5

Structure of hemagglutinin molecule. Sialic acid on host cells interacts with the binding cleft, which is bounded by regions—designated the loop and tip/interface—where antigenic drift is prevalent (blue areas). Antibodies to two of these regions are important in blocking viral infections. Continual changes in amino acid residues in these regions allow the influenza virus to evade the antibody response. Small black dots represent residues that exhibit a high degree of variation among virus strains. [Adapted from D. C. Wiley et al., 1981, *Nature* 289:373.]

in Chapter 18, a vaccine intended to maximize CTL activity must be infectious and capable of replicating within host cells to some extent. Thus, inactivated influenza preparations, which cannot replicate in host cells, are relatively ineffective at inducing CTL activity.

One of the cross-reactive influenza antigens, an internal viral protein called **nucleoprotein**, is recognized by a subset of CTLs that are indeed cross-reactive for all three human pandemic influenza A subtypes. Experimental vaccine trials have been performed in the ferret, the best animal model for human influenza. A plasmid DNA vaccine, encoding the hemagglutinin protein and two internal proteins (the nucleoprotein and matrix protein), was found to protect the ferrets against an antigenic drift variant of influenza. This experimental vaccine proved to be better than the licensed flu vaccine and suggests that a DNA vaccine, encoding internal proteins, might induce CTL activity that is cross-reactive for subtypes generated by antigenic drift.

TABLE 19-4

CROSS-REACTIVITY OF CTL RESPONSE TO INFLUENZA TYPE A VIRUS*

SUBTYPE USED TO CHALLENGE PRIMED LYMPHOCYTES IN VITRO	51CR RELEASE FROM INFECTED TARGET CELLS (%)				
	H2N1	H2N2	H3N2	H0N1	CONTROL (UNINFECTED)
H2N1	48	50	52	35	1
H2N2	45	53	53	40	2
H3N2	46	52	52	37	3
H0N1	34	52	45	42	1

* Mice were primed with an H2N1 subtype of influenza. The mouse splenic lymphocytes were isolated and challenged in vitro with macrophages infected with the influenza subtypes indicated. The CTL activity generated was then measured by monitoring 51Cr release from syngeneic 51Cr-labeled target cells infected with the indicated influenza subtypes.

SOURCE: Adapted from H. J. Zweernik et al., 1977, *Eur. J. Immunol.* **7**:630.

BACTERIAL INFECTIONS

Immunity to bacterial infections is achieved by means of antibody unless the bacterium is capable of intracellular growth, in which case delayed-type hypersensitivity has an important role. Bacteria enter the body either through a number of natural entry routes (e.g., the respiratory tract, the gastrointestinal tract, and the genitourinary tract) or through unnatural routes opened up by breaks in mucous membranes or skin. Depending on the number of organisms entering and the virulence of the organism, different levels of host defense are enlisted. If the inoculum size and the virulence are both low, then localized tissue phagocytes may be able to mount a nonspecific defense and eliminate the bacteria. Larger inoculums or organisms with increased virulence tend to induce an immune response.

Immune Response to Extracellular and Intracellular Bacteria

Infection by extracellular bacteria induces production of humoral antibodies, which are ordinarily secreted by plasma cells in regional lymph nodes and the submucosa of the respiratory and gastrointestinal tracts. The antibodies act at several levels to bring about destruction of the invading organisms, as illustrated in Figure 19-6.

Antibody that binds to accessible antigens on the surface of a bacterium can, together with the C3b component of complement, act as an opsonin that increases phagocytosis and thus clearance of the bacterium (see Figure 14-11). Antibody-mediated activation of the complement system can also induce localized production of immune effector molecules that help to develop an amplified and more effective inflammatory response. For example, the complement split products C3a, C4a, and C5a act as anaphylatoxins, inducing local mast cell degranulation and thus vasodilation and the extravasation of lymphocytes and neutrophils from the blood into tissue space. Other complement split products serve as chemotactic factors for neutrophils, thereby contributing to the buildup of phagocytic cells at the site of infection. In the case of some bacteria—notably the gram-negative organisms—complement activation can lead to lysis of the organism. If the bacterium secretes an exotoxin or endotoxin, antibody may bind to the toxin and neutralize it. The antibody-toxin complexes are then cleared by phagocytic cells in the same manner as any antigen–antibody complex.

Infections caused by bacteria that are capable of intracellular growth within phagocytic cells tend to induce a cell-mediated immune response, specifically, delayed-type hypersensitivity. In this response cytokines secreted by T_{DTH} cells are important—notably IFN-γ, which activates macrophages to achieve more effective killing of intracellular pathogens (see Figure 16-16).

Bacterial Evasion of Host-Defense Mechanisms

Host-defense mechanisms act at each of the four primary steps in bacterial infection, and many bacteria have evolved ways to circumvent these defenses (Table 19-5). Some bacteria have surface structures or molecules that enhance their ability to attach to host cells, the first step in infection. A number of gram-negative bacteria, for instance, have **pili** (long hairlike projections), which enable them to attach to the membrane of the intestinal or genitourinary tracts (Figure 19-7). Other bacteria, such as *Bordetella pertussis*, secrete adhesion molecules that attach to both the bacterium and the ciliated epithelial cells of the upper respiratory tract.

Secretory IgA antibodies, which can block bacterial attachment to mucosal epithelial cells, are the main host defense against the initial step of infection. However, some bacteria (e.g., *Neisseria gonorrhoeae*, *Haemophilus influenzae*, and *Neisseria meningitidis*) evade the IgA response by secreting proteases that cleave secretory IgA at the hinge region; the resulting Fab and Fc fragments have a shortened half-life in mucous secretions and are not able to agglutinate microorganisms.

Another way that bacteria evade the IgA response of the host and increase their ability to attach to epithelial cells is by changing their surface antigens. An example of this is provided by *N. gonorrhoeae*, which attaches to epithelial cells of the urethra or cervix by means of pili. In this organism, pilin, the protein component of the pili, has been shown to consist of constant, variable, and hypervariable amino acids. Variation in the pilin amino acid sequence is generated by gene rearrangements of the coding sequences. The pilin locus consists of one or two expression genes and 10–20 silent genes. Each gene is arranged into six regions called "minicassettes." Pilin variation is generated by a process of **gene conversion** in which one or more minicassettes from the silent genes replace a minicassette of the expression gene (Figure 19-8). This process generates enormous antigenic diversity of the pilin proteins, similar to that achieved by immunoglobulin-gene rearrangements. The continual changes in the structure of pilin may contribute to the pathogenicity of *N. gonorrhoeae* by increasing the likelihood of expression of pili that bind more firmly to epithelial cells. In addition, the continual changes in the pilin sequence allow the organism to evade neutralization by humoral antibody.

Some bacteria possess surface structures that serve to inhibit phagocytosis. A classic example is *Streptococcus*

Visualizing Concepts

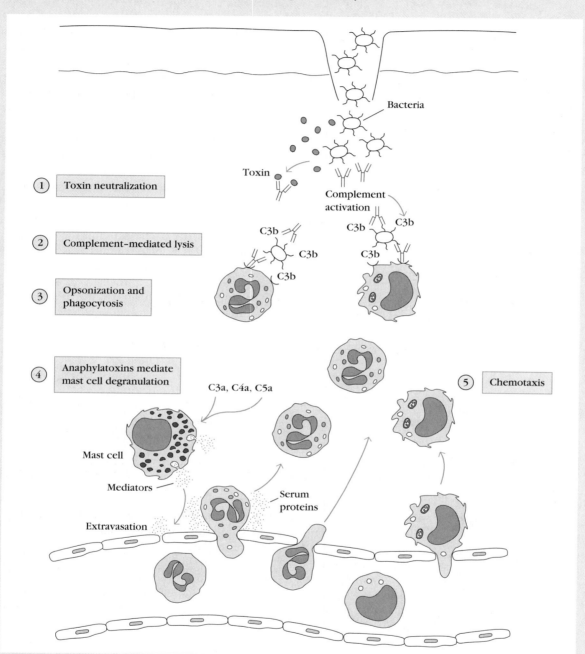

FIGURE 19-6

Antibody-mediated mechanisms for combating infection by extracellular bacteria. (1) Antibody neutralizes bacterial toxins (blue circles). (2) Complement activation on bacterial surfaces leads to complement-mediated lysis of bacteria. (3) Antibody and the complement split product C3b bind to bacteria, serving as opsonins to increase phagocytosis. (4) C3a and C5a, generated by antibody-initiated complement activation, induce local mast cell degranulation, releasing substances that mediate vasodilation and extravasation of lymphocytes and neutrophils. (5) Other complement split products are chemotactic for neutrophils.

pneumoniae, whose polysaccharide capsule is very effective in preventing phagocytosis. There are 84 serotypes of *S. pneumoniae* that differ from one another by distinct capsular polysaccharides. Infection with one serotype induces antibody that protects against re-infection with the same serotype but will not protect against infection by a different serotype. In this way *S. pneumoniae* can cause disease many times in the same individual. On other bacteria, such as *Streptococcus pyogenes*, a surface protein projection, called the M protein, inhibits phagocytosis. And some pathogenic staphylococci secrete a coagulase enzyme that produces a fibrin coat around the organism, shielding it from phagocytic cells.

Mechanisms for interfering with the complement system help other bacteria survive. In some gram-negative bacteria, for example, long side chains on the lipid A moiety of the cell-wall core polysaccharide help to resist complement-mediated lysis. *Pseudomonas* secretes an enzyme, elastase, that inactivates both the C3a and C5a anaphylatoxins, thereby diminishing the localized inflammatory reaction.

A number of bacteria escape host-defense mechanisms by their ability to survive intracellularly within phagocytic cells. Some, such as *Mycobacterium tuberculosis* and *Mycobacterium leprae*, do this by escaping the phagolysosome and growing within the more favorable environment of the cytoplasm. Other bacteria, such as *Mycobacterium avium* and *Chlamydia*, block lysosomal fusion with the phagolysosome; and some mycobacteria are resistant to the oxidative attack that takes place within the phagolysosome.

TABLE 19-5

HOST IMMUNE RESPONSES TO BACTERIAL INFECTION AND BACTERIAL EVASION MECHANISMS

INFECTION PROCESS	HOST DEFENSE	BACTERIAL EVASION MECHANISMS
Attachment to host cells	Blockage of attachment by secretory IgA antibodies	Secretion of proteases that cleave secretory IgA dimers *(Neisseria meningitidis, N. gonorrhoeae, Haemophilus influenzae)*
		Antigenic variation in attachment structures (pili of *N. gonorrhoeae*)
Proliferation	Phagocytosis (Ab- and C3b-mediated opsonization)	Production of surface structures (polysaccharide capsule, M protein, fibrin coat) that inhibit phagocytic cells
		Intracellular mechanisms for surviving within phagocytic cells
		Induction of apoptosis in macrophages *(Shigella flexneri)*
	Complement-mediated lysis and localized inflammatory response	Generalized resistance to complement-mediated lysis by gram-positive bacteria
		Insertion of membrane-attack complex prevented by long side chain in cell-wall LPS (some gram-negative bacteria)
		Secretion of elastase that inactivates C3a and C5a *(Pseudomonas)*
Invasion of host tissues	Ab-mediated agglutination	Secretion of hyaluronidase, which enhances bacterial invasiveness
Toxin-induced damage to host cells	Neutralization of toxin by antibody	

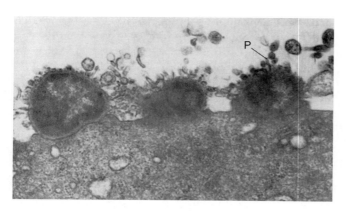

FIGURE 19-7

Electron micrograph of *Neisseria gonorrhoeae* attaching to urethral epithelial cells. Pili (P) extend from the gonococcal surface and mediate the attachment. [From M. E. Ward and P. J. Watt, 1972, *J. Inf. Dis.* **126**:601.]

Contribution of the Immune Response to Bacterial Pathogenesis

In some cases disease is caused not by the bacterial pathogen but by the immune response to the pathogen. As discussed in Chapter 13, pathogen-stimulated overproduction of cytokines leads to the symptoms of bacterial septic shock, food poisoning, and toxic-shock syndrome. For instance, cell-wall endotoxins of some gram-negative bacteria activate macrophages, resulting in release of high levels of IL-1 and TNF-α, which can cause septic shock. In the case of staphylococcal food poisoning and toxic-shock syndrome, exotoxins produced by the pathogens function as superantigens, which can activate all T cells expressing T-cell receptors with a particular V_β domain (see Table 12-5). The resulting overproduction of cytokines by activated T_H cells causes many of the symptoms associated with these diseases.

The ability of some bacteria to survive intracellularly within pathogenic cells can result in chronic antigenic activation of T_{DTH} cells, leading to tissue destruction by a delayed-type hypersensitivity reaction (see Chapter 16). Cytokines secreted by these activated T_{DTH} cells can lead to extensive accumulation and activation of macrophages, resulting in formation of a **granuloma**. The localized concentrations of lysosomal enzymes in these granulomas can cause extensive tissue necrosis. Much of the tissue damage seen with *M. tuberculosis* is due to a delayed-type hypersensitive response.

Diphtheria
(*Corynebacterium diphtheriae*)

Diphtheria is the prototype of a bacterial disease caused by a secreted exotoxin for which immunity can be induced by immunization with a **toxoid**. The causative agent, a gram-positive, rodlike organism called *Corynebacterium diphtheriae*, was first described by Klebs in 1883 and was shown a year later by Loeffler to cause diphthe-

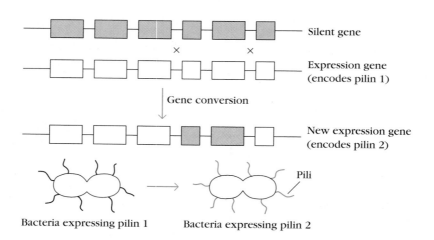

FIGURE 19-8

Variation of pilin sequences is generated by DNA rearrangements. The pilin locus consists of one or two expression genes and a series of 10–20 silent genes. Each gene contains a series of "minicassettes." One or more minicassettes of the expression gene can be replaced by a minicassette of one of the silent genes, a process termed gene conversion. [Modified from T. F. Meyer, 1990, *Annu. Rev. Microbiol.* **44**:460.]

ria in guinea pigs and rabbits. Autopsies on the infected animals revealed that while bacterial growth was limited to the site of inoculation, there was widespread damage to a variety of organs, including the heart, liver, and kidneys. This finding led Loeffler to speculate that the neurologic and cardiologic manifestations of the disease were caused by a toxic substance elaborated by the organism.

Loeffler's hypothesis was validated in 1888 when Roux and Yersin produced the disease in animals by injection of a sterile filtrate from a culture of *C. diphtheriae*. Two years later, von Behring showed that an antiserum to the toxin was able to prevent death in infected animals. He prepared a toxoid by treating the toxin with iodine trichloride and demonstrated that the toxoid could induce protective antibodies in animals. However, the toxoid was still quite toxic and therefore unsuitable for use in humans. In 1923 Ramon found that exposure of the toxin to heat and formalin rendered it nontoxic but did not destroy its antigenicity. Clinical trials showed that formalin-treated toxoid conferred a high level of protection against diphtheria.

As immunization with the toxoid increased, the number of cases of diphtheria decreased dramatically. In the 1920s there were approximately 200 cases of diphtheria per 100,000 population in the United States. In 1989 the Centers for Disease Control reported only three cases of diphtheria in the United States. Recently, there has been an alarming epidemic of diphtheria in the former Soviet Union due to a reduction in vaccination. The World Health Organization predicted that between 100,000 and 200,000 people would develop diphtheria in the former Soviet Union during 1995.

Natural infection with *C. diphtheriae* occurs only in humans. The disease is spread from one individual to another by airborne respiratory droplets. The organism colonizes the nasopharyngeal tract, remaining in the superficial layers of the respiratory mucosa. Growth of the organism itself causes little tissue damage, and only a mild inflammatory reaction develops. The virulence of the organism is completely dependent on its potent exotoxin. The toxin causes destruction of the underlying tissue resulting in the formation of a tough fibrinous membrane ("pseudomembrane") composed of fibrin, white blood cells, and dead respiratory epithelial cells. The membrane itself can lead to suffocation. The exotoxin also is responsible for widespread systemic manifestations. Pronounced myocardial damage (often leading to congestive heart failure) and neurologic damage (ranging from mild weakness to complete paralysis) are common.

The exotoxin that causes diphtheria symptoms is encoded by the *tox* gene carried by phage β. Within some strains of *C. diphtheriae* phage β can exist in a state of **lysogeny** in which the β-prophage DNA persists within the bacterial cell. Only strains carrying lysogenic phage β are able to produce the exotoxin. The diphtheria exotoxin contains two disulfide-linked chains, a binding chain and toxin chain. The binding chain interacts with ganglioside receptors on susceptible cells, facilitating internalization of the exotoxin. Toxicity results from the inhibitory effect of the toxin chain on protein synthesis. The diphtheria exotoxin is extremely potent; a single molecule has been shown to kill a cell. Removal of the binding chain prevents the exotoxin from entering the cell, thus rendering the exotoxin nontoxic. As discussed in Chapter 5, an immunotoxin can be prepared by replacing the binding chain with a monoclonal antibody specific for a tumor-cell surface antigen; in this way the toxin chain can be targeted to tumor cells (see Figure 5-23).

Today, diphtheria toxoid is prepared by treating diphtheria toxin with formaldehyde. The reaction with formaldehyde cross-links the toxin, resulting in an irreversible loss in its toxicity while enhancing its antigenicity. The toxoid is administered together with tetanus toxoid and inactivated *Bordetella pertussis* in a combined vaccine that is given to children beginning at 6–8 weeks of age. Immunization with the toxoid induces the production of antibodies (antitoxin), which can bind to the toxin and neutralize its activity. Because antitoxin levels decline slowly over time, booster doses are recommended at 10-year intervals to maintain antitoxin levels within the protective range. Interestingly, antibodies specific for epitopes on the binding chain of the diphtheria exotoxin are critical for toxin neutralization because these antibodies block internalization of the active toxin chain.

Tuberculosis
(Mycobacterium tuberculosis)

Tuberculosis is the leading cause of death in the world from a single infectious agent, killing about 3 million individuals every year and accounting for 18.5% of all deaths in adults between the ages of 15 and 59. About 1.7 billion people, roughly one-third of the world's population, are infected with the causative agent *M. tuberculosis* and are at risk of developing the disease. Long thought to have been eliminated as a public health problem in the United States, tuberculosis re-emerged in the early 1990s, particularly in the inner cities and in areas where HIV-infection levels are high. In 1992, 26,000 Americans were diagnosed with tuberculosis; this figure is the proverbial tip of the iceberg, because for every diagnosed case of tuberculosis, experts estimate that there are more than 600 infected individuals who have not yet developed symptoms. The situation is especially frightening because of the rapid emergence of *M. tuberculosis* strains that are resistant to antibiotics; some strains exhibit resistance to nine of the 11 antibiotics presently used in treating tuberculosis.

Although several *Mycobacterium* species can cause tuberculosis, *M. tuberculosis* is the principal causative agent. This organism is spread easily, and pulmonary infection usually results from inhalation of small droplets of respiratory secretions containing a few bacilli. The inhaled bacilli are ingested by alveolar macrophages and are able to survive and multiply intracellularly by inhibiting formation of phagolysosomes. When the infected macrophages lyse, as they eventually do, large numbers of bacilli are released. A cell-mediated response involving T_{DTH} cells, which is required for immunity to tuberculosis, may be responsible for much of the tissue damage in the disease. T_{DTH}-cell activity is the basis for the tuberculin skin test to the purified protein derivative (PPD) from *M. tuberculosis* (see Chapter 16).

One of two basic clinical patterns follows infection with *M. tuberculosis*. The most common clinical pattern, termed pulmonary tuberculosis, occurs in about 90% of those infected. In this pattern, T_{DTH} cells are activated within 2–6 weeks after infection, inducing the infiltration of large numbers of activated macrophages. These cells wall-off the organism inside a granulomatous lesion called a **tubercle** (Figure 19-9). A tubercle consists of a few small lymphocytes and a compact collection of activated macrophages, which sometimes differentiate into epithelioid cells or multinucleated giant cells. Because the activated macrophages suppress proliferation of the phagocytosed bacilli, infection is contained. Cytokines produced by T_{DTH} cells (T_H1 subset) play an important role in the response by activating macrophages, so that they are able to kill or inhibit growth of the organism. The role of IFN-γ in the immune response to mycobacteria has been demonstrated with knockout mice lacking IFN-γ. These mice died when they were infected with an attenuated strain of mycobacteria (BCG), whereas IFN-γ^+ normal mice survive.

Recent studies have revealed high levels of IL-12 in the pleural effusions of tuberculosis patients. The high levels of IL-12, produced by activated macrophages, are not surprising, given the decisive role of IL-12 in T_H1-mediated responses (see Figure 13-11). In mouse models of tuberculosis IL-12 has been shown to increase resistance to the disease. Not only does IL-12 stimulate development of T_H1 cells, but it also may contribute to resistance by inducing the production of chemokines that attract macrophages to the site of infection. When IL-12 is neutralized by antibody to IL-12, granuloma formation in tuberculous mice is blocked.

The massive activation of macrophages that occurs within tubercles often results in the concentrated release of lytic enzymes. These enzymes destroy nearby healthy

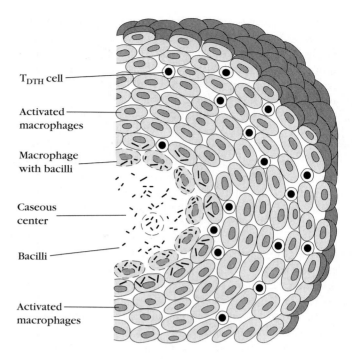

FIGURE 19-9

A tubercle formed in pulmonary tuberculosis. [Modified from A. M. Dannenberg, 1993, *Hosp. Prac.* (Jan. 15):51.]

cells, resulting in circular regions of necrotic tissue, which eventually form a lesion with a cheeselike consistency (see Figure 19-9). As these caseous lesions heal, they become calcified and are readily visible on x-rays, where they are called **Ghon complexes**.

The T_{DTH}-mediated immune response mounted by the majority of people exposed to *M. tuberculosis* controls the infection and later protects against re-infection. However, in about 10% of individuals infected with *M. tuberculosis*, the disease progresses to chronic pulmonary tuberculosis or extrapulmonary tuberculosis. This progression may occur years after the primary infection. In this clinical pattern accumulation of large concentrations of mycobacterial antigens within tubercles leads to extensive T_{DTH}-cell activation and ensuing macrophage activation. The resulting high concentrations of lytic enzymes cause the necrotic caseous lesions to liquefy, creating a rich medium that allows the tubercle bacilli to proliferate extracellularly. Eventually the lesions rupture, and the bacilli disseminate in the lung and/or are spread through the blood and lymphatic vessels to the pleural cavity, bone, urogenital system, meninges, peritoneum, or skin.

Tuberculosis is treated with several drugs, used in combination, including isoniazid, rifampin, streptomycin, pyrazinamide, and ethambutol. The combination therapy of isoniazid and rifampin has been particularly effective. The intracellular growth of *M. tuberculosis* makes it difficult for drugs to reach the bacilli. For this reason drug therapy must be continued for at least 9 months. Some patients with tuberculosis do not exhibit any clinical symptoms and some patients with symptoms begin to feel better within 2–4 weeks after treatment begins. The side effects associated with the usual antibiotic therapy leads many patients to stop taking the medications long before the recommended treatment period is completed. Because such brief treatment does not eradicate the organism, a multidrug-resistant strain can emerge. Noncompliance with required treatment regimes, one of the most troubling aspects of the recent surge in tuberculosis cases, clearly compromises efforts to contain the spread of the disease.

Presently, the only vaccine for *M. tuberculosis* is an attenuated strain of *M. bovis* called BCG (Bacillus Calmette-Guerin). The vaccine appears to provide fairly effective protection against extrapulmonary tuberculosis but has been inconsistent against pulmonary tuberculosis. In different studies, BCG has provided protection in anywhere from 0% to 80% of vaccinated individuals; in some cases, BCG vaccination has even increased the risk of infection. Moreover, following BCG vaccination, the tuberculin skin test cannot be used as an effective monitor of exposure to *M. tuberculosis*. Because of the variable effectiveness of the BCG vaccine and the inability to monitor for exposure with the skin test following BCG vaccination, this vaccine is not used in the United States. However, the alarming increase in multidrug-resistant strains has stimulated renewed efforts to develop a more effective tuberculosis vaccine.

Lyme Disease
(*Borrelia burgdorferi*)

In 1975 about 60 cases of a new and mysterious disease were reported in Lyme, Connecticut. The disease symptoms included unexplained "bull's-eye" rashes, headaches, and arthritis; in some cases severe neurologic complications developed, including excruciating headaches, meningitis, loss of memory, and mood swings. An epidemiologic study was initiated in the hope of identifying the causative agent. The disease was shown to have a higher incidence in individuals living in heavily wooded areas, and a close geographic clustering of infected individuals was found. In addition, the disease was shown to be contracted during the summer months between June and September. Finally in 1977, nine patients with the

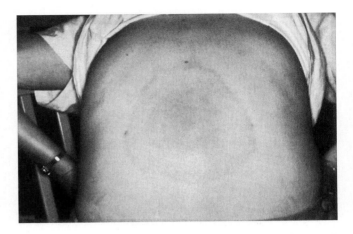

FIGURE 19-10

Bull's-eye rash is an early symptom of Lyme disease. [From A. Barbour and D. Fish, 1993, *The Biological and Social Phenomenon of Lyme Disease.* (June) **260**:1610–1616. © 1993 by A.A.A.S.]

disease remembered having been bitten by a tick at the site of the characteristic rash. Fortuitously, the tick had been saved by one patient and was examined by Willy Burgdorfer, a noted authority on tick-borne diseases. He found the tick (an *Ixodes* species) to be teeming with a new species of gram–negative spirochete, which was subsequently named *Borrelia burgdorferi* after its discoverer.

As an infected tick takes a blood meal, *B. burgdorferi* enters the bloodstream. Experiments with fluorescent antibodies to *B. burgdorferi* have revealed the presence of low numbers of the spirochete at the site of the bite and in various organs, including the kidneys, spleen, liver, cerebrospinal fluid, and brain. The clinical symptoms of Lyme disease generally begin with a characteristic rash, which first appears as a red papule and spreads to form what appears as a bull's-eye 10–50 cm in diameter (Figure 19-10). Following the rash, arthritic symptoms and neurologic symptoms often develop. Roughly 80% of individuals with Lyme disease develop some arthritic symptoms ranging from joint pain to chronic joint destruction. Neurologic symptoms develop in about 60% of Lyme patients. Most report headaches, and about 15% develop meningitis and encephalitis. The disease can be successfully treated with broad-spectrum antibiotics such as penicillin and tetracycline. Interestingly, though, soon after the antibiotic is administered, there is a temporary exacerbation of symptoms (called the Jarish-Herxheimer reaction).

Antibodies to a protein associated with the flagella of *B. burgdorferi* can often be detected after infection. However, these antibodies do not appear to confer protection against the spirochete and may even contribute to the pathogenesis of Lyme disease. Immune complexes, consisting of spirochete antigens and antibody, are thought to result in a type III hypersensitive reaction. Deposition of complexes near the original bite results in the characteristic rash; deposition of complexes in the joints is thought to induce an inflammatory response resulting in arthritic symptoms; deposition of the complexes in the vasculature and along the meninges leads to neurologic symptoms. These antigen-antibody complexes can activate the complement system, resulting in direct lytic damage to the joints or vasculature. Alternatively, complement split products, such as C3a and C5a, will induce neutrophil chemotaxis and activation. Some of the tissue damage may then result from lytic enzymes released by the activated neutrophils.

G. Habicht, G. Beck, and J. Benach have suggested that interleukin 1 (IL-1) is involved in the pathogenesis of Lyme disease. Like other gram-negative bacteria, *Borrelia* has a cell wall containing lipopolysaccharide (LPS). These researchers observed that when macrophages are cultured together with *B. burgdorferi*, the macrophages secrete high levels of IL-1. They suggested that high levels of IL-1 released by macrophages in Lyme disease may be responsible for many of the symptoms of the disease. For example, when IL-1 is injected into rabbit skin, a characteristic rash appears. Furthermore, when IL-1 is added to cultured synovial cells, the cells begin to secrete collagenase and prostaglandins. The release of collagenase in a joint could lead to the degradation of collagen and destruction of the joint. They have suggested that the exacerbation of symptoms seen with antibiotic treatment may result from massive killing of *B. burgdorferi*, releasing large quantities of LPS from the gram-negative cell wall. The LPS in turn is hypothesized to induce excessive release of IL-1, resulting in increased severity of symptoms, until the LPS levels subside.

Although mice are a major reservoir of *B. burgdorferi*, normal mice infected with *B. burgdorferi* do not develop Lyme disease, suggesting that they can mount a protective immune response. Comparison of the immune response to *B. burgdorferi* in normal mice and humans has shown that mice produce high levels of antibodies to two envelope outer-surface proteins, whereas humans fail to do so; instead, most infected humans produce antibodies to a flagellar antigen. The ability of the mice antibodies to protect against Lyme disease was studied in SCID mice, which are susceptible to the disease. Monoclonal antibodies to the outer-surface proteins protected SCID mice from disease, whereas monoclonal antibodies to the flagellar antigen did not. These results offer the possibility that a vaccine for Lyme disease consisting of the outer-surface proteins might induce protective antibodies in humans.

PROTOZOAN DISEASES

Protozoans are unicellular eukaryotic organisms. They are responsible for several serious diseases in humans, including amoebiasis, Chagas' disease, African sleeping sickness, malaria, leishmaniasis, and toxoplasmosis. The type of immune response that develops and the effectiveness of the response depends in part on the location of the parasite within the host. Many protozoans have stages in which they are free within the bloodstream, and it is during these stages that humoral antibody is most effective. Many of these same pathogens are also capable of intracellular growth, and during these stages cell-mediated immune reactions are effective in host defense. In the development of vaccines for protozoan diseases, the branch of the immune system that is most likely to confer protection must be carefully considered.

Malaria (*Plasmodium* Species)

Malaria, one of the most devastating diseases in the world today, is estimated to infect 600 million people worldwide and to cause 1–2 million deaths every year. Malaria is caused by various species of the genus *Plasmodium*, of which *P. falciparum* is the most virulent and prevalent. The alarming development of multiple drug resistance in *Plasmodium* and the increased resistance of its vector, the *Anopheles* mosquito, to DDT underscore the importance of developing new strategies to hinder the spread of malaria.

PLASMODIUM LIFE CYCLE AND PATHOGENESIS OF MALARIA

Plasmodium progresses through a remarkable series of developmental and maturational stages in its extremely complex life cycle. Female *Anopheles* mosquitoes, which feed on blood meals, serve as the vector for *Plasmodium*, and part of the parasite's life cycle takes place within the mosquito. (Because male *Anopheles* mosquitoes feed on plant juices, they do not transmit *Plasmodium*.)

Human infection begins when **sporozoites**, one of the *Plasmodium* stages, are introduced into an individual's bloodstream as an infected mosquito takes a blood meal (Figure 19-11). Within 30 min the sporozoites disappear from the blood as they migrate to the liver, where they infect hepatocytes. Sporozoites are long, slender cells that are covered by a 45-kDa protein called circumsporozoite (CS) antigen, which probably mediates adhesion of sporozoites to hepatocytes. Such adhesion has been demonstrated in vitro, and recombinant CS antigens have been shown to bind to hepatocytes in vitro.

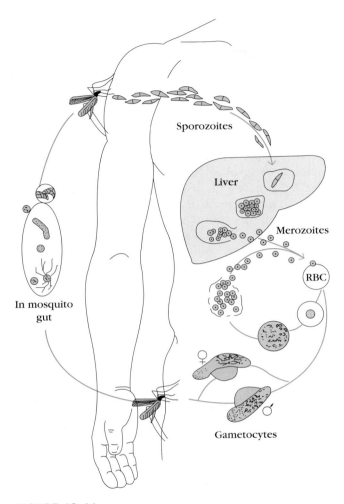

FIGURE 19-11

The life cycle of *Plasmodium*. Sporozoites enter the bloodstream when an infected mosquito takes a blood meal. The sporozoites migrate to the liver where they multiply, transforming liver hepatocytes into giant multinucleate schizonts, which release thousands of merozoites into the bloodstream. The merozoites infect red blood cells, which eventually rupture, releasing more merozoites. Eventually some of the merozoites differentiate into male and female gametocytes, which are ingested by a mosquito and differentiate into the sporozoite stage within the salivary gland of the mosquito.

The binding site on the CS antigen is a conserved region in the carboxyl-terminal end (called region II) that has a high degree of sequence homology with cell-adhesion molecules.

Within the liver, the sporozoites multiply extensively and undergo a complex series of transformations that culminate in the formation and release of **merozoites** in about a week. It has been estimated that a liver hepatocyte infected with a single sporozoite can release 5,000–10,000 merozoites. The released merozoites infect red blood cells, initiating the symptoms and pathology of malaria. Within a red blood cell, merozoites replicate and undergo successive differentiations; eventually the cell ruptures and releases new merozoites, which go on to infect more red blood cells. Eventually some of the merozoites differentiate into male and female **gameto- cytes**, which are ingested by a female *Anopheles* mosquito during a blood meal. Within the mosquito's gut, the male and female gametocytes fuse to form a zygote, which multiplies and differentiates into sporozoites within the salivary gland. The infected mosquito is now set to initiate the cycle once again.

The symptoms of malaria are recurrent chills, fever, and sweating. The symptoms peak roughly every 48 h, when successive generations of merozoites are released from infected red blood cells. An infected individual eventually becomes weak and anemic and shows spleno- megaly. The large numbers of merozoites formed can block capillaries, causing intense headaches, renal failure, heart failure, or cerebral damage—often with fatal conse- quences. There is speculation that some of the symptoms of malaria may be caused not by *Plasmodium* itself but instead by excessive production of cytokines. This hypo- thesis stemmed from the observation that cancer patients treated in clinical trials with recombinant tumor necrosis factor (TNF) developed symptoms that mimicked ma- laria. The relation between TNF and malaria symptoms was studied by infecting mice with a mouse-specific strain of *Plasmodium*, which causes rapid death by cere- bral malaria. Injection of these mice with antibodies to TNF was shown to prevent the rapid death.

HOST RESPONSE TO *PLASMODIUM* INFECTION

In regions where malaria is endemic, the immune response to *Plasmodium* infection is poor. Children less than 14 years old mount the lowest immune response and consequently are most likely to develop malaria. In some regions the childhood mortality rate for malaria reaches 50%, and worldwide the disease kills about a million children a year. The low immune response to *Plasmodium* among children can be demonstrated by measuring serum antibody levels to the sporozoite stage. Only 22% of the children living in endemic areas have detectable antibodies to the sporozoite stage, whereas 84% of the adults have such antibodies. Even in adults the degree of immunity is far from complete, however, and most people living in endemic regions have lifelong low-level *Plasmodium* infections.

A number of factors may contribute to the low levels of immune responsiveness to *Plasmodium*. The matura- tional changes from sporozoite to merozoite to gameto- cyte allow the organism to keep changing its surface molecules, resulting in continual changes in the antigens seen by the immune system. The intracellular phases of the life cycle in liver cells and erythrocytes also reduce the degree of immune activation generated by the pathogen and allow the organism to multiply while it is shielded from the attacking immune system. Furthermore, the most accessible stage, the sporozoite, circulates in the blood for only about 30 min before it infects liver hepatocytes; it is unlikely that much immune activation can occur in such a short period of time. And even when an antibody response does develop to sporozoites, *Plasmodium* has evolved a way of overcoming that response by sloughing off the surface CS-antigen coat, thus rendering the antibodies ineffective.

DESIGN OF MALARIA VACCINES

Clearly an effective vaccine for malaria should be designed to maximize the most effective immune defense mechanisms. Unfortunately, little is known of the roles that humoral and cell-mediated responses play in the development of protective immunity to this disease. Current approaches to design of malaria vaccines largely focus on the sporozoite stage. One experimental vaccine, for example, consists of *Plasmodium* sporozoites attenuated by x-irradiation. In one study nine volunteers were repeatedly immunized by the bite of *P. falciparum*–infected, irradiated mosquitoes. Later challenge by the bites of mosquitoes infected with virulent *P. falciparum* revealed that six of the nine recipients were completely protected. As encouraging as these results are, the need to breed mosquitoes to obtain *Plasmodium* sporozoites makes this approach impracticable for immunizing the millions of people living in endemic malaria regions. For example, an enormous insectory would be required to breed mosquitoes in which to prepare enough irradiated sporozoites to vaccinate just one small village in such regions.

Current vaccine strategies are aimed at producing synthetic subunit vaccines consisting of epitopes that can be recognized by T cells and B cells. One such vaccine, designated SPf66, consists of three epitopes from merozoite (blood-stage) proteins together with a conserved domain from the circumsporozoite protein. Clinical phase I trials have shown that the vaccine is safe and has a calculated efficacy of 75%. Presently this vaccine is being tested in clinical trials in Africa and in Latin America.

African Sleeping Sickness (*Trypanosoma* Species)

Two species of African trypanosomes, which are flagellated protozoans, can cause sleeping sickness, a chronic, debilitating disease transmitted to humans and cattle by the bite of the tsetse fly. In the bloodstream a trypanosome differentiates into a long, slender form that continues to divide every 4–6 h. The disease progresses through several stages, beginning with an early (systemic) stage in which trypanosomes multiply in the blood and progressing to a neurologic stage in which the parasite infects the central nervous system, causing meningoencephalitis and eventually the loss of consciousness.

As parasite numbers increase following infection, an effective humoral antibody response develops to the glycoprotein coat, called **variant surface glycoprotein** (VSG), that covers the trypanosomal surface. These antibodies eliminate most of the parasites from the bloodstream, both by complement-mediated lysis and by opsonization and subsequent phagocytosis. However, about 1% of the organisms, which bear an antigenically different VSG, escape the initial antibody response. These surviving organisms now begin to proliferate in the bloodstream, and a new wave of parasitemia is observed. The successive waves of parasitemia reflect a unique mechanism of antigenic shift by which the trypanosomes can evade the immune response to their glycoprotein antigens. This process is so effective that each new variant that arises in the course of a single infection is able to escape the humoral antibodies generated in response to the preceding variant, so that waves of parasitemia occur (Figure 19-12a).

Several unusual genetic processes generate the extensive variation in trypanosomal VSG that enables the organism to escape immunologic clearance, leading to successive waves of parasitemia. An individual trypanosome carries a large repertoire of VSG genes, each encoding a different VSG primary sequence. *Trypanosoma brucei*, for example, contains more than 1000 VSG genes in its genome, clustered at multiple chromosomal sites. A trypanosome expresses only a single VSG gene at a single time. Activation of a VSG gene results in duplication of the gene and its transposition to a transcriptionally active expression site (ES) at the telomeric end of specific chromosomes (Figure 19-12b). Activation of a new VSG gene displaces the previous gene from the telomeric expression site. A number of chromosomes in the trypanosome have transcriptionally active expression sites at the telomeric ends, so that a number of VSG genes can potentially be expressed, but unknown control mechanisms limit expression to a single VSG expression site at a time.

One interesting observation is that there appears to be some order to the VSG variation during infection. Each new variant arises not by clonal outgrowth from a single variant cell but instead from the growth of multiple cells that have activated the same VSG gene in the current wave of parasite growth. It is not known how this process is regulated among individual trypanosomes. Clearly the

Visualizing Concepts

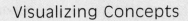

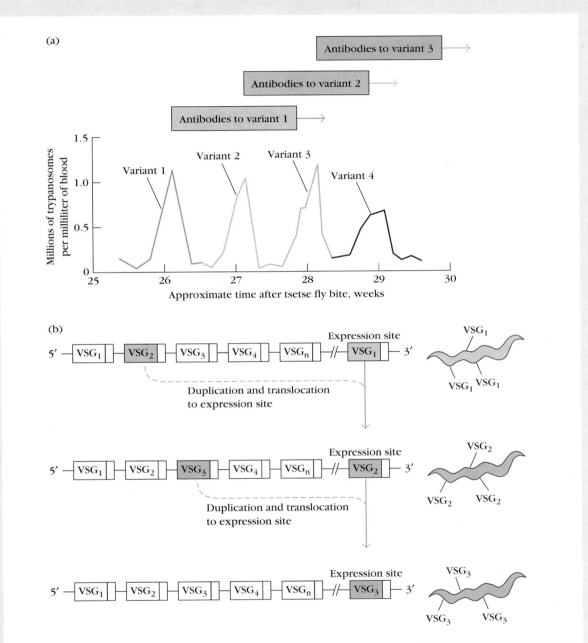

FIGURE 19-12

(a) Successive waves of parasitemia following infection with *Trypanosoma* result from antigenic shifts in the parasite's variable surface glycoprotein (VSG). Each variant that arises is unaffected by the humoral antibodies induced by the previous variant. (b) Antigenic shifts in trypanosomes occur by the duplication of gene segments encoding variant VSG molecules and their translocation to an expression site located close to the telomere. [Part (a) adapted from John Donelson, 1988, *The Biology of Parasitism*, Alan R. Liss.]

continual shifts in epitopes displayed by the VSG makes the development of a vaccine for African sleeping sickness extremely difficult.

DISEASES CAUSED BY PARASITIC WORMS (HELMINTHS)

Unlike protozoans, which are unicellular and often grow within human cells, helminths are large multicellular organisms that do not ordinarily multiply within humans and are not intracellular pathogens. Although helminths are more accessible to the immune system than protozoans, most infected individuals carry relatively few of these parasites; for this reason the immune system is not strongly engaged and the level of immunity generated to helminths is often very poor.

Parasitic worms are responsible for a wide variety of diseases in both humans and animals. More than a billion people are infected with *Ascaris*, a parasitic roundworm that infects the small intestine, and more than 300 million people are infected with *Schistosoma*, a trematode worm that causes a chronic debilitating infection. Several helminths are important pathogens of domestic animals and invade humans who ingest contaminated food. These helminths include *Taenia*, a tapeworm of cattle and pigs, and *Trichinella*, the roundworm of pigs that causes trichinosis.

Several *Schistosoma* species are responsible for the chronic, debilitating, and sometimes fatal disease **schistosomiasis** (formerly known as bilharzia). Three species, *S. mansoni*, *S. japonicum*, and *S. haematobium*, are the major pathogens in humans, infecting individuals in Africa, the Middle East, South America, the Caribbean, China, Southeast Asia, and the Philippines. A rise in the incidence of schistosomiasis in recent years has paralleled the increasing worldwide use of irrigation, which has expanded the habitat of the freshwater snail that serves as the intermediate host for schistosomes.

Infection occurs through contact with free-swimming infectious larvae, called **cercariae**, which are released from an infected snail at the rate of 300–3000 per day. When cercariae contact human skin, they secrete digestive enzymes that help them to bore into the skin, where they shed their tail and are transformed into **schistosomules**. The schistosomules enter the capillaries and migrate to the lungs, then to the liver, and finally to the primary site of infection, which varies with the species. *S. mansoni* and *S. japonicum* infect the intestinal mesenteric veins; *S. haematobium* infects the veins of the urinary

bladder. Once established in their final tissue site, schistosomules mature into male and female adult worms. The worms mate and the females produce at least 300 spiny eggs a day. Unlike protozoan parasites, schistosomes and other helminths do not multiply within their hosts. The eggs produced by the female worm do not mature into adult worms in humans; instead, some of them pass into the feces or urine and are excreted to infect more snails. The number of worms in an infected individual increases only through repeated exposure to the free-swimming cercariae, and so most infected individuals carry rather low numbers of worms.

Most of the symptoms of schistosomiasis are initiated by the eggs. As many as half of the eggs produced remain in the host, where they invade the intestinal wall, liver, or bladder and cause hemorrhage. A chronic state can then develop in which the adult worms persist and the unexcreted eggs induce cell-mediated delayed-type hypersensitive reactions, resulting in large granulomas that are gradually walled off by fibrous tissue. Although the eggs are contained by the formation of the granuloma, often the granuloma itself obstructs the venous blood flow to the liver or bladder.

Although an immune response does develop to the schistosomes, it is not sufficient to eliminate the adult worms in most individuals, even though the intravascular sites of schistosome infestation should make the worm an easy target for immune elimination. Instead the worms survive for up to 20 years. The schistosomules would appear to be the forms most susceptible to immune attack, but because they are motile, they can evade the localized cellular buildup of immune and inflammatory cells. Adult schistosome worms also possess several unique protective mechanisms that help them to escape immune defenses. The adult worm has been shown to decrease the expression of antigens on its outer membrane and also to enclose itself in a glycolipid and glycoprotein coat derived from the host, masking the presence of its own antigens. Among the antigens observed on the adult worm are the host's own ABO blood-group antigens and histocompatibility antigens! The immune response is of course diminished by this covering of the host's self-antigens, which probably contributes to the lifelong persistence of these organisms.

The relative role of humoral and cell-mediated responses in protective immunity to schistosomiasis is controversial. The humoral response following infection with *S. mansoni* is characterized by high titers of anti-schistosome IgE antibodies, localized increases in mast cells and their subsequent degranulation, and increased numbers of eosinophils (Figure 19-13, *top*). These manifestations suggest that cytokines produced by a T_H2-like

Visualizing Concepts

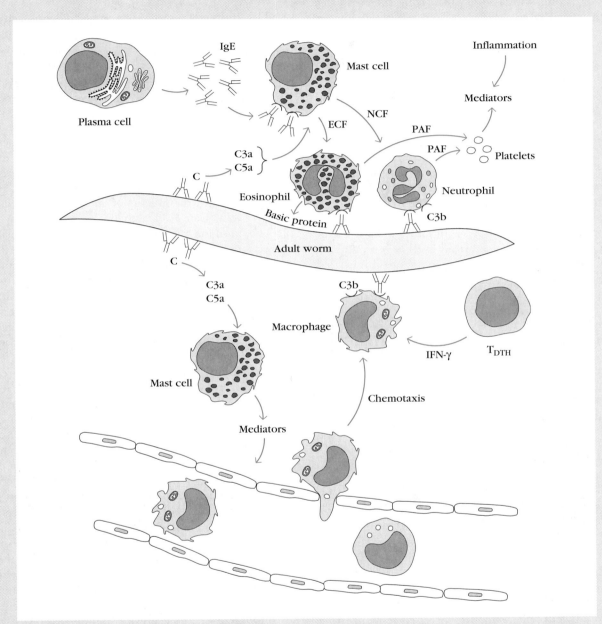

FIGURE 19-13

Overview of the immune response generated against *Schistosoma mansoni*. The response includes an IgE humoral component (*top*) and cell–mediated component involving T_DTH cells (*bottom*). C = complement; ECF = eosinophil chemotactic factor; NCF = neutrophil chemotactic factor; PAF = platelet–activating factor.

subset are important: IL-4, which induces B cells to class-switch to IgE production; IL-5, which induces bone marrow precursors to differentiate into eosinophils; and IL-3 (along with IL-4), which stimulates mast cell growth. Degranulation of mast cells releases mediators that increase the infiltration of such inflammatory cells as macrophages and eosinophils. The eosinophils express Fc receptors for IgE and IgG and bind to the antibody-coated parasite. Once bound to the parasite, an eosinophil can participate in antibody-dependent cell-mediated cytotoxicity (ADCC), releasing mediators from its granules that damage the parasite (see Figure 16-12). One eosinophil mediator, called basic protein, has been shown to be particularly toxic to helminths.

Immunization studies with mice, however, suggest that this humoral IgE response may not provide protective immunity. When mice are immunized with *S. mansoni* vaccine, the protective immune response that develops is not an IgE response, but rather is a cell-mediated T_{DTH} response characterized by IFN-γ production and macrophage accumulation (see Figure 19-13, *bottom*). Furthermore, inbred strains of mice with deficiencies in mast cells or IgE develop protective immunity following vaccination, whereas inbred strains with deficiencies in cell-mediated T_{DTH} responses fail to develop protective immunity in response to the vaccine. These studies suggest that the T_{DTH} response may be the most important in immunity to schistosomiasis. A. Sher and his colleagues have speculated that schistosomes may have evolved a clever defense mechanism by their ability to induce an ineffective T_H2-like response. This response would ensure that sufficient levels of IL-10 are produced to inhibit the effective response generated by the T_H1-like subset in the T_{DTH} response.

Antigens present on the membrane of cercariae and young schistosomules look promising as possible vaccine components because these stages appear to be most susceptible to immune attack. Monoclonal antibodies to cercariae and young schistosomules, shown to passively transfer resistance to mice and rats challenged with live cercariae, were used in affinity columns to purify schistosome membrane antigens from crude membrane extracts. When mice were immunized and boosted with these purified antigens, they exhibited increased resistance to a later challenge with live cercariae. Schistosome cDNA libraries were then established and screened with the monoclonal antibodies to identify those encoding the surface antigens. Experiments using cloned cercariae or schistosomule antigens are presently under way to assess their ability to induce protective immunity in animal models. However, in developing an effective vaccine for schistosomiasis a fine line separates a beneficial immune response, which at best limits the parasite load, from a detrimental response, which in itself may become pathologic.

SUMMARY

1. The immune response to viral infections involves both humoral and cell-mediated components (see Table 19-2). Antibody to the viral receptor can block viral infections of host cells. However, a number of viruses, including influenza, are able to mutate their receptor molecules and thus evade the humoral antibody response. Once a viral infection has been established, cell-mediated immunity appears to be more important. The cell-mediated response may develop in response to such internal viral proteins as the nucleoprotein of the viral core. These internal proteins are expressed together with class I MHC molecules on the membrane of infected host cells and serve to activate CTL activity.

2. The immune response to extracellular bacteria infections is generally mediated by antibody (see Figure 19-6). Antibody can induce localized production of immune effector molecules of the complement system, thus facilitating development of an inflammatory response. Antibody can also activate complement-mediated lysis of the bacterium, neutralize toxins, and serve as an opsonin to increase phagocytosis. Bacteria can evade the humoral antibody response by several mechanisms (see Table 19-5). Some bacteria secrete protease enzymes that cleave IgA dimers, thus reducing the effectiveness of IgA in the mucous secretions. Other bacteria escape phagocytosis by producing surface capsules or protein that inhibit adherence to phagocytes, by secreting toxins that kill phagocytes, or through their ability to survive within phagocytes. Host defense against intracellular bacteria depends largely on delayed-type hypersensitive responses.

3. Both humoral and cell-mediated immune responses have been implicated in immunity to protozoan infections. The effectiveness of the response depends in part on the site of the parasite. In general, humoral antibody is effective against blood-borne stages, but once protozoans infect host cells, cell-mediated immunity is necessary. Protozoans escape the immune response through several mechanisms. Some—notably *Trypanosoma brucei*—are covered by a glycoprotein coat that is constantly changed by a genetic-switch mechanism (see Figure 19-12). Others (including *Plasmodium*) slough off their glycoprotein coat after antibody has bound. In addition, the glycoprotein coat of *Plasmodium* contains few T-cell epitopes, and those that are present are in regions of the glycoprotein exhibiting the most variation among organisms.

4. Helminths are large parasites, which normally do not multiply within cells. Because relatively few of these

organisms are carried in an affected individual and because they do not multiply within the host, immune-system exposure to helminths is limited and consequently only a low level of immunity is induced. Although helminths generally are attacked by antibody-mediated defenses, a cell-mediated T$_{DTH}$ response plays a critical role in the response to *Schistosoma* (see Figure 19-13).

REFERENCES

BLOOM, B. R., AND C. J. L. MURRAY. 1992. Tuberculosis: commentary on a reemergent killer. *Science* **257**: 1055.

BODMER, H. C., ET AL. 1988. Enhanced recognition of a modified antigen by cytotoxic T cells specific for influenza nucleoprotein. *Cell* **52**:253.

BORST, P. 1991. Molecular genetics of antigenic variation. *Immunoparasit. Today* (March):A29.

BRAUN, R. 1988. Molecular and cellular biology of malaria. *BioEssays* **8**:194.

BRETSCHER, P. A. 1992. A strategy to improve the efficacy of vaccination against tuberculosis and leprosy. *Immunol. Today* **13**:342.

CAPRON, A., AND J. P. DESSAINT. 1992. Immunologic aspects of schistosomiasis. *Annu. Rev. Med.* **43**:209.

COOPER, A. M., AND J. L. FLYNN. 1995. The protective immune response to *Mycobacterium tuberculosis*. *Curr. Opin. Immunol.* **7**:512.

DOHERTY, P. C., ET AL. 1992. Roles of $\alpha\beta$ and $\gamma\delta$ T cell subsets in viral immunity. *Annu. Rev. Immunol.* **10**: 123.

GOOD, M. F. 1992. A malaria vaccine strategy based on the induction of cellular immunity. *Immunol. Today* **13**:126.

GOODING, L. R. 1992. Virus proteins that counteract host immune defenses. *Cell* **71**:5.

GREVE, J. M., ET AL. 1989. The major human rhinovirus receptor is ICAM-1. *Cell* **56**:839.

HABICHT, G. S., G. BECK, AND J. L. BENACH. 1987. Lyme disease. *Sci. Am.* **257**:78.

HALL, B. F., AND K. A. JOINER. 1991. Strategies of obligate intracellular parasites for evading host defences. *Immunoparasit. Today* (March):A22.

HUEBNER, R. E., AND K. G. CASTRO. 1995. The changing face of tuberculosis. *Annu. Rev. Med.* **46**:47.

KAUFMANN, S. H. E. 1993. Immunity to intracellular bacteria. *Annu. Rev. Immunol.* **11**:129.

LOCKSLEY, R. M., AND P. SCOTT. 1991. Helper T-cell subsets in mouse leishmaniasis: induction, expansion, and effector. *Immunoparasit. Today* (March):A58.

MAHMOUD, A. A. F. 1989. Parasitic protozoa and helminths: biological and immunological challenges. *Science* **246**:1015.

MCCONKEY, G. A., ET AL. 1990. The generation of genetic diversity in malarial parasites. *Annu. Rev. Microbiol.* **44**:479.

MEYER, T. F., C. P. GIBBS, AND R. HASS. 1990. Variation and control of protein expression in *Neisseria*. *Annu. Rev. Microbiol.* **44**:451.

MIMS, C. A. 1987. *Pathogenesis of Infectious Disease*. 2nd ed. New York: Academic Press.

MITCHELL, G. F. 1987. Cellular and molecular aspects of host-parasite relationships. In B. Cinander and R. G. Miller (eds.), *Progress in Immunology* VI. New York: Academic Press.

NARDIN, E. H., AND R. S. NUSSENZWEIG. 1993. T cell responses to pre-erythrocyte stages of malaria: role in protection and vaccine development against pre-erythrocyte stages. *Annu. Rev. Immunol.* **11**:687.

PLAYFAIR, H. L., ET AL. 1990. The malaria vaccine: antiparasite or anti-disease? *Immunol. Today* **11**:25.

ROBERTSON, B. D., AND T. F. MEYER. 1992. Genetic variation in pathogenic bacteria. *Trends Genet.* **8**:422.

ROTH, J. A. (ED.). 1988. *Virulence Mechanisms of Bacterial Pathogens*. American Society for Microbiology.

SHER, A., AND R. L. COFFMAN. 1992. Regulation of immunity to parasites by T cells and T-cell derived cytokines. *Annu. Rev. Immunol.* **10**:385.

SIMON, M. M., ET AL. 1991. A mouse model for *Borrelia burgdorferi* infection: approach to a vaccine against Lyme disease. *Immunol. Today* **12**:11.

STAUNTON, D. E., ET AL. 1989. A cell adhesion molecule, ICAM-1, is the major surface receptor for rhinoviruses. *Cell* **56**:849.

VIGNALI, D. A. A., ET AL. 1989. Immunity to *Schistosoma mansoni* in vivo: contradiction or clarification? *Immunol. Today* **10**:410.

WEISS, R. 1992. On the track of "killer" TB. *Science* **255**:148.

STUDY QUESTIONS

1. The effect of the MHC on the immune response to peptides of the influenza virus nucleoprotein was studied in H-2b mice that had been previously immunized with live influenza virions. The CTL activity of primed lymphocytes was determined by in vitro CML assays using H-2^k fibroblasts as target cells. The target cells had been transfected with different H-2^b class I MHC genes and were infected either with live influenza or incubated with nucleoprotein synthetic peptides. The results of these assays are shown in the table below.

For use with Question 1.

TARGET CELL (H-2^k FIBROBLAST)	TEST ANTIGEN	CTL ACTIVITY OF INFLUENZA-PRIMED H-2^b LYMPHOCYTES (% LYSIS)
(A) Untransfected	Live influenza	0
(B) Transfected with class I Db	Live influenza	60
(C) Transfected with class I Db	Nucleoprotein peptide 365–380	50
(D) Transfected with class I Db	Nucleoprotein peptide 50–63	2
(E) Transfected with class I Kb	Nucleoprotein peptide 365–380	0.5
(F) Transfected with class I Kb	Nucleoprotein peptide 50–63	1

a. Why was there no killing of the target cells in system A even though the target cells were infected with live influenza?

b. Why was a CTL response generated to the nucleoprotein in system C, even though it is an internal viral protein?

c. Why was there a good CTL response in system C to peptide 365–380, whereas there was no response in system D to peptide 50–63?

d. If you were going to develop a synthetic peptide vaccine for influenza in humans, how would these results obtained in mice influence your design of a vaccine?

2. Describe the nonspecific defenses that initially operate when a disease-producing microorganism enters the body.

3. Describe the various specific defense mechanisms that the immune system employs to combat various pathogens.

4. Discuss the role of the humoral and the cell-mediated responses in immunity to influenza.

5. Discuss the unique mechanisms each of the following pathogens has for escaping the immune response: (a) African trypanosomes, (b) *Plasmodium* species, and (c) influenza virus.

6. M. F. Good and coworkers analyzed the effect of MHC haplotype on the antibody response to a malarial circumsporozoite (CS) peptide antigen in several recombinant congenic mouse strains. Their results are shown in the table below.

For use with Question 6.

STRAIN	H-2 ALLELES					ANTIBODY RESPONSE TO CS PEPTIDE
	K	IA	IE	S	D	
B10.BR	k	k	k	k	k	<1
B10.A (4R)	k	k	b	b	b	<1
B10.HTT	s	s	k	k	d	<1
B10.A (5R)	b	b	k	d	d	67
B10	b	b	b	b	b	73
B10.MBR	b	k	k	k	q	<1

SOURCE: Adapted from M. F. Good et al., 1988, *Annu. Rev. Immunol.* **6**:633.

a. Based on the results of this study, which MHC molecule(s) serve(s) as restriction element(s) for this peptide antigen?

b. Since antigen recognition by B cells is not MHC restricted, why is the humoral antibody response influenced by the MHC haplotype?

7. The humoral response to influenza is subtype specific, whereas the cell-mediated response has been shown to cross-react with all influenza A subtypes.

a. Discuss the significance of this observation in terms of vaccine development for influenza.

b. Why might an internal viral protein, such as nucleo-protein, serve as a potential vaccine?

8. Fill in the blanks in the following statements.

a. The current vaccine for tuberculosis consists of an attenuated strain of *M. bovis* called _____.

b. Variation in influenza surface proteins is generated by _____ and _____.

c. Variation in pilin, which is expressed by many gram-negative bacteria, is generated by the process of _____.

d. The mycobacteria causing tuberculosis are walled off in granulomatous lesions called _____, which contain a small number of _____ and many _____.

e. The diphtheria vaccine is a formaldehyde-treated preparation of the exotoxin, called a _____.

f. A major contribution to nonspecific host defense against viruses is provided by _____ and _____.

g. The primary host defense against viral attachment and bacterial attachment to epithelial surfaces is _____.

h. Two cytokines of particular importance in the response to infection with *M. tuberculosis* are _____, which stimulates development of T_H1 cells, and _____, which promotes activation of macrophages.

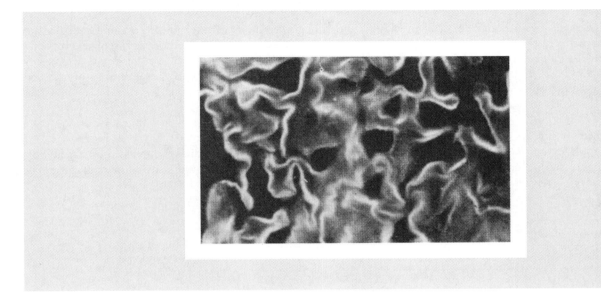

A U T O I M M U N I T Y

The response of the immune system against self-components is termed **autoimmunity**. Normally the mechanisms of self-tolerance protect an individual from potentially self-reactive lymphocytes. In the 1960s it was believed that all self-reactive lymphocytes were eliminated during their development and that a failure to eliminate these lymphocytes led to autoimmune consequences. Since the late 1970s a broad body of experimental evidence has countered that belief, revealing that not all self-reactive lymphocytes are deleted during T-cell and B-cell maturation. Instead normal healthy individuals have been shown to possess mature, recirculating self-reactive lymphocytes. Since the presence of these self-reactive lymphocytes does not inevitably result in autoimmune reactions, their activity must be regulated in normal individuals through clonal anergy or clonal suppression. A breakdown in this regulation can lead to activation of self-reactive clones of T or B cells, generating humoral or cell-mediated responses against self-antigens. These reactions can cause serious damage to cells or organs, sometimes with fatal consequences.

This chapter describes some common autoimmune diseases in humans. These can be divided into two broad categories: organ-specific and systemic autoimmune disease (Table 20-1). Such diseases affect 5%–7% of the human population, often causing chronic debilitating illnesses. Several experimental animal models used to study autoimmunity and various mechanisms that may contribute to induction of autoimmune reactions also are discussed. Finally, current and experimental therapies for treating autoimmune diseases are described.

ORGAN-SPECIFIC AUTOIMMUNE DISEASES

In an organ-specific autoimmune disease, the immune response is directed to a target antigen unique to a single organ or gland, so that the manifestations are largely limited to that organ. The target organs may be subjected to direct cellular damage by humoral or cell-mediated mechanisms; alternatively, the function of a target organ may be stimulated or blocked by autoantibodies.

Diseases Mediated by Direct Cellular Damage

Autoimmune diseases involving direct cellular damage occur when lymphocytes or antibodies bind to cell-membrane antigens, causing cellular lysis and/or an in-flammatory response in the affected organ. Gradually the cellular structure of an affected organ is replaced by connective tissue and the function of the organ declines. A few examples of this type of autoimmune disease are briefly discussed in this section.

HASHIMOTO'S THYROIDITIS

In **Hashimoto's thyroiditis**, which is most frequently seen in middle-aged women, an individual produces

TABLE 20-1

SOME AUTOIMMUNE DISEASES IN HUMANS

DISEASE	SELF-ANTIGEN	IMMUNE RESPONSE
ORGAN-SPECIFIC AUTOIMMUNE DISEASES		
Addison's disease	Adrenal cells	Autoantibodies
Autoimmune hemolytic anemia	RBC membrane proteins	Autoantibodies
Goodpasture's syndrome	Renal and lung basement membranes	Autoantibodies
Graves' disease	Thyroid-stimulating hormone receptor	Autoantibody (stimulating)
Hashimoto's thyroiditis	Thyroid proteins and cells	T_{DTH} cells, autoantibodies
Idiopathic thrombocytopenia purpura	Platelet membrane proteins	Autoantibodies
Insulin-dependent diabetes mellitus	Pancreatic beta cells	T_{DTH} cells, autoantibodies
Myasthenia gravis	Acetylcholine receptors	Autoantibody (blocking)
Myocardial infarction	Heart	Autoantibodies
Pernicious anemia	Gastric parietal cells; intrinsic factor	Autoantibody
Poststreptococcal glomerulonephritis	Kidney	Antigen-antibody complexes
Spontaneous infertility	Sperm	Autoantibodies
SYSTEMIC AUTOIMMUNE DISEASE		
Ankylosing spondylitis	Vertebrae	Immune complexes
Multiple sclerosis	Brain or white matter	T_{DTH} and T_C cells, autoantibodies
Rheumatoid arthritis	Connective tissue, IgG	Autoantibodies, immune complexes
Scleroderma	Nuclei, heart, lungs, gastrointestinal tract, kidney	Autoantibodies
Sjogren's syndrome	Salivary gland, liver, kidney, thyroid	Autoantibodies
Systemic lupus erythematosus (SLE)	DNA, nuclear protein, RBC and platelet membranes	Autoantibodies, immune complexes

(a)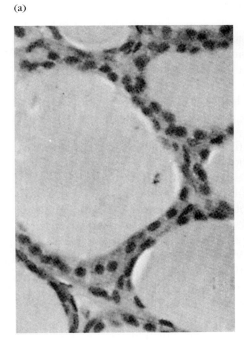

(b)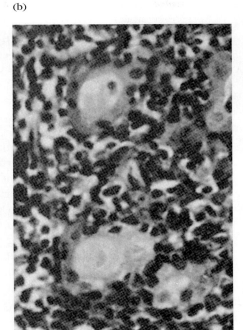

FIGURE 20-1

Photomicrographs of (a) normal thyroid gland and (b) gland in Hashimoto's thyroiditis showing intense lymphocyte infiltration. [From L. V. Crowley, 1983, *Introduction to Human Disease*, Wadsworth Health Sciences.]

autoantibodies and sensitized T_{DTH} cells specific for thyroid antigens. The DTH response is characterized by an intense infiltration of the thyroid gland by lymphocytes, macrophages, and plasma cells, which form lymphocytic follicles and germinal centers (Figure 20-1). The ensuing inflammatory response causes a **goiter**, or visible enlargement of the thyroid gland. Antibodies are formed to a number of thyroid proteins, including thyroglobulin and thyroid peroxidase, both of which are involved in the uptake of iodine. Binding of the autoantibodies to these proteins interferes with iodine uptake and leads to decreased production of thyroid hormones (**hypothyroidism**).

AUTOIMMUNE ANEMIAS

Autoimmune anemias include pernicious anemia, autoimmune hemolytic anemia, and drug-induced hemolytic anemia. **Pernicious anemia** is caused by autoantibodies to a membrane-bound intestinal protein, called **intrinsic factor**, that facilitates uptake of vitamin B_{12} from the small intestine. Binding of the autoantibody to intrinsic factor blocks the intrinsic factor–mediated absorption of vitamin B_{12}. In the absence of sufficient vitamin B_{12}, which is necessary for proper hematopoiesis, the number of functional mature red blood cells decreases below normal. Pernicious anemia is treated with injections of vitamin B_{12}, thus circumventing the defect in its absorption.

An individual with **autoimmune hemolytic anemia** makes autoantibody to RBC antigens, triggering complement-mediated lysis or antibody-mediated opsonization and phagocytosis of the red blood cells. The immunodiagnostic test for autoimmune hemolytic anemias generally involves a **Coombs test** in which the red cells are incubated with an anti-human IgG antiserum. If IgG autoantibodies are present on the red cells, the cells are agglutinated by the antiserum.

GOODPASTURE'S SYNDROME

In **Goodpasture's syndrome**, autoantibodies specific for certain basement-membrane antigens bind to the basement membranes of the kidney glomeruli and the alveoli of the lungs. Subsequent complement activation leads to direct cellular damage and an ensuing inflammatory response mediated by a buildup of complement split products. Damage to the glomerular and alveolar basement membranes leads to progressive kidney damage and pulmonary hemorrhage with death often within several months of the onset of symptoms. Staining of biopsies from patients with Goodpasture's syndrome with fluorescent-labeled anti-IgG and anti-C3b reveals linear deposits of IgG and C3b along the basement membranes (Figure 20-2).

INSULIN-DEPENDENT DIABETES MELLITUS

A disease afflicting 0.2% of the population, **insulin-dependent diabetes mellitus** (IDDM) is caused by an autoimmune attack on the pancreas. The attack is directed against specialized insulin-producing cells (beta

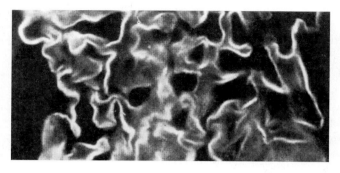

FIGURE 20-2

Fluorescent anti-IgG staining of a kidney biopsy from a patient with Goodpasture's syndrome reveals linear deposits of autoantibody along the basement membrane. [From J. A. Charlesworth and B. A. Pussell, 1986, in *Clinical Immunology Illustrated*, J. V. Wells and D. S. Nelson (eds.), Williams & Wilkins, p. 191.]

cells) that are located in spherical clusters, called the islets of Langerhans, scattered throughout the pancreas. The autoimmune attack destroys the beta cells resulting in decreased production of insulin and consequently increased levels of blood glucose.

This disease is characterized by **insulitis**, a condition in which a large numbers of T_{DTH} cells infiltrate the islets of Langerhans (Figure 20-3). A cell-mediated DTH response develops following the infiltration and activation of numerous macrophages. The subsequent beta-cell destruction is thought to be mediated by cytokines released during the DTH response and by lytic enzymes released from the activated macrophages. IFN-

γ, TNF-α, and IL-1 have each been implicated in destruction of the beta cells. Autoantibodies to beta cells may contribute to cell destruction by facilitating either antibody-plus-complement lysis or antibody-dependent cell-mediated cytotoxicity (ADCC).

Diseases Mediated by Stimulating or Blocking Autoantibodies

In some autoimmune diseases antibodies act as **agonists**, binding to hormone receptors in lieu of the normal ligand and stimulating inappropriate activity. This usually leads to an overproduction of mediators or an increase in cell growth. In other autoimmune conditions, autoantibodies bind to hormone receptors but act as **antagonists**, blocking receptor function. This generally causes impaired secretion of mediators and gradual atrophy of the affected organ.

GRAVES' DISEASE

The production of thyroid hormones is carefully regulated by thyroid-stimulating hormone (TSH), which is produced by the pituitary gland. Binding of TSH to a receptor on thyroid cells activates adenylate cyclase and stimulates the synthesis of two thyroid hormones, thyroxine and triiodothyronine. A patient with **Graves' disease** produces autoantibodies to the receptor for TSH. Binding of these autoantibodies to the receptor mimics the normal action of TSH, activating adenylate cyclase and resulting in production of the thyroid hormones. Unlike TSH, however, the autoantibodies are not

(a)

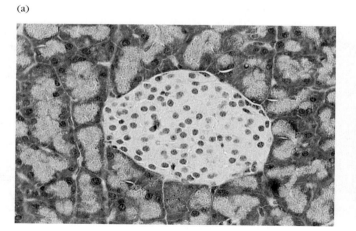

(b)

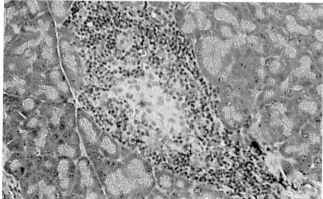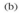

FIGURE 20-3

Photomicrographs of islet of Langerhans (a) in pancreas from a normal mouse and (b) in pancreas from a mouse with a disease resembling insulin-dependent diabetes mellitus. Note the lymphocyte infiltration into the islet (insulitis) in (b). [From M. A. Atkinson and N. K. Maclaren, 1990, *Sci. Am.* **263**(1):62.]

STIMULATING AUTOANTIBODIES (Graves' disease)

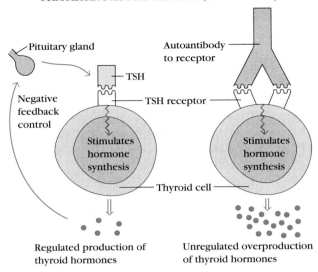

FIGURE 20-4

In Graves' disease, binding of autoantibodies to the receptor for thyroid-stimulating hormone (TSH) induces unregulated activation of the thyroid, leading to overproduction of the thyroid hormones (blue circles).

regulated, and consequently they overstimulate the thyroid. For this reason these autoantibodies are called **long-acting thyroid-stimulating (LATS) antibodies** (Figure 20-4).

Myasthenia Gravis

Myasthenia gravis is the prototype autoimmune disease mediated by blocking antibodies. A patient with this disease produces autoantibodies to the acetylcholine receptors on the motor end-plates of muscles. Binding of these autoantibodies to the receptors prevents binding by acetylcholine, thereby inhibiting muscle activation. The antibodies also induce complement-mediated degradation of the receptor, resulting in progressive weakening of the skeletal muscles (Figure 20-5).

SYSTEMIC AUTOIMMUNE DISEASES

In systemic autoimmune diseases, the response is directed toward a broad range of target antigens and involves a number of organs and tissues. These diseases reflect a generalized defect in immune regulation that results in hyperactive T cells and B cells. Tissue damage is widespread, both from cell-mediated immune responses and from direct cellular damage caused by autoantibodies or by accumulation of immune complexes.

Systemic Lupus Erythematosus

One of the best examples of a systemic autoimmune disease is **systemic lupus erythematosus** (SLE), which typically appears in women between 20 and 40 years of age with a female:male ratio of 10:1. SLE is

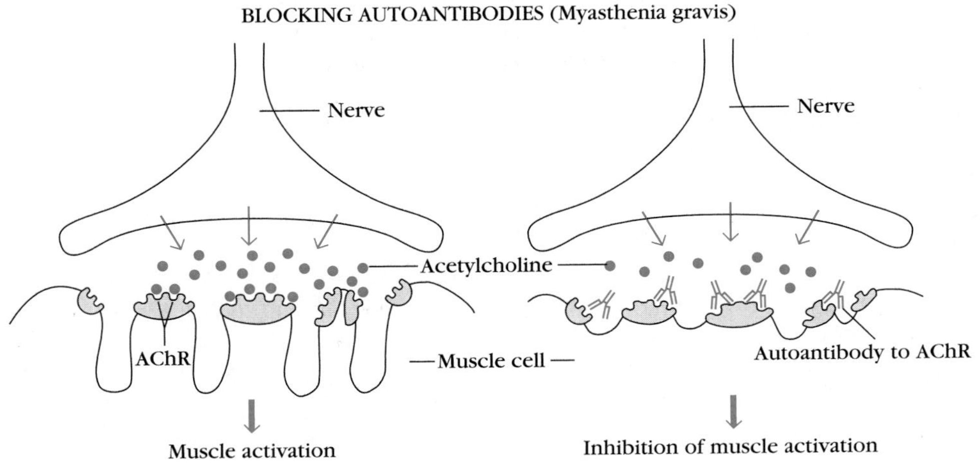

BLOCKING AUTOANTIBODIES (Myasthenia gravis)

FIGURE 20-5

In myasthenia gravis, binding of autoantibodies to the acetylcholine receptor (*right*) blocks binding of acetylcholine (blue circles) and subsequent muscle activation (*left*). In addition, the anti-AChR autoantibody induces complement activation resulting in damage to the muscle end-plate with a reduction in acetylcholine receptors as the disease progresses. AChR = acetylcholine receptor.

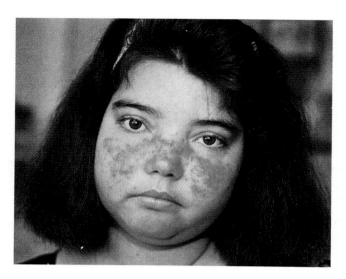

FIGURE 20-6

Characteristic "butterfly" rash over the cheeks of a young girl with systemic lupus erythematosus. [From L. Steinman, 1993, *Sci. Am.* **269**(3):80.]

characterized by fever, weakness, arthritis, skin rashes, pleurisy, and kidney dysfunction (Figure 20-6). Affected individuals may produce autoantibodies to a vast array of tissue antigens such as DNA, histones, RBCs, platelets, leukocytes, and clotting factors; interaction of these autoantibodies with their specific antigens produces various symptoms. Autoantibody specific for RBCs and platelets, for example, can lead to complement-mediated lysis, resulting in hemolytic anemia and thrombocytopenia, respectively. When immune complexes of autoantibodies with various nuclear antigens are deposited along the walls of small blood vessels, a type III hypersensitive reaction develops. The complexes activate the complement system and generate membrane-attack complexes and complement split products that damage the blood-vessel wall, resulting in vasculitis and glomerulonephritis.

Excessive complement activation in patients with severe SLE leads to elevated serum levels of the complement split products C3a and C5a, which may be three to four times higher than in normal individuals. C5a induces increased expression of the type 3 complement receptor (CR3) on neutrophils, facilitating neutrophil aggregation and attachment to the vascular endothelium. As neutrophils attach to small blood vessels, the number of circulating neutrophils declines (**neutropenia**) and various occlusions of the small blood vessels develop (**vasculitis**). These occlusions can lead to widespread tissue damage.

Laboratory diagnosis of SLE focuses on the characteristic antinuclear antibodies, which are directed against double-stranded or single-stranded DNA, nucleoprotein,

histones, and nucleolar RNA. Indirect immunofluorescent staining of serum from SLE patients produces various characteristic nuclei-staining patterns.

MULTIPLE SCLEROSIS

Multiple sclerosis (MS), an autoimmune disease affecting the central nervous system, is the most common cause of neurologic disability associated with disease in Western countries. Individuals with this disease produce autoreactive T cells that participate in the formation of inflammatory lesions along the myelin sheath of nerve fibers. The cerebrospinal fluid of patients with active MS contains activated T lymphocytes, which infiltrate the brain tissue and cause characteristic inflammatory lesions, destroying the **myelin**. Since myelin functions to insulate the nerve fibers, a breakdown in the myelin sheath leads to numerous neurologic dysfunctions.

RHEUMATOID ARTHRITIS

Rheumatoid arthritis is a common autoimmune disorder, most often affecting women from 40 to 60 years old. The major symptom is chronic inflammation of the joints, although the hematologic, cardiovascular, and respiratory systems frequently are also affected. Many individuals with rheumatoid arthritis produce a group of autoantibodies, called **rheumatoid factors**, that are reactive with determinants in the Fc region of IgG. The classical rheumatoid factor is an IgM antibody reactive to the Fc of IgG. Such autoantibodies bind to normal circulating IgG, forming IgM-IgG complexes that are deposited in the joints. These immune complexes can activate the complement cascade, resulting in a type III hypersensitive reaction leading to chronic inflammation of the joints.

ANIMAL MODELS FOR AUTOIMMUNE DISEASE

Animal models for autoimmune diseases have contributed valuable insights into the mechanism of autoimmunity; to our understanding of autoimmunity in humans; and to potential treatments. Autoimmunity develops spontaneously in certain inbred strains of animals; autoimmunity can also be induced by certain experimental manipulations (Table 20-2).

Spontaneous Autoimmunity in Animals

A number of autoimmune diseases that develop spontaneously in animals exhibit important clinical and pathologic similarities with certain autoimmune diseases in humans. Certain inbred mouse strains have been particularly valuable models for illuminating the immunologic defects involved in the development of autoimmunity.

New Zealand Black (NZB) mice and F_1 hybrids of NZB and **New Zealand White** (NZW) mice spontaneously develop autoimmune diseases closely paralleling systemic lupus erythematosus. These mice spontaneously develop autoimmune hemolytic anemia between 2 and 4 months of age at which time various autoantibodies can be detected, including antibodies to erythrocytes, nuclear proteins, DNA, and T lymphocytes. The animals develop glomerulonephritis from immune-complex deposits in the kidney and die prematurely by 18 months. As is true of SLE in humans, the incidence of autoimmunity in the **(NZB × NZW) F_1** hybrids is greater in females, a phenomenon apparently related to estrogen levels. The effect of androgens and estrogens on development of autoimmune symptoms in these mice was studied by N. Talal. In his study, male and female (NZB × NZW) F_1 mice were castrated before puberty and then given hormone replacements. In both male and female mice that received androgens, there was a delay in the onset of autoimmunity and a reduction in its severity. Estrogens had the opposite effect, promoting early onset of autoimmunity with increased severity.

An accelerated and severe form of systemic autoimmune disease resembling systemic lupus erythematosus (SLE) develops in a mouse strain called **MRL/*lpr*/*lpr***. These mice are homozygous for a gene called *lpr*, which has been identified as a defective *fas* gene. The *fas*-gene product is a cell-surface protein belonging to the TNF family of cysteine-rich membrane receptors (see Figure 13-5d). When the normal Fas protein interacts with its ligand, it transduces a signal that leads to apoptotic death of the Fas-bearing cells. This mechanism may operate in destruction of target cells by some CTLs (see Figure 16-8). It is hypothesized that Fas-induced apoptotic death may also be involved in the clonal deletion of self-reactive lymphocytes. If this is so, then a defect in the *fas* gene that prevents Fas-induced apoptosis may lead to inadequate clonal deletion and the persistence of autoreactive lymphocytes. Increased levels of a soluble form of the Fas protein, which might interfere with Fas-induced

TABLE 20-2

EXPERIMENTAL ANIMAL MODELS OF AUTOIMMUNE DISEASES

ANIMAL MODEL	POSSIBLE HUMAN DISEASE COUNTERPART	INDUCING ANTIGEN	DISEASE TRANSFERRED BY T CELLS
SPONTANEOUS AUTOIMMUNE DISEASE			
Nonobese diabetic (NOD) mouse	Insulin-dependent diabetes mellitus (IDDM)	Unknown	Yes
(NZB × NZW) F_1 mouse	Systemic lupus erythematosus (SLE)	Unknown	Yes
Obese-strain chicken	Hashimoto's thyroiditis	Thyroglobulin	Yes
EXPERIMENTALLY INDUCED AUTOIMMUNE DISEASE *			
Experimental autoimmune myasthenia gravis (EAMG)	Myasthenia gravis	Acetylcholine receptor	Yes
Experimental autoimmune encephalomyelitis (EAE)	Multiple sclerosis (MS)	Myelin basic protein (MBP); proteolipid protein (PLP)	Yes
Autoimmune arthritis (AA)	Rheumatoid arthritis	*M. tuberculosis* (proteoglycans)	Yes
Experimental autoimmune thyroiditis (EAT)	Hashimoto's thyroiditis	Thyroglobulin	Yes

* These diseases can be induced by injecting appropriate animals with the indicated antigen in complete Freund's adjuvant. Except for autoimmune arthritis, the antigens used correspond to the self-antigens associated with the human-disease counterpart. Rheumatoid arthritis involves reaction to proteoglycans, which are self-antigens associated with connective tissue.

apoptotic cell death, have recently been detected in the serum of some SLE patients.

Another important animal model is the **nonobese diabetic (NOD) mouse**, which spontaneously develops a form of diabetes that resembles human insulin-dependent diabetes mellitus (IDDM). Like the human disease, the NOD mouse disease begins with lymphocytic infiltration into the islets of the pancreas. Also, as in IDDM, there is a strong association between certain MHC alleles and development of diabetes in these mice. Experiments with these mice have shown that T cells from diabetic mice can transfer diabetes to nondiabetic recipients. For example, when the immune system of normal mice is destroyed by lethal doses of x-rays and then is reconstituted with an injection of bone marrow cells from NOD mice, the reconstituted mice develop diabetes. Conversely, when the immune system of still healthy NOD mice is destroyed by x-irradiation and then reconstituted with normal bone marrow cells, the NOD mice do not develop diabetes. Various studies have demonstrated a pivotal role for $CD4^+$ T cells in the NOD mouse, and recent evidence implicates the T_H1 subset in disease development.

Several other spontaneously occurring autoimmune diseases have been discovered in animals and have served as models for similar human diseases. Among these are **Obese-strain chickens**, which develop both humoral and cell-mediated reactivity to thyroglobulin resembling that seen in Hashimoto's thyroiditis.

Experimentally Induced Autoimmunity in Animals

Autoimmune dysfunctions similar to certain human autoimmune diseases can be induced experimentally in some animals (see Table 20-2). One of the first such animal models was discovered serendipitously in 1973 when rabbits were immunized with acetylcholine receptors purified from electric eels. The animals soon developed muscular weakness similar to that seen in myasthenia gravis. This **experimental autoimmune myasthenia gravis** (EAMG) was shown to result from antibodies to the acetylcholine receptor blocking muscle stimulation by acetylcholine in the synapse. Within a year this animal model had proved its value with the discovery that autoantibodies to the acetylcholine receptor were the cause of myasthenia gravis in humans.

Experimental autoimmune encephalomyelitis (EAE) is another animal model that has greatly improved understanding of autoimmunity. EAE can be induced in a variety of species by immunization with **myelin basic protein** (MBP) in complete Freund's adjuvant. Within 2–3 weeks the animals develop cellular infiltration of the myelin sheaths of the central nervous system, resulting in demyelination and development of paralysis. Most of the animals die. Those that recover are resistant to the development of disease after a subsequent injection of MBP and adjuvant. EAE is considered to be a good laboratory model for multiple sclerosis.

Experimental autoimmune thyroiditis (EAT) can be induced in a number of animals by immunization with thyroglobulin in complete Freund's adjuvant. Both humoral antibodies and T_{DTH} cells directed against the thyroglobulin develop, resulting in thyroid inflammation. EAT appears to best mimic Hashimoto's thyroiditis. In contrast to both EAE and EAT, which are induced by immunization with self-antigens, **autoimmune arthritis** (AA) is induced by immunization of rats with *Mycobacterium tuberculosis* in complete Freund's adjuvant. These animals develop an arthritis whose features are similar to those of rheumatoid arthritis in humans.

EVIDENCE IMPLICATING THE CD4+ T CELL, MHC, AND TCR IN AUTOIMMUNITY

The inappropriate response to self-antigens that characterizes all autoimmune diseases can involve either the humoral or the cell-mediated branch. Identifying the defect underlying human autoimmune diseases has been difficult, while characterizing the immune defect in the various animal models has been more successful. Surprisingly, each of the animal models has implicated the $CD4^+$ T cell as the primary mediator of autoimmune disease. T-cell recognition of antigen, of course, involves a trimolecular complex of the T-cell receptor, an MHC molecule, and antigenic peptide (see Figure 11-16). Thus an individual susceptible to autoimmunity must possess MHC molecules and T-cell receptors capable of binding self-antigens.

Role of CD4+ T-Cells and T_H1/T_H2 Balance

Autoimmune T-cell clones have been obtained from all of the animal models listed in Table 20-2 by culturing lymphocytes from the autoimmune animals in the presence of various T-cell growth factors and by inducing proliferation of specific autoimmune clones with the various autoantigens. For example, when lymph-node cells from EAE rats are cultured in vitro with myelin basic protein (MBP), clones of activated T cells emerge.

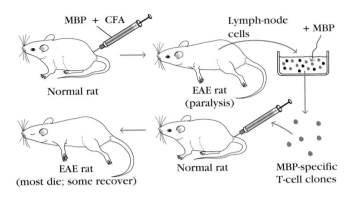

FIGURE 20-7

Experimental autoimmune encephalomyelitis (EAE) can be induced by injecting rats with myelin basic protein (MBP) in complete Freund's adjuvant (CFA). MBP-specific T-cell clones can be generated by culturing lymph-node cells from EAE rats with MBP. When these T cells are injected into normal animals, most develop EAE and die, although a few recover.

When sufficient numbers of these MBP-specific T-cell clones are injected intravenously into normal syngeneic animals, the cells penetrate the blood-brain barrier and induce demyelination; EAE develops within 5 days (Figure 20-7).

A similar experimental protocol has been used to isolate T-cell clones specific for thyroglobulin and for *M. tuberculosis* from EAT and AA animals, respectively. In each case the T-cell clone induces the experimental autoimmune disease in normal animals. Examination of these T cells has revealed that they bear the CD4 membrane marker. In a number of animal models for autoimmune diseases it has been possible to reverse the autoimmunity by depleting the T-cell population with antibody directed against CD4. For example, weekly injections of anti–CD4 monoclonal antibody abolished the autoimmune symptoms in (NZB × NZW) F_1 mice and in mice with EAE.

Most cases of organ-specific autoimmune disease develop as a consequence of self-reactive $CD4^+$ T cells. Analysis of these $CD4^+$ T cells has revealed that the **T_H1/T_H2 balance** can have an impact on whether autoimmunity develops or not. T_H1 cells have been implicated in the development of autoimmunity, whereas T_H2 cells not only protect against the induction of disease but also against progression of established disease. In EAE, for example, immunohistologic studies revealed the presence of T_H1 cytokines (IL-2, TNF-α, and IFN-γ) in the central nervous system tissues at the height of the disease. In addition, the MBP-specific $CD4^+$ T-cell

clones generated from animals with EAE, as shown in Figure 20-7, can be separated into T_H1 and T_H2 clones. Recent studies have shown that only the T_H1 clones transfer EAE to normal healthy mice, whereas the T_H2 clones not only do not transfer EAE to normal healthy mice but also protect the mice against induction of EAE following subsequent immunization with MBP plus adjuvant.

Experiments assessing the role of various cytokines or cytokine inhibitors on the development of EAE have provided further evidence for the differential role of T_H1 and T_H2 cells in autoimmunity. When mice were injected with IL-4 at the time of immunization with MBP plus adjuvant, the development of EAE was inhibited, whereas administration of IL-12 had the opposite effect, promoting the development of EAE. As noted in Chapter 13, IL-4 promotes development of T_H2 cells and IL-12 promotes development of T_H1 cells (see Figure 13-11). Thus the observed effects of IL-4 and IL-12 on EAE development are consistent with a role for T_H1 cells in the genesis of autoimmunity.

Association with the MHC

Several types of studies have supported an association between expression of a particular MHC allele and susceptibility to autoimmunity. Some of these studies have used the EAE animal model, whose inducing antigen— myelin basic protein (MBP)—has been well characterized and sequenced. Various MBP peptides have been assessed for their ability to activate T_H cells and elicit autoimmune encephalomyelitis reactions. The results of such experiments show that inbred mice expressing different MHC haplotypes develop EAE in response to different MBP peptides (Figure 20-8). Moreover, the same peptides that induce EAE in a given strain also induce maximal T_H–cell proliferation.

By typing the HLA alleles expressed by individuals with various autoimmune diseases, researchers have shown that some HLA alleles occur at a much higher frequency among autoimmune individuals than in the general population. The association between the expression of a given HLA allele and an autoimmune disease is expressed as the relative risk:

$$\text{Relative risk} = \frac{(\text{HLA allele}^+ / \text{HLA allele}^-)\ \text{Patients}}{(\text{HLA allele}^+ / \text{HLA allele}^-)\ \text{Controls}}$$

A relative risk value of 1 means that the HLA allele is expressed with the same frequency in the autoimmune and control subpopulations, whereas a relative risk value substantially above 1 indicates an association between the HLA allele and the autoimmune disease.

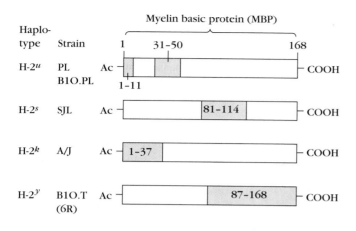

FIGURE 20-8

Experimental demonstration that the haplotype of the recipient mouse strain determines which MBP peptides are encephalitogenic. Injection of the MBP peptides (shown in blue) induced EAE and maximal T-cell proliferation in the indicated strains of mice. The haplotype of the mouse appears to determine which of the peptides is encephalitogenic.

The strongest association between an HLA allele and an autoimmune disease is seen in **ankylosing spondylitis**, an inflammatory disease of vertebral joints. Individuals who have HLA-B27 have a 90 times greater likelihood of developing ankylosing spondylitis than individuals with a different HLA-B allele. However, the existence of such an association should not be interpreted to imply that the expression of a particular MHC allele has caused the disease, because the relationship between MHC alleles and development of autoimmune disease is complex. That these diseases are not inherited via simple mendelian segregation of MHC alleles can be seen in identical twins when both inherit the MHC risk factor but only one develops autoimmunity. This finding suggests that multiple genetic factors and environmental factors have roles in the development of autoimmunity, with the MHC playing an important but not exclusive role. As the antigens inducing human autoimmune diseases are identified and sequenced, it will be possible to analyze the linkage between the MHC and various diseases more fully.

Table 20-3 lists a number of autoimmune diseases for which an association between a particular MHC allele and disease susceptibility has been demonstrated. One difficulty in associating a particular MHC allele with autoimmunity is the genetic phenomenon of **linkage disequilibrium** in which two alleles are inherited together with a higher frequency than normally expected. Initially class I MHC alleles were shown to be associated

with autoimmunity. But later most autoimmune diseases were shown to be much more strongly associated with class II MHC alleles. The fact that some of the class I MHC alleles were in linkage disequilibrium with the class II MHC alleles made their contribution to autoimmune susceptibility appear more pronounced than it actually was.

By using the polymerase chain reaction, H. McDevitt and his coworkers analyzed the nucleotide sequences of class II MHC genes from patients with different autoimmune diseases. They found that certain short sequences within the α_1 and β_1 domains of class II MHC molecules appear to play a major role in susceptibility and resistance to autoimmunity. These sequences are thought to be located within the peptide-binding groove of

TABLE 20-3

HLA ALLELES ASSOCIATED WITH INCREASED RISK FOR VARIOUS AUTOIMMUNE DISEASES

DISEASE	HLA ALLELE	RELATIVE RISK*
Ankylosing spondylitis	B27	90
Goodpasture's syndrome	DR2	16
Graves' disease	B8/DR3	3-4
Insulin-dependent diabetes mellitus	DR4/DR3 DR3/DQW8	20 100
Juvenile rheumatoid arthritis	B27/DR5	4
Multiple sclerosis	DR2	5
Myasthenia gravis	DR3	10
Pernicious anemia	DR5	5
Psoriatic arthritis (central)	B27	11
Reiter's syndrome	B27	37
Rheumatoid arthritis	Dw4/DR4	10
Sjogren's syndrome	Dw3	6
Systemic lupus erythematosus	DR3	5
Ulcerative colitis	B5	4

* Likelihood of developing disease compared to the general population, which is assigned a risk value of 1.

the class II MHC molecule. In patients with insulin-dependent diabetes mellitus (IDDM) and in the mouse model for diabetes (the NOD mouse), an aspartic residue at position 57 of the HLA-DQ β chain correlated with resistance to IDDM, whereas a valine, serine, or alanine at this position correlated with susceptibility to IDDM. Presumably the single-residue change at position 57 from a charged aspartic to an uncharged valine, serine, or alanine influences the binding of different self-peptides to the DQ molecule.

Association with the T-Cell Receptor

The presence of T-cell receptors containing particular V_α and V_β domains also has been linked to a number of autoimmune diseases including experimental EAE and its human counterpart, multiple sclerosis. In one approach, T cells specific for various encephalitogenic peptides of MBP were cloned and their T-cell receptors analyzed. In PL/J mice, for example, T-cell clones were obtained by culturing T cells with the acetylated amino-terminal nonapeptide of MBP presented in association with a class II IA^u MHC molecule. Analysis of the T-cell receptors on these clones revealed a restricted repertoire of V_α and V_β domains: 100% of the T-cell clones expressed V_α 4.3, and 80% of the T-cell clones expressed V_β 8.2.

In human autoimmune diseases, evidence for restricted TCR expression has been obtained in both multiple sclerosis and myasthenia gravis. The preferential expression of TCR variable-region genes in these autoimmune T-cell clones suggests that a single epitope might induce the clonal expansion of a small number of pathogenic T cells.

PROPOSED MECHANISMS FOR INDUCTION OF AUTOIMMUNITY

A variety of mechanisms have been proposed to account for the T-cell–mediated generation of autoimmune diseases (Figure 20-9). Evidence exists for each of these mechanisms, and it is likely that autoimmunity does not develop from a single event but rather from a number of different events.

Release of Sequestered Antigens

As discussed in Chapter 12, the induction of tolerance in self-reactive T cells is thought to occur through exposure of immature thymocytes to self-antigens and their subsequent clonal deletion. Any tissue antigens that are sequestered from the circulation, and therefore are not seen by the developing T cells in the thymus, will not induce self-tolerance. Exposure of mature T cells to such normally sequestered antigens at a later date might result in their activation.

Myelin basic protein is an example of an antigen normally sequestered from the immune system, in this case by the blood-brain barrier. In the EAE model, animals are injected directly with MBP, together with adjuvant, under conditions that maximize immune exposure. In this type of animal model, the immune system is exposed to sequestered self-antigens under nonphysiologic conditions; however, trauma to tissues following either an accident or a viral or bacterial infection might also release sequestered antigens into the circulation. A few tissue antigens are known to fall into this category. For example, sperm arise late in development and are sequestered from the circulation. However, after a vasectomy, some sperm antigens are released into the circulation and can induce autoantibody formation in some men. Similarly, the release of lens protein after eye damage or of heart-muscle antigens after myocardial infarction has been shown to lead to autoantibody formation on occasion.

Recent findings indicate that injection of normally sequestered antigens directly into the thymus can reverse the development of tissue-specific autoimmune disease in animal models. For instance, intrathymic injection of pancreatic islet beta cells prevented development of autoimmunity in NOD mice. Moreover, EAE was prevented in susceptible rats by prior injection of myelin basic protein (MBP) directly into the thymus. In these experiments, exposure of immature T cells to self-antigens that normally are not present in the thymus presumably led to tolerance to these antigens.

Molecular Mimicry

A number of viruses and bacteria have been shown to possess antigenic determinants that are identical or similar to normal host-cell components. Such **molecular mimicry** appears to occur in a wide variety of organisms (Table 20-4). In one study 600 different monoclonal antibodies, specific for 11 different viruses, were tested to evaluate their reactivity with normal tissue antigens. More than 3% of the virus-specific antibodies tested also bound to normal tissue, suggesting that molecular mimicry is a fairly common phenomenon.

Molecular mimicry has been suggested as one mechanism leading to autoimmunity. One of the best examples of this type of autoimmune reaction is post-rabies encephalitis, which used to develop in some individuals

Visualizing Concepts

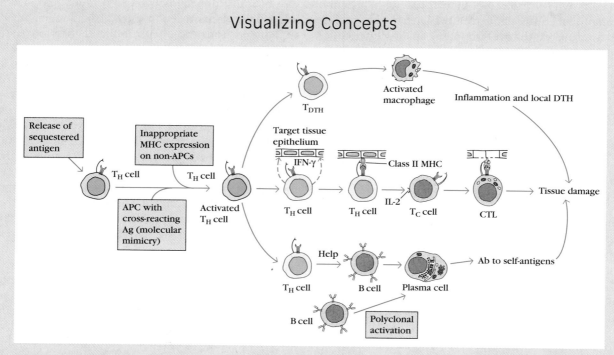

FIGURE 20-9

Proposed mechanisms for inducing autoimmune responses. Normal thymic selection appears to generate some self-reactive T_H cells; abnormalities in this process may generate even more self-reactive T_H cells. Activation of these self-reactive T cells in various ways, as well as polyclonal activation of B cells, is thought to induce an autoimmune response, in this case involving tissue damage. In all likelihood, several mechanisms are involved in each autoimmune disease. See text for details. [Adapted from V. Kumar et al., 1989, *Annu. Rev. Immunol.* **7**:657.]

who had received the rabies vaccine. In the past, the rabies virus was grown in rabbit brain-cell cultures, and preparations of the vaccine included antigens derived from the rabbit brain cells. In a vaccinated person these rabbit brain-cell antigens could induce formation of antibodies and activated T cells, which could cross-react with the recipient's own brain cells, leading to encephalitis. Cross-reacting antibodies are also thought to be the cause of heart damage in rheumatic fever, which usually develops after a *Streptococcus* infection. In this case the antibodies are to streptococcal antigens, but they cross-react with the heart muscle.

MIMICRY BETWEEN MBP AND VIRAL PEPTIDES

Since the encephalitogenic MBP peptides are known, the extent to which they are molecularly mimicked by proteins from other organisms can be assessed. For exam-

ple, one MBP peptide (61–69) is highly homologous with a peptide in the P3 protein of the measles virus (see Table 20-4). In one study, the sequence of another encephalitogenic MBP peptide (66–75) was compared with the known sequences of a large number of viral proteins. This computer analysis revealed sequence homologies between this MBP peptide and a number of peptides from animal viruses, including influenza, polyoma, adenovirus, Rous sarcoma, Abelson leukemia, poliomyelitis, Epstein-Barr, and hepatitis B viruses.

One peptide from the polymerase enzyme of the hepatitis B virus was particularly striking, exhibiting 60% homology with a sequence in the encephalitogenic MBP peptide. To test the hypothesis that molecular mimicry can generate autoimmunity, rabbits were immunized with this hepatitis B virus peptide. The peptide was shown to induce both the formation of antibody and the proliferation of T cells that cross-reacted with MBP; in addition, central nervous system tissue from the immunized rabbits showed cellular infiltration characteristic of that seen in EAE.

These findings suggest that infection with certain viruses expressing epitopes that mimic sequestered self-components, such as myelin basic protein, may induce autoimmunity to those components. Susceptibility to this type of autoimmunity may also be influenced by the MHC haplotype of the individual, since certain class I and class II MHC molecules may be more effective than others in presenting the homologous peptide for T-cell activation (see Figure 20-8).

MIMICRY INVOLVING HEAT-SHOCK PROTEINS

Another group of proteins implicated in autoimmunity through molecular mimicry are the **heat-shock proteins**, which are produced by mammalian cells in re-

sponse to elevated temperatures or other cellular stresses. These proteins, however, are not unique to mammalian cells and are found in a wide variety of bacterial and parasitic pathogens. These proteins exhibit remarkable evolutionary conservation: mammalian and microbial heat-shock proteins share more than 50% sequence identity. Despite their sequence homology, these proteins have been shown to serve as major immunodominant antigens in a variety of bacterial and parasitic infections. In human mycobacterial infection, for example, nearly 40% of the T-cell response is specific for microbial heat-shock protein (Hsp65). This has led to the suggestion that the high degree of sequence homology between microbial Hsp65 and the human heat-shock protein (Hsp60) may result in autoimmune consequences through molecular mimicry.

Several types of evidence support the role of heat-shock proteins in autoimmunity. For example, individuals

TABLE 20-4

MOLECULAR MIMICRY BETWEEN PROTEINS OF INFECTIOUS ORGANISMS AND HUMAN HOST PROTEINS

PROTEIN*	RESIDUE†	SEQUENCE‡
Human cytomegalovirus IE2	79	P D P L G R P D E D
HLA-DR molecule	60	V T E L G R P D A E
Poliovirus VP2	70	S T T K E S R G T T
Acetylcholine receptor	176	T V I K E S R G T K
Papilloma virus E2	76	S L H L E S L K D S
Insulin receptor	66	V Y G L E S L K D L
Rabies virus glycoprotein	147	T K E S L V I I S
Insulin receptor	764	N K E S L V I S E
Klebsiella pneumoniae nitrogenase	186	S R Q T D R E D E
HLA-B27 molecule	70	K A Q T D R E D L
Adenovirus 12 E1B	384	L R R G M F R P S Q C N
α-Gliadin	206	L G Q G S F R P S Q Q N
Human immunodeficiency virus p24	160	G V E T T T P S
Human IgG constant region	466	G V E T T T P S
Measles virus P3	13	L E C I R A L K
Corticotropin	18	L E C I R A C K
Measles virus P3	31	E I S D N L G Q E
Myelin basic protein	61	E I S F K L G Q E

* In each pair, the human protein is listed second. The proteins in each pair have been shown to exhibit immunologic cross-reactivity.

† Each number indicates the position in the intact protein of the amino-terminal amino acid in the indicated peptide.

‡ Amino acid residues are indicated by single-letter code. Identical residues are shown in blue.

SOURCE: Adapted from M. B. A. Oldstone, 1987, *Cell* **50**:819.

with rheumatoid arthritis have been shown to have T cells responsive to Hsp65, and antibodies to Hsp65 have been detected in NOD mice about 2 months before the onset of autoimmune destruction of pancreatic beta cells. In addition, T-cell clones reactive with Hsp65 have been isolated from prediabetic NOD mice. When these T-cell clones were injected into mice of an H-2 compatible, nondiabetic strain, the nondiabetic mice developed diabetes.

Perhaps the most compelling evidence that molecular mimicry between heat-shock proteins and tissue-specific proteins plays a role in autoimmunity comes from work by D. Jones, A. Coulson, and G. Duff on insulin-dependent diabetes mellitus (IDDM). These researchers found that individuals with IDDM have antibody specific for Hsp65; moreover, this anti-Hsp65 antibody was shown to cross-react with glutamic acid decarboxylase (GAD), a pancreatic enzyme localized in the insulin-producing beta cells of the islets of Langerhans. Sequence analyses revealed that microbial Hsp65, human Hsp60, and GAD exhibit striking sequence homology. Based on these results, Jones, Coulson, and Duff hypothesized that heat-shock proteins are homologous with a number of tissue-specific proteins.

To test this hypothesis, these researchers compared by computer analysis the known sequences of various human proteins with the overlapping sequences, each containing about 25 amino acid residues, that constitute the entire sequence of human Hsp60. As a control, computer analysis was performed with the overlapping 25-residue sequences of human albumin. The results of this study revealed that Hsp60 exhibited sequence homology with 86 human peptides, of which 19 were known autoantigens that had already been implicated in autoimmune pathogenesis (Table 20-5). Among the autoantigens that exhibited sequence homology with human Hsp60 were those implicated in IDDM, Hashimoto's thyroiditis, scleroderma, rheumatoid arthritis, multiple sclerosis, and Addison's disease. In contrast, the albumin control showed sequence homology with 138 human peptides, but of these, only 4 were known autoantigens.

Despite the evidence linking autoimmunity to heat-shock proteins, this association cannot be the whole story in the pathogenesis of autoimmunity. For instance, most normal individuals immunized with killed mycobacteria produce T cells reactive with Hsp65, but they do not develop autoimmunity. Several proposals have been suggested to account for this finding. One hypothesis is that although an immune response to heat-shock proteins occurs naturally, it is normally kept in check by a population of regulatory T cells specific for anti-Hsp T cells. Another hypothesis is that some MHC alleles bind to and present heat-shock peptides that do not mimic self-proteins, whereas other MHC alleles present heat-shock peptides that do mimic self-proteins, thus inducing autoimmune responses.

TABLE 20-5

MOLECULAR MIMICRY BETWEEN HUMAN HEAT-SHOCK PROTEIN HSP60 AND OTHER CELLULAR PROTEINS

ANTIGEN	AMINO ACID REGION	SEQUENCE*
Thyroglobulin	383–403	E K R W A S P R V A R
hsp60	65–75	E Q S W G S P K V T K
DNA-binding protein	73–82	E A G E A T T T T
hsp60	108–117	E A G D G T T T A T
Cytokeratin	545–555	G G M G G G L G G G
hsp 60	562–571	G G M G G G M G G G
Neurofilament triplet protein	727–749	V P E K K K A E S P V K E - E A V A E V V T I T
hsp60	152–175	I A E L K K Q S K P V T T P E E I A Q V A T I S

*Amino acid residues are indicated by single-letter code. Identical residues are in blue; conserved substitutions are underlined.

SOURCE: D. B. Jones et al., 1993, *Immunol. Today* **14**:115.

(a)

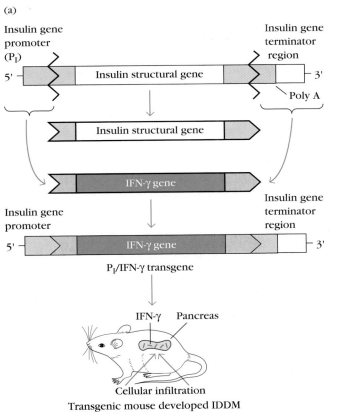

Insulin gene promoter (P$_I$)

Insulin gene terminator region

5' — Insulin structural gene — 3'

Poly A

Insulin structural gene

IFN-γ gene

Insulin gene promoter

Insulin gene terminator region

5' — IFN-γ gene — 3'

P$_I$/IFN-γ transgene

IFN-γ   Pancreas

Cellular infiltration
Transgenic mouse developed IDDM

(b)

FIGURE 20-10

Insulin-dependent diabetes mellitus (IDDM) in transgenic mice. (a) Production of transgenic mice containing an IFN-γ transgene linked to the insulin promoter (PI). The transgenics, which expressed the PI/IFN-γ transgene only in the pancreas, developed symptoms characteristic of IDDM. (b) Pancreatic islets of Langerhans from a normal BALB/c mouse (*left*) and from PI/IFN-γ transgenics at 3 weeks (*right*) showing infiltration of inflammatory cells. [Part (b) from N. Sarvetnick, 1988, *Cell* **52**:773.]

Inappropriate Expression of Class II MHC Molecules

The pancreatic beta cells of individuals with insulin-dependent diabetes mellitus (IDDM) express high levels of both class I and class II MHC molecules, whereas healthy beta cells express lower levels of class I and do not express class II at all. Similarly, thyroid acinar cells from those with Graves' disease have been shown to express class II MHC molecules on their membranes. This inappropriate expression of class II MHC molecules, which are normally expressed only on antigen-presenting cells, may serve to sensitize T$_H$ cells to peptides derived from the beta cells or thyroid cells, allowing activation of B cells or T$_C$ cells or sensitization of T$_{DTH}$ cells against self-antigens.

Other evidence suggests that certain agents can induce some cells that should not express class II MHC molecules to express them. For example, the T-cell mitogen phytohemagglutinin (PHA) has been shown to induce thyroid cells to express class II molecules. In vitro studies reveal that IFN-γ also induces increases in class II MHC molecules on a wide variety of cells, including pancreatic beta cells, intestinal epithelial cells, melanoma cells, and thyroid acinar cells. M. Feldman and G. F. Bottazzo hypothesized that trauma or viral infection in an organ may induce a localized inflammatory response, and thus increased concentrations of IFN-γ, in the affected organ. If IFN-γ induces class II MHC expression on non-antigen-presenting cells, inappropriate T$_H$-cell activation might follow, with autoimmune consequences. It is noteworthy that SLE patients with active disease have higher serum titers of IFN-γ than patients with inactive disease. Feldman and Bottazzo suggested that the increase in IFN-γ in these patients may lead to inappropriate expression of class II MHC molecules and thus to T-cell activation against a variety of autoantigens.

An interesting transgenic mouse system that implicates IFN-γ and inappropriate class II MHC expression in autoimmunity was developed by N. Sarvetnick. In this system an IFN-γ transgene was genetically engineered with the insulin promoter, so that the transgenic mice secreted IFN-γ from their pancreatic beta cells (Figure 20-10a). Since IFN-γ up-regulates class II MHC expression, these transgenic mice also expressed class II MHC molecules on their pancreatic beta cells. The mice developed diabetes, which was associated with cellular infiltration of lymphocytes and inflammatory cells similar to the infiltration seen in autoimmune NOD mice and in patients with insulin-dependent diabetes mellitus (Figure 20-10b).

Although inappropriate class II MHC expression on pancreatic beta cells may be involved in the autoimmune reaction in these transgenic mice, other factors also may play a role. For example, IFN-γ is known to induce production of several other cytokines, including IL-1 and TNF. Therefore, the development of autoimmunity in this transgenic system may involve antigen presentation by class II MHC molecules on pancreatic beta cells, together with a co-stimulatory signal, such as IL-1, that may activate self-reactive T cells. There is also some evidence to suggest that IL-1, IFN-γ, and TNF may directly impair the secretory function of human beta cells.

Polyclonal B-Cell Activation

A number of viruses and bacteria can induce nonspecific polyclonal B-cell activation. Gram-negative bacteria, cytomegalovirus, and Epstein-Barr virus (EBV) are all known to be such **polyclonal activators**, inducing the proliferation of numerous clones of B cells that express IgM in the absence of T_H cells. If B cells reactive to self-antigens are activated by this mechanism, autoantibodies can appear. For instance, during infectious mononucleosis, which is caused by EBV, a variety of autoantibodies are produced, including autoantibodies reactive to T and B cells, rheumatoid factors, and antinuclear antibodies. Similarly, lymphocytes from patients with SLE produce large quantities of IgM in culture, suggesting that they have been polyclonally activated. Many AIDS patients also show high levels of nonspecific antibody and autoantibodies to RBCs and platelets. These patients are often coinfected with other viruses such as EBV and cytomegalovirus, which may induce the polyclonal B-cell activation that results in autoantibody production.

TREATMENT OF AUTOIMMUNE DISEASES

Ideally, treatment for autoimmune diseases should be aimed at reducing only the autoimmune response while leaving the rest of the immune system intact. To date, this ideal has not been reached.

Current Therapies

Current therapies for autoimmune diseases are not cures but merely palliatives, aimed at reducing symptoms to provide the patient with an acceptable quality of life. For the most part these treatments provide nonspecific suppression of the immune system and thus do not distinguish between a pathologic autoimmune response and a protective immune response. Immunosuppressive drugs (e.g., corticosteroids, azathioprine, and cyclophosphamide) are often given with the intent of slowing proliferation of lymphocytes. By depressing the immune response in general, such drugs can reduce the severity of autoimmune symptoms. The general reduction in immune responsiveness, however, puts the patient at greater risk for infection or the development of cancer. A somewhat more selective approach employs **cyclosporin A** to treat autoimmunity. Since this agent blocks signal transduction mediated by the T-cell receptor (see Figure 12-13), it should inhibit only antigen-activated T cells while sparing nonactivated ones.

Another therapeutic approach that has produced positive results in some cases of myasthenia gravis is removal of the thymus. Because patients with this disease often have thymic abnormalities (e.g., thymic hyperplasia or thymomas), adult thymectomy often increases the likelihood of remission of symptoms.

Patients with Graves' disease, myasthenia gravis, rheumatoid arthritis, or systemic lupus erythematosus may experience short-term benefit from **plasmapheresis**. In this process plasma is removed from a patient's blood by continuous-flow centrifugation. The red blood cells are then resuspended in a suitable medium and returned to the patient. Plasmapheresis has been beneficial to patients with autoimmune diseases involving antigen-antibody complexes, which are removed with the plasma. Removal of the complexes, although only temporary, can result in a short-term reduction in symptoms.

Experimental Therapeutic Approaches

Studies with experimental autoimmune animal models have provided evidence that it is indeed possible to induce specific immunity to the development of autoimmunity. Several of these approaches are described in this section and outlined in Figure 20-11.

T-Cell Vaccination

I. R. Cohen and his coworkers have been pioneers in T-cell vaccination. The basis for this approach came from experiments with the EAE animal model. When rats were injected with low doses ($<10^4$) of cloned T cells specific for MBP, they did not develop symptoms of EAE and instead became resistant to the development of EAE when later challenged with a lethal dose of activated MBP-specific T cells or MBP in adjuvant. Later findings

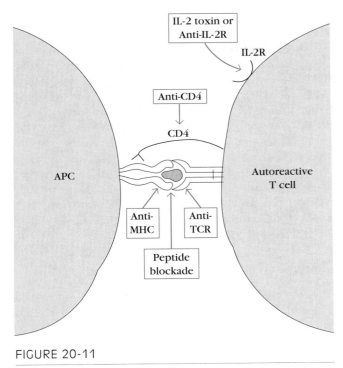

FIGURE 20-11

Some experimental agents for immunointervention in autoimmune disease. See text for discussion.

T-cell clones express V_β 8.2 almost exclusively. A synthetic peptide vaccine spanning the CDR2 region of the V_β 8.2 chain was shown to protect Lewis rats from developing EAE following an injection of MBP and adjuvant. When this same V-region peptide was injected into rats exhibiting severe EAE (characterized by hind-limb paralysis), disease progression was arrested and the animals recovered clinically within 3 days. Thus the synthetic TCR V-region peptide not only functioned as a vaccine to prevent clinical signs of EAE from developing, it also was an effective treatment for animals with established disease. As noted earlier, both multiple sclerosis and myasthenia gravis appear to be associated with restricted expression of TCR V-region genes, suggesting that a similar approach might be effective in patients with these diseases.

PEPTIDE BLOCKADE OF MHC MOLECULES

Identification and sequencing of various autoantigens has led to the development of new approaches to modulate autoimmune T-cell activity. In EAE, for example, the encephalitogenic peptides of MBP have been well characterized. Synthetic peptides differing by only one amino acid from their MBP counterpart have been shown to bind to the appropriate MHC molecule. Moreover, when sufficient amounts of such a peptide were administered along with the corresponding encephalitogenic MBP peptide, the clinical development of EAE was blocked. Presumably, the synthetic peptide acts as a competitor, occupying the antigen-binding cleft on MHC molecules and thus preventing binding of the MBP peptide.

In other studies blocking peptides complexed to soluble class II MHC molecules reversed the clinical progression of EAE in mice, presumably by inducing a state of clonal anergy in the autoimmune T cells. In a somewhat similar approach, a complex was formed between the blocking peptide, a class II MHC molecule, and the toxin adriamycin. This complex was shown to kill autoimmune EAE T cells in vitro.

MONOCLONAL-ANTIBODY TREATMENT

Monoclonal antibodies have been used successfully to treat autoimmune disease in several animal models. For example, a high percentage of (NZB × NZW) F_1 mice given weekly injections of high doses of monoclonal antibody specific for the CD4 membrane molecule recovered from their autoimmune lupus-like symptoms (Figure 20-12). Similar positive results were observed in NOD mice, in which treatment with an anti-CD4 monoclonal antibody led to disappearance of the lymphocytic infiltration and diabetic symptoms.

revealed that the efficacy of these autoimmune T-cell clones as a vaccine could be enhanced by cross-linking the cell-membrane components with formaldehyde or glutaraldehyde. When such cross-linked T cells were injected into animals with active EAE, permanent remission of symptoms was observed. The cross-linked T cells apparently elicit regulatory T cells specific for TCR variable-region determinants of the autoimmune clones. Presumably these regulatory T cells act to suppress the autoimmune T cells that mediate EAE.

Because of the effectiveness of T-cell vaccination in animal models, this approach has been tried with a few human patients. For example, a 42-year-old woman with severe progressive multiple sclerosis was injected subcutaneously with T cells that had been isolated from her own cerebrospinal fluid, cloned in vitro, and cross-linked with formaldehyde. The progression of her disease is currently being monitored. If this approach works, it represents a specific therapy that reduces only a specific autoimmune response without affecting overall immune responsiveness.

The finding that encephalitogenic T cells specific for MBP express T-cell receptors with a limited repertoire of V_α and V_β domains has led some researchers to use the restricted TCR V-region peptides as a possible vaccine. In the Lewis rat, for example, the encephalitogenic

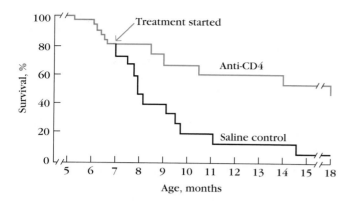

FIGURE 20-12

Weekly injections of anti-CD4 monoclonal antibody into (NZB × NZW) F_1 mice exhibiting autoimmune lupus-like symptoms significantly increased their survival rate. [Adapted from D. Wofsy, 1988, *Prog. Allergy,* **45**:106.]

Because anti-CD4 monoclonal antibodies block or deplete all T_H cells, regardless of their specificity, they can threaten the overall immune responsiveness of the recipient. One remedy for this disadvantage is to try to block antigen-activated T_H cells only, since these cells are involved in the autoimmune state. To do this, researchers have used monoclonal antibody directed against the α subunit of the high-affinity IL-2 receptor, which is expressed only by antigen-activated T_H cells. Because the IL-2R α subunit is expressed at higher levels on autoimmune T cells, monoclonal antibody to the α subunit (**anti-TAC**) might preferentially block autoreactive T cells. This approach was tested in adult rats injected with activated MBP-specific T cells in the presence or absence of anti-TAC. All the control rats died of EAE, whereas six of the nine treated with anti-TAC had no symptoms, and the symptoms in the other three were mild.

The association of autoimmune disease with restricted TCR expression in a number of animal models has prompted researchers to see if blockage of the preferred receptors with monoclonal antibody might be therapeutic. Injection of PL/J mice with monoclonal antibody specific for the V_β 8.2 T-cell receptor prevented induction of EAE by MBP in adjuvant. Even more promising was the finding that the anti-V_β 8.2 monoclonal antibody could also reverse the symptoms of autoimmunity in mice manifesting induced EAE (Figure 20-13) and that these mice manifested long-term remission. Clearly, the use of monoclonal antibodies as a treatment for human autoimmune diseases presents exciting possibilities.

Similarly, the association of various MHC alleles with autoimmunity (see Table 20-3), as well as the evidence for increased or inappropriate MHC expression in some

autoimmune disease, offers the possibility that monoclonal antibodies against appropriate MHC molecules might retard development of autoimmunity. Moreover, since antigen-presenting cells express many class II MHC molecules, it should theoretically be possible to selectively block an MHC molecule that is associated with autoimmunity, while sparing the other class II MHC molecules. In one study, injection of mice with monoclonal antibodies to class II MHC molecules prior to injection of myelin basic protein blocked the development of EAE. If, instead, the antibody was given after the injection of myelin basic protein, development of EAE was delayed but not prevented. In nonhuman primates, monoclonal antibodies to HLA-DR and HLA-DQ have been shown to reverse EAE.

TOLERANCE INDUCTION BY ORAL ANTIGENS

When antigens are administered orally, they tend to induce the state of immunologic unresponsiveness called **tolerance**. For example, mice fed MBP do not develop EAE following subsequent injection of MBP. This finding led H. Weiner, D. Hafler, and their colleagues to design a double-blind pilot trial in which 30 individuals with multiple sclerosis were fed either a placebo or 300 mg of bovine myelin every day for a year. The results of this study revealed that T cells specific for MBP were reduced in the myelin-fed group; there also was some suggestion that MS symptoms were reduced in the male

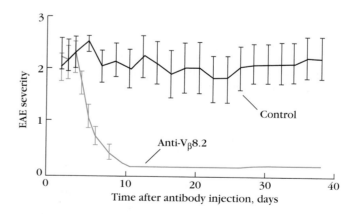

FIGURE 20-13

Injection of monoclonal antibody to the V_β 8.2 T-cell receptor into PL/J mice exhibiting EAE symptoms produced nearly complete remission of symptoms. EAE was induced by injecting mice with MBP-specific T-cell clones. EAE severity scale: 3 = total paralysis of lower limbs; 2 = partial paralysis of lower limbs; 1 = limp tail; 0 = normal (no symptoms). [Adapted from H. Acha-Orbea et al., 1989, *Annu. Rev. Immunol.* **7**:371.]

recipients (although the reduction fell short of statistical significance) but not in the female recipients. The difference in response between males and females may reflect differences in the HLA-DR phenotype: most of the males were HLA-DR2$^-$ and most of the females were HLA-DR2$^+$. (As noted earlier, this HLA allele has been associated with increased risk for multiple sclerosis.) Further investigation is needed to determine whether individuals with different HLA-DR phenotypes respond differently to the oral myelin. If further trials of this sort demonstrate the efficacy of this type of treatment, it will certainly prove to be a simple and risk-free treatment for patients with autoimmune disease.

SUMMARY

1. Human autoimmune diseases can be divided into organ-specific and systemic diseases (see Table 20-1). The organ-specific diseases involve an autoimmune response directed primarily against a single organ or gland. These include diseases in which autoreactive lymphocytes or autoantibodies bind to self-antigens, leading to direct cellular damage. Some organ-specific autoimmune disease are mediated by stimulating antibodies (Graves' disease) or blocking antibodies (myasthenia gravis). The systemic diseases are directed against a broad spectrum of tissues and have manifestations in a variety of organs resulting from cell-mediated responses and cellular damage caused by autoantibodies or immune complexes.

2. There are both spontaneous and experimental animal models for autoimmune diseases (see Table 20-2). Spontaneous autoimmune diseases resembling systemic lupus erythematosus occur in NZB and (NZB × NZW) F$_1$ mice and in MRL/*lpr*/*lpr* mice, which have a defective *fas* gene. Other spontaneous models include a thyroiditis seen in Obese-strain chickens that parallels Hashimoto's thyroiditis and a diabetes in NOD mice that resembles human insulin-dependent diabetes mellitus. Several experimental animal models have been developed by immunizing animals with self-antigens in the presence of adjuvant. In experimental autoimmune myasthenia gravis (EAMG), the antigen is the acetylcholine receptor; in experimental autoimmune encephalomyelitis (EAE), the antigen is myelin basic protein; in experimental autoimmune thyroiditis (EAT), the antigen is thyroglobulin.

3. Studies with experimental autoimmune animal models have revealed a central role for CD4$^+$ T$_H$ cells in the development of autoimmunity. In each of the experimentally induced autoimmune diseases, autoimmune T-cell clones can be isolated that induce the autoimmune disease in normal animals (see Figure

20-7). The relative number of T$_H$1 and T$_H$2 cells appears to play a pivotal role in determining whether autoimmunity develops: T$_H$1 cells promote the development of autoimmunity, whereas T$_H$2 cells appear to block development of autoimmune disease and also block the progression of the disease once established. The MHC haplotype of the experimental animal determines the ability to present various autoantigens to T$_H$ cells. In addition, some autoimmune animals utilize a restricted repertoire of TCR genes, which may predispose the animal toward T-cell activity in response to a given self-antigen.

4. A variety of mechanisms have been proposed for induction of autoimmunity, including release of sequestered antigens, molecular mimicry, inappropriate class II MHC expression on cells (in some cases stimulated by IFN-γ), and polyclonal B-cell activation (see Figure 20-9). Evidence exists for each of these mechanisms, reflecting the many different pathways leading to autoimmune reactions.

5. Current therapies for autoimmune diseases include treatment with immunosuppressive drugs, thymectomy, and plasmapheresis for diseases involving immune complexes. These therapies, which are relatively nonspecific, may have significant side effects. Several more specific approaches have shown some success in various animal models for autoimmune diseases (see Figure 20-11). These include vaccination with T cells specific for a given autoantigen, administration of synthetic blocking peptides that compete with autoantigen for binding to MHC molecules, treatment with monoclonal antibodies that react with some component specifically involved in an autoimmune reaction, and induction of tolerance to autoantigens by administering them orally.

REFERENCES

ADORINI, L., et al. 1993. Selective immunosuppression. *Immunol. Today* **14**:285.

BROCKE, S., ET AL. 1994. Infection and multiple sclerosis: a possible role for superantigens? *Trends Microbiol.* **2**: 250.

CHARLTON, B., AND K. J. LAFFERTY. 1995. The T$_H$1/T$_H$2 balance in autoimmunity. *Curr. Opin. Immunol.* **7**: 793.

COHEN, I. R. 1989. T cell vaccination against autoimmune disease. *Hosp. Prac.* (Feb. 15):57.

COHEN, I. R. 1991. Autoimmunity to chaperonins in the pathogenesis of arthritis and diabetes. *Annu. Rev. Immunol.* **9**:567.

FAUSTMAN, D., ET AL. 1991. Linkage of faulty major histocompatibility complex class I to autoimmune diabetes. *Science* **254**:1756.

FELDMANN, M., ET AL. 1992. T-cell-targeted immunotherapy. *Immunol. Today* **13**:84.

HASKINS, K., AND M. McDUFFIE. 1990. Acceleration of diabetes in young NOD mice with a CD4$^+$ islet-specific T cell clone. *Science* **249**:1433.

JONES, D. B., A. F. W. COULSON, AND G. W. DUFF. 1993. Sequence homologies between Hsp60 and autoantigens. *Immunol. Today* **14**:115.

KRONENBERG, M. 1991. Self-tolerance and autoimmunity. *Cell* **65**:537.

LIBLAU, R. S., S. M. SINGER, AND H. O. McDEVITT. 1995. T_H1 and T_H2 CD4$^+$ T cells in the pathogenesis of organ-specific autoimmune diseases. *Immunol. Today* **16**:34.

MARTIN, R., H. F. McFARLAND, AND D. E. McFARLIN. 1992. Immunological aspects of demyelinating disease. *Annu. Rev. Immunol.* **10**:153.

MUELLER, R., AND N. SARVETNICK. 1995. Transgenic/knockout mice—tools to study autoimmunity. *Curr. Opin. Immunol.* **7**:799.

NAPARSTEK, Y., AND P. H. PLOTZ. 1993. The role of autoantibodies in autoimmune disease. *Annu. Rev. Immunol.* **11**:79.

OFFNER, H., G. A. HASHIM, AND A. A. VANDENBARK. 1991. T cell receptor peptide therapy triggers autoregulation of experimental encephalomyelitis. *Science* **251**:430.

OKSENBERG, J. R., ET AL. 1989. T-cell receptor V_α and C_α alleles associated with multiple sclerosis and myasthenia gravis. *Proc. Nat'l. Acad. Sci. USA* **86**:988.

SHIZURU, J. A., AND N. SARVETNICK. 1991. Transgenic mice for the study of diabetes mellitus. *Trends Endocrinol. Metab.* **2**:97.

STEINMAN, L. 1991. The development of rational strategies for selective immunotherapy against autoimmune demyelinating disease. *Adv. Immunol.* **49**:357.

STEINMAN, L., J. R. OSKENBERG, AND C. C. A. BERNARD. 1992. Association of susceptibility to multiple sclerosis with TCR genes. *Immunol. Today* **13**:49.

THEOFILOPOULOS, A. N. 1995. The basis of autoimmunity. Part I: Mechanisms of aberrant self-recognition. *Immunol. Today* **16**:90.

THEOFILOPOULOS, A. N. 1995. The basis of autoimmunity. Part II: Genetic predisposition. *Immunol. Today* **16**:150.

WALDMANN, T. A. 1993. The IL-2/IL-2 receptor system: a target for rational immune intervention. *Immunol. Today* **14**:264.

WEINER, H. L., ET AL. 1993. Double-blind pilot trial of oral tolerization with myelin antigens in multiple sclerosis. *Science* **259**:1321.

WILDER, R. L. 1995. Neuroendocrine-immune system interactions and autoimmunity. *Annu. Rev. Immunol.* **13**:307.

WOFSY, D. 1988. Treatment of autoimmune diseases with monoclonal antibodies. *Prog. Allergy* **45**:106.

ZAMVIL, S. S., AND L. STEINMAN. 1990. The T lymphocyte in experimental allergic encephalomyelitis. *Annu. Rev. Immunol.* **8**:579.

STUDY QUESTIONS

1. For each of the following autoimmune diseases (a–l), select the most appropriate characteristic (1–12) listed below.

Diseases:

a. _____ Experimental autoimmune encephalitis (EAE)
b. _____ Goodpasture's syndrome
c. _____ Graves' disease
d. _____ Systemic lupus erythematosus (SLE)
e. _____ Insulin-dependent diabetes mellitus (IDDM)
f. _____ Rheumatoid arthritis
g. _____ Hashimoto's thyroiditis
h. _____ Experimental autoimmune myasthenia gravis (EAMG)
i. _____ Myasthenia gravis
j. _____ Pernicious anemia
k. _____ Multiple sclerosis
l. _____ Autoimmune hemolytic anemia

Characteristics:

1) Autoantibodies to intrinsic factor block vitamin B_{12} absorption
2) Autoantibodies to acetylcholine receptor
3) T_{DTH}-cell reaction to thyroid antigens
4) Autoantibodies to RBC antigens
5) T-cell response to myelin
6) Induced by injection of myelin basic protein + complete Freund's adjuvant
7) Autoantibody to IgG
8) Autoantibodies to receptor for thyroid-stimulating hormone
9) Autoantibodies to basement membrane

10) Autoantibodies to DNA and DNA-associated protein

11) Induced by injection of acetylcholine receptors

12) T_{DTH}-cell response to pancreatic beta cells

2. Experimental autoimmune encephalitis (EAE) has proved to be a useful animal model of autoimmune disorders.

a. Discuss how this animal model is generated.

b. What is unusual about the animals that recover from EAE?

c. How has this animal model indicated a role for T cells in the development of autoimmunity?

3. Molecular mimicry is one mechanism proposed to account for the development of autoimmunity. How has induction of EAE with myelin basic protein contributed to understanding of molecular mimicry in autoimmune disease?

4. Describe at least three different mechanisms by which a localized viral infection might contribute to the development of an organ-specific autoimmune disease.

5. In a system developed by Sarvetnik, transgenic mice expressing the IFN-γ transgene linked to the insulin promoter developed diabetes.

a. Why was the insulin promoter used?

b. What is the evidence that the diabetes in these mice is due to autoimmune damage?

c. What is unusual about MHC expression in this system?

d. How might this system mimic events that might be caused by a localized viral infection in the pancreas?

6. Monoclonal antibodies have been administered for therapy in various autoimmune animal models. Which monoclonal antibodies have been used and what is the rationale for these approaches?

7. Indicate whether each of the following statements is true or false. If you think a statement is false, explain why.

a. T_H1 cells have been associated with development of autoimmunity.

b. Exposure to mycobacterial heat-shock protein (Hsp65) induces an autoimmune response in humans.

c. Immunization of mice with IL-12 prevents induction of EAE by injection of myelin basic protein plus adjuvant.

d. The presence of the HLA B27 allele is diagnostic for ankylosing spondylitis, an autoimmune disease affecting the vertebrae.

e. Individuals with pernicious anemia produce antibodies to intrinsic factor.

f. A defect in the gene encoding Fas can reduce programmed cell death by apoptosis.

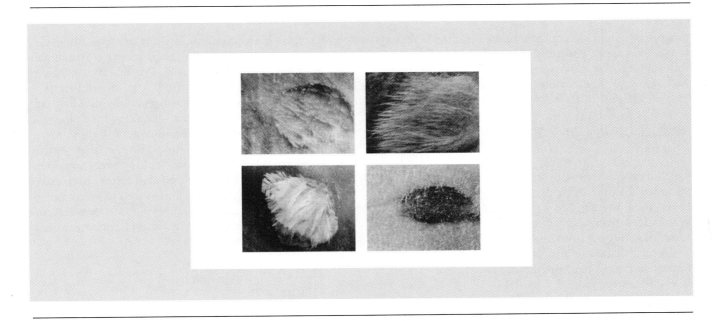

IMMUNODEFICIENCY DISEASES

PHAGOCYTIC DEFICIENCIES

HUMORAL DEFICIENCIES

CELL-MEDIATED DEFICIENCIES

COMBINED IMMUNODEFICIENCIES

COMPLEMENT DEFICIENCIES

The **immunodeficiency** diseases include a diverse spectrum of illnesses that stem from various abnormalities of the immune system. The basic clinical manifestations are frequent, prolonged, severe infections, which are often caused by organisms with normally low pathogenicity. An immunodeficiency disease may result from a primary congenital defect or may be acquired from a secondary cause, such as a viral or bacterial infection, malnutrition, or a drug treatment. Acquired immune deficiency syndrome (AIDS) is the most significant immunodeficiency arising from secondary causes, in this case a retrovirus named human immunodeficiency virus (HIV). Because of its worldwide impact and scientific importance, AIDS is covered separately in the next chapter.

Immunodeficiency diseases can result from congenital or acquired defects in hematopoietic stem cells, T cells, B cells, phagocytic cells, and the complement system. Each disease is caused by a congenital defect that interrupts hematopoiesis and development of leukocytes or results in impaired functioning of immune-system cells. Figure 21-1 outlines the nature of the defects associated with the immunodeficiency diseases discussed in this chapter. The prevalence of several of these diseases is given in Table 21-1.

PHAGOCYTIC DEFICIENCIES

Defects in phagocytic defense can result either from a reduction in the numbers of phagocytic cells or from a reduction in their function. Decreases in phagocyte production, extravasation, chemotaxis, and killing have each been implicated in immunodeficiencies (Table 21-2). In each case the hallmarks are recurrent bacterial or fungal infections. The clinical manifestations, which generally are related to the magnitude of the defect, range from mild skin infections to life-threatening systemic infections. The most common infectious organisms include *Staphylococcus aureus*, *Streptococcus pneumoniae*, *Escherichia coli*, and various species of *Pseudomonas*, *Candida*, and *Aspergillus*.

Reduction in Neutrophil Count

Quantitative deficiencies in neutrophils can range from an almost complete absence of cells, called **agranulocytosis**, to a reduction in peripheral blood neutrophils below 1500/mm^3, called **granulocytopenia** or **neutropenia**. These quantitative deficiencies may result from congenital defects or may be acquired through extrinsic factors. Acquired neutropenias are much more common than congenital ones.

Congenital neutropenias often involve a genetic defect affecting the myeloid progenitor stem cell that results in reduced production of neutrophils during hematopoiesis (see Figure 21-1). In **congenital agranulocytosis** myeloid stem cells are present in the bone marrow but rarely differentiate beyond the promyelocyte stage. As a result, children born with this condition show severe neutropenia with counts of less than 200 neutrophils/mm^3. These children frequently manifest bacterial infections as early as the first month of life. Experimental evidence suggests that this genetic defect results in decreased production of granulocyte colony-stimulating factor (G-CSF) and thus in a failure of the myeloid stem cell to differentiate along the granulocytic lineage (see Figure 3-2).

TABLE 21-1

PREVALENCE OF SELECTED IMMUNODEFICIENCY DISEASES

DISEASES	WORLDWIDE PREVALENCE
IgA immunodeficiency	1:700
Hereditary angioedema (deficiency in C1 inhibitor)*	1:1000
Common variable hypogammaglobulinemia	1:70,000
Severe combined immunodeficiency disease (SCID)—all forms	1:100,000
X-linked agammaglobulinemia	1:200,000

* Complement deficiencies are discussed in Chapter 14.

Because neutrophils have a short life span, their precursors divide rapidly in the bone marrow to maintain homeostatic levels of these cells. For this reason agents, such as radiation and certain drugs (e.g., chemotherapeutic drugs), that specifically damage rapidly dividing cells are likely to cause neutropenia. Occasionally neutropenia develops in such autoimmune diseases as Sjögren's syndrome or systemic lupus erythematosus; in these conditions, autoantibodies cause neutrophil destruction. Transient neutropenia often develops after certain bacterial or viral infections. It is not uncommon for children to manifest neutropenia after certain viral infections, but this neutropenia is transient, and neutrophil counts return to normal as the infection is cleared.

Defective Phagocytic Function

An effective phagocytic defense system involves a series of processes that interact in sequence to ingest and kill microorganisms. These processes include the adherence of phagocytes to vascular endothelial cells, emigration across the vascular endothelium, chemotaxis through subendothelial connective tissue to the site of immune reaction, attachment to the microorganism, phagocytosis, and subsequent killing and digestion. A dysfunction in any one of these processes may severely limit the effectiveness of the phagocytic defense system.

ADHERENCE DEFECTS

The development of an effective inflammatory response involves the adherence of neutrophils and monocytes to capillary endothelial cells near the site of the immune reaction. These adherent neutrophils and monocytes migrate through the capillary wall into extravascular sites, where an effective inflammatory response develops. A recently described autosomal recessive defect, called **leukocyte-adhesion deficiency** (LAD), involves an impairment of a variety of functions involving leukocyte adhesion. Included among the deficiencies is the inability of neutrophils, monocytes, and lymphocytes to adhere to vascular endothelial cells, thus preventing extravasation of these cells into the extravascular tissue spaces. Also impaired is the ability of CTLs and NK cells to adhere to their target cells and of T$_H$ cells and B cells to form conjugates. Individuals with this defect manifest recurrent bacterial infections and impaired wound healing.

The molecular basis of LAD has been shown to be defective biosynthesis of the β-chain component (CD18) of one subfamily of integrin adhesion molecules. The integrin molecules affected by this defect include the type 3 and type 4 complement receptors (CR3 and CR4), which bind the complement degradation product

Visualizing Concepts

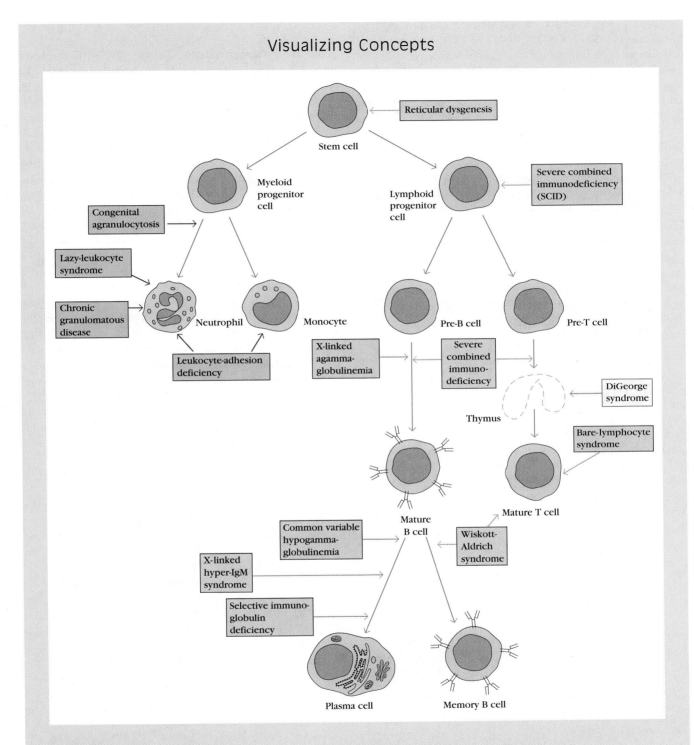

FIGURE 21-1

Congenital defects that interrupt hematopoiesis or impair functioning of immune–system cells result in various immuno-deficiency diseases. (Green boxes = phagocytic deficiencies, red = humoral deficiencies, yellow = cell-mediated deficien-cies, and purple = combined immunodeficiencies.)

C3bi, and LFA-1, which binds the intercellular adhesion molecule ICAM-1. CR3, CR4, and LFA-1 are all heterodimeric glycoproteins in which a unique α chain is noncovalently associated in the cell membrane with a common β chain (see Figure 15-2). The β-chain defect in LAD results in a near-total loss of all three membrane glycoproteins (Table 21-3).

Each of the three integrin receptors has its own role in leukocyte adhesion (Table 21-4). Monoclonal antibody to the β chain strongly inhibits adhesion of phagocytes to endothelial cells, random locomotion, and chemotaxis, suggesting that the β chain takes part in all these processes. Phagocytes from individuals with LAD show diminished in vitro adherence to cultured human endothelial cells. Activation of normal neutrophils with agents such as phorbol myristate acetate produces an increase in adherence from a baseline of 5%–10% to 50%–80% after activation; unactivated neutrophils from individuals with LAD exhibit 2%–5% adherence, and there is no appreciable increase in adherence after activation.

CHEMOTACTIC DEFECTS

A large number of clinical disorders reflect defects in neutrophil chemotaxis. These disorders may be caused by an intrinsic defect in the neutrophil itself or by an extrinsic defect such as a complement deficiency and a corresponding reduction in the chemotactic factors of the complement cascade (C3a, C5a, C5b67). One syndrome, called **lazy-leukocyte syndrome**, involves a congenital defect in which neutrophil migration is severely impaired.

KILLING DEFECTS

Chronic granulomatous disease (CGD) is the most prevalent defect associated with defective intracellular killing of ingested bacteria. The disease is inherited as an X-linked recessive disorder that is manifested in boys during the first 2 years of life. (A milder autosomal recessive form of this disease has been observed; this form can also occur in girls and often is not recognized until young adulthood.) Clinically, CGD is characterized by disseminated granulomatous lesions in various organs. Children with this disease often die of septicemia by 7 years of age.

The deficiency in CGD is in the bactericidal activity of neutrophils. Neutrophils from affected individuals can phagocytose bacteria but are unable to kill bacteria that contain the enzyme catalase. (Catalase-negative bacteria are not a problem because bacteria form H_2O_2 during their own metabolism; in the absence of catalase these bacteria cannot detoxify their own H_2O_2 and are unable to survive even in the defective phagocytes.) During normal phagocytosis there is a burst of respiratory oxidative activity, increased oxygen consumption, and a shift of glucose metabolism to the hexose monophosphate shunt. As glucose is metabolized, reduced pyridine nucleotides (NADH and NADPH) accumulate and convert O_2 into the bactericidal H_2O_2 and potent superoxides (see Table 3-5). The levels of H_2O_2 and superoxides are normally high enough to kill even catalase-positive bacteria. Neutrophils from CGD patients, however, show no increase in O_2 consumption, no increase in utilization of the hexose monophosphate shunt, and no H_2O_2 production during phagocytosis.

TABLE 21-2

PHAGOCYTIC DEFICIENCIES

DISEASE	IMMUNE-SYSTEM DEFICIENCY	POSSIBLE MECHANISM
Congenital agranulocytosis	Decreased neutrophil count	Decreased production of G-CSF
Leukocyte-adhesion deficiency (LAD)	Failure of neutrophils and monocytes to extravasate	Defective synthesis of β chain of integrin adhesion molecules
	Defective CTL killing	
	Defective T-cell help in B-cell activation	
Lazy-leukocyte syndrome	Decreased neutrophil chemotaxis	Not known
Chronic granulomatous disease (CGD)	Defective killing by neutrophils of phagocytosed bacteria	Decreased H_2O_2 production due to defective NADPH oxidase (cytochrome b)

The underlying defect in CGD appears to be in one of the genes encoding a subunit of cytochrome *b*, which is necessary for NADP recycling. The resulting decrease in the levels of reduced pyridine nucleotides leads to decreased H_2O_2 production; in this environment ingested catalase-positive bacteria can survive in neutrophils. The bacteria are carried by the cells into various organs, where the bacteria begin to grow, giving rise to the characteristic disseminated granulomatous lesions.

HUMORAL DEFICIENCIES

B-cell immunodeficiency disorders include a diverse spectrum of diseases ranging from the complete absence of mature recirculating B cells, plasma cells, and immunoglobulin to the selective absence of only certain classes of immunoglobulins (Table 21-5). Patients with these disorders usually are subject to recurrent bacterial infections but display normal immunity to most viral and fungal infections because the T-cell branch of the immune system is largely unaffected. The most common infections in patients with humoral immunodeficiencies involve such encapsulated bacteria as staphylococci, streptococci, and pneumococci because antibody is critical for the opsonization and clearance of these organisms. The severity of the disorder parallels the degree of antibody deficiency.

X-Linked Agammaglobulinemia

The first immunodeficiency disorder to be recognized, **X-linked agammaglobulinemia** (XLA), was originally described in 1952. Male infants with this disorder begin to manifest severe recurrent bacterial infections, especially of *Streptococcus pneumoniae, Staphylococcus aureus,* and *Haemophilus influenzae,* at about 6 months as the level of passively acquired maternal antibody declines and they are left unprotected.

The defect responsible for XLA, which has been mapped to the long arm of the X chromosome, is one of several X-chromosome defects that result in immunodeficiency diseases (Figure 21-2). These X-linked disorders exhibit several features in common: they each are recessive, occur with a frequency of 1 in 10^3–10^6 males, affect cells of the hematopoietic system, and occur in atypical forms in some patients; also, carriers of each disorder are normal by all immunologic criteria.

The defect causing XLA involves the maturation of pre-B cells to mature B cells in the bone marrow (see Figure 8-2). Patients have normal numbers of pre-B cells in their bone marrow but lack (or have severely reduced levels of) mature B cells and plasma cells. In normal individuals, for example, 5%–15% of peripheral-blood lymphocytes are B cells, whereas in XLA patients less than 0.1% of the peripheral lymphocytes are B cells. Afflicted males have extremely low concentrations of all classes of

T A B L E   2 1 - 3

PERCENTAGE OF GRANULOCYTES BEARING CR3, CR4, AND LFA-1 IN PATIENTS WITH LEUKOCYTE-ADHESION DEFICIENCY (LAD) AND IN NORMAL CONTROLS*

	PERCENTAGE OF CELLS BEARING				
LAD STATUS	CR3 M α CHAIN	LFA-1 L α CHAIN	CR4 X α CHAIN	COMMON β CHAIN	UNRELATED MOLECULE (CR1)
Severe					
Patient 1	0.1	0.15	0.1	0.15	94
Patient 2	0.0	0.0	0.3	0.1	100
Moderate					
Patient 3	6.0	11.0	7.0	4.4	92
Patient 4	4.0	31	3.5	2.5	99
Patient 5	4.0	26	4.0	6.0	87
Patient 6	3.0	24	2.0	4.0	109
Normal control	57.0	66.5	42.1	54.5	101

*Granulocytes were incubated with fluorochrome-labeled monoclonal antibody specific for the indicated receptor chains and then analyzed with a fluorescence-activated cell sorter (FACS) to determine the percentage of cells binding antibody.

SOURCE: D. C. Anderson et al., 1986, *J. Infect. Dis.* **152**:668.

serum immunoglobulins. Fluorescent antibody staining has revealed a complete absence of recirculating mature B cells and lack of cells in the B-cell–dependent areas of the peripheral lymphoid tissues in affected individuals. The lymph nodes are unusually small and lack germinal centers.

The defective gene in XLA was recently shown to encode a protein tyrosine kinase called Bruton's tyrosine kinase (BTK), after the researcher who first described the disorder. This kinase appears to be involved in B-cell signal transduction, coupling signal transduction to events that lead to B-cell maturation. In XLA patients B-cell maturation halts at the pre-B cell stage in which immunoglobulin heavy-chain genes are rearranged but light-chain genes remain in the germ-line configuration.

X-linked agammaglobulinemia can be diagnosed relatively easily by serum electrophoresis. IgG levels of affected individuals are usually 10%–20% of normal levels, and other isotypes are often not detectable. Treatment of patients with XLA requires periodic gamma-globulin

injections to passively protect them against common bacterial infections. Treated patients are still susceptible to sinopulmonary infections because secretory IgA is not transferred by gammaglobulin injections.

X-Linked Hyper-IgM Syndrome

A peculiar immunoglobulin deficiency, known as **X-linked hyper-IgM (XHM) syndrome**, is characterized by a deficiency of IgG, IgA, and IgE but markedly elevated levels of IgM as high as 10 mg/ml (normal IgM is 1.5 mg/ml). Like the other X-linked defects indicated in Figure 21-2, XHM syndrome is primarily an X-linked recessive disorder, but some forms appear to be acquired and affect both men and women. Affected individuals have high counts of IgM-secreting plasma cells in their peripheral blood and lymphoid tissue. In addition, XHM patients often have high levels of autoantibodies to neutrophils, platelets, and red blood cells. Children with XHM suffer recurrent infections, especially infec-

T A B L E   2 1 - 4

PROPERTIES OF INTEGRIN MOLECULES THAT ARE ABSENT IN LEUKOCYTE-ADHESION DEFICIENCY

PROPERTY	INTEGRIN MOLECULES*		
	LFA-1	CR3	CR4
CD designation	CD11a/CD18	CD11b/CD18	CD11c/CD18
Subunit composition	$\alpha L\beta 2$	$\alpha M\beta 2$	$\alpha X\beta 2$
Subunit molecular mass M_r (kDa)			
α chain	175,000	165,000	150,000
β chain	95,000	95,000	95,000
Cellular expression	Lymphocytes Monocytes Macrophages Granulocytes Natural killer cells	Monocytes Macrophages Granulocytes Natural killer cells	Monocytes Macrophages Granulocytes
Ligand	ICAM-1 ICAM-2	C3bi	C3bi
Functions inhibited with monoclonal antibody	Extravasation CTL killing T-B conjugate formation ADCC	Opsonization Granulocyte adherence, aggregation, and chemotaxis ADCC	Granulocyte adherence and aggregation

* CR3 = type 3 complement receptor, also known as Mac-1; CR4= type 4 complement receptor, also known as p 150,90. LFA-1, CR3, and CR4 are heterodimers containing a common β chain but different α chains designated L, M, and X, respectively.

tions caused by *Pneumocystis carinii*. The infections are more severe than expected for a deficiency characterized by low levels of immunoglobulins.

Although affected individuals exhibit normal counts of B cells expressing membrane-bound IgM or IgD, they appear to lack B cells expressing membrane-bound IgG, IgA, or IgE. The defect in XHM is in the gene encoding the CD40 ligand (CD40L), which maps to the X chromosome. T_H cells from patients with XHM fail to express functional CD40L on their membrane. Since an interaction between CD40 on the B cell and CD40L on the T_H cell is required for B-cell activation, the absence of this co-stimulatory signal inhibits the B-cell response to T-dependent antigens (see Figure 8-6). The B-cell response to T-independent antigens, however, is unaffected by this defect, accounting for the production of IgM antibodies.

As discussed in Chapter 8, class switching and formation of memory B cells both require contact with T_H cells via a CD40–CD40L interaction. The absence of this interaction in XHM results in the loss of class switching to IgG, IgA, or IgE isotypes and in a failure to produce memory B cells. In addition, XHM individuals fail to produce germinal centers during a humoral response, which highlights the role of the CD40–CD40L interaction in the generation of germinal centers.

Common Variable Hypogammaglobulinemia

Common variable hypogammaglobulinemia (CVH) refers to a heterogeneous group of disorders that cause late-onset hypogammaglobulinemia. Patients with this disorder typically develop recurrent bacterial infections beginning between 15 and 35 years of age because their serum immunoglobulin levels are severely reduced. A variety of immune deficiencies have been observed in affected individuals. In some cases the number of mature B cells is reduced; usually, however, B-cell levels are normal and the intrinsic defect appears to be in the differentiation of mature B cells into functional antibody-secreting plasma cells. To date, however, no definitive genetic basis has been demonstrated for CVH, although familial inheritance patterns have been reported.

A variety of defects could render plasma cells unable to synthesize the secreted form of the antibody molecule.

TABLE 21-5

HUMORAL AND CELL-MEDIATED DEFICIENCIES

DISEASE	IMMUNE-SYSTEM DEFICIENCY	POSSIBLE MECHANISM
HUMORAL DEFICIENCIES		
X-linked agammaglobulinemia (XLA)	Reduction in B-cell count Absence of immunoglobulins	Block in maturation of pre-B cells due to defective V-D-J gene rearrangement
X-linked hyper-IgM (XHM) syndrome	Low levels of IgG and IgA Very high levels of IgM	Defect in class switching
Common variable hypogammaglobulinemia (CVH)	Decreased plasma-cell levels but usually normal B-cell levels Variable reduction in secreted Ig of all isotypes	Defective differentiation of B cells to plasma cells due to defective processing of Ig transcripts, lack of cytokine receptors on B cells, or abnormal T-cell response
Selective immunoglobulin deficiencies	Decreased levels of one or more Ig isotypes	Defect in maturation of plasma cells or necessary T-cell–derived cytokines
CELL-MEDIATED DEFICIENCIES		
DiGeorge syndrome	Decreased T-cell counts	Lack of T-cell maturation due to absence of thymus
Nude mice	Decreased T-cell counts	Lack of T-cell maturation due to absence of thymus

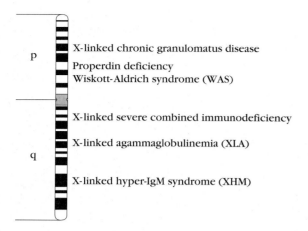

X-linked chronic granulomatus disease

Properdin deficiency

Wiskott-Aldrich syndrome (WAS)

X-linked severe combined immunodeficiency

X-linked agammaglobulinemia (XLA)

X-linked hyper-IgM syndrome (XHM)

FIGURE 21-2

Several X-linked immunodeficiency diseases result from defects in loci on the X chromosome. [Based on J. W. Belmont, 1995, *Trends Genet.* **11**:112.]

For example, a defect in polyadenylation of the primary Ig transcript might prevent the loss of the M1 and M2 exons, which is necessary for the expression of secreted antibody (see Figure 7-18). In other cases defective heavy-chain glycosylation may prevent secretion of antibodies by plasma cells. Another possibility is that B cells in CVH patients lack receptors for the cytokines that trigger the activation and differentiation of B cells into antibody-secreting cells (see Figure 8-19). Alternatively, the defect may be in the T cells that play a role in the humoral response. Some CVH patients, for example, have been shown to have defective T_H cells that cannot mediate B-cell activation and differentiation. In contrast, other patients have an excess of T cells that may act as suppressors and prevent plasma cells from secreting immunoglobulin.

Selective Immunoglobulin Deficiencies

Some immunodeficiency disorders involve a deficiency in a single immunoglobulin class or subclass. Most common is a **selective IgA deficiency**, which occurs in 1 in 600–800 people. Although some affected individuals are completely asymptomatic, many develop recurrent respiratory infections and gastrointestinal symptoms of malabsorption and infection. This is not surprising in view of the important protective role of secretory IgA in the mucous secretions of the respiratory and gastrointestinal tracts. Affected individuals also have an increased incidence of severe allergic reactions, presumably due to increased penetration of allergens through mucosal surfaces and subsequent stimulation of IgE production.

The B cells of patients with IgA deficiency generally bear membrane IgA; the defect appears to be in the maturation of these cells into IgA-secreting plasma cells. It is not known whether the defect is in the B cell itself or whether the defect is at the level of T-cell help. It has been suggested that there may be a decrease in IL-5 or TGF-β, which are known to mediate a class switch to IgA. The defect in some patients has been shown in vitro to be caused by T-cell–mediated suppression of IgA production by B cells.

CELL-MEDIATED DEFICIENCIES

Because of the central role of T cells in the immune system, a T-cell deficiency can affect both the humoral and the cell-mediated responses. The impact on the cell-mediated system can be severe, with a reduction in both delayed-type hypersensitive responses and cell-mediated cytotoxicity. Whereas defects in the humoral system are associated primarily with infections by encapsulated bacteria, defects in the cell-mediated system are associated with increased susceptibility to viral, protozoan, and fungal infections. Intracellular pathogens such as *Candida albicans* (Figure 21-3), *Pneumocystis carinii*, and *Mycobacteria* are often implicated, reflecting the importance of T cells in eliminating intracellular pathogens. Infections

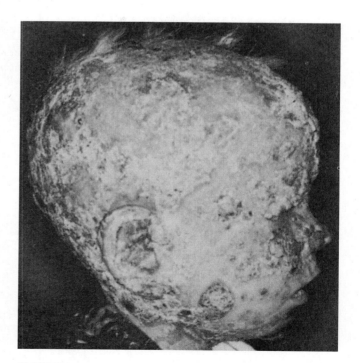

FIGURE 21-3

Chronic cutaneous candidiasis in a boy with defective cell-mediated immunity. [From R. J. Schlegel et al., 1970, *Pediatrics* **45**:926.]

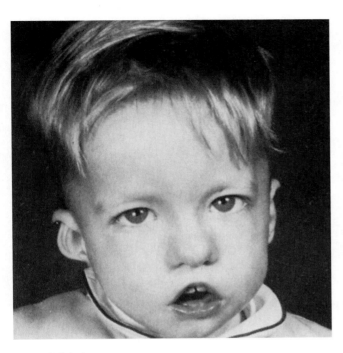

FIGURE 21-4

A child with DiGeorge syndrome showing characteristic dysplasia of ears and mouth and abnormally long distance between the eyes. [R. Kretschmer et al., 1968, *New Engl. J. Med.* **279**:1295; photograph courtesy of F. S. Rosen.]

with viruses that are rarely pathogenic for the normal individual (such as cytomegalovirus or even an attenuated measles vaccine) may be life-threatening for those with impaired cell-mediated immunity. Defects that cause decreased T-cell counts generally also affect the humoral system, because of the requirement for T_H cells in B-cell activation. Generally there is some decrease in antibody levels, particularly in the production of specific antibody following immunization.

DiGeorge Syndrome (Congenital Thymic Aplasia)

DiGeorge syndrome, first described in 1965, is characterized by the absence of a thymus, hypoparathyroidism, cardiovascular anomalies, characteristic facial features (Figure 21-4), and increased incidence of infections. The syndrome reflects a failure of the third and fourth pharyngeal pouches to develop between 10 and 12 weeks of gestation, a time when several organs, including the aortic arch of the heart, are developing.

Children born with this defect often have seizures on the first day of life due to low calcium in the blood, a result of the hypoparathyroid condition. Cardiac defects are the most common cause of death. If the child survives the neonatal period, increased susceptibility to vari-

ous opportunistic infections is observed. Generally these children have effective humoral immunity against common bacterial infections but are extremely susceptible to viral, protozoan, and fungal infections; even the common attenuated measles vaccine may be life-threatening to affected children.

Evaluation of children with complete DiGeorge syndrome reveals a severe decrease in the total number of T cells, which can be demonstrated by flow cytometry. Functionally, there is an absence of T_{DTH} skin-test reactivity to common antigens, a decreased response to T-cell mitogens such as PHA, and decreased responsiveness to allogeneic cells in the mixed-lymphocyte reaction (MLR). In partial DiGeorge syndromes, the thymus is abnormally situated or is extremely small. In these cases there can be intermediate counts of T cells and responsiveness to T-cell mitogens or antigens.

Treatment for DiGeorge syndrome involves the grafting of fetal thymus tissue. The age of the thymus tissue is important: fetal thymuses older than 14 weeks of gestation should not be used because they have T cells that can cause graft-versus-host disease in the immune-suppressed recipient. The grafted thymic tissue provides a source of thymic hormones and a cellular environment in which T-cell stem cells can mature and differentiate. Once mature T cells are formed, unfortunately, the grafted thymus can sometimes be rejected by the very cells it helped to mature.

Nude Mice

An autosomal recessive thymic defect in mice resembles DiGeorge syndrome. Among the many defects exhibited by these mice is an absence of hair follicles, and they are called **nude mice** because of their strange hairless state (Figure 21-5). What makes these mice interesting from an immunologic perspective is that they lack a thymus or have a vestigial thymus and show varying degrees of cell-mediated immunodeficiency. The defect is inherited and

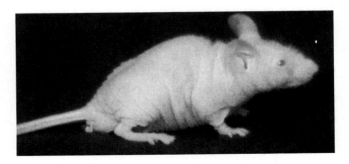

FIGURE 21-5

A nude mouse (*nu/nu*). This defect leads to absence of a thymus or a vestigial thymus and cell-mediated immunodeficiency. [Courtesy of Jackson Laboratories.]

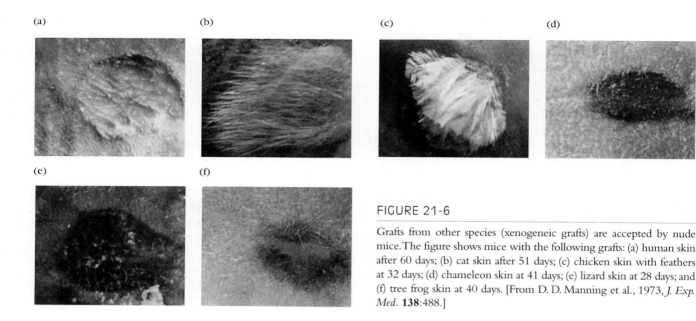

FIGURE 21-6

Grafts from other species (xenogeneic grafts) are accepted by nude mice. The figure shows mice with the following grafts: (a) human skin after 60 days; (b) cat skin after 51 days; (c) chicken skin with feathers at 32 days; (d) chameleon skin at 41 days; (e) lizard skin at 28 days; and (f) tree frog skin at 40 days. [From D. D. Manning et al., 1973, *J. Exp. Med.* **138**:488.]

controlled by a recessive gene on chromosome 11; *nu/nu* homozygotes are hairless and lack a thymus, whereas *nu/+* heterozygotes are normal.

Several inbred mouse strains homozygous for the recessive *nu* gene have been developed, and these animals have served as important model systems. Because these mice lack a thymus, the pre-T cells fail to mature and there is a marked absence of cell-mediated immunity. This lack of a functioning cell-mediated response is best demonstrated in these mice by their ability to accept foreign (**xenogeneic**) skin grafts. Even grafts of human skin or chicken skin, feathers and all, are accepted by nude mice (Figure 21-6).

COMBINED IMMUNODEFICIENCIES

As one might expect, combined deficiencies of the humoral and cell-mediated branches are the most serious of the immunodeficiency disorders (Table 21-6). The onset of infections begins early in infancy, and the prognosis for these infants is early death unless some therapeutic intervention reconstitutes their defective immune system. Considerable success has been achieved with bone marrow transplantation from HLA-matched donors.

Reticular Dysgenesis

Reticular dysgenesis is a rare, fatal congenital disease in which the lymphoid and myeloid stem cells fail to differentiate during hematopoiesis. Children born with this defect lack not only phagocytic cells of the monocyte and granulocyte series but also T and B lymphocytes. The developmental failure must therefore be at a very early stage in hematopoiesis, before the stem cell differentiates into separate lymphoid and myeloid lineages (see Figure 21-1). Children born with this disorder die shortly after birth.

Bare-Lymphocyte Syndrome

Several severe combined immunodeficiency diseases caused by a deficiency in expression of MHC molecules are collectively referred to as **bare-lymphocyte syndrome**. These disorders are classified into three types: type I bare-lymphocyte syndrome involves defective class I MHC expression; type II syndrome, defective class II MHC expression; and type III syndrome, defective class I and class II MHC expression. The absence or reduced levels of MHC molecules impairs antigen presentation to T cells. Consequently, individuals born with bare-lymphocyte syndrome suffer recurrent bacterial and viral infections and often die by 5 years of age.

The defect causing type I bare-lymphocyte syndrome in one family was found not to involve the class I MHC genes. Although family members failed to express class I MHC molecules on their cells, they had normal levels of mRNA encoding the class I α chain and normal intracellular levels of class I MHC molecules. The defect in these individuals was traced to the transporter protein (TAP), which normally transports antigenic peptides generated in the cytosolic processing pathway into the lumen of the endoplasmic reticulum for assembly with class I MHC molecules (see Figure 10-6a). In the absence of antigenic peptides, the class I MHC α chains fail to assemble with β_2-microglobulin and therefore are not expressed on the plasma membrane.

Researchers have begun to unravel the molecular defect causing type II bare-lymphocyte syndrome. Antigen-presenting cells (e.g., B cells, macrophages, dendritic cells), which normally express class II MHC molecules, do not do so in patients with the type II syndrome. Moreover, IFN-γ, which induces increased class II MHC expression in normal individuals, does not induce class II expression in patients with this syndrome. The observation that none of the three class II MHC molecules (DP, DQ, and DR) is expressed in affected individuals suggests that the genes encoding these molecules are regulated coordinately. As discussed in Chapter 9, regulation of MHC expression depends in part on DNA-binding proteins (transcription factors) that bind to the promoters associated with each MHC gene. The finding that the *DP, DQ,* and *DR* promoters contain several conserved motifs suggests that each of these class II genes is activated by binding of the same transcription factor(s). Evidence suggests that a defect in binding of this factor to the conserved class II MHC promoter motif leads to the coordinated loss of all three class II molecules observed in bare-lymphocyte syndrome.

Severe Combined Immunodeficiency Disease (SCID)

A group of diseases characterized by markedly depressed counts of T cells and B cells is referred to as **severe combined immunodeficiency disease** (SCID). This disorder is associated with increased susceptibility to viral, bacterial, fungal, and protozoan diseases; a failure to thrive and reduced weight gain are also usually observed.

TABLE 21-6

COMBINED IMMUNODEFICIENCIES

DISEASE	IMMUNE-SYSTEM DEFICIENCY	POSSIBLE MECHANISM
Reticular dysgenesis	Decreased numbers of all cells of lymphoid and myeloid lineages	Defective maturation of hematopoietic stem cells
Bare-lymphocyte syndrome	Some reduction in CDT4$^+$ T-cell counts	Failure to express class I and/or class II MHC molecules on cells
	Reduced B-cell and T$_c$-cell activation Decreased T$_{DTH}$-cell activity	
Severe combined immunodeficiency disease (SCID)	Marked reduction in T- and B-cell counts in all forms	Various mechanisms
X-linked SCID		Defective T- and B-cell maturation
Autosomal recessive SCID		Defective T- and B-cell maturation
ADA-deficiency SCID		Selective killing of lymphocytes by metabolites that accumulate in absence of adenosine deaminase (ADA)
PNP-deficiency SCID		Selective killing of lymphocytes by metabolites that accumulate in absence of purine necleoside phosphorylase (PNP)
CB-17 SCID mouse		Aberrant D-J joining of Ig heavy-chain and TCR β- and δ-chain gene segments
Wiskott-Aldrich syndrome (WAS)	Low levels of IgM Elevated levels of IgA and IgE Abnormal T-cell function with progressive dysfunction	Defective glycosylation of membrane glycoproteins (CD43) on lymphocytes

So severe is the immune compromise that organisms nonpathogenic for the normal individual can cause serious or even life-threatening infections in the SCID patient. Infants born with SCID generally develop recurrent infections at 3–6 months of age. The most common manifestations are pneumonia due to *Pneumocystis carinii*, prolonged diarrhea due to rotavirus or bacterial infections of the gastrointestinal tract, and moniliasis caused by the common yeast, *Candida albicans*. These children are so severely immunocompromised that even attenuated vaccines such as the oral Sabin polio vaccine or the measles vaccine can cause progressive infection and death. The disease received national attention in the 1970s when the plight of a boy named David, who lived inside a sterile plastic bubble, was much publicized.

Individuals with SCID exhibit structural and functional abnormalities in both the humoral and cell-mediated branches of the immune system. Generally, recirculating lymphocyte counts are dramatically reduced; the tonsils usually are absent; peripheral lymph nodes are absent or extremely small; and the usual thymic shadow does not show on an x-ray. Functional abnormalities in SCID patients generally include quite low antibody levels, negative skin test for delayed-type hypersensitivity, little if any proliferation in mitogen-stimulation assays, and markedly reduced cytokine production.

Over half of all SCID cases result from an X-linked recessive defect; the remaining cases are caused by autosomal recessive defects (see Table 21-6). The defect causing **X-linked SCID** (XSCID) lies in the gene encoding the common γ subunit of a number of cytokine receptors including the receptors for IL-2, IL-4, IL-7, IL-9, and IL-15 (see Figure 13-6c); this subunit may also be part of the IL-13 receptor. The γ-chain gene maps to the q arm of the X chromosome (see Figure 21-2).

Bone marrow transplantation from HLA-identical siblings has successfully reconstituted the immune system in some SCID children. Because 60% of SCID patients do not have HLA-identical siblings, marrow from haploidentical parental donors often is administered. The problem with HLA-mismatched bone marrow is that fatal graft-versus-host disease can develop. This fatal reaction can be avoided by treating the donor bone marrow with monoclonal anti-T-cell antibody plus complement to deplete T cells prior to transplantation.

ADA-DEFICIENCY AND PNP-DEFICIENCY SCID

The defects causing two autosomal recessive forms of SCID also have been established. In both cases the disease results from an inherited deficiency of an enzyme—either **adenosine deaminase** (ADA) or **purine nucleoside phosphorylase** (PNP). A PNP deficiency results in accumulation of dGTP and dATP, and an ADA deficiency leads to accumulation of dATP (Figure 21-7). Because both dATP and dGTP are selectively toxic to dividing B and T cells, individuals with either ADA or PNP deficiency have markedly reduced counts of mature B and T cells.

Patients with ADA-deficiency SCID have been treated successfully with infusions of the purified enzyme, and some have also received **gene therapy**. Indeed, the first gene therapy of any kind in humans was performed in 1990 on two young girls suffering from ADA-deficiency SCID. The gene therapy was accomplished with a retrovirus in which key retroviral genes had been replaced with the ADA gene. The patients' bone marrow cells or peripheral blood lymphocytes were removed and infected in vitro with the engineered retrovirus; the genetically altered bone marrow cells then were reinfused back into the little girls. A major limitation with this technique has been the inability to identify and isolate the pluripotent stem cell in humans (see Chapter 3). Because the hematopoietic cells carrying the engineered ADA gene are not pluripotent, they are not capable of self-renewal; for this reason this therapy was expected to have short-term effects. Contrary to these expectations, however, reports published in 1995 indicated that the transduced peripheral-blood lymphocytes and bone marrow progenitors still were surviving in the recipients 4 years after their introduction and that active ADA enzyme continued to be produced by these cells. Although both patients continued to receive weekly injections of the ADA enzyme throughout these trials, the amount of enzyme administered had been cut in half. In both trials, the patients remained free of infections, suggesting that their immune systems were functioning well.

More recently, similar gene therapy was used to treat a newborn baby boy born with ADA-deficiency SCID. In this case, however, cord blood was used since it contains a rich supply of stem cells. The 4-day-old infant was injected with cord blood cells containing the engineered ADA gene. If the gene was inserted into pluripotent stem cells, the researchers anticipated that a long-term cure might be achieved in this infant. A 1996 report on this infant revealed that T cells derived from the engineered stem cells were multiplying and supplanting the ADA-defective cells. The weekly ADA injections in this infant have been cut in half and he continues to thrive.

SCID MICE AND SCID-HUMAN MICE

An autosomal recessive mutation resulting in severe combined immunodeficiency disease developed spontaneously in CB-17 mice. Like humans with this disease, CB-17 SCID mice fail to develop mature T and B cells; these mice can be kept alive by housing them in a sterile environment. When normal mouse bone marrow cells are injected into SCID mice, normal T and B

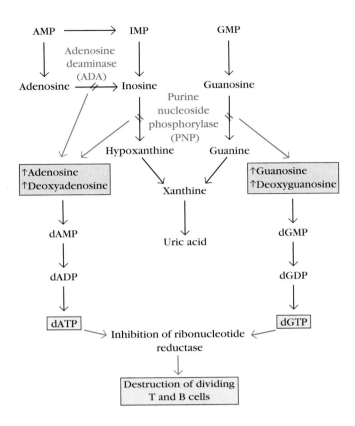

AMP ⟶ IMP   GMP

Adenosine deaminase (ADA)

Adenosine ⟶ Inosine   Guanosine

Purine nucleoside phosphorylase (PNP)

Hypoxanthine   Guanine

↑Adenosine
↑Deoxyadenosine

Xanthine

↑Guanosine
↑Deoxyguanosine

dAMP   Uric acid   dGMP

dADP   dGDP

dATP ⟶ Inhibition of ribonucleotide reductase ⟵ dGTP

Destruction of dividing T and B cells

FIGURE 21-7

Molecular basis of severe combined immunodeficiency disease resulting from genetic defect in adenosine deaminase (ADA) or purine nucleoside phosphorylase (PNP). The normal pathway of AMP and GMP degradation, which yields uric acid, involves steps catalyzed by ADA and PNP; the latter enzyme acts on both inosine and guanosine. The accumulation of dGTP and/or dATP in the absence of PNP or ADA, respectively, leads to inhibition of ribonucleotide reductase and the selective killing of dividing T and B cells.

cells develop. These mice have proven to be a valuable model system for the study of immunodeficiency and hematopoiesis.

The defect in CB-17 SCID mice is in the recombinase enzyme machinery that normally catalyzes functional rearrangements of variable-region gene segments in immunoglobulin and T-cell receptor DNA. As illustrated in Figure 7-9, SCID mice have a defect in joining of the D and J coding sequences resulting in the deletion of one or both of the coding sequences. Interest in SCID mice has mushroomed following the development of SCID-human mice (see Figure 2-1).

Wiskott-Aldrich Syndrome

Wiskott-Aldrich syndrome (WAS) is another of the X-linked recessive immunodeficiency diseases affecting

boys. Although the defective gene causing this disorder has not yet been identified, preliminary evidence suggests that it maps to the X chromosome and may encode a transcription factor. The defect appears to compromise the functioning of mature B and T cells (see Figure 21-1).

WAS patients exhibit a variety of abnormalities including eczema, thrombocytopenia (low platelet count), increased susceptibility to bacterial infections, and bloody diarrhea. These patients have normal levels of IgG, low levels of IgM, and elevated levels of IgA and IgE. They generally exhibit an absence of isohemagglutinins and fail to produce antibodies to polysaccharide antigens in general. The absence of antibodies to polysaccharide antigens leaves these patients at risk for infections with encapsulated pyogenic bacteria. T-cell function is variable and tends to get progressively worse as WAS patients grow older; most patients do not exhibit cutaneous delayed-type hypersensitivity. Lymphocytes from WAS patients are smaller and have fewer microvilli than normal lymphocytes. These morphologic abnormalities result from an alteration in or complete absence of a cell-membrane glycoprotein called sialophorin (CD43). WAS patients have been treated successfully with bone marrow transplantation.

COMPLEMENT DEFICIENCIES

Immunodeficiency diseases resulting from defects in the complement system are discussed in Chapter 14. Many complement deficiencies are associated with increased susceptibility to bacterial infections and/or immune-complex diseases. One of these complement disorders, a deficiency in properdin, which stabilizes the C3 convertase in the alternative complement pathway, is caused by a defect in a gene located on the X chromosome.

SUMMARY

1. Immunodeficiency diseases can affect any component of the immune system. Disorders involving the phagocytic system, complement system, humoral system, or cell-mediated system have all been reported. Many of the disorders result from defects that prevent normal hematopoiesis and leukocyte development. The developmental stage affected by a particular genetic defect determines the nature of the resulting disease (see Figure 22-1).

2. Phagocytic disorders can result from quantitative deficiencies (agranulocytosis or neutropenia) or from a functional defect in one of the steps of phagocytosis (leukocyte adhesion, chemotaxis, phagocytosis, or

killing). Examples include congenital agranulocytosis, leukocyte-adhesion deficiency, lazy-leukocyte syndrome, and chronic granulomatous disease (see Table 21-2).

3. Humoral immunodeficiencies can result from defects in B-cell maturation, intrinsic defects of mature B cells, ineffective T_H-cell activation, or inappropriate suppression by T cells. Examples of humoral deficiencies include X-linked agammaglobulinemia, X-linked hyper-IgM syndrome, common variable immunodeficiency, and selective IgA deficiency (see Table 21-5).

4. Cell-mediated immunodeficiencies can result from defective T-cell maturation due to thymic aplasia. DiGeorge syndrome is an example of a cell-mediated immune defect.

5. Because both humoral and cell-mediated immunity are deficient in combined immunodeficiencies, these disorders lead to early death unless treatment reconstitutes the defective immune system. Combined immunodeficiencies can result from defects in stem-cell differentiation (reticular dysgenesis), from failure to express MHC molecules (bare-lymphocyte syndrome), from defective T- and B-cell maturation (severe combined immunodeficiency disease), and from deficiencies in adenosine deaminase or purine nucleoside phosphorylase, which result in selective killing of T and B cells (see Table 21-6). These disorders are treated by bone marrow transplantation or gene therapy.

6. The defects responsible for several immunodeficiency diseases have been mapped to the X chromosome (see Figure 21-2). All of these disorders are recessive, affecting 1 in 10^3–10^6 males; carriers are immunologically normal.

REFERENCES

ANDERSON, D. C., AND T. A. SPRINGER. 1987. Leukocyte adhesion deficiency: an inherited defect in the Mac-1, LFA-1 and p150,95 glycoproteins. *Annu. Rev. Med.* **38**:175.

BELMONT, J. W. 1995. Insights into lymphocyte development from X-linked immune deficiencies. *Trends Genet.* **11**:112.

BLAESE, R.M., ET AL. 1995. T lymphocyte-directed gene therapy for ADA-SCID: initial results after 4 years. *Science* **270**:475.

BORDIGNON, C., ET AL. 1995. Gene therapy in peripheral blood lymphocytes and bone marrow for ADA-immunodeficient patients. *Science* **270**:470.

BOSMA, M. J., AND A. M. CARROLL. 1991. The SCID mouse mutant: definition, characterization, and potential uses. *Annu. Rev. Immunol.* **9**:323.

CONLEY, M. E. 1992. Molecular approaches to analysis of X-linked immunodeficiencies. *Annu. Rev. Immunol.* **10**:215.

CONLEY, M. E. 1995. Primary immunodeficiencies: a flurry of new genes. *Immunol. Today* **16**:313.

COURNOYER, D., AND C. T. CASKEY. 1993. Gene therapy of the immune system. *Annu. Rev. Immunol.* **11**:297.

DERRY, J. M. J., H.D. OCHS, AND U. FRANCKE. 1994. Isolation of a novel gene mutated in Wiskott-Aldrich syndrome. *Cell* **78**:635.

KANESHIMA, H., R. NAMIKAWA, AND J. M. MCCUNE. 1994. Human hematolymphoid cells in SCID mice. *Curr. Opin. Immunol.* **6**:327.

KARA, C. J., AND L. H. GLIMCHER. 1991. In vivo footprinting of MHC class II genes: bare promoters in the bare lymphocyte syndrome. *Science* **252**:709.

MALYNN, B. A., ET AL. 1988. The SCID defect affects the final step of the immunoglobulin VDJ recombinase mechanism. *Cell* **54**:453.

MCCUNE, J. M., ET AL. 1988. The SCID-Hu mouse: murine model for the analysis of human hematolymphoid differentiation and function. *Science* **241**: 1632.

SIDERAS, P., AND C. I. E. SMITH. 1995. Molecular and cellular aspects of X-linked agammaglobulinemia. *Adv. Immunol.* **59**:135.

THOMPSON, L. 1992. At age 2, gene therapy enters a growth phase. *Science* **258**:744.

TSUKADA, S., D. J. RAWLINGS, AND O. N. WITTE. 1994. Role of Bruton's tyrosine kinase in immunodeficiency. *Curr. Opin. Immunol.* **6**:623.

VERMA, I. M. 1990. Gene therapy. *Sci. Am.* **263**(5):68.

STUDY QUESTIONS

1. Indicate whether each of the following statements is true or false. If you think a statement is false, explain why.

a. DiGeorge syndrome is a congenital birth defect resulting in absence of the thymus.

b. X-linked agammaglobulinemia (XLA) is a combined B-cell and T-cell immunodeficiency disease.

c. The hallmark of a phagocytic deficiency is increased susceptibility to viral infections.

d. In chronic granulomatous disease, H_2O_2 produced by catalase-negative bacteria results in bacterial killing in the defective granulocytes.

e. Gamma-globulin injections are given to treat individuals with X-linked agammaglobulinemia.

f. D_H-J_H joining is defective in CB-17 SCID mice.

g. Mice with the SCID defect lack functional B and T lymphocytes.

h. A thymic transplant can restore the immune defect in CB-17 SCID mice.

i. Children born with DiGeorge syndrome often manifest increased infections with encapsulated bacteria.

j. Failure to express class II MHC molecules in bare-lymphocyte syndrome affects cell-mediated immunity only.

2. Granulocytes from patients with leukocyte-adhesion deficiency (LAD) express greatly reduced amounts of three integrin molecules designated CR3, CR4, and LFA-1.

a. What is the nature of the defect that results in decreased or in no expression of these receptors in LAD patients?

b. What is the normal function of the integrin molecule LFA-1? Give specific examples.

c. Would you expect LAD patients to exhibit normal levels of specific antibody following antigenic challenge? Explain your answer.

3. Immunologists have studied the defect in SCID mice in an effort to understand the molecular basis for severe combined immunodeficiency in humans. In both SCID mice and humans with this disorder, mature B and T cells fail to develop.

a. In what way do rearranged Ig heavy-chain genes in SCID mice differ from those in normal mice?

b. In SCID mice, rearrangement of κ light-chain DNA is not attempted. Explain why.

c. If you introduced a rearranged, functional μ heavy-chain gene into progenitor B cells of SCID mice, would the κ light-chain DNA undergo a normal rearrangement? Explain your answer.

d. If you compared gene rearrangements in TCR α- and β-chain DNA in T-cell thymomas derived from SCID mice and from normal CB-17 mice, what differences would you detect?

4. Four major classes of immunodeficiencies are discussed in this chapter. Identify each class and briefly describe the clinical manifestations commonly observed with diseases in each class.

5. The accompanying figure outlines some of the steps in development of immune-system cells. The numbered arrows indicate the cell type whose function is defective or the developmental step that does not occur in particular immunodeficiency diseases. Identify the defective cell type or developmental step associated with each of the following diseases. Use each number only once.

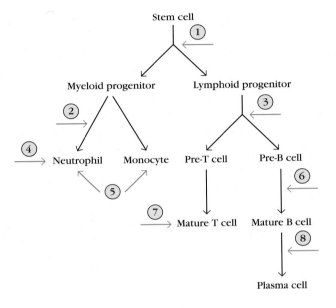

a. _____ Chronic granulomatous disease

b. _____ Severe combined immunodeficiency disease (SCID)

c. _____ Congenital agranulocytosis

d. _____ Reticular dysgenesis

e. _____ Common variable hypogammaglobulinemia

f. _____ X-linked agammaglobulinemia

g. _____ Leukocyte-adhesion deficiency (LAD)

h. _____ Bare-lymphocyte syndrome

6. As indicated in several chapters, SCID-human mice are a valuable experimental system for studying human lymphoid cells within an animal model.

a. Describe the procedure for preparing SCID-human mice.

b. Why are human fetal liver cells used in this procedure?

c. Why are the human cells not rejected by the recipient mouse?

d. Why does graft-versus-host disease not develop in the recipient mouse?

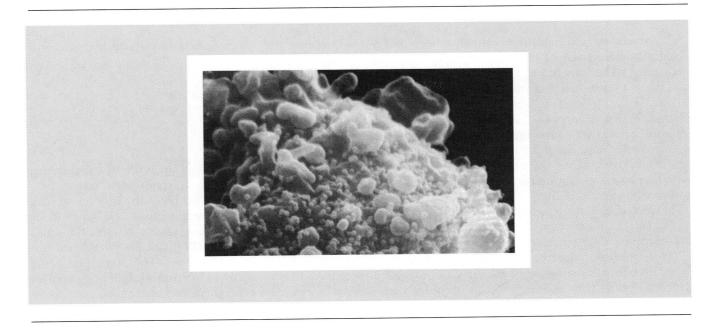

THE IMMUNE SYSTEM IN AIDS

DISCOVERY OF AIDS AND ITS CAUSATIVE AGENT

HUMAN IMMUNODEFICIENCY VIRUS (HIV)

DIAGNOSIS OF HIV INFECTION AND AIDS

DESTRUCTION OF CD4+ T CELLS

IMMUNOLOGIC ABNORMALITIES IN AIDS

DEVELOPMENT OF AN AIDS VACCINE

Since the early 1980s, the spread of the disease now known as acquired immunodeficiency syndrome (AIDS) has been dramatic. Many predict that AIDS eventually will cause millions of deaths and sorely stress health-care systems worldwide in the next decade or two. AIDS—the epitome of an acquired immunodeficiency disease—renders its victims susceptible to opportunistic infections and certain rare forms of cancer, which are the immediate cause of death. As the number of reported AIDS cases escalated, the acquisition of scientific information about AIDS exhibited a comparable surge, with reports in the scientific literature increasing logarithmically from 1982 to the present. Never has so much been learned about a

disease and its causative agent in such a short time. This explosion of information about AIDS has expanded our understanding of the immune system to such an extent that this entire chapter is devoted to AIDS, the immunodeficiencies associated with it, and efforts to develop AIDS vaccines.

DISCOVERY OF AIDS AND ITS CAUSATIVE AGENT

In the summer of 1981, five cases of *Pneumocystis carinii* pneumonia, all in young homosexual men from the same area of Los Angeles, were reported to the Centers for Disease Control (CDC), the agency of the U.S. Public Health Service responsible for monitoring infectious diseases in the United States. Soon thereafter, the CDC began to get reports of **Pneumocystis carinii pneumonia**, **Kaposi's sarcoma**, and various **opportunistic infections** clustered in young homosexual men living in New York City, San Francisco, and Los Angeles. *Pneumocystis carinii* had been known as a widespread, generally harmless protozoan rarely associated with pneumonia, and Kaposi's sarcoma had been recognized as a rare tumor of blood-vessel tissue associated with aging. What caught the attention of the CDC was that these diseases had previously been limited to individuals with impaired cell-mediated immunity. Such diseases might be expected in individuals born with immune deficiencies, in transplant recipients receiving immunosuppressive drugs, or in cancer patients receiving chemotherapy, but their presence in young men with no obvious condition that would impair immunity was puzzling and alarming.

In December 1981, reports in the *New England Journal of Medicine* indicated that the original victims of the still-unnamed disorder had decreased counts of CD4⁺ T cells, confirming the suspected linkage to a compromised immune system. In early 1982 the CDC suggested that this distinct new disorder be called **acquired immunodeficiency syndrome**, now commonly known as **AIDS**. The syndrome appeared to be a collection of symptoms associated with an immunodeficiency that was not inborn or imposed but somehow acquired.

Although first identified in homosexual men in the United States, AIDS was soon observed in other groups, including users of intravenous (IV) drugs, hemophiliacs, blood-transfusion recipients, sexual partners of AIDS patients, and eventually in infants of mothers with the disease. Because these findings suggested that AIDS was transmissible, the CDC asked in 1982 that all AIDS cases be reported in order to monitor the disease. Since that time the spectrum of clinical disease included in the definition of AIDS has broadened, and the number of reported cases has increased exponentially. What began as five cases reported in a CDC newsletter in 1981 mushroomed to staggering proportions within a few years.

According to CDC estimates, as of the mid-1990s, 1–2 million Americans had been infected with the virus that causes AIDS. Worldwide estimates are even more alarming with reports from the World Health Organization (WHO) suggesting that over 22 million people are infected worldwide. As shown in Figure 22-1, about 70% of those currently infected live in sub-Saharan Africa, but the incidence of infection is predicted to increase most dramatically in Asia during the remainder of this decade. The estimated rate of infection among women is substantially lower than that in men in the Americas and Western Europe, but not in sub-Saharan Africa. By the most conservative estimates, Michael Merson, AIDS chief of the World Health Organization, predicts that 40 million people will be infected with HIV by the end of the decade. Of these, he predicts that 10 million will be from Asia alone. The high rates of infection among men and the likely increase in infection rates among women and children portend widespread

economic and social disaster unless effective interventions are developed.

HUMAN IMMUNODEFICIENCY VIRUS (HIV)

In 1983 Luc Montagnier's group at the Pasteur Institute isolated a retrovirus from a lymph node biopsy of a patient with AIDS. In 1986 the retrovirus was named **human immunodeficiency virus**, or **HIV**. Following the discovery of an antigenic variant in 1986, the original virus was designated HIV-1 and the variant was designated HIV-2. Both HIV-1 and HIV-2 are genetically related to the **simian immunodeficiency viruses** (SIVs), which are found in African primates. Recently, a new variant, designated HIV-0, was identified in Cameroon.

Relation Between HIV and Other Retroviruses

The retroviruses can be divided into two groups: transforming and cytopathic. The **transforming retroviruses** induce changes in cell growth that lead to cancer. These viruses often carry genes, called **oncogenes**, that influence cellular growth. Included in this group are bovine leukemia virus, avian type C virus, mammalian type C virus, and human T-cell lymphotrophic virus type 1 and 2 (HTLV-1 and HTLV-2). The best studied of this group is HTLV-1, which causes T-cell leukemia. Although this retrovirus does not carry an oncogene, it nonetheless induces cancer by stimulating expression of the high-affinity receptor for IL-2 in infected T cells. As an infected cell secretes IL-2, it autostimulates its own division in an unregulated way, causing T-cell leukemia (see Figure 13-13).

The **cytopathic retroviruses** are members of the lentivirus family. Cytopathic retroviruses induce damage or death to cells. One branch of this group includes visna virus, caprine arthritis encephalitis virus, equine infectious anemia virus, and feline immunodeficiency virus. The other branch of this group includes human immunodeficiency virus (HIV-1, HIV-2, and HIV-0) and simian immunodeficiency virus (SIV). HIV-1 infects humans, chimpanzees, pigtailed macaques, and SCID-human mice but causes immune suppression with development of AIDS only in humans (Table 22-1). The majority of HIV infections worldwide involve HIV-1. HIV-2 was initially isolated from samples that originated in Senegal in West Africa. Infection with HIV-2 is endemic in many countries of West Africa, but is much rarer in other parts of the

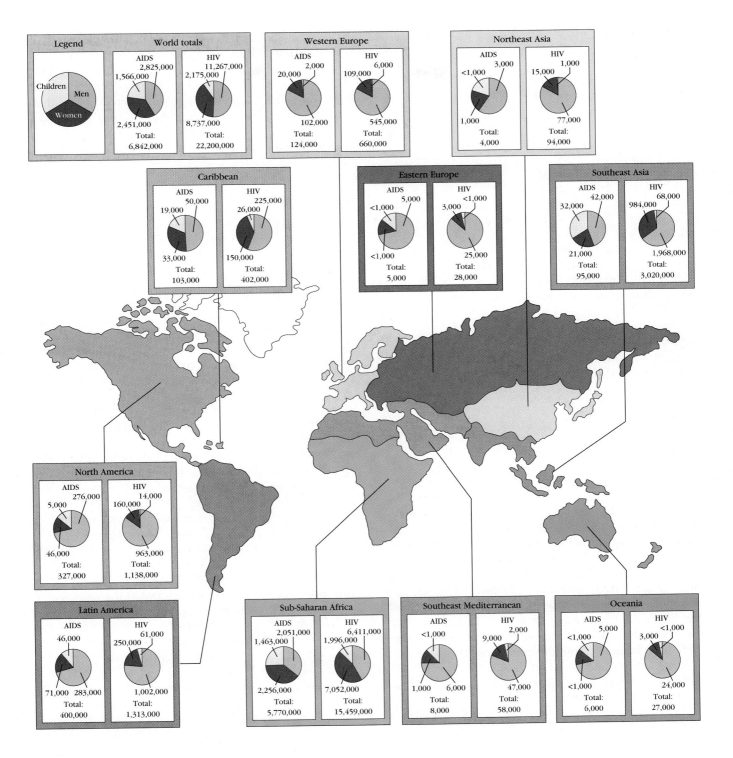

FIGURE 22-1

Estimated incidence and distribution of AIDS cases and infection with HIV, the virus causing AIDS. In the Americas and Western Europe about 80% of infected individuals are men, whereas in sub-Saharan Africa only about 40% of infected individuals are men. [Data from Global AIDS Policy Coalition, 1995, Harvard University.]

T A B L E   2 2 - 1

INFECTIVITY AND PATHOGENICITY OF HIV-1, HIV-2, AND SIV$_{AGM}$ IN VARIOUS ANIMALS

VIRUS	ANIMAL	INFECTION	AIDS
HIV-1	Human	+	+
	Chimpanzee	+	−
	SCID-human mouse	+	?
	Pigtailed macaque	+	?
HIV-2	Human	+	+
	Chimpanzee	+	−
	Macaque (rhesus) monkey	+	+
	Baboon	+	+
SIV$_{AGM}$	African green monkey	+	−
	Macaque (rhesus) monkey	+	+(SAIDS)

world. A small number of cases of HIV-2 infection have been reported in Europe and the Americas. Most HIV-2 strains appear to spread more slowly and to be less pathogenic than HIV-1. HIV-2, which infects humans, chimpanzees, macaque monkeys, and baboons, has a broader host range than HIV-1. Infection of macaque monkeys and baboons with some strains of HIV-2 results in symptoms of AIDS and holds promise as an animal model for AIDS.

Various strains of simian immunodeficiency viruses have been isolated from different African primates:

- SIV$_{AGM}$ from African green monkeys
- SIV$_{CPZ}$ from wild chimpanzees
- SIV$_{MAC}$ from captive macaque (rhesus) monkeys
- SIV$_{MND}$ from mandrills
- SIV$_{SM}$ from captive sooty mangabeys

SIV$_{AGM}$ is present in an estimated 40% of the African green monkey population in some parts of Africa. Although SIV$_{AGM}$ infection of African green monkeys does not cause immune suppression, injection of

SIV$_{AGM}$ into macaques leads to a fatal AIDS-like disease called **simian AIDS** (SAIDS) and to death within 3–36 months. Comparisons of the DNA sequences of various HIV-1, HIV-2, and SIV isolates have revealed that both HIV-1 and HIV-2 are more closely related to SIV than to each other. For example, HIV-1 and HIV-2 exhibit only 40%–50% DNA sequence homology, whereas HIV-2 has 75% homology with strains of SIV$_{SM}$, SIV$_{MAC}$, and SIV$_{AGM}$.

Structure of HIV

All members of the lentivirus family of retroviruses, including the three types of HIV and various SIVs, share numerous structural and molecular features. These viruses have an RNA genome and two associated molecules of **reverse transcriptase**, which catalyzes the "reverse transcription" of viral RNA into DNA. Other nucleoid proteins include the p10 protease and p32 integrase. Surrounding the viral genome and nucleoid proteins are two layers of core proteins; in HIV these core proteins are designated p17 and p24 (Figure 22-2).

The viral core, or **nucleocapsid**, is surrounded by an **envelope** derived from the host-cell membrane, which is modified by the insertion of two HIV glycoproteins, **gp120** and **gp41**. The gp41 glycoprotein spans the membrane; gp120 is noncovalently associated with gp41 but extends beyond the membrane. Both gp120 and gp41 have important roles in the binding of HIV to cells in the infection process. Researchers discovered quite early that the HIV envelope is studded with human proteins (including class I and class II MHC molecules) acquired by the virus as it buds from the human cell membrane. Subsequent studies revealed that the level of these human proteins is far greater than had initially been thought. In fact, the HIV envelope actually contains more molecules of human proteins than molecules of gp120! This startling finding is discussed later in the chapter.

HIV Infection of Target Cells

Entry of HIV into target cells involves two steps: **binding** of virions to receptors on target cells is followed by **fusion** of the viral envelope with the plasma membrane of the target cells. The two envelope glycoproteins that make up the surface projections on HIV play vital roles in these initial steps in HIV infection: gp120 in binding and gp41 in fusion. Once inside a target cell, the viral RNA is copied into DNA. The viral DNA is then integrated into the host-cell DNA, forming a **provirus**, which may remain in a latent state or may be activated and transcribed into viral proteins.

Visualizing Concepts

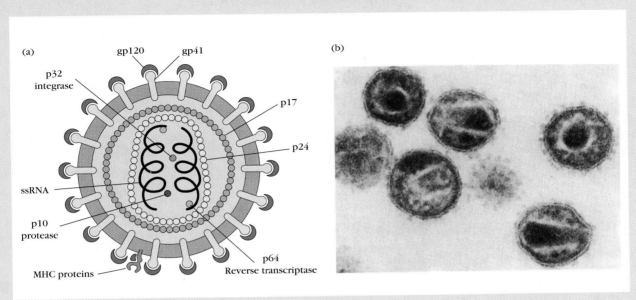

FIGURE 22-2

Structure of HIV. (a) Cross-sectional schematic diagram of HIV virion. Each virion expresses 72 glycoprotein projections composed of gp120 (orange) and gp41 (light blue). Gp41 is a transmembrane molecule that crosses the lipid bilayer of the envelope. Gp120 is noncovalently associated with gp41 and serves as the viral receptor for CD4 on host cells. The viral envelope also contains some host-cell membrane proteins such as class I and class II MHC molecules. Within the envelope is the viral core, or nucleocapsid, which includes a layer of a protein called p17 (green) and an inner layer of a protein called p24 (yellow). The HIV genome consists of two copies of ssRNA, which are associated with two molecules of reverse transcriptase (light red) and nucleoid proteins p10, a protease (red), and p32, an integrase (dark blue). (b) Electron micrograph of HIV virions magnified 200,000 times. The glycoprotein projections are faintly visible as "knobs" extending from the periphery of each virion. [Part (a) adapted from B. M. Peterlin and P. A. Luciw, 1988, *AIDS* **2**:S29; part (b) from micrograph by Hans Geldenblom of the Robert Koch Institute (Berlin) in R. C. Gallo and L. Montagnier, 1988, *Sci. Am.* **259**:40.]

ENTRY OF HIV INTO CELLS

The first step in HIV infection is binding of viral gp120 to receptors on target cells. The major cellular receptor for HIV is CD4. Because the T_H cell expresses the highest levels of CD4, T_H lymphocytes are the prime target for HIV, and the virus is said to be **lymphotrophic**. Other cells that bind HIV include macrophages, monocytes, dendritic cells, Langerhans cells, hematopoietic stem cells, certain rectal-lining cells, and microglial cells. Because these cells express lower levels of CD4 than

T_H cells, they can bind less HIV than T_H cells. HIV-1 has a 25-fold higher affinity for CD4 than does HIV-2. The lower binding affinity of HIV-2 for CD4 may account, in part, for its lower pathogenicity compared with HIV-1. The importance of CD4 in HIV binding can be demonstrated by transfecting the gene encoding CD4 into certain human cells in tissue culture that lack CD4; such cells, formerly resistant to HIV infection, sometimes become susceptible to HIV after the CD4 gene is transfected into them. After binding of HIV to its receptors, the viral envelope fuses with the target-cell plasma mem-

Visualizing Concepts

(a) Infection of target cell

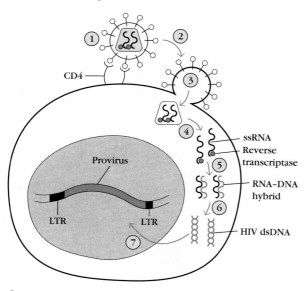

(b) Activation of provirus

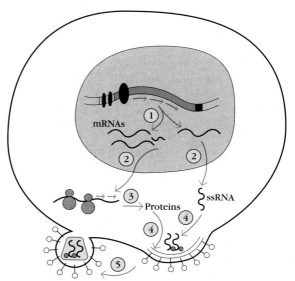

① HIV gp140 binds to CD4 on target cell.

② Fusogenic domain in gp41 and fusin, a G-protein–linked receptor in the target-cell membrane, mediate fusion.

③ Nucleocapsid containing viral genome and enzymes enters cells.

④ Viral genome and enzymes are released following removal of core proteins.

⑤ Viral reverse transcriptase catalyzes reverse transcription of ssRNA, forming RNA-DNA hybrids.

⑥ Original RNA template is partially degraded by ribonuclease H, followed by synthesis of second DNA strand to yield HIV dsDNA.

⑦ The viral dsDNA is then translocated to the nucleus and integrated into the host chromosomal DNA by the viral integrase enzyme.

① Transcription factors stimulate transcription of proviral DNA into genomic ssRNA and, after processing, several mRNAs.

② Viral RNA is exported to cytoplasm.

③ Host-cell enzymes catalyze synthesis of viral proteins.

④ HIV ssRNA and proteins assemble beneath the host-cell membrane, into which gp41 and gp140 are inserted.

⑤ The membrane buds out forming the viral envelope.

FIGURE 22-3

Overview of HIV infection of target cells and activation of provirus. (a) Following entry of HIV into cells and formation of dsDNA, integration of the viral DNA into the host-cell genome yields the provirus. (b) The provirus remains latent until events in the infected cell trigger its activation, leading to formation and release of viral particles.

brane (Figure 22-3a). The fusion event appears to involve a hydrophobic region—called the **fusogenic domain**—near the amino-terminal end of gp41 (see Figure 22-8).

Binding of gp120 to CD4 is not by itself sufficient to allow fusion by the gp41 component. When the gene for human CD4 is transfected into mouse cells, HIV will bind to the CD4 on the transfected mouse cells but fusion of the HIV envelope with the plasma membrane of the transfected cell will not occur. This finding led to speculation that another membrane molecule, present on certain human cells but missing from mouse cells, is required for HIV fusion and entry into cells.

The search for such a fusion cofactor was disappointing for several years. Recently, however, E. A. Berger and coworkers at the National Institute of Allergy and Infectious Disease discovered a membrane protein, which they called **fusin**, that has all the hallmarks of the putative cofactor. They showed that the mink or monkey cells engineered to express human CD4 on their membrane were resistant to HIV infection, even though HIV could bind to these cells. But when the mink or monkey cells were transfected with both human CD4 and fusin cDNA, HIV not only bound to the cells but it also fused with the plasma membrane, allowing the entry of viral RNA and the subsequent infection of the cell. Furthermore, the addition of anti-fusin antibodies before

exposure of the cells to HIV blocked fusion and infection (Figure 22-4). Fusin is a putative G-protein–coupled receptor with seven transmembrane segments similar to the chemokine receptors described in Chapter 13 (see Figure 13-5e).

Even before the discovery of fusin, certain chemokines were found to be potent suppressors of HIV's ability to infect cells, suggesting an intriguing tie between HIV infection and chemokines and their receptors. In view of the demonstrated requirement for fusin, it seems likely that these chemokines may suppress HIV infection by interacting with fusin, thereby blocking its activity in HIV fusion. Indeed, a recent study by R. Koup found that a small group of individuals who had repeatedly

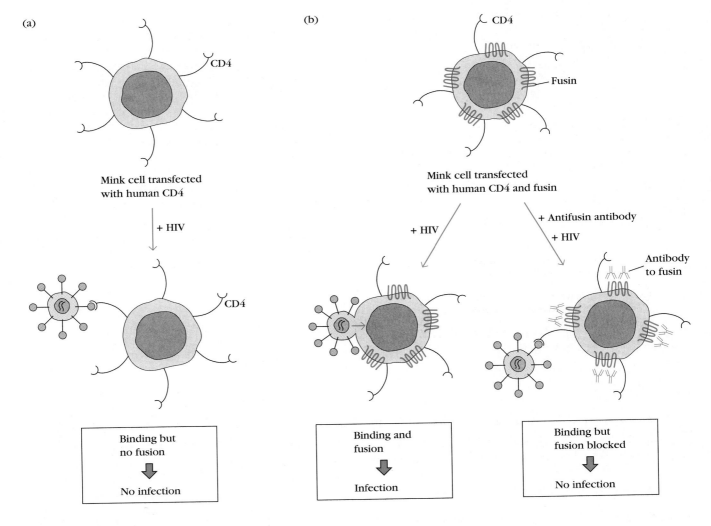

FIGURE 22-4

Experimental demonstration of requirement for fusin in fusion of HIV with host cells. Mink cells normally do not express either CD4 or fusin and thus are resistant to HIV infection. (a) Cells transfected with human CD4 bind HIV but are not infected. (b) Cells cotrans-

fected with both human CD4 and fusin become infected as both HIV binding and fusion occur. In the presence of antifusin antibody, cotransfected cells only bind HIV.

been exposed to HIV but did not become infected have higher levels of certain chemokines. Together these findings suggest that various methods of blocking fusin activity may offer new approaches for treating HIV-infected individuals.

INTEGRATION OF HIV INTO HOST GENOME

Following fusion, the HIV nucleocapsid is internalized, and the viral RNA is uncoated, establishing a productive infection (see Figure 22-3a). The HIV RNA is then transcribed into DNA by the viral reverse transcriptase enzyme. The viral DNA then integrates into the host-cell genome, forming a provirus. This process is mediated by a viral enzyme called **integrase**, which is in the nucleocapsid. Once integrated, the viral DNA is permanently associated with the host-cell DNA and is passed on to daughter cells as the cell divides. As long as the provirus remains in the latent state, the viral genes are not expressed, and therefore the virus is able to remain hidden from the host immune system.

ACTIVATION OF HIV PROVIRUS

The HIV provirus remains in the latent state within a virus-infected cell until it is activated by various factors, as discussed later. Proviral activation initiates transcription of the structural genes into mRNA, which is then translated into viral proteins, and synthesis of ssRNA (Figure 22-3b). As the viral proteins begin to assemble within the host cell, the host-cell plasma membrane is modified by insertion of gp41 and associated gp120. The viral ssRNA and core proteins assemble beneath the modified membrane, acquiring the modified host-plasma membrane as its envelope during a process called **budding**.

In some cases activation of the HIV provirus and budding of newly assembled viral particles lead to lysis of an infected cell, whereas in other cases an infected cell may survive these events. Infected T cells tend to produce massive amounts of HIV by budding, and the process generally leads to lysis of the T cell. On the other hand, macrophages tend to have lower levels of HIV budding and consequently the infected macrophage survives, continually producing low levels of the virus.

Transmission of HIV

It is now known that HIV not only binds to but also can infect a rather wide variety of cell types (Table 22-2). HIV can exist as a provirus and replicate in any of these cells; however, as indicated in the previous section, cells that express only low levels of CD4 tend to survive HIV infection. What this means is that other cells, notably macrophages and dendritic cells, can harbor the virus, protecting it from the immune system and serving as a reservoir from which the virus can be transmitted throughout the body or from one individual to another. Examination of lymph nodes from AIDS patients, for example, has shown that most of the HIV particles are in or near dendritic cells, not in T cells, suggesting that dendritic cells are a major site of HIV replication. The ability of HIV to infect microglial cells, which are macrophage-like cells located in the central nervous system, may lead to some of the neurologic manifestations in AIDS.

Normally the HIV level is quite low in semen and vaginal fluid, and the level of free virus is lower still in

TABLE 22-2

CELL TYPES THAT CAN BE INFECTED BY HIV

HEMATOPOIETIC/IMMUNE CELLS	BRAIN/GLIAL CELLS	OTHERS
T lymphocytes	Astrocytes and oligodentrocytes	Fibroblasts
B lymphocytes	Microglia	Sperm
Primary monocytes/macrophages	Glial cell lines	Liver sinusoid epithelium
Kuppfer cells (liver macrophages)	Fetal neural cells	Bowel epithelium
Monocyte cell lines	Brain capillary endothelium	Colon carcinoma cells
Bone marrow precursor cells		Osteosarcoma cells
Dendritic cells		Rhabdomyosarcoma cells
Langerhans cells		Fetal chorionic villi
		Rabbit macrophages

other body fluids, such as urine, saliva, breast milk, and tears. The major transmission routes are by sexual intercourse, transfusion of blood or blood products, IV drug use involving shared needles, and transplacental transfer from an infected mother to the fetus; each of these routes is likely to involve cell-associated virus. These findings and the results of other studies strongly suggest that the most important mode of HIV transmission from an infected to an uninfected individual is HIV-infected cells, in particular macrophages, dendritic cells, and lymphocytes.

HIV Genome

The HIV genome is more complex than that of other known retroviruses. The organization of the HIV-1 genome is diagrammed in Figure 22-5a. All retroviral proviruses are flanked by repetitive sequences called **long-terminal repeats** (LTRs). The 5′ LTR contains enhancer and promoter sequences essential for proviral transcription; the 3′ LTR is required for polyadenylation of the RNA transcripts.

The HIV provirus contains three genes common to all other retroviruses: *gag*, encoding the viral core proteins; *env*, encoding the surface envelope glycoproteins; and *pol*, encoding the nonstructural proteins required for replication. Each of these genes encodes a large polyprotein precursor that is cleaved to render the final gene products (Figure 22-5b). The polyprotein encoded by *pol* is cleaved to generate three enzymes: reverse transcriptase (p64 and p51), protease (p10), and integrase (p32). The *gag* gene encodes a 53-kDa polyprotein that is cleaved by the *pol*-encoded protease to yield p24, p7, p9, and p17. The inner and outer protein layers of the nucleocapsid are composed of p24 and p17, respectively. The *env* gene encodes a l60-kDa glycosylated polyprotein that is cleaved by a host-cell protease to yield gp120 and gp41.

In addition to *gag*, *env*, and *pol*, the HIV genome contains six additional genes: virion infectivity factor (*vif*), viral protein R (*vpr*), transactivator (*tat*), regulator of expression of virion proteins (*rev*), negative regulatory factor (*nef*), and either viral protein U (*vpu*) found in HIV-1 or viral protein X (*vpx*) found in HIV-2. Three of these genes—*tat*, *rev*, and *nef*—encode regulatory proteins that control the expression of the structural genes *gag*, *pol*, and *env*.

As indicated in Figure 22-5a, the coding sequences of several genes overlap. Differential RNA processing of the single primary transcript and translation of the resulting mRNAs in different reading frames yield the various gene products. Both *tat* and *rev* are split genes; the exons are spliced together during RNA processing, and depending on the reading frame during translation, either Tat or Rev is synthesized.

Factors That Promote Activation of HIV Provirus

Transcription of HIV proviral DNA into ssRNA and mRNA is catalyzed by RNA polymerase, which initially binds to the promoter in the 5′ LTR. The HIV promoter is relatively weak and has a low affinity for RNA polymerase. For this reason, once RNA polymerase has bound to the HIV promoter and begins to transcribe the proviral DNA, it tends to dissociate and thus generates only short, truncated RNA transcripts (Figure 22-6a). Synthesis of full-length HIV-1 transcripts can occur only after the weak promoter is converted into a strong, fully active promoter. Thus, activation of the HIV provirus and its progression from latency to the lytic state depends on this change in promoter activity.

Binding of the HIV regulatory protein Tat to the emerging RNA transcript mediates conversion of the weak HIV promoter into a strong one. Tat activates proviral expression by interacting with a short sequence of RNA located at the 5′ end of all transcripts just downstream of the start site (Figure 22-6b). The RNA sequence, known as the TAR element (for transacting responsive), forms a 59-nucleotide RNA stem-loop structure. The binding of Tat to this RNA stem-loop structure both increases the initiation of transcription and stabilizes the RNA polymerase complex as it moves along the proviral DNA, so that RNA transcription does not terminate prematurely. Thus, in the presence of Tat, transcription of the proviral genome increases by several thousandfold.

In addition, certain host-cell transcription factors, such as NF-kB, can bind to the HIV promoter, converting it from a weak to a strong promoter (Figure 22-6c). Interaction of T cells with antigen-presenting cells induces various transcription factors, including NF-κB, which promotes transcription of the gene encoding interleukin 2 (see Figure 12-12). Thus, antigen activation of an HIV-infected T cell leads to an increase in NF-κB, which then stimulates expression of the HIV proteins as well as host-cell encoded IL-2 and IL-2 receptors. Several viruses have been shown to enhance transcription of HIV proviral DNA, thus accelerating the progression of AIDS. These viruses include HTLV-1, cytomegalovirus, herpes simplex virus, Epstein-Barr virus, adenovirus, papovaviruses, and hepatitis B virus. Many of these viruses can infect an HIV-infected cell and induce production of transcription factors (e.g., NF-κB) that bind to the proviral promoter, converting it from a weak to an active promoter. These findings explain why many HIV-infected intravenous drug users progress to full-blown AIDS much more rapidly than HIV-infected individuals who do not use IV drugs. If an infected drug user continues to use IV drugs, antigens

(a)

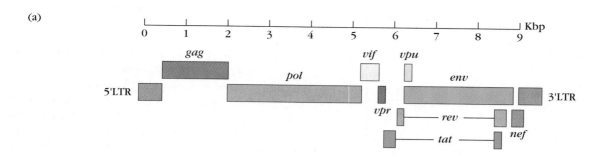

(b)

Gene	Protein product	Function of encoded proteins
gag	53-kDa precursor	*Nucleocapsid proteins*
	↓	
	p17	Forms outer core-protein layer
	p24	Forms inner core-protein layer
	p9	Is component of nucleoid core
	p7	Binds directly to genomic RNA
env	160-kDa precursor	*Envelope glycoproteins*
	↓	
	gp41	Is transmembrane protein associated with gp 120 and required for fusion
	gp120	Protrudes from envelope and binds CD4
pol	Precursor	*Enzymes*
	↓	
	p64	Has reverse transcriptase and RNase activity
	p51	Has reverse transcriptase activity
	p10	Is protease that cleaves *gag* precursor
	p32	Is integrase
vif	p23	Promotes infectivity of viral particle
vpr	p15	Weakly activates transcription of proviral DNA
tat	p14	Strongly activates transcription of proviral DNA
rev	p19	Allows export of unspliced and singly spliced mRNAs from nucleus
nef	p27	Increases viral replication; down-regulates host-cell CD4
vpu	p16	Is required for efficient viral assembly and budding

FIGURE 22-5

Genetic organization of HIV-1 (a) and functions of encoded proteins (b). The three major genes—*gag, pol,* and *env*—encode polyprotein precursors that are cleaved to yield the nucleocapsid core proteins, enzymes required for replication, and envelope core proteins. Of the remaining six genes, three (*tat, rev,* and *nef*) encode regulatory proteins that play a major role in controlling expression; two (*vif* and *vpu*) encode proteins required for virion maturation; and one (*vpr*) encodes a weak transcriptional activator. The 5′ long terminal repeat (LTR) contains sequences to which various regulatory proteins bind. The organization of the HIV-2 genome is very similar, except the *vpu* gene is replaced by *vpx* in HIV-2.

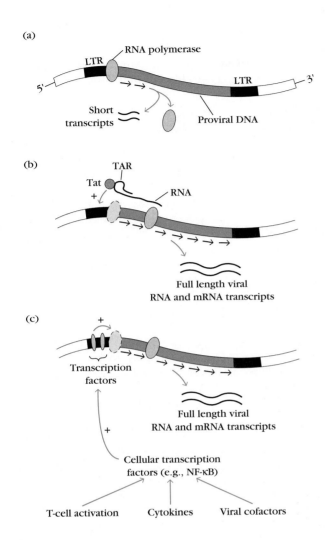

FIGURE 22-6

Factors that mediate activation of HIV provirus. (a) In the absence of activation, the HIV promoter binds RNA polymerase weakly. As a result, the enzyme dissociates before the entire proviral genome is transcribed, thus maintaining the latent state. (b) Conversion of the promoter to one that binds RNA polymerase strongly can be mediated by the HIV regulatory protein Tat, which binds to the TAR element in the nascent RNA transcript. (c) Promoter conversion is also induced by binding of certain transcription factors whose production is stimulated by antigen activation of HIV-infected T cells or by infection with other viruses. Promoter conversion leads to production of full-length viral transcripts and initiates the lytic cycle.

introduced into the bloodstream may cause T-cell activation and consequently transcription of HIV proviral DNA. In addition, IV drug users are often coinfected with other viruses such as hepatitis B virus or cytomegalovirus, which would have a similar effect.

Expression of HIV Proviral DNA

Transcription of HIV proviral DNA yields a single primary RNA transcript that is spliced in alternative ways to yield three sizes of mRNAs: a 9-kb unspliced mRNA; 4-kb single-spliced mRNAs, formed by removal of one intron; and 2-kb double-spliced mRNAs, formed by removal of two or more introns. All these mRNAs are exported from the nucleus to the cytoplasm where they are translated into viral proteins, which are assembled together with some of the full-length unspliced RNA to form new viral particles. However, only the 2-kb mRNAs, which encode the Tat, Nef, and Rev regulatory proteins, can be directly transported from the nucleus to the cytoplasm. Translocation of the unspliced and the single-spliced mRNAs requires the Rev protein, which binds to a region on the longer mRNAs, called the Rev response element (RRE), thereby facilitating their export from the nucleus.

Because of the difference in the exportability of HIV mRNAs, production of HIV proteins following activation occurs in two stages (Figure 22-7). The first viral proteins to appear are the regulatory proteins: Tat, Rev, and Nef. As long as Rev levels are low, only the 2-kb double-spliced mRNAs can be exported from the nucleus and translated into proteins. Later, as the level of Rev increases, it facilitates export of the full-length unspliced RNA and the 4-kb single-spliced mRNAs, which encode the structural proteins and the enzymes of the *gag, env,* and *pol* genes.

Genetic Variation in HIV

HIV is capable of tremendous genetic variation, with mutations in the viral genome occurring at rates millions of times faster than those observed in human DNA. The influenza virus causing the common flu also has a high mutation rate, which has hampered development of an effective flu vaccine. Yet the rate of mutation in HIV is 65 times that observed for influenza! Sequencing studies reveal that no two AIDS patients carry the identical virus; furthermore, HIV isolates taken from the same individual at different times also can differ substantially. The DNA sequence diversity seen in HIV is generated by its reverse transcriptase enzyme, which has been shown to be extremely error-prone and thus gives rise to numerous base substitutions, additions, and deletions. An estimated 5–10 errors are introduced into the HIV genome during each round of replication. As discussed in a later section, these changes make development of an HIV vaccine extremely difficult, because antibodies or cell-mediated immunity directed against one isolate may not recognize another isolate.

(a) Early HIV-1 gene expression

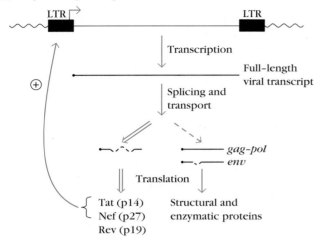

(b) Late HIV-1 gene expression

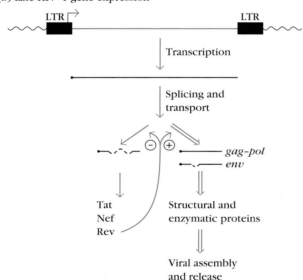

FIGURE 22-7

Stages in the expression of HIV-1 proviral DNA. (a) Early in expression the predominant products formed are the HIV regulatory proteins, including Tat, Rev, and Nef, which are encoded by 2-kb mRNAs. Tat and Nef act on the 5′ LTR to regulate HIV transcription. (b) Later, the increased level of Rev promotes transport of longer mRNAs, and there is a shift from production of regulatory proteins to production of the structural and enzymatic proteins encoded by *gag, env,* and *pol.* [Adapted from W. C. Greene, 1991, *New Engl. J. Med.* **324**:308.]

The genetic variation in HIV has led to generation of distinct strains exhibiting different biological activities in HIV isolates from different parts of the world. Some strains preferentially infect macrophages; other strains show a preference for T cells. A recent study of strains isolated from individuals in Thailand revealed that some strains were more likely to pass through mucous membranes and to be transmitted sexually, whereas other strains were unable to pass through mucous membranes and were more likely to be transmitted by IV drugs.

ROLE OF IMMUNE RESPONSE IN EMERGENCE OF HIV VARIANTS

The emergence of distinct HIV isolates in infected individuals results partly from immune-system selection of HIV variants. After an individual is infected with HIV, specific neutralizing antibodies are made to viral protein or glycoprotein components. These antibodies bind to HIV and have been shown to block its ability to infect T cells in vitro. However, when HIV is grown in T-cell lines in the presence of human serum containing neutralizing antibody, a viral population resistant to the neutralizing antibody emerges after 4–5 weeks in culture. What this means is that although an individual may initially produce antibody that can inactivate HIV, the high mutation rate, coupled with the high rate of viral replication, enables some viral progeny to become resistant to the effects of the antibody. These resistant viruses survive, replicate, and continue to infect additional cells, so that eventually a population of resistant viral particles emerges.

Comparison of HIV isolates obtained from a single individual at various times illustrates how HIV can change over time. In one study, HIV isolates obtained from peripheral-blood lymphocytes of an infected individual on two different occasions separated by 16 months showed an average of 13% variation in their DNA sequences. Such variation would be likely to change the viral isolates' biological activity. Indeed, J. Levy has shown that early in HIV infection the HIV isolates replicate slowly, infect macrophages preferentially, and do not induce syncytia. Later in HIV infection the isolates replicate rapidly, infect T cells, and induce syncytia.

VARIATION IN THE ENVELOPE GLYCOPROTEINS

The external presentation of gp120 and gp41 on the envelope of HIV makes these two glycoproteins potential targets for antibody-mediated neutralization of viral infectivity. For this reason considerable research has focused on the structure and antigenicity of these two envelope glycoproteins. Both gp120 and gp41 are derived from a common glycosylated precursor protein (gp160), which is synthesized in the rough endoplasmic reticulum of the infected cell. The precursor is cleaved, generating a carboxyl-terminal fragment (gp41), which spans the membrane, and a larger amino-terminal fragment (gp120), which remains noncovalently associated with gp41 on the membrane (see Figure 22-2a).

Of all the HIV proteins, gp120 shows the most sequence variation, with gp41 ranking second. When the gp120 and gp41 sequences of different isolates were compared, some regions were found to be constant and other regions were found to be hypervariable (Figure 22-8). The constant regions are thought to be conserved to preserve essential viral functions. For example, both the CD4-binding site in gp120 and the fusogenic domain in gp41 are conserved regions.

A number of research groups have focused on producing neutralizing antibodies to accessible, conserved regions of gp120 or gp41. Antibodies to the conserved

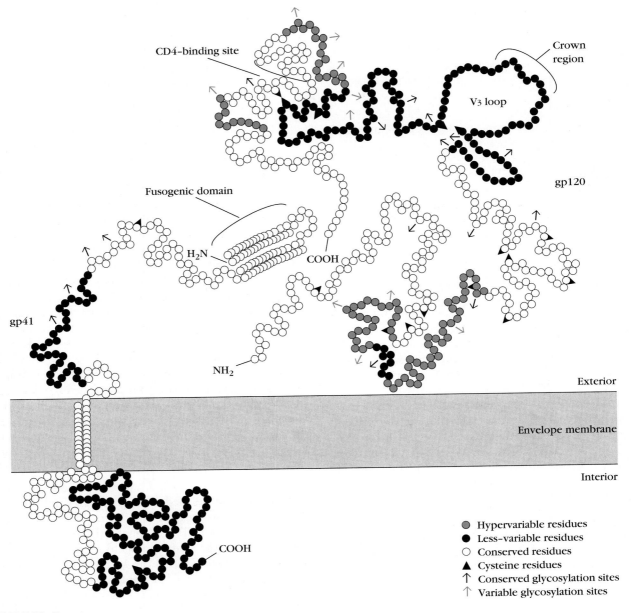

FIGURE 22-8

Schematic diagram of HIV-1 envelope glycoproteins showing hypervariable amino acid residues, less-variable residues, and conserved residues (see key). Because neutralizing antibodies are produced predominantly to an epitope in the hypervariable V3 loop of gp120, anti-HIV antibodies generally are strain specific. The crown region, however, is considerably less variable than the remainder of the V3 loop (see Figure 22-9). Note that the CD4-binding site on gp120 and the fusogenic domain in gp41, both of which mediate essential viral functions, have conserved amino acid sequences. [Adapted from R. C. Gallo, 1988, *J. Acquired Immune Deficiency Syndromes* **1**:521.]

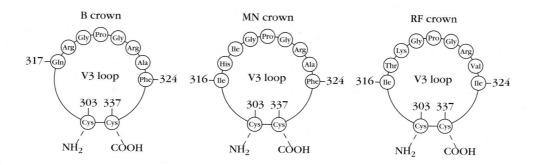

FIGURE 22-9

Amino acid sequences of three crown regions—designated B, MN, and RF—in the V3 loop of gp120 from HIV-1. Although the entire V3 loop exhibits extensive variation, the crown region exhibits much less (see Figure 22-8). Thus HIV isolates can be grouped into a small number of classes based on their crown sequence. The numbers refer to residue positions in the overall gp120 sequence.

region of gp120 that is the putative CD4-binding site have been shown to block binding of soluble gp120 to CD4. Unfortunately, these antibodies are not effective at blocking HIV infection. This may be because there are so many gp120-CD4 interactions at the interface of the virus and cell that they act cooperatively, increasing the likelihood of HIV binding to the target cell and rendering the neutralizing antibody ineffective. Antibodies to this conserved region on gp120 are present in HIV-infected individuals, but the titer is low.

Another conserved region that appears promising as a potential target for neutralizing antibody is a subregion within the third hypervariable region of gp120 known as the **V3 loop**, which spans residues 307 to 330 (see Figure 22-8). This region extends as a loop formed by two disulfide-linked cysteine residues at position 303 and 337. The two cysteines are highly conserved and are present in all HIV-1 isolates studied to date. Antibodies to the V3 loop have been shown to be quite effective at neutralizing viral infectivity. Unfortunately, the sequence of the V3 loop—the most variable region in gp120— differs by as much as 50% between HIV-1 isolates. Thus most neutralizing antibodies to the V3 loop are strain specific.

There is, however, a small subregion within the V3 loop that is largely conserved. This subregion, which was identified by sequencing the V3 loop of over 200 HIV isolates, is located at the crown of the loop and consequently called the **crown region**. HIV isolates can be grouped into a small number of classes based on the crown sequence. For example, 30% of HIV isolates in North America have a crown sequence designated MN (Figure 22-9). Antibodies to the MN crown sequence of the V3 loop have been shown to block infectivity of all MN viral isolates. There is a great deal of interest in producing antibodies to the different crown sequences of the V3 loop as a possible vaccine approach. This approach is discussed in the section on vaccines.

DIAGNOSIS OF HIV INFECTION AND AIDS

Most HIV-infected individuals develop symptoms of AIDS between 8 and 10 years after infection, but approximately 25% of infected individuals have remained symptom-free for some 10–12 years. Whether all HIV-infected individuals eventually will develop AIDS is not known; nor is it possible to predict how quickly any given infected individual will develop symptoms. By compiling detailed information about the various serologic events associated with HIV infection, clinicians hope to develop ways to predict, with some degree of accuracy, the likelihood of progression into AIDS. The $CD4^+$ T-cell count, although widely used clinically, is only a crude predictor of progression. In order to increase the accuracy of AIDS progression, several other serologic events are also being monitored.

Serologic Profile of HIV Infection

Following HIV infection a sequence of serologic events occurs that can be used to diagnose HIV infection and to predict the progression from latency to lytic infection, culminating in an AIDS diagnosis (Figure 22-10). Soon after infection, the virus appears to replicate actively and the viral core protein p24 can be detected in the serum by ELISA or RIA. The p24 antigen is detectable in the serum for only a few weeks following infection and then disappears as the antibody response (**seroconversion**) develops. In most cases the time between infection and seroconversion is 6 weeks, but in some individuals the lag period has lasted for more than 3 years.

At seroconversion IgM antibody to HIV antigens can be detected; within a few weeks of seroconversion these IgM antibodies decline and anti-HIV IgG antibodies

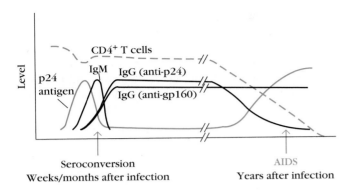

FIGURE 22-10

Serologic profile of HIV infection. Soon after infection, the HIV core protein p24 is detectable in the serum. HIV infection is most commonly detected by the presence of anti-HIV antibodies following seroconversion, which occurs at a variable interval after actual infection. Clinical symptoms indicative of AIDS, including very low T-cell counts generally do not appear for at least 8 years following infection, but this interval is also variable.

appear. The IgG antibodies are specific for many of the HIV structural proteins (e.g., gp160, gp120, gp41, p24, and p17). The appearance of antibody to the p24 core protein correlates with viral latency. As long as the antibody to p24 remains high, an individual remains asymptomatic. When the antibody to p24 begins to decline, there is a corresponding increase in the p24 antigen in the serum. This decline in antibody to p24 and increase in p24 antigen are associated with the progression of HIV from latency to lytic infection and have been used clinically to predict the onset of overt disease.

Progression from latent HIV infection to AIDS can be predicted more reliably by use of $CD4^+$ T-cell counts and p24 levels than by T-cell counts alone. For example, of HIV-infected individuals who have $CD4^+$ T-cell counts greater than $400/\mu l$ and also are positive for p24, about 45% will progress to AIDS within 3 years. However, of infected individuals who are p24 positive and have $CD4^+$ T-cell counts less than $400/\mu l$, 80% will progress to AIDS within 3 years.

Screening Tests for HIV Infection

The standard screening test for HIV infection is an indirect ELISA for serum antibody to HIV in which viral antigens are absorbed onto a solid phase (see Figure 6-14). The patient's serum is added, unbound antibody is washed away, and then an enzyme-conjugated goat antihuman immunoglobulin reagent is added. After excess reagent is washed away, the substrate for the enzyme is added. A colored reaction product indicates that the

patient has antibody to the HIV antigens and must therefore have been exposed to the virus.

There is a lag period between the time of HIV infection and the appearance of enough antibody to be detected in the ELISA assay. Because of the lag period, potentially infectious individuals may screen negative for HIV infection. The importance of the lag period between HIV infection and seroconversion was demonstrated in 1991 by a news report of the transmission of HIV from an infected organ donor to a number of transplant recipients. In this case, the organ donor had been infected with HIV but had not yet seroconverted. Thus when an ELISA test was performed prior to organ transplantation, the donor screened negative for HIV infection. The lag period, often referred to as a "window of opportunity," is a time when an HIV-infected individual will screen negative using an ELISA test for HIV-specific antibody. Also, AIDS patients often test negative for antibody in the late stages of the disease, when serum antibody levels drop as a result of depleted levels of T_H cells.

More sensitive and expensive tests, such as the Western blot and the polymerase chain reaction (PCR), are used to confirm HIV infection or to detect low-level infection. In a Western-blot assay, HIV proteins and glycoproteins are separated by electrophoresis and then transferred to a nitrocellulose membrane. The patient's serum is added to the nitrocellulose and allowed to react, and then a radiolabeled goat antihuman immunoglobulin reagent is added (see Figure 6-15). The presence of radioactive bands corresponding to the molecular weight of HIV antigens indicates the presence in the patient of antibody to HIV.

In 1987 the CDC recommended that a positive HIV ELISA test should be confirmed by another ELISA and then by a positive Western blot. The polymerase chain reaction can be used to amplify a small number of HIV proviral DNA copies in infected cells isolated from a large amount of cellular DNA (see Figure 2-7). The PCR technique has made it possible to demonstrate HIV infection in a number of individuals who had tested negative by the ELISA and Western-blot assays.

Clinical Diagnosis of AIDS

The disease manifestations initially recognized by the CDC as being indicative of AIDS were limited to a few opportunistic infections or Kaposi's sarcoma. It soon became apparent, however, that a much broader range of indicator diseases should be included in the diagnosis of AIDS. In an effort to reflect the diversity of disease symptoms in AIDS, the CDC has classified the indicator diseases into various categories. The CDC classification was initially published in 1986 and was revised in 1993 (Table 22-3). The revised classification consists of three clinical categories (A, B, and C), each of which is subdivided into three ranges of CD4$^+$ T-cell counts (>500/μl, 200–499/μl, and <200/μl).

Category A includes three general presentations of HIV infection. Initial HIV infection sometimes causes an acute mononucleosis-like illness, which is generally followed by an asymptomatic latency period. Often, however, individuals manifest no apparent symptoms at all upon initial HIV infection and pass without any indications into an asymptomatic latency period. Finally, a significant number of individuals infected with HIV have a persistent generalized lymphadenopathy, characterized by enlargement of multiple lymph nodes, but no concurrent illness. In all three cases, the individual is infected with HIV and is usually antibody positive in an ELISA or Western-blot test but is not diagnosed as having AIDS unless the CD4$^+$ T-cell count drops below 200/μl.

Category B includes various symptomatic conditions attributable to HIV infection that are not included in category C. These conditions develop due to diminished cell-mediated immunity and require clinical management that is complicated by HIV infection. Individuals manifesting any category B symptom and having a CD4$^+$ T-cell count below 200/μl are diagnosed as having AIDS. Category C includes the greatest number and most serious of the AIDS indicator conditions, including invasive cervical cancer, Kaposi's sarcoma, *Pneumocystis carinii* pneumonia, infections with various *Mycobacterium* species, and toxoplasmosis of the brain. HIV-infected individuals who manifest any category C symptom are diagnosed as having AIDS regardless of their CD4$^+$ T-cell count (see Table 22-3).

DESTRUCTION OF CD4$^+$ T CELLS

One of the early observations of immune-system impairment in HIV infection was a reduction in the number of CD4$^+$ T cells. Uninfected individuals have approximately 1100 CD4$^+$ T cells/μl of whole blood; in AIDS patients the numbers drop dramatically, often reaching levels below 200/μl. Normally the ratio of CD4$^+$ to CD8$^+$ T cells in the peripheral blood is about 2:0, but in AIDS patients the ratio is reversed, becoming less than 1:0 and sometimes reaching values below 0:2. When lymphocytes are stained with fluorescent anti-CD4 monoclonal antibody and passed through a fluorescence-activated cell sorter, the CD4$^+$ T cells appear as a distinct peak; in AIDS patients this peak is markedly reduced.

The number of CD4$^+$ cells in the peripheral blood has been shown to vary among clinical subgroups of AIDS patients (Figure 22-11). Although there is considerable variation in the counts among individuals in each group, the average count for the control group differs significantly from those of all the HIV-infected groups exhibiting symptoms. Once the CD4$^+$ T-cell count falls below 200/μl, an individual is quite susceptible to opportunistic infections and neoplasms. About 40% of AIDS patients manifesting opportunistic infections have no detectable CD4$^+$ T cells at all. The very low number or complete absence of CD4$^+$ T cells in these patients probably explains their susceptibility to opportunistic infections, and the finding that such patients have the shortest life expectancy of all AIDS patients.

After individuals are infected with HIV, their CD4$^+$ T-cell count drops very gradually over the first 8–10 years and then begins to drop very quickly in most cases (see Figure 22-10). Because there is little change in the CD4$^+$ T-cell numbers over these 8–10 years, it was assumed that there was little viral destruction of these T cells. This assumption has been undermined by recent studies that found CD4$^+$ T cells are indeed destroyed in large numbers before AIDS symptoms appear, but this destruction is coupled with a high rate of T-cell production. During this period, an estimated two billion (2 × 10^9) CD4$^+$ T cells are killed every day, and the immune system responds to this enormous cell destruction by producing about 2 × 10^9 new CD4$^+$ T cells every day!

The other interesting observation in these studies was that CD4$^+$ T-cell counts increased considerably when viral replication was inhibited with a protease inhibitor or a reverse transcriptase inhibitor. This increase was observed even in patients with very low T-cell counts. This finding suggests that it might be possible to restore T-cell counts in AIDS patients if viral replication could be halted. The problem, however, is how to effectively halt viral replication over an extended period. Because of the extreme genetic variation of the virus, drug-resistant strains begin to emerge within 2–4 weeks of antiviral drug treatment.

Depletion of HIV-Infected CD4$^+$ T Cells

As explained previously, as long as the HIV provirus in an infected CD4$^+$ T cell remains in the latent state, no damage to the cell is evident. However, once the provirus is activated and new HIV virions begin to assemble and bud from the infected cell, extensive damage to the cell membrane can occur, leading to death of the cell (Figure

TABLE 22-3

CLINICAL DIAGNOSIS OF HIV-INFECTED INDIVIDUALS

CD4+ T-CELL COUNT	CLINICAL CATEGORIES *		
	(A)	(B)	(C)
(1) ≥500/μl	A1	B1	**C1**
(2) 200–499/μl	A2	B2	**C2**
(3) <200/μl	**A3**	**B3**	**C3**

CLASSIFICATION OF AIDS INDICATOR DISEASES[†]

CATEGORY A

Asymptomatic: no symptoms at the time of HIV infection

Acute infection: glandular fever-like illness lasting a few weeks at the time of infection

Persistent generalized lymphadenopathy (PGL): lymph node enlargement persisting for 3 or more months with no evidence of infection

CATEGORY B

Bacillary angiomatosis

Candidiasis, oropharyngeal (thrush)

Candidiasis, vulvovaginal: persistent, frequent, or poorly responsive to therapy

Cervical dysplasia (moderate or severe)/cervical carcinoma in situ

Constitutional symptoms such as fever or diarrhea lasting ≥ 1 month

Hairy leukoplakia, oral

Herpes zoster (shingles) involving at least two distinct episodes or more than one dermatome

Idiopathic thrombocytopenic purpura

Listeriosis

Pelvic inflammatory disease, particularly by tubo-ovarian abscess

Peripheral neuropathy

CATEGORY C

Candidiasis of bronchi, tracheae, or lungs

Candidiasis, esophageal

Cervical cancer (invasive)

Coccidioidomycosis, disseminated or extrapulmonary

Cryptococcosis, extrapulmonary

Cryptosporidiosis, chronic intestinal (> 1 month's duration)

Cytomegalovirus disease (other than liver, spleen, or nodes)

Cytomegalovirus retinitis (with loss of vision)

Encephalopathy, HIV–related

Herpes simplex: chronic ulcer(s) (> 1 month's duration) or bronchitis, pneumonitis, or esophagitis

Histoplasmosis, disseminated or extrapulmonary

Isosporiasis, chronic intestinal (>1 month's duration)

Kaposi's sarcoma

Lymphoma, Burkitt's

Lymphoma, immunoblastic

Mycobacterium avium complex or *M. Kansasii*, disseminated or extrapulmonary

Mycobacterium, other species, disseminated or extrapulmonary

Pneumocystis carinii pneumonia

Progressive multifocal leukoencephalopathy

Salmonella septicemia (recurrent)

Taxoplasmosis of brain

Wasting syndrome due to HIV

---

* Categories in boldface are now reported as AIDS. For category A diagnosis, no condition in categories B or C can be present. For category B diagnosis, no condition in category C can be present.

[†] 1993 revision.

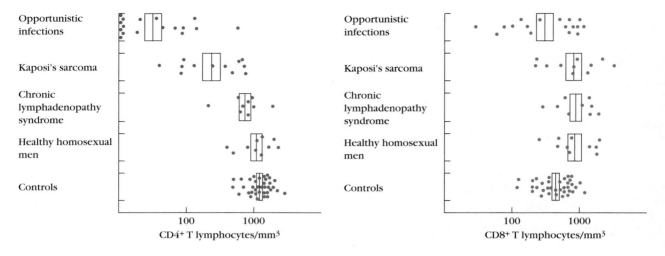

FIGURE 22-11

Quantitation of CD4$^+$ and CD8$^+$ T lymphocytes in normal controls and in clinical subpopulations of AIDS patients. There is a clear correlation between the severity of AIDS symptoms and CD4$^+$ T-cell counts. [From H. C. Lane and A. S. Fauci, 1985, *Annu. Rev. Immunol.* **3**:477.]

22-12). In addition, the humoral or cell-mediated response generated against HIV may lead to destruction of HIV-infected CD4$^+$ T cells. Those infected CD4$^+$ T cells expressing gp120 and gp41 on their membrane can be killed by antibody-plus-complement lysis; those that express viral peptides associated with class I MHC molecules can be killed by a CTL response against the altered self-cells. Both processes represent a normal immune response against a virus, a process that should serve to eliminate virus-infected cells and thus prevent further spread of the virus. The irony in the case of HIV is that the immune response to eliminate the virus kills off the central cells of the immune system itself.

The actual number of HIV-infected CD4$^+$ T cells present in both asymptomatic and symptomatic AIDS patients is somewhat controversial. Analyses of peripheral blood from infected but asymptomatic individuals indicate that only 0.01%–1.0% of CD4$^+$ cells is infected. As AIDS progresses, the proportion of infected CD4$^+$ T cells increases, reaching levels of 1% or greater. Recent evidence, however, suggests that the level of HIV infection in circulating CD4$^+$ cells may be substantially less than that in noncirculating T cells. For example, analyses of lymph node biopsies from HIV-infected individuals reveal that lymph node tissue contains 10–100 times as many HIV particles as do circulating CD4$^+$ T cells. Because antigen-activated T cells loose their homing receptors and cease circulating, such activated T cells are preferentially located in peripheral lymphoid tissue. Furthermore, as noted earlier, antigen activation of HIV-infected T cells stimulates the lytic cycle. For these reasons, the higher levels of HIV infection in lymph node T cells compared with recirculating T cells is not surprising.

The relatively small proportion of HIV-infected CD4$^+$ T cells observed in AIDS patients cannot account for the dramatic decline in T-cell counts that is a hallmark of this disease. As noted earlier, this decline often reaches levels of 90%. Thus the decline in CD4$^+$ T-cell numbers and function cannot result entirely from HIV-mediated damage to infected cells.

Depletion of Uninfected CD4$^+$ T Cells

In asymptomatic HIV-infected individuals, CD4$^+$ T cells begin to lose their capacity to respond to foreign antigen long before their numbers plummet. Various mechanisms other than direct virus-mediated damage have been proposed to account for the decline of CD4$^+$ T-cell function and the dramatic depletion of CD4$^+$ T cells seen in AIDS patients. Several of the proposed mechanisms involve soluble gp120. Because the noncovalent interaction of gp120 and gp41 is unstable, large quantities of free gp120 are shed into the surrounding fluid. The soluble gp120 present in the blood and lymph of HIV-infected individuals might mediate a decrease in the function and numbers of uninfected CD4$^+$ T cells in several ways.

DESTRUCTION MEDIATED BY ANTI-gp120 ANTIBODY

Because soluble gp120 has high affinity for CD4$^+$, it can bind to CD4 molecules on normal, uninfected

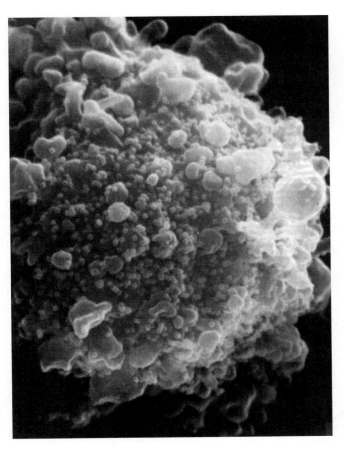

FIGURE 22-12

Once the HIV provirus is activated, buds representing newly formed viral particles can be observed on the surface of an infected T cell. The extensive cell damage resulting from budding and release of virions leads to death of infected cells. [Courtesy of R. C. Gallo, 1988, *J. Acquired Immune Deficiency Syndromes* **1**:521.]

CD4$^+$ T cells. Subsequent binding of anti–gp120 antibody may lead to destruction of these T cells by antibody-plus-complement lysis or by antibody-dependent cell-mediated cytotoxicity (ADCC), as illustrated in Figure 22-13. These mechanisms might be expected to cause destruction of the numerous other cell types expressing CD4 (see Table 22-2); yet these cell types are not extensively depleted in AIDS patients. However, T$_H$ cells express a much higher density of CD4 molecules than do macrophages and other CD4-bearing cells. For this reason, T$_H$ cells would be able to bind considerable soluble gp120, making them sensitive to antibody-plus-complement lysis and ADCC. Other cells that express low levels of CD4 probably cannot bind enough soluble gp120 to make them sensitive to these mechanisms of destruction.

gp120-INDUCED DISRUPTION OF T-CELL ACTIVATION

The binding of soluble gp120 to CD4 on uninfected cells may also block interaction of CD4 with class II MHC molecules on antigen-presenting cells, thereby preventing transduction of part of the activating signal (see Figure 22-13). This inhibition of T-cell activation would reduce the functional activity of T$_H$ cells. Alternatively, binding of soluble gp120 to CD4 may generate an inappropriate signal leading to programmed cell death, or apoptosis. As discussed in Chapter 12, in normal T-cell activation, the T-cell receptor first transmits a signal after recognizing an antigenic peptide–class II MHC complex on an antigen-presenting cell; then the CD4 molecule on the T cell binds to the class II MHC molecule and transmits a subsequent signal. Together these signals constitute activating signal 1 (Figure 22-14a).

The order in which the two components of activating signal 1 occur appears to be crucial. For example, T cells undergo programmed cell death when they are first incubated with anti-CD4 antibody, which stimulates the second half of signal 1, and then are exposed to antigen presented by antigen-presenting cells, which normally stimulates the first half of signal 1 (Figure 22-14b).

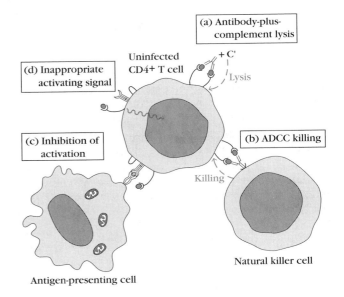

FIGURE 22-13

Four possible mechanisms by which soluble gp120 (blue) may induce depletion of uninfected CD4$^+$ T cells. Mechanisms (a) and (b) involve interaction of anti-gp120 antibodies with soluble gp120 bound to CD4 on uninfected T cells. Mechanisms (c) and (d) involve disruption of normal T-cell activation. See text for discussion. C′ = complement.

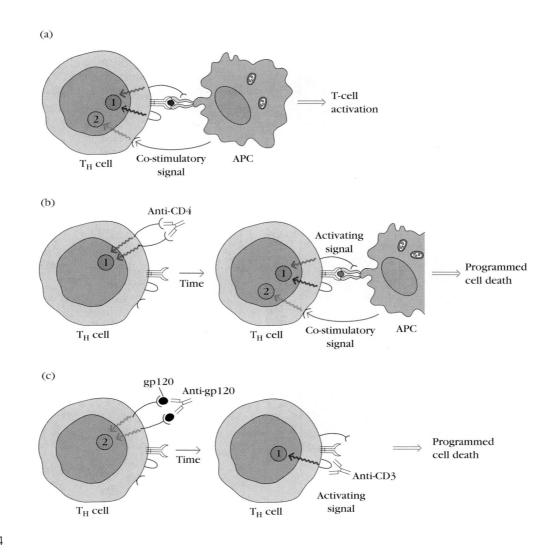

FIGURE 22-14

Experimental demonstration that inappropriate signal can prime T$_H$ cells for programmed cell death. (a) T-cell activation requires activating signal 1 (red and pink) generated by antigen recognition and a co-stimulatory signal 2 (purple). Signal 1 has two components: the TCR component (red) is transmitted when a T-cell receptor and associated CD3 molecule recognize a peptide–class II MHC complex; the CD4 component (pink) is transmitted when CD4 on the T cell interacts with the class II molecule. For normal T-cell activation, the TCR-mediated signal must occur before the CD4-mediated signal. (b, c) When normal T$_H$ cells are treated experimentally so as to induce the CD4 component of signal 1 and are then exposed to antigen or anti-CD3 to induce the TCR-mediated component, the cells undergo programmed cell death (apoptosis).

Similar results are obtained when normal CD4$^+$ T cells are first incubated with gp120 and anti–gp120, and subsequently exposed to anti–CD3, which normally can generate the first half of signal 1 (Figure 22-14c). Based on these findings, some have proposed that binding of gp120 to CD4 on uninfected T cells in AIDS patients primes these cells for programmed cell death when they are later activated by antigen. This hypothesis predicts that the rate of CD4$^+$ T-cell depletion depends on the level of T-cell activation.

gp120-STIMULATED SYNCYTIA FORMATION

In vitro experiments reveal that an HIV-infected CD4$^+$ T cell can form a giant multinucleated cell, called a **syncytium**, by fusing with as many as 500 uninfected CD4$^+$ T cells. These giant multinucleated cells produce large quantities of the virus for a short period of time and die within 48 h of their formation. Some evidence suggests that interaction of soluble gp120 with CD4 membrane molecules may induce cell fusion leading to syncytia formation. In one in vitro study, a recombinant vaccinia virus carrying the gp120 gene was able to cause syncytia formation and subsequent cell death in a CD4$^+$ T-cell line. Taken together, these findings suggest that the fusion of activated virus-infected CD4$^+$ T cells expressing gp120 with other, uninfected CD4$^+$ T cells may lead to the progressive depletion of CD4$^+$ T cells that is seen in AIDS patients.

INTERFERENCE WITH T-CELL MATURATION BY GP120

Depletion of T cells normally induces T-cell maturation within the thymus to restore the peripheral T-cell numbers. Some researchers have suggested that soluble gp120 in AIDS patients binds to CD4 on thymocytes, thus interfering with the positive selection of class II MHC–restricted cells that occurs during T-cell maturation (see Figure 12-5). In the experiments outlined in Figure 12-6, antibody to class II MHC molecules selectively interfered with maturation of CD4$^+$ T cells. By analogy, binding of soluble gp120 to CD4 might interfere with the maturation process. Destruction of mature CD4$^+$ T cells in the periphery, coupled with a lack of replacement by developing thymocytes, could explain the progressive CD4$^+$ T-cell depletion in AIDS patients.

IMMUNOLOGIC ABNORMALITIES IN AIDS

The total collapse of the immune system in AIDS reflects the central role of CD4$^+$ T cells in both humoral and cell-mediated responses. Not surprisingly, AIDS patients manifest a variety of immunologic abnormalities (Table 22-4). HIV infection initially leads to **viremia**, a condition in which viral particles can be readily detected in circulating lymphocytes. Shortly thereafter the virus largely disappears from the circulating lymphocytes; in most individuals, nearly a decade passes before large numbers of virus-infected cells are detected again in circulating lymphocytes. This observation initially led to the belief that following initial infection, HIV entered a long latency lasting nearly a decade. However, as mentioned previously, subsequent studies revealed that peripheral lymphoid tissue (e.g., lymph nodes, spleen, tonsils, and adenoids) exhibit active viral replication and HIV levels that are 10–100 times higher than that observed in circulating lymphocytes. Thus, although the CD4$^+$ T-cell count may remain high in the early years following infection, this count may not accurately reflect the impact of HIV on lymphocytes residing in peripheral lymphoid tissue.

Pathologic Changes in Lymph Nodes

Soon after an individual is infected with HIV, circulating antibodies are thought to form complexes with viral particles, and the virus appears to disappear from the bloodstream. Although some virions are eliminated by phagocytosis, others infect cells of the regional lymph nodes establishing a massive covert infection. The infection appears to occur as antibody-HIV complexes carried into a node are trapped by Fc receptors along the long cytoplasmic processes of follicular dendritic cells within the germinal center. Biopsies from patients with early HIV infection (those with CD4$^+$ T-cell counts $\geq 500/\mu$l) reveal millions of HIV viral particles along the long processes of the follicular dendritic cells. As CD4$^+$ T cells traffic through the lymph nodes, some probably become infected by the HIV particles associated with the follicular dendritic cells.

The peripheral lymph nodes of HIV-infected individuals undergo striking changes in structure as AIDS progresses. These changes begin with the HIV infection and subsequent death of the follicular dendritic cells; eventually the germinal center becomes involuted due to the loss of these cells. Lymph node biopsies of HIV-infected patients reveal a progression of structural changes. In patients with intermediate HIV infection (i.e., those with CD4$^+$ T-cell counts of 200–499/μl), the lymph nodes begin to show signs of disruption. Interdigitating dendritic cells are also infected and killed by HIV. Because these cells play a vital role in CD4$^+$ T-cell activation, a reduction in dendritic cell numbers may result in a corresponding reduction in T-cell activity. Finally, in patients with advanced disease (those with CD4$^+$ T-cell counts <200/μl), lymph nodes show extensive damage and tissue necrosis, with loss of follicular dendritic cells and consequently the loss of germinal centers. As the lymph node architecture is destroyed, the nodes are less able to trap HIV particles or provide a suitable environment for T-cell and B-cell activation. At this point there is a significant increase in detectable virus in the peripheral blood and a corresponding increase in manifestations of AIDS.

Reduced Antigen-Specific Responses by T$_H$ Cells

One of the earliest immunologic abnormalities associated with AIDS is the reduced ability of T cells to proliferate in vitro in response to mitogens or soluble antigens. This is illustrated by the data in Table 22-5, which compares the in vitro proliferative response to pokeweed mitogen and tetanus toxoid by T cells from AIDS patients and normal controls. The researchers conducting this study wanted to know if the decreased proliferation observed with unfractionated T cells from AIDS patients reflected reduced numbers of T cells compared with controls or some inherent defect in the T cells. They separated CD4$^+$ and CD8$^+$ T cells with a fluorescence-activated cell sorter, adjusted cell numbers so that comparable numbers of T-cells were present in the AIDS and control samples, and repeated the proliferation assays.

The results with these samples containing equal numbers of CD4$^+$ and CD8$^+$ cells showed that CD4$^+$ T cells from AIDS patients responded at near-normal levels to pokeweed mitogen. The low response to mitogen with the unfractionated cell sample reflected the smaller number of T cells in this sample compared with that of controls. On the other hand, the CD4$^+$ and the CD8$^+$ cells from AIDS patients, even when cell numbers were equalized, remained unable to respond to tetanus toxoid antigen (Table 22-5). This study demonstrates one of the earliest abnormalities seen in AIDS patients: the inability of CD4$^+$ T cells to proliferate in response to a specific antigen. The absence of antigen-specific T-cell proliferation lends support to various hypotheses suggesting that the CD4$^+$ T cells in AIDS patients may have received an inappropriate activating signal, inducing these cells to become anergic or programming the cells for death by apoptosis.

T A B L E   2 2 - 4

IMMUNOLOGIC ABNORMALITIES ASSOCIATED WITH HIV INFECTION

STAGE OF INFECTION	TYPICAL ABNORMALITIES OBSERVED
	LYMPH NODE STRUCTURE
Early	Infection and destruction of dendritic cells; some structural disruption
Late	Extensive damage and tissue necrosis; loss of folicular dendritic cells and germinal centers; inability to trap antigens or support activation of T and B cells
	T HELPER (T$_H$) CELLS
Early	Lack of in vitro proliferative response to specific antigen
Late	Marked decrease in T$_H$-cell numbers and corresponding helper activities
	ANTIBODY PRODUCTION
Early	Enhanced nonspecific IgG and IgA production but reduced IgM synthesis
Late	Lack of proliferation of HIV-specific B cells: absence of detectable anti-HIV antibodies in some patients
	CYTOKINE PRODUCTION
Early	Increased levels of some cytokines
Late	Shift in cytokine production from T$_H$1 subset to T$_H$2 subset
	DELAYED-TYPE HYPERSENSITIVITY
Early	Highly significant reduction in proliferative capacity of T$_{DTH}$ cells and reduction in skin-test reactivity
Late	Elimination of DTH response; complete absence of skin-test reactivity
	T CYTOTOXIC (T$_C$) CELLS
Early	Comparatively normal reactivity
Late	Reduction but not elimination of CTL activity due to impaired ability to generate CTLs from T$_C$ cells

Ineffective Antibody Response

Many HIV-infected individuals can produce antibodies to various HIV gene products, including envelope glycoproteins (gp160, gp41, and gp120) and core proteins (p55, p17, and p24). Unfortunately the presence of high titers of circulating antibody to HIV proteins in no way indicates protective immunity. One reason the antibody has so little effect seems to be the frequent antigenic drift in HIV. Furthermore, the decline of CD4$^+$ T$_H$ cells in AIDS patients eventually affects the functioning of B cells in the humoral response. As AIDS progresses, patients are increasingly unable, for lack of T$_H$ cells, to mount a humoral antibody response to new antigens. The decline in antibody levels as AIDS progresses can be so pronounced that some patients screen as antibody negative in the HIV ELISA test during advanced stages of the disease. Some studies have indicated that anti-HIV antibody may actually be detrimental because binding of antibody-HIV immune complexes to Fc receptors on macrophages and subsequent receptor-mediated endocytosis may lead to increased HIV infection of macrophages.

Cytokine Imbalance

Several findings suggest that an imbalance in expression of cytokines or of cytokine receptors may contribute to the pathogenesis of AIDS. Elevated levels of IL-1, IL-6, GM-CSF, OSM, TNF-α, and TNF-β have been reported in both serum and cerebrospinal fluid of AIDS patients. The higher levels of cytokines may also contribute to some of the symptoms seen in AIDS patients (Figure 22-15). For example, IL-1 is known to cause fever and may be responsible for the persistent fevers seen in AIDS patients. High levels of IL-1 have also been reported in patients with Alzheimer's disease; it is possible that some of the symptoms of dementia in AIDS patients may be due to similar effects caused by IL-1. Another cytokine, TNF, has been shown to cause weight loss and may play a role in AIDS wasting syndrome. Additionally, IL-1, IL-6, TNF-α, and OSM have been reported to induce proliferation of Kaposi's sarcoma cells. In vitro studies also suggest that elevated levels of cytokines may contribute to the progression of HIV from latency to lytic infection. For example, TNF-α, IL-6, and GM-CSF induce expression of HIV reverse transcriptase in infected monocytes, and TNF-α, TNF-β, and IL-1 induce HIV production in infected CD4$^+$ T cells.

M. Clerici and G. M. Shearer noted that as AIDS progresses IL-2 and IFN-γ levels decrease, whereas IL-4 and IL-10 levels increase (Figure 22-16). This observation suggests that the activity of the T$_H$1 subset decreases and that of the T$_H$2 subset increases during AIDS progression. The T$_H$1 response may reflect activity of T$_{DTH}$ cells

---

TABLE 22-5

IN VITRO PROLIFERATIVE RESPONSE OF PERIPHERAL-BLOOD LYMPHOCYTES FROM AIDS PATIENTS AND NORMAL CONTROLS*

| | [^{3}H] THYMIDINE INCORPORATED (CPM) | | | |
| | POKEWEED MITOGEN | | TETANUS TOXOID | |
CELL SAMPLE†	AIDS	CONTROL	AIDS	CONTROL
Unfractionated	1,400 ± 800	10,800 ± 1,900	<100	20,300 ± 6,400
CD4$^+$ T cells	17,800 ± 2,600	19,600 ± 2,200	<100	16,900 ± 1,200
CD8$^+$ T cells	3,100 ± 515	4,400 ± 680	<100	45,300 ± 600

* Lymphocytes were cultured in the presence of [^{3}H]thymidine and either pokeweed mitogen or tetanus toxoid. At the end of a 5-day culture period, the amount of radioactivity (CPM) incorporated into cells was determined.

† Cell numbers in the unfractionated sample were not equalized and represent the cell counts in peripheral blood. After separation of CD4 and CD8, cell numbers in the AIDS and control samples were equalized.

SOURCE: Data from H. C. Lane and A. S. Fauci, 1985, *Annu. Rev. Immunol.* **3**:477.

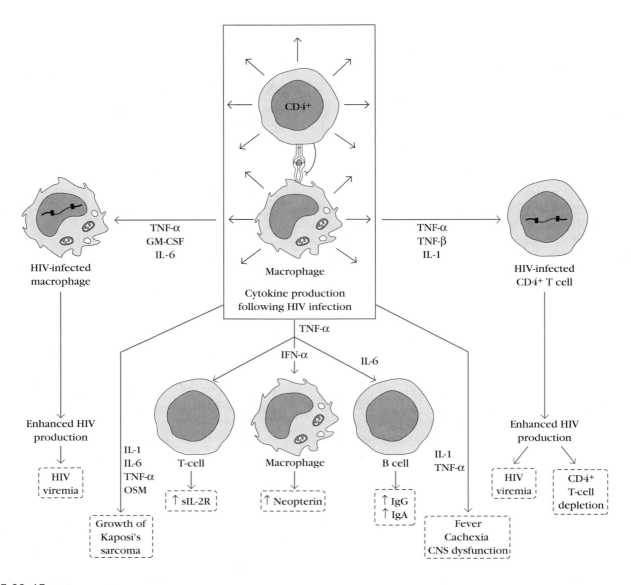

FIGURE 22-15

Effects of various cytokines that are present at elevated levels following HIV infection. IL = interleukin; IFN = interferon; OSM = oncostatin M; sIL-2R = soluble receptor for IL-2; TNF = tumor necrosis factor; GM-CSF = granulocyte-monocyte colony-stimulating factor. [Adapted from T. Matsuyama, N. Kobayashi, and N. Yamamoto, 1991, *AIDS* **5**:1405.]

and/or induce CTL activity. A T_H2 response, on the other hand, would lead to antibody production. Thus this shift from T_H1 to T_H2 activity may contribute to the progression of AIDS.

Decreased DTH Response

As noted, both IL-2 and IFN-γ have been shown to decrease with time following HIV infection (Figure 22-16). The decline in IFN-γ most likely reflects a decrease in T_{DTH}–cell function and is responsible for the significant reduction in skin-test reactivity in AIDS patients (Table 22-6). As discussed in Chapter 16, the delayed-type hypersensitive response is an important host–defense mechanism against intracellular pathogens such as *Pneumocystis carinii*, *Mycobacterium tuberculosis*, *Mycobacterium avium*, *Candida albicans*, *Histoplasma*, and *Cryptococcus*. Given the limited ability of AIDS patients to mount a DTH response, it is not surprising that they exhibit increased susceptibility to intracellular pathogens.

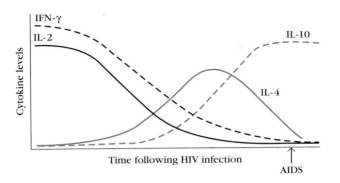

FIGURE 22-16

Following HIV infection there is a shift in cytokines that indicates progression into AIDS. IL-2 and IFN-γ levels are initially quite high but begin to drop with time following HIV infection. In contrast the levels of IL-4 and IL-10 begin to increase. This shift in cytokines suggests a shift from initial T_H1 activity following HIV infection to T_H2 activity as the disease progresses into full-blown AIDS. (Based on data from M. Clerici and G. M. Shearer, 1993, *Immunol. Today* **14**(3):107.)

Impaired CTL Activity

Although the level of CD8$^+$ T$_C$ cells is near normal in AIDS patients, their ability to generate CTLs from T$_C$ cells, which requires IL-2, is impaired, most likely due to reduced IL-2 levels. Therefore, despite the presence of adequate numbers of T$_C$ cells, AIDS patients have limited abilities to eliminate virus-infected cells and tumor cells. This was demonstrated in one study by measuring the cytolytic activity of CD8$^+$ T cells from AIDS patients infected with cytomegalovirus (CMV) and from CMV-infected controls in CML assays (see Figure 16-14b). The T cells from the AIDS patients showed lower ability to kill CMV-infected target cells than did T cells from the controls.

Because HIV antigens are not expressed on latently infected host cells, these cells are safe from CTL-mediated killing until activation of the provirus initiates expression of the viral antigens. Interestingly, long-term survivors of HIV infection have high counts of CD8$^+$ T cells, and these cells have been shown to produce a factor that promotes viral latency in HIV-infected CD4$^+$ T cells in vitro. What relation, if any, this cell antiviral factor (CAF) has to the chemokine suppressors of HIV infection discussed earlier currently is unknown.

TABLE 22-6

SKIN-TEST REACTIVITY IN AIDS PATIENTS AND NORMAL CONTROLS

	NO. RESPONDING/NO. TESTED (%)	
ANTIGEN	AIDS PATIENTS (N = 20)	CONTROLS (N = 20)
Control	0	0
Tetanus	10	90
Diphtheria	5	80
Streptococcus	15	70
Tuberculosis	0	60
Candida	10	90
Trichophyton	0	80
Proteus	40	50

SOURCE: Data from H. C. Lane and A. S. Fauci, 1985, *Annu. Rev. Immunol.* **3**:477.

DEVELOPMENT OF AN AIDS VACCINE

As discussed in Chapter 18, the development of a vaccine requires knowledge of the infectious agent, characterization of the immune response to the agent, and determination of what type of immune response is protective. There are no shortcuts, and the development of most vaccines has been a long and arduous process. For example, development and testing of the most recent hepatitis B vaccine took 17 years. Human clinical trials of a vaccine must be conducted according to guidelines set by the Food and Drug Administration (FDA). A vaccine is first tested in appropriate animals to determine whether it is safe.

Once a vaccine is deemed safe in animal trials, three phases of human clinical trials are then conducted. Phase I and phase II human trials are intended to evaluate the safety, dosage, and immunogenicity of a vaccine preparation. Normally, the major focus of phase I trials is safety. A relatively small sample is evaluated for detrimental effect. Phase II trails involving a larger sample are designed to extend the phase I findings on safety, dosage, and immunogenicity. Phase III trials, which are designed to determine the effectiveness of a vaccine, require much larger numbers of volunteers so that the degree of protection afforded by the vaccine can be assessed by statistical measures. Because of the high mortality of HIV infection, the FDA has tried to shorten some aspects of the review process. All AIDS-related drug treatments and vaccines have been given a special designation, 1-AA, that automatically moves them ahead in the review process. Before describing the various experimental

AIDS vaccines currently being evaluated, let's examine why development of an effective vaccine has proved so difficult.

Obstacles to Development of an AIDS Vaccine

Despite the extensive efforts to develop an AIDS vaccine and the actions of the FDA to hasten testing and review, several properties of HIV itself hamper vaccine development. For any vaccine to be successful it must be able to induce an immune response that renders the host protected against the pathogen. Unfortunately, the type of immune response that is protective against HIV is not yet known. Moreover, as was seen in the development of a vaccine for measles, some types of immune response actually may increase the likelihood of infection. J. Levy has shown that certain subclasses of antibody to HIV mediate uptake of the virus into macrophages via Fc receptors and thus enhance infection. Therefore, until the mechanisms of protective immunity to HIV are more fully understood, researchers will not be able to focus their energy on one type of immune response and may develop vaccines that do not elicit protective immunity.

As discussed earlier, HIV constantly mutates and changes its surface glycoproteins, allowing it to evade the immune response. Such antigenic shift, which occurs in a variety of other viruses, has been a major obstacle to development of an AIDS vaccine. The challenge facing researchers is to develop a single vaccine (or mixture of a small number of vaccines) that is effective against myriad antigenically diverse HIV strains. Although the results of some experimental vaccine trials in animals have been promising, the implications of these trials may be limited. In these studies a state of immunity that protects the animal against a later challenge with live SIV or HIV has been induced; however, to date the strain of the virus used for the subsequent challenge has been the same as the strain used for immunization. Knowing that HIV has such a high mutation rate, one must continually ask whether the animal will be protected against other strains of the virus that differ antigenically from the immunizing strain.

Before his death in 1993, Albert Sabin, the developer of the oral polio vaccine, raised another caution in regard to interpreting the effectiveness of the initial AIDS vaccine trials. Sabin pointed out that all animal vaccine trials to date have challenged the animal with the live virus, not with virus-infected cells. Since the HIV-infected cell has been shown to be the major vehicle of transmission, Sabin suggested that test animals should be challenged with virus-infected cells rather than with the free virus. He believed that it will be much more difficult to gener-ate immunity to HIV-infected cells than to the free virus and therefore cautioned against unwarranted optimism about the positive results of the early vaccine trials.

Another major hindrance to developing an AIDS vaccine has been the lack of a suitable animal model. The chimpanzee and the pigtailed macaque monkey are the only natural animal models for HIV-1 infection. Although HIV can produce a persistent infection in the chimpanzee, the infection does not lead to an immune deficiency (see Table 22-1). Testing of a potential vaccine in chimpanzees must therefore focus on inhibition of viral replication rather than on the immunodeficiency manifestations. Moreover, use of chimpanzees for AIDS-vaccine testing poses an increasing threat to the already dwindling chimpanzee population. The competing interests associated with use of chimpanzees for vaccine testing highlights the need for proper management of experimental animals, careful design of animal trials, and sharing of information among research laboratories involved in vaccine testing around the world.

Development of SCID-human mice has given AIDS researchers some optimism in their search for a practical animal model. Two distinct approaches to developing the SCID-human mouse have proved useful. In the approach developed by J. M. McCune, the immune system of CB-17 SCID mice is reconstituted with human fetal liver, mesenteric lymph node, and thymus (see Figure 2-1). In the other approach, developed by E. E. Mosier, SCID mice are reconstituted with human peripheral-blood mononuclear cells. In both systems the mice become populated with human T and B lymphocytes and with other white blood cells. When SCID-human mice are challenged with HIV, the human CD4$^+$ T cells and myeloid cells have been shown to become infected. Mosier, for example, found a significant depletion in the CD4$^+$ T cells of SCID-human mice within 8 weeks of HIV infection (Figure 22-17). These mice may prove to be a workable animal model for studying the mechanism of immune suppression in AIDS and for evaluating potential drug and vaccine therapies.

Indeed, SCID-human mice have already proved useful for in vivo evaluation of antiviral agents and AIDS vaccines. McCune, for example, demonstrated that azido-3′-deoxythymidine (AZT), the first therapeutic drug approved for AIDS patients, inhibits HIV infection in SCID-human mice developed by his method. Studies with these mice helped to define therapeutic levels of AZT and dideoxyinosine (ddI) for use in humans. Mosier also showed that SCID-human mice were protected from a later challenge with HIV when they were produced with peripheral-blood cells from human volunteers who had been immunized with a recombinant vaccinia virus vaccine expressing gp160.

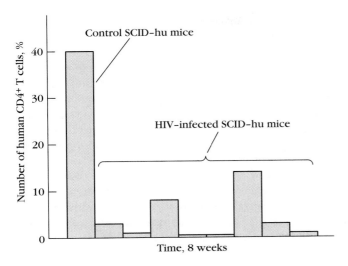

FIGURE 22-17

Depletion of CD4+ T cells in HIV-infected SCID-human mice 8 weeks after infection. [Data from E. E. Mosier et al., 1991, *Science* **251**:791.]

Experimental AIDS Vaccines

Ever since HIV was identified as the causative agent of AIDS, tremendous effort has been directed toward the development of a safe and effective vaccine. Several types of vaccines have been designed, including inactivated whole virus, live recombinant viruses, attenuated virus, recombinant DNA products, synthetic peptides, and anti-idiotype antibodies. A summary of human trials of AIDS vaccines is presented in Table 22-7.

INACTIVATED WHOLE VIRUSES

Inactivated preparations of HIV-1 and SIV have been produced by irradiating the virus and treating it with formaldehyde. This procedure, similar to that used to develop the Salk polio vaccine, inactivates the retroviral genome and releases much of the gp120 from the envelope. The noninfectious SIV or HIV preparation is then used as a vaccine.

Initial vaccine trials in animals with the inactivated whole virus looked promising. For example, in one trial nine macaques were vaccinated with inactivated SIV and subsequently challenged with live SIV. The results showed that eight of the nine test animals had no detectable SIV and no development of SAIDS. However, the results were soon challenged in 1992 when it was discovered that the SIV vaccine was prepared by growing SIV in human T-cell cultures. As SIV buds out of the human T cells, it acquires human MHC mole-

cules on its envelope. Subsequent experiments suggested that the vaccinated macaques actually responded to the human MHC antigens on the vaccine and on the live SIV challenge.

In humans trials, inactivated HIV-1 virus has been administered to HIV-infected volunteers with the objective of boosting their immune response to viral antigens and slowing disease progression. The results have been variable and disappointing overall.

CLONED ENVELOPE GLYCOPROTEINS

Several groups have applied gene-engineering techniques to clone the gp120 gene or the entire gp160 gene in order to produce large quantities of gp120 or gp160 for immunization. The first of the cloned gp160 vaccines, which was produced by MicroGeneSys, Inc., was administered to 140 healthy seronegative volunteers in September 1987. The vaccine induced largely humoral immunity to HIV. The antibodies elicited in the volunteers were shown to inhibit viral replication in vitro, but the inhibition was always strain specific—a result of the antigenic variation of gp160. As of mid-1994, phase II clinical trials of cloned gp120 vaccine were under way in patients with early HIV infection; phase I and II clinical trials were under way in uninfected volunteers; and phase I trials were under way in HIV-infected pregnant women, newborns, and children.

Phase I clinical trials of two genetically engineered gp120 vaccines began in the spring of 1993. One vaccine, produced by Genentech, consists of gp120 from the MN strain of HIV-1. The MN sequence is a conserved crown sequence present in a high proportion of HIV isolates in North America (see Figure 22-9). The other vaccine, produced by Chiron, contains gp120 from the SF-2 strain, which has another conserved crown sequence. Earlier animal trials of Genentech's recombinant gp120 vaccine were promising. In these animal trials four chimpanzees were immunized, two with recombinant gp160 and two with recombinant gp120, and then challenged with live HIV-1. The control unimmunized group and both chimpanzees immunized with gp160 became infected with HIV-1 within 7 weeks of challenge. However, the two chimpanzees that were immunized with the recombinant gp120 were reported to show no sign of HIV infection, even by the very sensitive PCR technique, for more than 6 months.

The results of the human trials with gp120 are not in yet, but a 1994 report raised concerns. Five recipients of the Genentech and Chiron vaccines were found to become HIV-positive after sexual exposure or IV drug use. This would suggest that the vaccine was not protective. What is particularly troubling was that one female vaccine recipient who became infected by her sexual partner (who already was infected) exhibited an accelerated decline in CD4$^+$ T cells. It is not known whether the vaccine put her at increased risk for this rapid T-cell decline.

ATTENUATED VIRUSES

In general, attenuated viral vaccines are produced by growing live viruses under unusual culture conditions that force the virus to mutate to survive in the new conditions. The Sabin polio vaccine, for example, was produced by growing the live polio virus in monkey kidney cell cultures. The majority of viral vaccines used today are attenuated vaccines; these include the measles, mumps, rubella, and polio vaccines. Because the vaccine is live, it is able to infect cells and grow for a limited amount of time before the immune response eliminates the virus. During this time, the attenuated virus is able to induce a potent immune response, often including gen-

eration of cell-mediated CTLs specific for the endogenously produced viral antigens. In addition, attenuated viral vaccines tend to induce a good memory cell response, which accounts for the life-long immunity generated by these vaccines. The limitation of these vaccines is the risk that the attenuated virus may be able to mutate back to a virulent strain.

Because of the high rate of mutation in HIV and its virulence, attenuated HIV strains were long considered too dangerous for use as vaccines. This prevailing opinion was called into question in 1992 by the work of R. Desrosiers and his colleagues. These researchers eliminated the regulatory gene *nef* from a highly virulent strain of SIV. When the *nef*-deleted strain of SIV was injected into six macaques, the animals did not develop symptoms of SAIDS. The macaques were then challenged with a small dose of infectious live SIV and remained healthy. Finally, the researchers challenged the animals with a huge dose of infectious SIV and found that the animals still continued to remain healthy. The

TABLE 22-7

SURVEY OF AIDS VACCINE TRIALS IN HUMANS IN PROGRESS IN MID-1994

TYPE OF VACCINE	COMPANY	RECIPIENT	STATUS
Inactivated HIV	Immunization Products, Ltd.	HIV-infected asymptomatic patients	Phase II/III
gp160	Immuno AG National Institutes of Health	AIDS patients	Phase I
gp160	MicroGeneSys	HIV-infected asymptomatic patients	Phase II
		HIV-negative volunteers	Phase I/II
		HIV-infected pregnant women, newborns, and children	Phase I
gp120 (MN crown)	Genentech	HIV-infected adults, pregnant women, newborns, and children	Phase I
gp120 (SF-2 crown)	Chiron, Ciba-Geigy	AIDS patients; HIV-infected pregnant women, newborns, and children	Phase I
p24	MicroGeneSys	AIDS patients	Phase I
p24 synthetic peptide	Viral technologies	Uninfected volunteers	Phase I
Vector vaccine (gp120 in canarypox virus)	Pasteur Merieux	Uninfected volunteers	Phase I
Anti-idiotype antibody	IDEC Pharmaceuticals	HIV-infected asymptomatic patients	Phase I

excitement about the attenuated vaccine soon began to wane when it was discovered that the attenuated SIV vaccine caused SAIDS in newborn macaques. The attenuated virus had not mutated back to a virulent form, but the low immunity of the newborn animals made them susceptible to the attenuated vaccine. This finding cast an air of caution on developing an attenuated HIV-1 vaccine for humans.

RECOMBINANT VIRUSES CARRYING HIV GENES

Recombinant vector vaccines are another approach that may prove useful in the search for an effective AIDS vaccine. Vaccinia virus and the Sabin polio virus are both live attenuated viruses that have proved to be safe and successful vaccines for smallpox and polio, respectively. Both of these viruses can be engineered to carry genes from HIV-1, and the recombinant virus can then be used as an HIV vaccine (see Figure 18-4). Because the recombinant virus is attenuated (not inactivated), it is able to infect host cells and would therefore be expected to induce CTL activity. As with any attenuated vaccine, the prolonged exposure to the viral antigens tends to induce a very good immune response without the need of additional boosters.

Vaccinia virus, which is a large virus, can be engineered to carry several dozen foreign genes without impairing its capacity to infect host cells and to replicate in them. A genetically engineered vaccinia virus can be administered simply by dermal scratching; the virus causes a limited localized infection in host cells. The foreign genes are expressed by the vaccinia, and if the foreign gene product is a viral envelope protein, it is inserted into the membrane of the infected host cell and there stimulates the development of T-cell–mediated immunity. Vaccinia virus carrying gp160 has been shown to infect host cells at the site of scarification; the gp160 is glycosylated, cleaved into gp120 and gp41, and inserted into the plasma membrane of the infected host cells. A number of HIV genes have been engineered into vaccinia virus, including *env, tat, pol,* and *gag.*

Trials using a recombinant vaccine were conducted by Daniel Zagury and coworkers of the Pasteur Institute. Healthy human volunteers (including Zagury himself) were immunized by scarification with recombinant vaccinia virus expressing the gp160 envelope glycoprotein. The primary response was weak, and the volunteers were subsequently boosted intramuscularly with their own cells, which had first been infected in vitro with the recombinant vaccinia virus. These individuals showed enhanced in vitro cell-mediated immunity to HIV following each booster immunization. Such an approach to large-scale clinical trials is limited logistically by the diffi-

culty of immunization with autologous cells infected in vitro with recombinant vaccinia virus.

Zagury's vaccinia-based HIV vaccine trials were criticized because of questions about the degree of informed consent in the test trials on human subjects in Zaire, which were conducted without the prior approval of a Zairian or French human-subjects ethics committee. Consequently, the French minister of health, Bruno Durieux, imposed a ban on these vaccine trials, and the National Institutes of Health in the United States rescinded permission for Robert Gallo at the National Cancer Institute to collaborate with Zagury. Adding to the controversy was the finding that three recipients of the vaccine died from disseminated vaccinia infection. Although vaccinia is a safe vaccine in healthy individuals, the attenuated virus can cause disseminated lesions in individuals with a compromised immune system. At the VIIth International Conference on AIDS in Florence, Zagury announced that he would discontinue the vaccinia vaccine trials. This case demonstrates the importance of ethical awareness in scientific research, particularly where the welfare of human subjects is involved.

In 1994 trials were begun using engineered canarypox vaccines. The canarypox virus has no known pathogenicity in humans, even in immunocompromised individuals. Like vaccinia, the canarypox virus should induce both humoral and cell-mediated immunity to HIV antigens. According to a 1995 report, engineered canarypox vaccines carrying the *gag, pol,* or *env* genes from HIV-1 could protect macaque monkeys challenged with live HIV-2. This is the first demonstration of cross-protection between HIV-1 and HIV-2 and adds a ray of hope to further studies with the engineered canarypox.

SYNTHETIC CROWN-SEQUENCE PEPTIDES

The principal neutralizing epitope of HIV overlaps with the V3 loop of gp120, and antibodies to the V3 loop have been shown to protect chimpanzees from HIV infection. Because of the high level of variation in the V3 loop, antibody neutralization is always strain specific. However, the so-called crown sequence in the V3 loop is coserved to a considerable degree (see Figure 22-8). Approximately 30% of North American HIV isolates, for example, have the crown sequence designated MN.

Synthetic peptides of different HIV crown sequences, including the MN sequence, have been prepared and tested for their ability to activate T-cell proliferation and cytotoxicity in vitro. These synthetic peptides appear to activate a population of T_H cells and to induce some cytotoxic activity; however, because these peptides are processed as exogenous antigens, the T cytotoxic cells induced were all CD4$^+$, class II restricted. These studies suggest that cocktails of synthetic peptides, representing the crown sequences of the predominant HIV isolates, might induce protective antibody or CD4$^+$ T cytotoxic cells.

SUMMARY

1. HIV is an enveloped retrovirus containing ssRNA that is the causative agent for AIDS. The virus infects host cells when its envelope glycoprotein gp120 binds to CD4 molecules on cell membranes. Upon entry into a cell, the virus copies its RNA into DNA with a viral reverse transcriptase. The DNA can then integrate into the host chromosomal DNA forming a provirus, which can remain in a latent state for varying periods of time (see Figure 22-3a).

2. Activation of an HIV-infected CD4$^+$ T cell also triggers activation of the provirus, resulting in transcription of the viral structural proteins and assembly of viral particles at the host cell's plasma membrane (see Figure 22-3b). Viral particles are released from the host cell by a process called budding, in which portions of the host-cell plasma membrane modified with viral glycoproteins become the viral envelope. Destruction of the host-cell plasma membrane in this process can lead to cell death. The HIV regulatory protein Tat, certain host-cell factors, and coinfection with some other viruses promote provirus activation and production of viral particles (see Figure 22-6b,c).

3. Following infection with HIV, it typically takes several weeks to a few months before antibodies against HIV antigens are detectable (seroconversion). The lag period between infection and seroconversion, however, may last up to 3 years in some individuals. It usually takes 8–10 years before HIV-infected individuals show significant disease manifestations; about 25% of infected individuals have remained symptom-free for considerably longer. A clinical diagnosis of AIDS includes documented HIV infection, the presence of one or more indicator diseases, and, in most cases, a CD4$^+$ T-cell count less than 500/μl (see Table 22-3).

4. HIV infection leads to numerous immunologic abnormalities (see Table 22-4) and eventually to severe depletion of CD4$^+$ T cells. As a result, both humoral and cell-mediated immunity is severely depressed in AIDS patients. Since less than 0.01% of the CD4$^+$ T cells in an HIV-infected individual are actually infected with the virus, the extensive depletion of T$_H$ cells that is observed means that uninfected CD4$^+$ T$_H$ cells also are destroyed. Several mechanisms proposed to account for destruction of uninfected T$_H$ cells involve gp120, a viral envelope protein that is shed into the blood and lymph of HIV-infected individuals. The binding of soluble gp120 to CD4 on uninfected cells may lead to their destruction, inhibit their functioning, or interfere with T-cell maturation (see Figure 22-13).

5. Several approaches are being tried in the extensive effort to develop an effective AIDS vaccine. Experimental vaccines that have been developed and tested to some extent include inactivated HIV strains, cloned envelope glycoproteins, recombinant vector viruses carrying HIV envelope-protein genes, and synthetic peptides of the gp120 crown sequence (see Table 22-7). Development of an effective AIDS vaccine has been hampered by the extensive antigenic variation exhibited by HIV; the ability of HIV to exist as a provirus in host cells, where it is inaccessible to the immune system; and the lack of a good animal model for AIDS.

REFERENCES

Abimiku, A. G., et. al. 1995. HIV-1 recombinant poxvirus vaccine induces cross-protection against HIV-2 challenge in rhesus macaques. *Nature Med.* **1**:321.

Ameisen, J. C., et al. 1995. The relevance of apoptosis to AIDS pathogenesis. *Trends Cell Biol.* **5**:27.

Arthur, L. O., et al. 1992. Cellular proteins bound to immunodeficiency viruses: implications for pathogenesis and vaccines. *Science* **258**:1935.

Ascher, M. S., and H. W. Sheppard. 1990. AIDS as immune system activation. *J. Acquired Immune Deficiency Syndromes* **3**:177.

Berzofsky, J. A. 1991. Approaches and issues in the development of vaccines against HIV. *J. Acquired Immune Deficiency Syndrome* **4**:451.

Bolognesi, D. P. 1994. Prospects for an HIV vaccine. *Sci. Am. Sci and Med.* (Mar/Apr):44.

Broder, C. C., et al. 1994. CD26 antigen and HIV fusion? *Science* **264**:1156.

Cao, Y., et al. 1995. Virologic and immunologic characterization of long-term survivors of human immunodeficiency virus type 1 infection. *New Engl. J. Med.* **332**:201.

Capon, D. J., and R. H. R. Ward. 1991. The CD4-gp120 interaction and AIDS pathogenesis. *Annu. Rev. Immunol.* **9**:649.

Clerici, M., and G. M. Shearer. 1994. The T$_H$1-T$_H$2 hypothesis of HIV infection: new insights. *Immunol. Today* **15**:575.

COHEN, J. 1994. At conference, hope for success is further attenuated. *Science* **266**:1154.

CONSTANTINE, N. T. 1993. Serologic tests for the retroviruses: approaching a decade of evolution. *AIDS* **7**:1.

DALGLEISH, A. G. 1995. The immune response to HIV: potential for immunotherapy. *Immunol. Today* **16**:356.

DANIEL, M., ET AL. 1992. Protective effects of a live attenuated SIV vaccine with a deletion in the *nef* gene. *Science* **258**:1938.

EIDEN, L. E., AND J. D. LIFSON. 1992. HIV interactions with CD4: a continuum of conformations and consequences. *Immunol. Today* 13:201.

FENG, Y., ET AL. 1996. HIV-1 entry cofactor: functional cDNA cloning of a seven-transmembrane G protein–coupled receptor. *Science* 272:872.

FOX, C. H., AND M. COTTLER-FOX. 1992. The pathobiology of HIV infection. *Immunol. Today* 13:353.

GREENE, W. C. 1991. The molecular biology of human immunodeficiency virus type I infection. *New Engl. J. Med.* **324**:308.

HABESHAW, J., E. HOUNSELL, AND A. DALGLEISH. 1992. Does the HIV envelope induce a chronic graft-versus-host-like disease? *Immunol. Today* **13**:207.

HASELTINE, W. A. 1991. Molecular biology of the human immunodeficiency virus type I. *FASEB* **5**: 2349.

HO, D., ET AL. 1995. Rapid turnover of plasma virions and CD4 lymphocytes in HIV-1 infection. *Nature* **373**:123.

MATSUYAMA, T., N. KOBAYASHI, AND N. YAMAMOTO. 1991. Cytokines and HIV infection: is AIDS a tumor necrosis factor disease? *AIDS* 5:1405.

MCCUNE, J. M., ET AL. 1990. Suppression of HIV infection in AZT-treated SCID-hu mice. *Science* **247**: 564.

MCCUNE, J. M., ET AL. 1991. The SCID-hu mouse: a small animal model for HIV infection and pathogenesis. *Annu. Rev. Immunol.* **9**:399.

MOSIER, E. E., ET AL. 1991. Human immunodeficiency virus infection of human-PBL-SCID mice. *Science* **251**:791.

MURPHEY-CORB, M., ET AL. 1989. A formalin inactivated whole SIV vaccine confers protection in macaques. *Science* **246**:1293.

PANTALEO, G., AND A. S. FAUCI. 1995. New concepts in the immunopathogenesis of HIV infection. *Annu. Rev. Immunol.* **13**:487.

PANTALEO, G., ET AL.1993. HIV infection is active and progressive in lymphoid tissue during the clinically latent stage of disease. *Nature* **362**:355.

PUTNEY, S. 1992. How antibodies block HIV infection: paths to an AIDS vaccine. *TIBS* **17**:191.

ROSENBERG, Z. F., AND A. S. FAUCI. 1991. Immunopathogenesis of HIV infection. *FASEB* **5**:2382.

SAFRIT, J. T., AND R. A. KOUP. 1995. The immunology of primary HIV infection: which immune responses control HIV replication? *Curr. Opin. Immunol.* **7**: 456.

WEI, X., ET AL. 1995. Viral dynamics in human immunodeficiency virus type 1 infection. *Nature* **373**:117.

STUDY QUESTIONS

1. Indicate whether each of the following statements is true or false. If you think a statement is false, explain why.

a. HIV-1 and HIV-2 are more closely related to each other than to SIV.

b. HIV-1 causes immune suppression in both humans and chimpanzees.

c. SIV is endemic in the African green monkey.

d. The Tat protein of HIV appears to increase proviral transcription.

e. T-cell activation increases transcription of the HIV proviral genome.

f. Patients with advanced stages of AIDS always have detectable antibody to HIV.

g. The polymerase chain reaction is a sensitive test that can be used to detect antibodies to HIV.

h. Production of antibody to HIV sometimes increases the likelihood of HIV infection.

2. Various mechanisms have been proposed to account for the decrease in the numbers and function of uninfected CD4[+] T cells in HIV-infected individuals.

a. Which HIV protein has been implicated in several of these mechanisms? In what form would it affect uninfected T_H cells.

b. Briefly describe three mechanisms by which uninfected CD4[+] T cells might be destroyed.

c. What mechanism might account for the decreased ability of T_H cells from asymptomatic AIDS patients to respond to foreign antigens?

3. Would you expect to see much p17 and p24 in the blood of HIV-infected individuals in the asymptomatic latency period?

4.   If p24 levels begin to increase dramatically in the blood of an HIV-infected individual, what would this indicate about HIV infection?

5.   Why do clinicians monitor the level of skin-test reactivity in HIV-infected individuals? What change might you expect to see in skin-test reactivity with progression into AIDS?

6.   What type of immune response would probably be induced by immunization with a recombinant vaccinia virus carrying the HIV gene encoding gp120?

7.   Certain chemokines have been shown to suppress infection of cells by HIV. Propose an explanation of this finding in terms of what's known about the fusion of HIV with target cells, a necessary step in the infection process.

8.   Suppose you are a physician who has two HIV-infected patients. Patient BW has a fungal infection (candidiasis) in the mouth region, and patient LS has a *Mycobacterium* infection. The CD4$^+$ T-cell count of both patients is in the range of 200 and 499 per μl. Would you diagnose either or both patients as having AIDS?

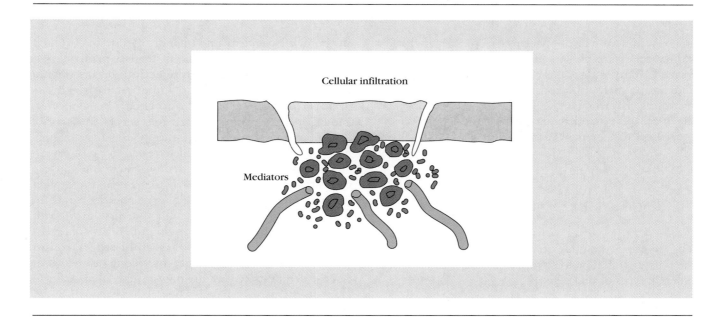

Cellular infiltration

Mediators

TRANSPLANTATION IMMUNOLOGY

Transplantation, as the term is used in immunology, refers to the act of transferring cells, tissues, or organs from one site to another. The surgical procedures for many kinds of transplantation were developed by turn of the century. With the surgical technology in place, scientists began to ask whether organs or tissues might be transplanted from one individual to another. In the early 1900s a Viennese surgeon observed that he could surgically remove a kidney from an animal and then transplant it back into the same animal and restore kidney function. When the kidney was transplanted to a different animal, however, it soon ceased to function. Experimental transplantation between animals continued through the 1920s and 1930s, but every attempt was a dismal failure. Autopsies revealed massive infiltration of white blood cells into the donated organ or tissue.

Several observations by P. B. Medawar in the early 1940s provided insight into the nature of graft rejection: While working with burn patients during World War II, he noticed that grafts of skin from one site to another on the same patient were readily accepted, whereas grafts from relatives were rejected. In one patient a skin graft from a brother had been rejected; when a second graft from the same donor was attempted, the rejection reaction occurred much faster and with much greater intensity. In subsequent animal experiments, Medawar discovered that prior sensitization with donor cells led to heightened rejection of a subsequent graft. In 1945 he published a paper suggesting that graft rejection resulted from an immunologic response to the donor organ.

Medawar's suggestion proved to be correct. Thus no matter how skilled the surgeon is, a surgically successful transplant can be thwarted by an immunologic attack. The very system that evolved to recognize and destroy altered self-cells is simply performing its function by recognizing and destroying the foreign cells of a graft. Since these early findings, the subdiscipline of transplantation immunology has developed to understand the immunologic basis of graft rejection and to find techniques for reducing immune-system activation, thereby promoting graft acceptance. Various immunosuppressive agents soon were developed to diminish the immunologic attack. Within 10 years of Medawar's 1945 paper, the first kidney transplantation in humans was successfully performed. Today, kidney, heart, lung, liver, bone marrow, and cornea transplantations are performed with ever-increasing frequency and success. This chapter describes the mechanisms underlying graft rejection and various procedures that are used to prolong graft survival.

IMMUNOLOGIC BASIS OF GRAFT REJECTION

The degree of immune response to a graft varies with the type of graft. The following terms are used to denote different types of transplants:

- **Autograft** is self-tissue transferred from one body site to another in the same individual. These grafts are often performed on patients with burns by transferring healthy skin to the burned area.
- **Isograft** is tissue transferred between genetically identical individuals. In inbred strains of mice an isograft can be performed from one mouse to another syngeneic mouse. In humans an isograft can be performed between genetically identical (monozygotic) twins.
- **Allograft** is tissue transferred between genetically different members of the same species. In mice an allograft is performed by transferring tissue or an organ from one inbred strain to another. In humans, unless an identical twin is available, most organ grafts from one individual to another are allografts.
- **Xenograft** is tissue transferred between different species (e.g., the graft of a baboon heart into a human).

Autografts and isografts are usually accepted, owing to the genetic identity between graft and host (Figure 23-1a). Because an allograft is genetically dissimilar to the host, it is often recognized as foreign by the immune system and is rejected in an allograft reaction. Obviously, xenografts exhibit the greatest genetic disparity and therefore engender the most vigorous graft rejection.

Specificity and Memory of the Rejection Response

The time sequence of allograft rejection varies according to the tissue involved. In general, skin grafts are rejected faster than more vascularized tissues such as kidney or heart. Despite these time differences, the immune response culminating in graft rejection always displays the attributes of specificity and memory. If a strain-A inbred mouse is grafted with skin from strain B, primary graft rejection, known as **first-set rejection**, occurs (Figure 23-1b). As the reaction develops, the vascularized transplant becomes infiltrated with lymphocytes, monocytes, and other inflammatory cells; there is decreased vascularization of the transplanted tissue by 6–9 days, visible necrosis by 10 days, and complete rejection by 14 days.

Immunologic memory is demonstrated when a second strain-B graft is transferred to a previously grafted strain-A mouse. In this case, a graft-rejection reaction develops more quickly than after the first graft, with complete rejection occurring within 5–6 days; this secondary response is designated **second-set rejection** (Figure 23-1c). The specificity of second-set rejection can be demonstrated by grafting an unrelated strain-C graft at the same time as the second strain-B graft. Rejection of the strain-C graft proceeds according to first-set rejection kinetics, whereas the strain-B graft is rejected in an accelerated second-set fashion.

Role of Cell-Mediated Responses

In the early 1950s A. Mitchison showed in adoptive-transfer experiments that lymphocytes, but not serum antibody, could transfer allograft immunity. Later studies began to implicate T cells in allograft rejection. For example, nude mice, which lack a thymus and consequently lack functional T cells, were found to be incapable of allograft rejection; indeed these mice even accept xenografts (see Figure 21-6). In other studies, T cells derived from an allograft-primed mouse were shown to transfer second-set allograft rejection to an unprimed syngeneic recipient, as long as that recipient was grafted with the same allogeneic tissue (Figure 23-2).

Analysis of the T-cell subpopulations involved in allograft rejection has implicated both $CD4^+$ and $CD8^+$ populations. In one study the role of $CD4^+$ and $CD8^+$ T-cell subpopulations in rejection of skin allografts was analyzed by injecting the recipient mice with monoclonal antibodies to deplete one or both types of T cells and then measuring the rate of graft rejection. As shown in Figure 23-3, removal of the $CD8^+$ population alone had no effect on graft survival, and the graft was rejected at the same rate as in control mice (15 days). Removal of the $CD4^+$ T-cell population alone prolonged graft survival from 15 days to 30 days. However, removal of both the $CD4^+$ and the $CD8^+$ T cells resulted in long-term survival (up to 60 days) of the allografts. This study indicated that both $CD4^+$ and $CD8^+$ T-cells participated in rejection and that the collaboration of both subpopulations resulted in more pronounced graft rejection.

Visualizing Concepts

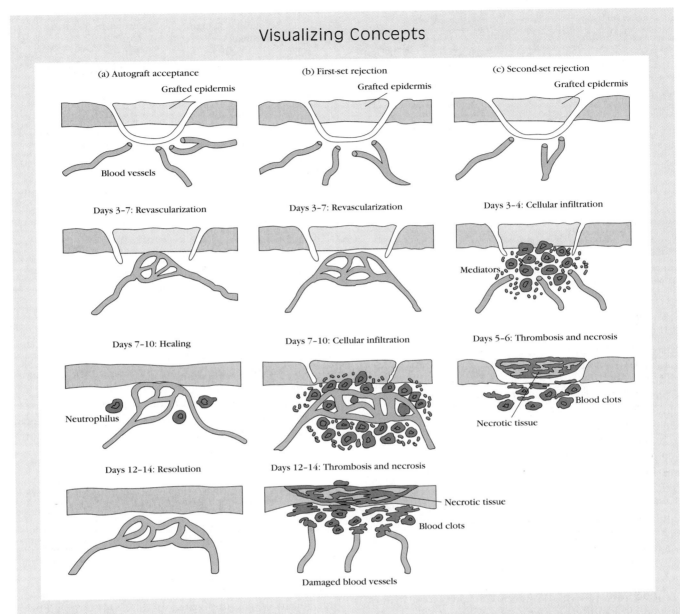

FIGURE 23-1

Schematic diagrams of the process of graft acceptance and rejection. (a) Acceptance of an autograft is completed within 12–14 days. (b) First-set rejection of an allograft begins 7–10 days after grafting, with full rejection occurring by 12–14 days. (c) Second-set rejection of an allograft begins within 3–4 days, with full rejection by 5–6 days. The cellular infiltrate that invades an allograft contains lymphocytes, phagocytes, and other inflammatory cells.

Transplantation Antigens

Tissues that are antigenically similar are said to be **histocompatible**; such tissues do not induce an immunologic response that leads to tissue rejection. Tissues displaying significant antigenic differences are **histoincompatible**; such tissues induce an immune response leading to tissue rejection. The various antigens that determine histocompatibility are encoded by more than 40 different loci, but the loci responsible for the most vigorous allograft-

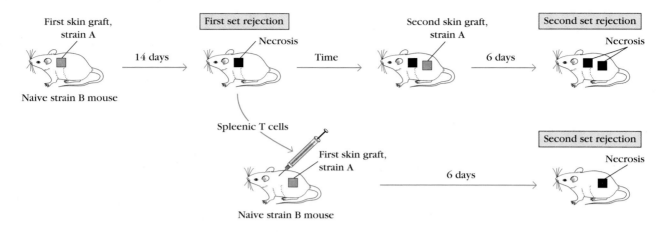

FIGURE 23-2

Experimental demonstration that T cells can transfer allograft rejection. When T cells derived from an allograft-primed mouse are transferred to an unprimed syngeneic mouse, the recipient mounts a second-set rejection to an initial allograft from the original allogeneic strain.

rejection reactions are located within the **major histocompatibility complex** (MHC). The organization of the MHC—called the H-2 complex in mice and the HLA complex in humans—was described in Chapter 9 (see Figure 9-1). Because the MHC loci are closely linked, they are usually inherited as a complete set, called the **haplotype**, from each parent.

Within an inbred strain of mice, all animals are homozygous at each MHC locus. When mice from two different inbred strains are mated, all the F_1 progeny inherit one haplotype from each parent (see Figure 9-2b); these F_1 offspring can accept grafts from either parent. MHC inheritance in outbred populations is more complex because the high polymorphism exhibited at each MHC locus gives a high probability of heterozygosity at most loci. In matings between outbred mice, there is only a 25% chance that any two offspring will inherit identical MHC haplotypes (see Figure 9-2c), unless the parents share one or more haplotypes in common. Therefore, for purposes of organ or bone marrow grafts, there is a 25% chance of identity within the MHC between siblings. With parent-to-child grafts, the donor and host will always have one haplotype in common but will be mismatched for the other haplotype.

MHC identity of donor and host is not the sole factor determining tissue acceptance. When tissue is transplanted between genetically different individuals, even if their MHC antigens are identical, the transplanted tissue is likely to be rejected because of differences at various **minor histocompatibility loci**. As discussed in Chapter 11, the major histocompatibility antigens are recognized directly by T_H and T_C cells, a phenomenon termed **alloreactivity**. In contrast, minor histocompatibility antigens are recognized only when they are presented in the context of self-MHC molecules. In addition, the tissue rejection induced by minor histocompatibility differences is usually less vigorous than that induced by major histocompatibility differences. Still, reaction to these minor tissue differences often results in graft rejection. For this reason, transplantation even between HLA–identical individuals requires some degree of immune suppression.

Mechanisms Involved in Graft Rejection

Graft rejection is caused principally by a cell–mediated immune response to **alloantigens** (primarily MHC molecules) expressed on cells of the graft. Both delayed-type hypersensitive and cell-mediated cytotoxicity reac-

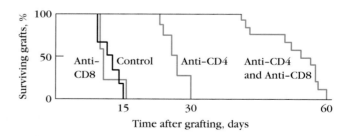

FIGURE 23-3

Experimental demonstration of the role of CD4+ and CD8+ T cells in allograft rejection in mice. Animals were treated with either anti-CD4 or anti-CD8 monoclonal antibody and then grafted with allogeneic skin; the rate of graft rejection was monitored and compared with that in untreated grafted controls. Removal of CD8+ T cells alone had no effect on graft survival, whereas removal of CD4+ T cells prolonged graft survival by about 15 days. However, removal of both T-cell populations resulted in much longer graft survival. [Adapted from S. P. Cobbold et al., 1986, *Nature* **323**:165.]

tions have been implicated. The process of graft rejection can be divided into two stages: (1) a **sensitization phase** in which antigen-reactive lymphocytes of the recipient proliferate in response to alloantigens on the graft and (2) an **effector stage** in which immune destruction of the graft takes place.

SENSITIZATION STAGE

During the sensitization phase, CD4$^+$ and CD8$^+$ T cells recognize alloantigens expressed on cells of the foreign graft and proliferate in response. Both major and minor histocompatibility alloantigens can be recognized. In general the response to minor histocompatibility antigens is weak, although the combined response to several minor differences can sometimes be quite vigorous. The response to major histocompatibility antigens involves recognition of both the MHC molecule and an associated peptide ligand in the cleft of the MHC molecule. The peptides present in the groove of allogeneic class I MHC molecules are derived from proteins synthesized within the allogeneic cell. The peptides present in the groove of allogeneic class II MHC molecules are generally proteins taken up and processed through the endocytic pathway of the allogeneic antigen-presenting cell. In some cases peptide fragments of allogeneic class I

MHC molecules can be presented within the groove of a class II molecule.

Activation of host T$_H$ cells requires the interaction with an antigen-presenting cell (APC) expressing an appropriate antigenic ligand–MHC molecule complex and providing the requisite co-stimulatory signal. Depending upon the tissue, different populations of cells within a graft may function as APCs. Because dendritic cells are found in most tissues and because they constitutively express high levels of class II MHC molecules, they generally serve as the major APC in grafts. APCs of host origin can also migrate into a graft and endocytose the foreign alloantigens (both major and minor histocompatibility molecules) and present them as processed peptides together with self-MHC molecules.

In some organ and tissue grafts (e.g., grafts of kidney, thymus, and pancreatic islets), a population of donor APCs called **passenger leukocytes** has been shown to migrate from the graft to the regional lymph nodes (Figure 23-4). These passenger leukocytes are dendritic cells, which express high levels of class II MHC molecules (together with normal levels of class I MHC molecules) and are widespread in most mammalian tissues with the exception of the brain. Because passenger leukocytes express the allogeneic MHC antigens of the donor graft, they are recognized as foreign and therefore

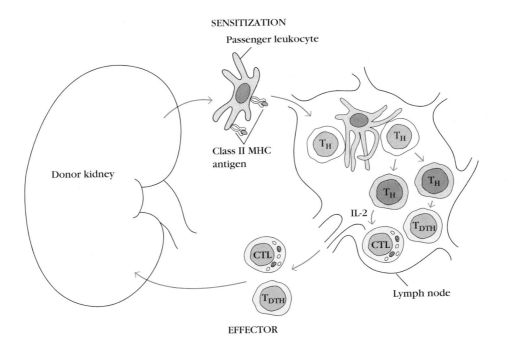

FIGURE 23-4

Migration of passenger leukocytes from a donor graft to regional lymph nodes of the recipient results in the activation of T$_H$ cells in response to different class II MHC antigens expressed by the passen-

ger leukocytes. These activated T$_H$ cells (gray) then induce generation of T$_{DTH}$ cells and/or CTLs (blue), both of which mediate graft rejection.

stimulate immune activation of T lymphocytes in the lymph node.

Passenger leukocytes are not the only cells in a graft that can present alloantigens to the immune system. In fact, in skin grafts and some other grafts, passenger leukocytes do not seem to play any role at all. Other cell types that have been implicated in alloantigen presentation to the immune system include Langerhans cells and endothelial cells lining the blood vessels. Both of these cell types express class I and class II MHC antigens.

Immunologic involvement varies with different types of transplants. When skin is grafted, for example, the graft at first does not contain functional blood vessels. Host lymphocytes, carried to the tissue by capillaries or lymphatics, encounter the foreign antigens of the skin graft and are carried by the afferent lymphatics to regional lymph nodes. Effector lymphocytes are generated in the regional nodes and are carried by the lymphatics back to the graft to mount an immunologic attack. In kidney or heart transplants the blood vasculature is immediately restored by suturing major blood vessels of the graft together with those of the host. Blood-borne lymphocytes encounter the alloantigens of the graft and are carried by blood vessels to the spleen or by the lymphatics to regional lymph nodes. Here, within the spleen or lymph nodes effector cells are generated and are then transported back to the graft by blood or lymph vessels.

Recognition of the foreign alloantigens expressed on the cells of a graft induces vigorous T-cell proliferation in the host. This proliferation can be demonstrated in vitro in a mixed–lymphocyte reaction (see Figure 16-13). Both dendritic cells and vascular endothelial cells from an allogeneic graft induce vigorous proliferation of host T cells in this reaction. The major proliferating cell is the CD4$^+$ T cell, which recognizes class II alloantigens directly or alloantigen peptides presented by host antigen-presenting cells. This amplified population of activated T$_H$ cells is thought to play a central role in inducing the various effector mechanisms of allograft rejection.

EFFECTOR STAGE

A variety of effector mechanisms participate in allograft rejection (Figure 23-5). The most common are cell-mediated reactions involving delayed-typed hypersensitivity and CTL-mediated cytotoxicity; less common mechanisms are antibody-plus-complement lysis and destruction by antibody-dependent cell-mediated cytotoxicity (ADCC). The hallmark of graft rejection involving cell-mediated reactions is an influx of T cells and macrophages into the graft. Histologically, the infiltration in many cases resembles that seen during a delayed-type hypersensitive response in which cytokines produced by T$_{DTH}$ cells promote macrophage infiltration (see Figure 16-15). Recognition of foreign class I alloantigens on the

graft by host CD8$^+$ cells can lead to CTL-mediated killing (see Figure 16-4). In some cases graft rejection is mediated by CD4$^+$ T cells that function as class II MHC–restricted cytotoxic cells.

In each of these effector mechanisms, cytokines secreted by T$_H$ cells play a central role (see Figure 23-5). For example, IL-2, IFN-γ, and TNF-β have each been shown to be important mediators of graft rejection. IL-2 promotes T-cell proliferation and generally is necessary for the generation of effector CTLs (see Figure 16-1). IFN-γ is central to the development of a DTH response, promoting the influx of macrophages into the graft and their subsequent activation into more destructive cells. TNF-β has been shown to have direct cytotoxic activity on the cells of a graft. A number of cytokines promote graft rejection by inducing expression of class I or class II MHC molecules on graft cells. The interferons (α, β, and γ), TNF-α, and TNF-β all increase class I MHC expression, and IFN-γ increases class II MHC expression as well. During a graft rejection episode, the levels of these cytokines increase, inducing a variety of cell types within the graft to express class I or class II MHC molecules. In rat cardiac allografts, for example, dendritic cells are initially the only cells that express class II MHC molecules, but as an allograft reaction begins, localized production of IFN-γ in the graft induces vascular endothelial cells and myocytes to begin to express class II MHC molecules as well.

CLINICAL MANIFESTATIONS OF GRAFT REJECTION

Graft rejection reactions have various time courses depending upon the type of tissue or organ grafted and the immune response involved. **Hyperacute** rejection reactions occur within the first 24 h after transplantation; **acute** rejection reactions usually begin in the first few weeks after transplantation; and **chronic** rejection reactions can occur from months to years after transplantation.

Hyperacute Rejection

In rare instances a transplant is rejected so quickly that the grafted tissue never becomes vascularized. These hyperacute reactions are caused by preexisting host serum antibodies specific for antigens of the graft. The antigen-antibody complexes that form activate the complement system, resulting in an intense infiltration of neutrophils into the grafted tissue. The ensuing inflammatory reaction causes massive blood clots within the capillaries, preventing vascularization of the graft (Figure 23-6).

Several mechanisms can account for the presence of preexisting antibodies specific for allogeneic MHC antigens. Recipients of repeated blood transfusions some-

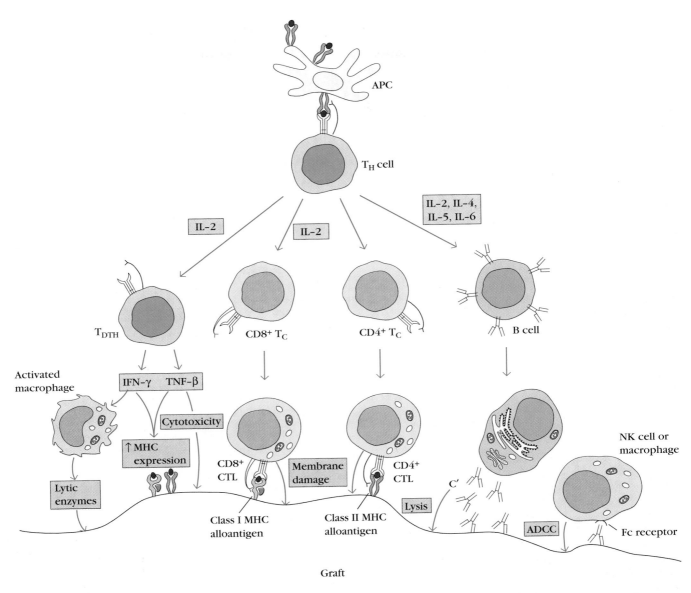

FIGURE 23-5

Effector mechanisms (purple blocks) involved in allograft rejection. The generation or activity of various effector cells depends directly or indi-rectly on cytokines (blue blocks) secreted by activated T_H cells. C′ = complement; ADCC = antibody-dependent cell-mediated cytotoxicity.

times develop significant levels of antibodies to MHC antigens expressed on white blood cells present in the transfused blood. If some of these MHC antigens are the same as those on a subsequent graft, then the antibodies can react with the graft, inducing a hyperacute rejection reaction. With repeated pregnancies women are exposed to the paternal alloantigens of the fetus and may develop antibodies to these antigens. If a woman receives a graft expressing any of these same MHC antigens, it is subject to a hyperacute rejection reaction. Finally, individuals who have had previous grafts sometimes have high levels

of antibodies to the allogeneic MHC antigens of this graft; these antibodies will mediate hyperacute rejection of any subsequent graft that expresses some of the same allogeneic antigens.

In some cases the preexisting antibodies participating in hyperacute graft rejection may be specific for blood-group antigens in the graft. If tissue typing and ABO blood-group typing are performed prior to transplanta-tion, these preexisting antibodies can be detected and grafts that would result in hyperacute rejection can be avoided.

① Pre-existing host antibodies are carried to kidney graft

Kidney graft

② Antibodies bind to antigens of renal capillaries and activate complement (C′)

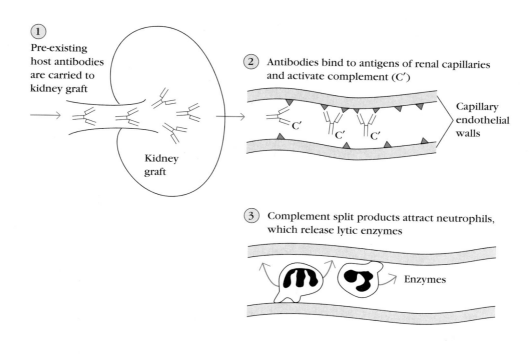

Capillary endothelial walls

③ Complement split products attract neutrophils, which release lytic enzymes

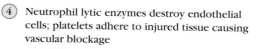

Enzymes

④ Neutrophil lytic enzymes destroy endothelial cells; platelets adhere to injured tissue causing vascular blockage

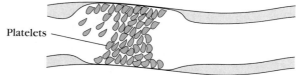

Platelets

FIGURE 23-6

Steps in the hyperacute rejection of a kidney graft. In this type of rejection reaction, the graft never becomes vascularized.

Acute Rejection

Cell-mediated allograft rejection manifests as an acute rejection of the graft beginning about 10 days after transplantation (see Figure 23-1b). Histopathologic examination reveals a massive infiltration of macrophages and lymphocytes at the site of tissue destruction, suggestive of T_H-cell activation and proliferation. Acute graft rejection is effected by the mechanisms described previously (see Figure 23-5).

Chronic Rejection

Chronic rejection reactions develop months or years after acute rejection reactions have subsided. The mechanisms of chronic rejection include both humoral and cell-mediated responses. Chronic rejection reactions are often difficult to manage with immunosuppressive drugs and may necessitate another transplantation.

TISSUE TYPING

Since differences in blood group and major histocompatibility antigens are responsible for the most intense graft rejection reactions, various tissue-typing procedures have been developed to screen potential donor and recipient cells and assess the likelihood of tissue compatibility. Initially, donor and recipient are screened for ABO blood-group compatibility by typing their red blood cell (RBC) antigens (see Figure 17-12). The A, B, and O antigens are expressed on donor RBCs, epithelial cells, and endothelial cells. Antibodies produced in the recipient to any of these antigens that are present on transplanted tissue will induce antibody plus complement lysis of the incompatible cells.

HLA typing of potential donors and a recipient can be accomplished with a microcytotoxicity test (Figure

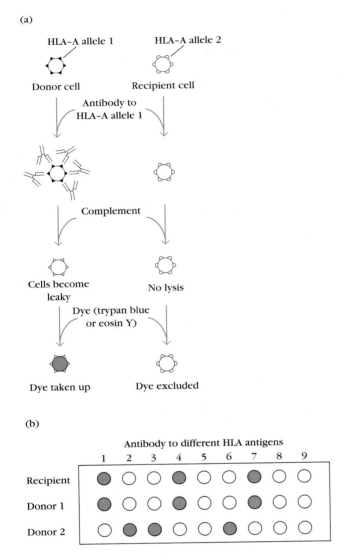

the uptake or exclusion of various dyes (e.g., trypan blue or eosin Y) by the cells. If the white blood cells express the MHC allele for which a particular monoclonal antibody is specific, then the cells will be lysed on addition of complement, and these dead cells will take up a dye such as trypan blue. HLA typing based on antibody-mediated microcytotoxicity can indicate the presence or absence of various MHC alleles.

Even when a fully HLA-compatible donor is not available, transplantation may be successful. In this situation, a one-way mixed-lymphocyte reaction (MLR) can be used to assess quantitatively the degree of class II MHC compatibility between potential donors and a recipient (see Figure 16-13). Lymphocytes from a potential donor that have been x-irradiated or treated with mitomycin C serve as the stimulator cells, and lymphocytes from the recipient serve as responder cells. Proliferation is indicated by the uptake of [^{3}H]thymidine. The greater the class II MHC differences between the donor and recipient cells, the more [^{3}H]thymidine uptake will be observed in an MLR assay. Intense proliferation of the donor lymphocytes indicates a poor prognosis for graft survival. The advantage of the MLR over microcytotoxicity typing is that it gives a better indication of the degree of T$_H$-cell activation generated in response to the class II MHC antigens of the potential graft. The disadvantage of the MLR is that it takes about 6 days to run the assay. If the potential donor is a cadaver, for example, it is not possible to wait 6 days for the results of the MLR, and in that case the microcytotoxicity test must be relied on.

GENERAL IMMUNO-SUPPRESSIVE THERAPY

Allogeneic transplantation requires some degree of immunosuppression if the transplant is to survive. Most of the immunosuppressive treatments that have been developed have the disadvantage of being nonspecific; that is, they result in generalized immunosuppression, which places the recipient at increased risk for infection. In addition, many immunosuppressive measures are aimed at slowing the proliferation of activated lymphocytes. However, because any rapidly dividing nonimmune cells (e.g., epithelial cells of the gut or bone-marrow hematopoietic stem cells) are also affected, serious or even life-threatening complications can occur.

Mitotic Inhibitors

Azathioprine (Imuran), a potent mitotic inhibitor, is often given just before and after transplantation to

FIGURE 23-7

Microcytotoxicity HLA typing. (a) White blood cells from potential donors and the recipient are added to separate wells of a microtiter plate. The example depicts only one HLA antigen on donor and recipient cells and shows the reaction sequence on addition of antibody to one of these antigens. (b) Because cells express numerous HLA antigens, they are separately tested with a battery of monoclonal antibodies specific for various HLA antigens. Here, donor 1 shares antigens 1, 4, and 7 with the recipient, whereas donor 2 has no antigens in common with the recipient.

23-7). In this test white blood cells from the potential donors and recipient are distributed into a separate series of wells on a microtiter plate, and then monoclonal antibodies specific for various class I and class II MHC alleles are added to different wells. After incubation, complement is added to the wells, and cytotoxicity is assessed by

diminish T-cell proliferation in response to the alloantigens of the graft. Azathioprine acts on cells in the S phase of the cell cycle to block synthesis of inosinic acid, which is a precursor of the purines adenylic and guanylic acid. Both B-cell and T-cell proliferation is diminished in the presence of azathioprine. Functional immune assays such as the MLR, CML, and skin test show a significant decline following azathioprine treatment, indicating an overall decrease in T-cell numbers.

Two other mitotic inhibitors that are sometimes used in conjunction with other immunosuppressive agents are cyclophosphamide and methotrexate. **Cyclophosphamide** is an alkylating agent that inserts into the DNA helix and becomes cross-linked, leading to disruption of the DNA chain. It is especially effective against rapidly dividing cells and therefore is sometimes given at the time of grafting to block T-cell proliferation. **Methotrexate** acts as a folic acid antagonist to block purine biosynthesis.

Corticosteroids

As discussed at the end of Chapter 15, corticosteroids are potent anti-inflammatory agents that exert their effects at many levels of the immune response. These drugs are often given to transplant recipients together with a mitotic inhibitor like azathioprine as a treatment for acute episodes of graft rejection.

Cyclosporin A, FK506, and Rapamycin

Cyclosporin A (CsA), FK506, and rapamycin are fungal metabolites with potent immunosuppressive properties. Although chemically unrelated, CsA and FK506 have similar actions. Both drugs block activation of resting T cells by inhibiting the transcription of genes encoding IL-2 and the high-affinity IL-2 receptor (IL-2R), which are essential for activation. As shown in Figure 12-13, CsA and FK506 exert this effect by binding to cytoplasmic proteins called immunophilins, forming a complex that blocks the phosphatase activity of calcineurin. This prevents the formation and nuclear translocation of the cytoplasmic subunit NF-ATc and its subsequent assembly into NF-AT, a DNA-binding protein necessary for transcription of the genes encoding IL-2 and IL-2R (see Figure 12-12). Rapamycin is structurally similar to FK506 and also binds to an immunophilin. However, the rapamycin-immunophilin complex does not inhibit calcineurin activity; instead it blocks the proliferation and differentiation of activated T_H cells in the G_1 phase of the cell cycle. All three drugs, by inhibiting T_H-cell proliferation and thus T_H-cell cytokine expression, reduce the subsequent activation of various effector populations involved in graft rejection, including T_{DTH} cells, T_C cells, NK cells, macrophages, and B cells.

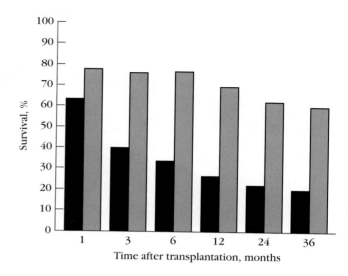

FIGURE 23-8

Comparison of survival rates of liver transplants in 84 patients who were immunosuppressed with azathioprine and corticosteroids (black) and in 55 patients who were immunosuppressed with cyclosporin A and corticosteroids (blue). [Adapted from S. M. Sabesin and J. W. Williams, 1987, *Hosp. Pract.* (July 15):75.]

The profound immunosuppressive properties of these three agents have made them a mainstay in heart, liver, kidney, and bone marrow transplantation. Cyclosporin A has been shown to prolong graft survival in kidney, liver, heart, and heart-lung transplants. In one study of 209 kidney transplants from cadaver donors, the 1-year survival rate was 64% among recipients receiving other immunosuppressive treatments and 80% among those receiving cyclosporin A. Similar results have been obtained with liver transplants (Figure 23-8). Despite these impressive results, cyclosporin A does have some negative side effects, the most notable of which is its toxicity to the kidneys. Acute nephrotoxicity is quite common, in some cases progressing to chronic nephrotoxicity and drug-induced kidney failure. FK506 and rapamycin are newer drugs and require longer experience in clinical trials before a full assessment of their merits can be made. They are 10–100 times more potent as immune suppressants than CsA and therefore can be administered at lower doses and consequently have fewer side effects than CsA.

Total Lymphoid Irradiation

Because lymphocytes are extremely sensitive to x-rays, x-irradiation can be used to eliminate recipient lymphocytes before grafting. In total lymphoid x-irradiation the recipient receives multiple x-ray exposures to the thymus, spleen, and lymph nodes and then receives the transplant. The typical protocol involves daily x-irradiation treatments of about 200 rads per day for several weeks until a total of 3400 rads has been administered. The recipient is grafted in this immunosuppressed state. Because the bone marrow is not x-irradiated, lymphoid stem cells proliferate and renew the population of recirculating lymphocytes. These newly formed lymphocytes appear to be more tolerant to the antigens of the graft.

SPECIFIC IMMUNO-SUPPRESSIVE THERAPY

The major limitation with each of the immunosuppressive treatments discussed thus far is that they lack specificity, thus producing a more-or-less generalized immunosuppression and increasing the recipient's risk for infection. Ideally what is needed is an antigen-specific immunosuppressant that will reduce the immune response to the alloantigens of the graft while preserving the response to unrelated antigens. Although this goal has not yet been achieved, steps are being made toward increasing the specificity of immunosuppression.

Monoclonal Antibodies to T-Cell Components or Cytokines

Thus far, monoclonal antibodies have been used successfully to suppress T-cell activity in general or to suppress the activity of broad subpopulations of T cells. The technology has not yet advanced to the point of using monoclonal antibodies to suppress only alloantigen-activated T cells, but animal models suggest that monoclonal antibodies are the immune suppressors of the future.

Monoclonal antibody to the CD3 molecule of the TCR complex has been shown in some cases to block T-cell activation. Injection of such monoclonal antibodies results in a rapid depletion of T cells from the circulation. This depletion appears to be caused by binding of antibody-coated T cells to Fc receptors on phagocytic cells, which then phagocytose and clear the T cells from the circulation. The success of anti-CD3 monoclonal antibody in reversing rejection episodes in animal models has led to its approval by the Food and Drug Administration for clinical trials. In some cases, anti-CD3 has reversed acute rejection in human patients.

Monoclonal antibodies specific for the high-affinity IL-2 receptor (anti-TAC) also have been used successfully to increase graft survival. Since the high-affinity IL-2 receptor is expressed only on activated T cells, exposure to anti-TAC following grafting should specifically block proliferation of T cells activated in response to the alloantigens of the graft. In one experiment, treatment of mice and rats with anti-TAC monoclonal antibody

TABLE 23-1

EFFECT OF TREATMENT WITH ANTI-TAC MONOCLONAL ANTIBODY* ON SURVIVAL OF CARDIAC ALLOGRAFTS IN RATS

ANTI-TAC DOSE (μG/KG/DAY)	TREATMENT PERIOD (DAYS AFTER GRAFTING)	MEAN GRAFT SURVIVAL IN DAYS (RANGE)
—	—	8 (4–9)
25	0–9	13 (12–14)
100	0–9	14 (13–16)
300	0–9	20 (20–21)
300	5–9	17 (15–26)
300	5–9/15–19	27 (26–28)

* Anti-TAC binds to the IL-2 receptor.

SOURCE: Data from J. W. Kupiec-Weglinski et al., 1986 *Proc. Nat'l. Acad. Sci. USA* **83**:2624.

markedly increased the acceptance of cardiac and kidney transplants from allogeneic donors (Table 23-1).

Both CD3 and the high-affinity IL-2 receptor are expressed on all activated T cells. Monoclonal antibodies specific for membrane molecules that are present only on particular T-cell subpopulations also have been developed. For example, monoclonal antibody to CD4 has been shown to prolong graft survival. In one study, monkeys were given a single large dose of anti-CD4 just before they received a kidney transplant. Graft survival in the anti-CD4–treated animals was markedly increased compared with that in untreated control animals. Interestingly, the anti-CD4 did not reduce the CD4$^+$ T-cell count but instead appeared to induce the T cells to enter an immunosuppressed state.

Simultaneous treatment for 6 days following transplantation with monoclonal antibodies to the adhesion molecules ICAM-1 and LFA-1 permitted indefinite survival of cardiac grafts between allogeneic mice. However, when either monoclonal antibody was administered alone, the cardiac transplant was rejected. The requirement that both monoclonal antibodies be given at the same time is thought to reflect the redundancy of adhesion molecules: LFA-1 is known to bind to ICAM-2 in addition to ICAM-1; and ICAM-1 is known to bind to Mac-1 and CD43 in addition to LFA-1. Only when both pairs are blocked at the same time will adhesion and signal transduction through this ligand pair be blocked.

Monoclonal antibody therapy, which usually is employed to deplete or inactivate T cells in graft recipients, also has been used to treat bone marrow before it is transplanted. Such treatment is designed to deplete the immunocompetent T cells in the bone marrow transplant, which can cause graft-versus-host disease (discussed later). The effectiveness of an anti–T-cell monoclonal antibody in reducing T-cell populations can be maximized by selecting monoclonal antibody isotypes that are good activators of the complement system.

One difficulty with monoclonal antibody intervention for prolonging graft survival is that the antibodies are generally of mouse origin. The recipient often develops an antibody response to the mouse monoclonal antibody, rapidly clearing it from the body. To avoid this limitation, human monoclonal antibodies and mouse-human chimeric antibodies (see Figure 5-25) are being evaluated in experimental trials.

Because cytokines appear to play an important role in allograft rejection, another strategy to prolong graft survival is to inject animals with monoclonal antibodies specific for the implicated cytokines, particularly TNF-α, IFN-γ, and IL-2. Monoclonal antibodies to TNF-α have been shown to prolong bone marrow transplants in mice and to reduce the incidence of graft-versus-host disease. Monoclonal antibodies to IFN-γ and to IL-2 have each been reported in some cases to prolong cardiac transplants in rats. Anti-cytokine antibodies have not yet been used in human transplantations.

Agents That Block the Co-stimulatory Signal

As discussed in Chapter 12, T_H-cell activation requires a co-stimulatory signal in addition to the signal mediated by the T-cell receptor. One such co-stimulatory signal is mediated by interaction of the B7 molecule on the membrane of antigen-presenting cells with the CD28 or CTLA-4 molecule on T cells (see Figure 12-14). In the absence of a co-stimulatory signal, antigen-activated T cells become anergic (see Figure 12-15). CD28 is expressed on both resting and activated T cells and binds B7 with a moderate affinity; CTLA-4 is expressed at much lower levels and only on activated T cells but binds B7 with a 20-fold higher affinity.

Demonstration of the B7-mediated co-stimulatory signal suggests that blocking the co-stimulatory signal following transplantation would cause the host's T cells to become anergic, thus enabling the grafted tissue to survive. D. J. Lenschow, J. A. Bluestone, and colleagues tested this approach by transplanting human pancreatic islets into mice that were injected with CTLA-4Ig, a soluble fusion protein consisting of the extracellular domains of CTLA-4 and the constant region of the IgG1 heavy chain. (Inclusion of the IgG1 heavy-chain constant region increases the half-life of the soluble fusion protein.) The xenogeneic graft exhibited long-term survival in

treated mice but was quickly rejected in untreated controls. Presumably, the soluble CTLA-4Ig binds to B7 on antigen-presenting cells, so the co-stimulatory signal is not generated when host T cells recognize the graft antigens.

Donor-Cell Microchimerism

Immunosuppressive drugs act not only by blocking T-cell activation but also by inducing host tolerance to the allogeneic cells. As a result of this tolerance, donor leukocytes can migrate from a graft and survive within the recipient, producing a state of long-term **microchimerism** in the recipient. Several studies have demonstrated that long-term transplant survivors exhibit donor-cell microchimerism, prompting the suggestion that graft acceptance depends upon establishment of a microchimeric state.

Evidence that microchimerism plays an important role in graft acceptance first came from studies of long-term survivors of kidney transplants. Five individuals who were among the original kidney transplant patients in the 1960s were examined in 1992. Biopsies on the still functioning kidney grafts revealed that the interstitial cells of the allograft were from the recipient, whereas the nephrons were from the donor. In addition, this study revealed the presence of dendritic cells from the donor in the skin and lymph nodes of the recipient. Another study conducted in 1992 involved 25 individuals who had received liver transplants 2–22 years previously and had been immunosuppressed with azathioprine or cyclosporin A. Examination of these individuals revealed donor-cell microchimerism in the skin, lymph nodes, heart, lungs, spleen, intestine, kidneys, bone marrow, and thymus. Although there were relatively few donor cells at each site, the widespread distribution of these donor cells suggests that substantial numbers of them survive within the recipient.

The growing awareness of the importance of microchimerism in graft acceptance suggests that administration of immunosuppressive drugs may be discontinued once a stable chimera is achieved. A 1993 report of 44 human liver transplant recipients who had survived 11–23 years revealed that 6 had stopped taking all immunosuppressive drugs and yet remained clinically stable. These findings led to initiation of clinical trials, which are currently under way, to determine if immunosuppressive drugs can be slowly eliminated without inducing graft rejection in liver transplant recipients after chimerism is established.

The mechanism by which microchimerism leads to immune suppression and graft acceptance remains to be determined. T. E. Starzl and coworkers believe that graft success depends upon both the migration of recipient leukocytes into the graft and the migration of donor leukocytes out from the graft. The net effect would be a two-directional immune reaction leading to immunologic tolerance to the alloantigens of the graft. Because dendritic cells are the major cell type in the chimeras, it has been suggested that they may function as APCs inducing a state of tolerance in the alloreactive T_H cells.

CLINICAL TRANSPLANTATION

The clinical results of transplantation of various cells, tissues, and organs in humans have improved considerably in the past few years, largely because of the use of immunosuppressive agents such as cyclosporin A. Nowadays, kidney and corneal transplantations are performed with high success rates; heart, lung, and liver transplantations are accomplished with somewhat lower, but still promising, success rates. In contrast, transplantations of bone marrow and pancreas exhibit even lower rates of success and are performed as a last resort only after other treatment possibilities have been exhausted.

Bone Marrow Transplants

Since the early 1980s bone marrow transplantation has been increasingly adopted as a therapy for a number of malignant and nonmalignant hematologic diseases, including leukemia, lymphoma, aplastic anemia, thalassemia major, and immunodeficiency diseases in general. In 1990, over 4000 allogeneic bone marrow transplantations were performed. The bone marrow, which is obtained from a donor by multiple needle aspirations, consists of erythroid, myeloid, monocytoid, megakaryocytic, and lymphocytic lineages. The graft, which usually consists of about 10^9 cells per kilogram of host body weight, is injected intravenously into the recipient. The first successful bone marrow transplantations were performed between identical twins. However, development of the tissue-typing procedures described earlier now makes it possible to identify allogeneic donors with identical or near-identical HLA antigens as the recipients.

In the usual procedure, the recipient of a bone marrow transplant is immunologically suppressed before grafting. Leukemia patients, for example, are often treated with cyclophosphamide and total-body irradiation to kill all cancerous cells. The immune-suppressed state of the recipient makes graft rejection rare; however, because the donor bone marrow contains immunocompetent cells, the graft may reject the host, causing **graft-versus-host disease** (GVHD). This is quite common in bone marrow transplantation, affecting between 50% and 70% of transplant patients. Graft-versus-host disease develops as

donor T cells recognize alloantigens on the host cells. The activation and proliferation of these T cells and the subsequent production of cytokines generate inflammatory reactions in the skin, gastrointestinal tract, and liver. If it is severe, GVHD can result in generalized erythroderma of the skin, gastrointestinal hemorrhage, and liver failure.

GVHD involves both an activation phase and an effector phase. In the activation phase, T_H cells from the donor bone marrow recognize recipient peptide-MHC complexes displayed on antigen-presenting cells. Antigen presentation, together with a co-stimulatory signal, induces donor T_H-cell activation, production of IL-2, and proliferation. Cytokines elaborated by the activated donor T_H cells induce the effector phase of GVHD by activating a variety of secondary effector cells including NK cells, CTLs, and macrophages. Although CTLs can act directly to cause tissue damage, cytokines such as TNF may play a more important role in the effector phase of GVHD. TNF, which is released by a variety of cells (e.g., T_H cells, CTLs, NK cells, and macrophages), has been shown to mediate direct cytolytic damage to cells. The role that TNF plays in GVHD in mice is demonstrated by the ability of monoclonal antibody to TNF to block the development of GVHD following bone marrow transplantation in mice.

Various treatments are used to prevent GVHD in bone marrow transplantation. The transplant recipient is usually placed on a regimen of immunosuppressive drugs, which often includes cyclosporin A and methotrexate. Another approach has been to treat the donor bone marrow with anti-T-cell antisera or monoclonal antibodies specific for T cells before transplantation, thereby depleting the offending T cells. Complete T-cell depletion from donor bone marrow, however, makes it more likely that the marrow will be rejected, and so the usual procedure now is a partial T-cell depletion. Apparently a low level of donor T-cell activity, which results in a low-level GVHD, is actually beneficial because it prevents any residual host T cells from becoming sensitized to the graft. In leukemia patients low-level GVHD also seems to result in destruction of leukemic cells, thus making it less likely for the leukemia to recur.

Organ Transplants

The impact of basic scientific research on clinical medicine is highlighted by the success rates for organ transplantation. In the case of kidney transplants, the survival rate in 1967 was 45%; by the early 1990s, the rate had been improved to about 90%. Currently more than 10,000 kidney transplantations are performed every year in the United States. Heart, heart-lung, and liver transplantations are also being done with remarkable success

TABLE 23-2

SURVIVAL RATES FOR ORGAN ALLOGRAFTS IN HUMANS

ORGAN ALLOGRAFT	1-YEAR SURVIVAL RATE (%)
Kidney (sibling)	90
Kidney (cadaver)	80
Heart	80
Heart-lung	74
Liver	70
Pancreas	40

SOURCE: J. R. Batchelor and Y. L. Chai, 1986, *Prog. Immunol.* **6**:1002.

(Table 23-2). A number of other experimental transplantations (e.g., of the pancreas and parts of the intestine) have been performed but have not yet attained a level of success that warrants widespread application.

Several factors have contributed to the increase in successful organ transplants, most notably HLA typing and immunosuppressive treatments. Comparisons of HLA antigen differences and graft survival have shown that matching of the class II D antigens is most important for success. The data in Figure 23-9, for example, reveal that survival of kidney grafts depends primarily on donor-recipient matching of the HLA-D antigens; matching or mismatching of the class I HLA-A and HLA-B antigens has little effect on graft survival unless there also is mismatching of the D antigens. In heart transplants, due to a shortage of transplantable organs and insufficient time, it is not possible to match HLA antigens prior to grafting. In order to assess the effect that differences in HLA antigens have on heart-transplant success, a number of studies have compared HLA antigen differences to graft-recipient survival rates. In one study of heart-transplant recipients, the 1000-day survival rate of the recipients was 90% when there was a single mismatch in HLA-DR antigens between the donor and recipient; the survival rate dropped to 65% when two HLA-DR antigens were mismatched.

An important finding that has emerged from experimental transplant models is that the critical period for graft rejection is from 2 to 4 weeks after grafting. If immunosuppressive drugs or monoclonal antibody therapy can prevent graft rejection during this critical period, when acute graft rejection would normally occur, then the prognosis for long-term graft survival improves dramatically. A number of reasons have been suggested for the decrease in immunogenicity shown by grafts that survive the critical period. One suggestion is that passenger leukocytes leave the graft, home to draining lymph nodes, and induce immune activation soon after grafting. If immune activation is decreased with immunosuppressive drugs or monoclonal antibodies until these allogeneic leukocytes die off, the potential for immune activation will dramatically decrease. There is also some speculation that, with time, continual alloantigen expression by the graft may induce a state of immunologic tolerance.

Transplantation of human pancreatic islet cells has been shown to reverse insulin-dependent diabetes mellitus, which is caused by degeneration of the insulin-producing islet cells of the pancreas. In the past, however, islet-cell allografts have often been rejected, even when the recipient is given potent immunosuppressive therapy. In an attempt to find a way to reduce rejection of islet-cell grafts, A. M. Posselt, A. Naji, and their colleagues injected rat pancreatic islet cells directly into the thymus of an allogeneic diabetic recipient rat. They found that the allogeneic islet cells survived indefinitely in the recipient, suggesting that the presence of alloantigens in the thymus induced the host's developing thymocytes to become tolerant to the alloantigens on the islet cells. This novel approach, reported in 1990, may well be applicable to other types of transplants and offers the promise of significantly improving graft survival rates without compromising the recipient's immune system.

Xenotransplants

In recent years, the supply of organs available for transplantation has fallen far short of the number of patients requiring transplants. As a result, nearly 60% of patients have died while still waiting for a transplant. The need for an alternative source of donor organs has focused attention on **xenotransplantation**. Primates (chimpanzees, monkeys, and baboons) have served as the main transplant donors, with the earliest xenotransplants of chimpanzee kidney into humans dating to 1964. To date kidney, heart, liver, and bone marrow xenotransplants from primates into humans have been performed.

Clinical results with primate transplants into humans have so far been disappointing. In 1993 T. E. Starzl performed two transplants from baboons into patients suffering from liver failure. Both patients died, one after 26 days and the other after 70 days. In 1994 a pig liver was transplanted into a 26-year-old suffering from acute hepatic failure. The liver functioned only 30 hours before it was rejected by a hyperacute rejection reaction. In 1995 baboon bone marrow was infused into an HIV-infected man with the aim of boosting his weakened immune system with immune cells that do not become infected with the virus. Although there were no complications from the

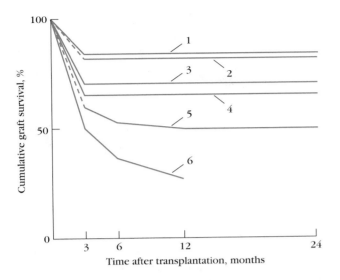

Curve no.	HLA mismatches (no.)	
	A,B	D
1	0	0
2	1 or 2	0
3	3 or 4	0
4	0	1 or 2
5	1 or 2	1 or 2
6	3 or 4	1 or 2

FIGURE 23-9

The effect of HLA-A, -B and -D antigen matching on survival of kidney grafts. Mismatching of HLA-A or HLA-B antigens has little effect on graft survival unless HLA-D is also mismatched. [Adapted from T. Moen et al., 1980, *N. Engl. J. Med.* **303**:850.]

transplant, the baboon bone marrow did not appear to establish itself in the recipient.

The major problem with xenotransplants is that immune rejection is often quite vigorous, even when recipients are treated with potent immunosuppressive drugs like FK506 or rapamycin. The major immune rejection response involves the production of humoral antibody and complement with the development of a hyperacute rejection reaction. One possible approach for limiting destruction mediated by antibody and complement is to produce transgenic donor animals expressing human decay-accelerating factor (DAF), which prevents activation of C3 and C5 (see Figure 14-8d). The presence of human DAF on donor cells should reduce the severity of the hyperacute rejection reaction to the graft. This approach is being tried with 35 transgenic pigs produced to express human DAF. Grafts from these animals will be evaluated in human clinical trials in the next few years.

There are other reasons why pigs are currently under consideration as potential transplant donors. They breed rapidly, have large litters, can be housed in pathogen-free environments, and share a considerable number of anatomic and physiologic similarities with humans. Although primates are more closely related to humans than pigs, the availability of primates as transplant donors is quite limited. One investment analyst predicts that within a few years there will be 50,000 pig heart transplants and 40,000 pig kidney transplants into humans each year.

A major concern with xenotransplantation is the potential for the spread of pathogens from the donor to the recipient. These diseases, called **xenozoonoses**, could potentially cause deadly infections in humans. A number of viral diseases, of limited pathogenicity in primates, have been shown to cause deadly infections in humans. Many scientists warn of the risk of introducing a new primate pathogen into the human population, through xenotransplantation, and caution against moving too rapidly into this new field of transplantation.

Transplants to Immunologically Privileged Sites

There are certain sites in the body, called **immunologically privileged sites**, where an allograft can be placed without engendering a rejection reaction. These sites include the anterior chamber of the eye, the cornea, the cheek pouch of the Syrian hamster, the uterus, the testes, and the brain. Each of these sites is characterized by an absence of lymphatic vessels and sometimes an absence of blood vessels as well. Consequently, the alloantigens of the graft are not generally able to sensitize the recipient's lymphocytes, and the graft shows an increased likelihood of acceptance, even when HLA antigens are not matched.

The privileged location of the cornea has allowed cornea transplants to be highly successful. The brain is another immunologically privileged site because the blood-brain barrier prevents the entry and exit of many molecules into or out of the brain. Transplantations of fetal brain-stem neurons into primates has shown some promise in reducing the symptoms of Parkinson's disease, and human fetal neurons have been transplanted into several patients with Parkinson's disease. The successful transplantation of allogeneic pancreatic islet cells into the thymus, discussed in the preceding section, has led to the speculation that the thymus may also be an immunologically privileged site.

Immunologically privileged sites fail to induce an immune response because they are effectively sequestered from the cells of the immune system. This suggests the possibility of experimentally sequestering grafted cells. In one study, pancreatic islet cells were encapsulated in semipermeable membranes (fabricated from an acrylic copolymer) and then transplanted into diabetic mice. The islet cells survived and produced insulin. The transplanted cells were not rejected because the recipient's immune cells could not penetrate the encapsulating semipermeable membrane. This novel transplant method enabled the diabetic mice to produce normal levels of insulin.

SUMMARY

1. Graft rejection is an immunologic response displaying the attributes of specificity, memory, and self/nonself recognition. In hyperacute rejection, preexisting host antibodies react with graft antigens, leading to an inflammatory response that prevents vascularization of the graft and its loss within a day. An acute rejection reaction, which is the most common type of graft rejection, involves the cell-mediated branch of the immune system with tissue damage mediated by T_{DTH} cells and/or CTLs (see Figure 23-5). Acute response to an allograft exhibits immunologic memory, with a more rapid second-set rejection than first-set rejection (see Figure 23-1), and can be transferred (see Figure 23-2).

2. The immune response is generated to tissue antigens on the transplanted tissue that differ from those of the host. Although more than 40 different loci encode such antigens, the loci responsible for the most vigorous graft-rejection reactions are contained within the major histocompatibility complex (MHC), called the HLA complex in humans. Even when a donor and a recipient have identical HLA antigens, differences in minor histocompatibility loci outside the MHC can contribute to graft rejection.

3. The process of graft rejection can be divided into a sensitization stage and an effector stage (see Figure 23-4). During the sensitization stage, passenger leukocytes, derived from the donor graft, migrate from the graft to the regional lymph nodes, where they are recognized as foreign by the recipient's T_H cells, stimulating T_H-cell proliferation. Following T_H-cell proliferation, a population of effector cells is generated, which migrates to the graft and mediates graft rejection.

4. The degree to which a recipient and potential graft donors are matched for MHC antigens can be assessed by tissue typing. In the microcytotoxicity test, monoclonal antibodies are used to detect the presence of various class I and class II MHC antigens on donor and recipient cells (see Figure 23-7). The more MHC antigens that a donor and recipient have in common, the more likely is a graft to survive. The mixed-lymphocyte reaction (MLR) can be used to quantitatively assess the class II MHC compatibility of a recipient and potential donors (see Figure 16-13).

5. Graft rejection can be suppressed by specific and nonspecific immunosuppressive agents. Nonspecific agents include mitotic inhibitors (purine analogs), corticosteroids, cyclosporin A, and total lymphoid x-irradiation. Experimental approaches using monoclonal antibodies offer the possibility of specific immunosuppression. These approaches include blocking proliferation of antigen-activated T cells with monoclonal antibodies to the IL-2 receptor or depletion of T-cell populations with monoclonal antibodies to CD3 or CD4. Another new approach that offers considerable promise is blocking the co-stimulatory signal by binding of inhibitors that interfere with the interaction of B7 and CD28 or CTLA-4. In the absence of this co-stimulatory signal, antigen-activated T_H cells become anergic.

6. A major complication in bone marrow transplantation is a graft-versus-host reaction mediated by the lymphocytes contained within the donor marrow. T-cell depletion from the donor marrow with antibody specific for T-cell populations reduces the risk of graft-versus-host disease. Transplantations of a variety of organs are being performed with remarkable success. HLA typing together with immunosuppressive therapy have contributed to the high success rate for organ transplants.

REFERENCES

COLVIN, R. B. 1990. Cellular and molecular mechanisms of allograft rejection. *Annu. Rev. Med.* **41**:361.

FERRARA, J. J. M., AND H. J. DEEG. 1991. Graft-versus-host disease. *N. Engl. J. Med.* **324**:667.

ISOBE, M., H. YAGITA, K. OKUMURA, AND A. IHARA. 1992. Specific acceptance of cardiac allograft after treatment with antibodies to ICAM-1 and LFA-1. *Science* **255**:1125.

KAUFMAN, C. L., B. GAINES, AND S. T. ILDSTAD. 1995. Xenotransplantation. *Annu. Rev. Immunol.* **13**:339.

LACY, P. E., ET AL. 1991. Maintenance of normoglycemia in diabetic mice by subcutaneous xenografts of encapsulated islets. *Science* **254**:1972.

LENSCHOW, D. J., ET AL. 1992. Long-term survival of xenogeneic pancreatic islets induced by CTLA-4Ig. *Science* **257**:789.

PARKMAN, R. 1991. The biology of bone marrow transplantation for severe combined immune deficiency. *Adv. Immunol.* **49**:381.

POSSELT, A. M., ET AL. 1990. Induction of donor-specific unresponsiveness by intrathymic islet transplantation. *Science* **249**:1293.

ROSENBERG, A. S., AND A. SINGER. 1992. Cellular basis of skin allograft rejection: an in vivo model of immune-mediated tissue destruction. *Annu. Rev. Immunol.* **10**:333.

SHERMAN, L. A., AND S. CHATTOPADHYAY. 1993. The molecular basis of allorecognition. *Annu. Rev. Immunol.* **11**:385.

SIGAL, N. H., AND F. J. DUMONT. 1992. Cyclosporin A, FK-506, and rapamycin: pharmacologic probes of lymphocyte signal transduction. *Annu. Rev. Immunol.* **10**:519.

STARZL, T. E., ET AL. 1993. Donor-cell chimerism permitted by immunosuppressive drugs: a new view of organ transplantation. *Immunol. Today* **14**:326.

STEELE, D. J., AND H. AUCHINCLOSS. 1995. Xenotransplantation. *Annu. Rev. Med.* **46**:345.

STUDY QUESTIONS

1. Indicate whether each of the following statements is true or false. If you think a statement is false, explain why.

a. Acute rejection is mediated by preexisting host antibodies specific for antigens on the grafted tissue.

b. Second-set rejection is a manifestation of immunologic memory.

c. Passenger leukocytes are host dendritic cells that migrate into grafted tissue and act as antigen-presenting cells.

d. All allografts between individuals with identical HLA haplotypes will be accepted.

e. Cytokines produced by host T_H cells activated in response to alloantigens play a major role in graft rejection.

2. You are a pediatrician treating a child who needs a kidney transplant. The child does not have an identical twin, but both parents and several siblings will donate a kidney if the MHC match with the patient is good.

a. What is the best possible MHC match that could be achieved in this situation?

b. In which relative(s) might you find it? Why?

c. What test(s) would you perform in order to find the best-matched kidney?

3. Indicate in the Response column in the accompanying table whether a skin graft from each donor to each recipient listed would result in a rejection (R) or an acceptance (A) response. If you believe a rejection reaction would occur, then indicate in the right-hand column whether it would be a first-set rejection (FSR), occurring in 12–14 days, or a second-set rejection (SSR), occurring in 5–6 days. All the mouse strains listed in the table have different H-2 haplotypes.

4. Graft-versus-host disease(GVHD) frequently develops after certain types of transplantations.

a. Briefly outline the mechanisms involved in GVHD.

b. Under what conditions is GVHD likely to occur?

c. Some researchers have found that GVHD can be diminished by prior treatment of the graft with monoclonal antibody plus complement or with monoclonal antibody conjugated to toxins. List at

For use with Question 3.

DONOR	RECIPIENT	RESPONSE	TYPE OF REJECTION
BALB/c	C3H		
BALB/c	Rat		
BALB/c	Nude mouse		
BALB/c	C3H, had previous BALB/c graft		
BALB/c	C3H, had previous C57BL/6 graft		
BALB/c	BALB/c		
BALB/c	(BALB/c × C3H)F_1		
BALB/c	(C3H × C57BL/6)F_1		
(BALB/c × C3H)F_1	BALB/c		
(BALB/c × C3H)F_1	BALB/c, had previous F_1 graft		

For use with Question 5a.

	ABO TYPE	HLA-A TYPE	HLA-B TYPE	HLA-C TYPE
RECIPIENT	O	A1/A2	B8/B12	CW3
POTENTIAL DONORS:				
Mother	A	A1/A2	B8/B12	Cw1/Cw3
Father	O	A2	B12/B15	Cw3
Sibling A	O	A1/A2	B8/B15	Cw3
Sibling B	O	A2	B12	Cw1/Cw3
Sibling C	O	A1/A2	B8/B12	Cw3
Sibling D	A	A1/A2	B8/B12	Cw3
Sibling E	O	A1/A2	B8/B15	Cw3

least two cell-surface antigens to which monoclonal antibodies could be prepared and used for this purpose, and give the rationale for your choices.

5. A child who requires a kidney transplant has been offered a kidney from both parents and from five siblings.

a. Cells from the potential donors are screened with monoclonal antibodies to the HLA-A, –B, and –C antigens in a microcytotoxicity assay. In addition, ABO blood-group typing is performed. Based on the results in the accompanying table, a kidney graft from which donor(s) is most likely to survive?

b. Now a one-way MLR is performed using various combinations of mitomycin-treated lymphocytes. The results, expressed as counts per minute of [3H]thymidine incorporated, are shown in the accompanying table; the stimulation index is listed below in parentheses. Based on these data, a graft from which donor(s) is most likely to be accepted?

For use with Question 5b.

RESPONDER CELLS	MITOMYCIN C-TREATED STIMULATOR CELLS					
	PATIENT	SIB A	SIB B	SIB C	SIB D	SIB E
Patient	1,672 (1.0)	1,800 (1.1)	13,479 (8.1)	5,210 (3.1)	13,927 (8.3)	13,808 (8.3)
Sib A	1,495 (1.6)	933 (1.0)	11,606 (12.4)	8,443 (9.1)	11,708 (12.6)	13,430 (14.4)
Sib B	25,418 (9.9)	26,209 (10.2)	2,570 (1.0)	13,170 (5.1)	19,722 (7.7)	4,510 (1.8)
Sib C	10,722 (6.2)	10,714 (5.9)	13,032 (7.5)	1,731 (1.0)	1,740 (1.0)	14,365 (8.3)
Sib D	15,988 (5.1)	13,492 (4.2)	18,519 (5.9)	3,300 (1.1)	3,151 (1.0)	18,334 (5.9)
Sib E	5,777 (6.5)	8,053 (9.1)	2,024 (2.3)	6,895 (7.8)	10,720 (12.1)	888 (1.0)

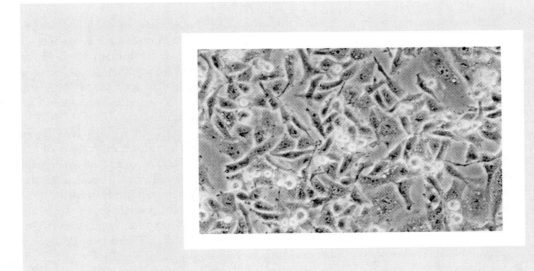

CANCER AND THE IMMUNE SYSTEM

As the death toll from infectious disease has declined in the Western world, cancer has become the second-ranking cause of death, led only by heart disease. Current estimates project that one person in three in the United States will develop cancer, and that one person in five will die from cancer. From an immunologic perspective, cancer cells can be viewed as altered self-cells that have escaped normal growth-regulating mechanisms. This chapter examines the unique properties of cancer cells, paying particular attention to those properties that can be recognized by the immune system. The immune

responses that develop to cancer cells, as well as the methods by which cancers manage to evade those responses, are then described. Finally, current clinical and experimental immunotherapies for cancer are discussed.

CANCER: ORIGIN AND TERMINOLOGY

In a mature animal, a balance is usually maintained between cell renewal and cell death in most organs and tissues. The various types of mature cells in the body have a given life span; as these cells die, new cells are generated by the proliferation and differentiation of various types of stem cells. Under normal circumstances, the production of new cells is so regulated that the numbers of any particular type of cell remain constant. Occasionally, though, cells arise that are no longer responsive to normal growth-control mechanisms. These cells give rise to clones of cells that can expand to a considerable size, producing a **tumor**, or **neoplasm**.

A tumor that is not capable of indefinite growth and does not invade the healthy surrounding tissue extensively is **benign**. A tumor that continues to grow and becomes progressively invasive is **malignant**; the term **cancer** refers specifically to a malignant tumor. In addition to uncontrolled growth, malignant tumors exhibit **metastasis**; in this process, small clusters of cancerous cells dislodge from a tumor, invade the blood or lymphatic vessels, and are carried to other tissues, where they continue to proliferate. In this way a primary tumor at one site can give rise to a secondary tumor at another site (Figure 24-1).

Malignant tumors are classified according to the embryonic origin of the tissue from which the tumor is derived. **Carcinomas** are tumors arising from endodermal or ectodermal tissues such as skin or the epithelial lining of internal organs and glands. **Sarcomas**, which arise less frequently, are derived from mesodermal connective tissues such as bone, fat, and cartilage. The **leukemias** and **lymphomas** are malignant tumors of hematopoietic cells of the bone marrow. Leukemias proliferate as single cells, whereas lymphomas tend to grow as tumor masses.

MALIGNANT TRANSFORMATION OF CELLS

Treatment of normal cultured cells with chemical carcinogens, irradiation, and certain viruses can alter the morphology and growth properties of the cells. In some cases this process, referred to as **transformation**, makes the cells able to induce tumors when they are injected into animals. Such cells are said to have undergone **malignant transformation**, and they often exhibit in vitro culture properties similar to those of cancer cells. For example, they have decreased requirements for growth factors and serum, are no longer anchorage-dependent, and grow in a density-independent fashion. Moreover, both cancer cells and transformed cells can be subcultured indefinitely; that is, they are **immortal**. Because of the similar properties of cancer and transformed cells, the process of malignant transformation has been studied extensively as a model of cancer induction.

Various chemical agents (e.g., DNA-alkylating reagents) and physical agents (e.g., ultraviolet light and ionizing radiation) that cause mutations have been shown to induce transformation. Induction of malignant transformation with such chemical or physical carcinogens appears to involve multiple steps and at least two distinct phases: **initiation** and **promotion**. Initiation involves changes in the genome but does not, in itself, lead to malignant transformation. Following initiation, promoters stimulate cell division and lead to malignant transformation.

The importance of mutagenesis in the induction of cancer is illustrated in certain diseases such as xeroderma pigmentosum. This rare disease in humans is caused by a defect in the gene encoding a DNA-repair enzyme called UV-specific endonuclease. Individuals with this disease are unable to repair UV-induced mutations and consequently develop skin cancers.

A number of DNA and RNA viruses have been shown to induce malignant transformation. Two of the best-studied DNA viruses known to cause malignant transformation are SV40 and polyoma. In both cases the viral genomes, which integrate randomly into the host chromosomal DNA, include several genes that are expressed early in the course of viral replication. SV40 encodes two early proteins called T and t, and polyoma encodes three early proteins called T, mid-T, and t. Each of these proteins plays a role in malignant transformation of virus-infected cells.

Most RNA viruses replicate in the cytoplasm and do not induce malignant transformation. The exceptions are retroviruses, which transcribe their RNA into DNA by means of a reverse transcriptase enzyme and then integrate the DNA transcript into the host's chromosomal DNA. This process is similar in the cytopathic retroviruses such as HIV-1 and HIV-2 and in the transforming retroviruses, which induce changes in the host cell that lead to malignant transformation. In some cases, retrovirus-induced transformation is related to the presence of **oncogenes**, or "cancer genes," carried by the retrovirus.

One of the best-studied transforming retroviruses is the **Rous sarcoma virus**. This virus carries an oncogene called v-*src*, which encodes a 60-kDa protein kinase (v-Src) that catalyzes the addition of phosphate to tyrosine residues on proteins. The first evidence that oncogenes alone could induce malignant transformation came from studies on the v-*src* oncogene from Rous sarcoma virus. When the v-*src* oncogene from Rous sarcoma virus was cloned and transfected into normal cells in culture, the cells underwent malignant transformation.

ONCOGENES AND CANCER INDUCTION

In 1971 Howard Temin suggested that oncogenes might not be unique to transforming viruses but might also be found in normal cells; indeed, he proposed that oncogenes might be acquired by a virus from the genome of an infected cell. He called these cellular genes **proto-oncogenes**, or **cellular oncogenes** (c-*onc*), to distinguish them from their viral counterpart (v-*onc*). In the

Visualizing Concepts

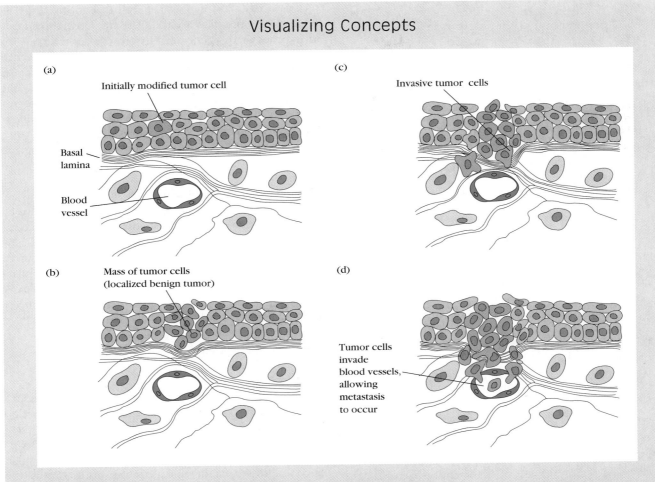

FIGURE 24-1

Tumor growth and metastasis. (a) A single cell develops altered growth properties at a tissue site. (b) The altered cell proliferates, forming a mass of localized tumor cells, or benign tumor. (c) The tumor cells become progressively more invasive, invading the underlying basal lamina. The tumor is now classified as malignant. (d) The malignant tumor metastasizes by generating small clusters of cancer cells that dislodge from the tumor and are carried by the blood or lymph to other sites in the body. [Adapted from J. Darnell et al., 1990, *Molecular Cell Biology*, 2d ed., Scientific American Books.]

mid–1970s J. M. Bishop and H. E. Varmus identified a homologous DNA sequence in normal chicken cells that is homologous to v-*src* from Rous sarcoma virus. This cellular oncogene was designated c-*src*. Since these early discoveries, numerous cellular oncogenes have been identified.

Sequence comparisons of viral and cellular oncogenes reveal that they are highly conserved in evolution. Although most cellular oncogenes consist of a series of exons and introns, their viral counterparts consist of uninterrupted coding sequences, suggesting that the virus might have acquired the oncogene sequence via an intermediate RNA transcript from which the intron sequences were removed during RNA processing. The actual coding sequences of viral oncogenes and the corresponding proto-oncogenes exhibit a high degree of homology; in some cases a single point mutation is all that distinguishes a viral oncogene from the corresponding

TABLE 24-1

FUNCTIONAL CLASSIFICATION OF ONCOGENES

TYPE/ NAME	NATURE OF GENE PRODUCT
CATEGORY I: ONCOGENES THAT INDUCE CELLULAR PROLIFERATION	
Growth factors	
sis	A form of platelet-derived growth factor (PDGF)
Growth-factor receptors	
fms	Receptor for colony-stimulating factor 1 (CSF-1)
erbB	Receptor for epidermal growth factor (EGF)
neu	Protein related to EGF receptor
erbA	Receptor for thyroid hormone
Signal transducers	
src	Tyrosine kinase
abl	Tyrosine kinase
Ha-*ras*	GTP-binding protein with GTPase activity
N-*ras*	GTP-binding protein with GTPase activity
K-*ras*	GTP-binding protein with GTPase activity
Transcription factors	
jun	Component of transcription factor AP1
fos	Component of transcription factor AP1
myc	DNA-binding protein
CATEGORY II: ONCOGENES THAT INHIBIT CELLULAR PROLIFERATION *	
RB	Suppressor of retinoblastoma
p53	Nuclear phosphoprotein that inhibits formation of small-cell lung cancer and colon cancers
DCC	Suppressor of colon carcinoma
APC	Suppressor of adenomatous polyposis
NF1	Suppressor of neurofibromatosis
WT1	Suppressor of Wilm's tumor
CATEGORY III: ONCOGENES THAT REGULATE PROGRAMMED CELL DEATH	
bcl-2	Suppressor of apoptosis

* The activity of the category II oncogene products is not well understood. However, loss or mutation in these oncogenes is associated with development of the indicated cancers.

proto-oncogene. It is now believed that most, if not all, oncogenes (both viral and cellular) are derived from cellular genes that encode various growth-controlling proteins. In addition, the proteins encoded by a particular oncogene and its corresponding proto-oncogene appear to have very similar functions. As discussed below, the conversion of a proto-oncogene into an oncogene appears in many cases to involve a change in the level of expression of a normal growth-controlling protein.

Function of Oncogenes

Homeostasis in normal tissue is maintained by a highly regulated process of cellular proliferation balanced by cell death. If there is an imbalance, either at the level of cellular proliferation or at the level of cell death, then a cancerous state will develop. Oncogenes have been shown to play an important role in this process, either by regulating cellular proliferation or by regulating cell death. Oncogenes can be divided into three categories reflecting these different activities (Table 24-1).

INDUCTION OF CELLULAR PROLIFERATION

One category of oncogenes encodes proteins that induce cellular proliferation. Some of these proteins function as growth factors or growth-factor receptors. Included among these are *sis*, which encodes a form of platelet-derived growth factor, and *fms*, *erbB*, and *neu*, which encode growth-factor receptors. In normal cells the expression of growth factors and their receptors is carefully regulated. Usually, one population of cells secretes a growth factor that acts on another population of cells carrying the receptor for that factor, thus stimulating proliferation of the second population. Inappropriate expression of either a growth factor or its receptor can result in uncontrolled proliferation.

Other oncogenes in this category encode products that function in signal-transduction pathways or as transcription factors. The *src* and *abl* oncogenes encode tyrosine kinases, and the *ras* oncogene encodes a GTP-binding protein. The products of these genes act as signal transducers. The *myc*, *jun*, and *fos* oncogenes encode transcription factors. Overactivity of any of these oncogenes may result in unregulated proliferation.

INHIBITION OF CELLULAR PROLIFERATION

A second category of oncogenes—called **tumor-suppressor genes**, or anti-oncogenes—function to inhibit excessive cell proliferation. Inactivation of these oncogenes abolishes their inhibitory activity, resulting in unregulated proliferation. The prototype of this category of oncogenes is *Rb*, the retinoblastoma gene. Hereditary retinoblastoma is a rare childhood cancer in which tumors develop from neural precursor cells in the immature retina. The affected child inherits a mutated *Rb* allele; somatic inactivation of the remaining *Rb* allele leads to tumor growth. Probably the single most frequent abnormality in human cancer is mutations in *p53*, which encodes a nuclear phosphoprotein. Over 90% of small-cell lung cancer and over 50% of breast and colon cancers have been shown to be associated with mutations in *p53*.

REGULATION OF PROGRAMMED CELL DEATH

A third category of oncogenes regulates programmed cell death. These genes encode proteins that either block or induce apoptosis. Included in this category of oncogenes is *bcl-2*, an anti-apoptosis gene. This oncogene was originally discovered from a chromosomal translocation associated with B-cell follicular lymphoma. Since its discovery, *bcl-2* has been shown to play an important role in regulating cell survival during hematopoiesis and in survival of selected B cells and T cells during maturation (see Chapters 8 and 12). Interestingly, the Epstein-Barr virus contains a gene that has sequence homology to *bcl-2* and may act in a similar manner to suppress apoptosis.

Conversion of Proto-Oncogenes to Oncogenes

In 1972 R. J. Huebner and G. J. Todaro suggested that mutations or genetic rearrangements of proto-oncogenes by carcinogens or viruses might alter the normal regulated function of these genes, converting them into potent cancer-causing oncogenes (Figure 24-2). Considerable evidence supporting this hypothesis accumulated in subsequent years. For example, some malignantly transformed cells contain multiple copies of cellular oncogenes, resulting in increased production of oncogene products. Such amplification of cellular oncogenes has been observed in cells from various types of human cancers. Several groups have identified c-*myc* oncogenes in homogeneously staining regions (HSRs) of chromosomes from cancer cells; these HSRs represent long tandem arrays of amplified genes.

In addition, some cancer cells exhibit chromosomal translocations, which usually involve movement of a proto-oncogene from one chromosomal site to another (Figure 24-3). In many cases of Burkitt's lymphoma, for example, c-*myc* is moved from its normal position on

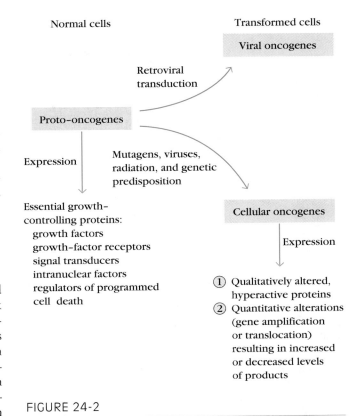

FIGURE 24-2

Conversion of proto-oncogenes into oncogenes can involve mutation, resulting in production of qualitatively different gene products, or DNA amplification or translocation, resulting in increased or decreased expression of gene products.

chromosome 8 to a position near the immunoglobulin heavy-chain enhancer on chromosome 14. As a result of this translocation, synthesis of the c-Myc protein, which functions as a transcription factor, increases.

Mutation in proto-oncogenes has also been associated with cellular transformation and may be a major mechanism by which chemical carcinogens or x-irradiation convert a proto-oncogene into a cancer-inducing oncogene. For instance, a single-point mutation in c-*ras* has been detected in human lung carcinoma, prostate carcinoma, bladder carcinoma, and neuroblastoma. This single mutation appears to reduce the GTPase activity of the Ras protein and may alter its function in the regulation of cellular growth.

Viral integration into the host-cell genome may in itself serve to convert a proto-oncogene into a transforming oncogene. For example, avian leukosis virus (ALV) is a retrovirus that does not carry any viral oncogenes and yet is able to transform B cells into lymphomas. This particular retrovirus has been shown to integrate within the c-*myc* proto-oncogene, which contains three exons.

(a) Chronic myelogenous leukemia

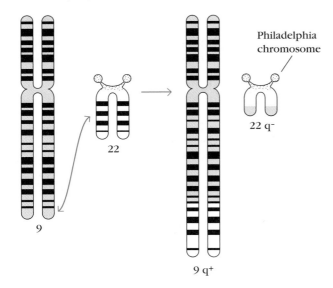

(b) Burkitt's lymphoma

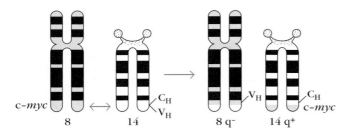

FIGURE 24-3

Chromosomal translocations in (a) chronic myelogenous leukemia (CML) and (b) Burkitt's lymphoma. Leukemic cells from all patients with CML contain the so-called Philadelphia chromosome, which results from a translocation between chromosomes 9 and 22. Cancer cells from some patients with Burkitt's lymphoma exhibit a translocation that moves part of chromosome 8 to chromosome 14. It is now known that this translocation involves c-*myc*, a cellular oncogene. Abnormalities such as these are detected by banding analysis of metaphase chromosomes. Normal chromosomes are shown on the left, and translocated chromosomes on the right.

Exon 1 of c-*myc* has an unknown function; exons 2 and 3 encode the Myc protein. Insertion of AVL between exon 1 and exon 2 has been shown in some cases to allow the provirus promoter to increase transcription of exons 2 and 3, resulting in increased synthesis of c-Myc.

A variety of tumors have been shown to express significantly increased levels of growth factors or growth-factor receptors. In adult T-cell leukemia, T cells infected with the HTLV-1 retrovirus show constitutive expres-

sion of IL-2 and the IL-2 receptor, enabling the cells to autostimulate their own proliferation in the absence of antigen activation (see Figure 13-13). Expression of the receptor for epidermal growth factor, which is encoded by c-*erbB*, has also been shown to be amplified in many cancer cells. And in breast cancer, increased synthesis of the growth-factor receptor encoded by c-*neu* has been linked with a poor prognosis.

One of the best examples of the association between increased expression of growth factors and cancer induction involves transforming growth factor (TGF-α). TGF-α, which is secreted by a variety of transformed cells, is similar in both structure and function to epidermal growth factor (EGF), and like EGF it is also able to bind to the EGF receptor on cells. Increased expression of both TGF-α and the EGF receptor have been observed in many cancer cells and in cells that have been transformed with retroviruses, viral oncogenes, and carcinogens.

TGF-α is thought to act as an autocrine activator of the EGF receptor. The effects of TGF-α overproduction have been studied by producing transgenic mice containing a TGF-α transgene linked to a metallothionine promoter. In these mice, the level of TGF-α expression could be controlled by adjusting their zinc intake. Experiments with these mice revealed that when TGF-α expression was high, they developed carcinomas of the liver and breast and also exhibited enlargement of the pancreas; however, when TGF-α expression was low, none of these changes was observed. Thus overexpression of the gene encoding TGF-α enables it to function as an oncogene in this system.

Induction of Cancer: A Multistep Process

The development from a normal cell to a cancerous cell is thought to be a multistep process of clonal evolution driven by a series of somatic mutations that progressively convert the cell from normal growth to a precancerous state and finally into a cancerous state.

The presence of myriad chromosomal abnormalities in precancerous and cancerous cells lends support to the role of multiple mutations in the development of cancer. This has been demonstrated in human colon cancer, which progresses in a series of well-defined morphologic stages (Figure 24-4). Colon cancer begins as small, benign tumors in the colorectal epithelium, called adenomas. These precancerous tumors grow, gradually becoming increasingly disorganized in their intracellular organization until they acquire the malignant phenotype. These well-defined morphologic stages of colon cancer have been correlated with a sequence of gene changes involving inactivation or loss of three anti-oncogenes

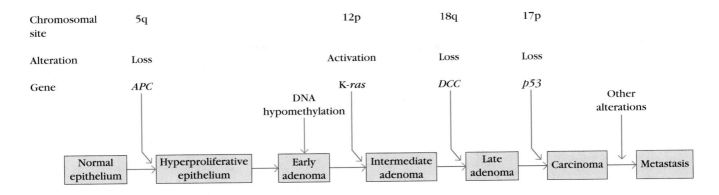

FIGURE 24-4

Model of sequential genetic alterations leading to metastatic colon cancer. Each of the stages indicated at the bottom is morphologically distinct, allowing researchers to determine the sequence of genetic alterations. [Adapted from B. Vogelstein and K. W. Kinzler, 1993, *Trends Genet.* **9**:138.]

(*APC*, *DCC*, and *p53*) and activation of one cellular proliferation oncogene (K-*ras*).

Studies with transgenic mice also support the role of multiple steps in the induction of cancer. Transgenic mice expressing high levels of Bcl-2 develop a population of small resting B cells, derived from secondary lymphoid follicles, that have greatly extended life spans. Gradually these transgenic mice develop lymphomas. Analysis of lymphomas in these transgenic mice have shown that approximately half have a c-*myc* translocation to the immunoglobulin H-chain locus. The synergism of Myc and Bcl-2 is highlighted in double-transgenic mice (produced by mating the *bcl-2*+ transgenic mice with *myc*+ transgenic mice). In this case the mice develop a very rapid onset leukemia.

TUMORS OF THE IMMUNE SYSTEM

Tumors of the immune system are classified as lymphomas or leukemias. Lymphomas proliferate as solid tumors within a lymphoid tissue such as the bone marrow, lymph nodes, or thymus; they include Hodgkin's and non–Hodgkin's lymphomas. Leukemias tend to proliferate as single cells and are detected by increased cell numbers in the blood or lymph. Leukemia can develop in lymphoid or myeloid lineages.

Historically the leukemias were classified as acute or chronic according to the clinical progression of the disease. The acute leukemias appeared suddenly and progressed rapidly, whereas the chronic leukemias were much less aggressive and developed slowly as mild, barely symptomatic diseases. These clinical distinctions apply to untreated leukemias; with current treatments the acute leukemias often have a good prognosis, and permanent remission can often be achieved. Now the major distinction between acute and chronic leukemias is the maturity of the cell involved. Acute leukemias tend to arise in less mature cells, whereas chronic leukemias arise in mature cells. The acute leukemias include **acute lymphocytic leukemia** (ALL) and **acute myelogenous leukemia** (AML); these diseases can develop at any age and have a rapid onset. The chronic leukemias include **chronic lymphocytic leukemia** (CLL) and **chronic myelogenous leukemia** (CML); these diseases develop slowly and are seen in adults.

A number of B- and T-cell leukemias and lymphomas have been shown to involve chromosomal translocations in which a proto-oncogene is translocated into the immunoglobulin genes or T-cell-receptor genes. One of the best-characterized involves the translocation of c-*myc* in Burkitt's lymphoma and in mouse plasmacytomas. In 75% of Burkitt's lymphoma patients, c-*myc* is translocated from chromosome 8 to the Ig heavy-chain gene cluster on chromosome 14 (see Figure 24-3b). In the remaining patients, c-*myc* remains on chromosome 8 and the κ or λ light-chain genes are translocated to a region 3′ of c-*myc*. Kappa-gene translocations from chromosome 2 to chromosome 8 occur 9% of the time, and λ-gene translocations from chromosome 22 to chromosome 8 occur 16% of the time.

Translocations of c-*myc* to the Ig heavy-chain gene cluster on chromosome 14 have been analyzed in some detail. In some cases the entire c-*myc* gene is translocated head-to-head to a region near the heavy-chain enhancer. In other cases exons 1, 2, and 3 or exons 2 and

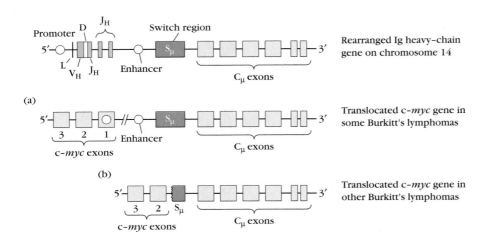

Promoter, D, J_H, Switch region, S_μ, Enhancer, C_μ exons, V_H, J_H, L

(a)

c-*myc* exons, Enhancer, S_μ, C_μ exons

(b)

c-*myc* exons, S_μ, C_μ exons

Rearranged Ig heavy-chain gene on chromosome 14

Translocated c-*myc* gene in some Burkitt's lymphomas

Translocated c-*myc* gene in other Burkitt's lymphomas

FIGURE 24-5

In many patients with Burkitt's lymphoma, the c-*myc* gene is translocated to the immunoglobulin heavy-chain gene cluster on chromosome 14. In some cases, the entire c-*myc* gene is inserted near the heavy-chain enhancer (a), but in other cases, only the coding exons (2 and 3) of c-*myc* are inserted at the S_m switch site (b). Only exons 2 and 3 of c-*myc* are coding exons. Translocation may lead to overexpression of c-Myc or to changes in the protein due to increased somatic mutation.

3 of c-*myc* are translocated head-to-head to the S_m or S_a switch site (Figure 24-5). In each case the translocation removes the *myc* coding exons from the regulatory mechanisms operating in chromosome 8 and places them in the immunoglobulin-gene region, a very active region that is expressed constitutively in these cells. The consequences of constitutive *myc* expression in lymphoid cells have been investigated in transgenic mice. In one study mice containing a transgene consisting of all three c-*myc* exons and the immunoglobulin heavy-chain enhancer were produced. Of 15 transgenic pups born, 13 developed lymphomas of the B-cell lineage within a few months of birth.

Various hypotheses have been suggested to account for *myc*-related oncogenesis. Some researchers have suggested that the presence of the immunoglobulin enhancer may result in overproduction of the c-Myc. Another hypothesis, based on the unusual level of mutations observed in exon 1 of c-*myc* after translocation, is that somatic mutation within the immunoglobulin V-region genes may induce mutations in the oncogene that lead to faulty regulation through its exon 1 or to changes in the function of its protein product.

TUMOR ANTIGENS

The subdiscipline of tumor immunology involves the study of antigens on tumor cells and the immune response to these antigens. Two types of tumor antigens have been identified on tumor cells: **tumor-specific transplantation antigens** (TSTAs) and **tumor-associated transplantation antigens** (TATAs). Tumor-specific antigens are unique to tumor cells and do not occur on normal cells in the body. They may result from mutations in tumor cells that generate altered cellular proteins; cytoso-

lic processing of these proteins would give rise to novel peptides that are presented with class I MHC molecules, inducing a cell-mediated response by tumor-specific CTLs (Figure 24-6). Tumor-associated antigens, which are not unique to tumor cells, may be proteins that are expressed on normal cells during fetal development when the immune system is immature and unable to respond but that normally are not expressed in the adult. Reactivation of the embryonic genes encoding these proteins in tumor cells results in their expression on the fully differentiated tumor cells. Tumor-associated antigens may also be proteins that are normally expressed at extremely low levels on normal cells but are expressed at much higher levels on tumor cells.

Characterization of tumor transplantation antigens is difficult because they do not generally elicit an antibody response and thus cannot be isolated by immunoprecipitation. Many tumor antigens are cellular proteins that give rise to peptides presented with MHC molecules; typically, these antigens have been identified by their ability to induce antigen-specific CTLs.

Tumor-Specific Antigens

Tumor-specific antigens have been identified on tumors induced with chemical or physical carcinogens and on some virally induced tumors. Demonstrating the presence of tumor-specific antigens on spontaneously occurring tumors is particularly difficult because the immune response to such tumors eliminates all of the tumor cells bearing recognizable antigens and in this way selects for cells bearing lower levels of tumor-specific antigens.

CHEMICALLY OR PHYSICALLY INDUCED TUMOR ANTIGENS

Methylcholanthrene and ultraviolet light are two carcinogens that have been used extensively to generate

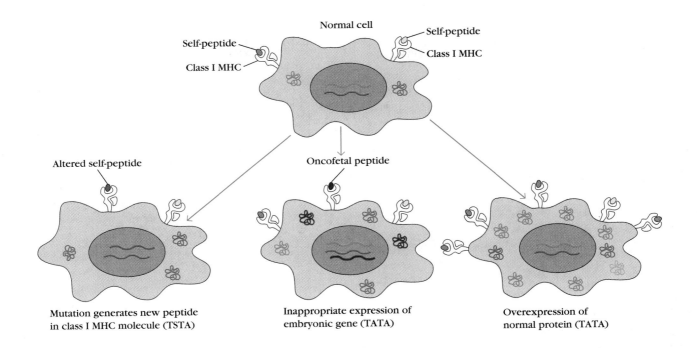

Normal cell

Self-peptide

Self-peptide

Class I MHC

Class I MHC

Altered self-peptide

Oncofetal peptide

Mutation generates new peptide
in class I MHC molecule (TSTA)

Inappropriate expression of
embryonic gene (TATA)

Overexpression of
normal protein (TATA)

FIGURE 24-6

Different mechanisms generate tumor-specific transplantation antigens (TSTAs) and tumor-associated transplantation antigens (TATAs). The latter are more common.

TABLE 24-2

IMMUNE RESPONSE TO METHYL-CHOLANANTHRENE (MCA) OR POLYOMA VIRUS (PV)*

TRANSPLANTED KILLED TUMOR CELLS	SOURCE OF LIVE TUMOR CELLS FOR CHALLENGE	TUMOR GROWTH
CHEMICALLY INDUCED		
MCA-induced sarcoma A	MCA-induced sarcoma A	−
MCA-induced sarcoma A	MCA-induced sarcoma B	+
VIRALLY INDUCED		
PV-induced sarcoma A	PV-induced sarcoma A	−
PV-induced sarcoma A	PV-induced sarcoma B	−
PV-induced sarcoma A	SV40-induced sarcoma C	+

* Tumors were induced either with MCA or PV, and killed cells from the induced tumors were injected into syngeneic animals, which were then challenged with live cells from the indicated tumor-cell lines. The absence of tumor growth after live challenge indicates that the immune response induced by tumor antigens on the killed cells provided protection against the live cells.

tumor-cell lines. When syngeneic animals are injected with killed cells from a carcinogen-induced tumor-cell line, the animals develop a specific immunologic response that can protect against later challenge by live cells of the same line but not other tumor-cell lines (Table 24-2). Even when the same chemical carcinogen induces two separate tumors at different sites in the same animal, the tumor antigens are distinct and the immune response to one tumor does not protect against the other tumor.

The tumor-specific transplantation antigens of chemically induced tumors have been difficult to characterize because they cannot be identified by induced antibodies but only by their T-cell–mediated rejection. One experimental approach that has allowed identification of genes encoding some TSTAs is outlined in Figure 24-7. When a mouse tumorigenic cell line (tum$^+$), which induces progressive tumor growth, is treated in vitro with a chemical mutagen, some cells are mutated so that they no longer are capable of inducing a tumor in syngeneic mice. These mutant tumor cells are designated as tum$^-$ variants. Most tum$^-$ variants have been shown to express TSTAs that are not expressed by the original tum$^+$ tumor-cell line. When tum$^-$ cells are injected into syngeneic mice, these unique TSTAs that the tum$^-$ cells

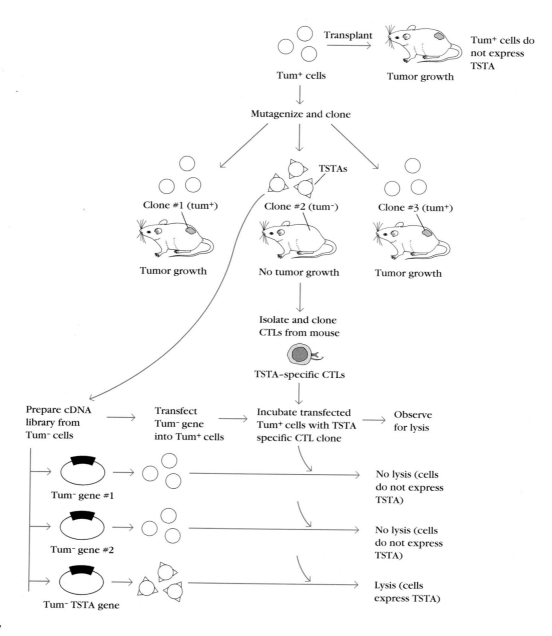

FIGURE 24-7

One procedure for identifying genes encoding tumor-specific transplantation antigens (TSTAs). Most TSTAs can be detected only by the cell-mediated rejection they elicit. In the first part of this procedure, a nontumorigenic (tum⁻) cell line is generated; this cell line expresses a TSTA that is recognized by syngeneic mice, which mount a cell-mediated response against it. To isolate the gene encoding the TSTA, a cosmid gene library is prepared from the tum⁻ cell line, the genes are transfected into tumorigenic tum⁺ cells, and the transfected cells are incubated with TSTA-specific CTLs.

express are recognized by specific CTLs. The TSTA-specific CTLs destroy the tum⁻ tumor cells, thus preventing tumor growth. To identify the genes encoding the TSTAs that are expressed on a tum⁻ cell line, a cosmid DNA library is prepared from the tum⁻ cells. Genes from the tum⁻ cells are transfected into the original tum⁺ cells. The transfected tum⁺ cells are tested for the expression of the tum⁻ TSTAs by their ability to activate cloned CTLs specific for the tum⁻ TSTA. A number of diverse TSTAs have been identified by this method.

In the past few years, two methods have facilitated the characterization of TSTAs (Figure 24-8). In one method peptides bound to class I MHC molecules on the membrane of the tumor cells are eluted with acid and puri-

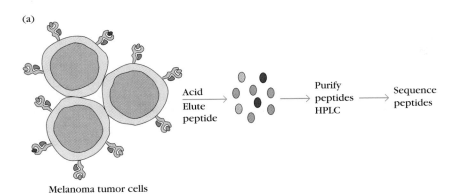

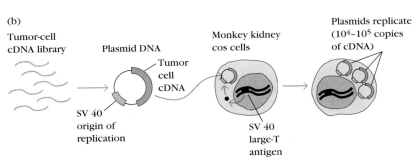

fied by high-pressure liquid chromatography (HPLC). In some cases sufficient peptide is eluted to allow its sequence to be deduced by Edman degradation. In a second approach cDNA libraries are prepared from tumor cells. These cDNA libraries are transfected transiently into COS cells, which are monkey kidney cells transfected with the gene coding for the SV40 large-T antigen. When these cells are later transfected with plasmids containing the tumor-cell cDNA and an SV40 origin of replication, the large-T antigen stimulates plasmid replication, so that up to $10^4–10^5$ plasmid copies are produced per cell. This results in high-level expression of the tumor-cell DNA.

The genes encoding some TSTAs have been shown to differ from normal cellular genes by a single-point mutation. Further characterization of TSTAs has demonstrated that many TSTAs are not cell-membrane proteins; rather, as indicated already, they are cytosolic proteins that are processed and presented as short peptides together with class I MHC molecules on the surface of tumor cells where they can be recognized by CTLs as altered self-cells.

VIRALLY INDUCED TUMOR ANTIGENS

In contrast to chemically induced tumors, virally induced tumors express tumor antigens shared by all tumors induced by the same virus. For example, when syngeneic mice are injected with killed cells from a particular polyoma-induced tumor, the recipients are protected against subsequent challenge with live cells from any polyoma-induced tumors (see Table 24-2). Likewise, when lymphocytes are transferred from mice with a virus-induced tumor into normal syngeneic recipients, the recipients reject subsequent transplants of all syngeneic tumors induced by the same virus. In the case of both SV40- and polyoma-induced tumors, the presence of tumor antigens is related to the neoplastic state of the cell. Although virally induced tumor antigens have not yet been established in human cancers, Burkitt's lymphoma cells have been shown to express a nuclear antigen of the Epstein-Barr virus that may indeed be a tumor-specific antigen for this type of tumor.

The potential value of these virally induced tumor antigens can be seen in animal models. In one experiment mice immunized with a preparation of genetically engineered polyoma virus tumor antigen were shown to be immune to subsequent injections of live polyoma-induced tumor cells. In another experiment mice were immunized with a vaccinia virus vaccine engineered with the gene encoding the polyoma tumor antigen. These mice also developed immunity, rejecting later injections of live polyoma-induced tumor cells (Figure 24-9). The first example of a virally induced tumor antigen associated with a human cancer is a peptide from human papilloma virus. This oncoviral peptide may prove useful for immunization of patients carrying virus-associated tumors.

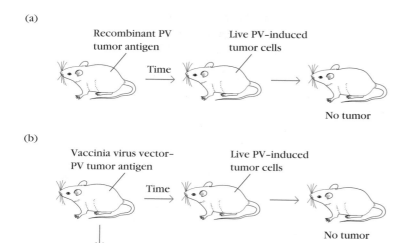

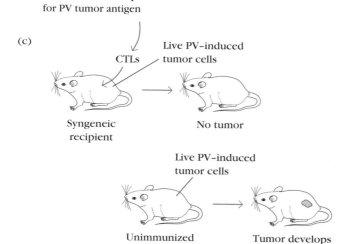

FIGURE 24-9

Experimental induction of immunity against tumor cells induced by polyoma virus (PV) has been achieved by immunizing mice with recombinant polyoma tumor antigen (a), with a vaccinia vector vaccine containing the gene encoding the PV tumor antigen (b), or with CTLs specific for the PV tumor antigen (c). Unimmunized mice (*bottom*) develop tumors when injected with live polyoma-induced tumor cells, whereas the immunized mice do not.

Tumor-Associated Antigens

The majority of tumor antigens are not unique to tumor cells but also are present on normal cells. These tumor-associated transplantation antigens may be proteins usually expressed only on fetal cells but not on normal adult cells, or they may be proteins expressed at low levels by normal cells but at much higher levels by tumor cells. The latter category includes growth factors and growth-factor receptors, as well as oncogene-encoded proteins.

Several growth-factor receptors are expressed at significantly increased levels on tumor cells and can serve as tumor-associated antigens. For instance, a variety of tumor cells express the EGF receptor at levels 100 times greater than that in normal cells. An example of an over-expressed growth factor serving as a tumor-associated antigen is a transferrin growth factor, designated p97, which aids in the transport of iron into cells. Whereas normal cells express less than 8,000 molecules of p97

per cell, melanoma cells express 50,000–500,000 molecules of p97 per cell. The gene encoding p97 has been cloned, and a recombinant vaccinia virus vaccine has been prepared carrying the cloned gene. When this vaccine was injected into mice, it induced both humoral and cell-mediated immune responses, which protected the mice against live melanoma cells expressing the p97 antigen. Results such as this highlight the importance of identifying tumor antigens as potential targets of tumor immunotherapy.

ONCOFETAL TUMOR ANTIGENS

Oncofetal tumor antigens, as the name implies, are found not only on cancerous cells but also on normal fetal cells. These antigens appear early in embryonic development, before the immune system acquires immunocompetence; if these antigens appear later on cancer cells, they are recognized as nonself and induce an immunologic response. Two well-studied oncofetal antigens are **alpha-fetoprotein** (AFP) and **carcinoembryonic antigen** (CEA).

Although the serum concentration of AFP drops from milligram levels in fetal serum to nanogram levels in normal adult serum, elevated AFP levels are found in a majority of patients with liver cancer (Table 24-3). CEA is a membrane glycoprotein found on gastrointestinal and liver cells of 2- to 6-month-old fetuses. Approximately 90% of patients with advanced colorectal cancer, and 50% of patients with early colorectal cancer have increased levels of CEA in their serum; some patients with other types of cancer also exhibit increased CEA levels. However, because AFP and CEA can be found in trace amounts in some normal adults and in some non-cancerous disease states, the presence of these oncofetal antigens is not diagnostic of tumors but rather serves to monitor tumor growth. If, for example, a patient has had surgery to remove a colorectal carcinoma, CEA levels are monitored following surgery. An increase in the CEA level is an indication of resumed tumor growth.

ONCOGENE PROTEINS AS TUMOR ANTIGENS

A number of tumors have been shown to express tumor-associated antigens encoded by cellular oncogenes. These antigens are also present in normal cells encoded by the corresponding proto-oncogene. In many cases there is no qualitative difference between the oncogene and proto-oncogene products; instead, the increased levels of the oncogene product can be recognized by the immune system. For example, as noted earlier, human breast-cancer cells exhibit elevated expression of the oncogene-encoded Neu protein, a growth-factor receptor, whereas normal adult cells express only trace amounts of Neu protein. Because of this difference in the Neu level, anti-Neu monoclonal antibodies can recognize and selectively eliminate breast-cancer cells without damaging normal cells.

A few tumors have been shown to express a proto-oncogene product that is qualitatively different from the normal protein. For example, single-point mutations in the *ras* proto-oncogene have been detected in a number of tumors including 17 out of 17 cases of malignant prostate cancer. If these qualitative changes can be recognized effectively by the immune system as tumor-specific antigens, they will lend themselves to various cancer immunotherapy approaches.

T A B L E   2 4 - 3

ELEVATION OF ALPHA-FETOPROTEIN (AFP) AND CARCINOEMBRYONIC ANTIGEN (CEA) IN SERUM OF PATIENTS WITH VARIOUS DISEASES

DISEASE	NO. OF PATIENTS TESTED	% OF PATIENTS WITH HIGH AFP OR CEA LEVELS *
AFP > 400 μg/ml		
Alcoholic cirrhosis	NA	0
Hepatitis	NA	1
Hepatocellular carcinoma	NA	69
Other carcinoma	NA	0
CEA >10 ng/ml		
Cancerous		
Breast carcinoma	125	14
Colorectal carcinoma	544	35
Gastric carcinoma	79	19
Noncarcinoma malignancy	228	2
Pancreatic carcinoma	55	35
Pulmonary carcinoma	181	26
Noncancerous		
Alcoholic cirrhosis	120	2
Cholecystitis	39	1
Nonmalignant disease	115	0
Pulmonary emphysema	49	4
Rectal polyps	90	1
Ulcerative colitis	146	5

* Although trace amounts of both AFP and CEA can be found in some healthy adults, none would have levels greater than those indicated in the table.

TATAs on Human Melanomas

Several tumor-associated transplantation antigens have been identified on human melanomas. Five of these—MAGE-1, MAGE-3, BAGE, GAGE-1,2—are oncofetal-type antigens. Each of these antigens is expressed on a significant proportion of human melanoma tumors, as well as on a number of other human tumors, but not on normal differentiated tissues except for the testis where it is expressed on germ-line cells. In addition, a number of differentiation antigens expressed on normal melanocytes—including tyrosinase, gp100, Melan-A or MART-1, and gp75—are overexpressed by melanoma cells, enabling them to function as tumor-associated transplantation antigens.

Several of the human melanoma tumor antigens are shared by a number of other tumors. About 40% of human melanomas are positive for MAGE-1, and about 75% are positive for MAGE-2 or 3. In addition to melanomas, a significant percentage of glioma cell lines, breast tumors, non-small cell lung tumors, and head or neck carcinomas express MAGE-1, 2 or 3. These shared tumor antigens could be exploited for clinical treatment. It might be possible to produce a tumor vaccine expressing the shared antigen for treatment of a number of these tumors, as discussed later in the chapter.

IMMUNE RESPONSE TO TUMORS

In experimental animals tumor antigens can be shown to induce both humoral and cell-mediated immune responses resulting in destruction of the tumor cells. In general, the cell-mediated response appears to play the major role in tumor elimination. A number of tumors have been shown to induce tumor-specific CTLs that recognize tumor antigens presented by class I MHC on the tumor cells. However, as discussed below, expression of class I MHC molecules is decreased in a number of tumors, thereby limiting the role of specific CTLs in destroying tumor cells.

Role of NK Cells and Macrophages

As noted in Chapter 16, recognition of tumor cells by NK cells is not MHC restricted. Thus the activity of these cells is not compromised by the decreased MHC expression exhibited by some tumor cells. In some cases Fc receptors on NK cells can bind to antibody-coated tumor cells leading to ADCC (see Figure 16-12). The importance of NK cells in tumor immunity is suggested by the mutant mouse strain called beige and by **Chediak-Higashi syndrome** in humans. In both cases,

a genetic defect causes marked impairment of NK cells and an associated increased incidence of certain types of cancer.

Numerous observations indicate that activated macrophages also play a significant role in the immune response to tumors. For example, macrophages are often observed to cluster around tumors, and their presence is often correlated with tumor regression. Like NK cells, macrophages are not MHC restricted and express Fc receptors, enabling them to bind to antibody on tumor cells and mediate ADCC. The antitumor activity of activated macrophages is probably mediated by lytic enzymes and reactive oxygen and nitrogen intermediates. In addition, activated macrophages secrete a cytokine called tumor necrosis factor (TNF-α) that has potent antitumor activity. When TNF-α is injected into tumor-bearing animals, it has been found to induce hemorrhage and necrosis of the tumor (see Figure 15-14a).

Immune Surveillance Theory

The immune surveillance theory was first conceptualized in the early 1900s by Paul Ehrlich. He suggested that cancer cells frequently arise in the body but are recognized as foreign and eliminated by the immune system. Some 50 years later Lewis Thomas suggested that the cell-mediated branch of the immune system had evolved to patrol the body and eliminate cancer cells. According to these concepts, tumors arise only if cancer cells are able to escape immune surveillance, either by reducing their expression of tumor antigens or by an impairment in the immune response to these cells.

Among the early observations that seemed to support the immune surveillance theory was the increased incidence of cancer in transplantation patients on immunosuppressive drugs. Other findings, however, were difficult to reconcile with this theory. Nude mice, for example, lack a thymus and consequently lack functional T cells. According to the immune surveillance theory, these mice should show an increase in cancer, but instead nude mice are no more susceptible to cancer than other mice. Furthermore, although individuals on immunosuppressive drugs do show an increased incidence of cancers of the immune system, other common cancers (e.g., lung, breast, and colon cancer) are not increased in these individuals, contrary to what the theory predicts. One possible explanation for the selective increase in immune-system cancers is that the immunosuppressive agents themselves may exert a direct carcinogenic effect on immune cells.

Experimental data concerning the effect of tumor-cell dosage on the ability of the immune system to respond also are incompatible with the immune surveillance theory. For example, animals injected with very low or very high doses of tumor cells develop tumors, whereas those injected with intermediate doses do not. The mechanism by which a low dose of tumor cells "sneaks through" is difficult to reconcile with the immune surveillance theory. Finally, this theory assumes that cancer cells and normal cells exhibit qualitative antigen differences. In fact, as discussed in previous sections, many types of tumors do not express tumor-specific antigens, and any immune response that develops must be induced by quantitative differences in antigen expression by normal cells and tumor cells.

The basic concept of the immune surveillance theory—that malignant tumors arise only if the immune system is somehow impaired or if the tumor cells lose their immunogenicity, enabling them to escape immune surveillance—at this time remains unproved. Nevertheless, it is clear that an immune response can be generated to tumor cells and therapeutic approaches aimed at increasing that response may serve as a defense against malignant cells.

TUMOR EVASION
OF THE IMMUNE SYSTEM

Although the immune system clearly can respond to tumor cells, the fact that so many individuals die each year from cancer suggests that the immune response to tumor cells is often ineffective. This section describes several mechanisms by which tumor cells appear to evade the immune system.

Immunologic Enhancement of Tumor Growth

Following the discovery that antibodies could be produced to tumor-specific antigens, attempts were made to protect animals against tumor growth by active immunization with tumor antigens or by passive immunization with antitumor antibodies. Much to the surprise of the researchers, these immunizations did not protect against tumor growth; in many cases they actually enhanced growth of the tumor.

The tumor-enhancing ability of immune sera subsequently was studied in cell-mediated lympholysis (CML) reactions in vitro. Serum taken from animals with progressive tumor growth was found to block the CML reaction, whereas serum taken from animals with regressing tumors had little or no blocking activity. K. E. and I. Hellstrom extended these findings by showing that children with progressive neuroblastoma had high levels of some kind of blocking factor in their sera and that children with regressive neuroblastoma did not have such factors. Since these first reports, blocking factors have been found to be associated with a number of human tumors.

In some cases, antitumor antibody itself acts as a blocking factor. Presumably the antibody binds to tumor-specific antigens and masks the antigens from cytotoxic T cells. In many cases the blocking factors are not antibodies alone but rather antibodies complexed to tumor antigens. Although these immune complexes have been shown to block the CTL response, the mechanism of this inhibition is not known. The complexes also may inhibit ADCC by binding to Fc receptors on NK cells or macrophages and blocking their activity.

Modulation of Tumor Antigens

Certain tumor-specific antigens have been observed to disappear from the surface of tumor cells in the presence of serum antibody and then to reappear after the antibody is no longer present. This phenomenon, called **antigenic modulation**, is readily observed when leukemic T cells are injected into mice previously immunized with a leukemic T-cell antigen (TL antigen). These mice develop high titers of anti-TL antibody, which binds to the TL antigen on the leukemic cells and induces capping, endocytosis, and/or shedding of the antigen-antibody complex. As long as antibody is present, these leukemic T cells fail to display the TL antigen and thus cannot be eliminated.

Reduction in Class I MHC Molecules

Since $CD8^+$ CTLs only recognize antigen associated with class I MHC molecules, any alteration in the expression of class I MHC molecules on tumor cells may exert a profound effect on the CTL-mediated immune response. Malignant transformation of cells is often associated with a reduction (or even a complete loss) of class I MHC molecules, and a number of tumors have been shown to express decreased levels of class I MHC molecules (Table 24-4). In many cases the decrease in class I MHC expression is accompanied by progressive tumor growth, and so the absence of MHC molecules on a tumor is generally an indication of a poor prognosis. As illustrated in Figure 24-10, the immune response itself may play a role in selecting tumor cells with decreased class I MHC expression.

Lack of Co-stimulatory Signal

T-cell activation requires an activating signal, triggered by recognition of a peptide–MHC molecule complex by the T-cell receptor, and a co-stimulatory signal triggered by the interaction of B7 on antigen-presenting cells with CD28 on the T cells (see Figure 12-14). Both signals are needed to induce IL-2 production and proliferation of T cells. The poor immunogenicity of many tumor cells may be due in large part to the lack of the co-stimulatory molecules. Without sufficient numbers of antigen-presenting

TABLE 24-4

SOME TUMORS WITH ALTERED MHC EXPRESSION
AND THE BIOLOGICAL CONSEQUENCES

EXPERIMENTAL TUMOR SYSTEMS	ALTERED MHC EXPRESSION	BIOLOGICAL CONSEQUENCES
AKR mouse leukemia	Absence of H-2K	Increased tumorigenicity
Murine D122 Lewis lung carcinoma	Reduced H-2K/H-2D ratio	Increased metastasis
Methylcholanthrene-induced murine T10 sarcoma	Absence of H-2K and increased H-2D	Increased metastasis
SV40-transformed mouse cells	Absence of H-2K	Increased tumorigenicity
Radiation leukemia virus (RadLV)– transformed mouse cells	Absence of class I	Lethal leukemogenesis
Herpes simplex virus type 2 (HSV-2)–infected cells	Reduced class I molecules	Resistance to lysis by CTLs
Human Burkitt's lymphoma	Absence of class I	Resistance to lysis by CTLs
Human urothelial cell line TGr III	Reduced class I	Increased tumorigenicity and invasiveness
Human small-cell lung cancer	Deficient class I	Increased tumorigenicity and early metastisis
Human neuroblastoma	Deficient class I	Increased N-*myc* expression
Human mucinous colorectal carcinoma	Reduced class I	Poor prognosis
Human melanomas	Reduced class I	Increased invasiveness and thicker primary form

SOURCE: From K. M. Hui, 1989, *BioEssays* **11**:23.

cells in the immediate vicinity of a tumor, the T cells will receive only a partial activating signal, which may lead to clonal anergy.

CANCER IMMUNOTHERAPY

Although various immune responses can be generated to tumor cells, the response frequently is not sufficient to prevent tumor growth. One approach to cancer treatment is to augment or supplement these natural defense mechanisms. Several types of cancer immunotherapy in current use or under development are described in this concluding section.

Manipulation of Co-stimulatory Signal

Several research groups have demonstrated that tumor immunity can be enhanced by providing the co-stimulatory signal necessary for activation of CTL precursors (CTL-Ps). When mouse CTL-Ps are incubated with melanoma cells in vitro, antigen recognition occurs, but in the absence of a co-stimulatory signal, the CTL-Ps do not proliferate and differentiate into effector CTLs. However, when the melanoma cells are transfected with the gene encoding the B7 ligand, then the CTL-Ps differentiate into effector CTLs.

These findings offer the possibility that B7-transfected tumor cells might be used to induce a CTL response in vivo. For instance, when P. Linsley, L. Chen, and their colleagues injected melanoma-bearing mice with B7$^+$ melanoma cells, the melanomas completely regressed in more than 40% of the mice. S. Townsend and J. Allison used a similar approach to vaccinate mice against malignant melanoma. Normal mice were first immunized with irradiated, B7-transfected melanoma cells and then challenged with unaltered malignant melanoma cells. The "vaccine" was found to protect a high percentage of the mice (Figure 24-11a). It is hoped that a similar vac-

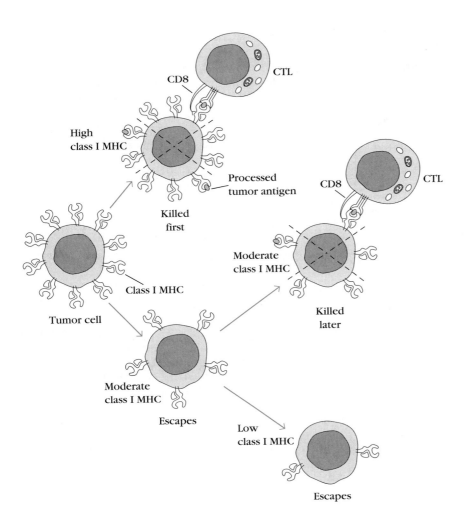

FIGURE 24-10

Down-regulation of class I MHC expression on tumor cells may allow a tumor to escape CTL-mediated recognition. The immune response may play a role in selecting for tumor cells expressing lower levels of class I MHC molecules by preferentially eliminating those cells expressing high levels of class I molecules. With time, malignant tumor cells may express progressively fewer MHC molecules and thus escape CTL-mediated destruction.

cine might prevent metastasis after surgical removal of a primary melanoma in human patients.

Because human melanoma antigens are shared by a number of different human tumors, it might be possible to generate a panel of B7-transfected melanoma cell lines that are typed for tumor antigen expression and for HLA expression. In this approach, the tumor antigen(s) expressed by a patient's tumor would be determined, and then the patient would be vaccinated with an irradiated B7-transfected cell line that expresses a similar tumor antigen(s).

Enhancement of APC Activity

Mouse dendritic cells cultured in GM-CSF and incubated with tumor fragments have been shown to activate both T_H cells and CTLs specific for the tumor antigens. When these mice were subsequently challenged with live tumor cells, they displayed tumor immunity. These experiments have led to a number of approaches aimed at expanding the population of antigen-presenting cells, so that these cells can activate T_H or CTLs specific for tumor antigens.

One approach that has been tried is to transfect tumor cells with the gene encoding GM-CSF. These engineered tumor cells, when reinfused back into the patient, will secrete GM-CSF, enhancing the differentiation and activation of host antigen-presenting cells, especially dendritic cells. As these dendritic cells accumulate around the tumor cells, the GM-CSF secreted by the tumor cells will enhance the presentation of tumor antigens to T_H and CTLs cells by the dendritic cells (Figure 24-11b). Clinical trials using melanoma cells transfected with GM-CSF are currently under way in melanoma patients.

Another way to expand the dendritic cell population is to culture dendritic cells from peripheral-blood progenitor cells in the presence of GM-CSF, TNF-α, and IL-4. These three cytokines allow the generation of large numbers of dendritic cells. If these dendritic cells are

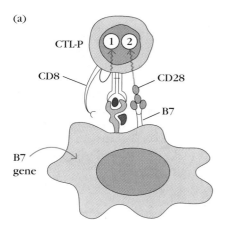

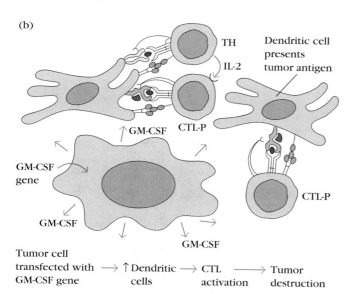

FIGURE 24-11

Use of transfected tumor cells for cancer immunotherapy. (a) Tumor cells transfected with the B7 gene express the co-stimulatory B7 molecule, enabling the tumor cells to provide both activating signal 1 and co-stimulatory signal 2 to CTL-Ps. As a result of the combined signals, the CTL-Ps differentiate into effector CTLs, which can mediate tumor destruction. In effect, the transfected tumor cell acts as an antigen-presenting cell. (b) Transfection of tumor cells with the gene encoding GM-CSF allows the tumor cells to secrete high levels of GM-CSF. This cytokine will activate dendritic cells in the vicinity of the tumor, enabling the dendritic cells to present tumor antigens to both T_H cells and CTL-Ps.

pulsed with tumor fragments and then reintroduced into the patient, they can now activate T_H and T_C cells specific for the tumor antigens.

A number of adjuvants, including the attenuated strain of *Mycobacterium bovis* called bacillus Calmette-Guerin (BCG) and *Corynebacterium parvuum,* have been used to boost tumor immunity. These adjuvants activate macrophages increasing their expression of various cytokines, class II MHC molecules, and the B7 co-stimulatory molecule. These activated macrophages are better activators of T_H cells, resulting in generalized increases in both humoral and cell-mediated responses. Although initially hailed as a "cancer cure," these adjuvants have shown only modest therapeutic results in melanoma patients and on the whole the clinical results with adjuvants have been disappointing.

Cytokine Therapy

The isolation and cloning of the various cytokine genes, mentioned in Chapter 13, has facilitated their large-scale production. A variety of experimental and clinical approaches have been developed to use recombinant cytokines, either singly or in combination, to augment the immune response against cancer. Among the cytokines that have been evaluated in cancer immunotherapy are interferons α, β, and γ; IL-1, IL-2, IL-4, IL-5, and IL-12; GM-CSF and TNF. Although these trials have produced occasional hopeful results, many obstacles remain to the successful use of this type of cancer immunotherapy.

The most notable obstacle is the complexity of the cytokine network itself (see Figure 13-4). This complexity makes it very difficult to know precisely how intervention with a given recombinant cytokine will affect the production of other cytokines. And since some cytokines act antagonistically, it is possible that intervention with a recombinant cytokine, designed to enhance a particular branch of the immune response, may actually lead to suppression. In addition, cytokine immunotherapy is plagued by difficulties with administering the cytokines in a localized fashion. In some cases systemic administration of high levels of a given cytokine has been shown to lead to serious and even life-threatening consequences. Although the results of several experimental and clinical trials of cytokine therapy for cancer are discussed here, it is important to keep in mind that this therapeutic approach is still in its infancy.

INTERFERONS

Large quantities of purified recombinant preparations of the interferons, IFN-α, IFN-β, and IFN-γ, are now available, each of which has shown some promise in the treatment of human cancer. To date, most of the clinical trials have involved IFN-α. Daily injections of recombinant IFN-α have been shown to induce partial or complete tumor regression in some patients with hematologic malignancies such as leukemias, lymphomas, and myelomas and with solid tumors such as melanoma, Kaposi's sarcoma, renal cancer, and breast cancer.

Interferon-mediated antitumor activity may involve several mechanisms. All three types of interferon have been shown to increase class I MHC expression on tumor cells; IFN-γ has also been shown to increase class II MHC expression on macrophages. Given the evidence for decreased levels of class I MHC molecules on malignant tumors, the interferons may act by restoring MHC expression, thereby increasing CTL activity against tumors. In addition, the interferons have been shown to inhibit cell division of both normal and malignantly transformed cells in vitro. It is possible that some of the antitumor effects of the interferons are related to this ability to directly inhibit tumor-cell proliferation. Finally, IFN-γ increases the activity of T_C cells, macrophages, and NK cells, all of which play a role in the immune response to tumor cells.

TUMOR NECROSIS FACTORS

The tumor necrosis factors, TNF-α and TNF-β, have been shown to exhibit direct antitumor activity, killing some tumor cells and reducing the rate of proliferation of others while sparing normal cells (Figure 24-12). In the presence of TNF-α or TNF-β a tumor undergoes visible hemorrhagic necrosis and tumor regression (see Figure 15-14a). TNF-α has also been shown to inhibit tumor-induced vascularization (angiogenesis) by damaging the vascular endothelial cells in the vicinity of a tumor, thereby decreasing the flow of blood and oxygen that is necessary for progressive tumor growth.

Phase I clinical trials of recombinant TNF-α in cancer patients appeared quite promising, and early news stories hailed TNF-α as the "cure for cancer." Further evaluation revealed that although TNF-α holds some promise, it is far from being an antitumor wonder drug. Injection of TNF-α directly into the tumor has led to complete tumor regression in some patients, but not in others.

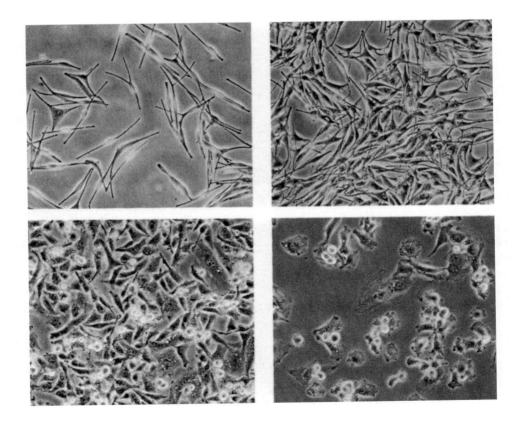

FIGURE 24-12

Photomicrographs of cultured normal melanocytes *(top)* and of cultured cancerous melanoma cells *(bottom)* in the presence and absence of tumor necrosis factor α (TNF-α). Note that in the presence of TNF-α, the cancer cells stop proliferating, whereas TNF-α has no inhibitory effect on proliferation of the normal cells. [From L. J. Old, 1988, *Sci. Am.* **258**(5):59.]

TNF-α therapy has several limitations: the short half-life of TNF-α necessitates frequent injections; and its adverse side effects include fever, chills, blood-pressure changes, and decreased counts of white blood cells.

IN VITRO–ACTIVATED LAK AND TIL CELLS

Animal studies have shown that lymphocytes can be activated against tumor antigens in vitro by culturing the lymphocytes with x-irradiated tumor cells in the presence of IL-2 and added tumor antigens. These activated lymphocytes mediate more effective tumor destruction than untreated lymphocytes when they are reinjected into the original tumor-bearing animal. It is difficult, however, to activate in vitro enough lymphocytes with antitumor specificity to be useful in cancer therapy.

While sensitizing lymphocytes to tumor antigens by this method, S. Rosenberg discovered that in the presence of high concentrations of cloned IL-2 and without the addition of tumor antigens, large numbers of activated lymphoid cells were generated that could kill fresh tumor cells but not normal cells. He called these cells **lymphokine-activated killer (LAK) cells**. In one study, for example, Rosenberg found that infusion of LAK cells plus recombinant IL-2 into tumor-bearing animals mediated effective tumor-cell destruction (Figure 24-13). LAK cells appear to be a heterogeneous population of lymphoid cells that includes natural killer (NK) cells and natural cytotoxic (NC) cells; the relative numbers of the two cell types depend on the source of the lymphocytes and the conditions of IL-2 activation.

Because large numbers of LAK cells can be generated in vitro and because these cells are active against a wide variety of tumors, their effectiveness in human tumor immunotherapy has been evaluated in several clinical trials. In these trials, peripheral-blood lymphocytes were removed from patients with various advanced metastatic cancers and were activated in vitro to generate LAK cells. Patients were then infused with their autologous LAK cells together with IL-2. A trial with 25 patients in 1985 resulted in cancer regression in some patients. A more extensive trial with 222 patients in 1987 resulted in complete regression in 16 patients. However, a number of undesirable side effects are associated with the high levels of IL-2 required for LAK-cell activity. The most noteworthy is vascular leak syndrome, which involves emigration of lymphoid cells and plasma from the peripheral blood into the tissues, leading to shock.

Tumors contain lymphocytes that have infiltrated the tumor and presumably are taking part in an antitumor response. By taking small biopsy samples of tumors, one can obtain a population of these lymphocytes and expand it in vitro with IL-2. These activated **tumor-infiltrating lymphocytes** are called **TIL cells**. Many

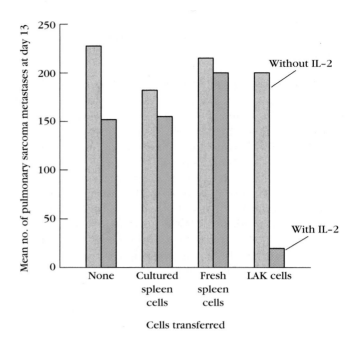

FIGURE 24-13

Experimental demonstration of tumor-destroying activity of LAK cells plus IL-2. Spleen cells or LAK cells, in the presence or absence of recombinant IL-2, were infused into mice with pulmonary sarcoma. The animals were evaluated 13 days later for the number of pulmonary sarcoma metastases. The LAK cells were prepared by isolating lymphocytes from tumor-bearing animals and incubating them in vitro with high concentrations of IL-2. Note that tumor regression occurred only when LAK cells and IL-2 were infused. [Data from S. Rosenberg et al., 1988, *Ann. Int. Med.,* **108**:853.]

TIL cells have a wide range of antitumor activity and appear to be indistinguishable from LAK cells. However, some TIL cells have specific cytolytic activity against their autologous tumor. These tumor-specific TIL cells are of interest because they have increased antitumor activity and require 100-fold lower levels of IL-2 for their activity than do LAK cells. In one study TIL cells were expanded in vitro from biopsy samples taken from patients with malignant melanoma, renal-cell carcinoma, and small-cell lung cancer. The expanded TIL cells were reinjected into autologous patients together with continuous infusions of recombinant IL-2. Renal-cell carcinomas and malignant melanomas showed partial regression in 29% and 23% of the patients, respectively.

Monoclonal Antibodies

Monoclonal antibodies have been used in various ways as experimental immunotherapeutic agents for cancer.

For example, anti–idiotype monoclonal antibodies have been used with some success in treating human B-cell lymphomas and T-cell leukemias. In one remarkable study, R. Levy and his colleagues successfully treated a 64-year-old man with terminal B-cell lymphoma. At the time of treatment the lymphoma had metastasized to the liver, spleen, bone marrow, and peripheral blood. Because this was a B-cell cancer the membrane-bound antibody on all the cancerous cells had the same idiotype. By the procedure outlined in Figure 24-14, these researchers produced mouse monoclonal antibody specific for the B-lymphoma idiotype. When this mouse monoclonal anti-idiotype antibody was injected into the patient, it bound specifically to the B-lymphoma cells

because these cells expressed that particular idiotype. Since B-lymphoma cells are susceptible to complement-mediated lysis, the monoclonal antibody activated the complement system and lysed the lymphoma cells without harming other cells. After four injections with this anti-idiotype monoclonal antibody, the tumors began to shrink, and as of the last report this patient has been in complete remission.

Monoclonal antibodies also have been used to prepare tumor-specific **immunotoxins.** These agents consist of the inhibitor chain of a toxin (e.g., diphtheria toxin) linked to an antibody against a tumor-specific or tumor-associated antigen (see Figure 5-23). In vitro studies have demonstrated that these "magic bullets" can kill tumor

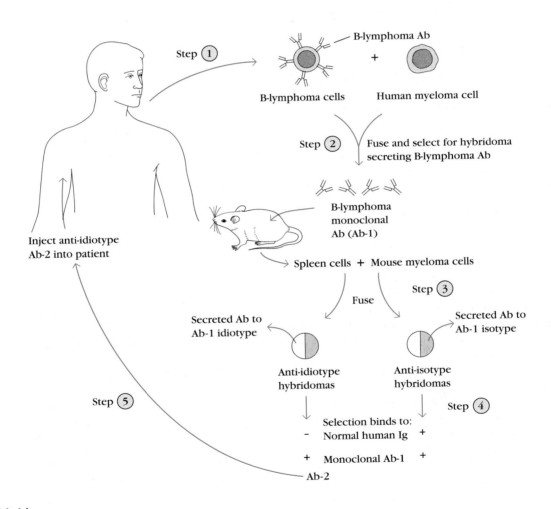

FIGURE 24-14

Treatment of B-cell lymphoma with monoclonal antibody specific for idiotypic determinants on the cancer cells. Because all the lymphoma cells are derived from a single transformed B cell, they all express membrane-bound antibody (Ab-1) with the same idiotype (i.e., the same antigenic specificity). In the procedure illustrated, monoclonal anti–idiotype antibody (Ab-2) against the B-lymphoma membrane-bound antibody was produced (steps 1–4). When this anti-idiotype antibody was injected into the patient (step 5), it bound selectively to B-lymphoma cells, which then were susceptible to complement-plus-antibody lysis.

cells without harming normal cells. Immunotoxins specific for tumor antigens in a variety of cancers (e.g., melanoma, colorectal carcinoma, metastatic breast carcinoma, and various lymphomas and leukemias) have been evaluated in phase I or phase II clinical trials. In eight separate trials, 12%–75% of leukemia and lymphoma patients exhibited partial or complete remission. In contrast, the clinical responses in patients with larger tumor masses were disappointing. In these patients, the tumor mass may render most of the tumor cells inaccessible to the immunotoxin.

Another cancer immunotherapy involves using monoclonal antibodies to bridge activated T cells directly to a tumor. In this approach two different monoclonal antibodies are produced: one specific for a tumor-cell membrane molecule and one specific for the CD3 membrane molecule of the TCR complex. A hybrid monoclonal antibody, or heteroconjugate, is then prepared with specificity for the tumor antigen and for CD3 (see Figure 5-25d). In vitro experiments with these heteroconjugates have revealed that they are able to cross-link and activate T cells directly on the surface of the tumor cell.

The finding that a variety of tumors express significantly increased levels of growth-factor receptors suggests that treatment with monoclonal antibodies against these receptors might inhibit tumor-cell activity. Monoclonal antibodies to the EGF receptor, to the p97 (transferrin) receptor, and to the IL-2 receptor have each been produced. In one study hundreds of mice with a lethal tumor were treated with chemotherapy alone or with chemotherapy plus monoclonal antibody to the EGF receptor. Chemotherapy alone failed to slow tumor growth in these mice, but every mouse that received the combined therapy recovered fully and the tumor did not recur following treatment. In a phase I clinical trial at Memorial Sloan-Kettering Cancer Center, patients with squamous-cell lung carcinoma are being treated with monoclonal antibody to EGF receptor. The results of this trial have not yet been published.

Tumor-Cell Vaccines

In a novel approach to developing tumor vaccines, a patient's own tumor cells are killed by x-irradiation, mixed with BCG, and reinjected into the patient. One woman treated in this way had been diagnosed with advanced malignant melanoma with literally hundreds of tumors on her right leg. Within 7 weeks after receiving this experimental vaccine, the tumors in her leg had disappeared, and the woman was still alive more than 3 years after treatment. Recent reports indicate that about 25% of patients with malignant melanoma have shown complete or partial remission after treatment with killed autologous tumor cells plus BCG.

SUMMARY

1. Tumor cells differ from normal cells in numerous ways. In particular, changes in growth regulation in tumor cells allow them to proliferate indefinitely, then invade the underlying tissue, and eventually metastasize to other tissues (see Figure 24-1). Normal cells can be transformed in vitro by chemical and physical carcinogens and by transforming viruses. Transformed cells exhibit altered growth properties and are sometimes capable of inducing cancer when they are injected into animals.

2. Proto-oncogenes encode proteins involved in control of cellular growth. It seems likely that conversion of a proto-oncogene to an oncogene may be involved in the induction of some kinds of cancer. This conversion may result from mutation in an oncogene, or its translocation or amplification (see Figure 24-2). A study of transformed cells has revealed the important role of cellular and viral oncogenes in the transformation process.

3. A number of B- and T-cell leukemias and lymphomas are associated with translocated proto-oncogenes. In its new site the translocated gene may come under the influence of an enhancer and be transcribed at higher levels than usual, or it may be subject to alteration by somatic mutation.

4. Tumor cells display tumor-specific antigens and the more comon tumor-associated antigens. Among the latter are oncofetal antigens, and increased levels of oncogene products. Several tumor-associated antigens expressed by melanoma cells are shared by other tumors; these common antigens might be useful clinically.

5. The immune response to tumors includes CTL-mediated lysis, NK-cell activity, macrophage-mediated tumor destruction, and destruction mediated by ADCC. Several cytotoxic factors, including TNF-α and TNF-β, help to mediate tumor-cell killing. Tumors may evade the immune response by modulating their tumor antigens, by reducing their expression of class I MHC molecules, and by antibody-mediated or immune-complex–mediated inhibition of CTL activity.

6. Experimental cancer immunotherapy has taken a variety of approaches. Enhancement of the co-stimulatory signal required for T-cell activation and of the activity of antigen-presenting cells has been achieved with transfected melanoma cells, leading to tumor destruction in experimental animals (see Figure 24-11). In some cases, injections of cytokines such as IFN-α and TNF-α have been shown to have beneficial effects. In another approach lymphocytes are activated in vitro

with high concentrations of IL-2, thereby inducing LAK cells or TIL cells with antitumor activity. Infusions of LAK cells plus IL-2 have reduced tumor development in experimental animals (see Figure 24-13). Some promising clinical results have been obtained in treating B-cell lymphomas and T-cell leukemias with monoclonal anti-idiotype antibodies (see Figure 24-14). Monoclonal antibodies specific for tumor antigens also have been used to produce immunotoxins. Vaccines of killed autologous tumor cells mixed with BCG have been somewhat effective in treatment of malignant melanomas.

REFERENCES

AISENBERG, A. C. 1993. Utility of gene rearrangements in lymphoid malignancies. *Annu. Rev. Med.* **44**:75.

ALLISON, J. P., A. A. HURWITZ, AND D. R. LEACH. 1995. Manipulation of costimulatory signals to enhance antitumor T-cell responses. *Curr. Opin. Immunol.* **7**:682.

BOON, T., ET AL. 1994. Tumor antigens recognized by T lymphocytes. *Annu. Rev. Immunol.* **12**:337.

CARBONE, D. P., AND J. D. MINNA. 1993. Antioncogenes and human cancer. *Annu. Rev. Med.* **44**:451.

COHEN, J. J. 1993. Apoptosis. *Immunol. Today* **14**:136.

COULIE, P. G., ET AL. 1994. A new gene coding for a differentiation antigen recognized by autologous cytolytic T lymphocytes on HLA-A2 melanomas. *J. Exp. Med.* **180**: 35.

COURNOYER, D., AND C. T. CASKEY. 1993. Gene therapy of the immune system. *Annu. Rev. Immunol.* **11**:297.

GEORGE, J. T., R. A. SPOONER, AND A. A. EPENETOS. 1994. Applications of monoclonal antibodies in clinical oncology. *Immunol. Today.* **15**:559.

JHAPPAN, C., ET AL. 1990. TGF-α overexpression in transgenic mice induces liver neoplasia and abnormal development of the mammary gland and pancreas. *Cell* **61**:1137.

KRADIN, R. L., ET AL. 1989. Tumor infiltrating lymphocytes and interleukin-2 treatment of advanced cancer. *Lancet* (March 18):577.

LIVINGSTONE, L. R., ET AL. 1992. Altered cell cycle arrest and gene amplification potential accompany loss of wild type *p53. Cell* **70**:923.

SUGIMURA, T. 1992. Multistep carcinogenesis: a 1992 perspective. *Science* **258**:603.

TOPALIAN, S. L., D. SOLOMON, AND S. A. ROSENBERG. 1989. Tumor-specific cytolysis by lymphocytes infiltrating human melanomas. *J. Immunol.* **142**:3714.

VAN DEN EYNDE, B., AND V. G. BRICHARD. 1995. New tumor antigens recognized by T cells. *Curr. Opin. Immunol.* **7**:674.

VOGELSTEIN, B., AND K. W. DINZLER. 1993. The multistep nature of cancer. *Trends Genet.* **9**:138.

WILLIAMS, G. T., C. A. SMITH, N. J. MCCARTHY, AND E. A. GRIMES. 1992. Apoptosis: final control point in cell biology. *Trends Cell Biol.* **2**:263.

STUDY QUESTIONS

1.   Indicate whether each of the following statements is true or false. If you think a statement is false, explain why.

a.   Hereditary retinoblastoma results from overexpression of a cellular oncogene.

b.   Translocation of c-*myc* gene is found in many patients with Burkitt's lymphoma.

c.   Multiple copies of cellular oncogenes are sometimes observed in cancer cells.

d.   Viral integration into the cellular genome may convert a proto-oncogene into a transforming oncogene.

e.   All oncogenic retroviruses carry viral oncogenes.

f.   The immune response against a virus-induced tumor protects against another tumor induced by the same virus.

g.   LAK cells are tumor specific.

2.   You are a clinical immunologist studying acute lymphoblastic leukemia (ALL). Leukemic cells from most patients with ALL have the morphology of lymphocytes but do not express cell-surface markers characteristic of mature B or T cells. You have isolated cells from ALL patients that do not express membrane Ig but do react with monoclonal antibody against a normal pre-B cell marker (B-200). You therefore suspect that these leukemic cells are pre-B cells. How would you confirm that the leukemic cells are committed to the B-cell lineage by means of genetic analysis?

3.   In a recent experiment melanoma cells were isolated from patients with early or advanced stages of malignant melanoma. At the same time T cells specific for tetanus toxoid antigen were isolated and cloned from each patient.

a.   When early-stage melanoma cells were cultured together with tetanus toxoid antigen and the tetanus toxoid–specific T-cell clones, the T-cell clones were observed to proliferate. This proliferation was blocked by addition of chloroquine or by addition of monoclonal antibody to HLA-DR. Proliferation was not blocked by addition of monoclonal antibody to HLA-A, -B, -DQ, or -DP. What might these findings indicate about the early-stage melanoma cells in this experimental system?

b. When the same experiment was repeated with advanced-stage melanoma cells, the tetanus toxoid T-cell clones failed to proliferate in response to the tetanus toxoid antigen. What might this indicate about advanced-stage melanoma cells?

c. When early and advanced malignant melanoma cells were fixed with paraformaldehyde and incubated with processed tetanus toxoid, only the early-stage melanoma cells could induce proliferation of the

tetanus toxoid T-cell clones. What might this indicate about early-stage melanoma cells?

d. How might you confirm your hypothesis experimentally?

4. What are three likely sources of tumor antigens?

5. Various cytokines have been evaluated for use in tumor immunotherapy. Describe four mechanisms by which cytokines mediate antitumor effects and the cytokines that induce each type of effect.

6. Infusion of transfected melanoma cells into cancer patients is a promising immunotherapy.

a. Which two genes have been transfected into melanoma cells for this purpose? What is the rationale behind use of each of these genes?

b. Why might use of such transfected melanoma cells also be effective in treating other types of cancers?

Abzyme a monoclonal antibody that has catalytic activity.

Acquired immunity host defenses that are mediated by B and T cells following exposure to antigen and that exhibit specificity, diversity, memory, and self/nonself recognition. See also **innate immunity**.

Acquired immunodeficiency syndrome (AIDS) a disease caused by human immunodeficiency virus (HIV) that is marked by significant depletion of CD4$^+$ T cells resulting in increased susceptibility to a variety of infections and cancers.

Active immunity acquired immunity that is induced by natural exposure to a pathogen or by **vaccination**.

Acute-phase response the systemic effects, associated with an acute **inflammatory response**, that include production of hepatocyte-derived serum proteins, fever, and increase in circulating leukocytes (see Figure 15-11).

Adjuvant a substance (e.g., Freund's adjuvant, alum, bacterial LPS) that nonspecifically enhances the immune response to an antigen (see Table 4-3).

Adoptive transfer an experimental technique in which lymphocytes from an antigen-primed donor are transferred to an x-irradiated recipient that lacks a functional immune system.

Affinity the binding strength between a single receptor site (e.g., one binding site on an antibody) and a ligand (e.g., an antigenic determinant). The association constant is a quantitative measure of affinity.

Affinity maturation the increase in average antibody affinity for an antigen that occurs during the course of an immune response.

Agglutinin any antibody that causes visible clumping (agglutination) of particulate antigens. A hemagglutinin is an antibody that causes clumping of red blood cells.

Agretope the region of a processed antigenic peptide that binds to an **MHC molecule** (see Figure 4-9).

Allele two or more alternative forms of a gene at a particular **locus** that confer alternative characters. The presence of multiple alleles results in **polymorphism**.

Allelic exclusion a process that permits expression of only one of the allelic forms of a gene. B and T cells exhibit allelic exclusion of the immunoglobulin and T-cell receptor genes, respectively (see Figure 7-13).

Allergen noninfectious antigens that induce **hypersensitivity** reactions, most commonly IgE-mediated type I reactions.

Allergy a **hypersensitivity** reaction that can involve various deleterious effects such as hay fever, asthma, **serum sickness**, systemic **anaphylaxis**, or contact dermatitis.

Allogeneic denoting members of the same species that differ genetically.

Allograft a tissue transplant between **allogeneic** individuals.

Allotype a set of **allotypic determinants** characteristic of some but not all members of a species.

Allotypic determinant an antigenic determinant that varies among members of a species. The constant regions of antibodies possess allotypic determinants (see Figure 5-14b).

Alpha-feto protein (AFP) see **Oncofetal tumor antigen**.

Alternative complement pathway activation of **complement** that is initiated by foreign cell-surface constituents; involves C3–C9, factors B and D, and properdin; and generates the **membrane-attack complex** (see Figure 14-1).

Anaphylatoxins the **complement** split products C3a and C5a, which mediate **degranulation** of mast cells and basophils, resulting in release of mediators that induce contraction of smooth muscle and increased vascular permeability.

Anaphylaxis an immediate type I hypersensitivity reaction, which is triggered by IgE-mediated mast cell **degranulation**. Systemic anaphylaxis leads to shock and is often fatal. Localized anaphylaxis involves various types of **atopic** reactions.

Antibody a protein (immunoglobulin), consisting of two identical heavy chains and two identical light chains, that recognizes a particular **epitope** on an antigen and facilitates clearance of that antigen (see Figure 5-3). Membrane-bound antibody is expressed by **B cells** that have not encountered antigen; secreted antibody is produced by **plasma cells**.

Antibody-dependent cell-mediated cytotoxicity (ADCC) a cell-mediated reaction in which nonspecific cytotoxic cells that express **Fc receptors** (e.g., NK cells, neutrophils, macrophages) recognize bound antibody on a target cell and subsequently cause lysis of the target cell (see Figure 16-12).

Antigen any substance (usually foreign) that binds specifically to an antibody or a T-cell receptor; often is used as a synonym for **immunogen**.

Antigenic determinant the site on an antigen that is recognized and bound by a particular antibody or T-cell receptor; also called **epitope**.

Antigenic drift a series of spontaneous point mutations that generate minor antigenic variations in pathogens and lead to strain differences.

Antigenic peptide see **Antigen processing**.

Antigenic shift sudden emergence of a new pathogen subtype possibly resulting from genetic reassortment leading to substantial antigenic differences.

Antigen processing degradation of antigens by one of two pathways yielding antigenic peptides that are displayed in association with MHC molecules on the surface of antigen-presenting cells or altered self-cells (see Figure 10-8).

Antigen-presenting cell (APC) any cell that can process and present antigenic peptides in association with **class II MHC molecules** and deliver a **costimulatory signal** necessary for T-cell activation. Macrophages, dendritic cells, and B cells constitute the professional APCs (see Figure 12-18). Nonprofessional APCs, which function in antigen presentation only for short periods, include thymic epithelial cells and vascular endothelial cells.

Anti-idiotype antibody a secondary antibody (Ab-2) that is specific for the **paratope** of a primary antibody (Ab-1) and thus mimics the **epitope** of the original antigen (see Figure 16-23). It represents an internal image of the original antigen and thus might be effective as a vaccine, avoiding immunization with a pathogen (see Figure 18-6).

Apoptosis morphologic changes associated with programmed cell death including nuclear fragmentation, blebbing, and release of apoptotic bodies, which are phagocytosed (see Figure 3-4). In contrast to **necrosis**, it does not result in damage to surrounding cells.

Atopic pertaining to clinical manifestations of type I (IgE-mediated) hypersensitivity including allergic rhinitis (hay fever), eczema, asthma, and various food allergies.

Autograft tissue grafted from one part of the body to another in the same individual.

Autoimmunity an abnormal immune response against self-antigens.

Autologous derived from the same individual.

Autosomal pertaining to all the chromosomes except the sex chromosomes.

Avidity the functional binding strength between two molecules that (unlike **affinity**) reflects the interaction of all the binding sites.

Basophil a nonphagocytic granulocyte that expresses Fc receptors for IgE (see Figure 3-14). Antigen-mediated cross-linkage of bound IgE induces **degranulation** of basophils.

B cell a lymphocyte that matures in the bone marrow and expresses membrane-bound antibody. Following interaction with antigen, it differentiates into antibody-secreting plasma cells and memory cells.

B-cell coreceptor a complex of three proteins (CR2, CD19, and TAPA-1) associated with the B-cell receptor (see Figure 8-9). It is thought to amplify the activating signal induced by cross-linkage of the receptor.

B-cell receptor (BCR) complex comprising a membrane-bound immunoglobulin molecule and two associated signal-transducing Ig-α/Ig-β molecules (see Figure 8-7).

BCG (Bacillus Calmette-Guerin) an attenuated form of *Mycobacterium bovis* used as a specific vaccine and as an adjuvant component.

β_2-Microglobulin invariant subunit that associates with the polymorphic α chain to form **class I MHC molecules**; it is not encoded by MHC genes.

Bursa of Fabricius a **primary lymphoid organ** in birds where B-cell maturation occurs. The bone marrow is the functional equivalent in mammals.

C (constant) gene segment the 3′ coding of a re-arranged immunoglobulin or T-cell receptor gene. There are multiple C gene segments in germ-line DNA, but as a result of gene rearrangement and, in some cases, RNA processing, only one segment is expressed in a given protein.

CAMs see **Cell-adhesion molecules.**

Carcinoma tumor arising from endodermal or ecto-dermal tissues (e.g., skin or epithelium).

Carrier an immunogenic molecule containing anti-genic determinants recognized by T cells. Conjugation of a carrier to a nonimmunogenic **hapten** renders the hap-ten immunogenic.

Carrier effect dependence of a **secondary immune response** to a hapten on both the **hapten** and **carrier** used in the initial immunization (see Table 16-6).

CD3 a polypeptide complex containing three dimers: a $\gamma\varepsilon$ heterodimer, a $\varepsilon\delta$ heterodimer, and either a $\zeta\zeta$ homodimer or $\zeta\eta$ heterodimer (see Figure 11-9). It is associated with the T-cell receptor and functions in signal transduction.

CD4 a monomeric membrane molecule, usually pres-ent on T_H cells that acts as a coreceptor. It binds to the β_2 domain of **class II MHC molecules** and functions in signal transduction during T-cell activation.

CD8 a heterodimeric membrane molecule, usually pres-ent on T_C cells that acts as a coreceptor. It binds to the α_3 domain of **class I MHC molecules** and functions in signal transduction during T-cell activation.

CD antigen cell-membrane molecule used to differ-entiate human leukocyte subpopulations and identified by monoclonal antibody. All monoclonal antibodies that react with the same membrane molecule are grouped into a common cluster of differentiation, or CD (see Table 3-4).

Cell-adhesion molecules (CAMs) a group of cell-surface molecules that mediate intercellular adhesion. Most belong to one of four protein families: the **inte-grins**, **selectins**, mucin-like proteins, and **immunoglob-ulin superfamily** (see Figure 15-2).

Cell line a population of cultured tumor cells or normal cells that have been subjected to chemical or viral **trans-formation** (see Table 2-2). Cell lines can be propagated indefinitely in culture.

Cell-mediated immune response host defenses that are mediated by antigen-specific T cells and various non-specific cells of the immune system. It protects against intracellular bacteria, viruses, and cancer and is responsible

for graft rejection. Transfer of primed T cells confers this type of immunity on the recipient. See also **Humoral immune response.**

Cell-mediated lympholysis (CML) in vitro lysis of allogeneic cells or virus-infected syngeneic cells by T cells (see Figure 16-14); can be used as an assay for CTL activity or class I MHC activity.

Chemokine any of several low-molecular-weight poly-peptides that mediate **chemotaxis** for different leuko-cytes and regulate the expression and/or adhesiveness of leukocyte **integrins** (see Table 15-2).

Chemotaxis directional movement of cells in response to the concentration gradient of some substance.

Chimera an animal or tissue composed of elements derived from genetically distinct individuals. The **SCID-human mouse** is a chimera (see Figure 2-1).

Class I MHC molecules heterodimeric membrane proteins that consist of an a chain encoded in the **MHC** associated noncovalently with β_2**-microglobulin** (see Figure 9-5a). They are expressed by nearly all nucleated cells and function in antigen presentation to CD8$^+$ T cells. The classical class I molecules are H-2 K, D, and L in mice and HLA-A, -B, and -C in humans.

Class II MHC molecules heterodimeric membrane proteins that consist of a noncovalently associated α and β chain, both encoded in the **MHC** (see Figure 9-5b). They are expressed by **antigen-presenting cells** and function in antigen presentation to CD4$^+$ T cells. The classical class II molecules are H-2 IA and IE in mice and HLA-DP, -DQ, and -DR in humans.

Class III MHC molecules various proteins encoded in the **MHC** but distinct from class I and class II MHC molecules. They include some complement components, two steroid 21-hydroxylases, and tumor necrosis factor α and β.

Class switching see **Isotype switching.**

Classical complement pathway activation of **com-plement** that is initiated by antigen-antibody complexes; involves C1–C9; and generates the **membrane-attack complex** (see Figure 14-1).

Clonal anergy a proposed mechanism for rendering peripheral antigen-reactive lymphocytes functionally in-active.

Clonal deletion proposed mechanism for eliminating, by **apoptosis,** self-reactive lymphocytes induced by their contact with self-antigens.

Clonal selection proposed mechanism whereby anti-gen binding to receptors (membrane antibody or T-cell receptor) on a lymphocyte stimulates the cell to undergo mitosis and develop into a **clone** of cells with the same **antigenic specificity** as the original parent cell.

Clone   cells arising from a single progenitor cell.

Colony-stimulating factors (CSFs) the group of factors that induces the proliferation and differentiation of hematopoietic cells and some other cells.

Complement   the group of serum proteins that participates in an enzymatic cascade, ultimately generating the cytolytic **membrane-attack complex** (see Tables 14-1 and 14-2).

Complementarity-determining region (CDR) see **Hypervariable region**.

Congenic   denoting individuals that differ genetically at a single genetic locus or region; also called coisogenic.

Constant (C) region   the nearly invariant portion of antibody heavy and light chains and of the polypeptide chains of the T-cell receptor.

Cortex   the outer or peripheral layer of an organ.

Co-stimulatory signal   additional signal that is required to induce proliferation of antigen-primed T cells and is generated by interaction of CD28 on T cells with B7 on antigen-presenting cells or altered self-cells (see Figures 12-17 and 16-2). In B-cell activation, an analogous signal (competence signal 2) is provided by interaction of CD40 on B cells with CD40L on activated T_H cells (see Figure 8-10).

Cross-reactivity   ability of a particular antibody or T-cell receptor to react with two or more antigens that possess a common **epitope**.

CTL   see **Cytotoxic T lymphocyte**.

Cytokine   any of numerous secreted, low-molecular-weight proteins that regulate the intensity and duration of the immune response by exerting a variety of effects on lymphocytes and other immune cells (see Table 13-1).

Cytotoxic   having the ability to kill cells.

Cytotoxic T lymphocyte (CTL)   an effector T cell (usually $CD8^+$) that can mediate the lysis of target cells bearing antigenic peptides associated with an MHC molecule (see Figure 16-4). It usually arises from an antigen-activated T_C cell (see Figure 16-1).

D (diversity) gene segment   that portion of a rearranged immunoglobulin heavy-chain gene or T-cell receptor gene that is situated between the V and J gene segments and encodes part of the hypervariable region. There are multiple D gene segments in germ-line DNA,

but gene rearrangement results in only one occurring in each functional rearranged gene.

Degranulation   discharge of the contents of cytoplasmic granules by **basophils** and **mast cells** following cross-linkage (usually by antigen) of bound IgE (see Figure 17-5). It is characteristic of type I **hypersensitivity**.

Delayed-type hypersensitivity (DTH)   a type IV hypersensitive response mediated by sensitized T_{DTH} **cells**, which release various **cytokines** and **chemokines** (see Figure 16-15). The response generally occurs 2–3 days after T_{DTH} cells interact with antigen. It is an important part of host defense against intracellular parasites and bacteria.

Dendritic cells   professional **antigen-presenting cells** that have long membrane processes. They are found in the lymph nodes, spleen, and thymus (follicular and interdigitating dendritic cells); skin (Langerhans cells); and other tissues (interstitial dendritic cells).

Differentiation antigen   a cell-surface marker that is expressed only during a particular developmental stage or by a particular cell lineage.

Domain   an independently folded structural unit within a protein. See also **Immunoglobulin fold**.

Edema   abnormal accumulation of fluid in intercellular spaces, often resulting from a failure of the lymphatic system to drain off normal leakage from the capillaries.

Effector cell   any cell capable of mediating an immune function (e.g., activated T_H cells, CTLs, and plasma cells).

ELISA (enzyme-linked immunosorbent assay)   an assay for quantitating either antibody or antigen by use of an enzyme-linked antibody and a substrate that forms a colored reaction product (see Figure 6-14).

Endocytosis   process by which cells ingest extracellular macromolecules by enclosing them in a small portion of the plasma membrane, which invaginates and is pinched off to form an intracellular vesicle containing the ingested material (see Figure 1-3).

Endogenous   originating within the organism or cell.

Endotoxins   certain lipopolysaccharide (LPS) components of the cell wall of gram-negative bacteria that are responsible for many of the pathogenic effects associated with these organisms. Some function as **superantigens**.

Eosinophil   a granulocyte that functions in **antibody-dependent cell-mediated cytotoxicity**, particularly of parasites, and also has some phagocytic ability (see Figure 3-14).

Epitope   see **Antigenic determinant**.

Epstein-Barr virus (EBV)   the causative agent of Burkitt's **lymphoma** and infectious mononucleosis. It can transform human B cells into stable **cell lines**.

Equilibrium dialysis   an experimental technique that can be used to determine the affinity of an antibody for antigen and its **valency** (see Figure 6-2).

Equivalence   a measure of the proportion of antibody to antigen that yields the maximum precipitate in liquids and gels (see Figure 6-4).

Erythema   redness of the skin caused by engorgement of capillaries during an **inflammatory response**.

Erythroblastosis fetalis   a type II hypersensitivity reaction in which maternal antibodies against fetal **Rh antigens** cause hemolysis of the erythrocytes of a newborn (see Figure 17-13); also called hemolytic disease of the newborn.

Erythropoiesis   the generation of red blood cells.

Exocytosis   process by which cells release molecules (e.g., cytokines, lytic enzymes, degradation products) contained within a membrane-bound vesicle by fusion of the vesicle with the plasma membrane (see Figure 3-13).

Exogenous   originating outside the organism or cell.

Exon   a continuous segment of DNA that encodes part of a gene product; also called coding sequence.

Exotoxins   toxic proteins secreted by gram-positive and gram-negative bacteria; some function as **superantigens**. They cause food poisoning, toxic-shock syndrome, and other disease states. See also **Immunotoxin**.

Extravasation   movement of blood cells through an unruptured vessel wall into the surrounding tissue, particularly at sites of inflammation (see Figures 15-3 and 15-7).

Exudate   fluid with a high content of protein, salts, and cellular debris that accumulates extravascularly, usually as a result of inflammation.

F(ab')$_2$ fragment   a bivalent antigen-binding fragment of an immunoglobulin molecule that consists of both light chains and part of both heavy chains. It is obtained by brief pepsin digestion (see Figure 5-2).

Fab fragment   a monovalent antigen-binding fragment of an immunoglobulin molecule that consists of one light chain and part of one heavy chain. It is obtained by brief papain digestion (see Figure 5-2).

Fc fragment   a crystallizable, non-antigen-binding fragment of an immunoglobulin molecule that consists of the carboxyl-terminal portions of both heavy chains and possesses binding sites for Fc receptors and the C1q component of complement. It is obtained by brief papain digestion (see Figure 5-2).

Fc receptor   cell-surface receptor specific for the Fc portion of certain classes of immunoglobulin. It is present on lymphocytes, mast cells, macrophages, and other accessory cells.

First-set graft rejection   process whereby an **allograft** is rejected following first exposure to the alloantigens of the donor. Complete rejection usually occurs within 12–14 days (see Figure 23-1b).

Fluorescent antibody   an antibody with a **fluorochrome** conjugated to its Fc region that is used to stain cell-surface molecules or tissues, a technique called **immunofluorescence**.

Fluorochrome   a fluorescent dye, which can be conjugated with an antibody or other protein. Two common fluorochromes used to tag antibodies are fluorescein isothiocyanate (FITC), which emits a yellow-green color, and rhodamine (Rh), which emits a red color. See also **Immunofluorescence**.

Framework region   a relatively conserved sequence of amino acids located on either side of the hypervariable regions in the variable domains of immunoglobulin heavy and light chains (see Figure 5-8).

Fusin   a G protein–linked receptor present on certain human cells, including CD4$^+$ T cells, that is thought to be required for fusion of **HIV** with target cells.

Gamma globulins   group of serum proteins originally characterized by having a greater electrophoretic mobility than other fractions and later shown to contain the immunoglobulins.

Gene locus   see **Locus**.

Genome   the total genetic material contained in the haploid set of chromosomes.

Genotype   the combined genetic material inherited from both parents; also, the **alleles** present at one or more specific loci.

Germ line   the unmodified genetic material that is transmitted from one generation to the next through the gametes.

Germinal center   a region within lymph nodes and the spleen where B-cell activation, proliferation, and differentiation occurs (see Figure 8-15).

Graft-versus-host disease (GVHD) a reaction that develops when a graft contains immunocompetent T cells that recognize and attack the recipient's cells.

Granulocyte any **leukocyte** that contains cytoplasmic granules, particularly the basophil, eosinophil, and neutrophil (see Figure 3-14).

Granuloma a tumor-like mass or nodule that arises due to a chronic **inflammatory response** and contains many activated macrophages, epithelioid cells (modified macrophages), T_{DTH} cells, and multinucleated giant cells resulting from fusion of macrophages (see Figure 16-16).

H-2 complex term for the **MHC** in the mouse.

Haplotype the set of **alleles** of linked genes present on one parental chromosome; commonly used in reference to the **MHC** genes.

Hapten a low-molecular-weight compound that is not immunogenic by itself but when coupled to a carrier can elicit anti-hapten antibodies (see Figure 4-12). Dinitrophenol (DNP) is a common hapten.

Heavy chain the larger polypeptide of an antibody molecule composed of one variable domain (V_H) and three or four constant domains (C_H1, C_H2, etc.). There are five major classes of heavy chains in humans, which determine the **isotype** of an antibody (see Table 5-1).

Hemagglutinin see **Agglutinin**.

Hematopoiesis formation and development of red and white blood cells (see Figure 3-2).

Hematopoietins family of proteins that includes many cytokines whose receptors share several conserved motifs (see Figure 13-5).

Hemolytic plaque assay in vitro technique for detecting **plasma cells** based on their ability to lyse antigen-sensitized erythrocytes in the presence of complement, thereby forming visible plaques (see Figure 16-20).

Heterologous originating from a different species; see also **Xenogeneic**.

High-endothelial venule (HEV) an area of a capillary venule composed of specialized cells with a plump, cuboidal ("high") shape through which lymphocytes migrate to enter various lymphoid organs (see Figure 15-4).

Hinge region the portion of immunoglobulin heavy chains between the **Fc** and **Fab** regions. It gives flexibility to the molecule and allows the two antigen-binding sites to function independently.

Histamine one of numerous mediators present in the cytoplasmic granules of basophils and mast cells. It is released during degranulation and causes increased vascular permeability and contraction of smooth muscle.

Histocompatible denoting individuals whose major histocompatibility antigens, which are encoded by the **MHC**, are identical. Grafts between such individuals generally are accepted.

HIV (human immunodeficiency virus) a **retrovirus** that infects human CD4$^+$ T cells and causes **acquired immunodeficiency syndrome (AIDS)**.

HLA (human leukocyte antigen) complex term for the **MHC** in humans.

Homologous originating from the same species; also refers to similarity in the sequences of DNA or proteins.

HTLV (human T lymphotrophic virus) a **retrovirus** that infects human CD4$^+$ T cells and causes adult T-cell leukemia.

Humoral pertaining to extracellular fluid including the plasma and lymph.

Humoral immune response host defenses that are mediated by antibody present in the plasma, lymph, and tissue fluids. It protects against extracellular bacteria and foreign macromolecules. Transfer of antibodies confers this type of immunity on the recipient. See also **Cell-mediated immune response**.

Hybridoma a **clone** of hybrid cells formed by fusion of normal lymphocytes with myeloma cells; it retains the properties of the normal cell to produce antibodies or T-cell receptors but exhibits the immortal growth characteristic of myeloma cells (see Figure 2-2). Hybridomas are used to produce **monoclonal antibody**.

Hypersensitivity exaggerated immune response that causes damage to the individual. Immediate hypersensitivity (types I, II, and III) is mediated by antibody or immune complexes, and delayed-type hypersensitivity (type IV) is mediated by T_{DTH} cells (see Table 17-1).

Hypervariable region one of three regions within the variable domain of each chain in immunoglobulins and T-cell receptors that exhibits the most sequence variability and contributes the most to the antigen-binding site; also called complementary-determining region (CDR).

Idiotope a single **antigenic determinant** in the variable domains of an antibody or T-cell receptor; also called idiotypic determinant. Idiotopes are generated by the unique amino acid sequence specific for each antigen (see Figure 5-14).

Idiotype the set of antigenic determinants (**idiotopes**) characterizing each unique antibody or T-cell receptor.

Immediate hypersensitivity an exaggerated immune response mediated by antibody (type I and II) or antigen-antibody complexes (type III) that manifests within minutes to hours following exposure of a sensitized individual to antigen (see Table 17-1).

Immune complex a macromolecular complex of antibody bound to antigen, which sometimes includes **complement** components. Deposition of immune complexes in various tissues results in type III **hypersensitivity**.

Immunization the process of producing a state of immunity in a subject. See also **Active immunity** and **Passive immunity.**

Immunoabsorption removal of antibody or antigen from a sample by adsorption to a solid-phase system to which the complementary antigen or antibody is bound.

Immunocompetent denoting a mature lymphocyte that is capable of recognizing a specific antigen and mediating an immune response.

Immunodeficiency any deficiency in the immune response. It may result from a defect involving phagocytosis, the humoral response, or the cell-mediated response. Combined immunodeficiencies affect both the humoral and cell-mediated immune response (see Figure 21-1).

Immunofluorescence technique of staining cells or tissue with **fluorescent antibody** and visualizing the section under a fluorescent microscope (see Figure 6-16).

Immunogen a substance capable of eliciting an immune response. All immunogens are **antigens**, but some antigens (e.g., haptens) are not immunogens.

Immunoglobulin (Ig) see **Antibody**.

Immunoglobulin fold characteristic **domain** structure present in immunoglobulins that consists of about 110 amino acids folded into two β pleated sheets, each containing three or four antiparallel β strands, and stabilized by an intrachain disulfide bond forming a loop of about 60 amino acids (see Figure 5-6).

Immunoglobulin superfamily group of proteins that contain **immunoglobulin-fold** domains, or structurally related domains, including immunoglobulins, T-cell receptors, MHC molecules, and numerous other membrane molecules (see Figure 5-19).

Immunotoxin an **exotoxin** or radioisotope conjugated to a monoclonal antibody, which usually is specific for a **tumor antigen** (see Figure 5-23).

Inflammatory response a localized tissue response to injury or other trauma characterized by pain, heat, redness, and swelling. The response, which includes both localized and systemic effects, consists of altered patterns of blood flow, an influx of phagocytic and other immune

cells, removal of foreign antigens, and healing of the damaged tissue (see Figures 15-10 and 15-11).

Innate immunity nonspecific host defenses that exist prior to exposure to an antigen and involve anatomic, physiologic, endocytic and phagocytic, and inflammatory mechanisms. See also **Acquired immunity**.

Integrins a group of heterodimeric cell-adhesion molecules (e.g., LFA-1, VLA-4, and Mac-1) present on various leukocytes that bind to Ig-superfamily CAMs (e.g., ICAMs, VCAM-1) on endothelium (see Figure 15-2).

Interferons (IFNs) several glycoprotein **cytokines** produced and secreted by certain cells that induce an antiviral state in other cells and also help to regulate the immune response (see Table 13-1).

Interleukins (ILs) a group of **cytokines** secreted by leukocytes that primarily affect the growth and differentiation of various hematopoietic and immune-system cells (see Table 13-1).

Intron noncoding sequence within a gene, which is transcribed into the primary transcript but is removed during processing and does not appear in mRNA.

In vitro referring to experiments involving living cells or cellular components performed outside the intact organism.

In vivo referring to experiments carried out in an intact, living organism.

Isograft graft between genetically identical individuals.

Isotype an antibody class, which is determined by the heavy-chain constant-region sequence. The five human isotypes, designated IgA, IgD, IgE, IgG, and IgM, exhibit structural and functional differences (see Table 5-4). Also refers to the set of **isotypic determinants** that is carried by all members of a species.

Isotype switching conversion of one antibody class (**isotype**) to another resulting from the genetic rearrangement of heavy-chain constant-region genes in B cells; also called class switching.

Isotypic determinant an **antigenic determinant** within the immunoglobulin constant regions that is characteristic of a species (see Figure 5-14).

J chain a polypeptide that joins subunits of polymeric IgA and IgM (see Figure 5-15).

J (joining) gene segment that portion of a rearranged immunoglobulin or T-cell receptor gene that joins the variable region to the constant region and encodes part of the **hypervariable region**. There are multiple J gene segments in germ-line DNA, but gene rearrangement results in only one segment occurring in each functional rearranged gene.

Kaposi's sarcoma a neoplastic lesion characterized by multiple bluish nodules in the skin and hemorrhages; it is common in AIDS patients.

Kappa (κ) chain see **Light chain**.

Karyotype the chromosomal constitution of a given cell.

Kinins group of peptides released during an **inflammatory response** that act as vasodilators, inducing smooth-muscle contraction and increased vascular permeability.

Knockout mouse a form of **transgenic mouse** in which a normal gene is replaced with a mutant allele or disrupted form of the gene; as a result the animal lacks a functional gene product (see Figures 2-12 and 2-13).

Lambda (λ) chain see **Light chain**.

Langerhans cell a type of **dendritic cell** that is found in the skin and bears Fc receptors.

Leukemia cancer originating in any class of hematopoietic cell that tends to proliferate as single cells within the lymph or blood.

Leukocyte any blood cell that is not an erythrocyte; white blood cell.

Leukopenia reduction in the number of circulating white blood cells.

Leukotrienes several lipid mediators of inflammation and type I hypersensitivity; also called slow reactive substance of anaphylaxis (SRS-A). They are metabolic products of arachidonic acid (see Figure 15-9).

Ligand any molecule recognized by a **receptor**.

Light chain the smaller polypeptide of an antibody molecule composed of one variable domain (V_L) and one constant domain (C_L). There are two major types (kappa and lambda) of light chains in humans.

Locus the specific chromosomal location of a gene.

LPS (lipopolysaccharide) a group of substances present in the cell wall of gram-negative bacteria that are B-cell **mitogens**, can induce an inflammatory response, and also function as an **adjuvant**.

Lymph a pale, watery, proteinaceous fluid that is derived from intercellular tissue fluid and circulates in lymphatic vessels.

Lymph node a small **secondary lymphoid organ** that contains lymphocytes, macrophages, and dendritic cells and serves as a site for filtration of foreign antigen and activation and proliferation of lymphocytes (see Figures 3-19 and 3-21). See also **Germinal center**.

Lymphoblast a cell stage that occurs in lymphocytes after activation and before cell division (see Figure 3-10). It is distinguished by a higher cytoplasm : nucleus ratio than in resting lymphocytes.

Lymphocyte a mononuclear leukocyte that mediates humoral or cell-mediated immunity. See also **B cell** and **T cell**.

Lymphokine a **cytokine** produced by activated lymphocytes, especially T_H cells.

Lymphoma a cancer of lymphoid cells that tends to proliferate as a solid tumor.

Lymphopoiesis the differentiation of lymphocytes from hematopoietic stem cells.

Lysogeny state in which a viral genome (**provirus**) is associated with the host genome in such a way that the viral genes remain unexpressed.

Lysosome a small cytoplasmic vesicle found in many types of cells that contains hydrolytic enzymes, which play an important role in the degradation of material ingested by **phagocytosis** and **endocytosis**.

Lysozyme an enzyme present in tears, saliva, and mucous secretions that digests mucopeptides in bacterial cells walls and thus functions as a nonspecific antibacterial agent.

Macrophage a large, leukocyte derived from a **monocyte** that functions in phagocytosis, antigen processing and presentation, secretion of cytokines, and antibody-dependent cell-mediated cytotoxicity.

MALT (mucosal-associated lymphoid tissue) collective term for **secondary lymphoid organs** located along various mucous membrane surfaces including Peyer's patches, tonsils, the appendix, as well as diffuse lymphoid follicles within the intestinal lamina propria.

Marginal zone a diffuse region of the spleen, located between the **red pulp** and **white pulp**, that is rich in B cells and contains lymphoid follicles, which can develop into **germinal centers** (see Figure 3-22).

Mast cell a bone marrow–derived cell present in a variety of tissues that resembles peripheral-blood basophils, bears **Fc receptors** for IgE, and undergoes IgE-mediated **degranulation**.

Medulla the innermost or central region of an organ.

Megakaryocyte a white blood cell that produces **platelets** by cytoplasmic budding.

Membrane-attack complex (MAC) the complex of complement components C5–C9, which is formed in the terminal steps of either the classical or alternative complement pathway, and mediates cell lysis by creating a membrane pore in the target cell.

Memory, immunologic the attribute of the immune system mediated by **memory cells** whereby a second encounter with an antigen induces a heightened state of immune reactivity.

Memory cell clonally expanded progeny of T and B cells formed during the **primary immune response** following initial exposure to an antigen. Memory cells are more easily activated than **naive** lymphocytes and mediate a **secondary immune response** on subsequent exposure to antigen.

MHC (major histocompatibility complex) a complex of genes encoding cell-surface molecules that are required for antigen presentation to T cells and for rapid graft rejection. It is called the H-2 complex in the mouse and the HLA complex in humans.

MHC molecules proteins encoded by the major histocompatibility complex and classified as class I, class II, and class III MHC molecules.

MHC restriction the characteristic of T cells that permits them to recognize antigen only after it is processed and the resulting antigenic peptides are displayed in association with either a **class I** or **class II MHC molecule**.

Minor histocompatibility loci genes outside of the MHC that encode antigens contributing to graft rejection.

Mitogen any substance that nonspecifically induces DNA synthesis and cell division, especially of lymphocytes. Common mitogens are concanavalin A, phytohemagglutinin, **LPS**, pokeweed mitogen, and various **superantigens**.

Mixed-lymphocyte reaction (MLR) in vitro T-cell proliferation in response to cells expressing allogeneic MHC molecules (see Figure 6-13); can be used as an assay for class II MHC activity.

Monoclonal derived from a single cell.

Monoclonal antibody homogeneous preparation of antibody molecules, produced by a hybridoma, all of which exhibit the same antigenic specificity (see Figure 5-22).

Monocyte a mononuclear phagocytic leukocyte that circulates briefly in the bloodstream before migrating into the tissues where it becomes a **macrophage**.

Naive denoting mature B and T cells that have not encountered antigen; synonymous with unprimed and virgin.

Natural killer (NK) cell a large, granular lymphocyte (null cell) that has cytotoxic ability but does not express antigen-binding receptors. It exhibits antibody-independent killer of tumor cells and also can participate in antibody-dependent cell-mediated cytotoxicity.

Necrosis morphologic changes associated with death of individual cells or groups of cells, leading to disruption and atrophy of tissue. See also **Apoptosis**.

Neoplasm any new and abnormal growth; a benign or malignant tumor.

Network theory the theory that the immune system is regulated by a network of idiotype and anti-idiotype reactions involving antibodies and T-cell receptors (see Figure 16-23). See also **Anti-idiotype antibody**.

Neutrophil a circulating, phagocytic granulocyte involved early in the **inflammatory response** (see Figure 3-14). It expresses **Fc receptors** and can participate in **antibody-dependent cell-mediated cytotoxicity**.

Northern blotting common technique for detecting specific mRNAs in which denatured mRNAs are separated electrophoretically and then transferred to a polymer sheet, which is incubated with a radiolabeled DNA probe specific for the mRNA of interest.

Nude mouse homozygous genetic defect (*nu/nu*) carried by an inbred mouse strain that results in the absence of the thymus and consequently a marked deficiency of T cells and cell-mediated immunity. The mice are hairless (hence, the name) and can accept grafts from other species.

Null cell a small population of peripheral-blood lymphocytes that lack the membrane markers characteristic of B and T cells. **Natural killer cells** are included in this group.

Oncofetal tumor antigen an antigen that is present during fetal development but generally is not expressed in tissues except by tumor cells. Alpha-feto protein (AFP) and carcinoembryonic antigen (CEA) are two examples that have been associated with various cancers (see Table 24-3).

Oncogene a gene encoding a protein capable of inducing cellular **transformation**. Oncogenes derived from viruses are termed v-onc, while their cellular counterparts (**proto-oncogenes**) are denoted c-onc.

Oncogenic   causing cancer.

Opsonin   a substance (e.g., an antibody or C3b) that binds to an antigen and enhances its phagocytosis.

Opsonization   deposition of opsonins on an antigen, thereby promoting a stable, adhesive contact with an appropriate phagocytic cell (see Figure 14-11).

Ouchterlony method   a double immunodiffusion technique involving the diffusion of antigen and antibody within a gel resulting in formation of a visible band of precipitate in the region of **equivalence** (see Figure 6-8).

PALS (periarteriolar lymphoid sheath)   see **White pulp**.

Paratope   the site in the variable (V) domain of an antibody or T-cell receptor that binds to an epitope on an antigen.

Passive immunity   acquired immunity conferred by the transfer of immune products, such as antibody or sensitized T cells, from an immune individual to a nonimmune one. See also **Active immunity**.

Pathogen   a disease-causing organism.

Perforin   cytolytic product of CTLs that, in the presence of Ca^{2+}, polymerizes to form transmembrane pores in target cells (see Figure 16-7).

Peyer's patches   lymphoid nodules located along the small intestine that function to trap antigens from the gastrointestinal tract and provide sites where B and T cells can interact with antigen.

Phagocytosis   a process by which certain cells (phagocytes) engulf microorganisms, other cells, and foreign particles (see Figure 3-13).

Phagosome   intracellular vacuole containing ingested particulate materials; formed by invagination of the cell membrane during **phagocytosis**.

Phylogeny   the evolutionary history of a species.

Pinocytosis   a type of **endocytosis** in which a cell ingests extracellular fluid and soluble materials contained within that fluid.

Plaque-forming count (PFC)   the number of plaques formed in the in vitro **hemolytic plaque assay**, which detects antibody-forming plasma cells.

Plasma   the cell-free, fluid portion of blood, which contains all the clotting factors.

Plasma cell   a differentiated antibody-secreting cell derived from an antigen-activated **B cell**.

Plasmacytoma   a plasma-cell tumor.

Plasmapheresis   a technique in which plasma is removed from an individual's blood and the erythrocytes are resuspended in a suitable medium and then returned to the individual.

Platelet   a small nuclear membrane-bound cytoplasmic structure derived from megakaryocytes, which contains vasoactive substances and clotting factors important in blood coagulation, inflammation, and allergic reactions; also called thrombocyte.

Polyclonal   pertaining to many different clones.

Polymorphism   presence of multiple **alleles** at a specific genetic locus. The major histocompatibility complex is highly polymorphic.

Precipitin   an antibody that aggregates a soluble antigen, forming a macromolecular complex that yields a visible precipitate.

Primary immune response   the immune response that is induced by initial exposure to an antigen, which activates naive lymphocytes. It is mediated largely by IgM antibody and sensitized T cells. It develops more slowly and to a lesser extent than a **secondary immune response** (see Figure 16-19).

Primary lymphoid organs   organs in which lymphocyte precursors mature into antigenically committed, immunocompetent cells. In mammals, the bone marrow and thymus are the primary lymphoid organs in which B-cell and T-cell maturation occur, respectively.

Prostaglandins   a group of biologically active lipid derivatives of arachidonic acid (see Figure 15-9). They mediate the inflammatory response and type I hypersensitivity reaction by inhibiting platelet aggregation, increasing vascular permeability, and inducing smooth-muscle contraction.

Proteasome   a large multifunctional protease complex responsible for degradation of intracellular proteins (see Figure 10-5).

Proto-oncogenes   genes that in normal cells encode various growth-controlling proteins (see Table 24-1). Under certain conditions, proto-oncogenes are converted into **oncogenes** (see Figure 24-2).

Provirus   viral DNA that is integrated into host-cell genome in a latent state and must undergo activation before it is transcribed, leading to formation of viral particles.

Pseudogene nucleotide sequence that is a stable component of the genome but is incapable of being expressed. They are thought to have been derived by mutation of ancestral active genes.

Pyrogen a fever-causing substance released by activated leukocytes.

Pyrogenic pus producing.

Radioimmunoassay (RIA) a highly sensitive technique for measuring antigen or antibody that involves competitive binding of radiolabeled antigen or antibody (see Figure 6-13).

Reagin IgE antibody that mediates type I immediate **hypersensitivity.**

Receptor, cell-surface molecule present on the cell membrane that has a high affinity for a particular ligand.

Recombination signal sequences (RSSs) conserved nucleotide sequences that flank gene segments in germ-line immunoglobulin and T-cell receptor DNA and direct joining of segments during gene rearrangement (see Figure 7-6).

Red pulp portion of the spleen consisting of a network of sinusoids populated by macrophages and erythrocytes (see Figure 3-22). It is the site where old and defective red blood cells are destroyed.

Retrovirus a type of RNA virus that uses a reverse transcriptase to produce a DNA copy of its RNA genome. HIV, causing AIDS, and HTLV, causing adult T-cell leukemia, are both retroviruses.

Rh antigen any of a large number of antigens present on the surface of blood cells that constitute the Rh blood group. See also **Erythroblastosis fetalis.**

Rheumatoid factor autoantibody found in the serum of individuals with rheumatoid arthritis and other connective-tissue diseases.

Rhogam antibody against **Rh antigen** that is used to prevent **erythroblastosis fetalis.**

Sarcoma tumor of supporting or connective tissue.

SCID-human mice experimental animal model in which human thymus and lymph node tissue is implanted in CB-17 mice, a strain carrying a mutation causing severe combined immunodeficiency (see Figure 2-1). The resulting chimeric mice are valuable for studies on lymphocyte development.

Second-set graft rejection acute, rapid rejection of an allograft in an individual who has received a previous graft from the same donor (see Figure 23-1). The reaction is mediated by primed T cells.

Secondary immune response the immune response that is induced following a second exposure to antigen, which activates memory lymphocytes. It occurs more rapidly and is stronger than the **primary immune response** (see Figure 16-19).

Secondary lymphoid organs organs and tissues in which mature, immunocompetent lymphocytes encounter trapped antigens and are activated into **effector cells**. In mammals, the **lymph nodes** and **spleen**, and mucosal-associated lymphoid tissue (**MALT**) constitute the secondary lymphoid organs.

Secretory component a protein derived from the poly-Ig receptor that forms part of the secretory IgA and IgM (see Figure 5-17).

Secretory IgA dimeric IgA linked to the **secretory component**; it is present in mucous secretions (see Figure 5-17).

Selectins a group of monomeric cell-adhesion molecules present on leukocytes (L-selectin) and endothelium (E- and P-selectin) that bind to mucin-like CAMs (e.g., GlyCam, PSGL-1) (see Figure 15-2).

Serum fluid portion of the blood, which is free of cells and clotting factors.

Serum sickness a type III hypersensitivity reaction that develops when antigen is administered intravenously, resulting in the formation and tissue deposition of large amounts of antigen-antibody complexes. It often develops when individuals are immunized with antiserum derived from other species.

Somatic mutation a mechanism by which point mutations are introduced into rearranged immunoglobulin variable-region genes during activation and proliferation of B cells. It contributes significantly to antibody diversity.

Southern blotting a common technique for detecting specific DNA sequences in which restriction-enzyme fragments are separated electrophoretically, then denatured and transferred to a polymer sheet, which is incubated with a radioactive probe specific for the sequence of interest (see Figure 2-6).

Specificity, antigenic capacity of antibody and T-cell receptor to recognize and interact with a single, unique **antigenic determinant.**

Spleen secondary lymphoid organ where old erythrocytes are destroyed and blood-borne antigens are trapped and presented to lymphocytes in the PALS and marginal zone (see Figure 3-22).

Stem cell a cell from which differentiated cells derive.

Superantigen a substance that binds to the V_β domain of the T-cell receptor and residues in the α chain of class II MHC molecules (see Figure 12-16). They induce activation of all T cells expressing T-cell receptors with a particular V_β domain. They function as potent T-cell **mitogens** and may cause food poisoning and other disorders.

Syngeneic denoting genetically identical members of the same species.

T cell a lymphocyte that matures in the thymus and expresses a T-cell receptor, CD3, and CD4 or CD8. Several distinct T-cell subpopulations are recognized.

T-cell receptor (TCR) antigen-binding molecule expressed on the surface of T cells and associated with **CD3**. It is a heterodimer consisting of either an α and β chain or a γ and δ chain (see Figures 11-3 and 11-9).

T cytotoxic (T_C) cell generally a CD8$^+$ class I MHC–restricted T cell, which differentiates into a **CTL** following interaction with altered self-cells (e.g., tumor cells, virus-infected cells).

T_{DTH} cell generally a CD4$^+$ lymphocyte derived from a T_H cell that mediates **delayed-type hypersensitivity**.

T_H1 subset subpopulation of activated CD4$^+$ T cells that secrete characteristic cytokines and function primarily in cell-mediated responses by promoting activation of T_{DTH} cells, macrophages, and T_C cells (see Table 13-2).

T_H2 subset subpopulation of activated CD4$^+$ T cells that secrete characteristic cytokines and function primarily in the humoral response (see Table 13-2).

T helper (T_H) cell generally a CD4$^+$ class II MHC–restricted T cell, which plays a central role in both humoral and cell-mediated immunity and secretes numerous cytokines when activated.

Thromboxane lipid inflammatory mediator derived from arachidonic acid (see Figure 15-9).

Thy-1 glycoprotein that is the earliest appearing surface marker of the T-cell lineage.

Thymocyte developing T cells present in the thymus.

Thymus a primary lymphoid organ, located in the thoracic cavity, where T-cell maturation occurs.

Thymus-dependent antigen a soluble protein that can induce antibody production only with help of T_H cells; response to such antigens involves isotype switching, affinity maturation, and memory-cell production.

Thymus-independent antigen an antigen (e.g., LPS, polymeric protein antigens, capsular polysaccharides) that does not require the presence of T_H cells to induce antibody production (see Table 8-2).

Titer a measure of the relative strength of an antiserum. The titer is the reciprocal of the last dilution of an antiserum capable of mediating some measurable effect such as precipitation or agglutination.

Tolerance state of immunologic unresponsiveness.

Toxoid a toxin that has been altered to eliminate its toxicity but that still can function as an **immunogen**.

Transfection experimental introduction of foreign DNA into cultured cells, usually followed by expression of the genes in the introduced DNA (see Figure 2-10).

Transformation change that a normal cell undergoes as it becomes malignant; also, permanent, heritable alteration in a cell resulting from the uptake and incorporation of foreign DNA into the genome.

Transgene a cloned foreign gene present in an animal or plant.

Transgenic mouse a mouse carrying a transgene, which has been introduced and stably incorporated into germ-line cells so that it can be passed on to progeny (see Figure 2-11). See also **Knockout mouse**.

Tuberculin crude protein fraction isolated from supernatant of *Mycobacterium tuberculosis* cultures. It can be used in a skin test for exposure to *M. tuberculosis*.

Tumor antigens cell-surface proteins present on the surface of tumor cells that can induce a cell-mediated immune response. Some are found only on tumor cells; others are also found on normal cells (see Figure 24-6).

Tumor necrosis factors (TNFs) Two related **cytokines** produced by macrophages (TNF-α) and some T cells (TNF-β). Both factors are cytotoxic to tumor cells but not to normal cells; they also play a role in inflammatory responses.

V (variable) gene segment the 5$'$ coding portion of rearranged immunoglobulin and T-cell receptor genes. There are multiple V gene segments in germ-line DNA, but gene rearrangement results in only one segment occurring in each functional rearranged gene.

Vaccination intentional administration of a harmless or less harmful form of a pathogen to induce a specific immune response that protects the individual against later exposure to the same pathogen.

Vaccine a preparation of antigenic material used to induce immunity against pathogenic organisms.

Valence, valency numerical measure of combining capacity, generally equal to the number of binding sites. Antibody molecules are bivalent or multivalent, whereas T-cell receptors are univalent.

Variable (V) region amino-terminal portion of immunoglobulin and T-cell receptor chains that are highly variable and responsible for the **antigenic specificity** of these molecules.

Virgin see **Naive**.

Virulence a measure of the infectious ability of a pathogen.

Western blotting a common technique for detecting a protein in a mixture in which the proteins are separated electrophoretically and then transferred to a polymer sheet, which is flooded with radiolabeled or enzyme-conjugated antibody specific for the protein of interest (see Figure 6-15).

Wheal and flare reaction characteristic type I hypersensitivity response that occurs in the skin involving a sharply delineated swelling of the skin (wheal) with surrounding redness (flare).

White pulp portion of the spleen that surrounds the arteries, forming a periarteriolar lymphoid sheath (PALS) populated mainly by T cells (see Figure 3-22).

Xenogeneic denoting individuals of different species.

Xenograft graft or tissue transplanted from one species to another.

CHAPTER 1

1. (a) CM. (b) H and CM. (c) H and CM. (d) H and CM. (e) CM. (f) CM. (g) H. (h) CM. (i) H. (j) H. (k) CM.

2. The four immunologic attributes are specificity, diversity, memory, and self/nonself recognition. Specificity refers to the ability of certain membrane-bound molecules on lymphocytes to recognize only a single antigen (or small number of closely related antigens). Rearrangement of the immunoglobulin genes during lymphocyte maturation gives rise to antigenic specificity, and also generates a vast array of different specificities, or diversity, among mature lymphocytes. The ability of the immune system to respond to nonself molecules, but (generally) not to self-molecules, results from the elimination during lymphocyte maturation of immature cells that recognize self-antigens. Following exposure to a particular antigen, mature lymphocytes reactive with that antigen proliferate and differentiate, generating a larger population of memory cells with the same specificity; this expanded memory cell population can respond more rapidly and intensely following a subsequent exposure to the same antigen, thus displaying immunologic memory.

3. The secondary immune response involves an amplified population of memory cells. The response is more rapid and achieves higher levels than the primary response.

4. (a) Both antibodies and T-cell receptors display fine specificity for antigen; subtle modifications in an antigen prohibit its binding to its corresponding antibody or T-cell receptor. MHC molecules do not possess such fine specificity, and a variety of unrelated peptide antigens can be bound by the same MHC molecule. (b) Antibodies are expressed only by cells of the B-cell lineage; T-cell receptors are expressed by cells of the T-cell lineage; class I MHC molecules are expressed by virtually all nucleated cells; class II MHC molecules are expressed only by specialized cells that function as antigen-presenting cells

(e.g., B cells, macrophages, and dendritic cells). (c) Antibodies can bind to protein or polysaccharide antigens; T-cell receptors recognize only peptides associated with MHC molecules; MHC molecules only bind processed peptides.

5. Endocytosis is the internalization of (1) extracellular macromolecules by (2) the infolding and pinching off of small regions of the plasma membrane, yielding (3) small endocytic vesicles; (4) most cells are capable of endocytosis. Phagocytosis is the internalization of (1) extracellular particulate material, including whole microorganisms, by (2) the extension of membrane processes (pseudopodia) around the material, yielding (3) relatively large vesicles called phagosomes; (4) only a few cell types (e.g., macrophages, neutrophils) are capable of phagocytosis.

6. (a) Macrophages, B cells, dendritic cells. (b) Co-stimulatory; T_H cells. (c) II; I. (d) Exogenous; endocytic processing pathway; II. (e) Endogenous; cytoplasm; I.

7. During the inflammatory response the diameter of the capillaries in the affected region increases (vasodilation), as does their permeability, which facilitates an influx of white blood cells, particularly phagocytes.

8. They can only recognize antigen that is associated with class I MHC molecules.

9. (a) 13. (b) 19. (c) 6. (d) 12. (e) 2. (f) 18. (g) 8. (h) 15. (i) 4. (j) 14. (k) 7. (1) 9. (m) 17. (n) 5. (o) 3. (p) 10.

CHAPTER 2

1. (a) The genomic clone contains intervening sequences (introns) that are removed during processing of the primary transcript and therefore do not specify any amino acid residues in the protein product. (b) DNA must be microinjected into a fertilized egg so that the DNA (transgene) will be passed on to all daughter cells. (c) Primary lymphoid cultures have a finite life span and contain a heterogeneous population of cells.

2. (a) Homozygous; syngeneic. (b) B, T. (c) Normal antigen-primed B cells, cancerous plasma cells (myeloma cells); unlimited; monoclonal antibodies. (d) Transformation; indefinite.

3.

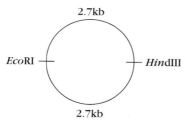

Primary transcript 5′

L E E E

mRNA

L E

AAA

Protein product

4. c.

5. a, b, d.

6. Transfected DNA integrates only into a small percentage of cells. If a selectable marker gene is also present, the small number of transfected cells will grow in the appropriate medium, whereas the much larger number of non-transfected cells will die.

7. The mouse would become a mosaic in which the transgene would have incorporated into some of the somatic cells but not all.

8. Since cleavage with each restriction enzyme alone produced a single band, the plasmid, which is circular, must contain one restriction site for each enzyme. Since simultaneous cleavage of the 5.4-kb plasmid with both enzymes yielded a single band, the fragments from each cleavage must have the same length. Thus the restriction sites must be equidistant from each other in both directions on the plasmid as shown in the diagram below.

2.7kb

EcoRI

HindIII

2.7kb

9. d.

10. Isolate mRNA from activated T cells and transcribe it into cDNA using reverse transcriptase. Insert cDNA into a suitable expression vector, such as plasmid DNA carrying an ampicillin selection gene. Transfer the recombinant plasmid DNA into E. coli and grow in the presence of ampicillin to select for bacteria containing the plasmid DNA. Test the bacterial culture supernatant for the presence of IL-2 by seeing if the monoclonal antibody to IL-2 reacts with the culture supernatant. Once a bacterial culture is identified that is secreting IL-2, the cDNA can be cloned.

11. Radiolabel the mRNA and used the labeled mRNA as a probe to screen the genomic library via in situ hybridization. Re-plate and culture the selected clone, isolate the cloned DNA from the host DNA, and treat the cloned DNA with a restriction enzyme. Analyze the resulting restriction fragments by Southern blotting using the labeled mRNA to identify the fragment containing the binding site. To further pinpoint the binding sequence in this fragment, perform a DNA footprinting experiment with the protein sample.

12. In production of transgenic mice a functional foreign gene is added to the genome; the process involves introduction of a cloned natural gene or cDNA into a fertilized egg, which then is implanted into a pseudopregnant female. In production of knockout mice a nonfunctional form of a mouse gene replaces the functional gene so that the animal does not express the encoded product; the process involves selection of transfected embryonic stem (ES) cells carrying the mutated gene and injection of the ES cells into a blastocyst, which then is implanted into a pseudopregnant female.

13. (a) 8. (b) 2. (c) 5. (d) 9. (e) 4. (f) 3. (g) 6. (h) 7. (i) 10.

CHAPTER 3

1. (a) In general CD4$^+$ T cells that recognize class II MHC molecules function as T_H cells, whereas CD8$^+$ T cells that recognize class I MHC molecules function as T_C cells. However, some functional T_H cells express CD8 and are class I restricted, and some functional T_C cells express CD4 and are class II restricted. But these are exceptions to the general pattern. (b) The bone marrow contains few pluripotent stem cells, which constitute only about 0.05% of all bone marrow cells. (c) T_H cells recognize antigen associated with class II MHC molecules. Activation of macrophages increases their expression of class II MHC molecules. (d) Organized lymphoid follicles are also present in the tonsils, Peyer's patches, and other mucosal-associated tissue. (e) In response to infection, T_H cells and macrophages are activated and secrete various cytokines that induce increased hematopoietic activity. This inducible hematopoiesis expands the population of white blood cells involved in fighting infection. (f) Unlike other types of dendritic cells, follicular dendritic cells do not express class II MHC molecules and thus do not function as antigen-presenting cells for T_H-cell activation. These cells, which are present only in lymph follicles, can trap circulating antibody-antigen complexes; this ability is thought to facilitate B-cell activation and development of memory B cells. (g) B and T lymphocytes pos-

sess antigen-binding receptors, but a small population of lymphoid cells, called null cells, do not.

2. (a) T_H cells in paracortical areas; B cells in germinal centers within secondary follicles located in the node cortex. (b) T_H cells in paracortical areas. (c) No areas of rapid cell proliferation, since T_H cells are required for B-cell activation. (d) B cells in secondary follicles and germinal centers.

3. Monocyte progenitor cells have receptors for M-CSF; they do not secrete it. If both M-CSF and its receptor were expressed by these cells, they could autostimulate their own proliferation.

4. The primary lymphoid organs are the bone marrow (bursa of Fabricius in birds) and the thymus. These organs function as sites for B-cell and T-cell maturation, respectively.

5. The secondary lymphoid organs are the spleen, lymph nodes, various mucosal-associated lymphoid tissue (MALT). MALT includes the tonsils, Peyer's patches, and appendix, as well as loose collections of lymphoid cells associated with the mucous membranes lining the respiratory, digestive, and urogenital tracts. All these organs trap antigen and provide sites where lymphocytes can interact with antigen and subsequently undergo clonal expansion.

6. Stems cells are capable of self-renewal and can give rise to more than one cell type, whereas progenitor cells have lost the capacity for self-renewal and are committed to a single cell lineage. Commitment of progenitor cells depends on their acquisition of responsiveness to particular growth factors.

7. Nude mice and people with DiGeorge's syndrome have a congenital defect that prevents development of the thymus. Both lack circulating T cells and cannot mount cell-mediated immune responses.

8. The thymic stroma contains epithelial cells, interdigitating dendritic cells, and macrophages, which form a three-dimensional network. These cells secrete various hormonal factors that are necessary for thymocyte growth and maturation into immunocompetent T cells. Thymic stromal cells also play a role in the selection of T cells in the thymus.

9. Antigenic commitment involves random rearrangements of genes encoding the antigen-binding receptors on T cells and B cells. As a result of this process, each mature B or T cell expresses receptors with a single specificity and thus can interact only with antigen of that specificity. Antigen is not involved in antigenic commitment, which takes place in the primary lymphoid organs. Mature, antigenically committed lymphocytes migrate from the primary lymphoid organs to the secondary lymphoid organs where they are exposed to antigen. Those lymphocytes whose specificity corresponds to a particular antigen interact with the antigen. This interaction stimulates proliferation and differentiation of the lymphocyte clone into memory cells and effector cells; that is, they undergo clonal selection. The long-lived memory cells are responsible for immunologic memory.

10. The thymus of an individual reaches its maximal size during puberty. During the adult years, the thymus gradually atrophies.

11. (a) The lethally irradiated mice serve as an assay system for pluripotent stem cells, since only mice injected with bone marrow samples containing pluripotent stem cells will survive. As pluripotent stem cells are successively enriched in a bone marrow sample, the total number of cells that must be injected to restore hematopoiesis decreases (see Figure 3-7). (b) Bone marrow cells are incubated with biotin-conjugated monoclonal antibody against CD34, a membrane molecule that is expressed by stem cells but not by other bone marrow cells. Cells that bind the conjugated anti-CD34 antibody will be retained on a column of avidin-coated beads, whereas $CD34^-$ cells will pass through the column. The $CD34^+$ stem cells can be removed from the column by agitation. See Figure 3-9.

12. In a neonatal mouse, thymectomy eliminates T-cell maturation, causing the animal to become immunodeficient and eventually to die. In an adult mouse, thymectomy does not have a profound effect because many of the recirculating T cells have a long life span and can respond to antigenic challenge by clonal selection.

13. The bursa of Fabricius in birds is the primary site where B lymphocytes develop. Bursectomy would result in a lack of circulating B cells and humoral immunity, and would probably be fatal.

14. Following phagocytosis by macrophages, most bacteria and fungi are destroyed and broken down; the resulting antigenic peptides are displayed along with class II MHC molecules on the cell surface, where they can induce T_H-cell activation and subsequent antibody (humoral) response. In contrast, intracellular bacteria and fungi have various mechanisms for surviving in macrophages following phagocytosis. These bacteria thus do not induce an antibody response.

15. (a) T. (b) F: The marginal zone is rich in B cells, and PALS is rich in T cells. (c) T. (d) T. (e) F: The spleen is not supplied with afferent lymphatics.

16. (a) 5. (b) 10. (c) 3. (d) 6. (e) 11. (f) 4. (g) 12. (h) 15. (i) 7. (j) 2. (k) 8. (l) 13.

CHAPTER 4

1. (a) True. (b) True. (c) False: A hapten cannot stimulate an immune response unless it is conjugated to a larger protein carrier. However, the hapten can combine with pre-formed antibody specific for the hapten. (d) True. (e) False: A T cell can only recognize peptides that have been processed and presented by MHC molecules. These epitopes tend to be internal peptides. (f) True. (g) True. (h) False: Each MHC molecule binds a number of different peptides. It is not yet known what features different peptides must have in common to be able to bind to the same MHC molecule. (i) False: Immunogens are capable of stimulating a specific immune response; antigens are capable of combining specifically with the antibodies or T-cell receptors induced during an immune response. Although all immunogens exhibit antigenicity, some antigens do not exhibit immunogenicity.

2. Probably not. In order to stimulate T_H-cell proliferation, the antigenic peptide must interact with class II MHC molecules expressed by the mice. Since IA^k and IA^d are encoded by allelic MHC genes and consequently exhibit allelic differences, they would most likely not bind the same hemagglutinin peptide. Thus, a peptide that is immunogenic for mice expressing IA^k probably would not be immunogenic for mice expressing IA^d.

3. (a) The UV-inactivated vaccine would be seen as an exogenous antigen. Exogenous antigens are internalized through phagocytosis or endocytosis and then are processed in the endocytic pathway. The resulting antigenic peptides are presented by class II MHC molecules on the surface of antigen-presenting cells. Since T_C cells are generally class I MHC restricted, they would not be activated by this type of vaccine, although class II MHC–restricted T_H cells might be. (b) Because the attenuated virus replicates within host cells, it is seen as an endogenous antigen. Endogenous antigens are processed within the cytoplasm or endoplasmic reticulum and are presented by class I MHC molecules, which are present on the membrane of most nucleated cells. Therefore, the attenuated virus would be likely to activate T_C cells, which are class I MHC restricted.

4. (a) Native BSA: Heat denaturation is likely to destroy B-cell epitopes in a globular protein, although the T-cell epitopes are generally stable to heat. (b) HEL: The immunogenicity of an antigen generally is related to its foreignness to the animal exposed. However, collagen and some other proteins highly conserved throughout evolution exhibit little foreignness across diverse species and thus often are weak antigens. (c) 150,000-MW protein: Other things being equal, larger proteins are more immunogenic than smaller ones. (d) Copolymer that includes tyrosine residues: The immunogenicity of synthetic copolymers is increased by inclusion of aromatic residues.

5. b, d.

6. T_4 could be coupled to a large protein to form an immunogenic hapten-carrier conjugate, which then could be used to induce production of anti-T_4 antibody in test animals. The ability of the anti-T_4 antibody to react with serum T_4 could form the basis for various sensitive immunoassays described in Chapter 6.

7. (a) T. (b) T. (c) B. (d) B. (e) T. (f) T. (g) BT. (h) B. (i) BT.

CHAPTER 5

1. (a) True. (b) False: An HGPRT$^-$ myeloma cell lacks the enzyme to utilize hypoxanthine. (c) True. (d) False: Multiple isotypes can appear on the surface of a single B cell. A mature B cell expresses both IgM and IgD. A memory B cell can express additional isotypes such as IgG. (e) True. (f) True. (g) True. (h) False: Secreted serum IgM is a pentamer. Because of its larger size and valency, IgM is more effective than IgG in cross-linking bacterial surface antigens, which leads to agglutination. (i) True. (j) False: Hypoxanthine allows cell growth by the salvage pathway. (k) True. (l) False: Both heavy- and light-chain variable regions contain approximately 110 amino acids. (m) False: The unfused revertant would grow in HAT medium, making it impossible to select for the hybridomas.

2. (a) The molecule would have to possess the following structural features: 2 identical heavy chains and 2 identical light chains (H_2L_2); interchain disulfide bonds joining the heavy chains (H–H) and the heavy and light chains (H–L); a series of intrachain domains containing approximately 110 amino acids and stabilized by an intra-domain disulfide bridge of about 60 amino acids; single constant domain in light chains and 3 or 4 constant domains in heavy chain. The amino-terminal domain of both the heavy and light chains should show sequence variation. (b) The antisera to both whole human IgG and human κ chain should cross-react with the new immunoglobulin class, since both of these antisera have antibodies specific for the light chain. The new isotype would be expected to contain either kappa or lambda light chains. (c) Reduce the interchain disulfide bonds of the new isotype with mercaptoethanol and alkylation. Separate the heavy and light chains. Immunize a rabbit with the heavy chain. The rabbit antisera should react with the new isotype but not with any other known isotypes.

3. IgM and IgD differ in their constant-region domains, whereas antigenic specificity is determined by the variable-region domains. Molecules of IgM and IgD that have different C domains but identical V_H and V_L domains are found on a given B cell; thus the cell is unspecific although it bears two isotypes.

4. Advantages of IgG compared with IgM are (1) its ability to cross the placenta and protect the developing fetus; (2) its higher serum concentration, which results in IgG antibodies binding to and neutralizing more antigen molecules and being more effective in antigen clearance; (3) its smaller size, which enables IgG to diffuse more readily into intercellular fluids. The disadvantages of IgG compared with IgM are its lower capacity to (1) agglutinate antigens and (2) activate the complement system, both of which are due to the lower valency of IgG.

5. (a) See Figures 5-2 and 5-3. The number of interchain disulfide bonds joining the heavy chains varies among IgG subclasses (see Figure 5-16). (b) Draw as a dimer containing α heavy chains. Add J chain and secretory component (see Figure 5-17a). (c) Draw as a pentamer containing μ heavy chains. The μ heavy chain contains five domains and no hinge region; the extra C_H domain replaces the hinge. Add J chain. Pentameric IgM also has additional interchain disulfide bonds joining C_H domains in the subunits and the J chain to two of the subunits (see Figure 5-15e).

6. [Answer to question 6 is shown below]

PROPERTY	WHOLE IGG	H CHAIN	L CHAIN	FAB	F(AB')2	FC
Binds antigen	+	+/−	+/−	+	+	−
Bivalent antigen binding	+	−	−	−	+	−
Binds to Fc receptors	+	−	−	−	−	+
Fixes complement in presence of antigen	+	−	−	−	−	−
Has V domains	+	+	+	+	+	−
Has C domains	+	+	+	+	+	+

7. (a) AL. (b) ID. (c) IS. (d) AL. (e) No antibodies will be formed.

8. [Answer to question 8 is shown below]

	RABBIT ANTISERA TO MOUSE ANTIBODY COMPONENT				
	γ CHAIN	κ CHAIN	IgG FAB FRAGMENT	IgG Fc FRAGMENT	J CHAIN
Mouse γ chain	Yes	No	Yes	Yes	No
Mouse κ chain	No	Yes	Yes	No	No
Mouse IgM whole	No	Yes	Yes	No	Yes
Mouse IgC/Fc fragment	Yes	No	No	Yes	No

9. Myeloma cells suitable for hybridoma production (1) exhibit immortal growth, enabling the hybridoma to be cultured indefinitely; (2) are Ab⁻, ensuring that the hybridoma only secretes antibody characteristic of the plasma-cell fusion partner; and (3) are HGPRT⁻, ensuring that unfused myeloma cells cannot grow in HAT-selection medium.

10. (a) Immunoglobulin-fold domains contain approximately 110 amino acid residues, which are arranged in two antiparallel β pleated sheets, each composed of multiple β strands separated by short loops of varying lengths (see Figure 5-6). Each Ig-fold domain is stabilized by an intra-domain disulfide bond between two conserved cysteine residues about 60 residues apart. (b) See Figure 5-19. The Ig-fold domain structure is thought to facilitate interactions between domains; such interactions between nonhomologous domains may allow different members of the immunoglobulin superfamily to bind to each other.

11. The hypervariable regions, also called complementarity-determining regions (CDRs), are located in the loops of the immunoglobulin folds constituting the V_H and V_L domains (see Figures 5-6 and 5-8). There are three hypervariable regions in each V_H domain, and three in each V_L domain. Residues in the hypervariable regions constitute most of amino acids involved in antigen binding.

12. In the absence of aminopterin, you could not select for the hybridoma because both the fused and unfused cells would grow using the de novo pathway.

13. (a) Some normal cells likely would be killed. Although an immunotoxin preferentially binds to tumor cells, the Fc region of the antibody component can bind to Fc receptors on various immune-system cells. If this

occurs, then the toxin would be endocytosed and kill the normal cell. One way to avoid damage to normal cells is to engineer an immunotoxin in which the toxin chain replaces the Fc region of the antibody (see Figure 5-25c). (b) No. In an immunotoxin, the binding chain of the toxin is replaced by a tumor-specific antibody, which targets the toxin to tumor cells (see Figure 5-23). Thus, if the antibody is degraded, the toxin will be unable to get into normal cells and kill them.

14. The antiserum would also contain antibodies to the kappa and lambda light chains, which are present in all isotypes. To prepare an IgG-specific antiserum, the technician needs to reduce the interchain disulfide bonds in the mouse IgG with mercaptoethanol and isolate the heavy chain. Rabbits immunized with the mouse heavy chains alone will be specific for the IgG isotype.

15. (a) Four different antigen-binding sites (indicated in boldface) and 10 different antibody molecules: $\mathbf{H_sL_s}/H_sL_s$, $\mathbf{H_mL_m}/H_mL_m$, $\mathbf{H_sL_m}/H_sL_m$, $\mathbf{H_mL_s}/H_mL_s$, H_sL_s/H_mL_m, H_sL_s/H_sL_m, H_sL_s/H_mL_s, H_mL_m/H_sL_m, H_mL_m/H_mL_s, and H_sL_m/H_mL_s. (b) Two different antigen-binding sites and three different antibody molecules: $\mathbf{H_sL_s}/H_sL_s$, $\mathbf{H_mL_s}/H_mL_s$, and H_sL_s/H_mL_s. (c) One binding site and one antibody molecule: $\mathbf{H_sL_s}/H_sL_s$.

16. (a) 3, 6, 10, 11. (b) 4. (c) 2, 9, 13. (d) 5, 12. (e) 1, 3, 4, 7, 8, 11, 12.

CHAPTER 6

1. (a) True. (b) True. (c) False: Papain digestion yields monovalent Fab fragments (see Figure 5-2), which cannot cross-link antigens. (d) True. (e) True. (f) True. (g) False: It is qualitative but not quantitative. (h) False: Agglutination tests are more sensitive.

2. Coat a microtiter plate with antigens from HIV. Add serum from a patient suspected of being infected with HIV. Incubate the plate, and then wash away unbound antibodies. Add a goat anti-human immunoglobulin reagent that has been conjugated with an enzyme. Incubate the plate and wash away unbound antibody. Add substrate and observe for a colored reaction.

3. (a) Whole bovine serum. (b) See figure below.

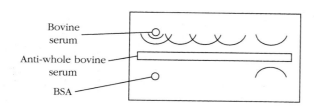

4. Bottle A: H1–C1. Bottle B: H2–C2. Bottle C: H2–C1. Bottle D: H1–C2.

5. ELISA and RIA can both be used to determine the concentration of a hapten.

6. (a) A. (b) D. (c) B. (d) E. (e) F. (f) C.

7. (a) Isolate the heavy chains from the myeloma proteins of known isotype. Immunize rabbits with the isolated heavy chains to obtain antisera specific for each heavy-chain class. Then determine which of these anti-isotype antisera reacts with myeloma protein X. (b) The level of myeloma protein X could be determined by radial immunodiffusion (Mancini method) or by a more sensitive assay such as ELISA.

8. (a) Rocket electrophoresis or Mancini radial immunodiffusion with goat anti-isotype serum specific for IgG. (b) ELISA or RIA with anti-insulin antibody and radioactively labeled or enzyme-linked insulin. (c) RIA with radiolabeled IgE. (d) Immunofluorescence with fluorochrome-labeled antibody to C3. (e) Agglutination test with type-A red blood cells. (f) Ouchterlony double immunodiffusion hamburger extract and antiserum to horsemeat. (g) Immunofluorescence with fluorochrome-labeled antibody to the syphilis spirochete.

9. b.

10. Affinity refers to the strength of the interaction between a *single* antigen-binding site in an antibody and the corresponding ligand. Avidity refers to the total effective strength of all the interactions between *multiple* antigen-binding sites in an antibody and multiple identical epitopes in a complex antigen. Because bacteria often have multiple copies of a particular epitope on their surface, the avidity of an antibody is a better measure than its affinity of its ability to combat bacteria.

11. (a) Antiserum #1 $K_0 = 1.2 \times 10^5$; antiserum #2 $K_0 = 4.5 \times 10^6$; antiserum #3 $K_0 = 4.5 \times 10^6$. (b) Each antibody has a valence of 2. (c) Antiserum #2. (d) The monoclonal antiserum #2 would be best because it recognizes a single epitope on the hormone and, therefore, would be less likely than the polyclonal antisera to cross-react with other serum proteins.

12. (a) Tube 1 contained $F(ab')_2$ fragments. Because these fragments contain two antigen-binding sites, they can cross-link and eventually agglutinate SRBCs. Activation of complement by IgG requires the presence of the Fc fragment, which is missing from $F(ab')_2$ fragments. (b) Tube 2 contained Fab fragments. Univalent Fab fragments can bind to SRBCs and inhibit subsequent agglutination by whole anti-SRBC. (c) Tube 3 contained intact antibody. (d) Tube 4 contained Fc fragments. These fragments lack antigen-binding sites and thus cannot mediate any antibody effector functions.

13. (a) In precipitation reactions, an excess of either antibody or antigen inhibits precipitate formation (see Figure 6-4). The formation of a precipitate when equal volumes of the original undiluted solutions were mixed indicates this reaction was in the equivalence zone. The absence of precipitate with the diluted anti-X indicates that this reaction had an antigen excess. (b) In the first (undiluted) reaction, little or no protein X or anti-X would be in the supernatant. In the second (diluted) reaction, the supernatant would contain protein X, which is in excess.

CHAPTER 7

1. (a) False: V_κ gene segments and C_λ are located on separate chromosomes and cannot be brought together during gene rearrangement. (b) True. (c) True. (d) True. (e) True. (f) True.

2. V_H and J_H gene segments cannot join because both are flanked by recombination signal sequences (RSSs) containing a 23-bp (2-turn) spacer (see Figure 7-6b). According to the one-turn/two-turn joining rule, signal sequences having a two-turn spacer can only join with signal sequences having a one-turn (12-bp) spacer.

3. Light chains: $500 V_L \times 4 J_L = 2 \times 10^3$

   Heavy chains: $300 V_H \times 15 D_H \times 4 J_H = 1.8 \times 10^4$

   Antibody molecules: $(2 \times 10^3 \text{ LCs}) \times (1.8 \times 10^4 \text{ HCs}) = 3.6 \times 10^7$

4. (a) 1, 2, 3. (b) 3. (c) 3. (d) 5. (e) 2, 3, 4. (f) 2. (g) 5.

5. Somatic mutation contributes to the variability of all three complementarity-determining regions. Additional variability is generated in the CDR3 of both heavy and light chains by junctional flexibility, which occurs during heavy-chain D-J and V-DJ rearrangements and light-chain V-J rearrangements, by P-nucleotide addition at heavy- and light-chain variable-region joints, and by N-nucleotide addition at the heavy-chain D-J and V-DJ joints. See Table 7-4.

6. (a) R: Productive rearrangement of heavy-chain allele 1 must have occurred since the cell line expresses heavy chains encoded by this allele. (b) G: Allelic exclusion forbids heavy-chain allele 2 from undergoing either productive or nonproductive rearrangement. (c) NP: The κ genes rearrange before the λ genes. Since the cell line expresses λ light chains, both κ alleles must have undergone nonproductive rearrangement, thus permitting λ-gene rearrangement to occur. (d) NP: Same reason as given in (c) above. (e) R: Productive rearrangement of λ-chain allele 1 must have occurred since the cell line ex-

presses λ light chains encoded by this allele. (f) G: Allelic exclusion forbids λ-chain allele 2 from undergoing either productive or nonproductive rearrangement (see Figure 7-13).

7. The κ-chain DNA must have the germ-line configuration because a productive heavy-chain rearrangement must occur before the light-chain (κ) DNA can begin to rearrange.

8. (a) No. (b) Yes. (c) No. (d) No. (e) Yes.

9. Random addition of N-nucleotides at the D-J and V-DJ junctions contributes to the diversity within the CDR3 of heavy chains, but this process can result in a nonproductive rearrangement if the triplet reading frame is not preserved.

10. The joints between variable-region gene segments (V_L-J_L and V_H-D_H-J_H) occur in CDR3. During formation of these joints, junctional flexibility, P-nucleotide addition, and N-nucleotide addition introduce diversity. Because these processes do not affect the rest of the variable region, CDR3 exhibits the greatest diversity.

11.

(a) Normal mice

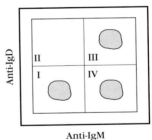

(b) *RAG-1⁻* mice

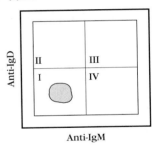

12. Four chances (see Figure 7-13).

13. (a) 5. (b) 5, 6, 9. (c) 1. (d) 4. (e) 2, 8. (f) 2, 11. (g) 3, 7. (h) 3, 10.

14. (a) 5. (b) 1. (c) 6. (d) 2. (e) 3. (f) 7. (g) 4.

CHAPTER 8

1. (a) False: The V_H-D_H-J_H rearrangement occurs during the pro-B cell stage; successful completion of heavy-chain rearrangement marks the beginning of the pre-B cell stage in which membrane-bound μ chains are expressed. (b) False: Immature B cells express only IgM. (c) False: TdT, which catalyzes N-nucleotide addition, is expressed only in pro-B cells. (d) True. (e) True. (f) False: Pro-B cells must interact with stromal cells to develop into pre-B

cells. Progression of pre-B cells into immature B cells requires IL-7 released from stromal cells, but not direct contact. (g). True. (See Figure 8-1.)

2. (a) Progenitor B cell: no cytoplasmic or membrane staining with either reagent. (b) Pre-B cell: anti-μ staining in cytoplasm and on membrane. (c) Immature B cell: anti-μ staining in cytoplasm and on membrane. (d) Mature B cell: anti-μ and anti-δ staining in cytoplasm and on membrane. (e) Plasma cell: anti-μ staining in cytoplasm; no membrane staining but pentameric IgM is secreted. (See Figure 8-3.)

3. The B-cell coreceptor consists of three membrane proteins: TAPA-1, CR2, and CD19; the latter belongs to the Ig superfamily. The CR2 component can bind to complement-coated antigen bound to the B-cell receptor (BCR). This binding permits interaction of CD19 with the Ig-α/Ig-β component of the BCR, leading to intensification of the activating signal induced by antigen binding (see Figure 8-9). In addition, interaction of CR2 on centrocytes with CD23 expressed by follicular dendritic cells, along with a signal provided by binding of IL-1, promotes formation of plasma cells within the germinal center (see Figure 8-20).

4. (a) Both single and double transgenics carried the anti-HEL transgene. Because the transgene is already rearranged, rearrangement of endogenous immunoglobulin heavy- and light-chain genes does not occur in pro-B and pre-B cells; therefore, the rearranged immunoglobulin encoded by the transgene is expressed preferentially by mature B cells. (b) Add radiolabeled HEL and see if it binds to the B-cell membrane using autoradiography. To determine the isotype on the membrane antibody (mIg) on these B cells, incubate the cells with fluorochrome-labeled antibodies specific for each isotype (e.g., anti-μ, anti-δ, etc.) and see which fluorescent antibodies stain the B cells. (c) So that the HEL transgene could be induced by adding Zn^{2+} to the mouse's water supply. (d) First, B cells and T cells from the double-transgenic mice and normal syngeneic mice must be separated from each other. This can be accomplished by treating a preparation of spleen cells with a fluorochrome-labeled antibody specific for CD3, which is expressed on the membrane of T cells but not B cells, and passing the treated preparation through a FACS (see Figure 6-17). This will yield a T-cell fraction and a residual fraction containing B cells and other spleen cells. After treating the residual fraction with fluorochrome-labeled anti-IgM, pass it through a FACS to obtain a B-cell fraction. Now, mix the transgenic B cells with normal syngeneic T cells (sample A), and mix the transgenic T cells with normal syngeneic B cells (sample B). Transfer each cell mixture to lethally x-irradiated, syngeneic adoptive-trans-

fer recipients, challenge the recipients with HEL, and determine if they produce anti-HEL serum antibodies. If the B cells are anergic, then no antibody response would occur with sample A.

5. (a) B-cell activation by soluble protein antigens requires the involvement of T_H cells. Cross-linkage of mIg on a naive B cell by thymus-dependent antigens provides competence signal 1; subsequent binding of CD40 on the B cell to CD40L on an activated T_H cell provides competence signal 2. The combined effect of these signals drives the B cell from G_0 to the G_1 stage of the cell cycle and up-regulates expression of cytokine receptors on the B cell. Binding of T_H-derived cytokines then provides a progression signal that stimulates proliferation of the activated B cells (see Figure 8-10). (b) Binding of LPS, a type 1 thymus-independent antigen, provides both competence signal 1 and 2 (see Figure 8-6). Efficient proliferation requires a cytokine-mediated progression signal.

6. (a) Sample B yields a single restriction fragment with each digest characteristic of unrearranged germ-line DNA. Thus this sample is from liver cells. (b) The two fragments obtained with the *Bam*HI digest of sample C indicates that both heavy-chain alleles are rearranged, whereas no κ-chain rearrangement has occurred. Thus this sample is from pre-B lymphoma cells. (c) The blots obtained with sample A indicate that one heavy-chain allele is rearranged and one light-chain allele is rearranged. This pattern indicates this sample is from IgM-secreting myeloma cells.

7. (a) Basal light zone. (b) Paracortex. (c) Centroblasts; dark zone. (d) Centrocytes; follicular dendritic cells. (e) Apical light zone; T_H cells. (f) Basal light zone. (g) Medulla. (h) Memory B cells; apical light zone. (i) Centroblasts.

8. (a) See Table 8-2. (b) TI antigens.

9. (a) Each mIg molecule is associated with two molecules of a heterodimer called Ig-α/Ig-β forming the B-cell receptor (BCR). Both Ig-α and Ig-β have long cytoplasmic tails, which are capable of mediating signal transduction to the cell interior (see Figure 8-8). (b) B-cell activating and differentiating signals—provided by antigen binding, interaction with T_H cells, or cytokine binding—trigger intracellular signal-transduction pathways that ultimately generate active transcription factors. These then translocate to the nucleus where they stimulate or inhibit transcription of specific genes.

10. (a) The recipient mice had a haplotype other than H-2^b. (b) The purpose of these experiments was to see the effect of a self-antigen, represented by the transgene-encoded K^b, that is expressed only in the periphery. Linking the K^b transgene to a liver-specific promoter assured

that the K^b class I molecule would be expressed in the periphery but not in the bone marrow where immature B cells could interact with it. (c) These results suggest that exposure to self-antigens in the periphery can lead to negative selection and apoptosis (clonal deletion) in some cases (see Figure 8-14).

CHAPTER 9

1. (a) True. (b) True. (c) False: Class III MHC molecules are soluble proteins that do not function in antigen presentation. They include several complement components, TNF-α, TNF-β, and two heat-shock proteins. (d) False: The offspring of heterozygous parents inherit one MHC haplotype from each parent and thus will express some molecules that differ from those of each parents; for this reason parents and offspring are histoincompatible. In contrast, siblings have a one in four chance of being histocompatible (see Figure 9-2c). (e) True. (f) False: Most nucleated cells express class I MHC molecules, but neurons, placental cells, and sperm cells at certain stages of differentiation appear to lack class I molecules. (g) True.

2. (a) S. (b) S and C. (c) S. (d) C. (e) S and C. (f) S. (g) C.

3. (a) Strain A. (b) Strain B. (c) Strain A. (d) To introduce strain-A parental alleles at all loci except for the selected MHC. (e) To achieve homozygosity within the MHC. (f) To identify progeny that are homozygous b/b within the MHC. This is achieved by selecting mice that reject grafts from strain A (see Figure 9-3).

4. (a) Liver cells: Class I Kb, Kk, Db, Dk, Lk, and Lb. (b) Macrophages: Class I Kb, Kk, Db, Dk, Lb, and Lk. Class II IAαkαk, IAαbβb, IAαkβb, IAαbβk, IEαkβk, IEαbβb, IEαkβb, and IEαbβk.

5. [Answer to question 5 is shown below]

Transfected gene	MHC MOLECULES EXPRESSED ON THE MEMBRANE OF THE TRANSFECTED L CELLS					
	D^k	D^b	K^k	K^b	IA^k	IA^b
None	+	−	+	−	−	−
K^b	+	−	+	+	−	−
$IA\alpha^b$	+	−	+	−	−	−
$IA\beta^b$	+	−	+	−	−	−
$IA\alpha^b$ and $IA\beta^b$	+	−	+	−	−	+

6. (a) SLJ macrophages express the following MHC molecules: Ks, Ds, Ls, and IAs. Because of the deletion of the IEα locus, IEs is not expressed by these cells. (b) The transfected cells would express one heterologous IE molecule, IEαkβs, and one homologous IE molecule, IEαkβk, in addition to the molecules listed in (a).

7. See Figures 9-5, 5-3, and 5-19.

8. (a) The polymorphic residues are clustered in short stretches primarily within the membrane-distal domains of the class I and class II MHC molecules (see Figure 9-14). These regions form the peptide-binding cleft of MHC molecules. (b) MHC polymorphism is thought to arise by gene conversion of short nearly homologous DNA sequences within unexpressed pseudogenes in the MHC to functional class I or class II genes.

9. (a) The proliferation of and IL-2 production by T_H cells is detected in assay 1, and the killing of LCM-infected target cells by cytotoxic T lymphocytes (CTLs) is detected in assay 2. (b) Assay 1 is a functional assay for class II MHC molecules, and assay 2 is a functional assay for class I molecules. (c) Class II IAk molecules are required in assay 1, and class I Dd molecules are required in assay 2. (d) You could transfect L cells with the IAk gene and determine the response of the transfected cells in assay 1. Similarly, you could transfect a separate sample of L cells with the Dd gene and determine the response of the transfected cells in assay 2. In each case, a positive response would confirm the identity of the MHC molecules required for LCM-specific activity of the spleen cells. As a control in each case, L cells should be transfected with a different class I or class II MHC gene and assayed in the appropriate assay. (e) The immunized spleen cells express both IAk and Dd molecules. Of the listed strains, only A.TL and (BALB/c × B10.A) F_1 express both of these MHC molecules, and thus these are the only strains from which the spleen cells could have been isolated.

10. It is not possible to predict. Since the peptide-binding cleft is identical, both MHC molecules should bind the same peptide. However, the amino acid differences outside the cleft might prevent recognition of the second MHC molecule by the T-cell receptor on the T_C cells.

11. Use a battery of monoclonal antibodies specific for the MHC molecules corresponding to each MHC haplotype to determine if both strains express the same set of MHC molecules. This approach is used in tissue typing to identify potential graft donors (see Figure 23-7).

12. If RBCs expressed MHC molecules, then extensive tissue typing would be required before a blood transfusion, and only a few individuals would be acceptable donors for a given individual.

CHAPTER 10

1. By convention, antigen-presenting cells are defined as those cells that can display antigenic peptides associated with class II MHC molecules and can deliver a co-stimulatory signal to $CD4^+ T_H$ cells. Target cells display peptides associated with class I MHC molecules to $CD8^+ T_C$ cells.

2. (a) Self-MHC restriction is the attribute of T cells that limits their response to antigen associated with self-MHC molecules on the membrane of antigen-presenting cells or target cells. In general, $CD4^+ T_H$ cells are class II MHC restricted, and $CD8^+ T_C$ cells are class I MHC restricted, although a few exceptions to this pattern occur. (b) Antigen processing involves the intracellular degradation of protein antigens into peptides that associate with class I or class II MHC molecules. (c) Endogenous antigens are synthesized within altered self-cells (e.g., virus-infected cells or tumor cells), are processed in the cytosolic pathway, and are presented by class I MHC molecules to $CD8^+ T_C$ cells. (d) Exogenous antigens are internalized by antigen-presenting cells, processed in the endocytic pathway, and presented by class II MHC molecules to $CD4^+ T_H$ cells.

3. (a) Class I MHC molecules only display peptides derived from endogenous antigens by the cytosolic processing pathway. Since the UV-inactivated (killed) influenza virus cannot replicate in the target cells, no endogenous viral proteins are synthesized. (b) Class II MHC molecules only display peptides produced in the endocytic processing pathway, which is inhibited by chloroquine. Thus, this compound inhibits the response of class II–restricted T cells. (c) Emitine inhibits protein synthesis and thus prevents synthesis of viral proteins in target cells infected with live influenza virus. As a result, class I–restricted T cells do not respond. Since the response of class II–restricted cells does not depend on protein synthesis, their response is not inhibited by emitine. (d) An exogenous antigen, like hemagglutinin, is processed in the cytosolic pathway and the resulting peptides displayed with class II MHC molecules. Thus, only class II–restricted cells can respond to hemagglutinin treatment.

4. (a) EN: Class I molecules associate with antigenic peptides and display them on the surface of target cells to $CD8^+ T_C$ cells. (b) EX: Class II molecules associate with antigenic peptides and display them on surface of APCs to $CD4^+ T_H$ cells. (c) EX: The invariant chain interacts with the peptide-binding cleft of class II MHC molecules in the rough endoplasmic reticulum, thereby preventing binding of peptides from endogenous antigens. It also assists in folding of the class II α and β chains and in movement of class II molecules from the RER to endocytic compartments. (d) EX: Lysosomal hydrolases degrade exogenous antigens into peptides; these enzymes also degrade the invariant chain associated with class II molecules, so that the peptides and MHC molecules can associate. (e) EN: TAP, a transmembrane protein located in the RER membrane, mediates transport of antigenic peptides produced in the cytosolic pathway into the RER lumen where they can associate with class I MHC molecules. (f) B: In the endogenous pathway, vesicles containing peptide–class I MHC complexes move from the RER to the Golgi complex and then on to the cell surface. In the exogenous pathway, vesicles containing the invariant chain associated with class II MHC molecules move from the RER to the Golgi and on to endocytic compartments. (g) EN: Proteasomes are large protein complexes with multiple peptidase activity that degrade intracellular proteins within the cytosol. When associated with LMP2 and LMP7, which are encoded in the MHC region, proteasomes preferentially generate peptides that associate with class I MHC molecules. (h) EX: Antigen-presenting cells internalize exogenous (external) antigens by phagocytosis or endocytosis. (i) EN: Calnexin is a protein within the RER membrane that acts as a molecular chaperone, assisting in the folding and association of newly formed class I α chains and β_2-microglobulin into a heterodimer. (j) EX: Following degradation of the invariant chain associated with a class II MHC molecule, a small fragment called CLIP remains bound to the peptide-binding cleft, presumably preventing premature peptide loading of the MHC molecule. Eventually, CLIP is displaced by an antigenic peptide.

5. (a) Chloroquine inhibits the endocytic processing pathway, so that the APCs cannot display peptides derived from native lysozyme. The synthetic lysozyme peptide will exchange with other peptides associated with class II molecules on the APC membrane, so that it will be displayed to the T_H cells and induce their activation. (b) Delay of chloroquine addition provides time for native lysozyme to be degraded in the endocytic pathway.

6. (a) Dendritic cells: constitutively express both class II MHC molecules and co-stimulatory signal. B cells: constitutively express class II molecules, but must be activated before expressing the B7 co-stimulatory signal. Macrophages: must be activated before expressing either class II molecules or the B7 co-stimulatory signal. (b) See Table 10-1. Many nonprofessional APCs function only during sustained inflammatory responses.

7. (a) R. (b) R. (c) NR. (d) R. (e) NR. (f) R.

CHAPTER 11

1. (a) False: The distance between CD4 and the TCR is too great for them to coprecipitate; however, CD3 and the TCR are close enough that they will coprecipitate in response to monoclonal anti-CD3. (b) True. (c) True. (d) False: The TCR variable-region genes are located on different chromosomes from the Ig variable-region genes. (e) False: All T-cell receptors have a single binding site for peptide-MHC complexes. (f) False: Because allelic exclusion is not complete for the TCR α chain, a T cell occasionally expresses two α chains resulting from rearrangement of both α-chain alleles. (g) False: The estimated TCR diversity is several orders of magnitude greater than Ig diversity (see Table 11-2). (h) True.

2. Functional $\alpha\beta$ TCR genes from a T_C clone specific for one hapten on an H-2^d target cell were transfected into another T_C clone specific for a second hapten on an H-2^k target cell. Cytolysis assays revealed that the transfected T_C cells only killed target cells that presented antigen associated with the original MHC restriction element. See Figure 11-15.

3. See Figure 11-3.

4. (a) CD3 is a complex of three dimers containing five different polypeptide chains. It is required for the expression of the T-cell receptor and plays a role in signal transduction across the membrane. CD3 and the T-cell receptor associate to form the TCR-CD3 membrane complex (see Figure 11-9). (b) CD4 and CD8 interact with the membrane-proximal domains of class II and class I MHC molecules, respectively, thereby increasing the avidity of the interaction between T cells and peptide-MHC complexes. CD4 and CD8 also play a role in signal transduction. (c) CD2 and other accessory molecules (LFA-1, CD28, and CD45R) bind to their ligands on antigen-presenting cells or target cells. The initial contact between a T cell and antigen-presenting cell or target cell probably is mediated by these cell-adhesion molecules. Subsequently, the T-cell receptor interacts with peptide-MHC complexes. These molecules also may function in signal transduction.

5. (a) TCR. (b) TCR. (c) Ig. (d) TCR/Ig. (e) TCR. (f) TCR/Ig. (g) Ig.

6. (a) The three assumptions were: 1) That TCR mRNA should be associated with polyribosomes, like the mRNAs encoding other membrane proteins; therefore, isolation of the polyribosomal mRNA fraction would significantly enrich the proportion of TCR mRNA in the preparations. 2) That B cells and T cells would express many common genes and the unique T-cell mRNAs would include those encoding the T-cell receptor; therefore, subtractive hybridization using B-cell mRNA would remove all the cDNAs common to both B and T cells, leaving the unique T-cell cDNA unhybridized. 3) That the TCR genes undergo DNA rearrangement and, therefore, can be detected by Southern blotting using cDNA probes. See Figure 11-4. (b) If they wanted to identify the IL-4 gene, they should perform subtractive hybridization using a T_H clone as an IL-4 producer and a T_C clone as a source of mRNA lacking the message for IL-4. In addition, the gene for IL-4 would not be expected to rearrange, and therefore could not be identified by Southern-blot analysis indicating gene rearrangement.

7. [Answer to question 7 is shown below]

GENE PRODUCT	cDNA SOURCE	mRNA SOURCE
IL-2	A	B
CD8	C	A or B
J chain	E	F
IL-1	D	G
CD3	A, B, or C	H

8. [Answer to question 8 is shown below]

SOURCE OF SPLEEN CELLS FROM LCM-INFECTED MICE	RELEASE OF ^{51}CR FROM LCM-INFECTED TARGET CELLS			
	B10.D2 (H-2^d)	B10 (H-2^b)	B10.BR (H-2^h)	(BALB/C × B10) F$_1$ (H-$2^{b/d}$)
B10.D2 (H-2^d)	+	−	−	+
B10 (H-2^b)	−	+	−	+
BALB/c (H-2^d)	+	−	−	+
BALB/b (H-2^b)	−	+	−	+

CHAPTER 12

1. (a) The immature thymocytes express both CD4 and CD8, whereas the mature CD8$^+$ thymocytes do not express CD4. To distinguish these cells, the thymocytes are double-stained with fluorochrome-labeled anti-CD4 and anti-CD8 and analyzed in a FACS. (b) See the table below.

TRANSGENIC MOUSE	IMMATURE THYMOCYTES	MATURE CD8$^+$ THYMOCYTES
H-2^h female	+	+
H-2^h male	+	−
H-2^d female	+	−
H-2^d male	+	−

(c) Because the gene encoding the H-Y antigen is on the Y chromosome, this antigen is not present in females. Thymocytes bearing the transgenic T-cell receptor, which is H-2^k restricted, would undergo positive selection in both male and female H-2^k transgenics. However, subsequent negative selection would eliminate thymocytes bearing the transgenic receptor, which is specific for H-Y antigen, in the male H-2^k transgenics (see Figure 12-8). (d) Because the H-2^d transgenics would not express the appropriate MHC molecules, T-cells bearing the transgenic T-cell receptor would not undergo positive selection.

2. Cyclosporin A blocks production of NF-ATc, one of the transcription factors necessary for proliferation of antigen-activated T$_H$ cells (see Figure 12-13).

3. (a) NF-κB and NF-ATc. (b) IL-2 enhancer. See Figure 12-12.

4.

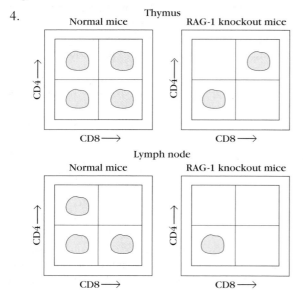

5. (a) Class I K, D, and L molecules and class II IA molecules. (b) Class I molecules only. (c) The normal H-2^b mice should have both CD4$^+$ and CD8$^+$ T cells because both class I and class II MHC molecules would be present on thymic stromal cells during positive selection. H-2^b mice with knock out of the *IA* gene would express no class II molecules; thus these mice would have only CD8$^+$ cells.

6. (a) Thymus donor in experiment A was H-2^d (BALB/c) and in experiment B was H-2^b (C57BL/6). (b) The haplotype of the thymus donor determines the MHC restriction of the T cells in the chimeric mice. Thus, H-2^b target cells were lysed in experiment B in which the thymus donor was H-2^b. (c) The H-2^k target cells were not lysed in either experiment because neither donor thymus expressed H-2^k MHC molecules; thus H-2^k–reactive T cells were not positively selected in the chimeric mice.

7. (a) Protein kinases. (b) CD45. (c) B7. (d) Protein phosphatase. (e) IL-2. (f) CD28; B7. (g) CD8. (h) Class II MHC, B7. (I) CD4. (j) Phospholipase. (k) Protein kinase.

8. (a) Because the pre-T cell receptor, which does not bind antigen, is associated with CD3, cells expressing the pre-TCR as well as the antigen-binding T-cell receptor would stain with anti-CD3. It is impossible to determine from this result, how many of the CD3-staining cells are expressing complete T-cell receptors. The remaining cells are even more immature thymocytes that do not express CD3. (b) No. Because some of the CD3-staining cells express the pre-TCR or the $\gamma\delta$ TCR instead of the complete $\alpha\beta$ TCR, you cannot calculate the number of T$_C$ cells by simple subtraction. To determine the number of T$_C$ cells, you need fluorescent anti–CD8 antibody, which will stain only the CD8$^+$ T$_C$ cells.

CHAPTER 13

1. (a) False: The high-affinity IL-2 receptor comprises three subunits—the α, β, and γ chains—all of which are transmembrane proteins. (b) False: Anti-TAC binds to the 55-kDa α chain of the IL-2 receptor. (c) False: Although all class I and class II cytokine receptors contain two or three subunits, the receptors for IL-1, IL-8, TNF-α, TNF-β, and some other cytokines have only one chain (see Figure 13-5). (d) False: Low levels of the IL-2R β chain are expressed in resting T cells, although expression is increased greatly following activation. The α chain is expressed only by activated T cells. (e) False: The cytosolic domains of class I and class II cytokine receptors appear to be closely associated with intracellular tyrosine kinases

but do not themselves possess tyrosine kinase activity. (f) Yes (see Figure 13-6).

2. Only antigen-activated T cells will proliferate, because they express the high-affinity IL-2 receptor, whereas resting T cells do not and therefore cannot respond to IL-2.

3. Cytokines, growth factors, and hormones are all secreted proteins that bind to receptors on target cells, eliciting various biological effects. Cytokines tend to be produced by a variety of cells, although their production is carefully regulated, and exert their effects on several cell types; most cytokines also act in an autocrine or paracrine fashion. Growth factors, unlike cytokines, are often produced constitutively. Hormones, unlike cytokines, generally act over long distances (endocrine effect) on one or a few types of target cells.

4. (a) γ chain and β chain (low level). (b) α, β, and γ chains. (c) γ chain and β chain (low level); cyclosporin A prevents the gene activation that leads to increased expression of the β and α chains. (d) γ chain and β chain (low level). (e) α, β, and γ chains. (f) β and γ chains (see Figure 13-8).

5. (a) Superantigens bind to class II MHC molecules outside of the normal peptide-binding cleft; unlike normal antigens, they are not internalized and processed by antigen-presenting cells but bind directly to class II molecules. Superantigens also bind to regions of the V_β domain of the T-cell receptor that are not involved in binding normal antigenic peptides (see Figure 4-14). Superantigens exhibit specificity for one or a few V_β domains; thus a given superantigen can activate all T cells that express the V_β domain(s) for which it is specific regardless of the antigenic specificity of the T cells. (b) A given superantigen can activate 5%–25% of T_H cells, leading to excessive production cytokines. The high levels of cytokines are thought to cause the symptoms associated with food poisoning and toxic-shock syndrome. (c) Yes. To exert their effect, superantigens must form a ternary complex with a class II MHC molecule and T-cell receptor.

6. The receptors for IL-3, IL-5, and GM-CSF contain a common signal-transducing β chain, designated KH97. Cytokine binding to each of these receptors probably triggers a similar signal-transduction pathway.

7. An HTLV protein called Tax has been shown to induce expression of a cellular transcription factor (or factors) that activates transcription of the genes encoding IL-2 and the IL-2 receptor. Thus a T cell infected with HTLV-1 expresses IL-2 and its receptor constitutively, rendering the cell responsive to IL-2–induced proliferation in the absence of antigen activation (see Figure 13-13).

8. (a) The T_H1 subset is responsible for classical cell-mediated functions (e.g., delayed-type hypersensitivity

and activation of T_C cells). Viral infections and intracellular pathogens are likely to induce a T_H1 response. (b) The T_H2 subset functions primarily as a helper for B-cell activation. This subset may be best suited to respond to freeliving bacteria and helminthic parasites and may mediate allergic reactions, since IL-4 and IL-5 are known to induce IgE production and eosinophil activation, respectively.

CHAPTER 14

1. (a) True. (b) True. (c) True. (d) True. (e) False: Enveloped viruses can be lysed by complement because their outer envelope is derived from the plasma membrane of a host cell. (f) True.

2. Serum IgM is in a planar form in which the complement-binding sites in the Fc region are not accessible. Only after binding to antigen does IgM assume a conformation in which the complement-binding sites are accessible (see Figure 14-3).

3. A C3 deficiency is more serious clinically because it impairs both the classical and alternative pathways. In contrast, with a C1 deficiency, the alternative pathway would still operate.

4. The degraded antibody would be less able to serve as an opsonin or to initiate complement activation.

5. (a) The classical pathway is initiated by immune complexes involving IgG or IgM; the alternative pathway generally is initiated by bacterial cell–wall components. (b) The initial reaction sequences generating C5 convertase differ in the two pathways. The terminal sequence leading from bound C5b to the MAC is the same in both pathways. See Figure 17-1. (c) Complement activation by either pathway has the *same* biological consequences because components mediating all the biological effects of complement are generated in both pathways.

6. (a) Innocent-bystander lysis may occur when free C5b67 binds to nearby healthy cells, including red blood cells. Binding of S protein to the free C5b67 prevents its insertion into the membrane of red blood cells and other healthy cells. In addition, red blood cells contain two membrane proteins, homologous restriction factor (HRF) and membrane inhibitor of reactive lysis (MIRL), which block the terminal sequence leading to MAC formation and thereby protect these cells from nonspecific complement-mediated lysis. (b) A defect in S protein, in the membrane-bound HRF and MIRL, or in the phospholipid membrane anchors that tether HRF and MIRL to the cell surface theoretically could lead to increased complement-mediated lysis of red blood cells. The presence of

defective membrane anchors has been associated with chronic hemolytic anemia in some individuals.

7. See Table 14-6.

8. (a) 4. (b) 5. (c) 6. (d) 2. (e) 7. (f) 11. (g) 3. (h) 1. (i) 8. (j) 10. (k) 9. (l) 12.

9. [Answer to question 9 is shown below]

	COMPONENT KNOCKED OUT						
	CLq	C4	C3	C5	C6	C9	FACTOR B
Complement activation							
Formation of C3 convertase in classical pathway	A	A	NE	NE	NE	NE	NE
Formation of C3 convertase in alternative pathway	NE	NE	A	NE	NE	NE	A
Formation of C5 convertase in classical pathway	A	A	A	NE	NE	NE	NE
Formation of C5 convertase in alternative pathway	NE	NE	A	NE	NE	NE	A
Effector functions							
C3b-mediated opsonization	D	D	A	NE	NE	NE	D
Neutrophil chemotaxis	D	D	D	D	D	NE	D
Cell lysis	D	D	A	A	A	A	D

CHAPTER 15

1. (a) False: Various chemokines are chemotactic for all types of leukocytes (see Table 15-2). (b) False: Integrins are expressed by various leukocytes but not by endothelial cells. (c) True. (d) True. (e) True. (f) False: Systemic effects, called the acute-phase response, are induced by cytokines generated in the localized acute inflammatory response. (g) True. (h) False: Granulomas may form in sites of chronic infection but are unlikely during an acute inflammatory response.

2. The increased expression of ICAMs on vascular endothelial cells near an inflammatory site facilitates ad-herence of leukocytes to the blood vessel wall, resulting in increased migration of leukocytes into the area.

3. (a) Rolling, activation, arrest/adhesion, and trans-endothelial migration (see Figures 15-3a and 15-7). (b) Neutrophils generally extravasate at sites of inflammation because they bind to the cell-adhesion molecules that are induced on vascular endothelium early in the inflammatory response. (c) Different lymphocyte subsets express homing receptors that bind to tissue-specific adhesion molecules (vascular addressins) on HEVs in different lymphoid organs, on inflamed endothelium, or on venules in tertiary sites. The homing of particular lymphocytes to certain sites is facilitated by chemokines that preferentially attract different lymphocytes. Thus, differences in (1) vascular addressins, (2) homing receptors, and (3) chemokines and their receptors determine the recirculation pattern of particular lymphocyte subsets.

4. IL-1, IL-6, and TNF-α (see Table 15-3).

5. TNF-α released by activated during a localized acute inflammatory response acts on vascular endothelial cells and macrophages inducing secretion of colony-stimulating factors (CSFs), which stimulate hematopoiesis in the bone marrow. This is part of the systemic acute-phase response.

6. (a) N. (b) 1. (c) N. (d) 3. (e) N. (f) 2. (g) 3 (see Figure 15-3).

7. IFN-γ stimulates activation of macrophages, resulting in increased expression of class II MHC molecules, increased microbicidal activity, and cytokine production. The accumulation of large numbers of activated macrophages is responsible for much of the tissue damage associated with chronic inflammation. TNF-α secreted by activated macrophages also contributes to the tissue wasting common in chronic inflammation. These two cytokines act synergistically to facilitate migration of large numbers of cells to sites of chronic inflammation.

8. Binding of all these cytokines to their receptors on hepatocytes induces formation of the same transcription factor, NF-16, which stimulates transcription of acute-phase proteins.

9. (a) 7. (b) 1, 6. (c) 10, 11. (d) 2. (e) 8. (f) 4. (g) 10. (h) 9.

CHAPTER 16

1. (a) False: The indirect hemolytic plaque assay detects both IgM- and IgG-secreting plasma cells. (b) True. (c) True. (d) True. (e) False: Antigenic competition will re-

duce the response to SRBC. (f) True. (g) True. (h) True. (i) True. (j) False: TEPC-15 is a myeloma-derived antibody specific for phosphorylcholine. It can serve as an antigen to which anti-idiotype antibody can bind.

2. The monoclonal antibody to LFA-1 should block formation of the CTL–target-cell conjugate. This should inhibit killing of the target cell and, therefore, should result in diminished ^{51}Cr release in the CML assay.

3. [Answer to question 3 is shown below]

POPULATION 1	POPULATION 2	PROLIFERATION
C57BL/6 (H-2^b)	CBA (H-2^k)	1 & 2
C57BL/6 (H-2^b)	CBA (H-2^k) mitomycin C-treated	1
C57BL/6 (H-2^b)	(CBA × C57BL/6) F$_1$	1
C57BL/6 (H-2^b)	C57L (H-2^b)	Neither

4. (a) Low affinity; IgM. (b) High affinity; IgG. (c) Low affinity; IgM. (d) Low affinity; IgG.

5. (a) CD4$^+$ T$_H$ cells. (b) To demonstrate the identity of the proliferating cells, you could incubate them with fluorescein-labeled anti-CD4 monoclonal antibody and rhodamine-labeled anti-CD8 monoclonal antibody. The proliferating cells will be stained only with the anti-CD4 reagent. (c) As CD4$^+$ T$_H$ cells recognize allogeneic class II MHC molecules on the stimulator cells, they are activated and begin to secrete IL-2, which then autostimulates T$_H$-cell proliferation. Thus, the extent of proliferation is directly related to the level of IL-2 produced.

6. (a) Direct hemolytic plaque assay for primary response (see Figure 16-20a); indirect hemolytic plaque assay for secondary response (see Figure 16-20b). (b) The direct PFC assay gives the number of IgM-secreting plasma cells. Subtract the direct PFCs from the indirect PFCs to obtain the number of IgG-secreting plasma cells. A = 310 IgM-secreting plasma cells and 33-IgG secreting plasma cells; B = 62 IgM-secreting plasma cells and 3998 IgG-secreting plasma cells; C = 366 IgM-secreting plasma cells and 20 IgG secreting plasma cells. (c) Group B illustrates the carrier effect. Only group B received a secondary immunization of both hapten and carrier, and therefore only group B has both memory B cells for DNP and memory T cells for the BSA carrier, allowing class switching from the IgM isotype to the IgG isotype, which is measured in the indirect assay.

7. (a) Neither. (b) Both. (c) CTL. (d) CTL. (e) T$_H$ cell. (f) CTL. (g) T$_H$ cell. (h) CTL. (i) T$_H$ cell. (j) T$_H$ cell. (k) Neither. (l) Both. (m) CTL. (n) Both. (o) Both. (p) T$_H$ cell. (q) Neither. (r) CTL. (s) T$_H$ cell.

8. [Answer to question 8 is shown below]

Source of primed spleen cells	[^{51}CR] RELEASE FROM LCM-INFECTED TARGET CELLS			
	B10.D2 (H-2^d)	B10 (H-2^b)	B10.BR (H-2^k)	(BALB/c × B10) F$_1$ (H-2$^{b/d}$)
B10.D2 (H-2^d)	+	−	−	+
B10 (H-2^b)	−	+	−	+
BALB/c (H-2^d)	+	−	−	+
(BALB/c × B10) (H-2$^{b/d}$)	+	+	−	+

9. To determine T$_C$ activity specific for influenza, perform a CML reaction by incubating spleen cells from the infected mouse with influenza-infected syngeneic target cells. To determine T$_H$ activity, incubate the spleen cells from the infected mouse with syngeneic APCs presenting influenza peptides, and measure IL-2 production.

CHAPTER 17

1. (a) False: IgE is increased. (b) False: IL-4 increases IgE production. (c) True. (d) False: Antihistamines are helpful in type I hypersensitivity, which involves release of histamine via mast cell degranulation. Because type III hypersensitivity primarily involves immune-complex deposition, antihistamines are ineffective. (e) False: Most pollen allergens contain multiple allergenic components. (f) False: Unlike IgG, IgE cannot pass through the placenta. (g) True. (h) True.

2. (a) The complete antibodies would cross-link FcεRI molecules on the membrane of mast cells and basophils, resulting in their activation and degranulation. The released mediators would induce vasodilation, smooth-muscle contraction, and a local wheal and flare reaction. Because the Fab fragment is monovalent, it cannot cross-link FcεRI molecules and thus cannot induce degranulation. However, this type of antireceptor antibody could bind to FcεRI and might thereby block binding of IgE to the receptors. (b) The response induced by complete anti-FcεRI antibodies does not depend on allergen-specific IgE and thus would be similar in allergic and nonallergic mice. Injection of Fab fragments of anti-FcεRI might prevent allergic mice from reacting to an allergen if these fragments block binding of IgE to mast cells and basophils.

3. Engineer chimeric monoclonal antibodies to snake venom that contain mouse variable regions but human

heavy- and light-chain constant regions (see Figure 5-24).

4. (a) Type I hypersensitivity: localized atopic reaction resulting from allergen cross-linkage of fixed IgE on skin mast cells inducing degranulation and mediator release. (b) Type III hypersensitivity: immune complexes of antibody and insect antigens form and are deposited locally, causing an Arthus-type reaction resulting from complement activation and complement split products. (c) Type IV hypersensitivity: sensitized T_{DTH} cells release their mediators inducing macrophage accumulation and activation. Tissue damage results from lysosomal enzymes released by the macrophage.

5. (a) IV. (b) All four types. (c) I and III. (d) IV. (e) I. (f) II. (g) I. (h) I. (i) II. (j) II. (k) I.

6. [Answer to question 6 is shown below]

CHAPTER 18

1. (a) True. (b) True. (c) True. (d) False: Because DNA vaccines allow prolonged exposure to antigen, they are likely to generate immunologic memory. (e) True. (f) False: A DNA vaccine contains the gene encoding an entire protein antigen, which most likely contains multiple epitopes.

2. Because attenuated organisms are capable of limited growth within host cells, they are processed by the cytosolic pathway and presented on the membrane of infected host cells together with class I MHC molecules. These vaccines, therefore, usually can induce a cell-mediated immune response. The limited growth of attenuated organisms within the host often eliminates the need for booster doses of the vaccine. Also, if the attenuated organism is able to grow along mucous membranes, then the vaccine will be able to induce the production of secretory IgA. The major disadvantage of attenuated whole-organism vaccines is that they may revert to a virulent form. They also are more unstable than other types of vaccines, requiring refrigeration to maintain their activity.

3. (a) The antitoxin was given to inactivate any toxin that might be produced if *Clostridium tetani* infected the wound. The antitoxin was necessary because the girl had not been previously immunized and, therefore, did not have circulating antibody to tetanus toxin or memory B cells specific for tetanus toxin. (b) Because of the treatment with antitoxin after the first injury, the girl would not develop immunity to tetanus as a result of this injury. Therefore, after the second injury 3 years later, she will require another dose of antitoxin. To develop long-term immunity, she should be vaccinated with tetanus toxoid.

IMMUNOLOGIC EVENT	TYPE I HYPERSENSITIVITY	TYPE II HYPERSENSITIVITY	TYPE III HYPERSENSITIVITY	TYPE IV HYPERSENSITIVITY
IgE-mediated degranulation of mast cells	+			
Lysis of antibody-coated blood cells by complement		+		
Tissue destruction in response to poison oak				+
C3a- and C5a-mediated mast-cell degranulation		(some)	+	
Chemotaxis of neutrophils			+	
Chemotaxis of eosinophils	+			
Activation of macrophages by IFN-g				+
Deposition of antigen-antibody complexes on basement membranes of capillaries			+	
Sudden death due to vascular collapse (shock) shortly after injection or ingestion of antigen	+			

4. The Sabin polio vaccine is attenuated, whereas the Salk vaccine is inactivated. The Sabin vaccine thus has the usual advantages of an attenuated vaccine compared with inactivated vaccines (see Answer #2). Moreover, since the Sabin vaccine is capable of limited growth along the gastrointestinal tract, it induces production of secretory IgA.

5. T-cell epitopes generally are internal peptides, which commonly contain a high proportion of hydrophobic residues. In contrast, B-cell epitopes are located on an antigen's surface, where they are accessible to antibody, and contain a high proportion of hydrophilic residues. Thus, synthetic hydrophobic peptides are most likely to represent T-cell epitopes and induce cell-mediated response, whereas synthetic hydrophilic peptides are most likely to represent accessible B-cell epitopes and induce an antibody response.

6. When the majority of a population is immune to a particular pathogen—that is, there is herd immunity—then the probability of the few susceptible members of the population contacting an infected individual is very low. Thus susceptible individuals are not likely to become infected with the pathogen. If the number of immunized individuals decreases sufficiently, most commonly because of reduction in vaccination rates, then herd immunity no longer operates to protect susceptible individuals and infection may spread rapidly in a population, leading to an epidemic.

7. The MHC molecules of the strain B mice are not able to bind the peptide and present it to T cells. You could test this hypothesis by transfecting the genes encoding the MHC molecules of the strain A and strain B mice into separate cultures of L cells and then incubating the transfected L cells with the peptide to see if they can bind the peptide and activate T cells.

8. Pathogens with a short incubation period (e.g., influenza virus) cause disease symptoms before a memory-cell response can be induced. Protection against such pathogens is achieved by repeated reimmunizations to maintain high levels of neutralizing antibody. For pathogens with a longer incubation period (e.g., polio virus), the memory-cell response occurs sufficiently rapidly to prevent development of symptoms, and high levels of neutralizing antibody at the time of infection are unnecessary.

9. Bacterial capsular polysaccharides, inactivated bacterial exotoxins (toxoids), and surface protein antigens. The latter two commonly are produced by recombinant DNA technology.

10. The attenuated Sabin vaccine can cause life-threatening infection in individuals, such as children with AIDS, whose immune systems are severely suppressed.

CHAPTER 19

1. (a) Because the infected target cells expressed H-2^k MHC molecules, but the primed T cells were H-2^b restricted. (b) Because the influenza nucleoprotein is processed by the endogenous processing pathway and the resulting peptides are presented by class I MHC molecules. (c) Probably because the transfected class I D^b molecule is only able to present peptide 365–380 and not peptide 50–63. Alternatively, peptide 50–63 may not be a T-cell epitope. (d) These results suggest that a cocktail of several immunogenic peptides would be more likely to be presented by different MHC haplotypes in humans and would provide the best vaccines for humans.

2. Nonspecific host defenses include ciliated epithelial cells; bactericidal substances in mucous secretions; complement split products activated by the alternative pathway that serve both as opsonins and as chemotactic factors; and phagocytic cells.

3. Specific host defenses include secretory IgA in the mucous secretions; IgG and IgM in the tissue fluids; the classical complement pathway; complement split products; the opsonins (IgM, IgG, and C3b); and phagocytic cells. Cytokines produced during the specific immune response, including IFN-γ, TNF, IL-1, and IL-6, contribute to the overall intensity of the inflammatory response.

4. Humoral antibody peaks within a few days of infection and binds to the influenza HA glycoprotein blocking viral infection of host epithelial cells. However, the antibody is strain specific and therefore its major role is in protecting against re-infection with the same strain of influenza. The cell-mediated response peaks about 8 days after infection and serves to kill virally infected self-cells. The CTL response is necessary to eliminate the virus. Unlike the humoral antibody response, which is strain specific, the CTL response is able to recognize epitopes shared by different influenza subtypes.

5. (a) African trypanosomes are capable of antigenic shifts in the variant surface glycoprotein (VSG). The antigenic shifts are accomplished as gene segments encoding part of the VSG are duplicated and translocated to transcriptionally active expression sites. (b) Plasmodium evades the immune system by continually undergoing maturational changes from sporozoite to merozoite to gametocyte, allowing the organism to continually change its surface molecules. In addition, the intracellular phases of its life cycle reduce the level of immune activation. Finally, the organism is able to slough off its circumsporozoite coat after antibody binds to it. (c) Influenza is able to evade the

immune response through frequent antigenic changes in its hemagglutinin and neuraminidase glycoproteins. The antigenic changes are accomplished by the accumulation of small point mutations (antigenic drift) or through genetic reassortment of RNA between influenza virions from humans and animals (antigenic shift).

6. (a) IA^b. (b) Because antigen-specific, MHC-restricted T_H cells participate in B-cell activation.

7. (a) The fact that the CTL response is cross-reactive means that it might be possible to induce an immune response to several human pandemic subtypes with a single vaccine. However, because the MHC haplotype determines which peptides are presented to the T cells, it will be necessary to identify immunodominant T-cell epitopes for individuals with different MHC haplotypes and then prepare a cocktail of synthetic peptides. (b) The nucleoprotein can serve as a potential vaccine because it will be processed by the endogenous processing pathway and presented together with class I MHC molecules on the membrane of the infected host cell.

8. (a) BCG (Bacillus Calmette-Guerin). (b) antigenic shift, antigenic drift. (c) gene conversion. (d) tubercles; T_{DTH} cells; activated macrophages. (e) toxoid. (f) interferon α and interferon β. (g) secretory IgA. (h) IL-12; IFN-γ.

CHAPTER 20

1. (a) 6. (b) 9. (c) 8. (d) 10. (e) 12. (f) 7. (g) 3. (h) 11. (i) 2. (j) 1. (k) 5. (l) 4.

2. (a) EAE is induced by injecting mice or rats with myelin basic protein in complete Freund's adjuvant. (b) The animals that recover from EAE are now resistant to EAE. If they are given a second injection of myelin basic protein in complete Freund's adjuvant, they no longer develop EAE. (c) If T cells from mice with EAE are transferred to normal syngeneic mice, the mice will develop EAE. See Figure 20-7.

3. A number of viruses have been shown to possess protein that share sequences with myelin basic protein (MBP). Since the encephalitogenic peptides of MBP are known, it is possible to test these peptides to see if they bear sequence homology to known viral protein sequences. Computer analysis has revealed a number of viral peptides that bear sequence homology to MBP. By immunizing rabbits with these viral sequences, it was possible to induce EAE. The studies on the encephalitogenic peptides of MBP also showed that different peptides

induced EAE in different strains. Thus the MHC haplotype will determine which cross-reacting viral peptides will be presented and, therefore, will influence the development of EAE.

4. (1) A virus might express an antigenic determinant that cross-reacts with a self-component. (2) A viral infection might induce localized concentrations of IFN-γ. The IFN-γ might then induce inappropriate expression of class II MHC molecules on non-antigen-presenting cells, enabling self-peptides presented together with the class II MHC molecules on these cells to activate T_H cells. (3) A virus may damage a given organ resulting in release of antigens that are normally sequestered from the immune system.

5. (a) So that the IFN-γ transgene would only be expressed by pancreatic beta cells. (b) There was a cellular infiltration of lymphocytes and macrophages similar to that seen in insulin-dependent diabetes mellitus. (c) The IFN-γ transgene induced the pancreatic beta cells to express class II MHC molecules. (d) A localized viral infection in the pancreas might result in the localized production of IFN-γ by activated T cells. The IFN-γ might then induce the inappropriate expression of class II MHC molecules by pancreatic beta cells as well as the production of other cytokines such as IL-1 or TNF. If self-peptides are presented by the class II MHC molecules, then IL-1 might provide the necessary co-stimulatory signal to activate T cells against the self-peptides. Alternatively, the TNF might also cause localized cellular damage. See Figure 20-10.

6. Anti-CD4 monoclonal antibodies have been used to block T_H activity. Monoclonal antibodies (anti-TAC) specific for the high-affinity IL-2 receptor have been tried to block activated T_H cells. The association of some autoimmune diseases with restricted T-cell receptor expression has prompted researchers to use monoclonal antibody specific for T-cell receptors carrying particular V domains. Finally, antibodies against specific MHC alleles associated with increased risk for autoimmunity have been tested in EAE models.

7. (a) True. (b) False: Although Hsp65 has been associated with certain autoimmune diseases, most normal individuals mount an immune response to mycobacterial Hsp65 without developing any autoimmune symptoms. (c) False: IL-2, which promotes the development of T_H1 cells, increases the autoimmune response to MBP plus adjuvant. (d) False: The presence of HLA B27 is strongly associated with susceptibility to ankylosing spondylitis but is not the only factor required for development of the disease. (f) True. (g) True.

CHAPTER 21

1. (a) True. (b) False: X-linked agammaglobulinemia is characterized by a reduction in B cells and an absence of immunoglobulins. (c) False: Phagocytic defects result in recurrent bacterial and fungal infections. (d) True. (e) True. (f) True. (g) True. (h) False: The mice need lymphoid stem cells containing the enzymes that catalyze rearrangement of variable-region gene segments in DNA encoding immunoglobulin and the T-cell receptor. (i) False: These children are usually able to eliminate common encapsulated bacteria with antibody plus complement but are susceptible to viral, protozoan, fungal, and intracellular bacterial pathogens, which are eliminated by the cell-mediated branch of the immune system. (j) False: Humoral immunity also is affected because class II–restricted T_H cells must be activated for an antibody response to occur.

2. (a) Leukocyte-adhesion deficiency results from biosynthesis of a defective β chain in LFA-1, CR3, and CR4, which all contain the same β chain. (b) LFA-1 plays a role in cell adhesion by binding to ICAM-1 expressed on various types of cells. Binding of LFA-1 to ICAM-1 is involved in the interactions between T_H cells and B cells, between CTLs and target cells, and between circulating leukocytes and vascular endothelial cells. (c) No: Formation of T_H-cell/B-cell conjugates is required for B-cell activation. This conjugate formation depends in part on interaction between LFA-1 present on T_H cells and ICAM-1 present on B cells. Because this interaction is deficient in LAD patients, their ability to produce specific antibody is impaired.

3. (a) The rearranged heavy-chain genes in SCID mice lack the D and/or J gene segments (see Figure 7-10). (b) According to the model of allelic exclusion discussed in Chapter 7, a productive heavy-chain gene rearrangement must occur before κ-chain genes are rearranged. Since SCID mice lack productive heavy-chain rearrangement, they do not attempt κ light-chain rearrangement. (c) Yes: The rearranged μ heavy-chain gene would be transcribed to yield a functional μ heavy chain. The presence of the μ heavy chain then would induce rearrangement of the κ-chain gene (see Figure 7-21). (d) In normal animals, rearranged TCR β-chain DNA contains both a D and J segment, whereas α-chain DNA lacks a D segment (see Figure 11-7). In SCID mice, the DNA encoding the β chain of the T-cell receptor would undergo defective gene rearrangement in which the D and/or J gene segments are deleted during the joining process. However,

gene rearrangements in the α-chain DNA would be the same in SCID and normal mice.

4. Phagocytic deficiencies: recurrent bacterial and fungal infections ranging from mild skin infections to life-threatening systemic infections. Humoral deficiencies: recurring bacterial infections particularly by encapsulated bacteria (e.g., staphylococci, streptococci, and pneumococci). Cell-mediated deficiencies: increased susceptibility to infections caused by viruses, protozoa, fungi, and intracellular bacteria. Combined immunodeficiencies: extreme susceptibility to all types of infections beginning early in infancy; early death is likely unless these conditions are treated successfully.

5. (a) 4. (b) 3. (c) 2. (d) 1. (e) 8. (f) 6. (g) 5. (h) 7.

6. (a) SCID-human mice are prepared by implanting portions of human fetal liver, thymus, and lymph nodes into SCID mice (see Figure 2-1). (b) The fetal liver is used to provide a source of hematopoietic lymphoid stem cells. (c) The human cells are not rejected because the mouse does not have functional immunocompetent B or T cells. (d) Graft-versus-host disease does not develop because as the human T cells mature within the human thymic tissue, they are exposed to mouse MHC molecules and mouse antigens. Therefore, the human T cells become tolerant to the mouse antigens during thymic processing.

CHAPTER 22

1. (a) False: HIV-2 and SIV are more closely related. (b) False: HIV-1 infects chimpanzees but does not cause immune suppression. (c) True. (d) True. (e) True. (f) False: Patients with advanced AIDS sometimes have no detectable serum antibody to HIV. (g) False: The PCR detects HIV proviral DNA in latently infected cells. (h) True.

2. (a) Soluble gp120. (b) Binding of soluble gp120 to CD4 on uninfected T_H cells could result in antibody-plus-complement lysis or ADCC mediated by anti-gp120 antibody (see Figure 22-13). Gp120 binding also may trigger an inappropriate activating signal leading to apoptosis of the T_H cell. In addition, soluble gp120 may induce fusion of infected CD4$^+$ T cells with uninfected T cells, forming large, multinucleated syncytia. After a brief period of viral replication, these cells die. (c) Binding of soluble gp120 to CD4 $^+$ may block interaction of T_H cells with antigen-presenting cells, thus

inhibiting T-cell activation and the ability of the cells to respond to antigen.

3. No. In the latency period the virus is not replicating, and therefore, the levels of p17 and p24 decline.

4. An increase in the levels of p24 indicates that HIV infection is progressing from the latent phase into lytic infection. Increased levels of p24 can be used to indicate that an HIV-infected individual is progressing into AIDS.

5. Skin-test reactivity is monitored to indicate the functional activity of T_{DTH} cells. As AIDS progresses and $CD4^+$ T cells decline, there is a decline in skin-test reactivity to common antigens.

6. Cell-mediated immunity.

7. Fusion of HIV with a target cell involves the fusogenic domain of the gp41 envelope protein on HIV and a newly discovered membrane protein, called fusin, present on certain human cells. Because fusin is a member of the chemokine family of receptors, binding of chemokines to fusin may block its ability to function in fusion, thereby suppressing HIV infection.

8. Patient LS fits the definition of AIDS, whereas patient BW does not. The clinical diagnosis of AIDS among HIV-infected individuals depends on both the T-cell count and the presence of various indicator diseases. See Table 22-3.

CHAPTER 23

1. (a) False: Acute rejection is cell mediated and probably involves the first-set rejection mechanism (see 23-1b and 23-5). (b) True. (c) False: Passenger leukocytes are donor dendritic cells that express class I MHC molecules and high levels of class II MHC molecules. They migrate from the grafted tissue to regional lymph nodes of the recipient, where host immune cells respond to alloantigens on them (see Figure 23-4). (d) False: A graft that is matched for the major histocompatibility antigens, encoded in the HLA, may be rejected because of differences in the minor histocompatibility antigens encoded at other loci. (e) True.

2. (a) The best possible match is identity in the MHC haplotypes of donor and recipient. (b) There is a 25% chance that siblings will share identical MHC haplotypes (see Figure 9-2c). (c) Perform HLA typing using a microcytotoxicity test with monoclonal antibody to class I and class II MHC antigens. In addition, a one-way MLR

can be performed using donor lymphocytes treated with mitomycin C as stimulator cells and untreated recipient lymphocytes as responder cells (see Figure 16-13).

3. [Answer to question 3 is shown below]

DONOR	RECIPIENT	RESPONSE	REJECTION
BALB/c	C3H	R	FSR
BALB/c	Rat	R	FSR
BALB/c	Nude mouse	A	
BALB/c	C3H, had previous BALB/c graft	R	SSR
BALB/c	C3H, had previous C57BI/6 graft	R	FSR
BALB/c	BALB/c	A	
BALB/c	(BALB/c × C3H) F_1	A	
BALB/c	(C3H × C57BI/6) F_1	R	FSR
(BALB/c × C3H) F_1	BALB/c	R	FSR
(BALB/c × C3H) F_1	BALB/c, had previous F_1 graft	R	SSR

4. (a) Graft-versus-host disease (GVHD) develops as donor T cells recognize alloantigens on cells of an immune-suppressed host. The response develops as donor T_H cells are activated in response to recipient peptide-MHC complexes displayed on antigen-presenting cells. Cytokines elaborated by these T_H cells activate a variety of effector cells including NK cells, CTLs, and macrophages, which damage the host tissue. In addition cytokines such as TNF may mediate direct cytolytic damage to the host cells. (b) GVHD develops when the donated organ or tissue contains immunocompetent lymphocytes and when the host is immune suppressed. (c) The donated organ or tissue could be treated with monoclonal antibodies to CD3, CD4, or the high-affinity IL-2 receptor to deplete donor T_H cells. The rationale behind this approach is to diminish T_H-cell activation in response to the alloantigens of the host. The use of anti-CD3 will deplete all T cells; the use of anti-CD4 will deplete all T_H cells; the use of anti-IL-2R will deplete only the activated T_H cells.

5. (a) Siblings A, C, and E are all potential donors, as they have the same ABO blood type and HLA antigens as the recipient. (b) Sibling A is the best donor as indicated by the low proliferative response in a one-way MLR with the recipient.

CHAPTER 24

1. (a) False: Hereditary retinoblastoma results from inactivation of both alleles of the *Rb* gene, a tumor-suppressor gene. (b) True. (c) True. (d) True. (e) False: Some oncogenic retroviruses do not have viral oncogenes. (f) True. (g) False: LAK cells kill a wide variety of tumor cells and are not specific for a single type of tumor.

2. Cells of the pre-B cell lineage have rearranged the heavy-chain genes and express the μ heavy chain in their cytoplasm (see Figure 8-3). You could perform Southern-blot analysis with a C_μ probe to see if the heavy-chain genes have rearranged. You could also perform fluorescent antibody staining utilizing methods to stain the cytoplasmic μ heavy chain.

3. (a) Early-stage melanoma cells appear to be functioning as antigen-presenting cells, processing the antigen by the exogenous pathway and presenting the tetanus toxoid antigen together with the class II MHC DR molecule. (b) Advanced-stage melanoma cells might have a reduction in the expression of class II MHC molecules, or they may not be able to internalize and process the antigen by the exogenous route. (c) Since the paraformaldehyde-fixed early melanoma cells could present processed tetanus toxoid, they must express class II MHC molecules on their surface. (d) Stain the early and advanced melanoma cells with fluorescent monoclonal antibody specific for class II MHC molecules.

4. See Figure 24-6.

5. IFN-α, IFN-β, and IFN-γ enhance the expression of class I MHC molecules on tumor cells, thereby increasing the CTL response to tumors. IFN-γ also increases the activity of CTLs, macrophages, and NK cells, each of which play a role in the immune response to tumors. TNF-α and TNF-β have direct antitumor activity inducing hemorrhagic necrosis and tumor regression. IL-2 activates LAK and TIL cells, which both have antitumor activity.

6. (a) Melanoma cells transfected with the B7 gene are able to deliver the co-stimulatory signal necessary for activation of CTL precursors to effector CTLs, which then can to destroy tumor cells. Melanoma cells transfected with the GM-CSF gene secrete this cytokine, which stimulates the activation and differentiation of antigen-presenting cells, especially dendritic cells, in the vicinity. The dendritic cells then can present tumor antigens to T_H cells and CTL precursors, enhancing the generation of effector CTLs (see Figure 24-11). (b) Because some of the tumor antigens on human melanomas are expressed by other types of cancers, transfected melanoma cells might be effective against other tumors carrying identical antigens.

Line illustrations rendered by Network Graphics.

Foreword Opener From R. L. Stanfield, T. M. Fieser, R. A. Lerner, I. A. Wilson, *Science,* 1990, **24:**712.

Preface Opener From D. H. Fremont, M. Pique, and I. A. Wilson, *Science,* 1992, **257:**891.

Preface Photo From J. H. Brown, T. S. Jardetzky, J. C. Gorga, L. J. Stern, R. G. Urban, J. L. Strominger, D. C. Wiley, *Nature,* 1993, **364:**33.

Cover and Frontispiece Colorized by Marie T. Dauenheimer; image © by Morris J. Karnovsky, President and Fellow Harvard College.

Table of Contents Opener From J. H. Brown, T. S. Jardetzky, J. C. Gorga, L. J. Stern, R. G. Urban, J. L. Strominger, D. C. Wiley, *Nature,* 1993, **364:**33.

Part I Opener From Peter Arnold, Inc. © Manfred Kage.

Chapter 1 Opener From N. Sharon and H. Lis, *Scientific American,* Volume 268, January 1993, p. 85. Photograph courtesy of Kazuhiko Fujita. Micrograph by Morten H. Nielsen and Ole Werdelin.

Figure 1-1 From *Harper's Weekly,* Volume 29, 1885, p. 836; courtesy of the National Library of Medicine.

Figure 1-2 From N. Sharon and H. Lis, *Scientific American,* Volume 268, January 1993, p. 85. Photograph courtesy of Kazuhiko Fujita.

Figure 1-7 From A. S. Rosenthal et al., *Phagocytosis—Past and Future,* Academic Press, 1982, p. 239. Reprinted by permission.

Figure 1-13 From *Immunology: Recognition and Response,* edited by W. E. Paul, W. H. Freeman and Company, 1991, p. 49. Originally from "How T Cells See Antigen," by H. M. Grey et al., *Scientific American,* November 1989, p. 57. Copyright © 1989 by Scientific American Inc. All rights reserved. Micrograph courtesy of Morten H. Nielsen and Ole Werdelin.

Table 2-1 Adapted from Federation of American Societies for Experimental Biology, *Biological Handbooks, Vol.*

III: Inbred and Genetically Defined Strains of Laboratory Animals, Pergamon Press Ltd., 1979.

Table 2-3 From J. D. Watson, J. Tooze, and D. T. Kurtz, *Recombinant DNA: A Short Course.* Copyright © 1983 by W. H. Freeman and Company.

Figure 2-3 Adapted from Harvey Lodish et al., *Molecular Cell Biology,* 3rd Edition. Copyright 1995 by Scientific American Books.

Figure 2-6 From J. Darnell, H. Lodish, and D. Baltimore, *Molecular Cell Biology,* 2nd Edition. Copyright © 1990 by Scientific American Books.

Figure 2-7 Adapted from Harvey Lodish et al., *Molecular Biology,* 3rd ed. Copyright © 1995 by Scientific American Books.

Figure 2-8 Adapted from J. D. Watson et al., 1992, *Recombinant DNA,* 2nd ed. Copyright © 1992 by W. H. Freeman and Company.

Figure 2-9 Adapted from J. D. Watson. et al., 1992, *Recombinant DNA: A Short Course,* 2nd ed. Copyright © 1992 by W. H. Freeman and Company.

Figure 2-12 Adapted from Harvey Lodish, et al., *Molecular Cell Biology,* 3rd ed. Copyright © 1995 by Scientific American Books.

Figure 2-13 Adapted from M. R. Capecchi, *Trends in Genetics,* Volume J, 1989, p. 70.

Chapter 3 Opener From Lennart Nilsson, "Our Immune System: The Wars Within," *National Geographic,* June 1986, p. 718 Copyright © by Boehringer Ingelheim International. GmpH, Stockholm. Photo by Lennart Nilsson.

Figure 3-3b From M. J. Cline and D. W. Golde, "Cellular Interactions in Hematopoiesis," reprinted by permission from *Nature,* 1979, Volume 277, p. 180. Copyright 1979 Macmillan Magazines Ltd. Micrograph courtesy of Shirley Quan.

Figure 3-10b From J. R. Goodman, Department of Pediatrics, University of California at San Francisco.

Figure 3-12 From Lennart Nilsson, "Our Immune System: The Wars Within," *National Geographic*, June 1986, p. 718. Copyright Boehringer Ingelheim International. GmpH, Stockholm. Photo by Lennart Nilsson.

Figure 3-14 Adapted from J. H. Peters et al.,1996, *Immunology Today*,Volume 17, p. 273.

Figure 3-15 From A. K. Szakal et al., "Isolated Follicular Dendritic Cells: Cytochemical Volume Antigen Localization, Momarski, SEM, and TEM Morphology," *Journal of Immunology*,Volume 134, 1985, p. 1353. Copyright 1985 American Association of Immunologists. Reprinted with permission.

Figure 3-17 From W. van Ewijk, adapted, with permission, from the *Annual Review of Immunology*, Volume 9, p. 591. Copyright 1991 by Annual Reviews Inc.

Figure 3-18 From M. M. Compton and J. A. Cidlowski, *Trends in Endocrinology and Metabolism*, Volume 3, 1992, p. 17.

Figure 3-20 From W. Bloom and D. W. Fawcett, *Textbook of Histology*, 10th ed., Copyright © 1975, W. B. Saunders Co.

Part II Opener From Peter Arnold, Inc. © David Scharf.

Chapter 4 Opener From G. J. V. H. Nossal, *Scientific American*,Volume 269, 1993, p. 22.

Figure 4-2 From K. C. Garcia, et al., 1992, *Science*,Volume 257, p. 502.

Figure 4-3 From A. G. Amit et al., 1986, *Science*,Volume 233, p.747.

Figure 4-4 From I. A. Wilson and R. L. Stanfield, 1993, *Current Opinions in Structural Biology*,Volume 3, Number 113.

Figure 4-5 Adapted from M. Sela, "Antigenicity: Some Molecular Aspects," *Science*, Volume 166, December 12, 1969, p. 1365. Copyright © 1969 by the American Association for the Advancement of Science.

Table 4-6 Based on K. Landsteiner, *The Specificity or Serologic Reaction,* 1962, Dover Press, Modified by J. Klein, *Immunology, The Science of Self-Nonself Discrimination,* 1988, John Wiley Publishers.

Figure 4-6 From G. J. V. H. Nossal, *Scientific American*,Volume 269, September 1993, p. 22.

Figure 4-7a Adapted from M. Z. Atassi, *Immunochemistry* (now *Molecular Immunology*), Volume 12, 1975, p. 423. Copyright © 1975 by Pergamon Press.

Figure 4-8abc Adapted from D. Benjamin, J. Bersofsky, I. East et al., adapted, with permission, from the *Annual*

Review of Immunology,Volume 2, p. 67. Copyright © 1984 by Annual Reviews Inc.

Figure 4-10 From J. Rothbard et al., Modern *Trends in Human Leukemia*,Volume 7, 1987. Reprinted by permission of Springer-Verlag Inc.

Figure 4-11 From H. M. Grey et al., *Scientific American*, Volume 261, November 1989, p. 59. Copyright © 1989 by Scientific American Inc. All rights reserved.

Figure 5-1 Adapted from A. Tiselius and E. A. Kabat, reproduced from the *Journal of Experimental Medicine*, 1939, Volume 69, p. 119, by copyright permission of the Rockefeller University Press.

Figure 5-4 Adapted from J. Darnell, H. Lodish, and D. Baltimore, *Molecular Cell Biology*, 2nd Edition. Copyright © 1990 by Scientific American Books. Reprinted by permission of W. H. Freeman and Company.

Figure 5-5 Image provided by the laboratory of Dr. Alexander McPherson. The immunoglobulin structure was determined by Harris et al., *Nature*, Volume 360, 1992, pp. 369-372. A special thank you to the American Computing and Graphics and Visual Imaging Lab, University of California, Riverside, for help with image. The image was generated using the computer program, RIBBONS. The RIBBONS reference is: M. Carson and C. E. Bugg, "An Algorithm for Ribbon Models of Proteins," *Journal of Molecular Graphics*, Volume 4, 1986, pp. 121–122.

Figure 5-6a Adapted from M. Schiffer et al., reprinted with permission from *Biochemistry*, Volume 12, 1973, p. 4620. Copyright © 1973 by the American Chemical Society.

Figure 5-6b Adapted from Williams and Barclay, *Annual Review of Immunology*,Volume 6, 1988, p. 381.

Figure 5-7a From E. W. Silverton et al., *Proceedings of the National Academy of Sciences U.S.A.,* Volume 74, 1977, p. 5140.

Figure 5-8 Based on E. A. Kabat et al., *Sequence of Immunoglobulin Chains*, U.S. Department of Health Education and Welfare, 1977.

Figure 5-9 From K. C. Garcia, P. M. Ronco, P. J.Verroust et al., *Science*,Volume 257, 1992, p. 502.

Figure 5-10 From J. M. Rini, W. Schulze-Gahmen, and I. A. Wilson, *Science*, Volume 255, 1992, p. 959. Photograph courtesy of J. M. Rini, W. Schulze-Gahmen, and I. A. Wilson.

Tables 5-2 and 5-3 Adapted from I. A. Wilson and R. L. Stanfield, *Current Opinion in Structural Biology*,Volume 3, Number 113, 1993.

Figure 5-12 abc Photograph from R. C. Valentine and N. M. Green, *Journal of Molecular Biology*, Volume 27, 1967, p. 615. Reprinted by permission of Academic Press Inc. (London) Ltd.

Figure 5-13 Adapted from A. D. Keegan and W. E. Paul, *Immunology Today*, Volume 13, 1992, p. 63, and M. E. Reth, *Annual Review of Immunology*, Volume 10, 1992, p. 97.

Table 5-6 Adapted from G. Winter and W. J. Harris, *Immunology Today*, Volume 14, 1993, p. 243.

Figure 5-24 Adapted from M. Verhoeyen and L. Reichmann, *BioEssays*, Volume 8, 1988, p.14. Reprinted by permission of Cambridge University Press.

Figure 5-26 Adapted from W. D. Huse et al., *Science*, Volume 246, 1989, p. 1275.

Table 6-1 Adapted from H. N. Eisen, *Immunology*, 3rd ed.1990, Harper and Row Publishers.

Table 6-3 Adapted from N. R. Rose et al. (eds.), *Manual of Clinical Laboratory Immunology*. Copyright © 1986 American Society for Microbiology.

Figure 6-5 From J. S. Garvey, N. E. Cremer, and D. H. Sussdorf, *Methods in Immunology*, 3rd ed. Copyright © 1977 by Addison-Wesley Publishing Company, Inc., Advanced Book Program. Reprinted by permission of the author.

Figure 6-7 From D. M. Weir, (ed.) *Handbook of Experimental Immunology, Volume 1: Immunochemistry*, 4th ed., 1986. Reprinted by permission of Blackwell Scientific Publications Ltd.

Figure 6-7 From J. S. Garvey, N. E. Cremer, and D. H. Sussdorf, *Methods in Immunology*, 3rd Edition. Copyright © 1977 by Addison-Wesley Publishing Company, Inc., Advanced Book Program. Reprinted by permission of the author.

Figures 6-10 and 6-11 From D. M. Weir, (ed.) *Handbook of Experimental Immunology, Volume 1: Immunochemistry*, 4th Edition, 1986. Reprinted by permission of Blackwell Scientific Publications Ltd.

Figure 6-12 From J. S. Garvey, N. E. Cremer, and D. H. Sussdorf, *Methods in Immunology*, 3rd Edition. Copyright © 1977 by Addison-Wesley Publishing Company, Inc., Advanced Book Program. Reprinted by permission of the author.

Figure 7-2 Adapted from N. Hozumi and S. Tonegawa, *Proceedings of the National Academy of Science*, Volume 73, 1976, p. 3628.

Figure 7-7 From K. Okazki et al., *Cell*, Volume 49, 1987, p. 477. Reprinted by permission of Cell Press.

Figure 7-10 Adapted from F. W. Alt, *Immunology Today*, Volume 13, 1992, p. 306. Elsevier Science Publishing Company, Inc. Reprinted by permission.

Figure 7-13 Adapted from G. D. Yancopoulos and F. W. Alt, adapted, with permission, from the *Annual Review of Immunology*, Volume 4, 1986, p. 339. Copyright © 1986 by Annual Reviews, Inc.

Figure 7-16 Adapted from C. Berek and C. Milstein, *Immunological Review*, Volume 96, 1987, p. 23. Copyright © Munksgaard International Publishers Ltd., Copenhagen, Denmark.

Chapter 8 Opener From V. M. Sanders et al., "Characterization of the Physical Interaction Between Antigen-Specific B and T cells," *Journal of Immunology*, Volume 337, 1989, p. 562.

Table 8-1 Adapted from D. A. Nemazee and K. Burki, reprinted from *Nature*, Volume 337, 1989, p. 562.

Figure 8-5 Adapted from D. A. Nemazee and K. Burki, reprinted from *Nature*, Volume 337, 1989, p. 562; S. L. Tiegs et al., *Journal of Experimental Medicine*, Volume 177, 1993, p. 1009.

Figure 8-11 From M. Matsumura, D. H. Fremont, P. A. Paterson, and I. A. Wilson, *Science*, Volume 257, 1992, p. 927. Photographs courtesy of D. H. Fremont, M. Matsumura, M. Pique, and I. A. Watson.

Figure 8-12 From W. J. Poo et al., reprinted from *Nature*, Volume 332, 1988, p. 378. Copyright © 1988 Macmillan Magazines Ltd.

Table 8-3 Adapted from C. C. Goodnow, *Annual Review of Immunology*, Volume 10, 1992, p. 489.

Table 8-4 Adapted with permission from H. N. Eisen and G. W. Siskind, *Biochemistry*, Volume 3, 1964, p. 966. Copyright © 1964 American Chemical Society.

Figure 8-21 Adapted from M. F. Nevrath, E. R. Stuber, and W. Strober, *Immunology Today*, Volume 16, 1995, p. 564.

Chapter 9 Opener From M. Matsumura, D. H. Fremont, P. A. Paterson, and I. A. Wilson, *Science*, Volume 257, 1992, p. 927. Photographs courtesy of D. H. Fremont, M. Matsumura, M. Pique, and I. A. Watson.

Figures 9-7 and 9-8ab Adapted from J. H. Brown, T. S. Jerdetzky, J. C. Gorga, L. J. Stern, R. G. Urban, J. L. Strominger, and D. C. Wiley, *Nature*, Volume 364, 1993, p. 33.

Figure 9-10a From W. E. Paul (ed.), *Immunology: Recognition and Response*. Copyright © 1991 by W. H. Freeman, p. 56.

Figure 9-10b Adapted from J. H. Brown T. S. Jerdetzky, J. C. Gorga, L. J. Stern, R. G. Urban, J. L. Strominger, and D. C. Wiley, *Nature*, Volume 364, 1993, p. 33.

Figure 9-11 Data from V. H. Engelhard, *Current Opinions in Immunology*, Volume 6, 1994, p. 13.

Figure 9-12 From M. Matsumura, D. H. Fremont, P. A. Paterson, and I. A. Wilson, *Science*, Volume 257, 1992, p. 927. Photographs courtesy of D. H. Fremont, M. Matsumura, M. Pique, and I. A. Watson.

Figure 9-13a Adapted from P. Parham, reprinted with permission from *Nature*, Volume 360, 1992, p. 300. Copyright © 1992 Macmillan Magazines Limited.

Figure 9-13b Adapted from M. L. Silver et al., reprinted with permission from *Nature*, Volume 360, 1992, p. 367. Copyright © 1992 Macmillan Magazines Limited.

Figure 9-13c Adapted from D. R. Madden et al., *Cell*, Volume 70, 1992, p. 1035. Reprinted by permission of Cell Press.

Figure 9-14a Adapted from R. Sodoyer et al., *EMBO Journal*, Volume 3, 1984, p. 879. Published by European Molecular Biology Organization. Reprinted by permission of Oxford University Press.

Figure 9-14b Adapted from P. Parham, reprinted with permission from *Nature*, Volume 342, 1989, p. 617. Copyright © 1989 Macmillan Magazines Limited.

Table 9-3 Adapted from D. J. Maudsley and J. D. Pound, *Immunology Today*, Volume 12, 1991, p. 429.

Table 9-5 Adapted from S. Buus et al., *Science*, Volume 235, 1987, p. 1353. Copyright © 1987 by the American Association for the Advancement of Science.

Figure 10-1 Adapted from A. Rosenthal and E. Shevach, *Journal of Experimental Medicine*, Volume 138, 1974, p. 1194, by copyright permission of the Rockefeller University Press.

Table 10-2 Adapted from T. J. Braciale, I. A. Morrison, M. T. Sweester, J. Sambrook et al., *Immunological Reviews*, Volume 98, 1987, p. 95. Copyright © Munksgaard International Publishers Ltd., Copenhagen, Denmark.

Chapter 11 Opener From S. J. Davis and P. A. von der Merve , *Immunology Today*, Volume 17, April 1996, p. 181.

Figure 11-2 Based on J. Kappler et al., *Journal of Experimental Medicine*, Volume 153, 1981, p. 1198.

Figure 11-4 Based on S. Hendrick et al., *Nature*, Volume 308, 1984, p. 153.

Figure 11-5 Adapted from D. Raulet, adapted, with permission, from the *Annual Review of Immunology*, Volume 7,

1989, p. 175; and adapted from M. Davis, with permission, from the *Annual Review of Biochemistry*, Volume 59, 1990, p. 475. Copyright © 1989 and 1990, respectively, by Annual Reviews Inc.

Figure 11-11 From S. J. Davis and P. A. von der Merve, *Immunology Today*, Volume 17, April 1996, p. 181.

Figure 11-13 Adapted from J. McClusky, R. Block, A. Brooks, W. Chen, D. Kanost, and L. Kjer-Nielsen, *The Biology of Antigen Processing and Presentation in Antigen Processing and Recognition,* edited by J. McCluskey, CRC Press, Boca Raton, Florida, 1992.

Chapter 12 Opener Data from E. A. Robey et al., *Cell*, Volume 69, 1992, p. 1089.

Figure 12-2 Adapted from B. J. Fowlkes and D. M. Pardoll, *Advances in Immunology*, Volume 44, 1989, p. 207. Reprinted by permission of Academic Press.

Figure 12-9 Data from E. A. Robey et al., *Cell*, Volume 69, 1992, p. 1089.

Figure 12-11 Adapted from M. Izquerdo and D. A. Cantrell, *Trends in Cell Biology*, Volume 2, 1992, p.268.

Figure 12-14 Adapted from P. S. Linsley and J. A. Ledbetter, *Annual Review of Immunology*, Volume 11, 1993, p.191.

Table 12-4 Adapted from G. Crabtree, *Science*, Volume 243, 1989, p. 357. Copyright © 1989 by the American Association for the Advancement of Science.

Part III Opener From P. M. Motta and T. Fujita/Science Photo Library.

Figure 13-3b From J. L. Boulay and W. E. Paul, *Current Biology*, Volume 3, 1993, p. 573.

Figure 13-6 Adapted from Sugamura et al., *Annual Review of Immunology*, Volume 14, 1996, p. 179.

Figure 13-7 Adapted from T. Kishimoto et al., *Science*, Volume 258, 1992, p. 593. Copyright © 1992 by the American Association for the Advancement of Science.

Table 13-2 Adapted from F. Powrie and R. L. Coffman, *Immunology Today*, Volume 14, 1993, p. 270.

Figure 13-12 From P. A. Sieling and R. L. Modlin, *Immunology*, Volume 191, 1994, p. 378.

Figure 14-2a From N. C. Hughes-Jones, "The Classical Pathway," *Immunobiology of the Complement System*, Academic Press, 1986. Originally published in H. R. Knobel et al., *European Journal of Immunology*, Volume 5, 1975, p. 78.

Figure 14-2c From N. C. Hughes-Jones, "The Classical Pathway," *Immunobiology of the Complement System*, Academic Press, 1986. Originally published in J. Tschopp et al.,

Proceedings of the National Academy of Science, Volume 77, 1980, p. 7014.

Figure 14-3 From A. Feinstein, E. Munn, and N. Richardson, *Monographs in Allergy,* Volume 17, 1981, p. 28, S. Karger AG, Basel; and from A. Feinstein, E. Munn, and N. Richardson, *Annals of the New York Academy of Science,* Volume 190, 1981, p. 1104.

Table 14-3 From M. K. Pangburn, "The Alternate Pathway," in *Immunology of the Complement System,* Academic Press, 1986.

Figure 14-7a From E. R. Podack, "Assembly and Functions of the Terminal Components," *Immunobiology of the Complement System,* Academic Press, 1986.

Figure 14-7b From J. Humphrey and R. Dourmashkin, *Advances in Immunology,* Volume 11, 1969, p. 75. Reprinted by permission of Academic Press.

Figure 14-10 From R. D. Schreiber et al., "Bacterial Activity of the Alternative Complement Pathway Generated from 11 Isolated Plasma Proteins," reproduced from the *Journal of Experimental Medicine,* Volume 149, 1979, p. 870 by copyright permission of the Rockefeller University Press.

Figure 14-11 From N. R. Cooper and G. R. Nemerow, "Complement-Dependent Mechanisms of Virus Neutralization," *Immunobiology of the Complement System,* Academic Press, 1986, p. 155.

Figure 14-12 From N. R. Cooper and G. R. Nemerow, "Complement-Dependent Mechanisms of Virus Neutralization," *Immunobiology of the Complement System,* Academic Press, 1986, p. 150.

Chapter 15 Opener From S. D. Rosen and I. M. Stoolman, *Vertebrate Lectins,* 1987, Van Norstrand Reinhold.

Figure 15-1 Adapted from A. Ager, *Trends in Cell Biology,* Volume 4, 1994, p. 326.

Figure 15-3 Adapted from S. Townsend and J. Allison, *Science,* Volume 259, 1993, p. 368. Copyright © 1993 by the American Association for the Advancement of Science.

Figure 15-4a Adapted from A. O. Anderson and N. D. Anderson, "Structure and Physiology of Lymphatic Tissues," in *Cellular Functions in Immunity and Inflammation,* edited by J. J. Oppenheim et al., Elsevier Science Publishing Company, Inc., 1981, p. 39. Reprinted with permission.

Figure 15-4b From S. D. Rosen and I. M. Stoolman, *Vertebrate Lectins,* 1987, Van Norstrand Reinhold.

Figure 15-4c From S. D. Rosen, *Current Opinion in Cell Biology,* Volume 1, 1989, p. 913. Reprinted by permission of Current Science.

Figure 15-13 Adapted from "Research News," *Science,* Volume 259, 1993, p. 1693. Copyright © 1993 by the American Association for the Advancement of Science.

Figure 15-14a From L. J. Old, "Tumor Necrosis Factor," *Scientific American,* Volume 258, May 1988, p. 59. Copyright © 1988 by Scientific American Inc. All rights reserved.

Figure 15-14b From B. Beutler, *Hospital Practice,* April 15, 1993, p. 45. Reprinted with permission. Illustration by Hospital Practice.

Table 15-4 Adapted from J. P. Girard and T. A. Springer, *Immunology Today,* Volume 16, 1995, p. 449.

Chapter 16 Opener From J. D. E. Young and Z. A. Cohn, *Scientific American,* January 1988, p. 38. Copyright © 1988 by Scientific American Inc. SEM by Dr. Gilla Kaplan, The Rockefeller University.

Figure 16-3 From J. D. E. Young and Z. A. Cohn, *Scientific American,* January 1988, p. 38. Copyright © 1988 by Scientific American Inc. SEM by Dr. Gilla Kaplan, The Rockefeller University.

Figure 16-4 Adapted, with permission, from P. A. Henkart, *Annual Review of Immunology,* Volume 3, 1985, p. 31. Copyright © 1985 by Annual Reviews Inc.

Figure 16-5 Based on M. L. Dustin and T. A. Springer, *Nature,* Volume 341, 1989, p. 619.

Figure 16-6 From J. R. Yannelli et al., "Reorientation and Fusion of Cytotoxic T Lymphocyte Granules After Interaction with Target Cells as Determined by High Resolution Cinemicrography," *The Journal of Immunology,* Volume 136, 1986, pp. 377-382. Reprinted by permission.

Figure 16-7a From J. D. E. Young and Z. A. Cohn, *Scientific American,* January 1988, p. 38. Copyright © 1988 by Scientific American Inc.

Figure 16-7b From E. R. Podack and G. Dennert, reprinted from *Nature,* Volume 301, 1983, p. 442. Copyright © 1983 Macmillan Magazines Ltd.

Figure 16-8 Adapted from M. J. Smyth and J. A. Trapani, *Immunology Today,* Volume 16, Number 4, 1995, p. 202.

Figure 16-10 Adapted from H. R. Rodewald et al., *Cell,* Volume 69, 1992, p. 139. Reprinted by permission of Cell Press.

Table 16-8 Adapted from D. N. Khansari, *Immunology Today,* Volume 11, 1990, p. 170.

Figure 16-17 Adapted from D. K. Dalton, *Science,* Volume 259, 1993, p. 1739. Copyright © 1993 by the American Association for the Advancement of Science.

Figure 20-6 From L. Steinman, *Scientific American,* Volume 269, September 1993, p. 80.

Figure 20-9 From V. Kumar et al., adapted, with permission, from the *Annual Review of Immunology,* Volume 7, p. 657. Copyright © 1989 by Annual Reviews Inc.

Table 20-4 Adapted from M. B. A. Oldstone, *Cell,* Volume 50, 1987, p. 819. Reprinted by permission of Cell Press.

Table 20-5 From D. B. Jones et al., *Immunology Today,* Volume 19, 1993, p. 115. Reprinted by permission of Elsevier Science Publishing Company, Inc.

Figure 20-10b From N. Sarvetnick et al., *Cell,* Volume 52, 1988, p. 773. Reprinted by permission of Cell Press.

Figure 20-12 From D. Wofsy, "Treatment of Autoimmune Diseases with Monoclonal Antibodies," *Monoclonal Antibody Therapy, Progress in Allergy,* edited by H. Waldmann, 1988. Reprinted by permission of S. Karger AG, Basel.

Figure 20-13 Adapted from H. Acha-Orbea, I. Steinman, and H. O. McDevitt, "T-cell Receptors in Murine Autoimmune Diseases," adapted, with permission, from *Annual Review of Immunology,* Volume 7, 1989, p. 371. Copyright © 1988 by Annual Reviews Inc. Originally published in *Cell,* Volume 54, 1988, p. 268.

Chapter 21 Opener From D. D. Manning et al., reproduced from the *Journal of Experimental Medicine,* Volume 138, 1973, p. 488, by copyright permission of the Rockefeller University Press.

Table 21-3 From D. C. Anderson et al., *Journal of Infectious Disease,* Volume 152, 1986, p. 668. Copyright © 1986. Reprinted by permission of The University of Chicago Press.

Figure 21-2 From M. E. Conley, reproduced, with permission, from the *Annual Review of Immunology,* Volume 10, 1992, p. 215. Copyright © 1992 by Annual Reviews Inc.

Figure 21-3 From R. J. Schegel et al., reproduced by permission of *Pediatrics,* Volume 45, 1970, p. 926. Copyright © 1970.

Figure 21-4 From F. S. Rosen and R. Kretschmer et al., "Congenital Aplasia of the Thymus Gland," reprinted, by permission of *The New England Journal of Medicine,* Volume 279, 1968, p. 1295.

Figure 21-5 Courtesy The Jackson Laboratory, Bar Harbor, ME.

Figure 21-6 From D. D. Manning et al., reproduced from the *Journal of Experimental Medicine,* Volume 138, 1973, p. 488, by copyright permission of the Rockefeller University Press.

Chapter 22 Opener From R. C. Gallo, "HIV—The Cause of AIDS," *Journal of Acquired Immune Deficiency Syndromes,* Volume 1, 1988, p. 521. Reprinted by permission of Raven Press Ltd.

Figure 22-1 Data from Global AIDS Policy Coalition, 1995, Harvard University.

Figure 22-2a From R. C. Gallo and L. Montagnier, "The AIDS Epidemic," *Scientific American,* Volume 259, 1988, p. 40. Copyright © 1988 by Scientific American Inc. All rights reserved. Micrograph courtesy of Hans Gelderbloom of the Robert Koch Institute, Berlin.

Figure 22-2b Adapted from B. M. Peterlin and P. A. Luciw, "Molecular Biology of HIV," *AIDS,* 2(suppl 1), 1988, pp. S29–S40. Reprinted by permission of Current Science.

Figure 22-7 Adapted from W. C. Greene, reprinted by permission of *The New England Journal of Medicine,* Volume 324, 1991, p. 308.

Figure 22-11 From H. C. Lane and A. S. Fauci, reproduced, with permission, from the *Annual Review of Immunology,* Volume 3, 1985 by Annual Reviews Inc.

Figures 22-8 and 22-12 From R. C. Gallo, "HIV—The Cause of AIDS," *Journal of Acquired Immune Deficiency Syndromes,* Volume 1, 1988, p. 533. Reprinted by permission of Raven Press Ltd.

Tables 22-5 and 22-6 Data from H. C. Lane and A. S. Fauci, *Annual Review of Immunology,* Volume 3, 1985, p. 477.

Figure 22-15 Adapted from T. Matsuyama, N. Kobayashi, and N. Yamamoto, *AIDS,* Volume 5, 1991, p. 1405.

Figure 22-16 Based on data from M. Clerici and G. M. Shearer, *Immunology Today,* Volume 14, Number 3, p. 107.

Figure 22-17 Data from D. E. Mosier et al., *Science,* Volume 251, 1001, p. 791.

Figure 23-3 Adapted from S. P. Cobbold, G. Martin, and H. Waldmann, reprinted by permission from *Nature,* Volume 323, 1986, p. 165. Copyright © 1986 Macmillan Magazines Ltd.

Figure 23-8 Adapted from S. M. Sabesin and J. W. Williams, "Current Status of Liver Transplantation," *Hospital Practice,* Volume 22, Issue 7, 1987, p. 75. Illustration by Albert Miller. Reprinted with permission.

Table 23-1 Data from J. W. Kupiec-Weglinski et al., *Proceedings of the National Academy of Sciences U.S.A.,* Volume 83, 1986, p. 2624.